PARKINSON'S DISEASE AND MOVEMENT DISORDERS

FOURTH EDITION

PARKINSON'S DISEASE AND MOVEMENT DISORDERS

FOURTH EDITION

Editors

JOSEPH J. JANKOVIC, M.D.

Professor of Neurology
Director, Parkinson's Disease Center and Movement Disorders Clinic
Baylor College of Medicine
The Methodist Hospital
Houston, Texas

EDUARDO TOLOSA, M.D.

Professor of Neurology
Director, Parkinson's Disease and Movement Disorders Unit
Hospital Clinic Universitari
Barcelona, Spain

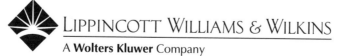

LIPPINCOTT WILLIAMS & WILKINS
A **Wolters Kluwer** Company
Philadelphia • Baltimore • New York • London
Buenos Aires • Hong Kong • Sydney • Tokyo

Acquisitions Editor: Anne M. Sydor
Developmental Editor: Marc Bendian
Production Editor: Thomas Boyce
Manufacturing Manager: Timothy Reynolds
Cover Designer: Christine Jenny
Compositor: Lippincott Williams & Wilkins Desktop Division
Printer: Edwards Brothers

© 2002 by LIPPINCOTT WILLIAMS & WILKINS
530 Walnut Street
Philadelphia, PA 19106 USA
LWW.com

Printed in the USA

Library of Congress Cataloging-in-Publication Data
Parkinson's disease and movement disorders / editors, Joseph J. Jankovic, Eduardo Tolosa.—4th ed.
   p. cm.
   Includes bibliographical references and index.
   ISBN 0-7817-3515-7
   1. Parkinson's disease. 2. Movement disorders. I. Jankovic, Joseph. II. Tolosa, Eduardo.
RC382 .P257 2002
616.8′3—dc21
                                                                 2002066093

Care has been taken to confirm the accuracy of the information presented and to describe generally accepted practices. However, the authors, editors, and publisher are not responsible for errors or omissions or for any consequences from application of the information in this book and make no warranty, expressed or implied, with respect to the currency, completeness, or accuracy of the contents of the publication. Application of this information in a particular situation remains the professional responsibility of the practitioner.

The authors, editors, and publisher have exerted every effort to ensure that drug selection and dosage set forth in this text are in accordance with current recommendations and practice at the time of publication. However, in view of ongoing research, changes in government regulations, and the constant flow of information relating to drug therapy and drug reactions, the reader is urged to check the package insert for each drug for any change in indications and dosage and for added warnings and precautions. This is particularly important when the recommended agent is a new or infrequently employed drug.

Some drugs and medical devices presented in this publication have Food and Drug Administration (FDA) clearance for limited use in restricted research settings. It is the responsibility of the health care provider to ascertain the FDA status of each drug or device planned for use in their clinical practice.

10   9   8   7   6   5   4   3   2   1

This book is dedicated to our loving families
in acknowledgment of their understanding and support

CONTENTS

CONTRIBUTING AUTHORS

Charles H. Adler, M.D., Ph.D. Chair, Division of Movement Disorders, Department of Neurology, Mayo Clinic Scottsdale, Scottsdale, Arizona

Catherine Bergeron, M.D., F.R.C.P.C. Centre for Research in Neurodegenerative Diseases, University of Toronto, Toronto, Ontario, Canada

Kevin M. Biglan, M.D. Department of Neurology, University of Rochester, Rochester, New York

David J. Brooks, M.D., D.Sc., F.R.C.P., F.Med.Sci. MRC Clinical Sciences Centre and Division of Neuroscience, Faculty of Medicine, Imperial College, Hammersmith Hospital, London, U.K.

Francisco Cardoso, M.D., Ph.D. Department of Psychiatry and Neurology, The Federal University of Minas Gerais, Belo Horizonte, MG, Brazil

Cynthia L. Comella, M.D. Associate Professor of Neurological Sciences, Rush Presbyterian-St. Luke's Medical Center, Chicago, Illinois

Günther Deuschl, M.D. Department of Neurology, Christian-Albrechts-Universität Kiel, Kiel, Germany

Dennis W. Dickson, M.D. Professor of Pathology, Mayo Clinic, Jacksonville, Florida

Bruno Dubois, M.D. INSERM E 007, Pavillon Claude Bernard, Hôpital de la Salpêtrière, Paris, France

Rodger J. Elble, M.D., Ph.D. Department of Neurology and The Center for Alzheimer Disease and Related Disorders, Southern Illinois University School of Medicine, Springfield, Illinois

Stanley Fahn, M.D. The Neurological Institute, Columbia University, New York, New York

Paul Foley Clinical Neurochemistry, Clinic for Psychotherapy and Psychiatry, University of Würzburg, Würzburg, Germany

Joseph H. Friedman, M.D. Director, Parkinson's Disease and Movement Disorders Center, Memorial Hospital of Rhode Island, Department of Neurology, Pawtucket, Rhode Island

Victor S. C. Fung, M.B.B.S., Ph.D., F.R.A.C.P Department of Neurology, Westmead Hospital, Westmead, New South Wales, Australia

Thomas Gasser, M.D. Department of Neurology, Klinikum Großhadern, Ludwig-Maximilians-Universität, München, Germany

Manfred Gerlach, M.D. Clinical Neurochemistry, Clinic for Psychotherapy and Psychiatry, University of Würzburg, Würzburg, Germany

Oscar S. Gershanik, M.D. Professor of Neurology, Sección Enfermedades Extrapiramidales, Centro Neurológico-Hospital Frances, Buenos Aires, Argentina

Sid Gilman, M.D., F.R.C.P William J. Herdman Professor and Chair, Department of Neurology, University of Michigan, Ann Arbor, Michigan

Santiago Giménez-Roldán, M.D. Professor of Neurology, Chairman and Head, Department of Neurology, Servicio de Neurología, Hospital General Universitario "Gregorio Marañon," Madrid, Spain

Christopher G. Goetz, M.D. Department of Neurological Sciences, Rush Presbyterian-St. Luke's Medical Center, Chicago, Illinois

Samuel M. Goldman, M.D., M.P.H. Clinical Research Scientist, The Parkinson's Institute, Sunnyvale, California

Francisco Grandas, M.D., Ph.D. Associate Professor of Neurology, Servicio de Neurología, Hospital General Universitario "Gregorio Marañon," Madrid, Spain

Marina Grisoli, M.D. Associate Chief, Department of Neuroradiology, Institute Nazionale Neurologie "C. Besta," Milano, Italy

Robert G. Grossman, M.D. Professor and Chairman, Department of Neurosurgery, Baylor College of Medicine, Houston, Texas

Peter Hagell Section of Restorative Neurology, Wallenberg Neuroscience Center, University Hospital, Lund, Sweden

Mark Hallett, M.D. Chief, Human Motor Control Section, NINDS, National Institutes of Health, Bethesda, Maryland

Yadollah Harati, M.D. Department of Neurology, Baylor College of Medicine, Houston, Texas

Stacy Horn, D.O. Department of Neurological Sciences, Rush Presbyterian-St. Luke's Medical Center, Chicago, Illinois

Michael W. Jakowec, Ph.D. Assistant Professor, Department of Cell Neurology and the Department of Cell and Neurobiology, Keck School of Medicine, University of Southern California, Los Angeles, California

Joseph J. Jankovic, M.D. Professor of Neurology, Director, Parkinson's Disease Center and Movement Disorders Clinic, Department of Neurology, Baylor College of Medicine, Houston, Texas

Peter Jenner, Ph.D., D.Sc. Neurodegenerative Diseases Research Centre, GKT School of Biomedical Sciences, King's College London, London, U.K.

Thomas Klockgether, M.D. Department of Neurology, University of Bonn, Bonn, Germany

William C. Koller, M.D. University of Miami Medical Center, Department of Neurology, Parkinson's Disease and Movement Disorder Center, Miami, Florida

Joachim K. Krauss, M.D. Professor and Vice-Chairman, Department of Neurosurgery, University Hospital, Klinikum Mannheim, Mannheim, Germany

Rajeev Kumar, M.D., F.R.C.P.C. Colorado Neurological Institute, Englewood, Colorado

Anthony E. Lang, M.D., F.R.C.P.C. Division of Neurology, Faculty of Medicine, University of Toronto, Toronto, Ontario, Canada

Myung Sik Lee, M.D., Ph.D. Department of Neurology, Yongdong Severance Hospital, Yonsei University College of Medicine, Kangnam-Koo, Seoul, South Korea

Peter LeWitt, M.D. Department of Neurology, Wayne State University, School of Medicine, The Clinical Neuroscience Center, Professional Village of West Bloomfield, West Bloomfield, Michigan

Olle Lindvall, M.D., Ph.D. Section of Restorative Neurology, Wallenberg Neuroscience Center, University Hospital, Lund, Sweden

Jill Marjama-Lyons, M.D. University of Florida Southside Specialty Care Center, Jacksonville, Florida

Steve G. Massaquoi, M.D. Department of Electrical Engineering and Computer Science, Massachusetts Institute of Technology, Cambridge, Massachusetts

Huw R. Morris, M.R.C.P. Clinical Neurology, National Hospital for Neurology and Neurosurgery, Queen Square, London, U.K.

Opas Nawasiripong, M.D. Department of Neurology, Baylor College of Medicine, Houston, Texas

C. W. Olanow, M.D., F.R.C.P.C. Department of Neurology, Mount Sinai Medical Center, New York, New York

Pau Pastor, M.D., Ph.D. Department of Psychiatry, Washington University School of Medicine, St. Louis, Missouri

John B. Penney, Jr. (deceased) Neurology Service, Massachusetts General Hospital, Boston, Massachusetts

Giselle M. Petzinger, M.D. Department of Neurology, Movement Disorders Section, Keck School of Medicine, University of Southern California, Los Angeles, California

Ronald Pfeiffer, M.D. Department of Neurology, University Health Science Center, University of Tennessee, Memphis, Tennessee

Bernard Pillon, Ph.D. INSERM E 007, Centre de Neuropsychologie, Fédération de Neurologie, Hôpital de la Salpêtrière, Paris, France

Werner Poewe, M.D. Universitätsklinik für Neurologie, Innsbruck, Austria

Peter Riederer, M.D. Clinical Neurochemistry, Clinic for Psychotherapy and Psychiatry, University of Würzburg, Würzburg, Germany

David E. Riley, M.D. Associate Professor, Case Western Reserve University School of Medicine, Director, Movement Disorders Center, University Hospitals of Cleveland, Cleveland, Ohio

Juha O. Rinne, M.D. Neurologist, Professor of Neurotransmission, Turku PET Centre, Turku, Finland

G. Webster Ross, M.D. Honolulu Department of Veterans Affairs, Honolulu, Hawaii

Evžen Růžička, M.D., Ph.D. Associate Professor of Neurology, Movement Disorders Center, Charles University, First School of Medicine, Prague, Czech Republic

Mario Savoiardo, M.D. Department of Neuroradiology, Istituto Nazionale Neurologico "C. Besta," Milano, Italy

Anette Schrag, M.D., Ph.D. Department of Motor Neurosciences and Movement Disorders, Institute of Neurology, University College London, London, U.K.

Kapil D. Sethi, M.D. F.R.C.P.(UK) Professor, Department of Neurology, Medical College of Georgia, Augusta, Georgia

Hiroshi Shibasaki, M.D., Ph.D. Department of Neurology, Kyoto University Graduate School of Medicine, Kyoto, Japan

Ira Shoulson, M.D. Department of Neurology, University of Rochester, Rochester, New York

Harvey S. Singer, M.D. Departments of Neurology and Pediatrics, Johns Hopkins University School of Medicine, Baltimore, Maryland

Caroline M. Tanner, M.D., Ph.D. Director of Clinical Research, The Parkinson's Institute, Sunnyvale, California

William G. Tatton, M.D., Ph.D., F.R.C.P.C. Department of Neurology, Mount Sinai School of Medicine, New York, New York

Philip D. Thompson, M.D., Ph.D. University Department of Medicine, University of Adelaide Department of Neurology, Royal Adelaide Hospital, Adelaide, South Australia

Eduardo Tolosa, M.D. Professor and Director, Department of Neurology, Hospital Clinic Universitari, Barcelona, Spain

Claudia Trenkwalder, M.D. Department of Clinical Neurophysiology, Georg-August University Göttingen, Göttingen, Germany

Alexander I. Troster, Ph.D. Associate Professor, Departments of Psychiatry and Behavioral Sciences and of Neurological Surgery, Director, Neuropsychology Clinics, University of Washington School of Medicine, Seattle, Washington

Francesc Valldeoriola, M.D. Movement Disorders Unit, Neurology Service, Institut Clínic de Malalties del Sistema Nerviós, Hospital Clínic, Barcelona, Spain

Jens Volkmann, M.D. Department of Neurology, Christian-Albrechts-Universität Kiel, Kiel, Germany

Gregor Wenning, M.D., Ph.D. Department of Neurology, University of Innsbruck, Innsbruck, Austria

Anne B. Young, M.D. Neurology Service, Massachusetts General Hospital, Boston, Massachusetts

PREFACE

Since the first edition of this book, published in 1988, extraordinary advances have been made in the treatment of Parkinson's disease and other movement disorders. The primary goal of this fourth edition is to update and critically review this progress.

Functional, biochemical, or structural abnormalities of the basal ganglia are responsible for the vast majority of the disorders discussed in this volume. The traditional models of the basal ganglia anatomy and function and their role in motor control, somatosensory function and behavior, however, are continuously being refined as a result of improvements in the histologic, neurochemical, and physiologic techniques. Our understanding of mechanisms underlying cell death and their relevance to neurodegeneration has also improved markedly as a result of new knowledge about cell biology and molecular genetics in certain forms of parkinsonism, cerebellar ataxias, Huntington's disease, and other neurodegenerative disorders. As a result of discoveries of new gene mutations and gene loci, parkinsonism, ataxias, dystonias, and paroxysmal dyskinesias are being reclassified. It is now generally accepted that there is no single cause of Parkinson's disease and the concept of "Parkinson's diseases" is now emerging to indicate multiple etiologies for a group of diseases with overlapping clinical and pathological features. New classes of diseases, such as synucleinopathies (e.g., Parkinson's disease, multiple system atrophy, dementia with Lewy bodies) and tauopathies (e.g., progressive supranuclear palsy, fronto-temporal dementia, and parkinsonism linked to chromosome 17) have evolved, largely based on studies of patients and families with these neurodegenerative diseases. As a result of these studies and new insights into the mechanisms of neuronal death, many neurodegenerative diseases, including Parkinson's disease, are now considered proteinopathies—due to abnormal protein processing in the affected cells.

In addition to the motor abnormalities associated with the various basal ganglia disorders, cognitive, emotional, and other behavioral aspects are increasingly recognized as important clinical features. More and more studies draw attention to the association of dementia and cognitive decline and various forms of parkinsonism as well as other movement disorders. Obsessive-compulsive disorders and abnormalities of attention are features not only of Tourette's syndrome, but also of a variety of other basal ganglia disorders. Similarly, the overlap between psychiatric disorders and movement disorders is a subject of many recent studies and is reviewed extensively in this new edition.

Advances in understanding mechanisms of neurodegeneration are now being translated into therapies that are not merely symptomatic, but also or solely neuroprotective. These putative neuroprotective strategies include caspase inhibitors (e.g., tetracycline derivatives), interactions with glyceraldehyde 3-phosphate dehydrogenase or GAPDH (e.g., TCH346), and inhibition of mixed lineage kinase-3 (MLK-3) pathway, critical in programmed cell death. Although levodopa continues to be the most effective symptomatic treatment for Parkinson's disease, the emergence of motor fluctuations and dyskinesias limits the usefulness of the drug. As a result of studies testing the usefulness of dopamine agonists as monotherapy in early stages of Parkinson's disease, most experts now advocate the use of dopamine agonists, rather than levodopa, as the earliest dopaminergic therapy in order to delay the onset of levodopa-induced motor complications. In addition, there is a growing body of evidence suggesting that dopamine agonists not only minimize the risk of adverse effects associated with chronic levodopa therapy and potentiate the effects of levodopa, they also may have disease-modifying effects. Other advances in symptomatic therapy of movement disorders, including botulinum toxin treatment of dystonia, tremor, tics, myoclonus, painful rigidity, and other movement disorders, are also highlighted in this volume. The renewed interest in surgical treatment, particularly high-frequency deep brain stimulation (DBS), of movement disorders such as Parkinson's disease, tremor, and dystonia, has been fueled in part by improved understanding of the functional anatomy underlying motor control, as well as refinement of methods and techniques in neurosurgery, neurophysiology, and neuroimaging.

It is the hope and wish of the editors that this new edition will serve as a testimony to the extraordinary progress that has been made in the area of Parkinson's disease, related neurodegenerative disorders, and movement disorders. Although not meant to be encyclopedic, the comprehensive volume highlights recent advances in basic and clinical sciences related to movement disorders and as such should be of interest not only to clinicians concerned with the care of those afflicted with Parkinson's disease and other movement disorders, but also to clinical and basic investigators pursuing answers to some of the unanswered questions about the pathogenesis of this challenging group of disorders. In addition to neurologists and neuroscientists, this book should be of value to neurosurgeons, psychiatrists, physiatrists, neurophysiologists, primary care physicians, nurses, and all health care professionals caring for patients with movement disorders.

We are extremely grateful to all the distinguished contributors for their scholarly reviews. Finally, we express our deep appreciation to the professional staff of Lippincott Williams & Wilkins, particularly Marc Bendian, Tom Boyce, and Anne Sydor, Ph.D. Without their tireless efforts, this volume could not be delivered in such a timely and professional way.

Joseph Jankovic, M.D., Houston
Eduardo Tolosa, M.D., Barcelona

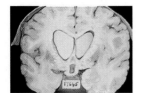

FIG. 14.3A

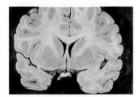

FIG. 14.3B

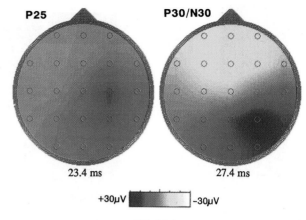

P25   P30/N30

23.4 ms   27.4 ms

+30μV   −30μV

FIG. 20.1

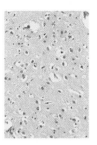

FIG. 41.3A

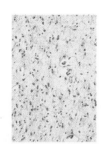

FIG. 41.3B

FIG. 41.3C

FIG. 41.3D

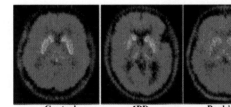

Control   IPD   Parkin   FIG. 42.1

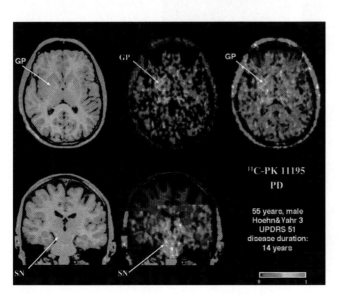

GP   GP   GP

11C-PK 11195
PD

55 years, male
Hoehn&Yahr 3
UPDRS 51
disease duration:
14 years

SN   SN

0   1

FIG. 42.2

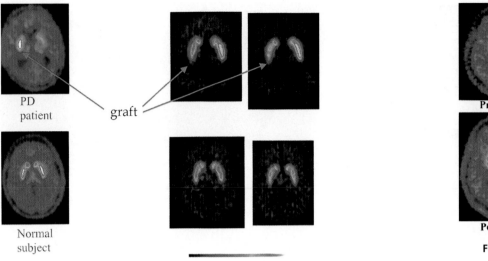

PD
patient

graft

Normal
subject

BP

FIG. 42.3

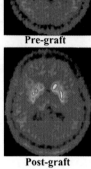

Pre-graft

Post-graft

FIG. 42.4

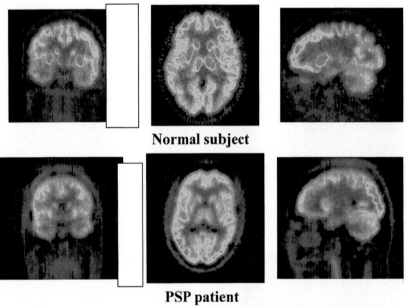

Normal subject

PSP patient

FIG. 42.5

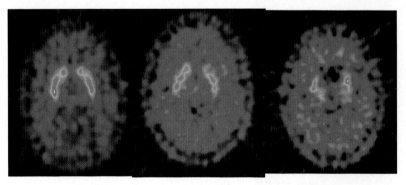

gene negative　　　**gene carrier**　　　**HD patient**　　　**FIG. 42.6**

BIOCHEMICAL AND FUNCTIONAL ORGANIZATION OF THE BASAL GANGLIA

ANNE B. YOUNG
JOHN B. PENNEY, JR.

The basal ganglia comprise a group of gray matter structures deep in the brain beneath the cerebral cortex surrounding the thalamus and hypothalamus. The anatomy and physiology of the basal ganglia are extremely complex; nevertheless, attempts to find the underlying principles of their organization can be used to formulate testable hypotheses about basal ganglia function. It is generally believed that they are responsible for modulating and facilitating various motor and cognitive programs (1,2).

Over the past 25 years much has been learned about the neurochemical anatomy and the internal organization of the striatum and its projections. The basal ganglia structures important in controlling movement include the caudate nucleus, the putamen, the globus pallidus (both internal and external segments), the subthalamic nucleus, and the substantia nigra (pars compacta and pars reticulata) (Fig. 1.1). During the past three to four decades the connections among these structures and between them and other brain regions have been defined in some detail. However, despite this extensive knowledge, questions about how these regions function remain unanswered.

Diseases of the basal ganglia result in a variety of abnormal movements ranging from extreme hypokinesia to hyperkinesia. Parkinson's disease (PD), the prototypical hypokinetic syndrome, is characterized by bradykinesia, rigidity, tremor, and loss of postural reflexes (see Chapter 7). In contrast, Huntington's disease, characterized by chorea, abnormal eye movements, slowed and irregular fine motor coordination, and, in advanced cases, dystonia, rigidity, and loss of postural reflexes (see Chapter 14), is the classic hyperkinetic syndrome. Other basal ganglia disorders include Wilson's disease, Hallervorden-Spatz disease, hemiballismus, cortical-basal ganglionic degeneration, and striatonigral degeneration; each results in some degree of movement abnormality, such as akinesia, bradykinesia, rigidity, chorea, dystonia, athetosis, and tremor. The dystonias, such as dystonia musculorum deformans and the focal dystonias (blepharospasm, torticollis, cranial dystonia), have no known pathology, but because their symptoms so resemble diseases with known basal ganglia neuropathology, they are thought to be due to unknown basal ganglia abnormalities. Although weakness is not a characteristic of most basal ganglia disorders, the speed, sequencing, and fluidity of individual movements and series of movements are greatly impaired.

Any hypothesis concerning the mechanism by which the basal ganglia influence motor function must incorporate information about the various pathologic states and how they can disrupt motor behavior. This chapter describes the basic anatomy of the basal ganglia and attempts to explain, within the framework of current anatomic and physiologic knowledge, some of the movement abnormalities seen in basal ganglia disorders.

ANATOMY OF THE BASAL GANGLIA

The basal ganglia were the subject of two entire issues of *Trends in Neuroscience* 1990 and 2000 (Oct; 23:S1–S126) and numerous reviews (2–8). Almost four decades ago, Carlsson (9) first demonstrated the existence of the biogenic amine dopamine in the brain; shortly afterward, investigators discovered a deficiency of dopamine in the brains of patients with PD (10). The next breakthrough came with the development of histofluorescence techniques, which showed that most of the dopamine in the brain was in the terminals of a pathway stretching from neuronal cell bodies in the substantia nigra pars compacta to the caudate and putamen (11). These discoveries led to the development of specific therapies for PD designed to correct this biochemical defect (12). Subsequent studies have demonstrated that the dopamine pathway modulates basal ganglia function by controlling the response of caudate and putamen neurons to cortical inputs (13,14).

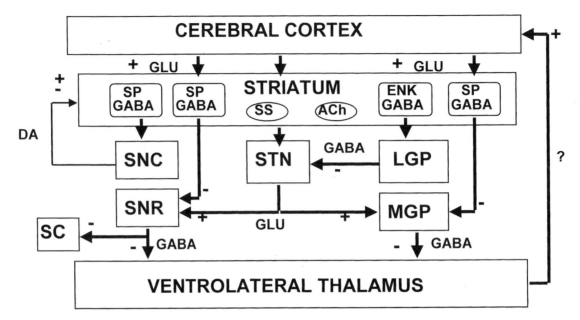

FIG. 1.1. A somewhat simplified diagram of the basal ganglia pathways involved in motor function. *Large letters* indicate the nuclei; *small letters* indicate the neurotransmitters and neuromodulators used by the pathways. *Arrowheads* indicate the direction of impulse flow. *Plus* and *minus* signs indicate the excitatory or inhibitory nature of the neurotransmitter of the pathway. The dopamine pathway from substantia nigra pars compacta to the striatum excites striatal substance P output cells and inhibits enkephalin output cells. ACh, acetylcholine; DA, dopamine; ENK, enkephalin; GABA, γ-aminobutyric acid; GLU, glutamate; LGP, lateral globus pallidus; MGP, medial globus pallidus; SC, superior colliculus; SNC, substantia nigra pars compacta; SNR, substantia nigra pars reticulata; SP, substance P; SS, somatostatin; STN, subthalamic nucleus.

Most afferents to the caudate and putamen come not from the substantia nigra but from the cerebral cortex, all areas of which send somatotopically organized excitatory projections to different clusters of neurons (matrisomes) in the neostriatum (the olfactory tubercle, the nucleus accumbens, the caudate nucleus, and the putamen) (15,16). Evidence suggests that this corticostriatal pathway uses glutamic acid as its neurotransmitter (17). The neostriatum also receives input from a variety of other structures, including the intralaminar nuclei of the thalamus (neurotransmitter unknown but probably glutamic acid) and the raphe nuclei (serotonin).

The caudate and putamen contain several neuronal types. The most abundant of these—close to 90% of the total—is the medium spiny neuron, which uses γ-aminobutyric acid (GABA) (17). The medium spiny neurons project to the major output regions of the basal ganglia, which are discussed later in this section. They also have many recurrent axon collaterals that are distributed primarily within each neuron's dendritic field (18). In addition to the medium spiny neurons, there are a few large cholinergic interneurons (large aspiny neurons); medium aspiny somatostatin-neuropeptide Y-nitric oxide synthase–positive interneurons; parvalbumin interneurons; GABA interneurons; and calretinin interneurons (17,19,20). Most of the

acetylcholine interneurons lie at the border between striosomes and striatal matrix (described later), are tonically active, have high concentrations of dopamine D2 receptors, and are involved in learning (3,21).

The neostriatal projection areas include the lateral globus pallidus (LGP), the medial globus pallidus (MGP), and the substantia nigra pars reticulata (SNr) (22,23). Each of the striatal regions (matrisomes) that receive input from a single region of cortex sends output to the same regions of LGP, MGP, and SNr. Thus there is divergence of cortical information in the striatum and reconvergence of this information in the pallidum (16). Most pallidal neurons are large GABAergic projection neurons with extremely large dendritic fields; interneurons in these areas are rare (17).

The LGP sends inhibitory projections to the caudate and putamen and prominent projections to the MGP, SNr, and substantia nigra pars compacta (SNc), but its major projection is to the subthalamic nucleus, which also receives a direct excitatory (presumably glutamatergic) projection from the motor cortex. An excitatory glutamatergic projection extends from the subthalamic nucleus to the LGP, with additional projections from the subthalamic nucleus to the MGP and SNr (17,23,24).

The MGP and SNr are the main output nuclei of the basal ganglia. They send major inhibitory GABAergic pro-

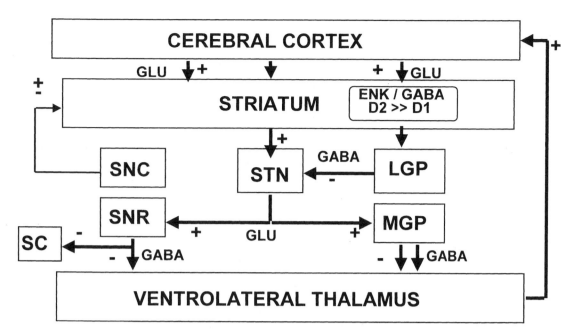

FIG. 1.3. The indirect motor circuit through the basal ganglia. In this pathway, excitatory cortical output stimulates striatal ENK and GABA neurons that project to LGP. The LGP is inhibited, so the STN is disinhibited. The excitatory STN drives the SNR and MGP to inhibit the thalamus. The STN can also be activated directly by the cortex. *Plus* and *minus* signs indicate the excitatory or inhibitory nature of the neurotransmitter of the pathway. This pathway is used to suppress inappropriate motor behaviors. It becomes hyperactive in Parkinson's disease, leading to inability to switch to new motor behaviors (akinesia). It is dysfunctional in early Huntington's disease, causing chorea, and totally destroyed in hemiballism. Pathway activity as in Figure 1.2. DA, dopamine; ENK, enkephalin; GABA, γ-aminobutyric acid; GLU, glutamate; LGP, lateral globus pallidus; MGP, medial globus pallidus; SC, superior colliculus; SNC, substantia nigra pars compacta; SNR, substantia nigra pars reticulata; STN, subthalamic nucleus.

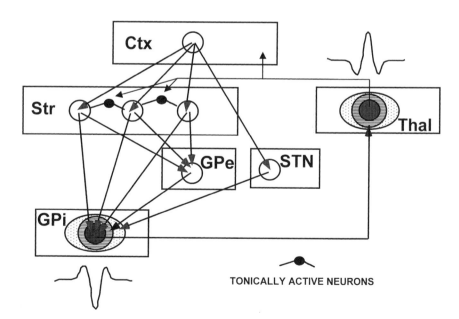

FIG. 1.4. How desired movements are focused through the basal ganglia. A single cortical area projects to several striatal areas whose outputs recombine in the globus pallidus. Tonically active neurons are involved in learning and probably pass information between related striatal areas. The indirect pathway operating via the LGP and STN produces a wide area of excitation in the MGP, and the direct pathway produces a narrow area of strong inhibition in this excited region. This pattern is reversed in the thalamus, resulting in a narrow area of disinhibition to support desired movements with a surrounding inhibition of competing movements. LGP, lateral globus pallidus; MGP, medial globus pallidus; STN, subthalamic nucleus.

The pattern by which striatal activity is transmitted to the MGP and SNr is different in the two pathways. The direct pathway causes inhibition of a relatively small region of MGP, and the indirect pathway acting via the STN produces a wider area of excitation of MGP (Fig. 1.5) (2,56). The result of these two activities is a focused center of decreased activity surrounded by a region of enhanced activity. In the thalamus this pattern of activity is transformed into a disinhibited center that facilitates desired activity with a surrounding periphery where undesired activities are suppressed.

The striatal neurons subserving the indirect pathway are inhibited by dopamine because they bear dopamine D2 receptors. Thus, in PD decreased inhibition of the indirect pathway should cause excessive subthalamic activity that results in excessive suppression of unwanted movements, a prediction consistent with known parkinsonian abnormalities (Fig. 1.4). DeLong and associates demonstrated the validity of this corollary by relieving parkinsonism in 1-methyl-4-phenyl-1,2,3,6-tetrahydropyridine (MPTP)–treated monkeys with subthalamic nucleus lesions (57). This finding is the theoretic justification for the revival of pallidotomy as a treatment for PD (58–60) and the new use of subthalamic stimulation (stimulation blockade) (61,62). Paradoxically, pallidotomies are most

effective at reducing levodopa-induced dyskinesias, although a simple interpretation of this theory predicts that dyskinesias should be worsened by pallidotomy (61,63). Perhaps this is because motor thalamus functions better with no information from MGP than with misinformation (58). An alternative possibility is that dyskinesias arise from inappropriate activation of the direct motor pathway (64) and that this activity is also blocked by pallidotomy. Interestingly, blockade of receptors for the glutamatergic subthalamic output also improves parkinsonism in animals, raising the hope that it is possible to do pharmacologic pallidotomies (65).

In the first edition of this book we predicted that Huntington's disease would be characterized by differential early loss of GABA- and enkephalin-containing striatal neurons projecting to the LGP. Loss of their inhibitory inputs would produce overactivity in LGP neurons, inhibiting (excessively) subthalamic nucleus neurons, much as would be seen in a direct subthalamic nucleus lesion. Since striatal outputs to the LGP are independent of other striatal outputs, a selective loss of these neurons could result in choreiform movements resembling those seen in local subthalamic nucleus lesions. Early in the disease, therefore, the patient encounters both difficulty suppressing unwanted movements and interruption of the normal sequence of

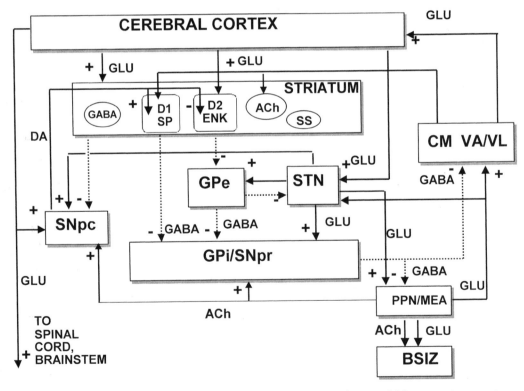

FIG. 1.5. Updated model of the basal ganglia. This more complete model incorporates recent data on the connections of the structures and includes both the pedunculopontine nucleus (PPN) and the bulbospinal inhibitory zone (BSIZ); the latter inhibits movement during sleep. Despite these improvements, this type of model neglects the functional, temporal, and plastic interactions of the neural structures.

motor programs by chorea. We predicted that later in the disease one might expect other striatal neurons, particularly those responsible for maintaining or facilitating motor behaviors, to be affected. Thus, later stages of Huntington's disease are characterized by a combination of unwanted abnormal involuntary movements and difficulty maintaining desired motor behaviors.

The striatolateral pallidal GABA-enkephalin neurons in the matrix are affected in Huntington's disease before the striatomedial pallidal GABA-substance P neurons (66). This process begins before the movement disorder becomes obvious (67). The exception to this rule is the juvenile or rigid form of Huntington's disease, in which the striatolateral pallidal and striatomedial pallidal pathways are equally affected (68). This involvement of the striatomedial pallidal pathway produces the rigid and dystonic features that are prominent in juvenile Huntington's disease. Hedreen and Folstein (69) provided evidence suggesting that striosomal neurons are affected even before the matrix GABA-enkephalin neurons. The loss of these neurons that normally inhibit the SNc dopamine neurons would cause a dopamine excess. This in turn would inhibit the dopamine D2 receptor–bearing enkephalin neurons, with resulting chorea and excitation of the dopamine D1 receptor–containing substance P neurons. Relative dopamine excess may explain why D2 receptor blockers are useful antichoreic agents early in the course of Huntington's disease. Loss of substance P neurons late in Huntington's disease would explain why DA blockers lose their effectiveness.

However, basal ganglia aficionados continue to challenge the simplified but classic model, noting exceptions to the predicted responses of particular pathways to drugs, lesions, and disease (3,8,62,70–72). Additional information about the anatomy of different pathways, their relative influence, and their pharmacology are being discovered. The notion that the subthalamic nucleus is just part of a side loop has changed. Indeed, inputs from cortex to subthalamic nucleus and thence to medial globus pallidus arrive at the pallidum before the inputs from cortex to striatum to pallidum do. The striatal circuit becomes a side pathway of the corticosubthalamopallidalthalamocortical loop. Furthermore, the subthalamic nucleus gives off excitatory projections not only to MGP and SNR but to LGP and striatum as well (71). In turn, the LGP projects not only to STN but also directly to MGP (73). There also appears to be dopamine influences on STN activity.

The output of MGP and SNR to thalamus does not synapse only on thalamocortical relay cells but also onto a complex web of GABAergic interneurons (74). Thalamus not only projects directly to various areas of cerebral cortex but to striatum, where it appears to preferentially excite cholinergic interneurons and also the medium spiny neurons of the direct pathway (75,76). In contrast, cerebral cortex appears to preferentially affect medium spiny neurons of the indirect pathway (77).

The brainstem connections to the basal ganglia are very rich and complex (78). At the midbrain pontine junction in the area of the pedunculopontine nucleus (PPN) there are clusters of neurons; one is the PPN proper and the other is the midbrain extrapyramidal area (MEA). Nearby are the dopaminergic neurons of A8. The PPN neurons are cholinergic, and they contain nitric oxide synthase, corticotropin releasing factor, and substance P. They have diffuse afferents (MGP, SNr, locus ceruleus, dorsal raphe, the orexin cells of the hypothalamus) (79) and efferents (SNR, MGP, VM [ventromedial nucleus], VL [ventrolateral nucleus], reticular thalamus, and the bulbospinal inhibitory zone). Their activity is state dependent. The MEA neurons are glutamatergic and also express parvalbumin. They receive projections from limbic/associative and sensorimotor cortices, MGP, and SNR and have projections to SNC, STN, and the bulbospinal inhibitory zone (80).

The PPN is involved in arousal, cardiorespiratory function, nociception, sleep, and eye movements and the MEA influences the reticulospinal and cerebellar-related motor pathways. Both the MEA and PPN converge onto the glycinergic inhibitory neurons of the bulbospinal inhibitory zone and thereby appear to play a role in atonia during sleep. At the same time the PPN appears to facilitate rapid eye movement sleep.

The pathways from basal ganglia to thalamus are more complex than previously appreciated in the classic model. MGP and SNR inputs not only contact thalamocortical relay neurons directly but also thalamic local circuit GABAergic interneurons (LCNs). The cortex sends excitatory afferents to both thalamocortical relay neurons and to LCNs. The LCNs, in turn, send inhibitory inputs to the thalamocortical relay neurons. Reticulothalamic GABAergic pathways also inhibit both thalamocortical relay neurons and LCNs, and the thalamocortical neurons send excitatory inputs to the reticulothalamic neurons.

Detailed electrophysiologic and pharmacologic studies suggest that the cellular response to a single neurotransmitter can vary greatly depending on the "state" of the cell (81–83). For example, medium spiny neurons in a slightly hyperpolarized state "downstate" may have no response or an inhibitory response to dopamine input but subsequently have a robust excitatory response when the medium spiny neuron is in the "upstate." Therefore, depending on the timing and strength of various inputs, the response of the cell to other inputs may be drastically different. When long-term plasticity is also taken into account, responses in a lesioned or disease circuit may be quite different from their responses in the intact state.

The plasticity of the system had also been underestimated, and such plasticity clearly has to be taken into account. The responses of individual neurons to altered inputs appear to be constantly modified (receptor desensitization, supersensitivity, redistribution). Data in the rat indicate that loss of dopamine input to the striatum alters the number and subunit constitution of N-methyl-D-aspartate receptor subunits in the cellular membrane. Stimulation by dopamine agonists tends to normalize these receptor changes (84). One transmitter can influence the makeup of other membranous receptors not only by phosphorylation but also by changing the number and composition of those receptors. These plastic changes have been observed as a result of the effects of dopamine lesions not only on striatal neurons but also on pallidal and thalamic neurons (8,74). These effects appear to be mediated not only via second-messenger systems that are linked directly to enzyme function but also via changes in transcriptional regulation of additional pathway components. Furthermore, membrane neurotransmitter receptors are connected to complex intracellular scaffolds that influence these secondary pathways and are also tightly regulated by cellular events (85,86).

SUMMARY

Future models will have to be displayed in four dimensions to reflect our current knowledge. The models must incorporate the additional pathways discovered to influence motor function such as the LGP to MGP inputs and the PPN and MEA influences. They need account for plastic changes in the connections themselves via sprouting and modification of local circuits and incorporate plastic changes in receptor composition, number, and distribution. The circuits subserving abnormal movements in primates and humans with specific lesions may be very different from those subserving normal movements in intact subjects. Defining and displaying these changes in new models will necessitate dynamic circuits that continually change in response to perturbations. These evolving models can be tested and challenged in the future.

REFERENCES

1. Marsden CD. The mysterious motor function of the basal ganglia: the Robert Wartenberg lecture. *Neurology* 1982;32:514–539.
2. Mink JW. The basal ganglia: focused selection and inhibition of competing motor programs. *Prog Neurobiol* 1996;50:381–425.
3. Graybiel AM, Aosaki T, Flaherty AW, et al. The basal ganglia and adaptive motor control. *Science* 1994;265:1826–1831.
4. Joel D, Weiner I. The organization of the basal ganglia–thalamocortical circuits: open interconnected rather than closed segregated. *Neuroscience* 1994;63:363–379.
5. Parent A, Hazrati LN. Functional anatomy of the basal ganglia: 1. The cortico-basal ganglia-thalamocortical loop. *Brain Res Rev* 1995;20:91–127.
6. Parent A, Hazrati LN. Functional anatomy of the basal ganglia: 2. The place of subthalamic nucleus and external pallidum in basal ganglia circuitry. *Brain Res Rev* 1995;20:128–154.
7. Calabresi P, Pisani A, Mercuri NB, et al. The corticostriatal projection: from synaptic plasticity to dysfunctions of the basal ganglia. *Trends Neurosci* 1996;19:19–24.
8. Chesselet MF, Delfs JM. Basal ganglia and movement disorders: an update. *Trends Neurosci* 1996;19:417–422.
9. Carlsson A. Occurrence, distribution, and physiological role of catecholamines in the nervous system. *Pharmacol Rev* 1959;11:300–304.
10. Ehringer H, Hornykiewicz O. Verteilung von Noradrenalin und Dopamin (3-Hydroxytyramin) im Gehirn des Menschen und ihr Verhalten bei Erkrankungen des extrapyramidalen Systems. *Klin Wochenschr* 1960;38:1238–1239.
11. Dahlstrom A, Fuxe K. Evidence for the existence of monoamine-containing neurons in the central nervous system. *Acta Physiol Scand* 1964;62:1–55.
12. Cotzias GC, Papavasiliou PS, Gellen R. Modification of parkinsonism: chronic treatment with L-dopa. *N Engl J Med* 1969;280:337–345.
13. Zigmond MJ, Abercrombie ED, Berger TW, et al. Compensations after lesions of central dopaminergic neurons: some clinical and basic implications. *Trends Neurosci* 1990;13:290–296.
14. Nisenbaum ES, Xu ZC, Wilson CJ. Contribution of a slowly inactivating potassium current to the transition to firing of neostriatal spiny projection neurons. *J Neurophysiol* 1994;71:1174–1189.
15. Alexander GE, Crutcher MD. Functional architecture of basal ganglia circuits: neural substrates of parallel processing. *Trends Neurosci* 1990;13:266–271.
16. Flaherty AW, Graybiel AM. Output architecture of the primate putamen. *J Neurosci* 1993;13:3222–3237.
17. Graybiel AM. Neurotransmitters and neuromodulators in the basal ganglia. *Trends Neurosci* 1990;13:244–254.
18. Bishop GA, Chang HT, Kitai ST. Morphological and physiological properties of neostriatal neurons: an intracellular horseradish peroxidase study in the rat. *Neuroscience* 1982;7:179–191.
19. Dawson TM, Bredt DS, Fotuhi M, et al. Nitric oxide synthase and neuronal NADPH diaphorase are identical in brain and peripheral tissues. *Proc Natl Acad Sci USA* 1991;88:7797–7801.
20. Figueredo-Cardenas G, Medina L, Reiner A. Calretinin is largely localized to a unique population of striatal interneurons in rats. *Brain Res* 1996;709:145–150.
21. Pisani A, Bonsi P, Picconi B, et al. Role of tonically active neurons in the control of striatal function: cellular mechanisms and behavioral correlates. *Prog Neuropsychopharmacol Biol Psychiatry* 2001;25:211–230.
22. Albin RL, Young AB, Penney JB. The functional anatomy of basal ganglia disorders. *Trends Neurosci* 1989;12:366–375.
23. Parent A. Extrinsic connections of the basal ganglia. *Trends Neurosci* 1990;13:254–258.
24. Nakanishi H, Kita H, Kitai ST. Intracellular study of rat substantia nigra pars reticulata neurons in an in vitro slice preparation: electrical membrane properties and response characteristics to subthalamic stimulation. *Brain Res* 1987;437:45–55.
25. Carpenter MB. Anatomy of the corpus striatum and brainstem integrating systems. In: Brooks VB, ed. *Handbook of physiology: the nervous system II*. Washington, DC: American Physiological Society, 1981:947.
26. Ilinsky IA, Jouandet ML, Goldman-Rakic PS. Organization of the nigrothalamocortical system in the rhesus monkey. *J Comp Neurol* 1985;236:315–330.
27. Hoover JE, Strick PL. Multiple output channels in the basal ganglia. *Science* 1993;259:819–821.
28. Kharazia VN, Weinberg RJ. Glutamate in thalamic fibers terminating in layer IV of primary sensory cortex. *J Neurosci* 1994;14:6021–6032.
29. Alexander GE, DeLong NR, Strick PL. Parallel organization of functionally segregated circuits linking basal ganglia and cortex. *Annu Rev Neurosci* 1986;9:351–357.
30. Haber SN, Lynd-Balta E, Spooren WPJM. Integrative aspects of

basal ganglia circuitry. In: Percheron G, ed. *The basal ganglia IV.* New York: Plenum, 1994:71–80.

31. Gerfen CR, Herkenham M, Thibault J. The neostriatal mosaic: 2. Patch- and matrix-directed mesostriatal dopaminergic and non-dopaminergic systems. *J Neurosci* 1987;7:3915–3934.

32. Jimenez-Castellanos J, Graybiel AM. Subdivisions of the dopamine-containing A8-A9-A10 complex identified by their differential mesostriatal innervation of striosomes and extrastriosomal matrix. *Neuroscience* 1987;23:223–242.

33. Gerfen CR, Young WS III. Distribution of striatonigral and striatopallidal peptidergic neurons in both patch and matrix compartments: an in situ hybridization histochemistry and fluorescent retrograde tracing study. *Brain Res* 1988;460:161–167.

34. Gimenez-Amaya JM, Graybiel AM. Compartmental origins of the striatopallidal projection in the primate. *Neuroscience* 1990; 34:111–126.

35. Gerfen CR. The neostriatal mosaic: compartmentalization of corticostriatal input and striatonigral output systems. *Nature* 1984;311:461–464.

36. Gerfen CR. The neostriatal mosaic: striatal patch—matrix organization is related to cortical lamination. *Science* 1989;246: 385–388.

37. Eblen F, Graybiel AM. Highly restricted origin of prefrontal cortical inputs to striosomes in the macaque monkey. *J Neurosci* 1995;15:5999–6013.

38. Selemon LD, Goldman-Rakic PSG. Longitudinal topography and interdigitation of corticostriatal projections in the rhesus monkey. *J Neurosci* 1985;5:776–794.

39. Gimenez-Amaya JM, Graybiel AM. Modular organization of projection neurons in the matrix compartment of the primate striatum. *J Neurosci* 1991;11:779–791.

40. Chen JF, Xu K, Petzer JP, et al. Neuroprotection by caffeine and A2a adenosine receptor inactivation in a model of Parkinson's disease. *J Neurosci* 2001;21(RC143):1–6.

41. Gerfen CR, McGinty JF, Young WS III. Dopamine differentially regulates dynorphin, substance P, and enkephalin expression in striatal neurons: in situ hybridization histochemical analysis. *J Neurosci* 1991;11:1016–1031.

42. Surmeier DJ, Kitai ST. Dopaminergic regulation of striatal efferent pathways. *Curr Opin Neurobiol* 1994;4:915–919.

43. Penney JB, Young AB. Speculations on the functional anatomy of basal ganglia disorders. *Annu Rev Neurosci* 1983;6:73–94.

44. Chevalier G, Deniau JM. Disinhibition as a basic process in the expression of striatal functions. *Trends Neurosci* 1990;13: 277–280.

45. Agid Y, Guyenet P, Glowinski J, et al. Inhibitory influence of the nigrostriatal dopamine system on the striatal cholinergic neurons in the rat. *Brain Res* 1975;86:488–492.

46. Mao CC, Cheney DL, Marco E, et al. Turnover times of gamma-aminobutyric acid and acetylcholine in nucleus caudatus, nucleus accumbens, globus pallidus, and substantia nigra effects of repeated administration of haloperidol. *Brain Res* 1977;132: 375–379.

47. Pan HS, Frey KA, Young AB, et al. Changes in [3H]muscimol binding in substantia nigra, entopeduncular nucleus, globus pallidus, and thalamus after striatal lesions as demonstrated by quantitative receptor autoradiography. *J Neurosci* 1983;3: 1189–1198.

48. Pan HS, Penney JB, Young AB. Gamma-aminobutyric acid and benzodiazepine receptor changes induced by unilateral 6-hydroxydopamine lesions of the medial forebrain bundle. *J Neurochem* 1985;45:1396–1404.

49. Wooten GF, Collins RC. Metabolic effects of unilateral lesion of the substantia nigra. *J Neurosci* 1981;1:285–291.

50. Robertson RG, Clarke CA, Boyce S, et al. The role of striatopallidal neurones utilizing gamma-aminobutyric acid in the patho-physiology of MPTP-induced parkinsonism in the primate: evidence from [3H]flunitrazepam autoradiography. *Brain Res* 1990; 531:95–104.

51. Trugman JM. D1/D2 actions of dopaminergic drugs studied with [14C]-2-deoxyglucose autoradiography. *Prog Neuropsychopharmacol Biol Psychiatry* 1995;19:795–810.

52. Berardelli A, Hallett M, Rothwell JC, et al. Single-joint rapid arm movements in normal subjects and in patients with motor disorders. *Brain* 1996;119:661–674.

53. DeLong MR. Primate models of movement disorders of basal ganglia origin. *Trends Neurosci* 1990;13:281–285.

54. Penney JB, Young AB. Striatal inhomogeneities and basal ganglia function. *Mov Disord* 1986;1:3–15.

55. McKenzie JS, Shafton AD, Stewart CA. Striatal output pathways involved in mechanisms of rotation in rats. *Curr Prob Neurol* 1989;9:195–206.

56. Hikosaka O, Matsumura M, Kojima J, et al. Role of the basal ganglia in initiation and suppression of saccadic eye movements. In: Mano N, Hamada I, DeLong MR, eds. *Role of the cerebellum and basal ganglia in voluntary movement.* Amsterdam: Elsevier, 1993:213–219.

57. Bergman H, Wichmann T, DeLong MR. Reversal of experimental parkinsonism by lesions of the subthalamic nucleus. *Science* 1990;249:1436–1438.

58. Baron MS, Vitek JL, Bakay RAE, et al. Treatment of advanced Parkinson's disease by posterior GPi pallidotomy: 1-year results of a pilot study. *Ann Neurol* 1996;40:355–366.

59. Laitinen LV, Bergenheim AT, Hariz MI. Ventroposterolateral pallidotomy can abolish all parkinsonian symptoms. *Stereotact Funct Neurosurg* 1992;58:14–21.

60. Lozano AM, Lang AE, Galvez-Jimenez N, et al. Effect of GPi pallidotomy on motor function in Parkinson's disease. *Lancet* 1995;346:1383–1387.

61. Marsden CD, Obeso JA. The functions of the basal ganglia and the paradox of stereotaxic surgery in Parkinson's disease. *Brain* 1994;117:877–897.

62. Obeso JA, Rodriguez MC, DeLong MR. Basal ganglia pathophysiology: a critical review. *Adv Neurol* 1997;74:3.

63. Bezard E, Brotchie JM, Gross CE. Pathophysiology of levodopa-induced dyskinesia: potential for new therapies. *Nat Rev Neurosci* 2001;2:577–588.

64. Hubbard CA, Trugman JM. Reversal of reserpine-induced catalepsy by selective D1 and D2 dopamine agonists. *Mov Disord* 1993;8:473–478.

65. Greenamyre JT. Pharmacological pallidotomy with glutamate antagonists? *Ann Neurol* 1996;39:557–558.

66. Reiner A, Albin RL, Anderson KD, et al. Differential loss of striatal projection neurons in Huntington disease. *Proc Natl Acad Sci USA* 1988;85:5733–5737.

67. Albin RL, Young AB, Penney JB, et al. Abnormalities of striatal projection neurons and N-methyl-D-aspartate receptors in presymptomatic Huntington's disease. *N Engl J Med* 1990; 322:1293–1298.

68. Albin RL, Reiner A, Anderson KD, et al. Striatal and nigral neuron subpopulations in rigid Huntington's disease: implications for the functional anatomy of chorea and rigidity—akinesia. *Ann Neurol* 1990;27:357–365.

69. Hedreen JC, Folstein SE. Early loss of neostriatal striosome neurons in Huntington's disease. *J Neuropathol Exp Neurol* 1995;54: 105–120.

70. Levy R, Hazerati L-N, Herrero M-T, et al. Re-evaluation of the functional anatomy of the basal ganglia in normal and parkinsonian states. *Neuroscience* 1997;76:335.

71. Parent A, Cicchitti F. The current model of basal ganglia organization under scrutiny. *Mov Disord* 1998;13:199.

72. Ruskin DN, Bergstrom DA, Kaneoke Y, et al. Multisecond oscil-

lations in firing rate in the basal ganglia: robust modulation by dopamine receptor activation and anesthesia. *J Neurophysiol* 1999;81:2046.

73. Kincaid AE, Penney JB Jr, Young AB, et al. Evidence for a projection from the globus pallidus to the entopeduncular nucleus in the rat. *Neurosci Lett* 1991;128:121.

74. Ilinsky IA, Yi H, Kultas-Ilinsky K. Mode of termination of pallidal afferents to the thalamus: a light and electron microscopic study with anterograde tracers and immunocytochemistry in Macaca mulatta. *J Comp Neurol* 1997;386:601–612.

75. Sidibe M, Smith Y. Differential synaptic innervation of striatofugal neurones projecting to the internal or external segments of the globus pallidus by thalamic afferents in the squirrel monkey. *J Comp Neurol* 1996;365:445.

76. Sidibe M, Smith Y. Thalamic inputs to striatal interneurons in monkeys: synaptic organization and co-localization of calcium binding proteins. *Neuroscience* 1999;89:1189.

77. Parthasarathy HB, Graybiel AM. Cortically driven immediate-early gene expression reflects modular influence of sensorimotor cortex on identified striatal neurons in the squirrel monkey. *J Neurosci* 1997;17:2477.

78. Rye DB, Saper CB, Lee HJ, et al. Pedunculopontine tegmental nucleus of the rat: cytoarchitecture, cytochemistry, and some extrapyramidal connections of the mesopontine tegmentum. *J Comp Neurol* 1987;259:483–528.

79. Kilduff TS, Peyron C. The hypocretin/orexin ligand–receptor system: implications for sleep and sleep disorders. *Trends Neurosci* 2000;23:359.

80. Bevan MD, Bolam JP. Cholinergic, GABAergic, and glutamate-enriched inputs from the mesopontine tegmentum to the subthalamic nucleus in the rat. *J Neurosci* 1995;15:7105–7120.

81. Hernandez-Lopez S, Bargas J, Surmeier DJ, et al. D1 receptor activation enhances evoked discharge in neostriatal medium spiny neurons by modulating an L-type Ca^{2+} conductance. *J Neurosci* 1997;17:3334.

82. Plenz D, Kitai ST. Up and down states in striatal medium spiny neurons simultaneously recorded with spontaneous activity in fast-spiking interneurons studied in cortex-striatum-substantia nigra organotypic cultures. *J Neurosci* 1998;18:266.

83. Galarraga E, Hernandez-Lopez S, Reyes A, et al. Cholinergic modulation of neostriatal output: a functional antagonism between different types of muscarinic receptors. *J Neurosci* 1999; 19:3629.

84. Dunah AW, Wang YH, Yasuda RP, et al. Alterations in subunit expression, composition, and phosphorylation of striatal NMDA glutamate receptors in the rat 6-OHDA models of Parkinson's disease. *Mol Pharmacol* 2000;57:242.

85. Kennedy MB. Signal transduction molecules at the glutamatergic postsynaptic membrane. *Brain Res Rev* 1998;26:243.

86. O'Brien RJ, Lau L-F, Huganir RL. Molecular mechanisms of glutamate receptor clustering at excitatory synapses. *Curr Opin Neurobiol* 1998;8:364.

2

MOTOR CONTROL AND MOVEMENT DISORDERS

RODGER J. ELBLE

This chapter provides an overview of motor control in the context of common movement disorders. To the extent possible, involuntary movements and their associated neurologic signs are divided into those of the basal ganglia and those of the cerebellum and its connections. Although somewhat artificial, this divisional classification has considerable experimental support and clinical tradition, and this classification is "anatomically correct" because there are no direct anatomic connections between the basal ganglia and cerebellum. However, the basal ganglia and cerebellum do not function in mutual isolation, and it is becoming increasingly clear, as in the case of tremor, that one structure can become secondarily involved when the primary disturbance is in the other. A more integrated and anatomically holistic discussion of motor control is provided in a brief review of locomotion, and this chapter concludes with a consideration of higher cortical function in motor control.

BASAL GANGLIA AND THEIR CONNECTIONS

The basal ganglia receive no input from ascending sensory pathways, and they have no direct spinal projections. The basal ganglia participate in a corticostriatopallidothalamocortical loop that is illustrated in Fig. 2.1 (1–3). Cortical projections to the basal ganglia are directed primarily to the striatum and subthalamic nucleus (STN). The striatum receives inputs from all areas of the cerebral neocortex, while the cortical inputs to subthalamus originate primarily from the frontal lobe. The striatum sends GABAergic inhibitory projections to the internal and external segments of the globus pallidus and to the substantia nigra pars reticulata (SNr). The SNr is functionally an extension of the globus pallidus interna (GPi). The globus pallidus externa (GPe) sends GABAergic inhibitory fibers to the GPi/SNr and to the STN, and the STN sends excitatory glutaminergic fibers to GPe and GPi/SNr (Fig. 2.1). Thus, there is a so-called direct pathway from the striatum to the GPi/SNr,

and there are two indirect pathways: striatum-GPe-STN-GPi/SNr and striatum-GPe-GPi/SNr.

The associative, sensorimotor (including oculomotor), and limbic areas of cerebral cortex project in a largely segregated manner to corresponding territories of the striatum. These territories are the anterior putamen and most of the caudate (associative); the postcommissural putamen and dorsolateral head of the caudate (sensorimotor); and the accumbens, olfactory tubercle, ventral putamen, and ventral caudate (limbic) (4). These three striatal territories project, respectively, to the dorsal, ventrolateral, and rostromedial areas of the internal and external pallidal segments. Similarly, the interconnections among GPe, GPi/SNr, and STN are organized in associative, sensorimotor, and limbic territories (4). The associative, sensorimotor, and limbic areas of GPi/SNr project, respectively, to ventralis anterior (VA) and medialis dorsalis (MD) (associative), ventralis lateralis (VL) and VA (sensorimotor), and posteromedial MD (limbic). In addition, SNr is involved in oculomotor control and projects to the superior colliculus.

Initially, striatum-GPe-STN-GPi/SNr was the only indirect pathway recognized in experimental models of the basal ganglia, but recent studies have demonstrated two interacting indirect pathways: striatum-GPe-GPi/SNr and striatum-GPe-STN-GPi/SNr (Fig. 2.1) (2). Excitatory corticostriate inputs to either pathway causes increased activity in GPi/SNr, which inhibits excitatory (glutaminergic) thalamocortical projections. GPe also projects to the thalamic reticular nucleus, which sends GABAergic inhibitory projections bilaterally to the VA and VL thalamus. Thus, the striatum-GPe-reticular nucleus pathway, like the other two indirect pathways, has a net inhibitory influence on excitatory thalamocortical projections from VA and VL. By contrast, cortical excitation of the direct striatum-GPi/SNr pathway has a net disinhibitory effect on VA and VL. The competing influences of these direct and indirect pathways are obvious, but the details of this competition and its physiologic significance are poorly understood. Additional competition exists in the excitatory projections from STN to

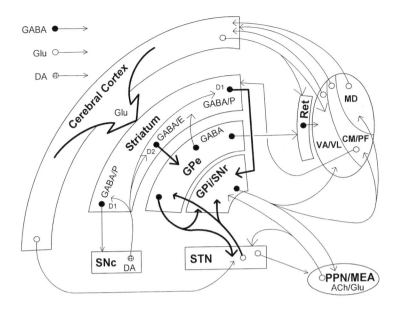

FIG. 2.1. Schematic diagram of the cortical–basal ganglia–thalamocortical loop. *Arrows* originating from *closed circles* represent inhibitory pathways with γ-aminobutyric acid (GABA) neurotransmission, and *arrows* originating from *open circles* represent excitatory pathways with glutaminergic neurotransmission. Ach, acetylcholine; DA, dopamine; Glu, glutamate; E, enkephalin; P, substance P; D1 and D2 are dopamine receptors. GPe and GPi, globus pallidus externa and interna; PPN/MEA, pedunculopontine nucleus/midbrain extrapyramidal area; SNr and SNc, substantia nigra pars reticulata and compacta; STN, subthalamus. Thalamic nuclei are the centromedian (CM), dorsal medial (MD), parafascicular (PF), ventrolateral (VL), ventroanterior (VA), and reticular (Ret).

GPi and GPe. STN neurons excite neurons in GPi, but they also indirectly inhibit GPi neurons through excitation of GPe neurons that project to GPi.

Many other basal ganglia pathways are important in motor control and are not shown in the simplified diagram in Fig. 2.1 (2,4). The microcircuits of the basal ganglia permit significant integration of the limbic, associative, and motor pathways, and these pathways are avenues whereby emotion and environment can influence motor function in normal people and in patients with Parkinson's disease (PD) and other basal ganglia disorders (3,4). Pathways between the cerebral hemispheres also exist. For example, GPi and SNr have small projections to the contralateral VA and VL thalamus, and STN, GPi, and SNr neurons project bilaterally to the mesopontine tegmentum, which contains the pedunculopontine nucleus (PPN), midbrain extrapyramidal area (MEA), and laterodorsal tegmental nucleus. These pathways possibly mediate the ipsilateral effect of pallidotomy and STN deep brain stimulation (DBS) in PD.

In this chapter, the PPN and MEA are collectively referred to as PPN/MEA because these two areas overlap anatomically and functionally (5). The PPN/MEA contains cholinergic, glutaminergic, and probably GABAergic neurons that participate in locomotor control and possibly in the integration of motor, associative, and limbic functions (5). The PPN/MEA has reciprocal connections with the STN, internal pallidum, and substantia nigra, and it also projects to the cerebellum and thalamus (5). Therefore, the PPN/MEA provides an avenue for the influence of emotion and environment on motor function and is believed to be an important site whereby the basal ganglia can influence locomotion.

The VL thalamus is divided into anterior and posterior parts (VLa and VLp) (6). VLa receives input from GPi and

corresponds to ventralis oralis posterior and anterior (Vop and Voa) by Hassler's nomenclature. Portions of ventralis anterior (VA) receive input from GPi and SNr. VLp receives input from the cerebellar nuclei and contains ventralis intermedius (Vim) by Hassler's nomenclature. Vim is the preferred target for thalamotomy and DBS in the treatment of essential, parkinsonian, cerebellar, rubral, and task-specific tremors. It is unclear why Vim should be the "Achilles heel" in so many tremor disorders with different pathophysiology.

Anderson and co-workers found that pallidal-receiving VLa neurons in monkeys exhibit roughly the same firing frequencies as cerebellar-receiving neurons in VLp (7). Most pallidal-receiving thalamic neurons increased their discharge prior to and during upper extremity movement, which is consistent with a phasic reduction in GPi discharge, a phasic increase in corticothalamic input, or both. Inactivation of GPi with muscimol increased neuronal firing frequencies in VLa, but the phasic movement-related modulation in thalamic discharge did not change qualitatively. Therefore, excitatory (glutaminergic) cortical inputs to VL thalamus must contribute significantly to the phasic movement-related modulation of thalamic discharge. The basal ganglia may be more involved in the facilitation and inhibition of thalamic discharge that is determined primarily by cortical inputs.

The discharge patterns of neurons in all parts of the basal ganglia correlate poorly with the kinematic and kinetic variables of movement (1). This suggests that the basal ganglia are not involved in programming the details of movement. Mounting evidence supports the hypothesis that the basal ganglia inhibit undesirable or competing movements and postural synergies and, at the same time, facilitate desired movements and postural synergies that are initiated by cerebral cortical mechanisms, with help from the cerebellum (1). The low-frequency discharge of dopaminergic nigrostriatal neurons correlates best with stimuli that predict the availability or attainment of reward, and dopaminergic nigrostriatal input enables cholinergic interneurons to coordinate striosomes and matrisomes, so as to facilitate behaviorally rewarding and contextually accurate movements (1).

The striatum is not the only nucleus that receives dopaminergic input. The STN, GPi, and SNr receive dopaminergic input from the substantia nigra pars compacta (SNc) and serotonergic input from the dorsal raphe nucleus (2). Therefore, dopaminergic neurons appear to modulate the input (i.e., striatal) and output pathways of the basal ganglia.

Parkinsonism

Rest tremor in the upper or lower extremities is the most specific feature of PD, but rigidity, akinesia, and bradykinesia are additional hallmarks of the disease. Action tremor in the upper extremities is common but rarely incapacitating. The MPTP (1-methyl-4-phenyl-1,2,3,6-tetrahydropyridine) model of PD suggests that loss of the dopaminergic nigrostriatal pathway is sufficient to produce these clinical signs.

Dopamine appears to facilitate the direct pathway and inhibit the indirect pathways from the striatum to GPi/SNr (2). The net result is increased and abnormally phasic activity in STN and GPi/SNr in patients with PD and in monkeys with MPTP-induced destruction of SNc. This observation provides a rationale for the treatment of PD with pallidotomy and STN DBS. However, it does not explain why the principal effect of pallidotomy is often a dramatic reduction in drug-induced hyperkinesias, which are associated with periods of reduced neuronal firing in GPi (2).

Multiple sites of tremor-related neuronal oscillation have been recorded within the cortical-basal ganglia-thalamocortical loop following damage to the nigrostriatal pathway in humans and monkeys. Neurons in the motor cortex, ventrolateral thalamus, GPi, and STN oscillate intermittently in correlation with tremor, and a stereotactic lesion or high-frequency stimulation in any of these locations suppresses tremor (8). The cerebellum is active in patients with Parkinson's tremor, but the cerebellum is not needed for the production of rest tremor (8). Thus, the principal source of oscillation in this complicated motor network is unclear. Many parts of the motor system are clearly involved, and their collective oscillation (rather than individual oscillation) may be necessary for Parkinson's rest tremor (8). This distributed network provides clinicians with multiple targets for treating Parkinson's tremor with drugs and stereotactic surgery.

Multiple striatal striosomes and matrisomes are coordinated by burst-pause-burst discharges of large cholinergic interneurons. This discharge could be the "go" signal for

movement, and its absence in dopamine-depleted animals could contribute to akinesia. Loss of dopaminergic and noradrenergic input to the frontal cortex may also contribute. Finally, the GPi and SNr project bilaterally to the PPN/MEA, and excessive inhibition of this brainstem region could contribute to the start hesitation and freezing in PD.

Abnormal coordination of the direct and indirect pathways through the basal ganglia is believed to be the basis for the erratic symptom fluctuations with dyskinesias (on–off phenomenon) that occur in advanced PD. The simplified view is that the indirect pathways are responsible for suppressing undesired movement or behavior, whereas the direct pathway is responsible for facilitating desired movement or behavior. Failure to coordinate the direct and indirect pathways leads to erratic motor function, which is woefully common in advanced PD. The dopaminergic nigrostriatal input to the striatal output neurons is clearly important in the control of these pathways, but the details are far from clear (9).

Chorea, Athetosis, and Ballism

Hemiballismus and hemichorea are produced by destructive lesions, most commonly strokes, in the STN (9). The slow writhing movements of athetosis are commonly seen in conjunction with chorea and probably have a similar mechanism. Glutaminergic subthalamic neurons excite GPi and SNr, which inhibit their projection sites in the VL and VA thalamus. Hemiballism and chorea are hypothesized to occur when subthalamic stimulation of the inhibitory pallidothalamic pathway is reduced, which is precisely opposite to the situation in parkinsonism. This simplified model is consistent with the clinical effect of subthalamic lesions but is not consistent with the observation that lesions in the internal pallidum do not cause ballism or chorea. In fact, internal pallidal lesions are an effective treatment for hemiballism (10) and for drug-induced hyperkinesias in patients with PD. The altered pattern of internal pallidal discharge (e.g., bursts and silent periods) may be more important in the production of chorea and ballism than the mean level of neuronal discharge (10).

Several authors have hypothesized a model in which the indirect striatum-GPe-STN-GPi/SNr and striatum-GPe-GPi/SNr pathways mediate the suppression of unwanted movement, whereas the direct striatum-GPi/SNr pathway disinhibits or facilitates desired movements and postural synergies (1). If true, a critical balance between the direct and indirect pathways is needed to produce normal movement and avoid parkinsonism and hyperkinesias. In accord with this hypothesis, the enkephalin-containing GABAergic striatal neurons that project to GPe are lost in Huntington's disease before the substance P–containing neurons that project directly to GPi and SNr, and this differential degeneration provides a plausible explanation for the chorea in this disease (9,11). In addition, the striatal striosomes throughout the caudate and putamen are selectively vulnerable in Huntington's disease, and loss of their inhibitory input to the SNc would create an enhanced dopaminergic state that promotes the occurrence of chorea (11).

Dystonia

Dystonia is an abnormal cocontraction of antagonistic muscles. Such cocontraction occurs in monkeys with pallidal lesions, causing reduced inhibition of ventrolateral thalamic neurons (1). Internal pallidal recordings in dystonic patients have revealed reduced mean firing rates and altered firing patterns (12). This association between reduced GPi activity and dystonia fits with the notion that dystonia is a hyperkinetic movement disorder. The use of VL thalamotomy and high-frequency thalamic stimulation in the treatment of dystonia follows logically from this hypothesis. However, thalamotomy is far more effective for tremor than for dystonia, and the efficacy of internal pallidotomy as a treatment for dystonia is at odds with the notion that dystonia is simply the result of reduced GPi activity (13).

Dystonia occurs in patients with strokes and other lesions in the striatum, pallidum, and thalamus (14,15), and peripheral nerve injuries and biomechanical trauma can cause focal dystonia (16). Lesion-induced dystonia usually develops after a delay of weeks or months. This delay suggests that secondary neuroplasticity in other brain regions is important in dystonia pathogenesis. Neuroplastic alteration of neuronal networks has been demonstrated in several investigations of dystonia. For example, monkeys that performed a task of highly repetitive hand opening and closure developed digital receptive fields in the sensory cortex (area 3b) that were roughly ten times larger than normal, and this cortical remapping was associated with hand dysfunction that resembled focal dystonia (17). In addition, expanded receptive fields for passive limb movement were found in the VL thalamus of dystonia patients (18).

The results of several experiments have indicated a disturbance of sensorimotor integration in patients with dystonia. Patients with dystonia have expanded, less specific sensory receptive fields in the internal pallidum and ventrolateral thalamus (10,18). Eleven patients with unilateral dystonia exhibited a diminished regional blood flow response in sensorimotor cortex when the affected hand was stimulated with a vibrator, and vibration induced a dystonic hand contraction in six patients (19). The dystonic hand response to vibration is blocked by intramuscular injection of lidocaine, which reduces muscle spindle activity (20). These experimental observations and the "sensory tricks" that suppress dystonia (e.g., *geste antagonistique* in cervical dystonia) are consistent with the notion that disturbed sensorimotor integration plays a fundamental role in the pathophysiology of dystonia (21).

Tics

Tics are brief, coordinated, stereotyped movements or vocalizations. Most tics are easily suppressed for short periods, but continued suppression causes anxiety and an urge to "let go." The distinction between voluntary and involuntary is particularly fuzzy for this disorder. An animal model does not exist.

Patients with Tourette's syndrome commonly have obsessive-compulsive behavior, hyperactivity, inattentiveness, impulsivity, and emotional lability. These abnormalities are consistent with dysfunction of lateral prefrontal, orbitofrontal, and limbic cortices and their subcortical connections (22). Patients with obsessive-compulsive disorder exhibit increased regional cerebral blood flow in the caudate nucleus, anterior cingulate cortex, and orbitofrontal cortex (23). Thus, one may hypothesize a disturbance of limbic indirect pathways through the basal ganglia, resulting in a failure to suppress undesired behavior (i.e., tics and compulsions). The efficacy of D2 antagonists supports this hypothesis.

CEREBELLUM

The microscopic anatomy of the cerebellar cortex is remarkably uniform across all functional divisions (24). The cerebellar cortex and deep cerebellar nuclei receive many excitatory inputs from sensory pathways and brainstem nuclei (Fig. 2.2). The inferior olive is the source of climbing fibers that project contralaterally to the cerebellum via the inferior cerebellar peduncle. These climbing fibers project to sagittal strips of cerebellar cortex, making strong one-to-one synapses with Purkinje cells. Most other inputs to the cerebellum are mossy fibers to the cerebellar granule cells, but there is also a multilayered neuromodulatory input from the locus ceruleus (norepinephrine), raphe nuclei (serotonin), and possibly the pedunculopontine nucleus (acetylcholine). The granule cells send parallel fibers along the cerebellar folia, perpendicular to the sagittal strips of climbing fiber input. Parallel fibers make excitatory synapses with multiple Purkinje cells, and each Purkinje cell receives input from numerous parallel fibers. The parallel fibers also synapse with inhibitory interneurons, called stellate, Golgi, and basket cells. The cortical response of this network is conveyed to the cerebellar nuclei by inhibitory GABAergic Purkinje cells. Since the cerebellar nuclei also receive excitatory climbing fiber and mossy fiber input, one can envision a process in which nuclear output is molded by competing inhibition (Purkinje cells) and excitation (climbing fibers and mossy fibers).

Many areas of cerebral cortex project to the contralateral cerebellum by way of the pontine nuclei, reticular formation, red nucleus, and inferior olive (24). These brainstem nuclei, except the olive, provide mossy fiber input to the

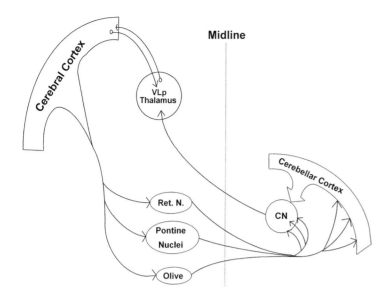

FIG. 2.2. Schematic diagram of corticobulbocerebellothalamocortical pathways. All *arrows* represent excitatory glutaminergic pathways except the projection from cerebellar cortex to the cerebellar nuclei (CN), which is inhibitory GABAergic. Ret. N., reticular nuclei; CN, cerebellar nuclei; VLp, ventralis lateralis posterior.

cerebellum. The pontine nuclei are the biggest source of mossy fibers. The premotor, supplementary motor, primary motor, somatosensory, posterior parietal, extrastriate visual and cingulate cortices are the main cortical inputs to the pontine nuclei, but inputs from auditory cortex also exist. Cortical inputs to the reticular nuclei originate mainly from sensorimotor cortex. The cerebellum also receives mossy fiber inputs from somatosensory pathways (e.g., the dorsal and ventral spinocerebellar tracts) and from the vestibulocerebellar pathway.

The cerebellar nuclei project to brainstem nuclei and the posterior ventrolateral thalamus (VLp), which contains the nucleus ventralis intermedius (VIM) by Hassler's nomenclature (6). The dentate and interposed (globose and emboliform) nuclei provide most of the cerebellothalamic afferents via the brachium conjunctivum. The fastigium contributes to this ventrolateral thalamic projection but also projects to the ventromedial thalamus, which provides widespread cortical activation. The sites of brainstem projection include the red nucleus, reticular formation, inferior olive, and lateral vestibular nucleus, which are discussed in greater detail under the headings "Guillain-Mollaret Triangle" and "Locomotion."

The dentate nucleus receives input from the lateral cerebellar cortex and is unique in its lack of direct somatosensory input. However, dentate and lateral cerebellar cortex receive abundant corticobulbocerebellar fibers that carry sensory information (25–27). Some dentate neurons fire before motor cortex neurons when monkeys perform abrupt, visually guided voluntary movements (25). Inactivation of the dentate nucleus in monkeys causes uncoordinated reaching and pinching with the ipsilateral upper extremity (25). Activation of the dentate and lateral cere-

bellum occurs during cognitive and sensory processing, and this activation is proportional to the complexity of the task. These observations and others suggest that the lateral cerebellum and dentate are involved in motor planning and learning, particularly when multiple body segments, multiple streams of information, and cognition are required (26).

The interposed nuclei receive input from the paramedian cerebellar cortex. These nuclei and cerebellar cortex receive abundant somatosensory feedback and corticopontocerebellar inputs from sensorimotor cortex. Consequently, this portion of the cerebellum responds to somatosensory reflex perturbations with short latencies and is involved in the control of muscle antagonists, whose activation is often delayed in patients with cerebellar pathology (25,28). Inactivation with muscimol of the interposed nuclei causes ipsilateral dysmetria and intention tremor in monkeys during reaching (25).

The fastigial nucleus receives input from the cerebellar vermis and flocculonodular lobe, which also projects directly to the lateral vestibular nucleus. The fastigium and midline cerebellar cortex participate in vestibulo-ocular control and locomotion, as discussed under the heading "Locomotion." Fastigial inactivation causes severe truncal dysequilibrium and gait ataxia in monkeys, with frequent falls to the side of the lesion.

When reaching for an object, feedforward control of movement utilizes current sensory information and prior experience to launch the hand in the correct direction and to decelerate the hand smoothly, as it approaches its target. The nervous system must initiate movement with appropriate force and direction, and this must be accomplished with due consideration of the complex mechanical properties of the limb. The segments and joints of an extremity have inertial, elastic, and viscous properties, and the motion of one limb segment influences other segments through so-called interaction torques and forces. Interaction torques and forces can facilitate or impede a desired movement, so the nervous system must generate muscle forces that are in harmony with the biomechanical properties of the body. Somatosensory and visual input are required to accomplish this feat, but a purely feedback mode of control would not have sufficient speed and sensitivity for rapid movements. Fortunately, the central nervous system learns the biomechanical characteristics of the body, and this knowledge is used to predict how body segments will interact during a particular movement. The cerebellum plays an important role in formulating and employing this model (26). Cerebellar patients execute limb movements with muscle torques that do not vary appropriately with interaction torques and forces. Consequently, cerebellar patients exhibit uncoordinated movement of limb segments, target overshoot, and decomposition of movement (26). Even when single joints are involved, cerebellar patients decelerate the limb segment with delayed, inappropriately sized antagonist muscle activity that contributes to target overshoot (28). The delayed antagonist activity is evident in the discharge of associated neurons in the motor cortex, and the transcortical sensorimotor loop behaves like a feedback control system that is devoid of anticipatory feedforward control. Each target overshoot necessitates a corrective response that is associated with yet another delayed deceleration and overshoot. Thus, dysmetria may lead to a terminal oscillation or so-called intention tremor.

A 3- to 5-Hz kinetic or intention tremor in the ipsilateral extremities occurs in laboratory primates with lesions in the deep cerebellar nuclei (globose and emboliform) or in the outflow tract of these nuclei (brachium conjunctivum) en route to the contralateral ventrolateral thalamus (27). This tremor is associated with oscillatory neuronal activity in the sensorimotor cortex, the interposed nuclei, and somatosensory afferents of monkeys but not in the dentate nucleus, which receives no somatosensory feedback. Tremor frequency is influenced by reflex arc length and by the inertia and stiffness of the body part. This influence of reflex dynamics and limb mechanics on the frequency of tremor is consistent with the hypothesis that cerebellar tremor is a mechanical-reflex oscillation that emerges from transcortical sensorimotor loops (27).

Somatosensory loops cannot be the sole source of tremor because upper extremity deafferentation in decerebellate monkeys does not eliminate their 2- to 4-Hz intention tremor (27). The involvement of a central source of oscillation in cerebellar intention tremor cannot be excluded. Any component of the Guillain-Mollaret triangle could contribute, as discussed in the following section of this chapter. However, somatosensory deafferentation does not preclude the influence of sensory feedback in tremorogenesis because visual feedback is preserved. Cerebellar action tremor is greatly reduced when voluntary movements are performed without visual feedback or without somatosensory feedback (27). One simple explanation for this phenomenon is that sensorimotor loops are devoid of feedforward control in patients with cerebellar lesions and that a purely feedback mode of control entails an excessive reliance on sensory feedback, which results in unstable oscillation.

Thalamotomy in the contralateral VIM suppresses cerebellar tremor. VIM is a cerebellar receiving nucleus and is a relay for short-latency proprioceptive feedback to the motor cortex (6). Therefore, VIM thalamotomy could interrupt an unstable transthalamocortical sensorimotor loop or could reduce the spread of oscillation from cerebellar-brainstem loops such as the Guillain-Mollaret triangle. Reverberation within the thalamocortical loop is one possible explanation for the disabling crescendo increase in cerebellar intention tremor, as the limb approaches its target. Thalamotomy reduces oscillation but has no effect on other aspects of cerebellar ataxia.

GUILLAIN-MOLLARET TRIANGLE

The Guillain-Mollaret triangle contains the dentate and interposed nuclei, the contralateral parvicellular red nucleus, the contralateral inferior olive, and their interconnecting fiber tracts. The anatomy of this loop is summarized in Fig. 2.3. Ataxia and tremor occur when this loop is damaged. This is one of several loops formed by excitatory projections from the deep cerebellar nuclei to nuclei in the contralateral mesodiencephalic junction, which include the red nucleus and the prerubral reticular formation (29). These mesodiencephalic nuclei project to the inferior olive, which projects via the inferior cerebellar peduncle to the deep cerebellar nuclei and Purkinje cells of the cerebellar cortex, and these projections are also excitatory. The tremor and ataxia caused by lesions in the cerebellar nuclei and brachium conjunctivum were discussed in the preceding section of this chapter. The remaining portions of this loop are considered here.

Rubral (midbrain) tremor is a striking combination of 2- to 5-Hz rest, postural, and kinetic tremor of an upper extremity (30). This unusual tremor is caused by lesions in the vicinity of the red nucleus. Ohye and co-workers performed serial stereotactic lesions in the parvicellular red nucleus, as well as decussation of the brachium conjunctivum and ventromedial mesencephalon (substantia nigra) in monkeys, and found that damage to all three areas was necessary for sustained tremor (31). This study confirmed earlier clinicopathologic observations in humans. Combined damage to the red nucleus and neighboring cerebellothalamic, cerebello-olivary, and nigrostriatal fiber tracts is required. The peculiar mixture of rest, postural, and kinetic tremor follows logically from this combination of pathology. However, rubral tremor usually begins weeks to

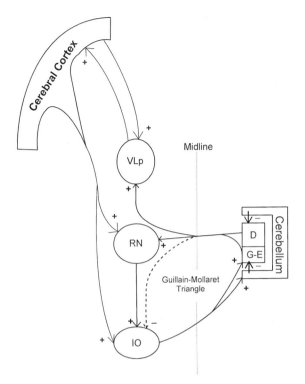

FIG. 2.3. Schematic diagram of the Guillain-Mollaret triangle and its connections with the cerebral cortex and thalamus. *Solid arrows* are excitatory glutaminergic pathways. The *broken arrow* is inhibitory GABAergic. The projections from cerebellar cortex to the dentate (D) and globose-emboliform (G-E) nuclei are also inhibitory GABAergic.

months after brainstem trauma or stroke, so that compensatory or secondary changes in nervous system function must contribute to tremorogenesis. Remy and co-workers recently demonstrated reduced striatal ^{18}F-fluorodopa uptake in six patients with rubral tremor (30). This finding explains why levodopa and dopaminergic agonists are occasionally beneficial. Rubral tremor, like many other tremors, responds to stereotactic thalamotomy in ventralis intermedius (VLp in Fig. 2.3).

Little insight into the function of the red nucleus has been gained from studies of rubral tremor, and data from animal studies are difficult to relate to humans because the anatomy in humans differs substantially from that in animals. In monkeys, the red nucleus consists of parvicellular and magnocellular divisions. Both divisions receive major inputs from motor cortex and the deep cerebellar nuclei. The magnocellular division is the origin of the rubrospinal tract, which is discussed under the heading "Locomotion." The existence of a significant rubrospinal tract in humans is doubtful because only a rudimentary magnocellularis is found in humans (32). In monkeys, neurons in the magnocellularis and motor cortex behave similarly, and the role of the magnocellularis appears to have been supplanted by the motor cortex in humans. Nearly all cells in the human red nucleus belong to the parvicellular division, which sends

most of its output to the inferior olive by way of the central tegmental tract (Fig. 2.3). The red nucleus also connects reciprocally with the cerebellar nuclei. The dentate and motor cortex provide most of the afferents to the parvicellularis, and both afferent projections are excitatory (gluta-minergic). The rubro-olivary and olivocerebellar projections are also excitatory. Thus, the Guillain-Mollaret triangle is a positive feedback system. This triangle and other positive feedback loops between the cerebellar nuclei and brainstem nuclei are prone to reverberation, and this reverberation is hypothesized to play a role in sustaining loop activity related to motor commands (29).

In addition to rubral and cerebellar input, the inferior olive receives descending input from motor and premotor cortex, and it receives sensory input from spinal cord, vestibular, and visual pathways. These anatomic connections provide the olive with a means for comparing expected outcomes, conveyed by neocortical inputs, with actual movement conveyed by sensory feedback. The olive tends to fire when a deviation from expected motor performance or sensory input occurs and is active during motor learning (26). It is unclear whether this comparator function is the main role of the olive.

Olivary neurons are capable of rhythmic discharge at 0.5 to 12 Hz, but they fire irregularly at roughly 1 Hz during arrhythmic movements and rest (33). By contrast, cerebellar mossy fibers fire at rates as high as 100 per second. The effect of climbing fiber discharge on Purkinje cells is to reduce the strength of the parallel-Purkinje cell synapse, thereby reducing Purkinje cell inhibition of the cerebellar nuclei. This synaptic interaction is believed to facilitate motor learning (26).

Olivary neurons are capable of synchronous rhythmic discharge, and they tend to fire rhythmically during rhythmic movements (33). Controversy surrounds the degree to which such rhythmic activity might function as a clock or timing device for coordinating movements (29). Olivary rhythmicity is mediated by the process of inhibition-rebound excitation in which a sodium action potential leads to a calcium-dependent potassium-mediated hyperpolarization that induces a low-threshold calcium spike. The low-threshold calcium spike may reach threshold and cause another sodium action potential, so the entire process of inhibition–rebound excitation can repeat itself in a rhythmic fashion. Synchrony of olivary discharge is facilitated by electrotonic dendrodendritic synapses (gap junctions) between olivary neurons (29). Synchronous oscillation of olivary neurons drives the cerebellar cortex and cerebellar nuclei into similar oscillation, which is facilitated by the inhibition–rebound properties of Purkinje cells (27).

The superior cerebellar peduncle contains dentate and globose-emboliform axons that project to the contralateral olive directly and indirectly, via the parvicellular red nucleus and neighboring mesodiencephalic nuclei (29). The nuclear axons in the indirect pathway are excitatory, while the axons in the direct pathway are inhibitory (GABAergic). These GABAergic neurons synapse near the electrotonic junctions between dendrites of olivary neurons, and this GABAergic input decreases the coupling between olivary neurons. Therefore, the red nucleus and deep cerebellar nuclei can increase the activity of olivary neurons and can control the extent to which these neurons fire in synchrony.

Abnormal olivary oscillation and synchrony is the hypothesized mechanism of *palatal myoclonus* (also termed palatal tremor). Palatal myoclonus is a vertical oscillation of the soft palate at 1 to 3 Hz. Two forms of palatal myoclonus, symptomatic and essential, differ clinically and pathophysiologically. Essential palatal myoclonus causes an annoying ear click but no other neurologic signs or symptoms, and the pathophysiology of essential palatal myoclonus is unknown (34). Symptomatic palatal myoclonus is produced by damage, usually ischemic, in the dentato-olivary pathway. Damage to fibers from the interposed nuclei may also be important. Fibers from these cerebellar nuclei pass through the brachium conjunctivum, into and around the contralateral red nucleus, and down the central tegmental tract to the olive. Lesions in this pathway cause vacuolar enlargement of olivary neurons and gross hypertrophy of the olivary nucleus (29). This olivary hypertrophy is a pathologic response to deafferentation and is visible with magnetic resonance imaging (MRI). Olivary hypertrophy and palatal myoclonus usually follow a stroke by several weeks or more, but microscopic changes occur within 12 to 20 days (35). Recent electrophysiologic studies of olivary hypertrophy have been performed in laboratory animals, but 1- to 3-Hz oscillation in association with palatal myoclonus has not been demonstrated (29).

A sizable body of experimental data incriminates enhanced olivocerebellar oscillation in the pathophysiology of *essential tremor* (ET), even though postmortem examinations have revealed no abnormalities (8,27). The enhancement of olivary rhythmicity with harmaline or serotonergic drugs produces an action tremor that is similar to ET. Lesions in the cerebellum and VIM thalamus greatly reduce ET. Positron emission tomography (PET) studies have revealed bilaterally increased olivary glucose utilization and bilaterally increased blood flow in the cerebellum, red nucleus, and thalamus of patients with ET. Functional MRI studies have disclosed increased blood flow bilaterally in the cerebellar hemispheres, dentate nucleus, and red nucleus and contralaterally in the globus pallidus, thalamus, and primary sensorimotor cortex (36). However, similar alterations in cerebellar blood flow occur in patients with parkinsonian, orthostatic, and primary writing tremors (36). All forms of tremor produce a mismatch between the intended movement (input from cerebral cortex) and actual movement (sensory feedback), and such a mismatch is known to cause increased olivocerebellar activity. Thus, PET evidence of increased olivocerebellar blood flow and glucose utilization is not proof of an olivocerebellar origin for tremor.

POSTURE AND LOCOMOTION

Basic Anatomy and Physiology

Cats with high cervical cord transections can walk on a treadmill with rudimentary locomotor activity that emerges from spinal cord networks, and similar functional capacity exists in patients with spinal cord lesions (37,38). The quality of treadmill walking improves with time, which is an observation of some relevance to the rehabilitation of spinal cord victims (38). However, the rhythmicity, interlimb coordination, and interjoint coordination remain abnormal, and patients and spinal animals require support with a body sling during treadmill walking because postural tonus and balance are not adequate.

Transection at the rostral pons or caudal midbrain (bulbospinal cat) leaves the cat with (a) no tendency to right itself when placed on its side or back (i.e., no righting reactions), (b) inappropriate foot placement when standing (abnormal placing reactions), (c) absence of effective postural responses to perturbations (e.g., absent hopping reactions), and (d) failure to shift the body's center of mass when the support surface is tilted (39). Transection rostral to the third cranial nerves (mesencephalic cat) permits spontaneous standing (righting), walking, running, and climbing, albeit abnormally. The decorticate cat is immediately able to right itself, stand, and walk, but posture and gait are still abnormal. Paw placing, supporting reactions, and hopping reactions are impaired, even after isolated removal of the frontal cortex. Complex postural adjustments (e.g., rescue responses) and skilled locomotion (e.g., walking on a beam or horizontal ladder) are not possible without the frontal lobes.

The spinal pattern generator of locomotion is integrated with complex motor pathways that include virtually all supraspinal motor centers. The ventrolateral spinal quadrant, containing the reticulospinal and vestibulospinal pathways, is important for the activation of spinal locomotor networks and for the recovery of locomotion after spinal cord injury (40). The vestibulospinal tract from the lateral vestibular nucleus is involved in the control of antigravity muscle tone, and this control of tone is shared by the nuclei reticularis gigantocellularis and pontis caudalis. These bulbospinal pathways are modulated in harmony with the support and swing (stepping) phases of the gait cycle, and this modulation is accomplished through connections with the cerebellar vermis and fastigial nuclei (Fig. 2.4). Thus, the cerebellum participates in the integrated control posture and movement. Lesions of the vermis produce truncal ataxia, as is seen in alcoholics with anterior vermis degeneration. Similarly, inactivation of the fastigium with muscimol causes severe truncal dysequilibrium with frequent falls to the side of the lesion (25). Damage to the flocculonodular lobe (vestibulocerebellum) and its connections with the vestibular nucleus produces truncal dysequilibrium and impaired head–eye coordination (vestibulo-ocular reflex).

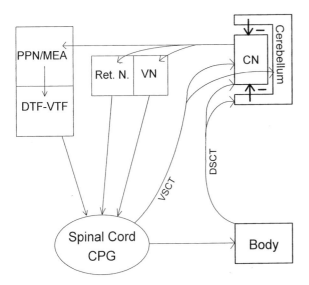

FIG. 2.4. Schematic diagram of the spinal cord central pattern generator (CPG) of locomotion and its connections with brainstem nuclei and the cerebellum. An efferent copy of the CPG output is sent to the cerebellar nuclei (CN) and cerebellar cortex by way of the ventral spinocerebellar tract (VSCT), and an afferent or sensory copy of body movement is carried to the cerebellum via the dorsal spinocerebellar tract (DSCT). The cerebellum interacts with the brainstem nuclei in the control of postural tonus and rhythmic coordination of limb segments. DTF and VTF, dorsal and ventral tegmental fields; PPN/MEA, pedunculopontine nucleus/midbrain extrapyramidal area; Ret. N., reticular nuclei; VN, lateral vestibular nucleus.

The lateral vermal and paravermal cerebellar cortex and the interposed (globose and emboliform) nuclei influence locomotor rhythmicity and phasic coordination of body segments through connections with rubrospinal, lateral pontomedullary reticulospinal, and vestibulospinal pathways (41). The ventral spinocerebellar pathway carries output (also termed spinal efferent copy) from the spinal pattern generator to the cerebellum, and the dorsal spinocerebellar pathway carries sensory feedback from the periphery (Fig. 2.4). The cerebellum also receives a cerebral efferent copy via corticobulbocerebellar pathways, involving the pontine, reticular, and olivary nuclei. With this information, the cerebellum assists in the production of rhythmic locomotor activity that is compatible with internal desires, environmental demands, and musculoskeletal constraints. Damage to the cerebellum or its afferent and efferent pathways causes postural instability and an arrhythmic, widebased, reeling or lunging gait with poorly coordinated limb segments.

The subthalamic locomotor region (SLR), PPN/MEA (also known as the mesencephalic locomotor region), ventral tegmental field (VTF), and dorsal tegmental field (DTF) are four anatomic loci in the brainstem and diencephalon that participate in the initiation of gait and in the control of postural tonus (Figs. 2.4 and 2.5) (41). The SLR is a poorly defined locus in the lateral hypothalamic area. Stimulation of this site in cats produces stooped, stealthy locomotion, as in the pursuit of prey. Brief stimulation of the PPN/MEA in cats induces rapid walking, followed by running. GABAergic inputs to the PPN/MEA from GPi/SNr have an inhibitory influence on locomotion. Therefore, the increased GPi/SNr activity in PD could cause akinesia and freezing through abnormal inhibition of PPN/MEA. Excitatory glutaminergic inputs to PPN/MEA from the STN and possibly motor cortex promote locomotion. Furthermore, cholinergic projections from the PPN/MEA to the "nonspecific" thalamic nuclei play a role in controlling arousal, which is important in all aspects of motor control.

The PPN/MEA and SLR connect with the VTF and DTF (41). The VTF corresponds to the rostral nucleus raphe magnus of the caudal midline pons. Stimulation of

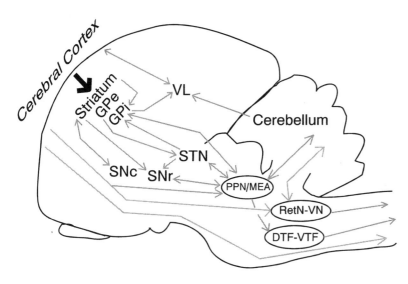

FIG. 2.5. Pathways involved in the supraspinal control of posture and movement. GPe and GPi, globus pallidus externa and interna; DTF and VTF, dorsal and ventral tegmental fields; PPN/MEA, pedunculopontine nucleus/midbrain extrapyramidal area; Ret. N., reticular nuclei; VN, lateral vestibular nucleus; SNr and SNc, substantia nigra pars reticulata and compacta; STN, subthalamus; VL, ventrolateral thalamus.

the VTF increases antigravity muscle tone. The DTF corresponds to the caudal nucleus raphe centralis superior of the caudal midline pons. Stimulation of the DTF decreases antigravity muscle tone. The DTF and VTF control postural tonus during locomotion in conjunction with neighboring reticulospinal and vestibulospinal pathways. Cholinergic agonists, excitatory amino acid agonists, GABAergic antagonists, and substance P facilitate locomotion when injected into the VTF and inhibit locomotion when injected into the DTF (42).

The frontal cortex participates in the purposeful modification and initiation of locomotion through connections with the PPN/MEA, SLR, basal ganglia, and spinal networks (Fig. 2.5) (41). Increased motor cortical discharge occurs in cats before and during the negotiation of obstacles (43), and the sensorimotor cortex interacts with the cerebellum in the feedforward control of posture and movement, as discussed under the heading "Cerebellum." Mammalian quadrupeds with pyramidal tract lesions are able to walk on smooth unobstructed surfaces but cannot adapt to environmental variations (37). Locomotion that requires precise foot placement (e.g., skilled locomotion such as walking on a horizontal ladder) is impossible without the frontal lobes (37,39).

Postural Control

Somatosensory, vestibular, and visual inputs to the central nervous system are utilized in the control of posture and balance. Somatosensory proprioception is the most important modality for generating protective postural reactions (44). Vestibular impairment produces poor control of the trunk and head, which leads to excessive motion of the body's center of mass and associated irregularities in stepping. Patients with somatosensory loss (e.g., due to peripheral neuropathy) exhibit increased reliance on vestibular, visual, and predictive mechanisms of postural control (44).

Modest mechanical perturbations of quiet stance (e.g., a nudge to the sternum) produce a synergistic distal-to-proximal activation of muscles in the lower extremities and torso. Opposing torques at the hips, knees, and ankles rotate the body about the ankles, in opposition to the perturbation. This coordinated sequence of reflex responses in muscles of the limbs and trunk has been called the ankle strategy of postural control and is preprogrammed by the nervous system, based on current sensory information, previous experience, and motor intent (44).

The amplitude and latency of postural reflexes are optimized by the nervous system, using previous experience in the context of current somatosensory, vestibular, and visual sensory information (i.e., using feedforward motor control) (44). Furthermore, the nervous system may generate postural activity in advance of a predictable perturbation, based on sensory feedback and previous experience. For example, muscles in the extremities are activated *before* impact during

a fall (45). Damage to the anterior lobe of the cerebellum impairs the feedforward control of postural responses (44).

The ankle strategy is inadequate for strong perturbations or a precarious base of support (e.g., a balance beam or slippery surface). Under these circumstances, hip rotation with appropriate arm motion *(hip strategy)* may be necessary to keep the body's center of mass over the base of support, or it may be necessary to establish an entirely new base of support through the execution of a so-called *rescue response.* Rescue responses require strength and agility that can easily exceed the neurological and musculoskeletal capabilities of neurologic patients. The frontal lobes and basal ganglia are necessary for the selection and execution of such skilled responses. Consequently, it is common to see patients with bilateral cerebral dysfunction "fall like a log," making no attempt to execute alternative rescue strategies (46).

Gait initiation is an important example of integrated postural control and movement. Normal adults exhibit three key events in gait initiation: (a) activation of tibialis anterior and inactivation of triceps surae produce bilateral ankle dorsiflexion; (b) abduction of the swing hip occurs simultaneously with event 1; and (c) abrupt 3- to 10-degree flexion of the support hip and knee occurs nearly simultaneously with events 1 and 2. Event 1 produces a sagittal moment of force (torque) that propels the body into forward motion. Events 2 and 3 propel the body laterally, toward the support limb, so that the swing foot can leave the ground. Thus, purposeful postural shifts of gait initiation propel the body from stable stance into forward motion, culminating in a forward step. A steady-state velocity of gait is attained in less than two steps. As walking proceeds, the COM must be carefully shifted from one support limb to another, resulting in a state of dynamic equilibrium. Rising on tiptoes, rising from a chair, and quickly bending forward require ankle moments of force and postural shifts in the sagittal plane that are similar to those in gait initiation (47). Each of these tasks entails postural shifts that move the body from one steady-state posture or movement to another. Patients with bilateral cerebral disease have particular difficulty with this type of task (48).

Role of Higher Cortical Function

Nutt and co-workers (46) divided gait disturbances into the following three categories:

1. *Lowest level disorders:* caused by diseases of the muscles, peripheral nerves, skeleton, peripheral vestibular system, and anterior visual pathway. Also included are the effects of secondary muscle deconditioning (type II atrophy), limb contractures, spinal ankylosis, and reduced pelvic mobility, which are common in older people.
2. *Middle-level disorders:* caused by ascending or descending sensorimotor tract lesions, cerebellar ataxia, bradykinesia, hyperkinesias, and dystonia.

3. *Highest level disorders:* caused by dysfunction of the frontal lobes and their connections with other cortical and subcortical structures.

The characteristics of middle and lowest level gait disturbances follow logically from the anatomy and physiology already reviewed in this chapter. The highest level gait disturbances have features that resemble the abnormal supporting, righting, and placing reactions in laboratory animals with resected frontal lobes. Patients with highest level gait disorders frequently exhibit variable performance, depending upon the environmental and emotional circumstances. Start hesitation, freezing, and absent rescue responses (falling like a log) are common. Also common are inappropriate or bizarre limb movements and postural synergies (e.g., leaning the wrong direction, abnormal foot placement). These characteristics of highest level gait disorders following logically from the notion that the cortical-basal ganglia-thalamocortical loop is involved in the facilitation of desired motor activity and the inhibition of undesired or inappropriate activity.

Locomotion in a familiar and friendly environment is performed effortlessly, with little conscious thought. However, the demands on cognitive function (e.g., attention, working memory) increase with the complexity of the locomotor act (walking > standing > sitting) and with the complexity of the environment (49). Cognitive demands are also increased when patients with motor or sensory impairment attempt to walk (49). Thus, even the most routine locomotor tasks require concomitant cognitive processing. Patients with frontal lobe and basal ganglia disease are less likely to meet these cognitive demands, and this may play a role in the freezing and variable performance exhibited by these patients (49).

Finally, cortical dementia can impair motor function without motor or sensory abnormalities in the neurologic examination (50). Consequently, Alzheimer patients exhibit an increased rate of falling. Declarative (explicit) memory is severely impaired, but motor learning (as in the pursuit rotor and serial reaction time tasks) is preserved as long as the Alzheimer patients are permitted to practice under constant conditions. Nevertheless, the *baseline* performance of Alzheimer patients in motor learning tasks is usually less than the performance of controls, and Alzheimer patients rarely achieve normal levels of motor performance, despite a normal *rate* of improvement with practice. Patients with mild Alzheimer's disease have prolonged reaction times and have difficulty making impromptu adjustments in a motor task. They are more likely to stumble over obstacles in their path, and Alzheimer patients who fall exhibit greater variability in stride length, which is a characteristic of disturbed locomotion. Alzheimer patients also have difficulty resolving conflicting visual and somatosensory information while trying to maintain stable stance.

CONCLUSION

Virtually the entire nervous system is involved in motor control. Many movement disorders cannot be explained in terms of pyramidal, extrapyramidal, or cerebellar function. Specialists in movement disorders enjoy ample reason to become broadly familiar with functions of the nervous system at all levels of the neuraxis, including higher cortical and limbic functions. This comprehensive approach will lead to improved diagnosis and treatment of patients with movement disorders.

REFERENCES

1. Mink JW. The basal ganglia: focused selection and inhibition of competing motor programs. *Progr Neurobiol* 1996;50(4):381–425.
2. Parent A, Cicchetti F. The current model of basal ganglia organization under scrutiny. *Mov Disord* 1998;13(2):199–202.
3. Bolam JP, Hanley JJ, Booth PA, et al. Synaptic organisation of the basal ganglia. *J Anat* 2000;196(Pt 4):527–542.
4. Nakano K, Kayahara T, Tsutsumi T, et al. Neural circuits and functional organization of the striatum. *J Neurol* 2000;247[Suppl 5]:V1–15.
5. Inglis WL, Winn P. The pedunculopontine tegmental nucleus: where the striatum meets the reticular formation. *Prog Neurobiol* 1995;47(1):1–29.
6. Hirai T, Jones EG. A new parcellation of the human thalamus on the basis of histochemical staining. *Brain Res Brain Res Rev* 1989;14(1):1–34.
7. Anderson ME, Turner RS. Activity of neurons in cerebellar-receiving and pallidal-receiving areas of the thalamus of the behaving monkey. *J Neurophysiol* 1991;66(3):879–893.
8. Elble RJ. Origins of tremor [comment]. *Lancet* 2000;355(9210):1113–1114.
9. Crossman AR. Functional anatomy of movement disorders. *J Anat* 2000;196(Pt 4):519–525.
10. Vitek JL, Chockkan V, Zhang JY, et al. Neuronal activity in the basal ganglia in patients with generalized dystonia and hemiballismus. *Ann Neurol* 1999;46(1):22–35.
11. Hedreen JC, Folstein SE. Early loss of neostriatal striosome neurons in Huntington's disease. *J Neuropathol Exp Neurol* 1995;54(1):105–120.
12. Hashimoto T, Tada T, Nakazato F, et al. Abnormal activity in the globus pallidus in off-period dystonia. *Ann Neurol* 2001;49(2):242–245.
13. Yoshor D, Hamilton WJ, Ondo W, et al. Comparison of thalamotomy and pallidotomy for the treatment of dystonia. *Neurosurgery* 2001;48(4):818–824.
14. Bhatia KP, Marsden CD. The behavioural and motor consequences of focal lesions of the basal ganglia in man. *Brain* 1994;117(Pt 4):859–876.
15. Lee MS, Marsden CD. Movement disorders following lesions of the thalamus or subthalamic region. *Mov Disord* 1994;9(5):493–507.
16. Jankovic J. Post-traumatic movement disorders: central and peripheral mechanisms. *Neurology* 1994;44(11):2006–2014.
17. Byl NN, Merzenich MM, Jenkins WM. A primate genesis model of focal dystonia and repetitive strain injury: I. Learning-induced dedifferentiation of the representation of the hand in the primary somatosensory cortex in adult monkeys. *Neurology* 1996;47(2):508–520.

18. Lenz FA, Jaeger CJ, Seike MS, et al. Thalamic single neuron activity in patients with dystonia: dystonia-related activity and somatic sensory reorganization. *J Neurophysiol* 1999;82(5):2372–2392.

19. Tempel LW, Perlmutter JS. Abnormal vibration-induced cerebral blood flow responses in idiopathic dystonia. *Brain* 1990;113(Pt 3):691–707.

20. Kaji R, Rothwell JC, Katayama M, et al. Tonic vibration reflex and muscle afferent block in writer's cramp. *Ann Neurol* 1995;38(2):155–162.

21. Naumann M, Magyar-Lehmann S, Reiners K, et al. Sensory tricks in cervical dystonia: perceptual dysbalance of parietal cortex modulates frontal motor programming. *Ann Neurol* 2000;47(3):322–328.

22. The Tourette Syndrome Classification Study Group. Definitions and classification of tic disorders. *Arch Neurol* 1993;50(10):1013–1016.

23. Rauch SL, Jenike MA, Alpert NM, et al. Regional cerebral blood flow measured during symptom provocation in obsessive-compulsive disorder using oxygen 15–labeled carbon dioxide and positron emission tomography. *Arch Gen Psychiatry* 1994;51(1):62–70.

24. Haines DE, Mihailoff GA, Bloedel JR. The cerebellum. In: Haines DE, ed. *Fundamental Neuroscience*. New York: Churchill Livingstone, 1997:379–398.

25. Thach WT, Goodkin HP, Keating JG. The cerebellum and the adaptive coordination of movement. *Annu Rev Neurosci* 1992;15:403–442.

26. Thach WT. On the specific role of the cerebellum in motor learning and cognition: clues from PET activation and lesion studies in man. *Behav Brain Sc* 1996;19:411–431.

27. Elble RJ. Animal models of action tremor. *Mov Disord* 1998;13[Suppl 3]:35–39.

28. Manto M. Pathophysiology of cerebellar dysmetria: the imbalance between the agonist and the antagonist electromyographic activities. *Eur Neurol* 1996;36(6):333–337.

29. De Zeeuw CI, Simpson JI, Hoogenraad CC, et al. Microcircuitry and function of the inferior olive. *Trends Neurosci* 1998;21(9):391–400.

30. Remy P, de Recondo A, Defer G, et al. Peduncular "rubral" tremor and dopaminergic denervation: a PET study. *Neurology* 1995;45:472–477.

31. Ohye C, Shibazaki T, Hirai T, et al. A special role of the parvocellular red nucleus in lesion-induced spontaneous tremor in monkeys. *Behav Brain Res* 1988;28(1–2):241–243.

32. Nathan PW, Smith MC. The rubrospinal and central tegmental tracts in man. *Brain* 1982;105(Pt 2):223–269.

33. Smith SS. Step cycle-related oscillatory properties of inferior olivary neurons recorded in ensembles. *Neuroscience* 1998;82(1):69–81.

34. Deuschl G, Mischke G, Schenck E, et al. Symptomatic and essential rhythmic palatal myoclonus. *Brain* 1990;113:1645–1672.

35. Jellinger K. Hypertrophy of the inferior olives: report on 29 cases. *Z Neurol* 1973;205(2):153–174.

36. Boecker H, Brooks DJ. Functional imaging of tremor. *Mov Disord* 1998;13[Suppl 3]:64–72.

37. Armstrong DM. The supraspinal control of mammalian locomotion. *J Physiol* 1988;405:1–37.

38. Dietz V, Colombo G, Jensen L, et al. Locomotor capacity of spinal cord in paraplegic patients. *Ann Neurol* 1995;37(5):574–582.

39. Henneman E. Motor functions of the brainstem and basal ganglia. In: Mountcastle VB, ed. *Medical physiology*, 13th ed. St. Louis: Mosby, 1974:678–721.

40. Eidelberg E, Walden JG, Nguyen LH. Locomotor control in macaque monkeys. *Brain* 1981;104(Pt 4):647–663.

41. Mori S, Matsuyama K, Mori F, et al. Supraspinal sites that induce locomotion in the vertebrate central nervous system. *Adv Neurol* 2001;87:25–40.

42. Kinjo N, Atsuta Y, Webber M, et al. Medioventral medulla-induced locomotion. *Brain Res Bull* 1990;24(3):509–516.

43. Widajewicz W, Kably B, Drew T. Motor cortical activity during voluntary gait modifications in the cat: II. Cells related to the hindlimbs. *J Neurophysiol* 1994;72(5):2070–2089.

44. Horak FB. Postural ataxia related to somatosensory loss. *Adv Neurol* 2001;87:173–182.

45. Dietz V, Noth J. Pre-innervation and stretch responses of triceps brachii in man falling with and without visual control. *Brain Res* 1978;142(3):576–579.

46. Nutt JG, Marsden CD, Thompson PD. Human walking and higher-level gait disorders, particularly in the elderly. *Neurology* 1993;43(2):268–279.

47. Schultz AB, Alexander NB, Ashton-Miller JA. Biomechanical analyses of rising from a chair. *J Biomech* 1992;25(12):1383–1391.

48. Elble RJ, Cousins R, Leffler K, et al. Gait initiation by patients with lower-half parkinsonism. *Brain* 1996;119:101–112.

49. Mesure S, Darmon A, Blin O. Imbalance of attentional and sensory inputs on gait. *Adv Neurol* 2001;87:243–250.

50. Elble RJ, Leffler K. Pushing and pulling with the upper extremities while standing: the effects of mild Alzheimer dementia and Parkinson's disease. [In process citation.] *Mov Disord* 2000;15(2):255–268.

NEUROTRANSMITTERS AND PHARMACOLOGY OF THE BASAL GANGLIA

PETER RIEDERER
MANFRED GERLACH
PAUL FOLEY

The basal ganglia are a group of subcortical brain nuclei long recognized to be crucial for the initiation, control, and integration of motor function in mammals, but which are also implicated in the modulation of cognitive and emotional functions. As the neuroanatomy of the basal ganglia in health and disease is described in other contributions to this volume, we will limit our discussion to those aspects required for our analysis of the localization of neurosubstances and their receptors in the basal ganglia.

DIRECT AND INDIRECT PATHWAYS IN THE BASAL GANGLIA

Despite the variety of connections between its structures, the passage of information through the basal ganglia can be described by a circuit: the cortex projects to the major input nucleus of the basal ganglia, the striatum (in humans consisting of putamen, nucleus caudatus, nucleus accumbens, and olfactory tubercle), which in turn projects via the globus pallidus (GP) and substantia nigra (SN) to the thalamus, which finally projects back to the cortex (1,2). The striatum is far from homogeneous, with regionalization of both activity and function being imposed by the major afferent pathways to the region. The various functions of the basal ganglia are reflected by parallel neural circuits passing through defined regions of the striatum, GP, and thalamus, thereby preserving striking somatotopic and functional specificity.

Neurotransmitters employed in this circuit have been identified; the corticostriatal efferents are glutamatergic and excitatory, whereas the striatopallidal and pallidofugal projections are GABAergic and inhibitory. In the striatum itself, D2 dopamine receptors negatively regulate met-enkephalin (ENK)/GABAergic neurons projecting to the external segment of the pallidum (GPe), whereas D1 receptors positively regulate substance P/dynorphin/GABAergic

projections to the internal segment of the pallidum (GPi) and the SN pars reticulata (SNr). The GPi and SNr are the major output nuclei of the basal ganglia and exert a tonic inhibitory influence on the excitatory premotor neurons of the ventral thalamus. Corticostriatal activation consequently results in disinhibition of the thalamus and of brainstem regions innervated directly by the striatum.

According to this model, the striatum projects to the SNr and GPi both directly and by an indirect route via the GPe and the subthalamic nucleus (STN). Both pathways are modulated by dopaminergic projections from the substantia nigra pars compacta (SNc) to the striatum, but in opposite directions by the two dopamine receptor types: D1 activation excites the direct striatonigral pathway, whereas D2 activation inhibits the output to the GPe. Attempts to explain movement disorders on the basis of basal ganglia architecture have generally focused on this dual innervation. As a result of reduced striatal dopamine levels in parkinsonism, striatal GABAergic fibers to the GPe are relieved from D2-mediated inhibition, leading to disinhibition of the STN and GPi and thus to a net increase in activity in the indirect pathway, whereas the reduced activation of D1 leads to reduced inhibition of SNr/GPi activity by the direct pathway.

There has recently been some criticism of this model of basal ganglia organization, and it is probable that it will require modification (e.g., ref. 3). However, this problem cannot be discussed here; the remainder of this chapter will instead restrict itself to describing the distribution of transmitters and receptors in the involved nuclei and pathways.

GABA IN THE BASAL GANGLIA

γ-Aminobutyric acid (GABA) can be regarded as the basic transmitter of the basal ganglia. GABAergic fibers are subject to the excitatory and inhibitory influences of other neuromodulators, but the GABAergic neurons constitute the basic circuits on which these other inputs act.

Striatal output neurons are mostly GABAergic medium spiny neurons and fall into two major classes defined by the copresence of peptides:

- Substance P– and dynorphin-containing projections from the striosomes ("patches") to the SNr, entopeduncular nucleus (EPN), and GPi (direct pathway); these neurons express D1 dopamine receptors. GABAergic neurons from these targets project to the ventral thalamus, which sends glutamatergic fibers to the cortex. The GPi also projects to the centromedial thalamus, which provides excitatory input to the sensorimotor striatum.
- ENK-positive efferents to the GPe (indirect pathway); these neurons express D2 receptor. The GPe sends a second GABAergic projection to the STN, which in turn projects (glutamate) to the SNr/GPi, which finally send GABAergic neurons to the thalamus.

Within the SNr, GABA release is modulated via D1 receptors by dendritically released dopamine; conversely, nigral dopaminergic neurons are inhibited by GABAergic projections from the SNr (via $GABA_A$ receptors) and by pallidonigral efferents (via $GABA_B$ receptors). Finally, intrinsic and extrinsic GABA neurons interact with dopaminergic and other neurons in the ventral tegmental area (VTA) (4–6).

In addition to striatal GABAergic outputs, there exist smaller populations of aspiny striatal GABAergic interneurons, the largest of which also express the calcium-binding protein parvalbumin (PV); they are innervated predominantly by cortical excitatory projections. Major targets of these interneurons appear to be spiny output neurons, so that they function as "feedforward" inhibitors of cortical input to GABAergic output cells (6).

Three major types of GABA receptor have been identified in the central nervous system (CNS). $GABA_C$ receptor appears to play no major role in the basal ganglia and will not be discussed further in this chapter. Until recently, most actions of GABA were attributed to the bicuculline-sensitive, ionotropic GABA receptor, $GABA_A$, found broadly distributed throughout the CNS. The G-protein-linked,

baclofen-sensitive $GABA_B$ receptor was defined in 1981 and is now recognized as important for fine-tuning of neuronal inhibition. Both receptor types are broadly distributed in the basal ganglia (Table 3.1) (7).

The central position of GABAergic transmission in extrapyramidal circuits has rendered it of great interest in the investigation of basal ganglia disease, especially as GABAergic activity has been reported to decline with age. ENK-positive GABAergic projections appear to be especially affected in Huntington's disease. It has been suggested that striatopallidal and striatonigral projections are lost in parkinsonism, as substance P levels decline in SN and GP, but metenkephalin levels are also reduced in these nuclei and in the putamen (4). Expression of mRNA for the GABA-synthesizing enzyme glutamate decarboxylase (GAD_{67}) was significantly increased in putamen, caudatus, and GPi of 1-methyl-4-phenyl-1,2,3,6-tetrahydropyridine (MPTP)–treated monkeys, one of the most popular animal models of parkinsonism, but not in the ventral striatum or GPe; the changes were reversed by L-dopa treatment, but not uniformly throughout the striatum. Similar changes are reported in the striatum of another animal model of parkinsonism, the 6-hydroxydopamine (6-OHDA)–lesioned rat, but GAD activity in these animals returned to normal levels within a few months. The levels in Parkinson's disease (PD) patients are either normal (both pallidal segments) or reduced (all striatal regions), whereas they are increased in progressive supranuclear palsy. The differences between the situation in parkinsonian patients and the MPTP-treated monkey could reflect real differences between model and disease or the effects of L-dopa therapy (3).

Effects of direct dopamine receptor stimulation on GABAergic activity have been mixed. The D2 receptor agonist quinpirole reduced GABA turnover in both intact and denervated rat striatum, consistent with an inhibitory effect of D2 activity. D1 agonists, on the other hand, have not produced consistent effects on GABAergic activity in animal models. Conversely, GABA agonists, such as muscimol and progabide, reduce dopamine synthesis and reverse neuroleptic-induced dopamine receptor supersensitivity (8,9).

GABA-related agents are not currently employed in the therapy of extrapyramidal disorders, although the $GABA_B$ agonist baclofen, which is used in the management of spas-

TABLE 3.1. GABA RECEPTORS IN THE BASAL GANGLIA

	Effector	Agonists	Antagonists	Basal Ganglia Location	Ref.
$GABA_A$	Intrinsic Cl channel	Muscimol isoguvacine	Bicuculline	General	11,12
$GABA_B$	$G_{i/o}$ (cAMP ↓, K^+ ↑, Ca^{2+} ↓)	Baclofen SR95531	2-OH-(–)saclofen	General	7,10

The $GABA_A$ receptor also includes a benzodiazepine binding site that modulates the response to activation of the actual GABA binding site. A third GABA receptor type ($GABA_C$) has not yet been found in the mammalian basal ganglia. As in all tables in this chapter, lists of agonists and antagonists cannot be comprehensive; for more details, see the *Trends in Pharmacological Sciences* annual "Receptor and ion channel nomenclature" supplement.
GABA, γ-aminobutyric acid; cAMP, cyclic adenosine monophosphate.

ticity, has been suggested as a candidate for modulation of the balance between direct and indirect pathways in parkinsonism. Progabide was seen earlier as possibly useful in managing L-dopa-induced dyskinesia (7,8).

GLUTAMATE IN THE BASAL GANGLIA

Glutamate receptors are found in all regions of the basal ganglia. Glutamatergic neurons project topographically from most regions of the cortex to the striatum, sensorimotor cortical areas projecting primarily to the putamen and associative areas to the caudatus, whereas the limbic cortex (as well as amygdala and the hippocampus) projects to the ventral striatum (ventral caudate-putamen, olfactory tubercle, and nucleus accumbens). In the striatum, glutamate acts via both NMDA (*N*-methyl-D-aspartate) and AMPA (α-amino-3-hydroxy-5-methyl-4-isoxazolepropionate) receptors, primarily at dendritic synapses, to elicit depolarization of spiny neurons.

Most studies to date have focused on the role of NMDA receptor–mediated mechanisms in the extrapyramidal system, principally because of problems regarding availability of suitable pharmacologic agents (Table 3.2). NMDA receptor concentration is greater in the ventral than the dorsal striatum, possibly reflecting greater cell density in this area; furthermore, ENK-positive projection neurons express greater levels of the NR-1 and NR-2 subunits than interneurons (6,13,14). Lower NMDA receptor levels are measured in the GP, EPN, and STN, but the presence of excitatory amino acid efferents to these nuclei supports

their physiologic significance. NMDA receptor levels are similarly low in the SN, which receives excitatory amino acid projections from both the cortex and the STN, but the infusion of NMDA receptor agonists or antagonists has been shown to elicit behavioral changes (5,14).

Activation of NMDA receptors in the caudate-putamen is implicated in the control of motor activity initiation; blockade of these receptors in rats is associated with reduced behavioral latency, increased locomotor activity, and stereotypy. It was thus hypothesized that reduced NMDA receptor stimulation might overcome akinesia subsequent to dopamine depletion; in rodent models of parkinsonism (reserpine, MPTP, 6-OHDA), however, this has not proved to be the case, suggesting that dopaminergic innervation must be intact for the activating effects of NMDA receptor blockade to be manifested. Similarly, the motor effects of L-dopa and anticholinergic agents are facilitated by NMDA receptor antagonists, although the latter are by themselves without marked effect. It has further been noted that intrastriatal NMDA receptor blockade reduced D2 receptor-induced motor activation in normal animals but facilitated the same in dopamine-depleted rats; D1 receptor–related activation was inhibited by NMDA receptor blockade in both paradigms (2,5).

It is clear that the response to NMDA receptor stimulation or blockade is complex, depending not only on the status of dopaminergic striatal innervation but also on the specific dopamine receptor type involved. This problem cannot be discussed in detail here; the reader is referred to recent reviews in refs. 5, 6, and 15. It should be noted, however, that in parkinsonism, glutamatergic hyperactivity in

TABLE 3.2. GLUTAMATE RECEPTORS IN THE BASAL GANGLIA

		Effector	Basal Ganglia Location		Ref.
NMDA	NR-1	Ionotropic: $Na^+/K^+/Ca^{2+}$	StrPr (Enk) Int (Ch, SST)		14,22, 26,27
Antagonists: MK-801 (dizocilpine), CGS19755	NR-2		StrPr (Enk) Int (Ch, SST)	SNc GP*i* STN	
AMPA	GluR-1 GluR-4	Ionotropic: $Na^+/K^+/Ca^{2+}$	StrPr GABA-Parv	Int (Ch) SNr	12,23,28
Antagonists: NBQX, CNQX	GluR-2 GluR-3		StrPr GABA-PV	SNr	
Kainate		Ionotropic: $Na^+/K^+/Ca^{2+}$	StrPr (Enk) GP*i*	STN	26
Agonists: ATPA, 4-methylglutamate *Antagonist: LY294486*					
Metabotropic	(mglu$_1$–mglu$_8$)	G-protein-linked ($G_{i/o}$ or $G_{q/11}$)	StrPr (Enk) GP*i*	STN SNr	24,26
Agonists, antagonists: see Roberts, 1995					

There are at least four distinct NR-2 subunits; for basal ganglia distribution, see ref. 14.
StrPr, striatal projection neurons; Int, striatal interneurons; Enk, enkephalin positive; SST, somatostatin positive; PV, parvalbumin positive; Ch, cholinergic; NBQX, 6-nitro-7-sulfamoylbenz(f)quinoxaline-2,3-dione; CNQX, 6-cyano-7-nitroquinoxaline-2,3-dione; ATPA, 2-amino-3-(3-hydroxy-5-*tert*-butylisoxazol-4-yl)propionate; other abbreviations as in text.

the striatum is accompanied by hypoactivity in the thalamocortical loop, so that systemic administration of antagonists has certain practical problems. The levels of glutamate, aspartate, and GABA are normal in all measured regions of the parkinsonian brain, whereas those of the NMDA receptor are normal in all areas except the caudate nucleus, where a small but significant decline is measured, although depletion of nigral NMDA binding sites in parkinsonism has also been reported. Declines in the concentrations of other glutamate receptor types (kainate and AMPA receptors) are also detected in the caudate nucleus; otherwise, these receptors are also normal in PD. CGP 39653 (NMDA receptor) binding is also normal in most regions apart from the putamen in PD but decreased in the GPi of patients who have experienced akinetic crises. Reduced pallidal NMDA receptor binding may reflect receptor down-regulation in response to increased STN activity (reviewed in 3, 16, 17).

Animal models of parkinsonism have suggested that NMDA receptor antagonists might be useful in relieving extrapyramidal symptoms of parkinsonism, including L-dopa-induced dyskinesia, and of Huntington's disease. The conflicting results in animal models of parkinsonism have hampered developments in this direction, but there is also a major problem in the fact that systemic administration of NMDA receptor antagonists has major side effects. The role of NMDA receptor antagonists in extrapyramidal therapy thus remains open (reviewed in 14, 18, 19). *Orphenadrine*, originally developed as an antihistamine/anticholinergic, is still used to a limited extent in antiparkinsonian therapy, and is now recognized to also be a noncompetitive NMDA receptor antagonist. The major NMDA receptor antagonists currently employed in antiparkinsonian therapy are *amantadine*—the antiparkinsonian properties of which were discovered long before its antiglutamatergic properties were recognized—and *budipine*, which is also anticholinergic, indirectly dopaminergic, noradrenergic, and serotonergic (20).

The employment of NMDA receptor antagonists to protect against excitotoxic damage has also been considered; for example, riluzole delays appearance of motor deficits in MPTP-treated monkeys. Intracerebral administration of NMDA receptor antagonists has also been found to relieve parkinsonian symptoms in this model; however, systemic administration of such drugs has not been as successful (14).

Elucidation of the role of striatal AMPA receptors in basal ganglia function has proved more elusive. Betarbet and colleagues (21 and references therein) reported that 75% of dopaminergic striatal cells express GluR1 and 25% NR1, but not GluR2/3 or group 1 metabotropic receptors (mGluR1, mGluR5), suggesting that these neurons express only calcium-permeable ionotropic glutamate receptors. AMPA receptor activation may reduce spontaneous motor activity in both rodents and primates, despite being present on the same striatal neurons as NMDA receptors (22). The distribution of the various AMPA and kainate-type glutamatergic receptors in human and rat pallidum and striatum suggests that antagonists of these receptors, particularly of the AMPA receptor GluR4, which dominates in the GPi neuropil, might be useful in antiparkinsonian treatment. The presence of glutamatergic receptors on striatal cholinergic interneurons means that antiglutamatergic agents might mimic the effect of antiparkinsonian anticholinergic drugs. Intrastriatal (but not systemic) application of AMPA receptor antagonists has been reported to be antiparkinsonian, but there are as yet no concrete suggestions that such agents be employed in the therapy of extrapyramidal motor disorders (15,23).

The significance of basal ganglia kainate and metabotropic glutamate receptors has been investigated even less. Vezina and Kim (24) have recently reviewed the evidence for a role of the latter in glutamate–dopamine interactions in the basal ganglia, including the sensitization of locomotor activity by psychotropic drugs. Smith et al. (7) proposed that the employment of antagonists to metabotropic glutamate receptors (particularly mGluR1 and mGluR5, located at STN synapses in the GPe, and mGluR4, located primarily at striatopallidal targets) might allow modulation of excitatory amino acid transmission in parkinsonism without the side effects of agents acting at ionotropic glutamate receptors. Changes in GluR1 levels in the MPTP model of parkinsonism have recently been reported, with increases in caudate and putamen (particularly in the striosomes), marked reductions in GP and SN, and little change in the STN (21).

Glutamate may also play a number of other significant roles in the function of the basal ganglia (14):

- Excitatory synaptic transmission at non-NMDA glutamate receptors in the striatum has been implicated in long-term depression (LTD), a form of neural plasticity. LTD requires the function of the dopaminergic nigrostriatal pathway and is thus lost in parkinsonism.
- NMDA receptor antagonists block striatal δ-opioid agonist (i.e., ENK-mediated)–induced dopamine release. δ-Opioid agonists also stimulate glutamate release.
- NMDA receptor stimulation increases striatal nitric oxide (NO) synthesis, either directly or via stimulation of acetylcholine (ACh) release by interneurons, leading to muscarinic activation of neuronal NO synthase–positive cells.
- Glutamate depresses striatal preproenkephalin mRNA levels (as does dopamine); ENK is employed as a neurosubstance in the indirect striatal pathway.
- Glutamate reduces D2 receptor affinity in striatal membranes by a non-NMDA mechanism.

There is finally some suggestion that some corticostriatal fibers may employ aspartate as an excitatory amino acid transmitter. Ungerstedt's laboratory has reported that activation of D1, κ-opioid, and cholecystokinin (CCK) receptors elicits striatal aspartate release, but its presence in presynaptic vesicles is yet to be demonstrated (25).

DOPAMINE IN THE BASAL GANGLIA

The caudate, putamen, and accumbens also receive prominent dopaminergic innervation via mesostriatal pathways (nigrostriatal path and elements of the mesolimbic system), and in particular accept afferents from the A9 region of the SN, particularly the SNc. The nigrostriatal pathway is of especial significance as it is this pathway which degenerates in parkinsonism, leading to reduced striatal dopamine levels and up-regulation of D2 receptor numbers. Its terminals form symmetric synapses with necks of dendrites on the spiny projection neurons. Dopaminergic innervation thus modulates excitatory cortical input, which generally interacts with heads of the same dendrites. Input from the retrorubral nucleus (A8) also modulates striatal output neuron activity; the density of the melanized cells in this region is also reduced in the parkinsonian brain. The ventral striatum receives its major dopaminergic innervation from the A10 cells of the VTA via the mesolimbic pathway. Dopaminergic fibers interact with GABAergic and substance P–containing medium spiny neurons projecting to the SN and GP (29).

The major modulator of striatal dopamine release is glutamate acting at both NMDA and AMPA receptors, although its basal release is largely a function of nigrostriatal activity levels. In addition, efferents from the ventral caudatus (which receives input from the limbic brain areas) modulate the activity of nigral dopamine neurons that innervate the dorsal striatum, which is primarily concerned with motor function. This implies that one part of the striatum is capable of modifying the activity of another, and also provides an interface between the limbic and motor areas of the brain. The dopaminergic elements of the striatum thus assume a vital role in the modulation of the integration of cortical input by this region (5,6,29).

It has also been established that a small number of intrastriatal dopaminergic small bipolar neurons exist, particularly in the rostrodorsal caudate nucleus and putamen, the density of which increases following destruction of the nigrostriatal tract. These neurons also bear NR-1 and AMPA GluR2/3 receptors (30).

Five distinct genes coding dopamine receptors have been identified, but the available receptor agonists and antagonists have until recently only allowed the pharmacologic distinction of two major receptor families, D1 and D2 (Table 3.3). Both classes are expressed on striatal efferents (medium spiny neurons). In situ hybridization investigations suggest that D1 receptors are principally (but not exclusively) located on substance P–positive striatonigral and striatopenduncular neurons, whereas D2 receptors are local to ENK-positive striatopallidal neurons. Neurons in the striatal matrix, strongly innervated by both glutamatergic cortical and dopaminergic nigral projections, express primarily D1 receptor, whereas the less densely innervated striosomes express D2 receptor. The significance of limited extent of coexpression of the two receptor types by some neurons remains unclear (31). On the other hand, reduced function of D2-bearing medium spiny neurons appears to be accompanied by increased activity of similar cells expressing D1 receptor. D2 receptors are also found on cholinergic interneurons, where they inhibit ACh release, and as autoreceptors on dopamine-releasing afferents. Interestingly, it is not established whether inhibitory D2 receptors are located presynaptically on cortical glutamatergic fibers. Of the minor dopamine receptor types, D5 receptor has been identified on striatal cholinergic interneurons, and on a few medium spiny cells, whereas D3/D4/D5 receptors

TABLE 3.3. DOPAMINE RECEPTORS IN THE BASAL GANGLIA

		Effector	Agonist	Antagonist	Basal Ganglia Location		Ref.
D1 family	D1	G_s (cAMP ↑)	SKF38393 dihydrexidine	SCH23390 SKF83566	StrPr SP Dyn	SNc SNr GPi STN	2,43,44
	D5	G_s	Similar to D1		Int-Ch		45
D2 family	D2	$G_{i/o}$ (cAMP ↓, K^+ ↑, Ca^{2+} ↓)	(+)PHNO quinpirole bromocriptine lisuride cabergoline	raclopride haloperidol sulpiride domperidone	StrPr Enk Int (Ch, GABA-Parv) SNc	GPi	11,43
	D3	$G_{i/o}$	7-OH-DPAT	nafadotride (+)S14297	Ventral striatum STN SNc		46
	D4	$G_{i/o}$	Same as D2 (lower affinity)	L741742 L745870 U101958	GPi Dorsal striatum Thalamus		47

PHNO, 9-hydroxy-4-propylnaphthoxamine; 7-OH-DPAT, 7-hydroxy-2-aminopropylaminotetralin; other abbreviations as in text and Table 3.2.

each occur together with D1/D2 receptors on striofugal cells (5,6).

The GPi expresses D1 receptor, consistent with its dense dopaminergic innervation, whereas the less innervated GPe expresses primarily D2 receptor. Both major classes of dopamine receptor are expressed in the STN and VTA. D1, but not D2, receptors have been identified in the EPN, but dopamine release has not been demonstrated, casting doubt on their function. Dopaminergic projections from the SNc to the SNr are presumed to regulate dopamine release and firing rate via D2 receptors and GABA release from afferents via D1 receptors. These latter receptors are also believed to be important for motor control and probably play an important role in the action of L-dopa in parkinsonian patients (4,5,29).

The action of dopamine in the basal ganglia cannot be discussed here in detail. Recognition of the crucial role of dopamine in extrapyramidal motor system was initiated by the discovery by Carlsson's and Sano's groups at the end of the 1950s that the amine was concentrated in the mammalian basal ganglia. This was followed by the discovery that striatal dopamine deficiency was central to parkinsonism and, conversely, that schizophrenia was relieved by reducing dopamine-mediated transmission.

A better understanding of the interaction of the effects mediated by D1 and D2 receptors (and possibly of their subtypes) appears necessary to properly appreciate the action of dopamine. For example: dyskinesia associated with long-term L-dopa administration is interpreted by the standard model as being indicative of an imbalance between the activity of the direct and indirect pathways. This has variously been attributed to various causes, but, interestingly, the D2 and mixed D2/D3 agonists employed in PD, such as lisuride, bromocriptine, ropinirole, and pramipexole, are less associated with this problem, whereas the mixed agonist D1/D2 pergolide is reported to be similar to L-dopa with respect to the induction of dyskinesia. Selective D1 stimulation with ABT-431 in patients with PD also elicited an improvement in motor symptoms comparable with that achieved by L-dopa, with significantly fewer problems with respect to dyskinesia (3,32).

It has been hypothesized that D2 receptor sensitivity might be regulated by the D1 receptor; indeed, the major characteristic that distinguishes post- from presynaptic striatal D2 is not one of structure but the fact that the former require concurrent D1 activation for full activity. Relations between the two receptor types in the CNS are complex; but activation of D1 receptor is generally reported to depress striatal D2 sensitivity, and the relationship depends on continued exposure to D2, but not necessarily D1, stimulation. The maintenance of this interaction has potential significance for normal CNS function; there is evidence that D2 sensitivity can be more dependent on this relationship than on D2 receptor concentration. For example, it is suggested that antipsychotic drugs with significant antagonist activity at D1 as well as at D2 are more effective than

pure D2 antagonists and avoid side effects produced by supersensitized striatal D2; the "atypical" antipsychotics exhibit such activity, in addition to activity at other receptor classes (33).

The role of dopaminergic SNc projections to the STN is not clear in either the normal or parkinsonian state. It has been noted that the motor response to L-dopa resembles that evoked by STN stimulation. The role of D1 receptors in L-dopa-induced dyskinesia is of particular interest; D1 receptor concentrations are elevated in striatum and putamen of PD patients, a change partially reversed by L-dopa treatment (34). Dopaminergic fibers that arborize directly in the STN and GPi and the dopamine released in the SNr by SNc dendrites are not considered by the standard model of basal ganglia function; in all three cases, D1 receptors are involved (3,35).

The situation is thus far from satisfactory and in need of a great deal of investigation. Experiments with "knockout mice" have underscored the significance of D2 receptors for motor control; mice lacking this receptor presented parkinsonian-like abnormalities of motor coordination, whereas those in which D1 receptor had been depleted were more affected with respect to their response to psychomotor stimulation (such as cocaine and amphetamine). Such drugs induce the expression of c-Fos and JunB, as well as of the peptide dynorphin, in D1 receptor–bearing neurons of the direct striatal pathway. On the other hand, induction of c-Fos and JunB can be elicited by stimulation of D2 receptor in the lateral striatum. D2 receptor stimulation in the caudate-putamen appears important for rapid initiation of movement (36).

D1 receptor–mediated activation of adenylyl cyclase leads to increased activation of protein kinase A (PKA), which phosphorylates the NMDA receptor NR1 and the dopamine- and cyclic adenosine monophosphate (cAMP)–regulated phosphoprotein (DARPP-32); the latter inhibits dephosphorylation of NR1, whereas activation of NR1 inhibits phosphorylation of DARPP-32, opposing dopamine receptor–mediated activity. There is thus an intimate interplay between glutamatergic and dopaminergic activity at the molecular level, leading to the suggestion that NMDA antagonists might thus be useful in facilitating dopaminergic transmission (37).

Because of its relevance to the therapy of PD, a final issue must be briefly mentioned here. It has been hypothesized that dyskinesias and other untoward effects of L-dopa therapy might result from the intermittent stimulation of dopamine receptors that would be expected to result from the typical dosing schedule, and that continuous receptor stimulation (e.g., by continuous infusion or the employment of antagonist with a long pharmacologic half-life) might circumvent such problems. While such therapeutic approaches have shown some promise in the clinic, it is also recognized that the duration of physiologic response to antiparkinsonian agents with short half-lives, such as lisuride and L-dopa itself, is much longer than might be expected from their plasma half-life. Further, there is evidence from animal studies that continuous dopamine receptor stimulation via indirect agonists (amphetamine, cocaine), in contrast to intermittent stimulation, leads to development of tolerance associated with D2 autoreceptor supersensitivity. Further evidence of the complicated nature of this situation is the fact that L-dopa therapy, in contrast to amphetamine use, does not normally lead to either tolerance or addiction; in fact, amphetamine dependency is not developed by parkinsonian patients (or in hyperkinetic children) unless they have been treated with L-dopa (38–41).

For other recent detailed reviews of the basal ganglia dopaminergic system, see refs. 29 and 42. The standard therapy of parkinsonism has been based since the 1970s on administration of the dopamine precursor L-dopa and/or direct dopamine receptor agonists. This broad field is discussed in detail elsewhere in this volume.

ACETYLCHOLINE IN THE BASAL GANGLIA

Acetylcholine has been intimately linked with striatal dopaminergic function, originally by observations that dopaminergic agonists and muscarinic antagonists both ameliorated parkinsonian symptoms. The neostriatum contains the highest concentrations in the CNS of all the cholinergic markers (ACh, choline acetyltransferase, high-affinity choline uptake, and muscarinic receptors). Cholinergic interneurons compose only 1% to 2% of striatal neurons but play an important role in the transfer of information from striatal input structures, the cortex and the SN, to striatal output systems. Dopaminergic fibers projecting from the brainstem interact both synaptically and extrasynaptically with the large aspiny cholinergic neurons; striatal D2 receptor localization largely corresponds to that of these cholinergic neurons. The degree of striatal dopamine–ACh interaction is greatest in the accumbal shell and the olfactory tubercle; in the accumbal core and caudate-putamen, the interaction is strongest in the matrix compartment (the striosomes are by definition poor in cholinergic markers). The extensive dendritic tree of the cholinergic neurons also receives GABAergic input from thalamic projections and from intrinsic neurons, with little (glutamatergic) cortical input, particularly in the ventral striatum. Cholinergic interneurons have extensive intrastriatal projections (about 0.5 mm), and synapse in turn on GABAergic efferents to the SN, and thus modulate the same fibers as dopaminergic input. There is also some evidence for extrastriatal cholinergic projections to the cortex (48).

Muscarinic ACh receptors are distributed in the basal ganglia in a highly specific fashion (Table 3.4). In the striatum, the m_2 receptor, perhaps acting as an autoreceptor, is found on large neurons throughout the caudate-putamen and accumbens, while the m_1 receptor is found on 80% of neurons in the rat striatum. The m_1 and m_4 receptors (the latter often colocated with D2 receptor) are implicated in control of both direct and indirect pathways and the coordination of spiny neural activity, although their precise roles (and, indeed, of ACh) in these capacities remain obscure. The intrastriatal segregation of m_1 and m_2 receptors to projection and local circuit neurons, respectively, suggests that m_1 receptors modulate extrinsic glutamatergic and monoaminergic afferents and intrinsic GABAergic inputs to projection neurons, whereas m_2 receptors regulate ACh release from cholinergic interneuron axons. In the SN, the m_4 receptor has been associated with a cholinergic projection from the pedunculopontine nucleus, whereas the m_5 receptor has been implicated in the control of dopaminergic transmission; in the rat, its mRNA is colocated with that for D2 receptor (49,50).

Dopaminergic agonists acting at D2 on the cholinergic interneurons tonically inhibit the depolarization-induced release of ACh, whereas D1 receptor activation enhances ACh release, probably by activation of glutamate release from corticostriatal projections. Dopaminergic terminals do not make synaptic contact with cholinergic interneurons in the striatum; instead, cholinergic and dopaminergic terminals provide parallel inputs to a third neuronal type, the medium spiny (GABAergic) neuron, whereas ACh- and dopamine-releasing neurons interact extrasynaptically, possibly by axo-axonic neuromodulation (51). Serotonergic agonists also inhibit the release of striatal ACh (52), but the significance of serotonergic innervation of the striatum remains relatively unexplored.

ACh regulates dopamine release in a complex manner (inhibition/stimulation), depending on striatal compartment. The m_1 muscarinic receptors distinct from ACh autoreceptors stimulate dopamine efflux (possibly by inhibiting nearby presynaptic dopamine autoreceptors), as do presynaptic nicotinic receptors, which also inhibit dopamine reuptake. Interestingly, chronic nicotine reduces striatal dopamine turnover and has positive effects on receptor binding, whereas acute nicotine potentiates the behavioral effects of haloperidol (44).

Despite the fact that anticholinergic (antimuscarinic) agents were long employed in antiparkinsonian therapy, their precise site of action has never been decisively established. It is generally reported that striatal muscarinic receptor levels are normal in parkinsonism but somewhat increased in the medial GP. Joyce (53) found that the greatest loss of striatal m_2 receptors in parkinsonism was in the dorsolateral striatum, whereas m_1 receptors were reduced in most regions; these changes were coordinated to some extent with loss of D2 receptor and dopamine uptake sites. Other workers have identified little or no change in striatal m_2 receptor levels (but increased binding in the cortex) together with reduced striatal m_1 receptor binding (16,54). None of this has thus far been related to the mechanism of action of anticholinergic antiparkinsonian drugs, most of which bind with high affinity to m_1 and with moderate affinity to m_2 muscarinic receptors. Izurieta-Sanchez et al. (55) recently reported that locally applied benzhexol had no effect on L-dopa-induced dopamine release in the rat striatum, also suggesting a site of action distal to this locus.

TABLE 3.4. ACH RECEPTORS IN THE BASAL GANGLIA

		Agonists	Antagonists	Effector	Basal Ganglia Location	Ref.
Nicotinic	Neuronal, α-bungarotoxin sensitive ($\alpha 7$, $\alpha 8$)	Anatoxin DMAC	α-bungarotoxin methyllycaconitine	Intrinsic Ca^{2+}/Na^+ channels	General	56,57, 61
	Neuronal, α-bungarotoxin insensitive ($\alpha 2$–6, $\beta 2$–4)	Nicotine cytisine ABT418	Dihydro-β-erythroidine	Intrinsic Ca^{2+}/Na^+ channels	General SN: esp. $\alpha 6$, $\beta 3$	
Muscarinic[a]	m_1		MT7 4-DAMP	$G_{q/11}$ (IP$_3$/DG)	StrPr Int-SOM	12,50, 59
	m_2		tripitramine AFDX384	$G_{i/o}$ (cAMP)	CaudPut NA StrPr Int-Ch	
	m_3		4-DAMP darifenacin	$G_{q/11}$ (IP$_3$/DG)	STN	60
	m_4		MT3 4-DAMP	$G_{i/o}$ (cAMP)	StrPr SN STN	
	m_5		4-DAMP darifenacin	$G_{q/11}$ (IP$_3$/DG)	SNc	

[a]Antagonists for muscarinic receptor subtypes are only relatively selective; given are those antagonists with the highest pA_2 listed in the 1998 edition of the "receptor and ion channel nomenclature" supplement of *Trends in Pharmacological Sciences*. Pirenzepine is the usual antagonist employed in binding experiments.
NA, nucleus accumbens; IP$_3$/DG, stimulates phosphoinositide metabolism; ABT418, (*S*)-3-methyl-2-pyrrolidinyl)isoxazole; DMAC, 3-(4)-dimethylaminocinnamylidine; MT3/MT7, black mamba toxins; 4-DAMP, 4-diphenylacetoxy-*N*-methylpiperidine methiodide. Other abbreviations as in text and Table 3.2.

This view is particularly supported by the fact that anticholinergic agents were relatively effective in the control of tremor, generally linked to oscillators located in the brainstem, but essentially ineffective with respect to akinesia. In general, however, the role of basal ganglia ACh in motor control remains relatively unexplored, to the extent that cholinergic neurons often merit no mention in discussions of the involved neural circuits. Calabresi and colleagues (48), however, have recently published an unusually detailed discussion of cholinergic function in the striatum, the major findings of which were as follows:

- ACh controls ACh release from cholinergic interneurons, principally via activation of m_2 receptors.
- ACh potentiates the activation of striatal efferents elicited by NMDA receptor activation, this potentiation being mediated by m_1 receptors and the activation of phospholipase C.
- ACh inhibits glutamate (via presynaptic m_2/m_3 receptors) and GABA release (m_1/m_2).

Nevertheless, the authors concluded that the precise role(s) of cholinergic transmission in the striatum remains "enigmatic," although the promotion of long-term potentiation via m_1 receptor activation may be involved.

The role of extrapyramidal nicotinic receptors is even less explored. Most studies until now have been restricted to determining the distribution of various nicotinic receptor subunits in animal brain. The $\alpha 6$ and $\beta 3$ subunits are concentrated in the basal ganglia (and medial habenula); $\alpha 4$ and $\beta 2$ is also found in the SN, as are $\alpha 5$ and $\alpha 7$, albeit at lower levels (56). Quik and colleagues detected mRNA for $\alpha 4$, $\alpha 6$, $\alpha 7$, and $\beta 2$–4 in monkey SN, with particularly high levels of $\alpha 6$ and $\beta 3$; the only changes following MPTP-induced nigral degeneration were the rise in $\alpha 6$ and decline in $\beta 3$ mRNA levels (57 and related papers). Basal ganglia nicotinic receptor levels have also been reported by some workers to be reduced in parkinsonism (58), but nicotinic agonists have historically proved to be of limited benefit in therapy; almost all classic anticholinergic antiparkinsonian drugs are antimuscarinic.

ADENOSINE IN THE BASAL GANGLIA

Adenosine is different to the neurosubstances thus far discussed in that it is not a true transmitter but rather a neuromodulator. It has long been recognized that adenosine was broadly present in synapses across the entire CNS but was nonetheless associated with specific physiologic actions in different regions, increasing the adenylyl cyclase response to neurotransmitter stimulation by other substances but also inhibiting release of the same transmitters. Adenosine is now regarded as an agent involved in fine-tuning synaptic transmission by other neurosubstances via direct receptor–receptor interaction and common signal pathways (62,63).

Three classes of adenosine have been identified in the CNS: A1 and A3, which inhibit cAMP formation, and

TABLE 3.5. ADENOSINE RECEPTORS IN THE BASAL GANGLIA

	Agonists	Antagonists	Effector	Basal Ganglia Location	Ref.
A_1	CPA CCPA	DPCPX	$G_{i/o}$ (cAMP ↓, K^+ ↑, Ca^{2+} ↓)	StrPr	69,72
A_{2A}	CGS21680 APEC	ZM241385 SCH58261	G_s (cAMP ↑)	StrPr	66
A_{2B}			G_s (cAMP ↑)	StrPr	69
A_3	2Cl-IB-MECA	MRS1220 L2268605	$G_{i/o}$ (cAMP ↓, PLC-C/D ↑)>	Not reported	

CPA, N^6-cyclopentyladenosine; CCPA, 2-chloro-N^6-cyclopentyladenosine; DPCPX, 8-cyclopentyl-1,3-dipropylxanthine; APEC, 2-(phenylethylamino)adenosine-5′-N-ethyluronamide; IB-MECA, N^6-(3-iodobenzyl)adenosine-5′-N-methyluronamide. Other abbreviations as in text and Table 3.2.

A2A/B, which enhances it (Table 3.5). In the striatum, A1 receptors are colocated with D1 receptors on direct pathway projections, while A2a receptors are found together with D2 on indirect output neurons; in each case, stimulation of adenosine receptor appears to counter the effect of dopaminergic stimulation on GABA release by these neurons (5). Among other suggested roles of striatal adenosine are the regulation of dopamine release (inhibition via A1 and stimulation via A2 receptors, the latter only significant at very high adenosine concentrations; A2 has not been reported on nigrostriatal terminals). Adenosine also modulates striatal ACh and GABA release via the same receptor classes, with A2 receptors playing a more significant role in these release of these transmitters; especially interesting is the high extracellular adenosine production that takes place at striatal cholinergic synapses (62,64).

A2 receptors also reduce D2 sensitivity by a direct receptor–receptor interaction in the striatal membrane, this direct modulation being enhanced in the 6-OHDA-denervated striatum. A similar interaction between A1 and D1 receptors has also been reported. For a recent review of this question, see ref. 63. Functional interaction of striatal A2A and NMDA receptors has also been reported, with the suggestion that NMDA might increase cAMP production via stimulation of adenosine receptors (65). At the molecular level, evidence has recently emerged that adenosine A2a receptors, in particular, regulate the expression of immediate early genes and of DARPP-32 in striatopallidal efferents (66).

Rather than acting alone, signal transduction systems can thus interact directly at the membrane level from an early stage of signal reception, and the potential influence of one signal on another is thereby enhanced. This interaction is superimposed on that of the second-messenger pathways activated by different transmitters and humoral factors, and of the different pathways activated by individual receptor types.

The action of adenosine receptor stimulation in other basal ganglia nuclei has not been as extensively investigated (62,66,67).

Evidence for a role of striatal adenosine in motor initiation includes the observation that stimulation of central adenosine A2a receptors by intraventricular or intrastriatal CGS 21680 elicits akinesia in rats, and that intrastriatal blockade of A2a receptors by a water-soluble adenosine A2a receptor antagonist reversed akinesia induced by systemic dopamine D1 and D2 antagonists, as did systemic administration of selective adenosine A2a receptor antagonists (5). Blockade of striatal A2a receptors might thus be useful in parkinsonian akinesia, especially as L-dopa-induced dyskinesia is less severe in monkey models of parkinsonism when the animals are treated with the A2a receptor antagonist KW-6002 (68). On the other hand, evidence suggests that stimulation of striatal adenosine A1 receptors produces motor inhibition; indeed, systemic adenosine A1 agonists induce akinesia and reversed motor activation induced by a dopamine D1 receptor agonist in reserpinized animals (5). A2 receptor levels were reported to be normal in the parkinsonian striatum but markedly reduced in Huntington's disease (69).

Adenosine A2a receptor antagonists have been proposed recently as new potential antiparkinsonians (70,71). The nonselective adenosine antagonist theophylline has occasionally been reported to improve major parkinsonian motor symptoms.

STRIATAL NEUROPEPTIDES

Specific peptide distribution in the striatum is employed to classify neuronal populations in this region, and many are implicated in the direct receptor–receptor modulation of D2 receptor sensitivity (73). In fact, two of the major striatal peptides down-regulating dopaminergic activity, neurotensin and CCK, have been suggested to be "endogenous antipsychotics" (74). The negative effect of CCK on D2 receptor persists when the latter is hypersensitized, and antagonizes many dopamine-induced stereotypies and the inhibition by dopamine of striatal dopamine release. Neurotensin has similar effects, but is itself positively regulated by D1 receptor activation (74). Hökfelt's group has also presented evidence that CCK potentiates striatal excitatory amino acid transmission via stimulation of the CCK$_B$ receptor (24).

The differentiation of striatal GABAergic neurons according to opioid peptide and substance P coexpression has been discussed above. It has been hypothesized that the function of dynorphin and ENK in the striatal output pathways is to dampen excessive excitation of these cells by the classical transmitters (75). Levels of these peptides are influenced by dopamine receptor activity—chronic apomorphine induces increased expression of substance P and dynorphin, but not of ENK in striosomes, whereas lesions of the nigrostriatal tract elicit the opposite changes—but the functional significance of the peptide changes is unclear; it is probable that dopamine receptor stimulation regulates peptide expression (76). Interestingly, the muscarinic antagonist and former antiparkinsonian agent scopolamine was found to block haloperidol-induced increases in ENK and D2 receptor expression (77). Also interesting is the finding that the motor effects elicited by dynorphin in mice are not blocked by naloxone but are opposed by NMDA receptor antagonists, suggesting that the peptide is also active at this receptor. It has been reported that dynorphin potentiates NMDA-activated currents, probably via the glycine site of the NMDA receptor (75).

Striatal GABAergic interneurons have also been classified according to their neuropeptide content (6):

- Parvalbumin (a calcium-binding protein), innervated via AMPA receptors from sensory and motor cortex.
- Somatostatin, usually together with NADPH-diaphorase and NO synthase. Striatal somatostatin is reduced in parkinsonism and increased in Huntington's disease.
- Calretinin (another calcium-binding protein).

Expression of preproenkephalin A (PPE-A; peptide marker of striatal indirect pathway) gene was increased in striatum of MPTP-treated monkeys, which effect was not reversed by L-dopa treatment, and striatal expression of preprotachykinin (PPT; substance P precursor, direct pathway) gene was decreased, an effect partially relieved by L-dopa. Both changes were related to the degree of MPTP-induced impairment. A similar effect of MPTP on the two peptides in marmosets, and also for the effect of L-dopa, has also been reported, as was the fact that the D2 agonists bromocriptine and ropinirole reversed the effect of MPTP on PPE-A but not on PPT—the opposite of what was achieved with L-dopa. The dissociation of expression of the two peptides in MPTP monkeys may be relevant both to the benefit of L-dopa therapy and to the complications associated with its long-term use. It also suggests that the predominant effect of L-dopa in the MPTP striatum is via the direct pathway. In PD, striatal expression of mRNA for neither ENK nor substance P is significantly different from that in normal persons. This contrasts with the antiparallel changes in the concentrations of these two peptides associated with acute nigrostriatal denervation in the rat, an effect reversed by the D2 receptor agonist quinpirole, as well as with reports of reduced substance P protein levels in stria-

tum and its output nuclei in parkinsonism. The absence of changes in PD could be the result of compensatory mechanisms in response to chronic nigrostriatal denervation or the result of L-dopa therapy. Nevertheless, altered activity of striatal projections might be expected to be reflected in the levels of the corresponding peptides (3).

Dopaminergic transmission is also subject to modulation by corticotropin-releasing factor (CRF)–, progesterone-, and gonadotropin-releasing hormone (GnRH)–associated peptide; these peptides appear to particularly modify dopamine release. Prolactin elevates striatal D2 receptor levels (78).

CANNABINOID RECEPTORS

The high levels of the $G_{i/o}$-protein-linked CB1-type cannabinoid receptors in the basal ganglia and cerebellum of both primates and rodents—indeed, the highest levels in the brain—have attracted attention in recent years. This interest has been supported by significant motor effects exerted by cannabinoid compounds, both natural and synthetic. In particular, the specific localization of such receptors on striatal output terminals in the GP and SN has been noted, with a slight preference for substance P–containing projections. mRNA for the receptor is also found in the STN.

Distribution of the putative endogenous ligand for cannabinoid receptors, *anandamide* (arachidonoylethanolamide), has thus far not been as thoroughly investigated, but it has been found in the striatum; the synthetic enzyme *amidase* is somewhat nonspecific and is thus also found in regions without known cannabinoid significance (79). Di Marzo et al. (80) found that the highest levels in rat brain of anandamide and another natural CB1 ligand, 2-arachidonoylglycerol (2-AG), were in the GP and SN; pallidal 2-AG levels were increased sevenfold in the reserpine-treated rat, whereas levels of both 2-AG and anandamide were reduced by treatment with D1 or D2 receptor agonists. More dramatically, total reversal of motor depression in reserpinized rats was achieved by combination of the D2 receptor agonist quinpirole and the CB1 receptor agonist SR141716A.

Effects of cannabinoid substances on neurotransmission in the basal ganglia has been demonstrated for a number of substances (79,81):

- Cannabinoids (such as Δ^9-tetrahydrocannabinol and WIN55,212-2) increased GABAergic transmission in the SNr and GP (where it may be involved in the induction of catalepsy), probably by inhibition of reuptake.
- Cannabinoid receptors are colocated in the striatum with both D1 and D2 receptors, and appear to oppose the action of each on adenylyl cyclase activity. Cannabinoid agonists also oppose dopamine reuptake but are not located on dopamine-releasing terminals (82).

- There is evidence that cannabinoid receptor activation opposes glutamate release (in the hippocampus); this was also demonstrated recently in the basal ganglia (83,84).
- CB1 and μ-opioid receptors are partly colocalized on caudate-putamen output neurons in the rat, suggesting a common pathway in the eliciting of motor depression by exogenous cannabinoids and opioids (85).

In summary, it has been suggested that cannabinoid receptors have a long-term role in the maintenance of basal ganglia tone. It would appear that the action of exogenously applied cannabinoids depends on the activity status of the basal ganglia; for example, they block the excitatory effect of the STN on the SN following stimulation of the former (86).

Unfortunately, there is little information regarding the effects of cannabinoid receptor–active agents in human extrapyramidal disease. Cannabis was employed in antiparkinsonian therapy in the 19th century, but more recent work has indicated little benefit for parkinsonian symptoms. On the other hand, cannabinoids have shown some promise in the management of L-dopa-associated dyskinesia, as well as management of tics associated with Tourette's syndrome (87). Changes in extrapyramidal disorders include the finding that cannabinoid receptor on medium spiny striatal neurons and on projection neurons is selectively depleted in Huntington's disease, changes that occur prior to terminal losses in the SN (79). Reduced striatal cannabinoid receptor levels, possibly due to increased endocannabinoid levels, have also been identified in the reserpine-treated rat, leading to the suggestion that cannabinoid receptor *antagonists* might be useful in parkinsonism: for example, the CB1 antagonist SR141716 reduces L-dopa-induced dyskinesia in primate models of parkinsonism (88).

For recent reviews of the role of cannabinoids in the basal ganglia, see refs. 79, 89, and 90.

STEROID HORMONES AND THE STRIATUM

There are corticosteroid binding sites in the striatum, as well as thyroid hormone binding sites (91). Corticosterone increases dopamine turnover in the mesolimbic system, dopamine release in rat accumbens and cortex, and dopamine uptake in caudatus/putamen. Stress and high corticosterone produce a brief (20 minute) increase in dopamine release in rat caudatus; uptake by synaptosomal preparations is increased following stress but not corticosterone treatment, whereas incubation with prednisolone decreases uptake. D1 receptor concentrations drop in most dopaminergic regions (including the striatum) in adrenalectomized rats, whereas D2 receptor levels fall in part of the striatum (91). Similarly, adrenalectomy decreases D1 receptor concentrations in the striatum and SN of the ovariectomized female rat, whereas D2 receptor levels decreased only in parts of the putamen; these changes are reversible by

corticosteroids, which also increased D1 receptor affinity (92).

Moreover, estrogen elevates striatal D2 and D1 receptor levels, converts D2 sites from low to high affinity, increases the density of GTP-resistant D2 in the lateral striatum, potentiates stereotypic responses to apomorphine, potentiates amphetamine-induced dopamine release, increases striatal dopamine uptake sites, and decreases D1 and D2 degradation rates (93). Estrogen has also been found to depress dopaminergic transmission, especially if administered from early in the animal's development (94); the opposition of acute and chronic treatment may be explained by differences between genomic and nongenomic effects of estrogen. This neuroprotective role for estrogen—women generally develop schizophrenia later than men (as estrogen levels decline), require lower neuroleptic doses, and experience more extrapyramidal (motor) side effects—underscores the need to consider endocrine parameters in neuropathology. For recent review of estrogen and movement disorders, see ref. 95.

THYROID HORMONES AND THE STRIATUM

Psychiatric and motor symptoms associated with abnormal thyroid hormone status suggest that the striatum may be involved; it is one of the brain regions most susceptible to damage by perinatal hypothyroidism. Reduced striatal concentrations of both D1 and D2 receptors and reduced dopamine uptake have been reported in hypothyroid animals, as has increased striatal D2 receptor sensitivity (96). Behavioral changes suggestive of increased striatal dopamine receptor sensitivity have also been observed in hypothyroid animals. Conversely, triiodothyronine (T_3) treatment has been associated with enhanced behavioral responses in both the nigrostriatal and mesolimbic pathways. In chronically thyroxine (T_4)–treated rats, neither apomorphine-induced stereotypies nor the effect of intraaccumbal dopamine were affected, nor was dopamine release, although dopamine synthesis was increased (97).

Increased extracellular adenosine synthesis in various brain regions (including the striatum), due to correlative changes in the activities of 5′-nucleotidase, adenosine deaminase, and adenosine kinase, reduced reuptake of adenosine, and the increased responsiveness of adenylyl cyclase to A1 receptor and guanosine triphosphate stimulation have been reported in the hypothyroid rat (98). Hypothyroidism might therefore lead to enhanced inhibition of dopamine release and thereby induce D2 receptor supersensitivity.

OTHER CLASSICAL TRANSMITTERS

Adrenoceptor modulation of dopamine release in rat accumbens slices has been described; β-adrenoceptor agonists enhance K^+-evoked release, whereas α_2-receptor agonists decrease it. Apomorphine also has a significant affinity for α_2 receptors, indeed greater than for D1 receptor. However, the significance of adrenergic transmission in the striatum has not been extensively investigated; in any case, noradrenergic innervation of this region (projections from the locus ceruleus, which, interestingly, also degenerates in PD) is exceedingly sparse. It has, however, been hypothesized that noradrenergic mechanisms might be significant in situations of compensatory dopamine release, such as follows chronic antipsychotic treatment (reviewed in ref. 5). Marien et al. (99) found that lesioning of the locus ceruleus was associated with reduced striatal dopamine release, but the physiologic basis for this effect is unknown. Noradrenergic innervation of the VTA has some impact on the SNc, as noradrenergic receptors are found here (reviewed in refs. 5, 99). Although systemic (nor)adrenaline exacerbates parkinsonian symptoms, it has been reported that intrastriatal application could be of benefit (100).

Significant *serotonergic* projections from the dorsal raphe and caudal linear nucleus to the striatum, SN and pallidum have been identified (reviewed in ref. 101), and several 5-hyroxytryptamine (5-HT) receptor types (including 5-HT_2 and 5-HT_6) are colocalized with peptides of both the direct and indirect paths in the striatum (102). 5-HT_1 receptors are especially abundant in the SNc, which receives afferents from the dorsal and medial raphe. 5-HT reuptake inhibitors increase akinesia in parkinsonism, whereas 5-HT_{1A} agonists relieve D1 and D2 antagonist–induced catalepsy. Serotonergic input to the striatum is involved in behavioral suppression (as opposed to facilitation), so that 5-HT_1 receptor agonists might assist motor initiation and thus relief of akinesia (5).

Histaminergic projections from the tuberomamillary nucleus of the hypothalamus innervate most areas of the brain, including the basal ganglia. H_2 and H_3 receptors are present in striatum in high concentrations; the former are postsynaptic and stimulate adenylyl cyclase activity, whereas H_3 receptors are located presynaptically, inhibiting the release of histamine and other neurotransmitters (103). The significance of this phenomenon for basal ganglia function is largely unexplored, but antihistaminergic agents (such as diphenhydramine) were long employed in the therapy of parkinsonism.

2,3-BENZODIAZEPINES

Members of the 2,3-benzodiazepine family, such as tofisopam, girisopam, and nerisopam, have neuroleptic and anxiolytic properties and may be involved in opioid signal transduction. Horvath et al. (104) recently reported that these substances bind exclusively in the basal ganglia, principally to striatal output neurons, via which they are transported to the SN and EPN.

CONCLUDING REMARKS: CONSEQUENCES FOR THE CLINIC

There are many issues in the pharmacology of basal ganglia function and disease that remain to be clarified. Of the biochemical changes associated with PD, best described are the reduced dopamine levels in most basal ganglia nuclei (but not in the GPi) and increased dopamine turnover, and this has determined antiparkinsonian therapy for the past 30 years. But it is not known, for example, why L-dopa leads to dyskinesias more frequently than other antiparkinsonian agents, especially when compared with D1 and D2 receptor agonists. It has been proposed that such dyskinesia resulted from glutamatergic hyperstimulation of striatal medium spiny efferent neurons, possibly secondary to nonphysiologic stimulation of coexpressed dopamine receptors. Furthermore, positive effects on parkinsonian symptoms in animal models have been associated with inhibition of glutamatergic transmission in the STN or its efferents to the GPi, so that administration of glutamate antagonists might be expected to be of benefit in PD. In fact, they have proved especially beneficial in cases of akinetic crisis, a severe form of clinical deterioration in PD (16,105). Metman et al. (106) examined the effect of three NMDA receptor antagonists (dextrorphan, dextromethorphan, and amantadine) in PD and found that all three were generally effective as adjuvant therapy to L-dopa in the reduction of the associated dyskinesia and motor fluctuations, without altering the symptomatic effect of L-dopa itself. Amantadine was most consistent in this respect, possibly as a result of its low affinity, rapid binding, concurrent binding of σ-receptors, or the binding of a specific, regional population of NMDA receptors.

On the other hand, current basal ganglia models do not explain why amantadine is such a weak antiparkinsonian agent in L-dopa-compensated cases of PD, in contrast to its efficacy in patients suffering from akinetic crises, at which stage the degeneration of the nigrostriatal system is presumed to be almost complete. Noteworthy is the fact that NMDA receptor concentration is reduced in the GPi of akinetic crisis–stage PD patients, who derive the most benefit from amantadine therapy; in particular, GluR1 receptor levels are specifically reduced in the GPi in both animal models of parkinsonism and in PD. A plausible explanation would be the already suggested selective distribution of receptors that amantadine blocks, perhaps combined with the loss of a particular input that overrides the dampening effect of amantadine. The absence of akinesia in most amantadine-treated patients may also be associated with a more complex arrangement or plasticity of basal ganglia function than currently assumed (3).

This one example underscores the need for an even greater understanding of the neurochemistry and pharmacology of the basal ganglia in both health and disease. The development of more effective therapies for extrapyramidal disorders will not rely on manipulation of individual transmitter systems, as the complex interplay of factors (transmitters, neuromodulators, hormones, growth factors) in several nuclei that regulates normal basal ganglia function must be addressed in an equally sophisticated manner if advances on current approaches are to be achieved. It should also be noted that a certain degree of "transmitter–receptor mismatch" (discrepancies between the location of transmitter release sites and their receptors) will also play a significant role in CNS function and thus the response to exogenous neuroactive substances (107). Furthermore, Parent and Cicchetti (108) and Joel and Weiner (109) have pointed to significant differences between rodent and primate brains that render the extrapolation of a basal ganglia model from one type to the other a dubious matter; for example, in contrast to rats, substance P– and ENK-positive terminals are equally abundant at SNr levels in primates, consistent with the direct innervation of the SNr by both major classes of striatal GABAergic neurons. Recognition of this fact means investigation of human brain tissue (from both healthy persons and from those with basal ganglia disease) and primate models are more likely to bring advances in knowledge of basal ganglia neurochemistry and organization than rodent model alternatives.

The multiple levels of integration in the extrapyramidal system which have been identified and which remain to be identified allow the smooth execution of motor activities in the healthy state, as well as allowing the considerable degree of neural plasticity observed in various neurodegenerative disorders. Further exploration of this system and cognizance of the interdependence of its various components are required for the development of better strategies in the management and cure of extrapyramidal disease.

REFERENCES

1. Albin RL, Young AB, Penney JB. The functional anatomy of basal ganglia disorders. *Trends Neurosci* 1989;12:366–376.
2. Starr MS. Glutamate/dopamine D1/D2 balance in the basal ganglia and its relevance to Parkinson's disease. *Synapse* 1995; 19:264–293.
3. Riederer P, Foley P. The motor circuit of the human basal ganglia reconsidered. *J Neural Transm* 2000;[Suppl 58]:97–110.
4. Mello LEAM, Villares J. Neuroanatomy of the basal ganglia. *Psychiatr Clin North Am* 1997;20:691–704.
5. Hauber W. Involvement of basal ganglia transmitter systems in movement initiation. *Prog Neurobiol* 1998;56:507–540.
6. Bolam JP, Hanley JJ, Booth PAC, et al. Synaptic organisation of the basal ganglia. *J Anat* 2000;196:527–542.
7. Smith Y, Charara A, Hanson JE, et al. GABA$_B$ and group I metabotropic glutamate receptors in the striatopallidal complex in primates. *J Anat* 2000;196:555–576.
8. Lloyd KG, Morselli PL. Psychopharmacology of GABAergic drugs. In: Meltzer HY, ed. *Psychopharmacology: a third generation of progress.* New York: Raven Publishers, 1987:183–195.
9. Gerfen CR, Wilson CJ. Basal ganglia. In: Bjorklund A, Hokfelt T, Swanson LW, eds. *The handbook of chemical neuroanatomy: integrated systems of the CNS,* part 3, vol 12. Amsterdam: Elsevier Science, 1996:369–466.
10. Stefani A, Spadoni F, Giacomini P, et al. The modulation of calcium current by GABA metabotropic receptors in a sub-population of pallidal neurons. *Eur J Neurosci* 1999;11:3995–4005.
11. Emson PC, Augood SJ, Senaris R, et al. Chemical signalling and striatal interneurons. *Prog Brain Res* 1993;89:155–165.
12. Kawaguchi Y, Wilson CJ, Augood SJ, et al. Striatal interneurons chemical physiology and morphological characterization. *Trends Neurosci* 1995;18:527–538.
13. Parent A, Hazrati LN. Functional anatomy of the basal ganglia: 1. The cortico-basal ganglia-thalamic-cortical loop. *Brain Res Brain Res Rev* 1995;20:91–127.
14. Ravenscroft P, Brotchie J. NMDA receptors in the basal ganglia. *J Anat* 2000;196:577–585.
15. Schmidt WJ, Kretschmer BD. Behavioural pharmacology of glutamate receptors in the basal ganglia. *Neurosci Biobehav Rev* 1997;21:381–392.
16. Lange KW, Kornhuber J, Riederer P. Dopamine/glutamate interactions in Parkinson's disease. *Neurosci Biobehav Rev* 1997; 21:393–400.
17. Gerlach M, Gsell W, Kornhuber J, et al. A post mortem study on neurochemical markers of dopaminergic, GABA-ergic and glutamatergic neurons in basal ganglia-thalamocortical circuits in Parkinson syndrome. *Brain Res* 1996;741:142–152.
18. Blandini F, Greenamyre JT. Prospects of glutamate antagonists in the therapy of Parkinson's disease. *Fund Clin Pharmacol* 1998;12:4–12.
19. Blanchet PJ, Papa SM, Metman LV, et al. Modulation of levodopa-induced motor response complications by NMDA antagonists in Parkinson's disease. *Neurosci Biobehav Rev* 1997; 21:447–453.
20. Eltze M. Multiple mechanisms of action: the pharmacological profile of budipine. *J Neural Transm* 1999;[Suppl 56]:83–105.
21. Betarbet R, Porter RH, Greenamyre JT. GluR1 glutamate receptor subunit is regulated differentially in the primate basal ganglia following nigrostriatal dopamine denervation. *J Neurochem* 2000;74:1166–1174.
22. Bernard V, Bolam JP. Subcellular and subsynaptic distribution of the NR1 subunit of the NMDA receptor in the neostriatum and globus pallidus of the rat: co-localization at synapses with the GluR2/3 subunit of the AMPA receptor. *Eur J Neurosci* 1998;10:3721–3736.
23. Bernard V, Gardiol A, Faucheux B, et al. Expression of glutamate receptors in the human and rat basal ganglia: effect of the dopaminergic denervation on AMPA receptor gene expression in the striatopallidal complex in Parkinson's disease and rat with 6-OHDA lesion. *J Comp Neurol* 1996;368:553–568.
24. Vezina P, Kim JH. Metabotropic glutamate receptors and the generation of locomotor activity: interactions with midbrain dopamine. *Neurosci Biobehav Rev* 1999;23:577–589.
25. Herrera-Marschitz M, Goiny M, You ZB, et al. Release of endogenous excitatory amino acids in the neostriatum of the rat under physiological and pharmacologically-induced conditions. *Amino Acids* 1998;14:197–203.
26. Albin RL, Makowiec RL, Hollingsworth ZR, et al. Excitatory amino acid binding sites in the basal ganglia of the rat: a quantitative autoradiographic study. *Neuroscience* 1992;46:35–48.
27. Landwehrmeyer BG, Standaert DG, Testa CM, et al. NMDA receptor subunit mRNA expression by projecting neurons and interneurons in the rat striatum. *J Neurosci* 1995;15:5297–5307.
28. Betarbet R, Greenamyre JT. Differential expression of glutamate receptors by the dopaminergic neurons of the primate striatum. *Exp Neurol* 1999;159:401–408.
29. Smith Y, Kieval JZ. Anatomy of the dopamine system in the basal ganglia. *Trends Neurosci* 2000;23[Suppl]:S28–S33.

30. Betarbet R, Turner R, Chockkan V, et al. Dopaminergic neurons intrinsic to the primate striatum. *J Neurosci* 1997;17:6761–6768.

31. Surmeier DJ, Song WJ, Yan Z. Coordinated expression of dopamine receptors in neostriatal medium spiny neurons. *J Neurosci* 1996;16:6579–6591.

32. Bezard E, Brotchie JM, Gross CE. Pathophysiology of levodopa-induced dyskinesia: potential for new therapies. *Nat Rev Neurosci* 2001;2:577–588.

33. LaHoste GJ, Marshall JF. The role of dopamine in the maintenance and breakdown of D_1/D_2 synergism. *Brain Res* 1993;611:108–116.

34. Guttman M. Dopamine receptors in Parkinson's disease. *Neurol Clin* 1992;10:377–386.

35. Levy R, Hazrati LN, Herrero MT, et al. Re-evaluation of the functional anatomy of the basal ganglia in normal and parkinsonian states. *Neuroscience* 1997;76:335–343.

36. Moratalla R, Xu M, Tonegawa S, et al. Cellular responses to psychomotor stimulant and neuroleptic drugs are abnormal in mice lacking the D1 dopamine receptor. *Proc Natl Acad Sci USA* 1996;93:14928–14933.

37. Snyder GL, Fienberg AA, Huganir RL, et al. A dopamine/D1 receptor/protein kinase A/ dopamine- and cAMP-regulated phosphoprotein (M_r 32kDa)/protein phosphatase-1 pathway regulates dephosphorylation of the NMDA receptor. *J Neurosci* 1998;18:10297–10303.

38. Nutt JG, Obeso JA, Stocchi F. Continuous dopamine-receptor stimulation in advanced Parkinson's disease. *Trends Neurosci* 2000;23[10 Suppl]:S109–S115.

39. Olanow W, Schapira AH, Rascol O. Continuous dopamine-receptor stimulation in early Parkinson's disease. *Trends Neurosci* 2000;23[10 Suppl]:S117–S126.

40. King GR, Ellinwood EH, Silvia C, et al. Withdrawal from continuous or intermittent cocaine administration: changes in D2 receptor function. *J Pharmacol Exp Ther* 1994;269:743–749.

41. Vanderschuren LJMJ, Kalivas PW. Alterations in dopaminergic and glutamatergic transmission in the induction and expression of behavioral sensitization: a critical review of preclinical studies. *Psychopharmacology* 2000;151:99–120.

42. Joel D, Weiner I. The connections of the dopaminergic system with the striatum in rats and primates: an analysis with respect to the functional and compartmental organization of the striatum. *Neuroscience* 2000;96:451–474.

43. Palacios JM, Landwehrmeyer B, Mengod G. Brain dopamine receptors: characterization, distribution, and alteration in disease. In: Jankovic J, Tolosa E, eds. *Parkinson's disease and movement disorders,* 2nd ed. Baltimore: Williams & Wilkins, 1993:35–54.

44. Gerfen CR. The neostriatal mosaic multiple levels of compartmental organization in the basal ganglia. *Annu Rev Neurosci* 1992;15:285–320.

45. Bergson C, Mrzljak L, Smiley JF, et al. Regional, cellular, and subcellular variations in the distribution of D1 and D5 dopamine receptors in primate brain. *J Neurosci* 1995;15:7821–7836.

46. Sokoloff P, Giros B, Martres MP, et al. Molecular cloning and characterization of a novel dopamine receptor (D3) as a target for neuroleptics. *Nature* 1990;347:146–151.

47. Van Toi HHM, Bunzow JR, Guan HC, et al. Cloning of the gene for a human D4 receptor with high affinity for clozapine. *Nature* 1991;350:610–614.

48. Calabresi P, Ceentonze D, Gubellini P, et al. Acetylcholine-mediated modulation of striatal function. *Trends Neurosci* 2000;23:120–126.

49. Hersch SM, Gutekunst CA, Rees HD, et al. Distribution of m1-m4 muscarinic receptor proteins in the rat striatum: light and electron microscopic immunocytochemistry using subtype-specific antibodies. *J Neurosci* 1994;14:3351–3363.

50. Alcantara AA, Mrzljak L, Jakab RL, et al. Muscarinic m1 and m2 receptor proteins in local circuit and projection neurons of the primate striatum: anatomical evidence for cholinergic modulation of glutamatergic prefronto-striatal pathways. *J Comp Neurol* 2001;434:445–460.

51. Lehmann J, Langer SZ. The striatal cholinergic interneuron: synaptic target of dopaminergic terminals? *Neuroscience* 1983;10:1105–1120.

52. Jackson D, Stachowiak MK, Bruno JP, et al. Inhibition of striatal acetylcholine release by endogenous serotonin. *Brain Res* 1988;457:259–266.

53. Joyce JN. Differential response of striatal dopamine and muscarinic cholinergic receptor subtypes to the loss of dopamine: III. Results in Parkinson's disease cases. *Brain Res* 1993;600:156–160.

54. Asahina M, Suhara T, Shinotoh H, et al. Brain muscarinic receptors in progressive supranuclear palsy and Parkinson's disease: a positron emission tomographic study. *J Neurol Neurosurg Psychiatry* 1998;65:155–163.

55. Izurieta-Sanchez P, Sarre S, Ebinger G, et al. Effect of trihexyphenidyl, a non-selective antimuscarinic drug, on decarboxylation of L-dopa in hemi-Parkinson rats. *Eur J Pharmacol* 1998;353:33–42.

56. Han ZY, Le Novere N, Zoli M, et al. Localization of nAChR subunit mRNAs in the brain of Macaca mulatta. *Eur J Neurosci* 2000;12:3664–3674.

57. Quik M, Jeyarasasingam G. Nicotinic receptors and Parkinson's disease. *Eur J Pharmacol* 2000;393:223–230.

58. Durany N, Zöchling R, Boissl KW, et al. Human post-mortem striatal α4β2 nicotinic acetylcholine receptor density in schizophrenia and Parkinson's syndrome. *Neurosci Lett* 2000;287:109–112.

59. Ince E, Ciliax BJ, Levey AI. Differential expression of D1 and D2 dopamine and m4 muscarinic acetylcholine receptor proteins in identified striatonigral neurons. *Synapse* 1997;27:357–366.

60. Weiner DM, Levey AI, Brann MR. Expression of muscarinic acetylcholine and dopamine receptor mRNAs in rat basal ganglia. *Proc Natl Acad Sci USA* 1990;87:7030–7034.

61. Court AJ, Perry EK. Distribution of nicotinic receptors in the CNS. In: Stone TW, ed. *CNS neurotransmitters and neuromodulators: acetylcholine.* Boca Raton, FL: CRC Press, 1995:85–104.

62. Sebastião AM, Ribeiro JA. Adenosine A2 receptor–mediated excitatory actions on the nervous system. *Prog Neurobiol* 1996;48:167–189.

63. Fuxe K, Ferré S, Zoli M, et al. Integrated events in central dopamine transmission as analyzed at multiple levels: evidence for intramembrane adenosine A2a/dopamine D2 and adenosine A1/dopamine D1 receptor interactions in the basal ganglia. *Brain Res Rev* 1998;26:258–273.

64. James S, Richardson PJ. Production of adenosine from extracellular ATP at the striatal cholinergic synapse. *J Neurochem* 1993;60:219–227.

65. Nash JE, Brotchie JM. A common signaling pathway for striatal NMDA and adenosine A2a receptors: implications for the treatment of Parkinson's disease. *J Neurosci* 2000;20:7782–7789.

66. Svenningsson P, Le Moine C, Fisone G, et al. Distribution, biochemistry, and function of striatal adenosine A2A receptors. *Prog Neurobiol* 1999;59:355–396.

67. Cunha RA. Adenosine as a neuromodulator and as a homeostatic regulator in the nervous system: different roles, different sources, and different receptors. *Neurochem Int* 2001;38:107–125.

68. Kanda T, Jackson MJ, Smith LA, et al. Combined use of the adenosine A(2A) antagonist KW-6002 with L-dopa or with

selective D1 or D2 dopamine agonists increases antiparkinsonian activity but not dyskinesia in MPTP-treated monkeys. *Exp Neurol* 2000;162:321–327.

69. Martinez-Mir M, Probst A, Palacio JM. Adenosine A2 receptors selective localization in the human brain and alterations with disease. *Neuroscience* 1991;42:697–706.

70. Richardson PJ, Kase H, Jenner P. Adenosine A2A receptor antagonists as new agents for the treatment of Parkinson's disease. *Trend Pharmacol Sci* 1997;18:338–344.

71. de Mendonca A, Sebastiao AM, Ribeiro JA. Adenosine: does it have a neuroprotective role after all? *Brain Res Rev* 2000;33:258–274.

72. Rivkees SA, Price SL, Zhou FC. Immunohistochemical detection of A1 adenosine receptors in rat brain with emphasis on localization in the hippocampal formation, cerebral cortex, cerebellum, and basal ganglia. *Brain Res* 1995;677:193–203.

73. Fuxe K, Agnati LF, von Euler G, et al. Neuropeptides, excitatory amino acid, and adenosine A2 receptors regulate D2 receptors via intramembrane receptor–receptor interactions: relevance for Parkinson's disease and schizophrenia. *Neurochem Int* 1992;20 [Suppl]:215S–224S.

74. Kinkead B, Binder EB, Nemeroff CB. Does neurotensin mediate the effects of antipsychotic drugs? *Biol Psychiatry* 2000;46:340–351.

75. Steiner H, Gerfen CR Role of dynorphin and enkephalin in the regulation of striatal output pathways and behavior. *Exp Brain Res* 1998;123:60–76.

76. Gerfen CR, McGinty JR, Young WS. Dopamine differentially regulates dynorphin substance P and enkephalin in striatal neurons: in situ hybridization histochemical analysis. *J Neurosci* 1991;11:1016–1031.

77. Hong JS, Yang HYT, Gillin JC, et al. Effect on long term administration of antipsychotic drugs on enkephalinergic neurons. *Adv Biochem Psychopharmacol* 1980;24:223–232.

78. Gobert A, Guibert B, Lenoir V, et al. GnRH-associated peptide (GAP) is present in the rat striatum and affects the synthesis and release of dopamine. *J Neurosci Res* 1992;31:359–364.

79. Glass M, Brotchie JM, Maneuf YP. Modulation of neurotransmission by cannabinoids in the basal ganglia. *Eur J Neurosci* 1997;9:199–203.

80. Di Marzo V, Hill MP, Bisogno T, et al. Enhanced levels of endogenous cannabinoids in the globus pallidus are associated with a reduction in movement in an animal model of Parkinson's disease. *FASEB J* 2000;14:1432–1438.

81. Romero J, de Miguel R, Ramos JA, et al. The activation of cannabinoid receptors in striatonigral GABAergic neurons inhibited GABA uptake. *Life Sci* 1998;62:351–363.

82. Szabo B, Muller T, Koch H. Effects of cannabinoids on dopamine release in the corpus striatum and the nucleus accumbens in vitro. *J Neurochem* 1999;73:1084–1089.

83. Gerdeman G, Lovinger DM. CB1 cannabinoid receptor inhibits synaptic release of glutamate in rat dorsolateral striatum. *J Neurophysiol* 2001;85:468–471.

84. Huang CC, Lo SW, Hsu KS. Presynaptic mechanisms underlying cannabinoid inhibition of excitatory synaptic transmission in rat striatal neurons. *J Physiol* 2001;532:731–748.

85. Rodriguez JJ, Mackie K, Pickel VM. Ultrastructural localization of the CB1 cannabinoid receptor in mu-opioid receptor patches of the rat caudate putamen nucleus. *J Neurosci* 2001;21:823–833.

86. Sanudo-Pena MC, Tsou K, Walker JM. Motor actions of cannabinoids in the basal ganglia output nuclei. *Life Sci* 1999;65:703–713.

87. Müller-Vahl KR, Kolbe H, Schneider U, et al. Cannabis in movement disorders. *Forschende Komplementärmedizin* 1999;6:23–27.

88. Silverdale MA, McGuire S, McInnes A, et al. Striatal cannabi-

noid CB1 receptor mRNA expression is decreased in the reserpine-treated rat model of Parkinson's disease. *Exp Neurol* 2001;169:400–406.

89. Rodriguez de Fonseca F, Del Arco I, Martin-Calderon JL, et al. Role of the endogenous cannabinoid system in the regulation of motor activity. *Neurobiol Dis* 1998;5:483–501.

90. Giuffrida A, Piomelli D. The endocannabinoid system: a physiological perspective on its role in psychomotor control. *Chem Phys Lipids* 2000;108:151–158.

91. Joëls M, de Kloet ER. Mineralocorticoid and glucocorticoid receptors in the brain: implications for ion permeability and transmitter systems. *Prog Neurobiol* 1994;43:1–36.

92. Biron D, Dauphin C, Di Paolo T. Effects of adrenalectomy and glucocorticoids on rat brain dopamine receptors. *Neuroendocrinology* 1992;55:468–476.

93. Lévesque D, Di Paolo T. Modulation by estradiol and progesterone of the GTP effect on striatal D-2 dopamine receptors. *Biochem Pharmacol* 1993;45:723–733.

94. Häfner H, Behrens S, De Vry J, et al. An animal model for the effects of estradiol on dopamine-mediated behavior: implications for sex differences in schizophrenia. *Psychiatry Res* 1991;38:125–134.

95. Kompoliti K. Estrogen and movement disorders. *Clin Neuropharmacol* 1999;22:318–326.

96. Foley PB, Cracker A. Dopamine agonist-mediated inhibition of acetylcholine release is modified by thyroid hormone status. *J Neurochem* 1993;61:812–817.

97. Baumgartner A, Campos-Barros A. Schilddrüsenhormone und depressive Erkrankungen—Kritische Übersicht und Perspektiven. Teil 1: Klinik; Teil 2: Schilddrüsenhormone und ZNS—Ergebnisse der Grundlagenforschung. *Nervenarzt* 1993;64:1–20.

98. Fideu MD, Arce A, Esquifino AI, et al. Thyroid hormones modulate both adenosine transport and adenosine A1 receptors in rat brain. *Am J Physiol* 1994;267:C1651–C1656.

99. Marien M, Lategan A, Colpaert F. Noradrenergic control of striatal dopamine release. In: Briley M, Marien M, eds. *Noradrenergic mechanisms in Parkinson's disease,* vol 9. Boca Raton, FL: CRC Press, 1994:139–158.

100. Richardson DE, Heath RG. Treatment of Parkinson's disease by injection of norepinephrine into the corpus striatum. *Acta Neurochir* 1992;117:141.

101. Halliday G, Harding A, Paxinos G. Serotonin and tachykinin systems. In: Paxinos G, ed. *The rat nervous system,* vol 34. San Diego: Academic Press, 1995:929–974.

102. Ward RP, Dorsa DM. Colocalization of serotonin receptor subtypes 5-HT2A, 5-HT2C, and 5-HT6 with neuropeptides in rat striatum. *J Comp Neurol* 1996;370:405–414.

103. Brown RE, Stevens DR, Haas HL. The physiology of brain histamine. *Prog Neurobiol* 2001;63:637–672.

104. Horvath EJ, Horvath K, Hamori T, et al. Anxiolytic 2,3-benzodiazepines, their specific binding to the basal ganglia. *Prog Neurobiol* 2000;60:309–342.

105. Danielczyk W. Die Behandlung von akinetischen Krisen. *Medizinische Welt* 1973;24:1278–1282.

106. Metman LV, Del Dotto P, Blanchet PJ, et al. Blockade of glutamatergic transmission as treatment for dyskinesias and motor fluctuations in Parkinson's disease. *Amino Acids* 1998;14:75–82.

107. Zoli M, Jansson A, Syková E, et al. Volume transmission in the CNS and its relevance for neuropsychopharmacology. *Trends Pharmacol Sci* 1999;20:142–150.

108. Parent A, Cicchetti F. The current model of basal ganglia organization under scrutiny. *Mov Disord* 1998;13:199–202.

109. Joel D, Weiner I. The connections of the dopaminergic system with the striatum in rats and primates: an analysis with respect to the functional and compartmental organization of the striatum. *Neuroscience* 2000;96:451–474.

MECHANISMS OF CELL DEATH IN PARKINSON'S DISEASE

C. WARREN OLANOW
WILLIAM G. TATTON
PETER JENNER

Parkinson's disease (PD) is an age-related and progressive neurodegenerative disorder that is characterized pathologically by preferential degeneration of dopaminergic neurons in the substantia nigra pars compacta (SNc) combined with the appearance of intracytoplasmic inclusions composed of protein aggregates known as Lewy bodies (1). Neurodegeneration in PD also occurs in other brain regions, including locus ceruleus, raphe nuclei, nucleus basalis of Meynert, hypothalamus, cerebral cortex, cranial nerve motor nuclei, and central and peripheral components of the autonomic nervous system. Current treatment of the motor symptoms of PD primarily consists of dopamine replacement therapy with levodopa or a dopamine agonist drug (2). Treatment is highly effective in the early stages of the disease, but with continued treatment the majority of patients develop adverse effects, such as motor fluctuations, dyskinesia, and psychosis. Furthermore, PD is associated with features such as freezing, autonomic dysfunction, and dementia, which do not respond to dopaminergic therapy. Thus, the majority of PD patients eventually experience disability that cannot be controlled with currently available therapies (2,3). Accordingly, there has been a concerted effort aimed at developing a neuroprotective therapy that will slow or stop disease progression. Toward this end, it is critical to understand the nature of the cell death process in PD. Nerve cell death can be considered from the standpoint of etiology, pathogenesis, and the pattern of cell death. Etiologic factors have been extensively covered elsewhere in this book and will only be touched on in this chapter. Pathogenetic factors and apoptotic mechanisms have been extensively reviewed in the previous version of this textbook as well as in other major reviews (4–6). In the present chapter we will present an overview of these topics and provide new information suggesting that defects in the capacity of the ubiquitin-proteasome system to clear unwanted cellular proteins may be a common theme in the different forms of PD.

ETIOLOGIC FACTORS

The specific cause of most cases of PD is not known, but there are important clues pointing to the involvement of genetic and environmental factors. An epidemiologic study utilized the World War II United States Veteran Twin Registry maintained by the National Academy of Science to assess the concordance of PD in monozygotic and dizygotic twins (7). Concordance for PD was significantly greater in monozygotic than dizygotic twins for patients under 50 years of age, consistent with the notion that genes play a major role in younger patients. In contrast, concordance between the two groups was not different for patients over the age of 50 years, suggesting that environmental and not genetic factors are the more important in the majority of patients with sporadic PD. However, it should be appreciated that preclinical changes in the nigrostriatal system that can be detected on positron emission tomography may not be recognized on clinical examination and may therefore fail to identify the true concordance rate in older individuals.

Epidemiologic studies indicate that a number of environmental factors are associated with an increased risk of developing PD (8–11). These include exposure to well water, farming, pesticides, herbicides, industrial chemicals, wood pulp mills, and a rural residence. Interestingly, there is also epidemiologic evidence of an inverse correlation between PD and smoking (12,13) or caffeine (14). A number of exogenous toxins have been reported to be associated with the development of parkinsonism, including trace metals, cyanide, lacquer thinner, organic solvents, carbon monoxide, and carbon disulfide. Endogenous toxins, such as tetrahydroisoquinolines and β-carbolines, formed as a result of the condensation of monoamines and acetaldehyde, may also have a role in the development of PD. However, the relationship between toxic exposure and the development of parkinsonism is poorly defined, and in many instances the clinical picture is not typical of Lewy body PD. Furthermore, no specific toxin has been identified in the brain of PD patients.

The most compelling evidence for an environmental component came from the discovery of the selective nigral toxicity of 1-methyl-4-phenyl-1,2,3,6-tetrahydropyridine (MPTP) (15). In the brain, MPTP is converted to 1-methyl-4-phenylpyridine (MPP+) by monoamine oxidase B (MAO-B) (16) and is selectively taken up by dopamine neurons where it inhibits complex I of the mitochondrial respiratory chain (17). The precise mechanism of cell death associated with MPTP toxicity is still debated but may be related to reduced ATP production, oxidative stress, or impaired proton pumping from mitochondria with a consequent fall in mitochondrial membrane potential and apoptosis. Interestingly, a Parkinson-like syndrome with nigral pathology and inclusion bodies has been induced by chronic administration of the widely available pesticide rotenone (18), another complex I inhibitor.

There is also evidence that genetic factors play a major role in the etiology of some cases of PD (see Chapter 7). Approximately 5% to 10% of PD patients have a familial pattern of inheritance, and PD syndromes have now been linked to a number of different gene loci (19,20). Specifically, gene mutations encoding for the proteins α-synuclein (21,22), parkin (23,24), and UCH-L1 (25) have been reported in association with the development of PD. These mutations have not been found in the general population, but demonstrate that a single-gene mutation can cause a PD syndrome. While parkin mutations may be found in as many as half of patients with early-onset PD (26), gene mutations do not account for the vast majority of cases of PD. However, they do provide an opportunity to develop transgenic and knockout models that can provide insight into the mechanisms responsible for cell death in PD and to test putative neuroprotective therapies.

It is also possible that PD results from a complex interaction between multiple gene mutations and/or environmental factors. Specifically, PD might develop as a result of a mutant gene that impairs the body's capacity to metabolize an exogenous toxin coupled with exposure to that toxin. A number of candidate genes have been screened in an attempt to find a genetic predisposition for PD. Some, but not all, studies have detected an increased incidence of mutations in the genes encoding for the CYP2D6, NAT-2, and MAO-A, and MAO-B proteins in PD patients (19,27–29). Other candidate genes that have been screened and appear not to be associated with an increase risk of PD are those that encode for Apo-ε4, tyrosine hydroxylase, glutathione peroxidase (GPX), catalase, copper-zinc superoxide dismutase, and the dopamine D2, D3, and D4 receptors (30).

Mutations in the mitochondrial genome have also been sought in view of the complex I defect that has been detected in MPTP-induced parkinsonism and PD. Complex I is composed of 43 subunits, 7 of which are encoded by mitochondrial DNA, which is more likely to undergo mutation than nuclear DNA. A 5-kb deletion has been detected in PD, but this defect is identical to that found in normal aging (31). Sequencing of total mitochondrial DNA has uncovered different point mutations in subunits of complex I, but no disease-specific mutation has been identified and it remains to be determined if these mutations constitute risk factors for the development of PD.

PATHOGENESIS

Numerous factors, including oxidative stress, excitotoxicity, mitochondrial dysfunction, and inflammatory factors, have been implicated in the pathogenesis of PD. These have been extensively reviewed in a supplement to *Annals of Neurology* dedicated to this topic (5). A review of the evidence for each of these factors is provided below.

Oxidative Stress

The notion that oxidant stress contributes to the pathogenesis of nigral cell death in PD derives from the fact that dopamine normally undergoes oxidative metabolism and has the potential to generate cytotoxic free radicals and other reactive oxygen species (ROS) (Fig. 4.1A) (32–34). A pathologic excess of free radicals might be formed under circumstances in which there is (a) increased dopamine metabolism with excess hydrogen peroxide (H_2O_2) formation; (b) glutathione (GSH) deficiency with failure to adequately clear H_2O_2; or (c) increased ferrous iron (Fe^{2+}) iron, which can interact with H_2O_2 to form the hydroxyl radical (OHz). In addition, dopamine auto-oxidation can lead to the formation of quinones and ROS (Fig. 4.1B).

Antioxidant defenses are normally available to protect against free-radical-mediated oxidant damage. GSH, GPX, and catalase clear peroxides and prevent their reaction with iron. Superoxide dismutase (SOD) clears the superoxide radical (O_2^-) by catalyzing its conversion to H_2O_2, thereby preventing O_2^--mediated tissue damage. Finally, free-radical scavengers, such as ascorbic acid (vitamin C) and α-tocopherol (vitamin E), react directly with free radicals, thereby preventing oxidation of more critical molecules and inhibiting chain reactions, such as lipid peroxidation. The evidence supporting a role for oxidative stress has primarily come from the examination of brain material demonstrating alterations in iron content and antioxidant defenses in the SNc of PD patients. What is not clear is which factor is primary and drives the development of oxidant stress or

(a) Dopamine enzymatic oxidation

i) $$DA + O_2 + H_2O \xrightarrow{MAO} 3,4\ DHPA + NH_3 + H_2O_2$$

ii) $$H_2O_2 + 2GSH \longrightarrow GSSG + 2H_2O$$

iii) $$H_2O_2 + Fe^{+2} \longrightarrow OH^\bullet + OH^- + Fe^{+3}$$

(b) Dopamine auto-oxidation

iv) $$DA + O_2 \longrightarrow SQ^\bullet + {}^\bullet O_2^- + H^+$$

$$DA + {}^\bullet O_2^- + 2H^+ \longrightarrow SQ^\bullet + H_2O_2$$

FIG. 4.1. The enzymatic (a) and chemical (b) metabolism of dopamine. Under normal circumstances, H_2O_2 generated by dopamine metabolism (i) is detoxified by GSH (ii). However, H_2O_2 has the potential to react with ferrous iron and generate the cytotoxic OHz radical (iii).

whether the oxidant stress that is found in the SNc in PD occurs secondary to an alternate etiologic event.

Iron

A consistent finding in the SNc of PD patients is an increase in the total iron content (35). Earle reported a generalized increase in brain iron in PD using x-ray fluorescence spectroscopy (36). Subsequently, studies using a variety of analytic techniques have demonstrated that iron levels are increased in the SNc in PD (37–41). The form in which iron is stored in PD is not known, but the issue is important because ferrous iron is much more reactive and prone to produce ROS than ferric iron, which tends to be unreactive and stored in ferritin molecules. There are conflicting reports in the literature as to the level of brain ferritin in PD (42,43). A study using antibodies against specific isoforms of ferritin showed no compensatory increase in neuronal ferritin in the SNc in PD (44). This raises the possibility that the increased iron is unbound and reactive, and therefore in a form in which it might contribute to the pathogenesis of PD. Infusion of iron into the SNc of the rodent induces a model of PD characterized by a progressive loss of striatal dopamine content, degeneration of SNc neurons, and apomorphine-induced behavioral changes (45–48). However, iron levels are elevated in other neurodegenerative illnesses, including multiple system atrophy, progressive supranuclear palsy, and Huntington's disease. Furthermore, iron accumulation in the SNc can be observed after MPTP treatment in monkeys and 6-hydroxydopamine (6-OHDA) lesions of the median forebrain bundle in rats (49,50), suggesting that iron can accumulate as a secondary and nonspecific response to cell degeneration. Furthermore, iron levels are not increased in the SNc of patients with incidental Lewy body disease (ILBD) who are thought to have a presymptomatic form of PD (51).

This suggests that the accumulation of iron in the parkinsonian nigra is unlikely to be the initiating event in the degenerative process. Nonetheless, these observations do not negate the potential importance of iron as even secondary accumulation may contribute to the cascade of events leading to cell death in PD. How iron accumulates in PD is not understood. Transferrin receptors are reduced on SNc neurons (52), but lactoferrin receptors are increased (53) and may permit iron to enter into, and accumulate in, nigral neurons.

Antioxidant Defenses

A defect in one or more of the naturally occurring antioxidant defenses could lead to a state of oxidant stress and consequent neurodegeneration. In PD, there are no changes in levels or activity of ascorbic acid, α-tocopherol, catalase, or GPX (42,54,55). SOD activity is reported to be elevated and, although debate exists, there does appear to be a selective increase in brain and cerebrospinal fluid (CSF) levels of the Mn-SOD isoform that is predominantly found in mitochondrial membranes (56,57). This finding is consistent with an adaptive increase in the inducible form of the SOD enzyme as a result of excess superoxide radical formation. Indeed, transgenic mice that overexpress the Cu-Zn isoform of SOD are resistant to MPTP toxicity (58).

More striking is the reduction in levels of GSH in the SNc of PD patients (59–61). A reduction in GSH could impair H_2O_2 clearance and promote OH• radical formation, particularly in the presence of increased iron. Reduced levels of GSH have not been detected in any other brain area in PD and, to date, have not been reported in other neurodegenerative disorders. The decrease in GSH is not associated with a corresponding increase in levels of oxidized glutathione (GSSG), which is surprising as one might expect that an increase in peroxides would shift the

GSH:GSSG ratio in favor of GSSG. However, in hepatic tissues, oxidative stress can deplete GSH without inducing a corresponding increase in GSSG (62). In addition, hepatocytes exposed to MPP$^+$ show a loss of GSH through efflux that is not associated with a change in the level of GSSG (63). The importance of the decrease in GSH levels lies in its selectivity to PD. It is noteworthy that patients with ILBD have a reduction in GSH in the SNc comparable to that seen in PD (51), suggesting that this is an early component of the degenerative process.

The cause of the decrease in GSH is unknown. There are no defects in the major enzymes associated with GSH synthesis (55). In particular, there is no change in the level of γ-glutamylcysteine synthetase, the rate-limiting enzyme for GSH formation, or in the activities of GPX or glutathione transferase. However, there is a significant increase in the level of γ-glutamyltranspeptidase (γ-GTT), an enzyme responsible for the cellular degradation and translocation of precursors of GSH and metabolism of GSSG. Increased γ-GTT may reflect an attempt by surviving cells to recruit GSH precursors into the cell to replenish diminished levels of GSH or a compensatory mechanism necessary for removing potentially toxic GSSG. Increased γ-GTP activity can also lead to the formation of glutathionyl or cysteinyl complexes with L-dopa, dopamine, or dihyrophenylacetic acid (DOPAC) (64). These complexes may exert toxicity by reacting with and irreversibly removing GSH, so depleting the cell of a major antioxidant defense. It is possible that decreased GSH in PD may be a secondary event and reflect cellular damage with leakage from neurons. Importantly, it is mitochondrial GSH that is most important for the integrity of neurons, and this has not as yet been directly measured.

Buthionine sulfoximine (BSO) is a selective inhibitor of γ-glutamylcysteine synthetase that inhibits GSH formation. BSO induces a dose-dependent degeneration of cultured dopaminergic neurons, but high levels of GSH depletion (approximately 80%) are required for cell death to occur (65). In contrast, BSO administration to rats or mice sufficient to induce a 40% to 60% decline in basal ganglia GSH levels paralleling that which occurs in PD had no effect on the number of tyrosine hydroxylase–positive cells (66). It is possible that the dose of BSO employed in these studies was inadequate as BSO mainly depletes cytosolic GSH levels and initially has relatively little effect on mitochondrial GSH content, which is preferentially conserved. However, BSO infusion into the ventricle sufficient to deplete GSH levels by 80% to 90% did not induce nigral degeneration (Mytilineou and Olanow et al., unpublished observation). Nonetheless, depletion of GSH to a level that does not itself induce cell death may render cells vulnerable to other toxins. Indeed, BSO enhances the nigral degeneration in rodents induced by 6-OHDA or MPP$^+$ (67,68). It may be that the decrease in nigral GSH levels found in individuals with ILBD has little effect alone, but renders nigral cells vulnerable to toxins to which the normal population is largely immune.

It is possible that the decrease in GSH in PD is secondary to a glial defect. GSH is primarily located within glia and actively transported to neurons. Using mercury orange staining and immunocytochemical techniques, there is a loss of GSH in neuronal cells, processes, and neuropil in the SNc neurons in PD (69). However, the magnitude of GSH loss that is found in PD is more than can be accounted for by a loss of neuronal GSH alone. This raises the possibility that glia might also be affected and contribute to the loss of GSH. We have demonstrated that BSO is more toxic in mixed rather than neuronally enriched mesencephalic cultures, suggesting that glia play a role in the degenerative process (66). Indeed, BSO damage to dopamine neurons can be ameliorated by agents that inhibit glial-derived nitric oxide (NO) and cytokines. This suggests that GSH deficiency may act initially by activating glial cells, which then in turn exert toxicity on neurons (see below).

Oxidative Damage

Postmortem studies in PD patients indicate that a variety of biomolecules have undergone oxidative damage, further supporting a role for free radicals and ROS in the pathogenesis of cell death in PD. Oxidative damage to lipids is suggested by the finding of increased levels of malondialdehyde (MDA) in the SNc but not the cerebellum of patients with PD compared to age-matched control individuals (70). MDA is an intermediate product formed during the chain reaction of lipid peroxidation. However, homogenization of brain tissue in the presence of excess iron can promote postmortem oxidative change and confound interpretation of studies. Similarly, levels of lipid hydroperoxides, another product of lipid peroxidation, are increased in the SNc of PD patients by tenfold in comparison with controls (71). Increased immunohistochemical staining for 4-hydroxy-2-nonenal (HNE) has also been detected in surviving dopaminergic neurons in PD patients (72). HNE is another product of lipid peroxidation that is highly reactive and forms stable adducts with nucleophilic groups on proteins, such as thiols and amines. HNE is highly toxic and when added to cultured cells induces apoptosis with DNA fragmentation and activation of caspases-8, 9, and 3 (73). HNE also inhibits NF-κB signaling pathways, induces poly(ADP-ribose)polymerase (PARP) cleavage, decreases GSH levels, and inhibits complexes I and II of the mitochondrial respiratory chain (74,75). Furthermore, HNE enhances cross-linking of proteins and formation of HNE-protein adducts, and inhibits proteasomal function (76). Very recently, we showed that low concentrations of HNE added to cell cultures produced inhibition of proteasomal activity while not affecting cell viability. In the presence of overexpression of wild-type or mutant proteins, HNE further inhibits proteasomal function to a point where cell death occurs. These actions of HNE are associated with an accumulation of ubiquitinated proteins and inclusion formation. Interestingly, HNE also enhances the formation of nitrated proteins suggesting that inhibition of proteasomal function also induces both oxygen and nitrogen radical formation (see section on ubiquitin-proteasome system below).

Protein carbonyl levels, a product of protein oxidation, are also increased in the SNc in PD, although increased levels were detected in all brain areas examined (77). This suggests that oxidative damage in PD may be widespread. Oxidative damage to DNA also appears to occur in PD as evidenced by an increase in levels of 8-hydroxy-2-deoxyguanosine (8-OHDG) (78). Here, too, increases were detected in the SNc as well as in other brain regions. We examined products of oxidative damage to the four DNA bases and found no increase in oxidative products other than those derived from guanine as previously reported (79,80). A selective increase in 8-hydroxyguanine products suggests damage is due to singlet oxygen or peroxy radicals. Damage by hydroxyl radicals would be expected to damage products arising from all DNA bases and NO-mediated damage should also cause alterations in the levels of xanthine and hypoxanthine that were not observed. Recent studies question whether there actually is any increase in oxidative damage to DNA in PD as the increase in 8-hydroxyguanine levels is associated with a corresponding decrease in levels of Fapy-guanine, another product of guanine oxidation. These two products (8-hydroxyguanine and Fapy-guanine) are the result of the respective oxidation and reduction of an intermediate oxidized form of guanine. Summation of both guanine oxidation products reveals no difference in total guanine damage between patients with PD and controls. The results found in PD may thus reflect an alteration in intracellular redox conditions rather than a direct increase in oxidative damage to guanine itself. Since the increase in 8-hydroxyguanine is localized to the cytosol rather than the nucleus, it may be indicative of alterations in mitochondrial (rather than nuclear) DNA.

There is thus evidence that oxidative damage occurs in PD, but the extent of this damage, and whether it is a primary or secondary phenomenon, remains to be clarified. The majority of PD patients receive levodopa that can be metabolized to yield a variety of oxidizing species and may thus contribute to the oxidative damage detected at postmortem in PD patients. In addition, there is concern that oxidant stress induced by levodopa may accelerate neuronal degeneration in PD. Levodopa can be chemically oxidized to produce aminochrome derivatives on the pathway to melanin formation or be decarboxylated to dopamine and thereby promote peroxide and hydroxyl radical formation. Levodopa can also form conjugates with GSH or cysteine and thereby aggravate the GSH deficiency in PD. However, it has proven difficult to establish whether levodopa treatment is or is not toxic in PD. In vitro studies indicate that levodopa can have both antioxidant and pro-oxidant characteristics in that it can promote free-radical formation on the one hand and up-regulate antioxidant defense systems and prevent damage from free radicals and other toxins on the other hand (81,82). That both of these effects occur by way of levodopa-generated ROS is apparent from the observation that both can be attenuated by ascorbate (81,83). In vivo, levodopa is reported to induce increased oxidized GSH levels (84), hydroxyl radical formation (85), and DNA damage (86); to interfere with mitochondrial respiratory chain activity (87); and to increase neuronal loss and oxidative damage in 6-OHDA-lesioned rodents (88,89). However, administration of large doses of levodopa has not resulted in a decrease in the numbers of dopaminergic neurons in normal rodents, primates, and humans (90–93). Furthermore, levodopa did not reduce the number of SNc dopamine neurons in 6-OHDA treated rodents in a carefully performed study (94). Indeed, there was a suggestion that levodopa may even have induced a trophic effect. These studies suggest that levodopa is not toxic to SNc neurons despite in vitro findings. However, the situation may be different in PD where the SNc is in a state of oxidant stress and defense mechanisms are impaired. To test this hypothesis, we treated mesencephalic cultures and newborn rat pups with levodopa combined with BSO, an inhibitor of GSH synthesis (95). In mesencephalic cultures, levodopa toxicity was enhanced by GSH depletion. In contrast, neither BSO nor levodopa nor their combination altered the number of nigral dopaminergic neurons in rat pups despite a profound reduction in GSH. This protection may relate to trophic factors, glia, and the high levels of ascorbate that are present in the PD patient. In addition, microdialysis studies have demonstrated that levodopa administration is not associated with free-radical production in dopamine-lesioned rodents (96). Current studies suggest that despite the potential of levodopa to induce neurodegenerative changes in in vitro models, it is not likely to be toxic to dopamine neurons in PD. Levodopa toxicity certainly cannot explain the reduction in GSH in ILBD patients who never received levodopa or the reduction in complex I activity found in PD patients as it is not found in levodopa-treated patients with other disorders, such as multiple system atrophy (MSA). Based on these considerations, most clinicians continue to routinely use levodopa for the symptomatic treatment of PD (97).

Mitochondrial Dysfunction

Examination of postmortem brain material from patients dying with PD has shown a decrease in complex I activity in the SNc (98,99). This defect is not found in other brain areas in PD patients or in the SNc or elsewhere in brains of patients with MSA and other neurodegenerative disorders who also experience extensive degeneration of nigrostriatal neurons. A similar defect in complex I has been reported in platelets, fibroblasts, and muscle of patients with PD, although these findings are less consistent (100,101).

The cause of the decreased complex I activity in PD remains a mystery. Systemic administration of MPTP or rotenone can induce nigral cell death with selective inhibition of complex I, but the relevance to routine cases of PD remains uncertain (17,18). The possibility of a primary mutation in mitochondrial or nuclear DNA has been suspected, but none has been identified to date despite complete mitochondrial genome screening (102). Studies involving the construction of cybrids using mitochondrial DNA obtained from PD patients with low complex I activity indicate that the defect persists through multiple generations and is therefore likely to be encoded (103). The cybrids continue to show low complex I activity as well as increased formation of ROS, susceptibility to MPP$^+$, increased antioxidant enzyme levels, increased levels of anti-apoptotic proteins, and abnormal calcium handling (104,105). Similarly, persistent mitochondrial defects in respiration have been noted in cloned fibroblasts taken from PD patients (106). These findings suggest that the complex I defect is determined by an abnormality of mitochondrial DNA, although DNA damage might be inherited or acquired. Mitochondrial DNA defects are maternally inherited, and rare families with a maternal inheritance pattern have been described. Oxidative stress can damage mitochondria, but changes typically are not confined to complex I, suggesting an alternate explanation for the mitochondrial damage found in PD.

It also remains to be determined how the complex I defect in PD contributes to cell degeneration. A defect in complex I activity could result in a reduction in ATP synthesis and a bioenergetic deficiency with weak excitotoxicity (see below). Indeed, studies of mitochondrial function in mouse brain synaptosomes indicate that complex I inhibition by MPTP or MPP$^+$ leads to a depletion of cellular ATP with calcium influx (107). However, not all PD patients express a defect in complex I, and it is not yet known to what degree the 30% to 40% reduction in complex I activity found in others can induce a bioenergetic defect. In this regard, it is noteworthy that decreased immunoreactivity for α-ketoglutarate dehydrogenase has been observed in both PD patients and following MPTP toxicity (108,109). A reduction in α-ketoglutarate dehydrogenase activity could impair compensatory electron entry into the respiratory cycle at complex II and magnify the effects of a complex I defect. A combination of a complex I defect and decreased α-ketoglutarate dehydrogenase activity is more likely to adversely affect cellular energy metabolism than is a defect in either enzyme alone.

Attention has also focused on the possibility that a complex I defect could lead to cell degeneration through free-radical production. A defect in complex I could promote respiration through complex II with a resultant increase in

the release of free radicals. Studies in cloned PD fibroblasts indicate that respiration using pyruvate, a substrate for complex I, is impaired whereas it is normal with succinate, a substrate for complex II (106). New studies have also begun to challenge the significance of the complex I inhibition found with MPP$^+$ (110,111). These studies demonstrate that MPP$^+$ preferentially binds to the vesicular monoamine transporter–2 (VMAT-2) and may cause cell death by promoting the release of stored dopamine with consequent oxidative damage rather than by a complex I defect per se. Indeed, rotenone produces markedly less neuronal degeneration than MPP$^+$ in these experiments despite being used in concentrations that produce much higher levels of complex I inhibition.

Finally, it is possible that mitochondrial dysfunction could cause cell death by promoting signaling mechanisms that lead to apoptosis (6). Complex I is a major contributor to proton pumping. Increasing evidence now indicates that impaired proton pumping with a consequent reduction in the mitochondrial membrane potential can lead to opening of the mitochondrial permeability transition pore and release of mitochondrial factors that signal for the onset of apoptosis (see below).

Excitotoxicity

Excitotoxicity is an established cause of neurodegeneration (112) occurring in response to a rise in glutamate or glutamatergic transmission (113). Excessive glutamatergic activity results in an increase in calcium flux into the cell with a rise in cytosolic free calcium and activation of calcium-dependent enzymes such as proteases, lipases, and endonucleases, with consequent damage to cytoskeletal proteins, membrane lipids, and DNA, respectively. There are natural defenses that protect against excitotoxicity largely linked to ATP production. A voltage-dependent Mg^{2+} blockade blocks the *N*-methyl-D-aspartate (NMDA) receptor and limits glutamate-mediated calcium influx. In addition, there are mechanisms to extrude calcium from the cell and to sequester calcium in endoplasmic reticulum, mitochondria, or the cell nucleus (114). Glial cells also have an energy-dependent uptake mechanism for glutamate that significantly limits its actions. Interestingly, this becomes impaired when glial cells are deficient in GSH. Finally, stimulation of glutamatergic receptors has the potential to induce protective as well as toxic effects.

Excitotoxicity has been implicated in PD based on two possible mechanisms. The first involves direct excitotoxicity by way of excessive glutamatergic activity through enhanced release of glutamate or through the actions of an exogenous or endogenous excitotoxin, such as quinolinic acid. Nigral dopaminergic neurons are rich in glutamate receptors and receive glutamatergic innervation from the cortex and the subthalamic nucleus (STN). Loss of striatal dopamine input results in disinhibition of the STN with a resultant increase in its excitatory output to SNc (115) that might conceivably promote excitotoxic cell death in target structures and so contribute to the progression of PD (116). In support of this hypothesis, STN lesions that block its excitatory output protect nigral neurons in rodents from the toxic effects of 6-OHDA (117). Furthermore, there are reports indicating that NMDA receptor antagonists can inhibit dopamine cell loss due to MPP⁺ infusion into the substantia nigra of rats (118).

The second explanation for how glutamate might be involved in cellular degeneration in PD invokes a "weak" excitotoxic mechanism (119,120). This theory hypothesizes that a primary defect in mitochondrial energy function causes cells to become susceptible to physiologic concentrations of glutamate to which they are normally immune. The bioenergetic defect results in a loss of the ATP-dependent Mg blockade of the NMDA receptor and permits normal concentrations of glutamate to mediate an excessive calcium influx into the cell. The bioenergetic consequence of the complex I and α-ketoglutarate dehydrogenase defects in PD are not known, but it is possible that they are sufficient to induce weak excitotoxicity. It can also be speculated that impaired α-ketoglutarate dehydrogenase activity may lead to an accumulation of metabolic glutamate, which could then exert an excitotoxic action.

Nitric Oxide, Peroxynitrite, and Protein Nitration

There is considerable evidence to suggest that excitotoxicity is mediated, at least in part, via nitric oxide (121), which is formed by the conversion of arginine to citrulline in a reaction catalyzed by nitric oxide synthase (NOS). A glutamate-mediated rise in cytosolic calcium results in activation of NOS and increased NO production. NO can react with superoxide radical to form peroxynitrite and subsequently hydroxyl radicals, both powerful oxidizing agents (122). NO might also contribute to cell degeneration by displacing iron from ferritin (123), thereby promoting oxidative damage and inhibition of mitochondrial function such that a reversible inhibition of complex I could be converted to an irreversible action by the effect of NO at the level of complex IV. Indeed, there is evidence that the neuronal mitochondrial respiratory chain is damaged by sustained exposure to NO and that GSH is an important defense against such damage (124,125). The mechanism of action of NO remains uncertain but may involve S-nitrosylation of thiol groups in the enzyme complex. NO may also affect GSH levels by selectively inhibiting GSH reductase, which recycles GSSG to GSH (126). All of this has implications for PD where there is evidence that NO is generated and GSH levels are decreased.

NO is toxic to mesencephalic dopaminergic cells in culture, and this toxicity is enhanced by GSH depletion. Decreased GSH levels cause an increase in neuronal NOS

expression and enhanced degeneration of dopamine neurons secondary to MPTP lesions (127). A role for NO in MPTP toxicity is also suggested by studies in mice in which the NOS inhibitor 7-nitroindazole (7-NI) protects dopaminergic neurons from MPTP toxicity (128). Similarly, in knockout mice with a defect in neuronal NOS production, MPTP toxicity is significantly reduced in comparison to wild type littermates (129). However, the removal of neuronal NOS only partially protects against NO toxicity compared to 7-NI, suggesting that other isoforms of NOS may also be involved. Indeed, MPTP toxicity is more inhibited in mice with a knockout of inducible NOS, suggesting the involvement of glial-derived NO and the proliferation of inducible NOS–positive glial cells following MPTP treatment. In contrast to the substantia nigra, there was no significant protection against MPTP's actions on striatal dopaminergic terminals as judged by measurement of dopamine and its metabolites. This suggests the differential involvement of neuronal and inducible NOS in MPTP toxicity based on brain area. Studies in baboons support the idea that NO is important for MPTP toxicity (130). Treatment with 7-NI during and following MPTP treatment markedly reduced the loss of nigral tyrosine hydroxylase–positive cells and improved motor performance in comparison with animals receiving MPTP treatment alone. Interestingly, the nonselective NOS inhibitor N^G-nitro-L-arginine methyl ester (L-NAME) did not inhibit MPTP toxicity in marmosets (131). The reason for this discrepancy may relate to the different specificities of the NOS inhibitors. L-NAME is a nonspecific long-lasting and irreversible NOS inhibitor that may affect constitutive NOS and reduce cerebral blood flow. In contrast, 7-NI is a specific, short-acting, reversible, neuronal NOS inhibitor that may or may not have an effect on blood flow (132). It is also possible that 7-NI exerts actions other than those related to its ability to inhibit neuronal NOS. Indazole compounds can interact with a variety of heme- and iron-sulfur centers and may also directly influence enzymes such as hemoxygenase, cytochrome P450, and mitochondrial complex I. Initial reports suggested that 7-NI had no effect on MAO activity in brain and did not alter the levels of MPP⁺ derived from MPTP treatment (133). However, a subsequent report suggested that 7-NI exerts significant inhibition of MAO-B (134). If this is of functional significance, it raises the possibility that 7-NI may inhibit MPTP toxicity by blocking its conversion to MPP⁺ and not through an antiexcitotoxic mechanism.

Damage due to NO can be estimated by measuring the formation of 3-nitrotyrosine (3-NT). Peroxynitrite can interact with, and nitrate, tyrosine residues on cellular proteins (135). 3-NT is a byproduct and marker of this reaction. In mice and monkeys treated with MPTP, increased levels of 3-NT have been reported using high-performance liquid chromatography (133); however, this technique is associated with false-positives peaks. Using mass spectrometric analysis, the presence of 3-NT has been convincingly shown in the brain of MPTP-treated mice (136). In addition, the nitration of tyrosine hydroxylase has also been demonstrated in MPTP-treated mice (137). Nitration may also be important in the toxic effects of 6-OHDA to dopaminergic neurons in vivo since we have demonstrated that intrastriatal injection leads to large increases in the levels of nitrotyrosine and nitrophenylalanine (138).

Using more reliable immunocytologic techniques, increased 3-NT staining has been detected in SNc dopamine neurons of MPTP-treated baboons (139) as well as in neurofibrillary tangles in the brains of AD patients (140) and in the core of Lewy bodies in PD patients (141). These findings implicate NO in these neurodegenerative processes, and indeed direct injection of free 3-NT into the striatum causes neurodegeneration (142). However, the precise role of NO in nigral cell death remains to be defined.

As discussed elsewhere in this chapter, oxidative damage and nitration of proteins, coupled with impairment in the ability of the 26S proteasome to degrade them, may underlie Lewy body formation and nigral cell degeneration. Indeed, nitrated forms of α-synuclein and other proteins have been detected in Lewy bodies in PD, suggesting that these proteins have not been recognized or properly degraded by the ubiquitin-proteasome system. This contrasts with the finding that the nitrated products of Cu-Zn SOD and tyrosine hydroxylase are directed to proteasomal degradation and are more rapidly degraded than the parent molecules (143).

Toxic effects of NO/peroxynitrite can also involve damage to DNA leading to products such as 8-hydroxyguanine and 8-nitrodeoxyguanosine and increases in DNA single-strand breakage (144). The latter is a trigger for the activation of PARP (145). Activation of PARP is highly energy dependent and leads to the cleavage of NAD$^+$ into ADP-ribose and nicotinamide. PARP also catalyzes the formation of poly(ADP-ribose) attached to a variety of proteins. PARP activation rapidly depletes NAD$^+$ stores, thus impairing mitochondrial function, glycolysis, and ATP formation (146). This may be relevant to MPTP toxicity because PARP inhibitors prevent striatal dopamine depletion and the ability of MPTP to decrease NAD$^+$ and ATP levels in mouse brain, although this is disputed (147). Furthermore, PARP knockout mice appear resistant to the neurotoxic effects of MPTP (148).

Glial Cell Involvement in Nigral Cell Death

PD is usually viewed as a neuronal disorder, but a body of information suggests that there is also glial cell involvement (149). A reactive gliosis with activation of microglia is apparent in the substantia nigra in PD as demonstrated by an increase in HLA-DR immunoreactivity (150). Elevated levels of interleukin-2 (IL-2) have been noted in the striatum of PD patients and levels of IL-2 and IL-6 are increased in the ventricular cerebrospinal fluid (151,152). In addition, the presence of immunoreactivity for CD23, inducible NOS, and COX-2 illustrate the presence of activated glial cells in the SNc in PD (153–155). The density of glial cells expressing tumor necrosis factor α (TNF-α), IL-1β, and interferon-γ (IFN-γ) on immunostaining is also increased in the PD nigra, and levels of TNF-α and IL-1β are increased in the cerebrospinal fluid in PD (149). It remains uncertain whether these changes are primary or secondary and develop in response to cell injury. However, the 70-fold increase in nuclear staining for NF-κB in nigral neurons in PD reported by Hunot et al. suggest that TNF-α and other cytokines have induced functional changes in PD (156). Further, an immune model of PD has been created based on antibodies generated against a hybrid line of dopaminergic neurons (157). Immunized animals exhibited hypokinesia, a significant loss of SNc neurons, and activated microglia, suggesting that loss of appropriate central nervous system nuclei via immune targeting could potentially contribute to human PD.

There is also evidence of gliosis involving both microglia and astrocytes following the destruction of nigral dopaminergic cells by MPTP (158). Glial cell activation is presumed to occur as a response to dopaminergic cell death in PD rather than the reverse, although this has not been proven. However, the toxicity of MPTP in mice can be attenuated by treatment with either aspirin or selective COX-1 and COX-2 inhibitors (158a,159), suggesting a role for both glial cells and inflammatory toxins in its mechanism of action. Furthermore, glial cell activation removes trophic support from neurons and is associated with the release of cytotoxic substances (160). For example, activation of astrocytes with lipopolysaccharide (LPS) causes the release of cytokines, glutamate, NO, and ROS (161,162). At the same time, the normal trophic support provided by glial cells to neurons is impaired and there is decreased release of brain-derived neurotrophic factor (BDNF) and glial-derived neurotrophic factor (GDNF) (160). These factors may have important consequences for cell survival. Indeed, trophic factors, such as GDNF, protect rat SNc neurons from transection of the nigrostriatal pathway (163). BDNF and GDNF also increase the survival of dopaminergic neurons after exposure to toxins like 6-OHDA and MPP$^+$/MPTP both in vitro and in vivo in rodents and primates (164–166). In addition, lentiviral delivery of GDNF has been demonstrated to provide marked behavioral and protection/rescue against nigral cell death in MPTP-treated rhesus monkeys (167). Whether a reduction in GDNF production plays a role in the pathophysiology of PD is not clear, but it is noteworthy that a recent in situ hybridization study found no detectable levels of GDNF mRNA in brains obtained from PD patients or age-matched controls (168).

LPS-induced activation of glial cells is known to result in an adverse effect on dopaminergic neurons. In vitro the addition of activated glial cells to primary dopaminergic mesencephalic cultures leads to the selective destruction of tyrosine hydroxylase–positive cells (169,170). The intranigral injection of LPS in rats also causes glial cell activation as shown by increases in GFAP, inducible NOS, and NADPH-diaphorase staining (171–173). This results in a selective loss of nigral tyrosine hydroxylase positive cells that is partially prevented by administration of a selective inducible NOS inhibitor (Jenner, unpublished data). Formation of NO appears to be important for the toxicity exerted by activated glial cells as there is a selective up-regulation of inducible NOS and marked immunoreactivity for 3-NT. The toxic actions of activated glial cells are further enhanced by a depletion of GSH (174–176). We have shown that the degeneration of cultured dopamine neurons associated with GSH depletion is dependent on activated glia and can be prevented by inhibitors of arachidonic acid and NO (66). Interestingly, we have shown that LPS is also capable of inducing up-regulation of SOD and thereby promoting enhanced survival of dopaminergic neurons after exposure to a variety of toxins (83). This effect is similar to what is seen following exposure to levodopa, where high doses induce degeneration but low doses may be associated with protective effects. This illustrates the difficulty in attempting to understand what is going on in PD based on in vitro and in vivo laboratory studies.

Apoptosis and Dopaminergic Nerve Cell Death

A body of information now suggests that cell death in PD occurs, at least in part, by way of an apoptotic process. This has great importance for developing therapies that might interfere with pro-apoptotic signals and provide neuroprotection for PD patients. Details of apoptosis are provided in the previous version of this chapter and in several cited reviews and will only be highlighted in this section.

Necrosis and Apoptosis

Neuronal death can be broadly divided into two processes: necrosis and apoptosis (4,6). Morphologically, necrosis involves rapidly progressive cellular disruption marked by cell swelling, organelle disintegration, plasma membrane fracture, and cytoplasmic extrusion. In contrast, apoptosis proceeds more slowly and involves cellular degradation rather than disruption. Apoptotic degradation features cell shrinkage, plasma membrane blebbing, nuclear chromatin condensation, nuclear DNA fragmentation, maintenance of plasma membrane integrity but a loss of phospholipid asymmetry, cytoskeletal digestion, and the formation of membrane-wrapped cytoplasmic and nuclear bodies. Apoptotic degradation primes dying cells for macrophage inges-

tion and avoids the spilling of cytoplasmic contents into the extracellular space, thus preventing inflammatory and immune responses that might injure intact neighboring cells.

Apoptotic degradation was originally described 30 years ago as a means of regulating the number of developing neurons (177). It is now appreciated that apoptosis can occur in several neurodegenerative disorders as well as in response to a variety of toxins that are relevant to PD. For example, neuronal apoptosis can be induced by levodopa, dopamine, GSH depletion, excessive iron levels, excitatory amino acids, MPTP, MPP$^+$, 6-hydroxydopamine, mitochondrial complex I inhibitors, and pro-oxidants (178–189). In general, low doses/concentrations of a toxic agent, particularly when delivered slowly, induce apoptosis whereas high levels or rapid delivery of the same toxin induce necrosis (190). Cell death due to apoptosis can vary in morphology, but is largely independent of cell type and the insult that initiates the process (191).

Classically, DNA gel electrophoresis was used to identify apoptosis based on detecting a "ladder" pattern typical of oligonucleosomal DNA digestion (192). However, this method permits detection only of relatively short pieces of fragmented DNA, which are not present in all forms of apoptosis. In addition, the method requires large amounts of tissue and therefore does not lend itself to the study of postmortem tissues. Furthermore, degenerating nerve cells are most likely to enter apoptosis in a desynchronized manner, and the life span of nuclei with fragmented DNA is only a matter of hours. Therefore, only small numbers of dopaminergic nerve cells might be undergoing apoptosis at any time. The development of in situ end labeling (ISEL) fluorescent stain techniques (also termed TdT dUTP nick end labeling or TUNEL), in which staining medium binds to the 3′ cut ends of DNA, provided the initial means to recognize apoptotic nuclear DNA cleavage in postmortem histologic brain sections (193). Using ISEL techniques, evidence of apoptosis has been described in AD (194,195), Huntington's disease (196,197), amyotrophic lateral sclerosis (198), and AIDS encephalitis (199).

The initial evidence demonstrating neuronal apoptosis in the PD postmortem brain was based on finding nuclear DNA cleavage with ISEL techniques (200). Furthermore, electron microscopic studies demonstrated occasional cells with nuclear ultrastructural changes typical of apoptosis (201). However, interpretation of these studies was confounded by the findings in some studies that large numbers of ISEL-positive nuclei were present in control brains (202), that the numbers of ISEL-positive nuclei were similar in PD and control brains (203), and that many ISEL-positive nuclei were likely glia rather than neurons (204). This disparate evidence probably resulted from technical problems with the terminal deoxynucleotidyltransferase (TdT) used in ISEL (205–207). TdT can label both single-strand and double-strand DNA breaks and therefore has the potential to label nuclei in necrotic as well as apoptotic cells (208). Depending on tissue preparation and ion concentrations, ISEL techniques can thus provide either false negatives or false positives that confound interpretation of these studies.

These difficulties have largely been overcome by the application of dual labeling techniques that allow for the simultaneous detection of both DNA cleavage and chromatin condensation in the same nucleus. Nuclear DNA cleavage and chromatin condensation are mediated by different signaling events (209,210), and both DNA cleavage and chromatin condensation can be readily visualized with fluorescent DNA binding dyes. The joint use of fluorescence ISEL and fluorescent DNA binding dyes allows for the demonstration of nuclear DNA fragmentation and chromatin condensation in the same nucleus (211,212). The presence of both provides strong evidence that the cell is undergoing apoptotic degradation. Using this combined approach, we did not find high levels of apoptotic degradation in control brains or apoptosis in the glia of PD brains as had been found with ISEL techniques alone. Rather, we detected both DNA fragmentation and chromatin clumping in the same nucleus in a significantly higher proportion of nigral neuromelanin-containing neurons in PD patients than in age-matched controls (211,212). While the number of apoptotic nuclei detected in the PD brain may seem unduly high as their existence is thought to be measured in hours, we have argued that these are vulnerable cells that have been pushed into an apoptotic state as a consequence of the agonal events associated with dying.

Although DNA cleavage and chromatin fragmentation can be used to recognize apoptosis, it does not define the numerous signaling pathways, which differentiate one form of apoptosis from another. A number of genes and their protein products have been found capable of influencing or even determining the progression of the apoptotic process (213,214). The genes *bax, bcl-x$_S$, bad, bak, ice* (IL-1β converting enzyme), *price*, and *ich-1$_L$* promote entry into the early stages of apoptosis, whereas *bcl-2, bcl-x$_L$, bcl-x$_\beta$ A1, mcl-1, bag-1, abl, raf-1,* and *ich-1$_S$* decrease or block the progression of apoptosis. Several of these are mammalian homologs of the *ced-3, ced-4,* and *ced-9* genes that respectively inhibit and promote apoptosis in the worm *C. elegans*. Thus, increased expression of bax and a variety of cysteine proteases (known as caspases) promotes neuronal apoptosis, whereas increased expression of bcl-2, bcl-x$_L$, or ich-1$_S$ promotes survival.

Mitochondrial factors are critical to some forms of neuronal apoptosis (6). There is normally an electrochemical proton gradient across the mitochondrial inner membrane known as the mitochondrial membrane potential ($\Delta\Psi_M$). Three mitochondrial complexes (I, III, and IV) use electron energy transferred from the carrier molecules NADH, ubiquinone, and cytochrome *c*, respectively, to pump protons across the mitochondrial inner membrane to generate

a $\Delta\Psi_M$ of approximately -150 mV. Flow cytometry studies indicate that $\Delta\Psi_M$ begins to decrease early in apoptosis, well before the onset of chromatin condensation or nuclear DNA strand breaks (215–217). A decrease in $\Delta\Psi_M$ leads to opening of a permeability transition pore (PTP) in the mitochondrial membrane, which allows for the free exchange of solutes across the mitochondrial membrane. This in turn is followed by mitochondrial swelling, fracture of the mitochondrial membrane, and release of molecules from within mitochondria such as holocytochrome *c* that signal the initiation of apoptosis (218). The importance of mitochondrial signaling in the initiation of at least some types of apoptosis is illustrated by studies showing that mitochondrial factors initiate apoptosis in cell-free systems (219) and that the mitochondrial protein cytochrome *c* can promote apoptosis when released into the cellular cytoplasm (220).

The PTP includes an ADP-ATP exchanger (the adenine nucleotide translocator, or ANT), a voltage-dependent anion channel, and a 70 K protein that binds peripheral benzodiazepine agonists and is therefore termed the mitochondrial benzodiazepine receptor. Increases in free cytosolic Ca^{2+}, increased levels of ROS, or a partial failure of mitochondrial proton pumping, acting individually or together, can promote opening of the PTP and dissipation of $\Delta\Psi$. Pro-apoptotic molecules, such as BAX, promote opening of the PTP, whereas anti-apoptotic molecules, such as BCL-2, promote closure of the PTP (222). Over the last several years a myriad of molecules have been shown to operate within subcellular decisional networks that can be either pro- or anti-apoptotic (223).

Additional evidence supporting the presence of apoptosis in PD has been provided by studies measuring alterations or translocation of signals involved in apoptosis. They demonstrated increased neuronal levels of activated caspase-3 in PD postmortem nigra (212,224). Activation of caspase-3 depends on the release of signaling proteins from mitochondria and is the critical event in many forms of apoptosis (225,226). Increased levels or pathologic distribution of other key pro-apoptotic signaling proteins have also been demonstrated in PD nigral neurons, including Bax (212,227), caspase-8 (228), p53 (229), and glyceraldehyde-3-phosphate dehydrogenase (212). Together these findings strongly support the view that apoptosis contributes to neuronal loss in PD and open the door to studies that fully define the specific apoptosis signaling pathways that are operative in PD. A complete understanding of the signaling pathways may provide insights into the cellular insults or defects that initiate the disease. Modulation of apoptosis signaling pathways may also offer new therapeutic approaches in PD as they have the potential to provide benefit to patients suffering from PD resulting from a variety of different etiologic factors (see below). Indeed, studies of apoptosis-based therapies for a variety of diseases, including PD, are now in clinical trial (230).

Protein Handling Dysfunction

Since the last edition of this chapter, a body of evidence has emerged suggesting that impairment in the capacity of the ubiquitin-proteasome system to clear abnormal intracellular proteins may be a common factor in the various etiopathologic forms of PD (231). This theory proposes that failure of the ubiquitin-proteasome to clear cytotoxic proteins underlies the neurodegenerative process and accounts for the development of both sporadic and familial cases of PD. The theory is attractive as it has the potential to link the different genetic, environmental, and pathogenetic features that have been identified in PD.

Ubiquitin-Proteasome System

The ubiquitin-proteasome system (UPS) is the primary system responsible for the degradation and clearance of unwanted proteins in eukaryotic cells (232). These include proteins that are mutant, damaged by excitotoxic or oxidative injury, or misplaced. Protein clearance is accomplished by way of a series of enzymatic reactions that label abnormal proteins with multiple ubiquitin molecules that signal for their degradation by the 26/20S proteasome (Fig. 4.2). Activated ubiquitin is generated from ubiquitin monomers by a ubiquitin-activating enzyme (E1), transferred to a ubiquitin-conjugating enzyme (E2), and attached to a protein substrate by one of hundreds of relatively specific ubiquitin ligases (E3) (233). Once proteins have been conjugated to ubiquitin, they translocate to the 26/20S proteasome where they are degraded by several protease enzymes (chymotryptic, tryptic, and postacidic) into constituent peptides or amino acids, which can then be recycled into the formation of new proteins. Finally, ubiquitin monomers are removed from ubiquitin-protein adducts immediately prior to their entry into the 20S proteasomal core by deubiquitinating enzymes. This permits monomeric ubiquitin to reenter the ubiquitin-proteasome cycle at E1 and aid in the clearance of additional unwanted proteins.

The 26/20SS proteasome itself is comprised of a 20S core, in which all enzyme activity occurs, and two 19S (PA700) or two 12S (PA28) regulatory caps or activators that unfold and deliver proteins to the 20S proteasomal core for degradation (Fig. 4.3). The 20S core is composed of two heptameric α rings and two β rings which are each made up of seven different subunits. All protease enzyme activity takes place within specific subunits of the β rings of the proteasomal core. The precise role of the α rings is not known; however, they are essential for the normal assembly and function of the proteasome. The combination of the 20S proteasome core with its 19S (PA700) activator is known as the 26/20S proteasome. Together they act to promote the clearance of ubiquitinated proteins in an ATP-dependent manner. The 11S activator clears nonubiquitinated proteins and is of particular importance because it does not depend on ATP availability and plays an important role in clearing oxidized proteins, which are increased in the SNc in PD. There is also some evidence indicating that the 20S proteasome can itself clear some proteins. The accumulation of intracellular proteins is regulated by heat-shock proteins (e.g., HsP70), which increase in response to cell stresses. They act as molecular chaperones to promote protein refolding and facilitate their proteasomal degradation. The existence of proteins that inhibit proteasomal function, such as P131, has also recently been appreciated. Such proteins presumably regulate proteasomal activity and

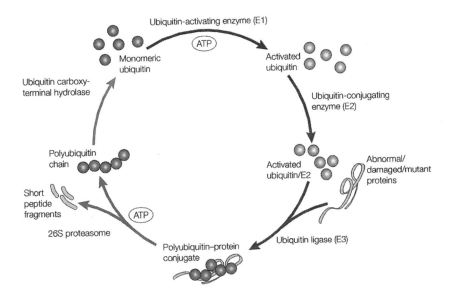

FIG. 4.2. Clearance of abnormal proteins by the ubiquitin-proteasome system. Proteins are ubiquitinated as a signal for proteasomal degradation by a series of enzymatic reactions as shown above: E1 enzymes activate ubiquitin monomers, E2 enzymes conjugate ubiquitin to proteins or to E3 enzymes, which are in turn a series of ubiquitin ligases and attach chains of ubiquitin to specific protein substrates. Labeling of proteins with multiple ubiquitin molecules (ubiquitination) is a signal for ATP-dependent degradation by the 26S proteasome complex. Prior to entry into the proteasomal core, deubiquitinating enzymes cleave ubiquitin monomers from ubiquitin-protein adducts so that they can be recycled in order to clear additional abnormal proteins. (Adapted with permission from McNaught KStP, Olanow CW, Halliwell, et al. Failure of the ubiquitin-proteasome system in Parkinson's disease. *Nat Rev Neurosci* 2001;2:89–94.)

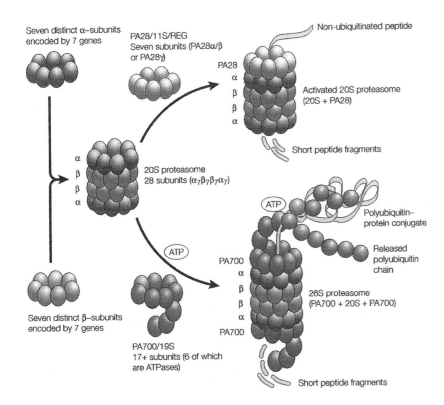

Seven distinct α–subunits encoded by 7 genes

PA28/11S/REG Seven subunits (PA28α/β or PA28γ)

PA28
α
β
β
α

Activated 20S proteasome (20S + PA28)

Non-ubiquitinated peptide

Short peptide fragments

α
β
β
α

20S proteasome 28 subunits ($\alpha_7\beta_7\beta_7\alpha_7$)

Seven distinct β–subunits encoded by 7 genes

PA700/19S 17+ subunits (6 of which are ATPases)

ATP

ATP

PA700
α
β
β
α
PA700

Polyubiquitin–protein conjugate

Released polyubiquitin chain

26S proteasome (PA700 + 20S + PA700)

Short peptide fragments

FIG. 4.3. Composition of the 20S proteasome and the PA700 and PA28 activators. The 20S proteasome is a multicatalytic protease found in the cytosol, perinuclear regions, and nucleus of eukaryotic cells. It is composed of two outer α rings and two inner β rings, which are stacked axially to form a hollow cylindrical structure in which proteolysis occurs. The β ring is composed of seven different subunits that host the three sites for protein catalysis. The α ring also comprises seven different subunits. It does not have enzymatic activity but serves as an anchor for the ATPase-containing PA700 (19S) regulator. The proteasome and the 19S regulator are collectively referred to as the 26/20S proteasome. The 19S regulatory complex opens the channel of the 20S proteasome and unfolds ubiquitinated proteins so that they can be metabolized in the catalytic core. These processes are ATP dependent. The PA28 (11S) regulatory complex may also bind to the 20S proteasome and open the channel for protein degradation, but it acts in an ATP-independent manner and primarily mediates the degradation of nonubiquitinated short peptides. (Adapted with permission from McNaught KStP, Olanow CW, Halliwell, et al. Failure of the ubiquitin-proteasome system in Parkinson's disease. *Nat Rev Neurosci* 2001;2: 89–94.)

prevent excessive and undesired destruction of native proteins. It is important to appreciate that, in addition to clearing unwanted proteins, the UPS system helps to regulate important transcriptional and transmitter proteins within the cell.

An increase in levels of intracellular proteins is also associated with a compensatory up-regulation of the proteasomal components and activity as well as the formation of aggresomes. These are composed of large numbers of proteasomes and are thought to be protective structures formed in response to increased intracellular levels of abnormal misfolded proteins so as to promote their clearance and to segregate them presumably to protect the cell from their cytotoxic properties (234). These tend to translocate and cluster in centrosomes near the cell nucleus, possibly to afford maximal protection to the most critical cell components. It is interesting to consider that Lewy bodies seen in PD are a type of aggresome that form in response to the accumulation of cytotoxic proteins and thus have a protective role in nigral dopaminergic neurons.

The accumulation of abnormal proteins due to failure of the UPS ultimately leads to the death of the cell. There is considerable evidence to suggest that this involves up-regulation of the pro-apoptotic protein Jun kinase (JNK), which in turn promotes the release of cytochrome *c* from mitochondria, increases FAS ligand formation, and inhibits the phosphorylation and activation of anti-apoptotic proteins such as bcl-2 (232). Heat-shock proteins function as anti-apoptotic agents by activating phosphatases that cleave

JNK, thereby preventing its up-regulation. However, intracellular proteins bind heat-shock proteins and, if excessive, can interfere with their capacity to block JNK activation. Other mechanisms, such as impaired axonal transport, might also have a role in the degenerative process.

UPS and Parkinson's Disease

There are many reasons to consider that defects in the capacity of the UPS to clear misfolded proteins play an important role in PD. PD is characterized by the presence of the Lewy body in degenerating neurons. The Lewy body is an intracytoplasmic inclusion that accumulates a wide range of free and ubiquitinated proteins, including neurofilament, monomeric ubiquitin, components of the UPS, protein adducts of 3-NT and HNE, torsin A, and α-synuclein (141,235–239). In addition, in PD the SNc as well as other brain regions have high levels of oxidized proteins (77) that may have accumulated as a consequence of a defect in the UPS. Finally, and of perhaps greatest importance in implicating the UPS in PD, is the finding that each of the gene mutations that have been detected in the various familial forms of PD can be linked to a failure of the UPS to clear abnormal proteins. Indeed, we have recently shown that there are defects in the UPS in patients with the sporadic form of PD and that interference with proteasomal function in model systems induces selective degeneration of dopamine neurons and inclusion bodies (240–242). Each of these will be reviewed in the ensuing text (Fig. 4.4).

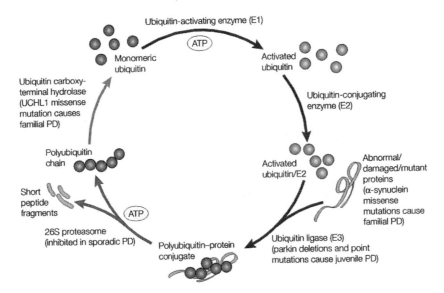

FIG. 4.4. Impairment of the ubiquitin-proteasome system in the different types of Parkinson's disease (PD). Defects in several of the components of the ubiquitin-proteasome system are associated with the development of PD. Defects in parkin may prevent ubiquitination of substrate proteins and cause them to accumulate. Defects in UCH-L1 may inhibit deubiquitination and limit the number of ubiquitin monomers available for clearing additional unwanted proteins. Defects in α-synuclein may cause the protein to misfold and resist clearance by the ubiquitin-proteasome system. Finally, defects in the structure and function of the proteasome in sporadic PD may inhibit normal protein clearance. Each of these defects has the potential to cause abnormal proteins to accumulate and interfere with normal cellular functions leading to neurodegeneration. (Adapted with permission from McNaught KStP, Olanow CW, Halliwell, et al. Failure of the ubiquitin-proteasome system in Parkinson's disease. *Nat Rev Neurosci* 2001;2:89–94.)

Abnormal Protein Clearance in Familial Forms of PD

Approximately 10% of PD cases display a familial pattern of inheritance. In recent years, several gene mutations have been discovered to cause or be associated with familial PD. As described below, each of these has the capacity to interfere with the normal degradation of proteins by way of the UPS and to cause the production and/or accumulation of abnormal and potentially cytotoxic proteins.

α-Synuclein

A large Italian-American family (the Contursi kindred) was discovered to have a PD syndrome linked to the q21-23 region of chromosome 4 (21,243). Patients had a typical levodopa-responsive clinical picture of PD, except for a slightly younger age of onset, and pathologic features that included nigral degeneration with Lewy bodies. Sequence analysis demonstrated a mutation in the gene that encodes for the protein α-synuclein consisting of a single base pair change from G to A at position 209 (G209A) with a resultant alanine to threonine substitution at position 53 (Ala53Thr) (22). A second α-synuclein mutation (Ala30Pro) was described in a German family (244). Eighty-five percent of patients who carried the mutant gene had clinical features of PD whereas the mutation was not

detected in any controls, indicating that a single mutation in the human α-synuclein gene could cause the development of a PD phenotype. These mutations were not detected in patients with sporadic PD or in most patients with other types of familial PD.

α-Synuclein is widely distributed in the brain, but little is known about its normal function. In tissue culture, α-synuclein expression leads to degeneration of cultured dopaminergic neurons and enhances their vulnerability to toxins; however, knockout mice showed no evidence of neurologic dysfunction. Transgenic mice that overexpress α-synuclein experience a progressive cytoplasmic accumulation of the protein with terminal degeneration and Lewy body–like inclusions in nigral dopaminergic neurons (245). However, they do not demonstrate behavioral abnormalities or neuronal degeneration. In contrast, overexpression of wild-type or mutant α-synuclein in *Drosophila* leads to a motor impairment (loss of the negative geotactic reflex) that responds to dopaminergic agents and degeneration of brainstem dopaminergic neurons with inclusion bodies (246). The mechanism by which α-synuclein accumulation might lead to dopaminergic neuronal death is not known. However, it is noteworthy that α-synuclein is a natively unfolded protein that tends to spontaneously aggregate and form fibrils, and that the mutant protein is more likely to misfold and resist or be unavailable for degradation by the

26/20S proteasome (247). Indeed, recent studies demonstrate that at least some types of α-synuclein are cleared through the 20S proteasome (248) and that synuclein accumulation has the potential to damage the proteasome.

UCH-L1

A missense mutation in the gene encoding for ubiquitin carboxy-terminal hydrolase-L1 (UCH-L1) (Ile93Met) has been identified in two German siblings with typical levodopa-responsive parkinsonism (25). UCH-L1 is a deubiquitinating enzyme that cleaves ubiquitin-peptide conjugates to provide monomeric ubiquitin, necessary for the degradation of additional abnormal proteins (233). Mutant UCH-L1 has reduced deubiquitinating activity in *Escherichia coli* (25), and inhibition of UCHs leads to degeneration of cultured dopamine neurons with the formation of inclusion bodies that stain for α-synuclein (240).

These observations suggest that impairment of UCH-L1 activity could lead to neuronal degeneration by reducing the availability of monomeric ubiquitin and decreasing the functional activity of the UPS. Postmortem brain tissue is not yet available from patients with this mutation, but neuronal death with inclusion bodies has been found in rodents with gracile axonal dystrophy (GAD), an autosomal recessive neurodegenerative disease associated with a mutation in UCH-L1 (249).

Parkin

A large number of deletions and point mutations in the *parkin* gene (chromosome 6q25.2-q27) have been described in young-onset (approximately age 20 years) Japanese patients with an autosomal recessive form of juvenile familial parkinsonism (AR-JP) (23,24). Patients have levodopa-responsive parkinsonism and degeneration of pigmented neurons in the SNc and locus ceruleus without Lewy bodies (250), although Lewy bodies have now been reported in a case with an older age of onset. *Parkin* mutations are a common cause of young onset parkinsonism, occurring in as many as half of the cases (26). Of particular importance is the finding that parkin is a ubiquitin ligase (E3), a protein that ubiquitinates proteins so as to prepare them for proteasomal degradation (251). In patients with AR-JP, both mRNA and protein levels for parkin are markedly reduced in the striatum and SNc (252). The specific substrates for parkin are now being determined and appear to include a glycosylated isoform of α-synuclein and the putative G-protein-coupled transmembrane polypeptide named the Pael receptor (parkin-associated endothelin-like receptor). Indeed, these are found to have accumulated without having been ubiquitinated in the substantia nigra of patients with AR-JP (253,254). The α-synuclein interacting protein synphilin-1 and the synaptic vesicle–associated protein CDCrel-1 (cell division control–related protein 1) might also be substrates for parkin, but it is not yet known if the levels of these proteins are altered in AR-JP (255,256). The

absence of Lewy bodies and early onset of symptoms in AR-JP patients may relate to the possibility that these potentially cytoprotective inclusions require the presence of ubiquitinated adducts to form insoluble aggregates.

Abnormal Protein Clearance in Toxic Forms of Parkinsonism

The role of toxins in the etiology of PD is not well defined, but parkinsonian syndromes have been described with MPTP and more recently with the widely available pesticide rotenone (18). Both agents are selective inhibitors of complex I of the mitochondrial respiratory chain and can cause a selective degeneration of nigral dopaminergic neurons. The precise mechanism as to precisely how a complex I defect causes cell death is not yet established, but the observation that cell death with rotenone is associated with protein accumulation and inclusion bodies suggests that protein accumulation plays a role (18). The direct effect of mitochondrial inhibition on proteasomal function has not yet been assessed, but impaired ATP production and oxidative stress associated with mitochondrial dysfunction could contribute to both proteasomal dissembly and dysfunction and result in impaired clearance of abnormal proteins.

Abnormal Protein Clearance in Patients with Sporadic PD

Although there is direct evidence implicating the UPS in patients with familial PD, the large majority of patients suffer from a sporadic form of the disease. A body of evidence now suggests that impaired protein handling plays a role in patients with sporadic PD as well. Autopsy studies demonstrate an increase in protein carbonyl levels in the SNc of PD patients, indicating that these proteins have undergone oxidative damage (77,257). In addition, Lewy bodies contain aggregated and poorly degraded proteins, including α-synuclein, ubiquitin, proteasomal components, and a variety of oxidized and nitrated proteins.

We have recently performed a study comparing the expression and function of proteasomes and their components in PD and control brains. We found that levels of the α subunits of the 20S proteasome are significantly reduced in the SNc in PD (241,242). A reduction in α subunits leads to impaired proteasomal assembly and function. Indeed, we also observed that in comparison to controls levels of all three of the 26S proteasome enzyme activities (chymotryptic, tryptic, and postacidic) are reduced (by approximately 40%) in the SNc of PD patients (242). These observations indicate that there is both an increase in oxidized proteins and an impairment in proteasomal function in the SNc in PD in comparison with controls. Furthermore, levels of the PA28 proteasomal activator are markedly low in the SNc of both PD patients and controls. As this regulator functions in an ATP-independent manner and has an important role in clearing oxidized proteins, this finding might account for the selective vulnerability of the SNc in PD.

The consequences of proteasomal inhibition on dopaminergic cells can be documented in laboratory studies. The proteasome inhibitor lactacystin induces a dose-dependent neuronal degeneration in PC12 cells and mesencephalic cultures, which is specific for dopamine neurons and associated with the formation of inclusion bodies in dopamine neurons that stain positively for both α-synuclein and ubiquitin (240,258). Moreover, supranigral infusion of lactacystin induces levodopa-responsive behavioral abnormalities with degeneration of dopamine neurons and inclusion bodies in rodents. Thus, proteasomal dysfunction in laboratory models can recapitulate the features of sporadic PD by inducing levodopa-responsive behavioral abnormalities and a selective loss of SNc dopamine neurons with inclusion bodies. Furthermore, we have recently shown that oxidative stress, such as exists in PD, enhances the loss of dopaminergic neurons induced by proteasome inhibitors (Olanow et al., unpublished observation). It is noteworthy that α-synuclein is an abundant component of Lewy bodies in patients with sporadic PD and colocalizes with ubiquitin, indicating that the protein has been prepared for degradation. We speculate that that α-synuclein and other proteins accumulate in sporadic PD because the proteins are not satisfactorily cleared by the UPS due to environmentally or genetically induced damage to either the UPS or to the proteins themselves.

CONCLUSION

Rare cases of PD have been identified to occur in association with gene mutations, but these do not account for the large number of sporadic cases. However, they have provided insight into the nature of the cell death process by permitting the development of model systems and studies of the proteins they regulate. Based on these studies there is convincing evidence to suggest that failure of the UPS with a consequent alteration in protein handling may represent a common link that underlies the nigrostriatal degeneration that occurs in the various forms of PD. Gene mutations in parkin and UCH-L1 could lead to protein accumulation by way of defects in enzymes required for ubiquitinating and deubiquitinating proteins. Mutations in α-synuclein could cause the protein to misfold and thereby resist clearance by the UPS. Toxins that target mitochondria might also induce degeneration by way of oxidative stress or by depriving the UPS of ATP necessary for its normal function and assembly. Finally, defects in proteasomal assembly and function have been found in the SNc in patients with sporadic PD. The basis of the proteasomal inhibition that occurs in sporadic PD is unknown. The integrity of the genes that encode critical proteins needs to be determined. It is also possible that a reduction in proteasomal function could result from damage induced by oxidizing species such as hydroxyl radical, peroxynitrite, and end products of lipid peroxidation such as HNE since markers of oxidative stress and excess nitration are present in the SNc in PD. Further, since the UPS is an energy-dependent pathway, impairment of mitochondrial function, as occurs in the SNc of some PD patients, may contribute to a reduction in the degradation of abnormal proteins. As nitrated α-synuclein and numerous other proteins are found in Lewy bodies, it is interesting to speculate on the possibility that genetic or oxidative damage to these and other widely expressed proteins might prevent their clearance and induce a sequence of events that includes protein accumulation, aggregation, and degeneration of dopaminergic neurons. The highly oxidative environment of the SNc might increase the possibility that proteins will undergo oxidative damage with consequent cross-linking, misfolding, and failure to be degraded through normal proteasomal mechanisms. Furthermore, levels of the PA28 regulator, which is important for the clearance of oxidized proteins, are low in the SNc and may deprive neurons of an important mechanism for clearing damaged proteins. Together, these changes may account for the preferential vulnerability of degeneration of SNc dopaminergic neurons in PD. Moreover, nerve cells in the brain do not turn over. This may result in the continuous accumulation of abnormal proteins over the life of an individual and account for why neurodegenerative disorders such as PD tend to be age related. We have speculated that Lewy bodies represent an attempt by the cell to segregate cytotoxic proteins and represent a neuroprotective mechanism. This may account for why approximately 10% of clinically normal individuals have incidental Lewy bodies at postmortem and may have a preclinical form of PD. This hypothesis proposes that a protein handling dysfunction is the basis of the cell death that occurs in PD and suggests that agents that prevent the formation and accumulation of cytotoxic proteins or enhance proteasomal function might be neuroprotective in PD.

REFERENCES

1. Forno S. Pathology of Parkinson's disease. In: Marsden CD, Fahn S, eds. *Movement disorders, neurology 2.* Cornwall: Butterworth Scientific, 1981:21–40.
2. Olanow CW, Watts RL, Koller WC. An algorithm (decision tree) for the management of Parkinson's disease (2001): treatment guidelines. *Neurology* 2001;56[Suppl 5]:1–88.
3. Lang AP, Lozano AE. Parkinson's disease. *N Engl J Med* 1998;339;1044–1053.
4. Olanow CW, Tatton WG. Etiology and pathogenesis of Parkinson's disease. *Ann Rev Neurosci* 1999;22:123–144.
5. Olanow CW, Jenner P, Beal F. Neurodegeneration and neuroprotection in Parkinson's disease. Supplement to *Ann Neurol* 1998;44(3).
6. Tatton WG, Olanow CW. Apoptosis in neurodegenerative dis-

ease: the role of mitochondria. *Biochim Biophys Acta* 1999; 1410:195–213.

7. Tanner CM, Ottman R, Goldman SM, et al. Parkinson disease in twins: an etiologic study. *JAMA* 1999;281:341–346.

8. Tanner CM, Langston JW. Do environmental toxins cause Parkinson's disease? A critical review. *Neurology* 1990;40:17–30.

9. Koller W, Vetere-Overfield B, Gray C, et al. Environmental risk factors in Parkinson's disease. *Neurology* 1991;40:1218–1221.

10. Hubble JP, Cao T, Hassanein RES, et al. Risk factors for Parkinson's disease. *Neurology* 1993;43:1693–1697.

11. Rajput AH, Uitti RJ, Stern W, et al. Geography, drinking water chemistry, pesticides and herbicides and the etiology of Parkinson's disease. *Can J Neurol Sci* 1987;14:414–418.

12. Baron JA. Cigarette smoking and Parkinson's disease. *Neurology* 1986;36:1490–1496.

13. Morens DM, Grandinetti A, Reed D, et al. Cigarette smoking and protection from Parkinson's disease: false association or etiologic clue? *Neurology* 1995;45:1041–1051.

14. Ross GW, Abbott RD, Petrovitch H, et al. Association of coffee and caffeine intake with the risk of Parkinson's disease. *JAMA* 2000;283:2674–2679.

15. Langston JW, Ballard PA, Tetrud JW, et al. Chronic parkinsonism in humans due to a product of meperidine analog synthesis. *Science* 1983;219:979–980.

16. Singer TP, Castagnoli N Jr, Ramsay RR, et al. Biochemical events in the development of parkinsonism induced by 1-methyl-4-phenyl-1,2,3,6-tetrahydropyridine. *J Neurochem* 1987;49:1–8.

17. Nicklas WJ, Vyas I, Heikkila RE. Inhibition of NADH-linked oxidation in brain mitochondria by 1-methyl-4-phenyl-pyridine, a metabolite of the neurotoxin 1-methyl-4-phenyl-1,2,5,6-tetrahydropyridine. *Life Sci* 1985;36:2503–2508.

18. Betarbet R, Sherer TB, MacKenzie G, et al. Chronic systemic pesticide exposure reproduces features of Parkinson's disease. *Nat Neurosci* 2000;3:1301–1306.

19. Wood N. Genetic risk factors in Parkinson's disease. *Ann Neurol* 1998;44(3 Suppl 1):S58–S62).

20. Gasser T. Genetics of Parkinson's disease. *J Neurol* 2001;248: 833–840.

21. Polymeropoulos MH, Higgins JJ, Golbe LI, et al. Mapping of a gene for Parkinson's disease to chromosome 4q21-q23. *Science* 1996;274:1197–1199.

22. Polymeropoulos MH, Lavedan C, Leroy E, et al. Mutation in the alpha-synuclein gene identified in families with Parkinson's disease. *Science* 1997;276:2045–2047.

23. Kitada T, Asakawa S, Hattori N, et al. Mutations in the parkin gene cause autosomal recessive juvenile parkinsonism. *Nature* 1998;392:605–608.

24. Hattori N, Kitada T, Matsumine H, et al. Molecular genetic analysis of a novel parkin gene in Japanese families with autosomal recessive juvenile parkinsonism: evidence for variable homozygous deletions in the parkin gene in affected individuals. *Ann Neurol* 1998;44:935–941.

25. Leroy E, Boyer R, Auburger G, et al. The ubiquitin pathway in Parkinson's disease. *Nature* 1998;395:451–452.

26. Lucking CB, Durr A, Bonifati V, et al. Association between early-onset Parkinson's disease and mutations in the parkin gene. *N Engl J Med* 2000;342:1560–1567.

27. Armstrong M, Daly AK, Cholerton S, et al. Mutant debrisoquine hydroxylation genes in Parkinson's disease. *Lancet* 1992; 339:1017–1018.

28. Kurth JH, Kurth MC, Poduslo SE, et al. Association of a monoamine oxidase B allele with Parkinson's disease. *Ann Neurol* 1993;33:368–372.

29. Hotamisligil GS, Girmen AS, Fink JS, et al. Hereditary variations in monoamine oxidase as a risk factor for Parkinson's disease. *Mov Disord* 1994;9:305–310.

30. Gasser T, Wszolek ZK, Trofatter J, et al. Genetic studies in autosomal dominant parkinsonism: evaluation of seven candidate genes. *Ann Neurol* 1994;36:387–396.

31. Ikebe S, Tanaka M, Ozawa T. Point mutations of mitochondrial genome in Parkinson's disease. *Mol Brain Res* 1995;28: 281–295.

32. Olanow CW. A radical hypothesis for neurodegeneration. *TINS* 1993;16:439–444.

33. Jenner P, Schapira AHV, Marsden CD. New insights into the cause of Parkinson's disease. *Neurology* 1992;42:2241–2250.

34. Jenner P, Olanow CW. Oxidative stress and the pathogenesis of Parkinson's disease. *Neurology* 1996;47:161–170.

35. Olanow CW, Youdim MHB. Iron and neurodegeneration: prospects for neuroprotection. In: Olanow CW, Jenner P, Youdim MHB, eds. *Neurodegeneration and neuroprotection in Parkinson's disease.* London: Academic Press, 1996:55–67.

36. Earle KM. Studies in Parkinson's disease including X-ray fluorescence spectroscopy of formalin fixed brain tissue. *J Neuropathol Exp Neurol* 1968;27:1–14.

37. Dexter DT, Wells FR, Lees AJ, et al. Increased nigral iron content and alterations in other metal ions occurring in brain in Parkinson's disease. *J Neurochem* 1989;52:1830–1836.

38. Sofic E, Riederer P, Heinsen H, et al. Increased iron (III) and total iron content in post mortem substantia nigra of parkinsonian brain. *J Neural Trans* 1988;74:199–205.

39. Hirsch EC, Brandel JP, Galle P, et al. Iron and aluminum increase in the substantia nigra of patients with Parkinson's disease: an x-ray microanalysis. *J Neurochem* 1991;56:446–451.

40. Olanow CW. Magnetic resonance imaging in parkinsonism. *Neurol Clin North Am* 1992:405–420.

41. Good P, Olanow CW, Perl DP. Neuromelanin-containing neurons of the substantia nigra accumulate iron and aluminum in Parkinson's disease: a LAMMA study. *Brain Res* 1992;593: 343–346.

42. Riederer P, Sofic E, Rausch W-D, et al. Transition metals, ferritin, glutathione, and ascorbic acid in parkinsonian brains. *J Neurochem* 1989;52:515–520.

43. Dexter DT, Carayon A, Vidailhet M, et al. Decreased ferritin levels in brain in Parkinson's disease. *J Neurochem* 1990;55: 16–20.

44. Connor JR, Snyder BS, Arosio P, et al. Quantitative analysis of isoferritins in select regions of aged, Parkinsonian, and Alzheimer diseased brains. *J Neurochem* 1995;65:717–724.

45. Ben-Schachar D, Youdim MBH. Intranigral iron injection induces behavioral and biochemical "parkinsonism" in rats. *J Neurochem* 1991;57:2133–2135.

46. Sengstock G, Olanow CW, Dunn AJ, et al. Iron induces degeneration of nigrostriatal neurons. *Brain Res Bull* 1992;28: 645–649.

47. Sengstock GJ, Olanow CW, Dunn AJ, et al. Infusion of iron into the rat substantia nigra: nigral pathology and dose-dependent loss of striatal dopaminergic markers. *J Neurosci Res* 1993; 35:67–82.

48. Sengstock G, Olanow CW, Dunn AJ, et al. Progressive changes in striatal dopaminergic markers, nigral volume, and rotational behavior following iron infusion into the rat substantia nigra. *Exp Neurol* 1994;130:82–94.

49. Temlett JA, Landsberg JP, Watt F, et al. Increased iron in the substantia nigra compacta of the MPTP-lesioned hemiparkinsonian African Green monkey: evidence from proton microprobe elemental microanalysis. *J Neurochem* 1994;62:134–146.

50. Oestreicher E, Sengstock GJ, Riederer P, et al. Degeneration of nigrostriatal dopaminergic neurons increases iron within the substantia nigra: a histochemical and neurochemical study. *Brain Res* 1994;660: 8–18.

51. Dexter DT, Sian J, Rose S, et al. Indices of oxidative stress and

mitochondrial function in individuals with incidental Lewy body disease. *Ann Neurol* 1994;35:38–44.

52. Faucheux BA, Hauw JJ, Agid Y, et al. The density of ^{125}I-transferrin binding sites on perikara of melanized neurons of the substantia nigra is decreased in Parkinson's disease. *Brain Res* 1997; 749:170–174.

53. Faucheux B, Nillesse N, Damier P, et al. Expression of lactoferrin receptors is increased in the mesencephalon of patients with Parkinson's disease. *Proc Natl Acad Sci USA* 1995;92: 9603–9607.

54. Dexter DT, Ward RJ, Wells FR, et al. α-Tocopherol levels in brain are not altered in Parkinson's disease. *Ann Neurol* 1992; 32:591–593.

55. Sian J, Dexter DT, Lees AJ, et al. Glutathione-related enzymes in brain in Parkinson's disease. *Ann Neurol* 1994;36:356–361.

56. Saggu H, Cooksey J, Dexter DT, et al. A selective increase in particulate superoxide dismutase activity in parkinsonian substantia nigra. *J Neurochem* 1989;53:692–697.

57. Yoshida E, Mokuno K, Aoki S-I, et al. Cerebrospinal fluid levels of superoxide dismutases in neurological diseases detected by sensitive enzyme immunoassays. *J Neurol Sci* 1994;124:25–31.

58. Przedborski S, Kostivc V, Jackson-Lewis V, et al. Transgenic mice with increased Cu/Zn-superoxide dismutase activity are resistant to MPTP-induced neurotoxicity. *J Neurosci* 1992;12: 1658–1667.

59. Perry TL, Godin DV, Hansen S. Parkinson's disease: a disorder due to nigral glutathione deficiency. *Neurosci Lett* 1982;33: 305–310.

60. Sofic E, Lange KW, Jellinger K, et al. Reduced and oxidized glutathione in the substantia nigra of patients with Parkinson's disease. *Neurosci Lett* 1992;142:128–130.

61. Sian J, Dexter DT, Lees AJ, et al. Alterations in glutathione levels in Parkinson's disease and other neurodegenerative disorders affecting basal ganglia. *Ann Neurol* 1994;36:348–355.

62. DeLeve LD, Kaplowitz N. Glutathione metabolism and its role in hepatotoxicity. *Pharmacol Ther* 1991;52:287–305.

63. Mithöfer K, Sandy MS, Smith MT, et al. Mitochondrial poisons cause depletion of reduced glutathione in isolated hepatocytes. *Arch Biochem Biophys* 1992;295:132–136.

64. Spencer JPE, Jenner P, Halliwell B. Superoxide-dependent depletion of reduced glutathione by L-DOPA and dopamine: relevance to Parkinson's disease. *Neuroreport* 1995;6:1480–1484.

65. Mytilineou C, Leonardi EK, Radcliffe P, et al. Deprenyl and desmethylselegiline protect mesencephalic neurons from toxicity induced by glutathione depletion. *J Pharmacol Exp Ther* 1998;284:700–706.

66. Mytilineou C, Kokotos Leonardi E, Kramer BC, et al. Glial cells mediate toxicity in glutathione depleted mesencephalic cultures. *J Neurochem* 1999;73:112–119.

66. Toffa S, Kunikowska GM, Zeng B-Y, et al. Chronic glutathione depletion in rat brain does not cause nigrostriatal pathway degeneration. *J Neural Transm [PDSect]* 1997;104:67–75.

67. Pileblad E, Magnusson T, Fornstedt B. Reduction of brain glutathione by L-buthionine sulfoximine potentiates the dopamine-depleting action of 6-hydroxydopamine in rat striatum. *J Neurochem* 1989;52:978–980.

68. Wüllner U, Löschmann P-A, Schulz JB, et al. Glutathione depletion potentiates MPTP and MPP+ toxicity in nigral dopaminergic neurones. *Neuroreport* 1996;7:921–923.

69. Pearce RKB, Owen A, Daniel S, et al. Alterations in the distribution of glutathione in the substantia nigra in Parkinson's disease. *J Neural Transm* 1991;104:661–677.

70. Dexter DT, Carter CJ, Wells FR, et al. Basal lipid peroxidation in substantia nigra is increased in Parkinson's disease. *J Neurochem* 1989;52:381–389.

71. Dexter DT, Holley AE, Flitter WD, et al. Increased levels of lipid hydroperoxides in the parkinsonian substantia nigra: an HPLC and ESR study. *Mov Disord* 1994;9:92–97.

72. Yoritaka A, Hattori N, Uchida K, et al. Immunohistochemical detection of 4-hydroxynonenal protein adducts in Parkinson's disease. *Proc Natl Acad Sci USA* 1996;93:2696–2713.

73. Liu W, Kato M, Akhand AA, et al. 4-hydroxynonenal induces a cellular redox status-related activation of the caspase cascade for apoptotic cell death. *J Cell Sci* 2000;113:635–641.

74. Camandola S, Poli G, Mattson MP. The lipid peroxidation product 4-hydroxy-2,3-nonenal inhibits constitutive and inducible activity of nuclear factor kappa B in neurons. *Mol Brain Res* 2000;85:53–60.

75. Picklo MJ, Amarnath V, McIntyre JO, et al. 4-Hydroxy-2(E)-nonenal inhibits CNS mitochondrial respiration at multiple sites. *J Neurochem* 1999;72:1617–1624.

76. Okada K, Wangpoengtrakul C, Osawa T, et al. 4-Hydroxy-2-nonenal-mediated impairment of intracellular proteolysis during oxidative stress: identification of proteasomes as target molecules. *J Biol Chem* 1999;274:23787–23793.

77. Alam ZI, Daniel SE, Lees AJ, et al. A generalized increase in protein carbonyls in the brain in Parkinson's but not incidental Lewy body disease. *J Neurochem* 1997;69:1326–1329.

78. Sanchez-Ramos J, Overvik E, Ames BN. A marker of oxyradical-mediated DNA damage (8-hydroxy-2′-deoxyguanosine) is increased in nigro-striatum of Parkinson's disease brain. *Neurodegeneration* 1994;3:197–204.

79. Alam ZI, Jenner A, Daniel SA, et al. Oxidative DNA damage in the parkinsonian brain: a selective increase in 8-hydroxyguanine in substantia nigra? *J Neurochem* 1997;69:1196–1203.

80. Shimura-Miura H, Hattori N, Kang D, et al. Increased 8-oxo-dGTPase in the mitochondria of substantia nigral neurons in Parkinson's disease. *Ann Neurol* 1999;46:920–924.

81. Mytilineou C, Han S-K, Cohen G. Toxic and protective effects of L-DOPA on mesencephalic cell cultures. *J Neurochem* 1993; 61:1470–1478.

82. Walkinshaw G, Waters CM. Induction of apoptosis in catecholaminergic PC12 cells by L-DOPA: implications for the treatment of Parkinson's disease. *J Clin Invest* 1995;95:2458–2464.

83. Kramer BC, Yabut JA, Cheong J, et al. Lipopolysaccharide prevents cell death caused by glutathione depletion; possible mechanisms of protection. *Neuroscience* 2002 (in press).

84. Spina MB, Cohen G. Exposure of striatal synaptosomes to L-dopa elevates levels of oxidized glutathione. *J Pharmacol Exp Ther* 1988;247:502–507.

85. Spencer Smith T, Parker WD Jr, Bennett JP. L-DOPA increases nigral production of hydroxyl radicals in vivo: potential L-DOPA toxicity? *Neuroreport* 1994;5:1009–1011.

86. Spencer JPE, Jenner A, Aruoma OI, et al. Intense oxidative DNA damage promoted by L-DOPA and its metabolites: implications for neurodegenerative disease. *FEBS Lett* 1994;353:246–250.

87. Przedborski S, Jackson-Lewis V, Muthane U, et al. Chronic levodopa administration alters cerebral mitochondrial respiratory chain activity. *Ann Neurol* 1993;34:715–723.

88. Blunt SB, Jenner P, Marsden CD. Suppressive effect of L-dopa on dopamine cells remaining in the ventral tegmental area of rats previously exposed to the neurotoxin 6-hydroxydopamine. *Mov Disord* 1993;8:129–133.

89. Ogawa N, Asanuma M, Kondo Y, et al. Differential effects of chronic L-DOPA treatment on lipid peroxidation in the mouse brain with or without pretreatment with 6-hydroxydopamine. *Neurosci Lett* 1994;171:55–58.

90. Hefti F, Melamed E, Bhawan J, et al. Long term administration of L-dopa does not damage dopaminergic neurons in the mouse. *Neurology* 1981;31:1194–1195.

91. Perry TL, Young VW, Ito M, et al. Nigrostriatal dopaminergic neurons remain undamaged in rats given high doses of L-dopa and carbidopa chronically. *J Neurochem* 1984;43:990–993.

92. Quinn N, Parkes JD, Janota I, et al. Preservation of substantia nigra neurons and locus ceruleus in patients receiving levodopa (2 gm) plus decarboxylase inhibitor over a four year period. *Mov Disord* 1986;1:65–68.

93. Pearce RKB, et al. L-Dopa and dyskinesias in normal monkeys. *Mov Disord* 1999;14[Suppl 1]:9–12.

94. Murer MG, Dziewczapolski G, Menalled LB, et al. Chronic levodopa is not toxic for remaining dopamine neurons, but instead promotes their recovery, in rats with moderate nigrostriatal lesions. *Ann Neurol* 1998;43:561–575.

95. Mytilineou C, Walker R, JnoBaptiste R, et al. Levodopa is toxic to dopamine neurons in an *in vitro* but not an *in vivo* model of oxidative stress. (Submitted.)

96. Camp DM, Loeffler DA, LeWitt PA. L-DOPA does not enhance hydroxyl radical formation in the nigrostriatal dopamine system of rats with a unilateral 6-hydroxydopamine lesion. *J Neurochem* 2000;74:1229–1240.

97. Agid Y, Ahlskog E, Albanese A, et al. Levodopa in the treatment of Parkinson's disease: a consensus meeting. *Mov Disord* 1999; 14:911–913.

98. Schapira AHV, Cooper JM, Dexter D, et al. Mitochondrial complex I deficiency in Parkinson's disease. *J Neurochem* 1990; 54:823–827.

99. Mizuno Y, Ohta S, Tanaka M, et al. Deficiencies in complex I subunits of the respiratory chain in Parkinson's disease. *Biochem Biophys Res Commun* 1989;163:1450–1455.

100. Schapira AHV. Evidence for mitochondrial dysfunction in Parkinson's disease: a critical appraisal. *Mov Disord* 1994;9: 125–138.

101. DiMauro S. Mitochondrial involvement in Parkinson's disease: the controversy continues. *Neurology* 1993;43:2170–2172.

102. Lestienne P, Nelson J, Riederer P, et al. Normal mitochondrial genome in brain from patients with Parkinson's disease and complex I defect. *J Neurochem* 1990;55:1810–1812.

103. Swerdlow RH, Parks JK, Miller SW, et al. Origin and functional consequences of the complex I defect in Parkinson's disease. *Ann Neurol* 1996;40:663–671.

104. Veech GA, Dennis J, Keeney PM, et al. Disrupted mitochondrial electron transport function increases expression of anti-apoptotic bcl-2 and bcl-X(L) proteins in SH-SY5Y neuroblastoma and in Parkinson disease cybrid cells through oxidative stress. *J Neurosci Res* 2000;61:693–700.

105. Cassarino DS, Bennett JP Jr. An evaluation of the role of mitochondria in neurodegenerative diseases: mitochondrial mutations and oxidative pathology, protective nuclear responses, and cell death in neurodegeneration. *Brain Res* 1999;29:1–25.

106. Mytilineou C, Werner P, Molinari S, et al. Impaired oxidative decarboxylation of pyruvate in fibroblasts from patients with Parkinson's disease. *J Neural Transm* 1994;8:223–228.

107. Scotcher KP, Irwin I, DeLanney LE, et al. Effects of 1-methyl-4-phenyl-1,2,3,6-tetrahydropyridine and 1-methyl-4-phenyl-pyridinium ion on ATP levels of mouse synaptosomes. *J Neurochem* 1990;54:1295–1301.

108. Mizuno Y, Matuda S, Yoshino H, et al. An immunohistochemical study on α-ketoglutarate dehydrogenase complex in Parkinson's disease. *Ann Neurol* 1994;35:204–210.

109. Mizuno Y, Saitoh T, Sone N. Inhibition of mitochondrial alpha-ketoglutarate dehydrogenase by 1-methyl-4-phenylpyridinium ion. *Biochem Biophys Res Commun* 1987;143:971–976.

110. Lotharius J, O'Malley KL. The parkinsonism-inducing drug 1-methyl-4-phenylpyridinium triggers intracellular dopamine oxidation: a novel mechanism of toxicity. *J Biol Chem* 2000; 275:38581–38588.

111. Nakamura K, Bindokas VP, Marks JD, et al. The selective toxicity of 1-methyl-4-phenylpyridinium to dopaminergic neurons: the role of mitochondrial complex I and reactive oxygen species revisited. *Mol Pharmol* 2000;58:271–278.

112. Choi D. Glutamate neurotoxicity and diseases of the nervous system. *Neuron* 1988;1:623–634.

113. Beal F. Excitoxicity and nitric oxide in Parkinson's disease pathogenesis. *Ann Neurol* 1998;44:110–114.

114. Nicotera P, Orrenius S. Calcium ions in necrotic and apoptotic cell death. In: Olanow CW, Jenner P, Youdim M, eds. *Neurodegeneration and neuroprotection in Parkinson's disease.* London: Academic Press, 1996:143–158.

115. DeLong MR. Primate models of movement disorders of basal ganglia origin. *TINS* 1990;13:281–289.

116. Rodriguez MC, Obeso JA, Olanow CW. Subthalamic nucleus-mediated excitotoxicity. In: Parkinson's disease: a target for neuroprotection. *Ann Neurol* 1998;44(3):175–188.

117. Piallat B, Benazzouz A, Benabid AL. Subthalamic nucleus lesion on rats prevents dopaminergic nigral neuron degeneration after striatal 6-OHDA injection: behavioural and immunohistochemical studies. *Eur J Neurosci* 1996;8:1408–1414.

118. Turski L, Bressler K, Rottig KJ, et al. Protection of substantia nigra from MPP+ neurotoxicity by NMDA antagonists. *Nature* 1991;349:414–418.

119. Beal MF. Does impairment of energy metabolism result in excitotoxic neuronal death in neurodegenerative illnesses? *Ann Neurol* 1992;31:119–130.

120. Greene JG, Greenmayre JT. Bioenergetics and excitotoxicity: the weak excitotoxic hypothesis. In: Olanow CW, Jenner P, Youdim M, eds. *Neurodegeneration and neuroprotection in Parkinson's disease.* London: Academic Press, 1996:125–142.

121. Dawson VL, Dawson TM, London ED, et al. Nitric oxide mediates glutamate neurotoxicity in primary cortical cultures. *Proc Natl Acad Sci USA* 1991;88:6368–6371.

122. Beckman JS, Beckman TW, Chen J, et al. Apparent hydroxyl radical production by peroxynitrite: implications for endothelial injury from nitric oxide and superoxide. *Proc Natl Acad Sci USA* 1990;87:1620–1624.

123. Reif DW, Simmons RD. Nitric oxide mediates iron release from ferritin. *Arch Biochem Biophys* 1990;283:537–541.

124. Bolanos JP, Heales SJR, Peuchen S, et al. Nitric oxide-mediated mitochondrial damage: a potential neuroprotective role for glutathione. *FRBM* 1996;21:995–1001.

125. Clementi E, Brown GC, Feelisch M, et al. Persistent inhibition of cell respiration by nitric oxide: crucial role of S-nitrosylation of mitochondrial complex I and protective action of glutathione. *Proc Natl Acad Sci USA* 1998;95:7631–7636.

126. Barker JE, Heales SJ, Cassidy A, et al. Depletion of brain glutathione results in a decrease of glutathione reductase activity: an enzyme susceptible to oxidative damage. *Brain Res* 1996; 716:118–122.

127. Liberatore GT, Jackson-Lewis V, Vukosavic S, et al. Inducible nitric oxide synthase stimulates dopaminergic neurodegeneration in the MPTP model of Parkinson's disease. *Nat Med* 1999;5:1403–1409.

128. Schulz JB, Matthews RT, Muqit MMK, et al. Inhibition of neuronal nitric oxide synthase by 7-nitroindazole protects against MPTP-induced neurotoxicity in mice. *J Neurochem* 1995;64: 936–939.

129. Przedborski S, Jackson Lewis V, Yokoyama R, et al. Role of neuronal oxide in 1-methyl-4-phenyl-1,2,3,6-tetrahydropyridine (MPTP)-induced dopaminergic neurotoxicity. *Proc Natl Acad Sci USA* 1996;93:4565–4654.

130. Hantrave P, Brouillet E, Ferrante R, et al. Inhibition of neuronal nitric oxide synthase prevents MPTP-induced parkinsonism in baboons. *Nat Med* 1996;2:1017–1021.

131. MacKenzie GM, Jackson MJ, Jenner P, et al. Nitric oxide synthase inhibition and MPTP-induced toxicity in the common marmoset. *Synapse* 1997;26:301–316.

132. Kelly PAT, Ritchie IM, Arbuthnott GW. Inhibition of neuronal nitric oxide synthase by 7-nitroindazole: effects upon local cerebral blood flow and glucose use in the rat. *J Cerebral Blood Flow Metab* 1995;12:311–317.

133. Schulz JB, Matthews RT, Miratul M, et al. Inhibition of neuronal nitric oxide synthase by 7-nitroindazole protects against MPTP-induced neurotoxicity in mice. *J Neurochem* 1995;64:936–939.

134. Castagnoli K, Palmer S, Anderson A, et al. The neural nitric oxide synthase inhibitor 7-nitroindazole also inhibits the monoamine oxidase-B-catalyzed oxidation of 1-methyl-4-phenyl-1,2,3,6-tetrahydropyridine. *Chem Res Toxicol* 1997;10:364–368.

135. Ischiropoulos H, Zhu L, Chen J, et al. Peroxynitrite-mediated tyrosine nitration catalyzed by superoxide dismutase. *Arch Biochem Biophys* 1992;298:431–437.

136. Pennathur S, Jackson-Lewis V, Przedborski S, et al. Mass spectrometric quantification of 3-nitrotyrosine, ortho-tyrosine, and o,o′-dityrosine in brain tissue of 1-methyl-4-phenyl-1,2,3,6-tetrahydropyridine-treated mice, a model of oxidative stress in Parkinson's disease. *J Biol Chem* 1999;274:34621–34628.

137. Ara J, Przedborski S, Naini AB, et al. Inactivation of tyrosine hydroxylase by nitration following exposure to peroxynitrite and 1-methyl-4-phenyl-1,2,3,6-tetrahydropyridine (MPTP). *Proc Natl Acad Sci USA* 1998;95:7659–7663.

138. Ferger B, Themann C, Rose S, et al. 6-hydroxydopamine increases the hydroxylation and nitration of phenylalanine in vivo: implication of peroxynitrite formation. *J Neurochem* 2001;78:509–514.

139. Ferrante RJ, Hantraye P, Brouillet E, et al. Increased nitrotyrosine immunoreactivity in substantia nigra neurons in MPTP treated baboons is blocked by inhibition of neuronal nitricoxide synthase. *Brain Res* 1999;823:177–182.

140. Good PF, Werner P, Hsu A, et al. Evidence for neuronal oxidative damage in Alzheimer's disease. *Am J Pathol* 1996;149:21–28.

141. Good PF, Hsu A, Werner P, et al. Protein nitration in Parkinson's disease. *J Neuropath Exp Neurol* 1998;57:338–342.

142. Mihm MJ, Schanbacher BL, Wallace BL, et al. Free 3-nitrotyrosine causes striatal neurodegeneration in vivo. *J Neurosci* 2001;21:RC149.

143. Souza JM, Choi I, Chen Q, et al. Proteolytic degradation of tyrosine nitrated proteins. *Arch Biochem Biophys* 2000;380:360–366.

144. Byun J, Henderson JP, Mueller DM, et al. 8-Nitro-2′-deoxyguanosine, a specific marker of oxidation by reactive nitrogen species, is generated by the myeloperoxidase-hydrogen peroxide-nitrite system of activated human phagocytes. *Biochemistry* 1999;38:2590–2600.

145. Szabo C, Zingarelli B, O'Connor M, et al. DNA strand breakage, activation of poly(ADP-ribose) synthetase, and cellular energy depletion are involved in the cytotoxicity of macrophages and smooth muscle cells exposed to peroxynitrite. *Proc Natl Acad Sci USA* 1996;93:1753–1758.

146. Ying W, Sevigny MB, Chen Y, et al. (ADP-ribose) glycohydrolase mediates oxidative and excitotoxic neuronal death. *Proc Natl Acad Sci USA* 2001;98:12227–12232.

147. Cosi C, Colpaert F, Koek W, et al. Poly(ADP-ribose) polymerase inhibitors protect against MPTP-induced depletions of striatal dopamine and cortical noradrenaline in C57B1/6 mice. *Brain Res* 1996;729:264–269.

148. Mandir AS, Przedborski S, Jackson-Lewis V, et al. Poly(ADP-ribose) polymerase activation mediates 1-methyl-4-phenyl-1, 2,3,6-tetrahydropyridine (MPTP)-induced parkinsonism. *Proc Natl Acad Sci USA* 1999;96:5774–5779.

149. Hirsch EC, Hunot S, Damier P, et al. Glial cells and inflammation in Parkinson's disease: a role in neurodegeneration. *Ann Neurol* 1998:S115–S120.

150. McGeer PL, Itagaki S, McGeer EG. Expression of the histocompatibility glycoprotein HLA-DR in neurological disease. *Acta Neuropathol* 1988;76:550–557.

151. Mogi M, Harada M, Kondo T, et al. Interleukin-2 but not basic fibroblast growth factor is elevated in parkinsonian brain: short communication. *J Neural Trans* 1996;103:1077–1081.

152. Mogi M, Harada M, Narabayashi H, et al. Interleukin (IL)-1 beta, IL-2, IL-4, IL-6 and transforming growth factor-alpha levels are elevated in ventricular cerebrospinal fluid in juvenile parkinsonism and Parkinson's disease. *Neurosci. Lett* 1996;211:13–16.

153. Hunot S, Dugas N, Faucheux B, et al. FcepsilonRII/CD23 is expressed in Parkinson's disease and induces, in vitro, production of nitric oxide and tumor necrosis factor-alpha inglial cells. *J Neurosci* 1999;19:3440–3447.

154. Hunot S, Boissiere F, Faucheux B, et al. Nitric oxide synthase and neuronal vulnerability in Parkinson's disease. *Neuroscience* 1996;72:355–363.

155. Knott C, Stern G, Wilkin GP. Inflammatory regulators in Parkinson's disease: iNOS, lipocortin-1, and cyclooxygenases-1 and -2. *Mol Cell Neurosci* 2000;16:724–739.

156. Hunot S, Brugg B, Ricard D, et al. Nuclear translocation of NFκB is increased in dopaminergic neurons of patients with Parkinson's disease. *Proc Natl Acad Sci* 1997;94:7531–7536.

157. Crawford GD, Le W-D, Smith RG, et al. A novel N18TG2 x mesencephalon cell hybrid expresses properties that suggest a dopaminergic cell line of substantia nigra origin. *J Neurosci* 1992;12:3392–3398.

158. Przedborski S, Vila M. MPTP: a review of its mechanisms of neurotoxicity. *Clin Neurosci Res* 2001;1:407–418.

158a. Aubin N, Curet O, Deffois A, et al. Aspirin and salicylate protect against MPTP-induced dopamine depletion in mice. *J Neurochem* 1998;71:1635–1642.

159. Teismann P, Ferger B. Inhibition of the cyclooxygenase isoenzymes COX-1 and COX-2 provide neuroprotection in the MPTP-mouse model of Parkinson's disease. *Synapse* 2001;39:167–174.

160. McNaught KStP, Jenner P. Dysfunction of rat forebrain astrocytes in culture alters cytokine and neurotrophic factor release. *Neurosci Lett* 2000;285:61–65.

161. McNaught KStP, Jenner P. Extracellular accumulation of nitric oxide, hydrogen peroxide, and glutamate in astrocytic cultures following glutathione depletion, complex I inhibition, and/or lipopolysaccharide-induced activation. *Biochem Pharmacol* 2000;60:979–988.

162. Park LC, Zhang H, Sheu KF, et al. Metabolic impairment induces oxidative stress, compromises inflammatory responses, and inactivates a key mitochondrial enzyme in microglia. *J Neurochem* 1999;72:1948–1958.

163. Lin WW, Doherty DH, Lile JD, et al. GDNF: a glial cell-line derived neurotrophic factor for midbrain dopaminergic neurons. *Science* 1993;260:1130–1132.

164. Hyman C, Hofer M, Barde Y-A, et al. BDNF is a neurotrophic factor for dopaminergic neurons of the substantia nigra. *Nature* 1991;350:230–232.

165. Tomac A, Lindqvist E, Lin LFH, et al. Protection and repair of the nigrostriatal dopaminergic system by GDNF in vivo. *Nature* 1995;373:335–339.

166. Tsukahara T, Takeda M, Shimohama S, et al. Effects of brain-derived neurotrophic factor on 1-methyl-4-phenyl-1,2,3,6-tetrahydropyridine-induced parkinsonism in monkeys. *Neurosurgery* 1995;37:733–739.

167. Kordower J, Emborg ME, Bloch J, et al. Neurodegeneration prevented by lentiviral vector delivery of GDNF in primate models of Parkinson's disease. *Science* 2000;290:767–773.

168. Hunot S, Bernard V, Faucheux B, et al. Glial cell line-derived neurotrophic factor (GDNF) gene expression in the human brain: a post mortem in situ hybridization study with special reference to Parkinson's disease. *J Neural Trans* 1996;103: 1043–1052.

169. McNaught KStP, Jenner P. Altered glial function causes death and increases neuronal susceptibility to 1-methyl-4-phenylpyridinium- and 6-hydroxydopamine-induced toxicity in astrocytic/ventral mesencephalic co-cultures. *J Neurochem* 1999;73: 2469–2476.

170. Le W-D, Rowe D, Xie W, et al. Microglial activation and dopaminergic cell injury: an in vitro model relevant to Parkinson's disease. *J Neurosci* 2001;21:8447–8455.

171. Castano A, Herrera AJ, Cano J, et al. Lipopolysaccharide intranigral injection induces inflammatory reaction and damage in nigrostriatal dopaminergic system. *J Neurochem* 1998;70: 1584–1592.

172. Yamada K, Komori Y, Tanaka T, et al. Brain dysfunction associated with an induction of nitric oxide synthase following an intracerebral injection of lipopolysaccharide in rats. *Neuroscience* 1999;88:281–294.

173. Possel H, Noack H, Putzke J, et al. Selective upregulation of inducible nitric oxide synthase (iNOS) by lipopolysaccharide (LPS) and cytokines in microglia: in vitro and in vivo studies. *Glia* 2000;32:51–59.

174. Ibi M, Sawada H, Kume T, et al. Depletion of intracellular glutathione increases susceptibility to nitric oxide in mesencephalic dopaminergic neurons. *J Neurochem* 1999;73:1696–1703.

175. Canals S, Casarejos MJ, de Bernardo S, et al. Glutathione depletion switches nitric oxide neurotrophic effects to cell death in midbrain cultures: implications for Parkinson's disease. *J Neurochem* 2001;79:1183–1195.

176. Chen Y, Vartiainen NE, Ying W, et al. Astrocytes protect neurons from nitric oxide toxicity by a glutathione-dependent mechanism. *J Neurochem* 2001;77:1601–1610.

177. Kerr JF, Wyllie AH, Currie AR. Apoptosis: a basic biological phenomenon with wide-ranging implications in tissue kinetics. *Br J Cancer* 1972;26:239–257.

178. Tatton NA, Kish SJ. In situ detection of apoptotic nuclei in the substantia nigra compacta of 1-methyl-4-phenyl-1,2,3,6-tetrahydropyridine-treated mice using terminal deoxynucleotidyl transferase labelling and acridine orange staining. *Neuroscience* 1997;77:1037–1048.

179. Walkinshaw G, Waters CM. Induction of apoptosis in catecholaminergic PC12 cells by L-DOPA: implications for the treatment of Parkinson's disease. *J Clin Invest* 1995;95: 2458–2464.

180. Ziv I, Melamed E, Nardi N, et al. Dopamine induces apoptosis-like cell death in cultured chick sympathetic neurons. *Neurosci Lett* 1994;170:136–140.

181. Farinelli SE, Greene LA. Cell cycle blockers mimosine, ciclopirox, and deferoxamine prevent the death of PC12 cells and postmitotic sympathetic neurons after removal of trophic support. *J Neurosci* 1996;16:1150–1162.

182. Mitchell IJ, Lawson S, Moser B, et al. Glutamate-induced apoptosis results in a loss of striatal neurons in the parkinsonian rat. *Neuroscience* 1994;63:1–5.

183. Portera-Cailliau C, Hedreen JC, Price DL, et al. Evidence for apoptotic cell death in Huntington disease and excitotoxic animal models. *J Neurosci* 1995;15:3775–3787.

184. Dipasquale B, Marini AM, Youle RJ. Apoptosis and DNA degradation induced by 1-methyl-4-phenylpyridinium in neurons. *Biochem Biophys Res Commun* 1991;181:1442–1448.

185. Mutoh T, Tokuda A, Marini AM, et al. 1-Methyl-4-phenylpyridinum kills differentiated PC12 cells with a concomitant change in protein phosphorylation. *Brain Res* 1994;661:51–55.

186. Hartley A, Stone JM, Heron C, et al. Complex I inhibitors induce dose-dependent apoptosis in PC12 cells: relevance to Parkinson's disease. *J Neurochem* 1994;63:1987–1990.

187. Slater AF, Nobel CS, Orrenius S. The role of intracellular oxidants in apoptosis. *Biochim Biophys Acta* 1995;1271:59–62.

188. Mukherjee SK, Yasharel R, Klaidman LK, et al. Apoptosis and DNA fragmentation as induced by tertiary butylhydroperoxide in the brain. *Brain Res Bull* 1995;38:595–604.

189. Mytilineou C, Leonardi EK, Radcliffe P, et al. Deprenyl and desmethylselegiline protect mesencephalic neurons from toxicity induced by glutathione depletion. *J Pharmacol Exp Ther* 1998;284:700–706.

190. Bonfoco E, Krainc D, Ankarcrona M, et al. Apoptosis and necrosis: two distinct events induced, respectively, by mild and intense insults with N-methyl-D-aspartate or nitric oxide/superoxide in cortical cell cultures. *Proc Natl Acad Sci USA* 1995;92:7162–7166.

191. Leist M, Jaattela M. Four deaths and a funeral: from caspases to alternative mechanisms. *Nat Rev Mol Cell Biol* 2001;2: 589–598.

192. Batistatou A, Greene LA. Internucleosomal DNA cleavage and neuronal cell survival/death. *J Cell Biol* 1993;122:523–532.

193. Migheli A, Cavalla P, Marino S, et al. A study of apoptosis in normal and pathologic nervous tissue after in situ end-labeling of DNA strand breaks. *J Neuropathol Exp Neurol* 1994;53: 606–616.

194. Anderson AJ, Su JH, Cotman CW. DNA damage and apoptosis in Alzheimer's disease: colocalization with c-Jun immunoreactivity, relationship to brain area and the effect of postmortem delay. *J Neurosci* 1996;16:1710–1719.

195. Lassmann H, Bancher C, Breitschopf H, et al. Cell death in Alzheimer's disease evaluated by DNA fragmentation in situ. *Acta Neuropathol Berl* 1995;89:35–41.

196. Dragunow M, Faull RL, Lawlor P, et al. In situ evidence for DNA fragmentation in Huntington's disease striatum and Alzheimer's disease temporal lobes. *Neuroreport* 1995;6: 1053–1057.

197. Thomas LB, Gates DJ, Richfield EK, et al. DNA end labeling (TUNEL) in Huntington's disease and other neuropathological conditions. *Exp Neurol* 1995;133:265–272.

198. Yoshiyama Y, Yamada T, Asanuma K, et al. Apoptosis related antigen, Le(Y) and nick-end labeling are positive in spinal motor neurons in amyotrophic lateral sclerosis. *Acta Neuropathol Berl* 1994;88:207–211.

199. Petito CK, Roberts B. Evidence of apoptotic cell death in HIV encephalitis. *Am J Pathol* 1995;146:1121–1130.

200. Mochizuki HK, et al. Histochemical detection of apoptosis in Parkinson's disease. *J Neurological Sci* 1996;137:120–123.

201. Anglade P, Vyas S, Javoy-Agid F, et al. Apoptosis and autophagy in nigral neurons of patients with Parkinson's disease. *Histol Histopathol* 1997;12:25–31.

202. Kingsbury AE, Mardsen CD, Foster OJ. DNA fragmentation in human substantia nigra: apoptosis or perimortem effect? *Mov Disord* 1998;13:877–884.

203. Kosel S, Egensperger R, von Eitzen U. On the question of apoptosis in the parkinsonian substantia nigra. *Acta Neuropathologica* 1997;93:105–108.

204. Banati RB, Daniel SE, Blunt SB. Glial pathology but absence of apoptotic nigral neurons in long-standing Parkinson's disease. *Mov Disord* 1998;13:221–227.

205. Charriaut-Mariangue C, Ben-Ari Y. A cautionary note on the use of the TUNEL stain to determine apoptosis. *Neuro Report* 1995;7:61–64.

206. Petito CK, Roberts B. Effect of postmortem interval on in situ end-labelling of DNA oligonucleosomes. *J Neuropathol Exp Neurol* 1995;54:761–765.

207. Tatton NA, Rideout HJ. Confocal microscopy as a tool to examine DNA fragmentation, chromatin condensation and other apoptotic changes in Parkinson's disease. *Parkinsonism and Rel Disord* 1999;5:179–186.

208. Grosse F, Manns A. Terminal deoxyribonucleotidyl transferase (EC 2.7.7.31). In: Burrell, ed. *Methods in molecular biology.* Totowa, NJ: Humana Press, 1993:95–105.

209. Kass GEN, Eriksson JE, Weiss M, et al. Chromatin condensation during apoptosis requires ATP. *Biochem J* 1996;318:749–752.

210. Susin SA, et al. Two distinct pathways leading to nuclear apoptosis. *J Exp Med* 2000;192:571–580.

211. Tatton NA, Maclean-Fraser A, Tatton WG, et al. A fluorescent double-labeling method to detect and confirm apoptotic nuclei in Parkinson's disease. *Ann Neurol* 1998;44[3 Suppl 1]:S142–S148.

212. Tatton NA. Increased caspase 3 and Bax immunoreactivity accompany nuclear GAPDH translocation and neuronal apoptosis in Parkinson's disease. *Exp Neurol* 2000;166:29–43.

213. Bredesen DE. Neural apoptosis. *Ann Neurol* 1995;38:839–851.

214. Kroemer G, Petit P, Xamzami N, et al. The biochemistry of programmed cell death. *FASEB* 1995;9:1277–1287.

215. Vayssiere JL, Petit PX, Risler Y, et al. Commitment to apoptosis is associated with changes in mitochondrial biogenesis and activity in cell lines conditionally immortalized with simian virus 40. *Proc Natl Acad Sci USA* 1994;91:11752–11756.

216. Petit PX, Lecoeur H, Zorn E, et al. Alterations in mitochondrial structure and function are early events of dexamethasone-induced thymocyte apoptosis. *J Cell Biol* 1995;130:157–167.

217. Zamzami N, Marchetti P, Castedo M, et al. Sequential reduction of mitochondrial transmembrane potential and generation of reactive oxygen species in early programmed cell death. *J Exp Med* 1995;182:367–377.

218. Zamzami N, Marchetti P, Castedo M, et al. Inhibitors of permeability transition interfere with the disruption of mitochondrial transmembrane potential during apoptosis. *FEBS Lett* 1996;384:53–57.

219. Newmeyer DD, Farschon DM, Reed JC. Cell-free apoptosis in Xenopus egg extracts: inhibition by Bcl-2 and requirement for an organelle fraction enriched in mitochondria [see comments]. *Cell* 1994;79:353–364.

220. Liu XS, Kim CN, Yang J, et al. Induction of apoptotic program in cell-free extracts: requirement for dATP and cytochrome c. *Cell* 1996;86:147–157.

221. Richter C. Pro-oxidants and mitochondrial Ca2+: their relationship to apoptosis and oncogenesis. *FEBS Lett* 1993;325:104–107.

222. Susin SA, Zamzami N, Castedo M, et al. Bcl-2 inhibits the mitochondrial release of an apoptogenic protease. *J Exp Med* 1996;184:131.

223. Ferri KF, Kroemer G. Organelle-specific initiation of cell death pathways. *Nat Cell Biol* 2001;3:255–263.

224. Hartmann, et al. Caspase-3: a vulnerability factor and final effector in apoptotic death of dopaminergic neurons in Parkinson's disease. *Proc Natl Acad Sci USA* 2000;97:2875–2880.

225. Reed JC, Kroemer G. Mechanisms of mitochondrial membrane permeabilization. *Cell Death Differ* 2000;7:1145.

226. Jacotot E, Costantini P, Laboureau E, et al. Mitochondrial membrane permeabilization during the apoptotic process. *Ann NY Acad Sci* 1999;887:18–30.

227. Hartmann A, Michel PP, Troadec JD, et al. Is Bax a mitochondrial mediator in apoptotic death of dopaminergic neurons in Parkinson's disease? *J Neurochem* 2001;76(6):1785–1793.

228. Hartmann A, Troadec JD, Hunot S, et al. Caspase-8 is an effector in apoptotic death of dopaminergic neurons in Parkinson's disease, but pathway inhibition results in neuronal necrosis. *J Neurosci* 2001;21:2247–2255.

229. de la Monte SM, Sohn YK, Ganju N, et al. P53- and CD95-associated apoptosis in neurodegenerative diseases. *Lab Invest* 1998;78:401–411.

230. Reed JC. Apoptosis-based therapies. *Nat Rev Drug Discovery* 2002;1:111–121.

231. McNaught KStP, Olanow CW, Halliwell, et al. Failure of the ubiquitin-proteasome system in Parkinson's disease. *Nat Rev Neuroscience* 2001;2:89–94.

232. Sherman MY, Goldberg AL. Cellular defenses against unfolded proteins: a cell biologist thinks about neurodegenerative diseases. *Neuron* 2001;29:15–32.

233. Pickart CM. Ubiquitin in chains. *TIBS* 2000;25;544–548.

234. Johnston JA, Ward CL, Kopito RR. Aggresomes: a cellular response to misfolded proteins. *J Cell Biol* 1998;143:1883–1898.

235. Forno LS. Neuropathology of Parkinson's disease. *J Neuropathol Exp Neurol* 1996;55:259–272.

236. Ii K, Ito H, Tanaka K, et al. Immunocytochemical co-localization of the proteasome in ubiquitinated structures in neurodegenerative diseases and the elderly. *J Neuropathol Exp Neurol* 1997;56:125–131.

237. Yoritaka A, Hattori N, Uchida K, et al. Immunohistochemical detection of 4-hydroxynonenal protein adducts in Parkinson disease. *Proc Natl Acad Sci USA* 1996;93:2696–2701.

238. Shashidharan P, Good PF, Hsu A, et al. Torsin A accumulation in Lewy bodies in sporadic Parkinson's disease. *Brain Res* 2000;877:379–381.

239. Spillantini MG, Crowther AR, Jakes R, et al. α-Synuclein in filamentous inclusions of Lewy bodies from Parkinson's disease and dementia with Lewy bodies. *Proc Natl Acad Sci USA* 1997;95:6469–6473.

240. McNaught KStP, Mytilineou C, JnoBaptiste R, et al. Impairment of the ubiquitin-proteasome system causes dopaminergic cell death and inclusion body formation in ventral mesencephalic cultures. *J Neurochem* 2002 (in press).

241. McNaught KStP, Jenner P, Isaacson O, et al. Defects in proteasomal α-subunits in patients with sporadic Parkinson's disease. *Neurosci Lett* 2002 (in press).

242. McNaught KS, Jenner P. Proteasomal function is impaired in substantia nigra in Parkinson's disease. *Neurosci Lett* 2001;297:191–194.

243. Golbe LI, Giuseppe DI, Bonavita V, et al. A large kindred with autosomal dominant Parkinson's disease. *Ann Neurol* 1990;27:276–282.

244. Kruger R, Kuhn W, Muller T, et al. Ala30Pro mutation in the gene encoding alpha-synuclein in Parkinson's disease. *Nat Genet* 1998;18:106–108.

245. Masliah E, Rockenstein E, Veinbergs I, et al. Dopaminergic loss and inclusion body formation in α-synuclein mice: implications for neurodegenerative disorders. *Science* 2000;287:1265–1269.

246. Feany MB, Bender WW. A Drosophila model of Parkinson's disease. *Nature* 2000;404:394–398.

247. Conway KA, Herper JD, Lansbury PT. Accelerated in vitro fibril formation of mutant α-synuclein linked to early-onset Parkinson's disease. *Nat Med* 1998;4:1318–1320.

248. Bennet CM, Bishop JF, Leng Y, et al. Degradation of α-synuclein by proteasome. *J Biol Chem* 1999;274:33855–33858.

249. Saigoh K, et al. Intragenic deletion in the gene encoding ubiquitin carboxy-terminal hydrolase in GAD mice. *Nat Genet* 1999;19:47–51.

250. Hattori N, Shimura H, Kubo S, et al. Autosomal recessive juvenile parkinsonism: a key to understanding nigral degeneration in sporadic Parkinson's disease. *Neuropathology* 2000;20[Suppl]:S85–S90.

251. Shimura H, Hattori N, Kubo S, et al. Familial Parkinson's disease product, parkin, is a ubiquitin-protein ligase. *Nat Gen* 2000;25:302–305.

252. Shimura H, Hattori N, Kubo S-I, et al. Immunohistochemical and subcellular localization of parkin protein: absence of protein in autosomal recessive juvenile parkinsonian patients. *Ann Neurol* 1999;45:668–672.

253. Shimura H, Schlossmacher MG, Hattori N, et al. Ubiquitination of a new form of α-synuclein by parkin from human brain: implications for Parkinson's disease. *Science* 2001;28:28.

254. Imai Y, Soda M, Inoue H, et al. An unfolded putative transmembrane polypeptide, which can lead to endoplasmic reticulum stress, is a substrate of parkin. *Cell* 2001;105:891–902.

255. Chung KK, Zhang Y, Lim KL, et al. Parkin ubiquitinates the alpha-synuclein-interacting protein, synphilin-1: implications for Lewy-body formation in Parkinson disease. *Nat Med* 2001; 7:1144–1150.

256. Zhang Y, Gao J, Chung KK, et al. Parkin functions as an E2-dependent ubiquitin-protein ligase and promotes the degradation of the synaptic vesicle–associated protein, CDCrel-1. *Proc Natl Acad Sci USA* 2000;97:13354–13359.

257. Halliwell B, Jenner P. Impaired clearance of oxidised proteins in neurodegenerative disease. *Lancet* 1998;351:1510.

258. Rideout HJ, Larsen KE, Sulzer D, et al. Proteasomal inhibition leads to formation of ubiquitin/alpha-synuclein–immunoreactive inclusions in PC12 cells. *J Neurochem* 2001;78:899–908.

ANIMAL MODELS OF MOVEMENT DISORDERS

GISELLE M. PETZINGER
MICHAEL W. JAKOWEC

Since the late 19th century, lesions created by surgical, thermal, electrolytic, and toxic processes have been used for scientific study of the effect of central nervous system (CNS) injury on brain function. Significant advancements in our understanding of the underlying mechanisms and treatment of movement disorders have resulted from the use of models involving neurotoxicant and pharmacologic agents. Identification of spontaneous genetic mutations in animals with stereotypic movement disorders as well as the development of important transgenic mouse lines derived from the isolation of human genes in familial forms of movement disorders have provided significant research tools to investigate the underlying disease mechanism(s). Characterization of the neurochemical, molecular, behavioral, and anatomic changes occurring in different models provides an important tool to study etiology, pathophysiology, and treatment of movement disorders.

This chapter focuses on those animal models of movement disorders that have well-defined behavioral features resembling the human condition. Animal models with either subtle or uncharacterized behavioral manifestations are addressed for their significant insight they provide. Highlighted are some of the different approaches used to generate a model for the same human disorder. This chapter features models of both hypokinetic (Parkinson's disease and its variants) and hyperkinetic (Huntington's disease) movement disorders.

MODELS OF HYPOKINETIC DISORDERS

Hypokinetic movement disorders include Parkinson's disease (PD), striatonigral degeneration (SND), multiple system atrophy (MSA), and progressive supranuclear palsy (PSP) and other tau-related disorders.

Parkinson's Disease

Parkinson's disease is characterized by bradykinesia, rigidity, postural instability, and resting tremor. The primary patho-logic features of PD are the loss of dopaminergic neurons in the substantia nigra, the depletion of striatal dopamine, and the appearance of intracellular inclusions called Lewy bodies. Clinical features become apparent when striatal dopamine depletion reaches 80% despite the fact that 40% to 60% of substantia nigra dopaminergic neurons remain. Since the destruction of the nigrostriatal system and consequent depletion of striatal dopamine are key features in the human condition, attempts have been made to lesion analogous anatomic areas through neurotoxic or surgical approaches in animals. In addition, naturally occurring spontaneous mutations in rodents (*weaver* mouse and *ASAGU* rat) and transgenic mice targeting recently identified genes from familial forms of movement disorders (*parkin, α-synuclein*) provide new models and insights into the development, plasticity, and maintenance of the basal ganglia.

Toxin-induced Models for Parkinson's Disease

Reserpine

Carlsson developed the first animal model for PD in the 1950s using rabbits he treated with reserpine. Reserpine, a catecholamine-depleting agent, blocks vesicular storage of monoamines. The akinetic state induced by reserpine, similar to that seen in PD, and the dopamine depletion found in the caudate nucleus and putamen (areas implicated in motor control of the animals) led Carlsson to speculate that PD resulted from striatal dopamine depletion. This hypothesis was further supported by the discovery of striatal dopamine depletion in postmortem brain tissue from PD patients. Observations derived from this animal model also led to the subsequent use of L-dopa (in conjunction with a peripheral dopa-decarboxylase inhibitor) as the gold standard treatment for PD (7,14). Though reversible in its effect, the insight gained from the reserpine-treated rabbit model of PD led to the development of other models of dopamine depletion using site-specific neurotoxicant injury.

α-Methylparatyrosine

Although less commonly used, α-methylparatyrosine (AMPT), like reserpine, serves as an effective catecholamine-depleting agent. It directly inhibits the enzyme tyrosine hydroxylase, the rate-limiting step in dopamine biosynthesis, and therefore prevents the nascent synthesis of dopamine in neurons including those of the substantia nigra pars compacta and ventral tegmental area. Like reserpine, the systemic administration of AMPT leads to a transient akinetic state in animals lasting only hours or days.

Reserpine and AMPT have been used to discover new dopaminomimetics for the management of PD, but since their effects are transient this model is primarily useful for acute studies. In addition, neither agent can duplicate the extensive biochemical and pathologic changes seen in PD. Consequently, other models with long-lasting behavioral alterations have been sought.

6-Hydroxydopamine

6-Hydroxydopamine (6-OHDA, or 2,4,5-trihydroxyphenylethylamine) is a specific catecholaminergic neurotoxin that is structurally analogous to both dopamine and noradrenaline. Acting as a "false substrate" 6-OHDA is rapidly accumulated in catecholaminergic neurons. The mechanism of 6-OHDA toxicity is complex and involves (a) alkylation, (b) rapid autoxidation (leading to the generation of hydrogen peroxide, superoxide, and hydroxyl radicals), and (c) impairment of mitochondrial energy production. Ungerstedt initially carried out administration of 6-OHDA to rats as a model of PD in 1968 using stereotactic bilateral intracerebral injections into the substantia nigra or lateral hypothalamus (medial forebrain bundle) (55). Animals lesioned with 6-OHDA displayed catalepsy, generalized inactivity, aphagia, and adipsia. Lesioned animals also had a high degree of morbidity and mortality, making use of this model in an experimental design involving large numbers of animals and extended time courses difficult. Modification of the regimen to a unilateral intracerebral lesion targeting the substantia nigra and/or medial forebrain bundle resulted in a more manageable animal model having (a) minimal postoperative morbidity, (b) behavioral asymmetry, and (c) a nonlesioned side to serve as a control (56,57). To more closely replicate the human condition, researchers have developed another model utilizing striatal injections of 6-OHDA. This regimen leads to progressive dopaminergic cell death (as seen in PD) unlike the acute cell death induced through medial forebrain bundle injections (49).

A distinctive behavioral feature of the unilateral 6-OHDA-lesioned rat model is rotation (50,51). This motor feature is due to the asymmetry in dopaminergic neurotransmission between the lesioned and intact sides. Specifically, the direction of rotation is contralateral to the side with greater dopaminergic activity. Initial reports of behavioral analysis examined (a) spontaneous, (b) amphetamine-induced, and (c) apomorphine-induced rotation. Rats with greater than 80% depletion of striatal dopamine display spontaneous ipsilateral rotation (toward the lesioned side) with the rate of rotation correlating with the severity of the lesion. Animals with more extensive lesioning are less likely to show behavioral recovery of spontaneous rotation. The ipsilateral rotational behavior in lesioned animals can be enhanced with administration of *d*-amphetamine phenylisopropylamine (AMPH). AMPH blocks dopamine reuptake on the nonlesioned side increasing dopamine receptor activity and causing the animal to rotate toward the lesioned side. Interestingly, AMPH-induced rotation is contralateral to the lesioned side during the first week after lesioning indicating a transient period of dopaminergic hyperactivity of the lesioned side. Conversely, the administration of apomorphine, a dopamine agonist, induces contralateral rotation due to dopamine supersensitivity on the lesioned side. Similar to spontaneous rotation, some rats show recovery dependent on the site of lesioning (striatal vs. nigral lesioning) and the degree of injury (partial vs. complete dopamine depletion). This simple model of rotation away from the side with the most dopamine receptor occupancy has recently proven much more complex and less predictable than previously thought, especially in the context of various pharmacologic treatments and neuronal transplantation.

Major contributions utilizing the 6-OHDA-lesioned rat include (a) evaluating pharmacological agents (agonists and antagonists) that act on dopamine receptors; (b) investigating neuroplasticity of the basal ganglia in response to nigrostriatal injury; and (c) evaluating neuronal transplantation as a therapeutic strategy for the treatment of PD.

There is extensive literature describing pharmacologic studies that utilize the 6-OHDA-lesioned rat to investigate various dopamine receptor (D1 through D5) agonists and antagonists, and other neurotransmitter systems (including glutamate, adenosine, nicotine, or opioids) that regulate dopamine neurotransmission. Numerous studies describe the effects of these compounds on electrophysiologic, behavioral, and molecular (signal transduction) pathways within the basal ganglia. A review of the vast amount of pharmacologic literature in this model is beyond the scope of this chapter.

In the context of neuroplasticity, the 6-OHDA-lesioned rat has been instrumental in characterizing the neurochemical, molecular, and morphologic alterations within the basal ganglia in response to nigrostriatal dopamine depletion (60). In surviving dopaminergic neurons these mechanisms include (a) increased turnover of dopamine and its metabolites, (b) alterations in the expression of tyrosine hydroxylase (the rate-limiting step in dopamine biosynthesis), (c) decreased dopamine uptake through altered dopamine transporter expression, (d) alterations in the electrophysiologic phenotype, such as firing rate, and (e) sprouting of new striatal dopamine terminals. These molecular mechanisms may provide new targets for novel therapeutic interventions such as growth factors and regulators of transcription to enhance the function of surviving dopaminergic neurons.

The 6-OHDA-lesioned rat has been important for establishing indicators of successful transplantation (8). The nearly complete depletion of striatal dopamine in conjunction with behavioral rotation has been used to study the expression of the dopamine phenotype of different tissue sources, including fetal mesencephalon, engineered cell lines, and progenitor cells. The near-absence of tyrosine hydroxylase immunoreactivity in the striatum allows for the assessment of transplant innervation and degree of dopaminergic phenotype expression. The reversal of rotational behavior has been used as an indicator of transplant success. Other motor behaviors in the 6-OHDA-lesioned rat do not appear to be sensitive to transplantation. This model has also allowed for investigation of other parameters important for transplantation, including (a) target site (striatum vs. substantia nigra), (b) volume of innervation, (c) number of cells transplanted, (d) age of host and donor tissues, (e) pretreatment of transplant tissue with neurotrophic factors, antioxidants, or other neuroprotective pharmacologic agents, and (f) surgical techniques including needle type, cell suspension, and other delivery methods. These advancements, made in the 6-OHDA-lesioned rat, permit further testing of transplantation in nonhuman primates and human clinical trials. The 6-OHDA-lesioned rat model continues to make significant contributions in neuronal transplantation by examining new techniques and cell lines including human progenitor and stem cells.

The 6-OHDA-lesioned rat primarily serves as a model of dopamine dysfunction since it is highly specific for catecholaminergic neurons and does not replicate many of the behavioral, neurochemical, and pathologic features of human PD. For example, the 6-OHDA-lesioned rat fails to display alterations in several neurotransmitter systems that are affected in PD, including cholinergic and serotonergic. Stereotactic injections of 6-OHDA to precise targets fail to replicate the extensive pathology of PD where other regions of the brain (locus ceruleus, nucleus basalis of Meynert, and raphe nuclei) are affected. Lewy body formation, a pathologic hallmark of PD, has not been reported. A recent report using a regimen of long-term administration of 6-OHDA into the third ventricle has shown more extensive lesioning reminiscent of the human PD (39). Despite the fact that the 6-OHDA-lesioned rat is the most common species used, other species, including the nonhuman primate, have been lesioned with 6-OHDA (2). Lesioning in nonhuman primates provides for the analysis of behaviors

such as quantifying arm and hand movements through targeting and retrieval tasks not possible in rats.

Overall, lesioning with 6-OHDA has provided a rich source of information regarding the consequences of precise dopamine depletion and its effects on rotational behavior, dopamine biosynthesis, biochemical and morphological aspects of recovery. It also serves as an excellent template to study both pharmacologic and transplantation treatment modalities for PD.

1-Methyl-4-phenyl-1,2,3,6-tetrahydropyridine

The meperidine analog 1-methyl-4-phenyl-1,2,3,6-tetrahydropyridine (MPTP) is converted to 1-methyl-4-pyridinium (MPP+) by monoamine oxidase B (MAO-B). MPP+ acts as a substrate of the dopamine transporter (DAT) leading to inhibition of mitochondrial complex I, the depletion of ATP, and dopaminergic neuron cell death. Self-administration of MPTP by heroin addicts induced clinical symptoms indistinguishable from idiopathic PD and identified a neurotoxicant useful for the development of animal models of PD (13,27). Subsequent administration to mice and nonhuman primates showed that MPTP selectively destroys dopaminergic neurons of the substantia nigra pars compacta (SNc), the same neurons affected in PD (46,47). Similar to PD, the ventral tegmental area and locus ceruleus are affected by MPTP lesioning but to a lesser extent than SNc. In addition, dopamine depletion occurs in the putamen and caudate nucleus with the putamen more affected depending on species (squirrel monkey) and mode of administration (long term, low dose). Unlike PD, Lewy bodies have not been reported; however, eosinophilic inclusions (reminiscent of Lewy bodies) have been described in aged nonhuman primates. The time course of MPTP-induced neurodegeneration is rapid, being completed within a few days. However, in humans affected by MPTP the time course of neurodegeneration may be protracted. Details of MPTP toxicity and utility are described in refs. 34 and 48.

The injection of MPTP into mice results in subtle behavioral deficits. However, administration of MPTP to nonhuman primates results in parkinsonian symptoms, including bradykinesia, postural instability, and rigidity. In some species resting or action/postural tremor has been observed (53). Similar to PD, the MPTP-lesioned nonhuman primate responds to traditional antiparkinsonian therapies such as L-dopa and dopamine receptor agonists. Following the administration of MPTP, the nonhuman primate progresses through acute (hours), subacute (days), and chronic (weeks) behavioral phases of symptom progression that are due to the peripheral and central effects of MPTP. The acute phase is characterized by sedation and a hyperadrenergic state, the subacute phase by the development of varying degrees of parkinsonian features, and the chronic phase by initial recovery (by some but not all animals) followed by the stabilization of motor deficits. Near-complete behavioral recovery has been described in all nonhuman primate species and is dictated by age, species, mode of MPTP administration, and the severity of the parkinsonian state at the end of the subacute phase.

The sensitivity to MPTP-mediated dopamine depletion in nonhuman primates is both age and species dependent, with older animals and Old World monkeys (such as rhesus, *Macaca mulatta*, or African green, *Cercopithecus aethiops*) being more sensitive than young and New World monkeys (such as the squirrel monkey, *Saimiri sciureus*, or marmoset, *Callithrix jacchus*), respectively.

Over the years, the different routes and dosing regimens of MPTP administration have led to a number of different nonhuman primate models with distinct biochemical and behavioral characteristics (32). With the investigation of novel therapeutic strategies (fetal, genetically engineered cell transplant, growth factors, and neuroprotective agents) it is critical that the proper model be selected to provide the most appropriate condition(s) for evaluating experimental results. For example in the *hemilesioned* model, the internal carotid injection of MPTP leads to the depletion of striatal dopamine and nearly complete destruction of nigrostriatal dopaminergic neurons ipsilateral to the injection (3). An advantage of this model is that the severely dopamine depleted ipsilateral side can serve as a template for evaluating the success of tissue transplantation. In this setting, the presence of any tyrosine hydroxylase–expressing cells and/or sprouting would be due to transplanted tissue survival alone with the contralateral side acting as control. In the *systemic MPTP-lesioned* model, administration of MPTP via intramuscular, intravenous, intraperitoneal, or subcutaneous injection leads to a bilateral depletion of striatal dopamine and nigrostriatal cell death. A feature of this model is that the degree of lesioning can be titrated, resulting in parkinsonian symptoms ranging from mild to severe. An advantage of the *systemic MPTP-lesioned* nonhuman primate is that remaining nigrostriatal dopaminergic neurons and axons, as wells as compensatory mechanisms, are likely to be present, and the effects of growth factor (for sprouting) or neuroprotective factors (for cell survival) can be evaluated. The *bilateral intracarotid* model (through sequential administration of MPTP injections into the carotid arteries), the *overlesioned* model (intracarotid infusion followed by a systemic administration of MPTP), and the chronic low dose model (chronic systemic administration of MPTP over months to years) also have unique neurochemical, behavioral, and pathologic advantages (32).

Similar to the human condition, the administration of levodopa (plus a peripheral dopa decarboxylase inhibitor) or a dopamine agonist in monkeys with MPTP-induced parkinsonism leads to motor complications such as wearing off (end-of-dose deterioration) and dyskinesia (chorea and dystonia). Although the etiology of dyskinesia is unknown, results of electrophysiologic, neurochemical, molecular, and neuroimaging studies in both rodent (6-OHDA) and nonhuman primate models suggest that (a) changes in the neuronal firing rate and pattern of the globus pallidus and subthalamic nucleus, (b) enhancement of D1 receptor–mediated signal transduction pathways, (c) alterations in the phosphorylation state and subcellular localization of glutamate (*N*-methyl-D-aspartate, or NMDA, subtype) receptors, (d) modifications in the functional links between dopamine receptor subtypes (D1 and D2, and D1 and D3), and (e) enhancement of opioid peptide–mediated neurotransmission may be involved in the expression of dyskinesia (6).

Behavioral recovery (varying in degree and time course) has been reported in most models of MPTP-induced parkinsonism in nonhuman primates and MPTP-lesioned rodents. Although it may present as a confounding parameter in some studies, recovery after MPTP lesioning may provide important insight into neuroplasticity of the basal ganglia. A number of adaptive mechanisms may account for behavioral recovery, including (a) alterations in dopamine biosynthesis (increased tyrosine hydroxylase protein and mRNA expression) and turnover; (b) down-regulation of dopamine transporter; (c) sprouting and branching of tyrosine hydroxylase fibers; (d) alterations of other neurotransmitter systems, including glutamate and serotonin; and (e) alterations of signal transduction pathways and transcription factors. An example of the time course of behavioral recovery in the MPTP-lesioned squirrel monkey and the expression of tyrosine hydroxylase immunoreactivity in the caudate nucleus is illustrated in Fig. 5.1. An understanding of the intrinsic neuroplasticity of the basal ganglia will support the identification of novel therapeutic targets for the management of neurodegenerative disease.

In addition to transplant studies in the 6-OHDA-lesioned rat, the MPTP-lesioned nonhuman primate model provides another valuable tool to test transplantation since it has behavioral features that closely resemble human PD. For example, prior to human clinical trials, new transplantation strategies, such as stem cells, can be assessed by determining functional benefit in nonhuman primates.

The systemic effects of MPTP have not been extensively studied. The peripheral conversion of MPTP to MPP$^+$ can occur in the liver resulting in transient injury to the liver and heart. It is not uncommon for researchers to experience a high degree of acute death of MPTP-injected mice and nonhuman primates within the first 24 hours. To address the potential peripheral effects of MPTP in the squirrel monkey, we conducted a toxicologic study examining biochemical markers of liver function. Core body temperature, heart rate, blood pressure, and body weight were also measured (Petzinger et al., manuscript in preparation). Squirrel monkeys administered MPTP (a series of six subcutaneous injections of 2 mg/kg, free base, 2 weeks apart) were given a comprehensive examination 1, 4, and 10 days after each injection. Biochemical markers of hepatocellular toxicity

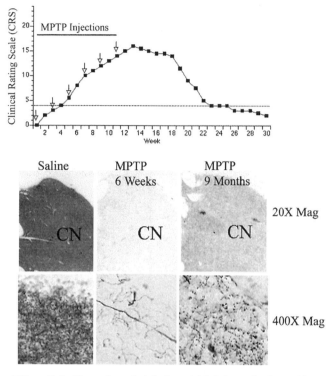

FIG. 5.1. The 1-methyl-4-phenyl-1,2,3,6-tetrahydropyridine (MPTP)–lesioned squirrel monkey shows behavioral recovery. The graph depicts the time course of motor behavior quantified using a Clinical Rating Scale (CRS). Animals were administered MPTP (2 mg/kg, free-base) by subcutaneous injection at 2-week intervals *(arrows)*. A CSR score of 4 or less (out of a possible score of 24) is considered normal motor behavior. The CRS time course shows that animals return to near normal motor behavior 12 weeks after the last injection of MPTP. The lower panels show immunohistochemical staining with an antibody against tyrosine hydroxylase protein. The upper row shows staining in the caudate nucleus at low magnification whereas the lower row shows staining at high magnification. Six weeks after the last injection of MPTP there is a severe depletion of tyrosine hydroxylase protein compared with saline controls, with staining seen in a few large fibers. However, at 9 months after the last injection of MPTP there is an increase in immunostaining but still below that of saline-injected controls.

were evident during the time course of MPTP lesioning. Markers of liver injury (hepatic enzymes) persisted for several weeks after the last injection of MPTP before returning to normal prelesioned levels. Measurement of core body temperature during the time course of MPTP lesioning showed significant hypothermia that persisted for up to 10 days after MPTP injection. These results indicate that the administration of MPTP leads to systemic changes that may be responsible for acute toxicity and death of some animals as well as influencing the pharmacologic parameters of experimental therapeutics under investigation.

Similar to nonhuman primates, rodents also show species, strain, and age differences with respect to MPTP sensitivity. Rats are much less sensitive to the effects of MPTP than mice. Mice show different degrees of lesioning

depending on the strain and its vendor source. Equal amounts of MPTP administered to C57BL/6 mice can lead to severe dopamine depletion and nigrostriatal dopaminergic neuron cell death, whereas strains such as Swiss Webster and CD-1 appear almost resistant. The background strain of any transgenic line (and their controls) to be investigated must be considered prior to the design of experiments involving MPTP lesioning.

Methamphetamine

Derivatives of the amphetamines have been the focus of neuroscientific research because they lead to the depletion of dopamine and serotonin. Epidemiologic studies have suggested that abusers of these drugs may be prone to developing movement disorders. When administered to rodents and nonhuman primates, methamphetamine (METH), one of the most potent amphetamine derivatives, leads to the severe depletion of striatal dopamine and degeneration of dopaminergic nigrostriatal terminals. There is evidence of METH-induced cell death in the substantia nigra (52). The effects of severe METH lesioning are long-lasting. However, there is evidence of recovery of dopaminergic innervation (18). The precise mechanism(s) mediating METH neurotoxicity involve a number of distinct processes, including (a) inhibition of tyrosine hydroxylase and dopamine transporter activity, (b) formation of reactive oxygen/nitrogen species, (c) overwhelming and/or damaging antioxidant enzymes (such as catalase or glutathione peroxidase), and (d) METH-induced hyperthermia (22). Despite the severe depletion of striatal dopamine, the motor behavioral alterations seen in rodents and nonhuman primates are subtle. Further studies of the effects of METH and substituted amphetamines, including methylenedioxymethamphetamine (MDMA, "ecstasy"), will provide the evidence of the effects of long-term striatal dopamine depletion on the induction of movement disorders.

Rotenone

Epidemiologic studies have suggested that environmental factors, such as pesticides, may increase the risk for PD. Specific neurochemical and pathologic damage to dopaminergic neurons by the acute application of some pesticides, such as rotenone, however, have generated mixed results in animals. Studies from Greenamyre and colleagues used a 5-week, low-dose infusion of rotenone (an inhibitor of mitochondrial complex I) into the jugular vein of the rat (5). This chronic infusion model resulted in selective death of a subset of nigrostriatal dopaminergic neurons, the formation of cytoplasmic inclusions, and the development of parkinsonian behavioral features (including hunched posture, rigidity, unsteady movement, and paw tremor) in some animals.

Genetic Models of Parkinson's Disease

Parkin

An autosomal recessive form of juvenile parkinsonism (AR-JP) led to the identification of a gene on chromosome 6q27 called *parkin*. Parkin protein has a large N-terminal ubiquitin-like domain and C-terminal cysteine ring structure. Mutations in *parkin* may account for the majority of autosomal recessive familial cases of PD. Recent biochemical studies indicate that parkin protein may play a critical role in mediating interactions with a number of different proteins involved in the proteasome-mediated degradation pathway. Mutations of the *parkin* gene have been introduced into transgenic mice. At present there is very little known about pathologic or behavioral alterations due to mutations in parkin protein. However, *parkin* transgenic models enable investigation of the ubiquitin-mediated protein degradation pathways and its relationship to neurodegenerative disease.

α-Synuclein

Rare cases of autosomal dominant familial forms of PD (the Contursi and German kindreds) have been linked to point mutations in the gene encoding α-synuclein (33). The normal function of α-synuclein is unknown, but its localization and developmental expression suggests a role in neuroplasticity (24). The disruption of normal neuronal function may lead to the loss of synaptic maintenance and subsequent degeneration. It is interesting that mice with knockout of α-synuclein are viable, suggesting that a "gain-in-function" phenotype or other protein–protein interactions may contribute to neurodegeneration. Although no mutant forms of α-synuclein have been identified in idiopathic PD, its localization to Lewy bodies (including PD and related disorders) has suggested a pathophysiologic link between α-synuclein aggregation and neurodegenerative disease. To investigate these potential mechanisms several groups have developed transgenic mouse models. An interesting caveat is that the mutant allele of α-synuclein in the Contursi kindred is identical to the wild-type mouse, suggesting that protein expression and/or protein–protein interactions may be more important than loss of function due to missense mutation. Therefore, transgenic mouse models developed for α-synuclein focus on altered protein expression through the use of different promoters and gene cassette constructs. Some transgenic mouse lines show pathologic changes in dopaminergic neurons (including inclusions, decreased striatal dopamine, and loss of striatal tyrosine hydroxylase immunoreactivity), behavioral deficits (rotorod and attenuation of dopamine-dependent locomotor response to amphetamine), whereas other lines show no deficit (1,25,29). No studies have reported the loss of substantia nigra dopaminergic neurons. This range of results with different α-synuclein constructs from different laboratories underscores the important link between protein expression (mutant vs. wild-type alleles) and pathologic and behavioral outcome.

Other Spontaneous and Transgenic Models for Parkinson's Disease

There are several natural spontaneous genetic animal models as well as new transgenic models that may provide insight into the mechanisms involved in movement disorders and neurodegenerative disease. The relationship between polymorphisms of ubiquitin carboxy-terminal hydrolase L1 (UCH-L1) and PD has implicated another protein involved in the ubiquitin-proteasome protein degradation pathway. In addition, transgenic mouse lines have employed knockout or knockin strategies that target genes such as superoxide dismutase (SOD), monoamine oxidase (MAO), dopamine receptors, dopamine transporter, caspases, neurotrophic factors, and neurotransmitter receptors. These transgenic lines will provide insight to mechanisms involved in basal ganglia movement disorders. Spontaneous genetic rodent models, including the *weaver*, *lurcher*, *reeler*, *Tshr*[hyt], *tottering*, *coloboma* mice and the *ASAGU* and *circling (ci)* rats, possess features that may also prove important to understanding neurodegenerative diseases. Several of these spontaneous rodent models display altered dopaminergic function or neurodegeneration, and have deficits in motor behavior (19). For example, the *weaver* mouse displays cell death of dopaminergic neurons whereas the *tottering* mouse displays tyrosine hydroxylase hyperinnervation. The *ASAGU* rat is a spontaneous model characterized by progressive rigidity, staggering gait, tremor, and difficulty in initiating movements (31). Microdialysis has revealed that prior to dopaminergic neuronal cell death, dysfunction in dopamine production correlates with behavioral deficits. Another potentially interesting rodent model is the *circling (ci)* rat, which displays spontaneous rotational behavior as a result of an imbalance in dopaminergic neurotransmission without asymmetric nigral cell death (36). Other genetic model of PD that represents the only model of age-related, progressive dopaminergic nigral neuronal degeneration is the heterozygote Nurr1 model (37). Nurr1 is a member of the nuclear receptor superfamily and is highly expressed in midbrain dopaminergic neurons beginning in embryonic stages and continuing into adulthood. Nurr1 is absolutely required for the induction and development of dopaminergic phenotype in the midbrain. In the Nurr1 heterozygote model a selective nigral dopaminergic neuron degeneration is produced by "knocking out" the *Nurr1* gene in mouse. Disruption of the gene induces massive apoptosis of dopaminergic precursor neurons in substantia nigra (38). Interestingly, the homozygous *Nurr1* gene knockout (Nurr1−/−) mice display a selective and complete loss of dopaminergic neurons in substantia nigra and dopamine levels in the striatum (39) and die in 24 hours, whereas the heterozygous *Nurr1* gene knockout (Nurr1+/−) mice are more vulnerable to dopaminergic neurotoxin MPTP compared with the wild-type (Nurr1+/+) mice (40). Most importantly, Nurr1+/− mice displayed progressive deficiency of nigral dopaminergic function, whereas Nurr1+/+ mice showed partial recovery several months after MPTP treatment. Le et al. (41) demonstrated that aged Nurr1+/− mice develop slower spontaneous locomotor activity, significantly slower traction reflex, and longer apomorphine-induced climbing behavior. These behavioral changes are associated with remarkable reduction of striatal DA levels and nigral DA neurons (41). Thus, the Nurr1+/− mice have behavioral and biochemical features similar to the progressive course seen in PD, and may serve as an ideal animal model to study the mechanisms of nigral degeneration and neuroprotection.

In addition to rodent genetic models, there is a growing interest in *Drosophila* models with directed expression of α-synuclein. In one study of a *Drosophila* model with directed expression of α-synuclein, directed expression of the molecular chaperone Hsp70 prevented dopaminergic neuronal loss (42). Since chaperone proteins, which are heat-shock proteins that are up-regulated during stress, help misfolded proteins to refold, chaperone therapies may hold the potential for preventing the progression of the disease.

Multiple System Atrophy and Striatonigral Degeneration

Multiple system atrophy (MSA) is a disorder characterized by a combination of clinical symptoms involving cerebellar, extrapyramidal, and autonomic systems. The predominant subtype of MSA is striatonigral degeneration (SND), a form of L-dopa-unresponsive parkinsonism. Neuropathologic changes of SND included degeneration of the nigrostriatal pathway, medium spiny striatal GABAergic projection pathways (putamen greater then caudate), as well as other regions of the brainstem, cerebellum, and spinal cord. Inclusion-like aggregates that immunostain for ubiquitin and α-synuclein are seen in oligodendrocytes and neurons.

The basis for developing an animal model for SND emerged from established animal models for both Parkinson's disease (having SNc pathology) and Huntington's disease (HD) (having striatal pathology). Rodent models for SND have been generated through sequential stereotactic injections of 6-OHDA and quinolinic acid (QA) into the medial forebrain bundle and striatum, respectively, or striatal injections of MPP+ and 3-nitropropionic acid (3-NP). These double-lesioning models are characterized morphologically by neuronal degeneration in the SNc and ipsilateral striatum. The order of neurotoxic lesioning may influence the degree of nigral or striatal pathology. For example, animals receiving 6-OHDA prior to QA exhibit predominantly nigral pathology, whereas animals receiving QA prior to 6-OHDA show predominantly striatal pathology. This

may be due to QA-induced terminal damage or other complex interactions after lesioning that reduces terminal uptake of 6-OHDA. Glial inclusions have not been reported in any of these models, indicating a significant difference in comparison with the human condition.

Motor deficits in models for SND are assessed by ipsilateral and contralateral motor tasks (including stepping response, impaired paw reaching, and balance) and drug-induced circling behavior. Characteristic drug-induced circling behavior occurs after 6-OHDA lesioning, resulting in ipsilateral rotation in response to amphetamine and contralateral rotation in response to apomorphine. The subsequent striatal lesioning with QA diminishes (or has no affect on) amphetamine-induced ipsilateral rotation and reduces (or abolishes) apomorphine-induced contralateral rotation. This observation may be mediated by dopamine release on the intact side (in response to amphetamine) and/or the loss of dopamine receptor activation on the lesioned side (in response to apomorphine). The lack of response to apomorphine (a dopamine agonist) has been shown to correlate with the striatal lesion volume and is analogous to the diminished efficacy of L-dopa therapy observed in the majority of SND patients.

A nonhuman primate (*Macaca fascicularis*) model of SND has been generated through the sequential systemic administration of MPTP and 3-NP (15,16). The parkinsonian features after MPTP lesioning are L-dopa responsive; however, subsequent administration of 3-NP exacerbates motor symptoms and nearly eliminates the L-dopa response. L-dopa occasionally induces facial dyskinesia as sometimes seen in human MSA. Similar to SND morphologic changes include cell loss in the SNc (typical of MPTP lesioning) and severe circumscribed (nondiffuse) degeneration of striatal GABAergic projection neurons (typical of 3-NP lesioning). Despite similarities to the human condition, the putamen and caudate nucleus show equal degrees of lesioning in the MSA model, whereas the putamen is more affected than the caudate nucleus in human SND. In addition, inclusion bodies that may underlie the pathogenesis of SND have not been reported in the nonhuman primate model.

The Tauopathies, Including Progressive Supranuclear Palsy and Other Tau-related Disorders

The low molecular weight microtubule associated protein tau has been implicated in a number of neurodegenerative diseases, including Alzheimer's disease, progressive supranuclear palsy (PSP), Pick's disease, frontotemporal dementia with parkinsonism (FTDP), and amyotrophic lateral sclerosis/parkinsonism-dementia complex (ALS/PDC) of Guam. Together these neurodegenerative diseases constitute what is referred to as the tauopathies because they share common neuropathologic features, including abnormal hyperphosphorylation and filamentous accumulation of aggregated tau proteins. Reports in the literature have implicated either alternative RNA splicing (generating different isoforms) or missense mutations as mechanisms underlying many of the tauopathies. Therefore, transgenic mice have been developed that overexpress specific splice variants or missense mutation of tau. One such transgenic line generated overexpressed the shortest human tau isoform (23). These mice showed progressive motor weakness, intraneuronal and intra-axonal inclusions (detectable by 1-month postnatal), and reduced axonal transport. Fibrillary tau inclusions developed in the neocortical neurons after 18 months of age implicating age-specific processes in the pathogenesis of fibrous tau inclusions. An interesting tau transgenic has been developed in *Drosophila melanogaster* where expression of a tau missense mutation showed no evidence of large filamentous aggregates (neurofibrillary tangles). However, aged flies showed evidence of vacuolization and degeneration of cortical neurons (59). These observations suggest that tau-mediated neurodegeneration is age dependent and may occur independent of protein aggregation.

MODELS OF HYPERKINETIC DISORDERS

Huntington's Disease

Huntington's disease (HD) is an autosomal dominant neurodegenerative disease that is clinically characterized by cognitive dysfunction, dementia, depression, abnormal involuntary movements (chorea), abnormal eye movements, and dystonia. Early motor features include chorea and parkinsonism. As the disease progresses bradykinesia remains, chorea deceases, and dystonia with rigidity appears. Juvenile-onset HD (JHD) progresses more rapidly then adult-onset HD and consists primarily of dystonia and bradykinesia. The predominant pathologic features of HD consist of neuronal loss of striatal medium spiny projection γ-aminobutyric acid (GABA) neurons and astrogliosis in the caudate nucleus, putamen, and, to a lesser degree, in the globus pallidus, thalamus, hippocampus, and cerebellum. Large cholinergic aspiny interneurons and medium (NADPH-diaphorase and somatostatin and neuropeptide Y containing) aspiny projection neurons are relatively less affected. Other cortical and subcortical regions are involved, including projection neuron targets in the globus pallidus and substantia nigra, but the degree of atrophy and degeneration varies. Nuclear inclusions may be seen in JHD. Mapping of the HD locus identified an unstable CAG trinucleotide repeat on chromosome 4p16.3 in exon-1 of what is now known as the *huntingtin* gene. The precise mechanism of neurodegeneration is unclear, but it is believed that the mutation in *huntingtin* leads to an increase in excitatory neurotransmission and/or impaired energy metabolism of striatal neurons.

Toxin-induced Models of HD

Since the first report in 1976 implicating an excitotoxic mechanism underlying HD, animal models for HD have been produced by intrastriatal injections of excitatory amino acids, including kainic acid (KA), quinolinic acid (QA), and ibotenic acid, or the systemic administration of the mitochondrial neurotoxin 3-NP (12,30). Administration of either excitatory amino acids or 3-NP has been shown to mimic the HD pattern of neurodegeneration and behavioral changes with some subtle differences in these models. In general, QA is thought to generate a more specific neurotoxic effect than other excitatory amino acids and to resemble the early stage of adult HD. Widely spread metabolic depression (defined by reduced cytochrome oxidase activity), minimal necrosis, and hyperlocomotion (similar to chorea) are observed. On the other hand, 3-NP is thought to resemble advanced HD or the JHD because it produces a severe effect with necrotic cavities in the striatum and delayed onset of dyskinetic movements.

Rodent Model of Huntington's Disease Using Excitatory Amino Acids

Excitatory amino acids, including QA, are potent agonists at the NMDA subtype of glutamate receptor. Stereotactic administration (unilateral) of QA into rat striatum results in a lesion similar in neuropathology and neurochemistry to that seen in HD. QA causes widespread metabolic depression, as well as destruction of GABA and substance P–containing cholinergic neurons. Dopaminergic fibers and striatal aspiny neurons containing neuropeptide Y and somatostatin that colocalize with NADPH diaphorase are spared. Many of the histopathologic features of excitatory amino acid lesioning are both dose dependent and age dependent, and may account for variability between studies. Typical motor-related behavioral deficits include drug-induced turning, hyperlocomotion, and impaired skilled-paw use. Rats with bilateral lesions show deficits in spatial learning function (water maze). Lesioned rodents do not show features of chorea or dystonia (the hallmarks of HD) but do show spontaneous locomotive activity that increases with the administration of dopamine agonists, including apomorphine.

Nonhuman Primate Model of Huntington's Disease Using Quinolinic Acid

The administration of excitatory amino acids to nonhuman primates may provide a model of HD that more closely resembles the human condition with respect to anatomy, neurochemistry, and behavior. Striatal lesions tend to be unilateral to avoid high mortality. Post lesion chorea- and dystonic-like movements do not occur spontaneously but can be induced by apomorphine and drugs that increase dopaminergic activity. Lesioned animals may show improvement in movement behavior with time, suggesting neuroplasticity in response to the injury.

Rodent Model of Huntington's Disease Using 3-NP

Noninvasive imaging techniques (including nuclear magnetic resonance and positron emission tomographic scanning) have shown a deficit in mitochondrial energy metabolism in HD patients. This finding suggested that the impairment in energy metabolism could be exploited as another means to generate an HD animal model. A compound to generate a model of HD through energy impairment was discovered through the ingestion of contaminated sugar cane. These patients developed selective damage to the putamen that led to delayed onset of chorea and dystonia resembling HD. The contaminating agent was identified as the succinate dehydrogenase inhibitor 3-NP. The systemic administration of 3-NP to animals leads to progressive striatal atrophy several weeks after injection. Similar to HD, medium spiny neurons are affected but NADPH diaphorase and cholinergic neurons and dopaminergic terminals similar are spared. The injection regimen is typically a chronic low dosage (over several months) to avoid mortality that often accompanies an acute high-dose injection. Initial motor symptoms include hyperactivity with loss of coordination. Wobbly gait is observed in the first few weeks followed by hypokinesia, dystonic posturing, and rigidity of the hindlimbs. Cognitive dysfunction in skilled-paw use learning (a measure of cognitive function) is impaired. Chorea or dystonia is not observed in the lesioned rodent. Symptoms may progress after stopping 3-NP administration and eventually behavioral recovery may occur in some animals.

Nonhuman Primate Model of Huntington's Disease Using 3-NP

The acute systemic injection of 3-NP in nonhuman primates leads to primarily bilateral putamen necrosis but may also affect the caudate nucleus and hippocampus. The degree of striatal neuronal loss and severity of behavioral deficits are dependent on the rate and duration of 3-NP administration and the age of the animal. Spontaneous neuronal symptoms include loss of muscle tone, general bradykinesia, and dystonia. The clinical and pathologic features resemble JHD. The chronic administration of 3-NP is carried out over a period of 4 to 6 months. During the presymptomatic phase (4 to 6 weeks from the first injection) animals may manifest limb dyskinesia, oral facial dyskinesia, leg dystonia, and hyperkinetic movements with apomorphine administration. After 10 to 12 weeks from the first injection animals develop spontaneous dyskinesia,

dystonia, and hypokinesia. Apomorphine increases the severity of these motor features. Cognitive deficits have been reported in both symptomatic and presymptomatic animals.

Transgenic Models of HD

The identification of mutations in the *huntingtin* gene has resulted in the development of numerous transgenic and knockout mouse lines. Genetic mutation of *huntingtin* in these strains and the subsequent pathologic and behavioral changes that occur provide insight into the underlying mechanisms of HD. Variability in behavior and pathology between different transgenic mouse HD models may be due to differences in mouse strains, construct types (with respect to promoters, exons, and vector type), and CAG triplet repeat length (11). One of the first HD transgenic mouse lines established was R6 (28). This construct used the entire exon-1 containing a CAG repeat (initially 130 repeats) plus 1-kb of the HD promoter. At 2 months of age, R6 transgenic mice develop tremor, shuttering movements, stereotypic grooming, and seizures upon handling. The phenotype progresses with a 60% weight loss and 20% reduction in brain size and brain weight without neuronal cell loss compared with normal littermates. Striatal and deep cortical cell death have also been observed. Death typically occurs at around 12 weeks of age. Neuropathologic analysis using immunohistochemical staining revealed cortical neuronal inclusions by 6 weeks that contained exon-1 of huntingtin and ubiquitin proteins. Similar to HD, decreased glutamatergic (AMPA and KA subtypes of glutamate receptors) and dopaminergic (D1 and D2) receptor subtype expression is detectable prior to the onset of symptoms when inclusions are observed. This observation led researchers to reevaluate the pathology of the human condition. In JHD, nuclear inclusions in cortical neurons (up to 50%) that are typically more widespread then the degree of neurodegeneration have since been identified. Furthermore, axonal inclusions (called dystrophic neurites) have subsequently been detected in adult HD. These inclusions also immunostain for ubiquitin and the N-terminal huntingtin. The time course of these observations in the transgenic mouse suggests a possible mechanism underlying the pathogenesis of HD where neuronal dysfunction (due to nuclear localization of the truncated huntingtin protein) leads to the disease phenotype prior to cell loss.

More recently, other transgenic mouse lines for HD have been established using the full-length *huntingtin* gene construct (20,35). Some lines show progressive motor abnormalities consisting of hyperactivity, stereotypic rotations, and excessive grooming. The hyperkinetic behavior is occasionally followed by hypokinetic behavior and death. Changes in behavior are seen before neuronal cell loss with either the absence of or a modest number of nuclear inclusions. Compared to truncated gene constructs, transgenic lines carrying the full-length cDNA for huntingtin show more significant and widespread neuronal loss (displaying apoptotic-like features) with reactive gliosis in the striatum, hippocampus, thalamus, and deep cortical region. Analysis of transgenic mice carrying either the truncated or full-length *huntingtin* gene has shown a decrease in the diameter and density of striatal dendrites. Unlike the human condition, the extent of the polyglutamine expansion does not directly correlate with the onset and severity of progression. Mice, homozygotic for *huntingtin* mutations, show an earlier onset of symptoms than heterozygotes. In contrast, rare homozygotes of HD do not differ significantly from HD heterozygotes. Similar to the human condition, *huntingtin* transgenic mice display alterations in specific subtypes of striatal receptors for glutamate, dopamine, and acetylcholine before the onset of behavioral changes (10). It is interesting to note that introduction of CAG expansion into the mouse *huntingtin* gene analog does not result in the same behavioral or pathologic features seen in other transgenic mouse lines. Furthermore, knockout of the mouse *huntingtin* gene is embryonic lethal in the homozygotic but not heterozygotic state (with no behavioral changes).

Dystonia

Dystonia is an autosomal dominant syndrome of sustained muscle contraction leading to twisting, abnormal posture, and repetitive movements. Dystonia can be classified according to etiology, age of onset, or anatomic distribution. Primary or idiopathic dystonia manifests in the absence of CNS lesions, whereas secondary dystonia is a manifestation of a variety of neurologic diseases or brain lesions often involving the basal ganglia. The etiology of idiopathic torsion dystonia (ITD) is presently unknown.

Spontaneous autosomal recessive genetic models of ITD in rodents have been identified and may provide insight into human dystonia (43,44). These models include (a) the wriggle mouse, (b) the dystonic rat, and (c) the dystonic hamster. Rodent models share common features, including (a) onset of dystonia within the first 10 to 16 days postnatal, which becomes generalized with time; (b) improvement of dystonia with sleep and worsening with stress; (c) the absence of CNS lesions; and (d) altered electrophysiologic and neurochemical properties of the cerebellum and brainstem nuclei. Behavioral and physiologic differences exist between these models. The wriggle mouse (allele identified to chromosome 11) is considered similar to idiopathic myoclonic dystonia with clinical features including tremor, dystonia, and myoclonus. Neurochemical data in this model suggest widespread overactivity of the serotonergic system with alterations in striatal and cerebellar noradrenergic, dopaminergic, and GABAergic systems. The dystonic Sprague-Dawley rat model has been proposed as a model of ITD. Primary dysfunction may involve abnormal cerebellar GABAergic output that leads to abnormal activity in the red nucleus and thalamus. Dysfunction of the basal ganglia may be secondary. Similar to the human condition, this rat model responds to benzodiazepine and anticholinergic treatment. The dystonic hamster (DT^{sz}), initially described as a model of seizures with tonic spasms, may actually represent a model of idiopathic paroxysmal dystonia. Dystonic attacks consisting of limb and trunk twisting occur spontaneously or in response to stress. These attacks progress in stages of severity, persist for several hours, and are not associated with loss of consciousness or electroencephalographic abnormalities. Administration of antiepileptic drugs is not beneficial, but diazepam and dopamine receptor antagonists show significant antidystonic effects. Abnormalities in 2-deoxyglucose and cytochrome oxidase I activity in the basal ganglia have been reported. These abnormalities result in decreased GABAergic activity, hyperdopaminergic activity, and alterations in cerebellar output.

The recent identification of genes and their proteins involved in human dystonia, including the *DYT1* gene and the torsin A protein, provides a new opportunity to develop transgenic mice models of idiopathic generalized dystonia. In addition to the spontaneous genetic models discussed above, these new transgenic models will provide valuable insight into the mechanisms underlying dystonia.

Experimental models of secondary dystonia have been generated in rodents and nonhuman primates and include (a) surgical lesioning of the thalamus and basal ganglia, (b) MPTP lesioning followed by L-dopa (or dopamine agonist) administration as a model of iatrogenic dystonia, (c) neuroleptic induced dystonia, and (d) other neurotoxic lesioning models (including 3-NP) that, in addition to a range of behavioral abnormalities, have a component of dystonia.

Tremor

Animal models of tremor have been developed from (a) application of tremorogenic drugs, (b) surgical lesions, and (c) genetic models (58). Tremorogenic drugs include harmaline and MPTP. Harmaline induces a postural/kinetic tremor in a wide variety of animal species and is analogous to essential or enhanced physiologic tremor. Studies suggest that harmaline may exert its effect on the inferior olive nucleus by inducing enhanced electric coupling of olivary neurons through GABA receptor–controlled gap junctions. MPTP has been reported to induce either a postural or resting tremor in the nonhuman primate (4). The variable expression of tremor after MPTP administration may be due to a number of factors including species and age of the animal. In addition to MPTP, lesioning of the substantia nigra with 6-OHDA in nonhuman primates leads to a resting tremor similar to that seen in humans. Surgical lesioning of most areas of the basal ganglia can also lead to tremor, but are not easily reproduced. In the brainstem, surgical targeting of the ventral medial tegmentum and the cerebellum has led to more reproducible induction of tremor. Experimental destruction of the ventral medial tegmentum in nonhuman primates results in a tremor with features similar to Holmes tremor (a symptomatic tremor with a combination of rest, intention, and occasionally postural tremor). Cooling of the lateral cerebellar nuclei in nonhuman primates creates an intention tremor. Finally, there are a number of spontaneous genetic animal models of tremor including mice *(trembler, wobbler, jimpy,* and *shiverer)*, Springer Spaniel dogs *(shaking pups)*, and the Pietrain pig *(Campus syndrome)*. The tremulous pig, as a model of human orthostatic tremor, is similar to the human condition since it does not show any pathologic abnormality. Many of the animal models of tremor have tremor frequencies that are different from that seen in the human condition. Despite these differences, the molecular changes characterized in these models may provide insight into the pathophysiology of tremor in humans.

Myoclonus

Myoclonus is characterized by sudden shock-like involuntary movements that consist of either muscle contractions (positive myoclonus) or inhibitions (negative myoclonus). The most common cause of myoclonus in humans is cerebral hypoxia-ischemia, secondary to transient cardiac arrest. The underlying mechanism of myoclonus may involve altered serotonergic neurotransmission. Treatments that increase serotonergic neurotransmission, such as 5-hydroxytryptophan (5-HTP), are reported to be beneficial. Many animal models for myoclonus have been developed through the systemic administration of pharmacologic or toxic substances (26). Of the toxin-induced models 1,1,1-trichloro-2,2-bis(*p*-chlorophenyl)ethane (DDT) has been the most widely studied (21). In mice, DDT produces persistent stimulus sensitive myoclonic movements that evolve over a 5-hour period. Similar to the human condition, myoclonus in this model is improved with administration of 5-HTP and other serotonergic agonists. A pharmacological model of transient myoclonus that targets serotonergic neurotransmission in guinea pig is through the administration of 5,7-dihydroxytryptamine (5,7-DHT) (9). Although posthypoxic myoclonus is the most common form of myoclonus in humans, it has been a difficult model to create due to high mortality. Two different approaches have utilized either potassium chloride with cessation of ventilation or mechanical carotid obstruction with cardiac compression to induced cardiac arrest (54). Studies from these models have supported that enhanced serotonergic neurotransmission may have therapeutic benefit for the treatment of myoclonus.

Tardive Dyskinesia

Tardive dyskinesia (TD) is a syndrome characterized by repetitive involuntary movements involving the mouth, face, tongue, limbs, and trunk. TD occurs after long-term administration of neuroleptics, may persist for months or longer after termination of treatment, and may even be permanent. Animal models for TD have been described in both rodents and nonhuman primates (17). Nonhuman primates, following long-term treatment (over several years) with neuroleptics, develop either focal (head or neck) or generalized (limbs and truck) dystonic and choreiform movements. Similar to the case of humans, treatment with dopamine or acetylcholine receptor antagonists, or GABA agonists alleviates TD symptoms. Rodent models of TD generated through shorter neuroleptic treatment in comparison with nonhuman primates manifest only vacuous chewing movements. Studies from these animal models of TD have supported dopamine receptor hypersensitivity and insufficient GABA neurotransmission as mechanisms underlying TD.

CONCLUSION

Animal models allow investigation of aspects of movement disorders not possible in humans or through in vitro studies. The utility of these models is dependent on how closely they replicate the human condition with respect to behavior, neurochemistry, or pathology. Researchers have attempted to develop or identify animal models that mimic some, if not most, of the features seen in the human. Characterization of the neurochemical, molecular, behavioral, and anatomic changes occurring in different models provides insight into the underlying mechanisms involved in normal CNS function, neurodegeneration, and neuroplasticity. Models of rodents, cats, pigs, and nonhuman primates allow for efficacy and evaluation testing of new therapeutic modalities. It must be appreciated that these models have limitations because the behavioral repertoire and brain anatomy are not identical to that of humans. In addition, many neurotoxic and pharmacologically induced models are generated in an acute fashion and generally not progressive as are the chronic progressive neurodegenerative diseases they mimic. Despite these limitations animal models continue to make significant contributions to the management and cure of many movement disorders.

ACKNOWLEDGMENTS

We thank our colleagues at the University of Southern California for their support. Thanks to Beth Fisher, Mickie Welsh, Mark Liker, Kerry Nixon, and Mark Lew for their helpful discussions. Studies in our laboratory were made possible through the generous support of the Parkinson's Disease Foundation, the Baxter Foundation, the Zumberge Foundation, and the Akerberg Foundation. Special thanks to the friends of the Division of Movement Disorders for their generous support. Thanks also to Nicolaus, Pascal, and Dominique for their patience.

REFERENCES

1. Abeliovich A, Schmitz Y, Farinas I, et al. Mice lacking alpha-synuclein display functional deficits in the nigrostriatal dopamine system. *Neuron* 2000;25:239–252.
2. Annett LE, Rogers DC, Hernandez TD, et al. Behavioral analysis of unilateral monoamine depletion in the marmoset. *Brain* 1992;115:825–856.
3. Bankiewicz KS, Oldfield EH, Chiueh CC, et al. Hemiparkinsonism in monkeys after unilateral internal carotid infusion of 1-methyl-4-phenyl-1,2,3,6-tetrahydropyridine. *Life Sci* 1986; 39:7–16.
4. Bergman H, Raz A, Feingold A, et al. Physiology of MPTP tremor. *Mov Disord* 1998;13:29–34.
5. Betarbet R, Sherer TB, MacKenzie G, et al. Chronic systemic pesticide exposure reproduces features of Parkinson's disease. *Nat Neurosci* 2000;3:1301–1306.
6. Bezard E, Brotchie JM, Gross CE. Pathophysiology of levodopa-induced dyskinesia: potential for new therapies. *Nat Rev Neurosci* 2001;2:577–588.
7. Birkmayer W, Hornykiewicz O. Der 1-3,4-dioxy-phenylanin (l-DOPA)-effek bei der Parkinson-akinesia. *Klin Wochenschr* 1961; 73:787.
8. Brundin P, Emgard M, Mundt-Petersen U. Grafts of embryonic dopamine neurons in rodent models of Parkinson's disease. In: Tuszynski MH, Kordower J, ed. *CNS regeneration: basic and clinical applications.* San Diego: Academic Press, 1999: 299–320.
9. Carvey P, Paulseth JE, Goetz CG, et al. L-5-HTP-induced myoclonic jumping behavior in guinea pigs: an update. *Adv Neurol* 1986;43:509–517.
10. Cha JH, Kosinski CM, Kerner JA, et al. Altered brain neurotransmitter receptors in transgenic mice expressing a portion of an abnormal human Huntington disease gene. *Proc Natl Acad Sci USA* 1998;95:6480–6485.
11. Chesselet M-F, Levine MS. Mouse models of Huntington's disease. In: Chesselet M-F, ed. *Molecular mechanisms of neurodegenerative diseases.* Totowa, NJ: Humana Press, 2000:327–346.
12. Coyle JT, Schwarcz R. Lesion of striatal neurones with kainic acid provides a model for Huntington's chorea. *Nature* 1976; 263:244–246.
13. Davis GC, Williams AC, Markey SP, et al. Chronic parkinsonism secondary to intravenous injection of meperidine analogues. *Psychiatry Res* 1979;1:249–254.
14. Ehringer H, Hornykiewicz O. Verteilung von noradrenalin und dopamin (3-hydroxytyramin) in gehrindes menschen und ihr verhalten bei erkrankungen des extrapyramidalen systems. *Klin Wochenschr* 1960;38:1238–1239.
15. Ghorayeb I, Fernagut PO, Aubert I, et al. Toward a primate model of L-dopa-unresponsive parkinsonism mimicking striatonigral degeneration. *Mov Disord* 2000;15:531–536.
16. Ghorayeb I, Puschban Z, Fernagut PO, et al. Simultaneous intrastriatal 6-hydroxydopamine and quinolinic acid injection: a model of early-stage striatonigral degeneration. *Exp Neurol* 2001;167:133–147.
17. Gunne LM, Haggstrom JE. Experimental tardive dyskinesia. *J Clin Psychiatry* 1985;46:48–50.
18. Harvey DC, Lacan G, Melega WP. Regional heterogeneity of dopaminerigc deficits in vervet monkey striatum and substantia nigra after methamphetamine exposure. *Exp Brain Res* 2000; 133:349–358.
19. Heintz N, Zoghbi HY. Insights from mouse models into the molecular basis of neurodegeneration. *Annu Rev Physiol* 2000; 62:779–802.
20. Hodgson JG, Agopyan N, Gutekunst CA, et al. A YAC mouse model for Huntington's disease with full-length mutant *huntingtin*, cytoplasmic toxicity, and selective striatal neurodegeneration. *Neuron* 1999;23:181–192.
21. Hwang EC, Van Woert MH. DDT-induced myoclonus: serotonin and alpha noradrenergic interaction. *Res Commun Chem Pathol Pharmacol* 1979;23:257–266.
22. Imam SZ, el-Yazal J, Newport GD, et al. Methamphetamine-induced dopaminergic neurotoxicity: role of peroxynitrite and neuroprotective role of antioxidants and peroxynitrite decomposition catalysts. *Ann NY Acad Sci* 2001;939:366–380.
23. Ishihara T, Hong M, Zhang B, et al. Age-dependent emergence and progression of a tauopathy in transgenic mice overexpressing the shortest human tau isoform. *Neuron* 1999;24:751–762.
24. Jakowec MW, Donaldson DM, Barba J, et al. The postnatal expression of α-synuclein in the substantia nigra and striatum of the rodent. *Dev Neurosci* 2001;23:91–99.
25. Kahle PJ, Neumann M, Ozmen L, et al. Subcellular localization of wild-type and Parkinson's disease–associated mutant alpha-synuclein in human and transgenic mouse brain. *J Neurosci* 2000;20:6365–6373.
26. Kanthasamy AG, Nguyen BQ, Truong DD. Animal model of posthypoxic myoclonus: II. Neurochemical, pathologic, and pharmacologic characterization. *Mov Disord* 2000;15:31–38.
27. Langston JW, Ballard P, Tetrud JW, et al. Chronic parkinsonism in humans due to a product of meperidine-analog synthesis. *Science* 1983;219:979–980.
28. Mangiarini L, Sathasivam K, Seller M, et al. Exon 1 of the *HD* gene with an expanded CAG repeat is sufficient to cause a progressive neurological phenotype in transgenic mice. *Cell* 1996; 87:493–506.
29. Masliah E, Rockenstein E, Veinbergs I, et al. Dopaminergic loss and inclusion body formation in alpha-synuclein mice: implications for neurodegenerative disorders. *Science* 2000;289: 1265–1269.
30. McGeer EG, McGeer PL. Duplication of biochemical changes of Huntington's chorea by intrastriatal injections of glutamic and kainic acids. *Nature* 1976;263:517–519.
31. Payne AP, Campbell JM, Russell D, et al. The AS/AGU rat: a spontaneous model of disruption and degeneration in the nigrostriatal dopaminergic system. *J Anat* 2000;196:629–633.
32. Petzinger GM, Langston JW. The MPTP-lesioned non-human primate: a model for Parkinson's disease. In: Marwah J, Teitelbaum H, eds. *Advances in neurodegenerative disease,* vol 1: *Parkinson's disease.* Scottsdale, AZ: Prominent Press, 1998: 113–148.
33. Polymeropoulos M, Lavendan C, Leroy E, et al. Mutation in the α-synuclein gene identified in families with Parkinson's disease. *Science* 1997;276:2045–2047.
34. Przedborski S, Jackson-Lewis V, Naini AB, et al. The parkinsonian toxin 1-methyl-4-phenyl-1,2,3,6-tetrahydropyridine (MPTP): a technical review of its utility and safety. *J Neurochem* 2001;76:1265–1274.
35. Reddy PH, Charles V, Williams M, et al. Transgenic mice expressing mutated full-length HD cDNA: a paradigm for locomotor changes and selective neuronal loss in Huntington's disease. *Phil Trans R Soc London B Biol Sci* 1999;354:1035–1045.
36. Richter A, Ebert U, Nobrega JN, et al. Immunohistochemical and neurochemical studies on nigral and striatal functions in the circling (ci) rat, a genetic animal model with spontaneous rotational behavior. *Neuroscience* 1999;89:461–471.
37. Saucedo-Cardenas O, Quintana-Hau JD, Le WD, et al. Nurr1 is essential for the induction of the dopaminergic phenotype and

the survival of ventral mesencephalic late dopaminergic precursor neurons. *Proc Natl Acad Sci USA* 1998;95:4013–4018.

38. Saucedo-Cardenas O, Conneely OM. Comparative distribution of Nurr1 and Nur77 nuclear receptors in the mouse central nervous system. *J Mol Neurosci* 1996;7:51–63.

39. Le WD, Zou LL, Conneely OM, et al. Selective agenesis of mesencephalic dopaminergic neurons in Nurr1 deficient mice. *Mov Disord* 1998;13[Suppl 2]:184.

40. Le WD, Conneely OM, He Y, et al. Reduced Nurr1 expression increases the vulnerability of mesencephalic dopamine neurons to MPTP-induced injury. *J Neurochem* 1999;73:2218–2221.

41. Le WD, Dong ZJ, He Y, et al. Aged Nurr1+/− mice develop behavioral and biochemical changes consistent with parkinsonism. *Parkinsonism Rel Disord* 2001;7:S39.

42. Auluck PK, Chan HYE, Trojanowski JQ, et al. Chaperon suppression of α-synuclein toxicity in a *Drosophila* model for Parkinson's disease. *Science* 2002;295:865–868.

43. Richter A, Loscher W. Pathophysiology of idiopathic dystonia: findings from genetic animal models. *Prog Neurobiol* 1998;54: 633–677.

44. Richter A, Loscher W. Animal models of dystonia. *Func Neurol* 2000;15:259–267.

45. Rodriguez MB-CP, Abdala P, Obeso J, et al. Dopamine cell degeneration induced by intraventricular administration of 6-hydroxydopamine in the rat: similarities with cell loss in Parkinson's disease. *Exp Neurol* 2001;169:163–181.

46. Vila M, Jackson-Lewis V, Vukosavic S, et al. Bax ablation prevents dopaminergic neurodegeneration in the 1-methyl-4-phenyl-1,2,3,6-tetrahydropyridine mouse model of Parkinson's disease. *PNAS* 2001;98:2837–2842.

47. Vila M, Wu DC, Przedborski S. Engineered modeling and the secrets of Parkinson's disease. *Trends Neurosci* 2001;24[Suppl 1]: S49–S55.

48. Royland JE, Langston JW. MPTP: a dopamine neurotoxin. In: Kostrzewa R, ed. *Highly selective neurotoxins.* Totowa, NJ: Humana Press, 1998:141–194.

49. Sauer H, Oertel WH. Progressive degeneration of nigrostriatal dopamine neurons following intrastriatal terminal lesions with 6-hydroxydopamine: a combined retrograde tracing and immunocytochemical study in the rat. *Neuroscience* 1994;59: 401–415.

50. Schwarting RK, Huston JP. The unilateral 6-hydroxydopamine lesion model in behavioral brain research: analysis of functional deficits, recovery and treatments. *Prog Neurobiol* 1996;20: 275–331.

51. Schwarting RK, Huston JP. Unilateral 6-hydroxydopamine lesions of meso-striatal dopamine neurons and their physiological sequelae. *Prog Neurobiol* 1996;49:215–266.

52. Sonsalla PK, Jochnowitz ND, Zeevalk GD, et al. Treatment of mice with methamphetamine produces cell loss in the substantia nigra. *Brain Res* 1996;738:172–175.

53. Taylor JR, Elsworth JD, Roth RH, et al. Severe long-term 1-methyl-4-phenyl-1,2,3,6-tetrahydropyridine-induced parkinsonism in the vervet monkey *(Cercopithecus aethiops sabaeus). Neuroscience* 1997;81:745–755.

54. Truong DDKA, Nguyen B, Matsumoto R, et al. Animal models of posthypoxic myoclonus: I. Development and validation. *Mov Disord* 2000;15:26–30.

55. Ungerstedt U. 6-Hydroxy-dopamine induced degeneration of central monoamine neurons. *Eur J Pharmacol* 1968;5:107–110.

56. Ungerstedt U. Postsynaptic supersensitivity after 6-hydroxy-dopamine induced degeneration of the nigro-striatal dopamine system. *Acta Physiol Scand [Suppl]* 1971;367:69–93.

57. Ungerstedt U, Arbuthnott GW. Quantitative recording of rotational behavior in rats after 6-hydroxydopamine lesions of the nigrostriatal dopamine system. *Brain Res* 1970;24:485–493.

58. Wilms H, Sievers J, Deuschl G. Animal models of tremor. *Mov Disord* 1999;14:557–571.

59. Wittmann CW, Wszolek MF, Shulman JM, et al. Tauopathy in *Drosophila:* neurodegeneration without neurofibrillary tangles. *Science* 2001;293:711–714.

60. Zigmond MJ, Abercrombie ED, Berger TW, et al. Compensations after lesions of central dopaminergic neurons: some clinical and basic implications. *Trends Neurosci* 1990;13:290–295.

EPIDEMIOLOGY OF MOVEMENT DISORDERS

ANETTE SCHRAG

Epidemiology serves several purposes: to describe the occurrence of disorders, time trends, and geographic differences in their frequency; to identify risk factors that may give clues to the etiology of disorders; to provide information for the planning of health care resources; and to give estimates for the prognosis of a disorder. However, epidemiologic studies are usually time consuming and expensive, and restrictions in resources therefore often limit the methodologic rigor that is crucial to the validity of such studies. Differences in the study design, especially case ascertainment methods and inclusion criteria, have important influence on the results of these studies. Epidemiologic studies of movement disorders are particularly complicated by the lack of diagnostic markers that allow an unequivocal diagnosis and by the differences in diagnostic criteria for most movement disorders. As a consequence, there are variations in diagnostic accuracy, which are reflected in prevalence rates (number of persons affected at a particular time in a defined population) and incidence rates (number of new cases developing over a defined period of time in a defined population at risk). Furthermore, many epidemiologic studies require large numbers, which will not be easily achieved for some of the rarer disorders. Conclusions from epidemiologic studies should therefore consider the methodology used, particularly in comparisons across studies.

A number of studies have been performed in Parkinson's disease, and great advances in genetic and epidemiologic studies in this disorder have been made in recent years. Few epidemiologic data exist for some of the rarer movement disorders, such as paroxysmal movement disorders. However, there is also increasing knowledge about the epidemiology of other akinetic movement disorders, tremor, dystonia, and other hyperkinetic movement disorders, which will be reviewed in this chapter.

PARKINSONISM

Parkinson's Disease

Prevalence

When comparing the results of prevalence studies across geographically and temporally different populations, a number of caveats require consideration to avoid erroneous conclusions. In particular, the method of ascertainment has dramatic influence on the results obtained, as do the choice of diagnostic criteria, the amount of information lost because of nonresponse, the age distribution of the population studied, and survival time. Door-to-door studies, the most time- and cost-intensive of prevalence studies, generally yield higher prevalence rates than studies based on review of medical records and previously made diagnosis, with the percentage of previously undiagnosed cases ranging from 10% to 50%, depending on the health care system in each country (1).

Although the prevalence rates of Parkinson's disease (PD) vary between 18 and 418 per 100,000 worldwide (2), the variations are much less marked when the differences between study methodology are considered. Age-adjustment and restriction to studies using similar methodology reduce the variation between prevalence rates to between 102 and 190 per 100,000 population, at least in Western countries. Using unified diagnostic criteria, relative similarity of ascertainment methods, and age adjustment of results, the Europarkinson study (1) reported the prevalence rates from five European countries within a similar range. However, clusters with a high prevalence of PD have been reported, e.g., in Iceland (2) or on the Faeroe Islands, where prevalence of PD was considerably higher than on the Danish mainland or a neighboring island when the same ascertainment methods were used (3). Similarly, in India and Sicily high prevalence rates of PD have been reported, even when adjustment for differences in age distribution were made (4,5). Conversely, low prevalence rates were reported in other populations, such as in Romanian Gypsies (6) and in northern Africa (7). Although such differences may in large part reflect the sometimes marked differences in methodology, they may also indicate actual differences in the occurrence of PD, which may be due to differences in genetic background or, alternatively, in environmental exposures. This question has been further addressed by a small number of studies comparing prevalence of PD in bi- or multiethnic populations, but the results are conflicting. In a study in New York City over a 4-year period

(1988–1991), the age-adjusted prevalence rates were lower for blacks than for whites and Hispanics, although cumulative incidence was higher for blacks, and more deaths occurred among incident black cases, suggesting that in black patients survival with PD is shorter (8). In a door-to-door survey in Cuba, prevalence rates of PD were higher in white than nonwhite subjects (9). Schoenberg et al. conducted two comparative studies with similar case ascertainment methods and identical diagnostic criteria (10). In the biracial population of Copiah County, Mississippi, the prevalence rates of PD in the white and the black population were similar. In Nigeria, on the other hand, the age-adjusted prevalence of PD was five times lower (11), suggesting that geographic differences not due to ethnic differences may influence the risk of PD. Along the same lines are the results of prevalence studies in China and Taiwan, populations that share a genetic background but have different levels of industrialization, which have yielded markedly different prevalence rates (14.6 versus 119 per 100,000) (12–14). The results of these latter studies suggest that environmental factors play an important role in the occurrence of PD in populations of similar genetic background.

Incidence

A better indicator for the frequency of a chronic disorder in the population than prevalence is the incidence rate, as it is independent of survival, which may vary in temporally or geographically separated populations. However, such studies require larger study populations and/or longer observation times and are therefore much rarer. Reported annual incidence rates of PD range from 4.9 to 26 per 100,000 (15–19). The longitudinal epidemiologic study in Rochester, Minnesota, using review of detailed medical records, reported an annual incidence rate of parkinsonism of 114.7 per 100,000 in the age group 50–99, increasing from 0.8 in the age group 0 to 29 years to 304.8 in the age group 80 to 99 years (17). In an Italian study, the reported annual incidence of PD was 326.3 per 100,000 in those aged 64 to 84 (20). However, the same caveats regarding comparability as for prevalence rates apply.

Association of Sex and Age with Prevalence and Incidence Rates

PD is rare before age 50 years and increases with age to affect approximately 2% in those aged 65 and above (21). Although many record-based studies reported lower prevalence rates in the eldest age group (22), door-to-door studies have not confirmed this drop in prevalence rate in those over 80 (21,23). It appears likely that PD is less frequently diagnosed in older patients, in part due to the difficulties in differentiating features of PD from those of ageing, such as postural instability and a small-stepped gait (24,25). Simi-

lar ascertainment bias may in part be responsible for the slight male predominance of PD, reported by many record- and clinic-based studies, as few door-to-door studies could confirm this. However, one prospective cohort study in an Italian population aged 65 to 84 also found a 2.13-fold increased risk of PD in men compared with women using screening and personal examination (20). As suggested by Tanner and Aston, a male preponderance, if confirmed in future population-based studies, could suggest an increased X-linked genetic disposition or influence of sex hormones on disease risk or, alternatively, greater exposure to a causative environmental factor in men (26).

Time Trends

Although it has been suggested that PD was rare before the 19th century, recent prevalence data indicate no marked change overall in occurrence over time. However, analysis of mortality and prevalence data suggests that age-specific mortality increased in older and decreased in younger age groups (27). Two recent incidence studies have directly investigated the pattern of PD incidence over time. In Rochester, Minnesota, no significant change in incidence rates from 1976 to 1990 was identified in a well-documented medical record system (28). In contrast, in a Finnish study, Kuopio et al. found an increase in prevalence of PD from 1971 to 1992 from 139 to 166 and in annual incidence of PD from 14.9 to 15.7 per 100,000, which was associated with male predominance and rural living (18), and suggested that an increased susceptibility in men and/or a greater exposure to an environmental risk factor in men may account for this increase in the incidence of PD.

Analytic Epidemiology

Genetic Factors

Family history has consistently been reported to be associated with an increased risk of PD compared with controls, suggesting that genetic factors play a role in the etiology of PD (29–31). However, it is uncertain whether this reflects an increased genetic susceptibility, pure genetic inheritance, shared familial exposure, or biased recall in families of patients with PD (26). Twin studies are of particular value to address this question. If genetic factors play an important role in the etiology of a disorder, the concordance rates in monozygotic twins are higher than in dizygotic twins. However, most twin studies have not confirmed an overall increased risk of PD in monozygotic twins compared with dizygotic twins (32,33). Tanner et al. conducted the largest of such twin studies in a cohort of World War II veterans in the United States (34). They found no overall difference in concordance rates in monozygotic twins compared with dizygotic twins, arguing for a lack of genetic causation of PD. However, in twins with age of onset below 50 years, the concordance rate in monozygotic twins was significantly increased with 1.0 compared with 0.167 in dizygotic twins. The relative risk was 6.0 (95% confidence interval, 1.69–21.26). These results suggested that genetic factors contribute significantly to the development of PD in those with young onset but do not play a major role in causing typical PD. Positron emission tomography (PET) studies in twins have also been used to assess the genetic contribution to PD. In a PET study in 9 monozygotic twins and 12 dizygotic twins, Vieregge et al. found that the concordance rates in both groups were similar when assessed 8 years apart, arguing against a genetic contribution to PD (35). In contrast, Piccini et al. found that the concordance for subclinical striatal dopaminergic dysfunction was significantly higher in 18 monozygotic than in 16 dizygotic twin pairs. In addition, the asymptomatic monozygotic cotwins all showed progressive loss of dopaminergic function over 7 years and 4 developed clinical PD, whereas none of the dizygotic twin pairs became clinically concordant, arguing for an underlying susceptibility in monozygotic twins of patients with PD (36).

One of the greatest discoveries in the last years in PD research has been the recognition that there are families in whom PD is genetically determined. However, mutations in the α-synuclein gene, inherited in an autosomal dominant pattern, account for only a small number of cases (37). The autosomal recessively inherited *parkin* gene, on the other hand, appears to account for a substantial minority of cases of sporadic PD (38). Although the typical phenotype of *parkin*-related parkinsonism differs from typical PD, the phenotype related to *parkin* mutations is wide and includes typical cases of PD (39). Nevertheless, it appears that in the great majority of PD cases such gene defect is not an etiologic factor. These results suggest that there is a genetic contribution to PD, but whether this contribution is restricted to a small number of cases or a smaller contribution relevant to the majority of cases is unclear. For a detailed discussion of the genetics of PD see Chapter 7.

Environmental Factors

The discovery that 1-methyl-4-phenyl-1,2,3,6-tetrahydropyridine (MPTP), a street drug contaminant, can cause human parkinsonism similar to that in PD has lend strong momentum to the hypothesis that PD may be caused by a single environmental toxin. In addition, infectious disease as a cause of PD has been implicated by the endemic encephalitis lethargica leading to postencephalitic parkinsonism. However, the lack of convincing marked geographic or temporal differences in prevalence and incidence rates does not strongly support an environmental exposure as the major cause of PD. Case-control studies in patients with PD, which have attempted to identify potential risk factors for the development of PD, have despite their abundance also not identified strong evidence for a single environmental cause. The most consistent finding in these studies has been the negative association of smoking with the development of PD (40,41),

but the exact nature of this relationship is unclear. Possible reasons for this association range from selective survival of nonsmokers (which is unlikely as this negative association is also seen in early-onset cases) to protective effects of smoking to the existence of a common predisposing factor, including personality (22). Other life exposures that have less consistently been found to be associated with PD are working on a farm or having a job that involves head trauma (30), exposure to pesticides (29,42), well-water drinking, and rural living (43). More recently, frequency of bowel movements, coffee drinking, alcohol consumption, and hypertension (44–47) have also been reported to be inversely related to PD, independent of smoking history (48). Furthermore, it has been reported that individuals working as teachers or those occupied in health care in Greater Vancouver had a 2- to 2.5-fold risk of PD compared with controls (49). The likelihood that a single environmental factor causes PD is therefore small, and it has been proposed that several environmental causes contribute to the development of PD (50), or that genetic and environmental factors act synergistically to cause PD (30,51).

Prognosis

Controversy exists with respect to the prognosis of PD. It appears clear that even patients with typical PD may present with considerable variation in phenotype and rate of progression. Some studies have described that presence of gait disturbance is associated with faster disease progression and an increased risk of death (25,52), and other studies have reported that those with older age at onset have a faster rate of progression and a higher incidence of dementia (52–55), but a lower rate of motor complications (55,56). However, with the exception of parkinsonism associated with the mutations described, no pathologic, genetic, or environmental factor has been identified to explain the variation in rate of progression and complications.

Life expectancy is decreased in patients with PD compared with the general population but reported mortality ratios vary considerably between 1.2 and 3.1 compared with age-matched controls or the general population (5,25, 53,57–59). Whether mortality has decreased as a result of dopaminergic treatment remains a matter of controversy. Although few data are available from the pre-levodopa era, mortality data appear to have remained the same, indicating that treatment has not resulted in an improved mortality despite the improvements in quality of life (60). In contrast to control populations, the most common cause of death is pneumonia (5,61).

Atypical Parkinsonism

Pathologic studies suggested that up to 35% of patients with a clinical diagnosis of PD coming to autopsy suffered from a different disorder, most commonly progressive supranuclear palsy (PSP), Alzheimer's disease, multiple system atrophy (MSA), and vascular disease (62–64). Until recently, few studies existed on prevalence and incidence rate of the atypical forms of parkinsonism, including PSP, MSA, and corticobasal degeneration, and these disorders, if differentiated from PD, were often excluded from epidemiologic studies. However, it has become increasingly clear that these disorders are more common than previously thought (65–69).

Progressive Supranuclear Palsy

The first prevalence study of PSP, conducted in New Jersey (70), yielded a prevalence rate of 1.4 per 100,000, approximately 1% of the prevalence of PD. However, the authors emphasized that this was likely to be an underestimate as only diagnosed cases were ascertained and the rate of unrecognized cases was assumed to be high. Since this early study, two population-based studies using standardized diagnostic criteria have reported higher prevalence rates compared with that previously believed, with 5 to 6 cases of PSP per 100,000, a large proportion of which were undiagnosed prior to the studies (65,66). The incidence of PSP has been reported from 0.3 to 1.1 per 100,000 (71). The most recent study from Olmsted county, Minnesota, which retrospectively analyzed a detailed medical record system and used standardized diagnostic criteria, reported an incidence rate of 5.3 cases per 100,000 in the ages 50 to 99 (72), which corresponds to the reported prevalence rates in this age group (7). Although few data from different geographic regions are available, PSP has been described in ethnically different populations (73–75), and in the French West Indies atypical parkinsonism and PSP have been reported to be overrepresented compared with European and North American populations (76). It has been hypothesized that this high prevalence is due to alimentary causes, such as the consumption of neurotoxic alkaloids contained in herbal teas and tropical fruit (76). It has also been speculated that atypical parkinsonism is more common in individuals of Afro-Caribbean and Indian origin in the PD population in London, England (77), but no epidemiologic data on differential frequency of atypical parkinsonism in these populations are available. Most clinic- and population-based studies reported a slight male preponderance in PSP (72,78,79), but confidence intervals in epidemiologic studies are wide, due to relatively small numbers. The incidence of PSP increases with advancing age (80) with a mean age at onset in the seventh decade. No case of PSP with onset before age 40 has been reported (79,81). Reported mean survival time ranges from 5.3 to 9.7 years (70,72,79,82) with pathologically confirmed survival time up to 18 years (83). Although the majority of cases with PSP are sporadic, several families with at least two members with PSP have been reported (80). Genetic studies have shown that PSP is associated with inheritance of a specific genotype (H1/H1)

in the *tau* gene. Litvan et al. investigated whether the genotype independently or in conjunction with selected environmental risk factors influences the age at onset, severity, or survival in patients with PSP, but found that tau genotyping did not appear to predict the prognosis of PSP (84). Similarly, two other studies did not find any effect of tau genotype on the age of onset of PSP (85,86). Despite the discovery that *tau* dysfunction is somehow involved in the pathogenesis of PSP, it is also possible that nongenetic factors contribute to neuronal degeneration in PSP. Two case-control studies have been conducted to date that show conflictual results with regard to education and residence in rural areas. Davis et al. (87) conducted a case-control study of 50 cases in New Jersey. The results suggested that rural residence and greater educational attainment but not history of smoking may be significant risk factors for PSP. On the other hand, in a subsequent study of 91 patients, the same authors reported that patients with PSP were found to be less likely to have completed at least 12 years of school. The authors hypothesized that lower level of education may be a proxy for poor early-life nutrition or for occupational or residential exposure to an unknown toxin (88).

Multiple System Atrophy

Multiple system atrophy accounts for 8% to 22% of patients diagnosed with PD coming to pathologic examination (63,64). Although pathologic studies are likely to be biased toward more frequent atypical cases (24), this indicates that MSA is less rare than previously thought. Two recent epidemiologic studies have found that it affects four to five people in a population of 100,000 people (65,68). However, these data are likely to be conservative, as patients not initially presenting with parkinsonism but autonomic failure or ataxia may not have been included in these studies. An incidence study in Olmsted County, Minnesota, using specific criteria, found 9 cases in the years 1976 to 1990 (72), yielding an annual incidence rate of 3.0 per 100,000 for the ages 50 to 99. Given a median survival of 5 to 9 years (89–93), this is comparable to the prevalence rates found in Europe. Symptoms of MSA most commonly begin in the sixth decade with an average age at onset of 54 (90,91,93), but the age of onset ranges between the fourth and eighth decade (90). MSA has been more commonly reported in men, but few population-based data are available to confirm this. Only one case-control study of MSA was performed more than 10 years ago (94). It included 60 MSA patients and 60 controls, and reported a greater exposure to metal dusts and fumes, plastic monomers and additives, organic solvents, and pesticides in the MSA compared with controls. In addition, symptoms of MSA in relatives were reported by a significantly larger group of patients' relatives than controls (23% vs. 10%). The authors hypothesized that MSA develops as a result of a genetically determined selective vulnerability in the nervous system.

However, in contrast to PSP, no case of familial MSA has been reported, and evidence for an association of genetic factors and MSA is scarce (85,95). A second case-control study is under way (69). An inverse relationship of MSA and smoking habits, similar to that in PD, has also been reported (96).

Distribution of Parkinsonism

The population prevalence of parkinsonism due to vascular disease or use of dopamine receptor–blocking drugs are not well known as these are often excluded from prevalence and incidence studies. They also strongly depend on the frequency on such drug use and the age distribution of the population studied. In the incidence study from Olmsted County, Minnesota, Bower et al. reported that only 42% of all cases of parkinsonism in the years 1976 to 1991 had PD (17). The main differential diagnosis included drug-induced parkinsonism (20%), unspecified parkinsonism (17%), parkinsonism in dementia (14%), and parkinsonism due to other causes (7%). Four percent had PSP, 2% had MSA, and only one patient had a diagnosis of vascular parkinsonism (less than 1%). This is in contrast to the study by Rajput et al. who, using the same hospital record system during the preceding decade, reported that 86% of patients with parkinsonism had PD, 7% drug-induced parkinsonism, and 1% to 2% had PSP, MSA, and vascular parkinsonism, respectively (16). More recent studies from other geographic areas have reported patterns of distribution in between the results of the two studies from Olmsted County. Baldereschi et al. (20) found that 62% of incident cases of parkinsonism in an elderly population had PD, 10% drug-induced parkinsonism, 12% parkinsonism in dementia, 12% vascular parkinsonism, and 6% unspecified parkinsonism. Morgante et al. in Sicily reported 69% had PD, 9% drug-induced parkinsonism, and 8% vascular parkinsonism (5), and Schrag et al. (97) found that 66% of all patients with parkinsonism had PD, 18% drug-induced parkinsonism, 7% vascular parkinsonism, 6% atypical parkinsonism, and 2% parkinsonism in dementia (but dementia clearly starting before onset was an exclusion criterion). Postencephalitic parkinsonism, once representing a large proportion of patients with parkinsonism following the worldwide epidemic of encephalitis lethargica between 1916 and 1927, is now rare, as no new epidemics have occurred. However, it is believed that occasional cases of postencephalitic parkinsonism continue to occur.

HYPERKINETIC MOVEMENT DISORDERS

Essential Tremor

Essential tremor (ET) is probably the most common movement disorder. However, prevalence rates vary widely as epidemiologic studies of ET are hampered by the lack of a bio-logic marker or a clearly delineated clinical phenotype. It is likely that ET is clinically, pathophysiologically, and genetically a heterogeneous condition (98,99), and phenotypic overlap in the phenotype with other conditions exists. The most difficult differential diagnoses are (a) enhanced physiologic tremor, (b) tremor occurring in association with other conditions, such as dystonia, PD, and peripheral neuropathy, and (c) isolated tremor syndromes, such as voice tremor, which may be either a form fruste of ET or a different condition. A particularly controversial area is the differentiation of ET from tremor in dystonia. Dubinski et al. found that, although typical ET was found in only 8 of 296 patients in a record review of patients with focal or generalized dystonia (100), a type of tremor was found in 46 (15.5%). Singer et al. reported in a recent prevalence study of dystonia that tremor occurred in approximately 40% of patients with adult-onset idiopathic focal and segmental dystonia. Eighteen percent had dystonic tremor (tremor in a body part affected by dystonia) and 21% had tremor associated with dystonia (tremor in a different body part) (101). Conversely, in a large study of 678 patients diagnosed with ET, 6.9% also had a coexisting dystonia (102), whereas in another study of 350 patients with ET from a movement disorders clinic, half of all patients (47%) had associated dystonia (103). Electrophysiologic studies reveal differences between tremor in dystonia in some tests between patients with isolated tremor and those with tremor and dystonia (98,104,105). However, a reliable clinical differentiation of individual patients is currently not possible. Some epidemiologic studies therefore excluded patients with dystonia from their analysis, whereas others included them. Another difficulty is the controversy on an association of ET with PD. Some authors contend that ET may predispose to the development of PD (106), whereas others (107) have not been able to confirm an increased association between ET and PD. Various types of neuropathy can be associated with tremor, but the mechanism of this association is poorly understood (108). Finally, an association of tremor with migraine has been demonstrated in familial and sporadic ET (109). Epidemiologic studies of ET are also complicated by the fact that the majority of individuals with tremor have mild symptoms, which may not lead to consultation with a physician or even remain unnoticed by affected subjects and their families. In addition, in many cases there is no positive family history of tremor, even when all family members are examined. Whether these sporadic cases have the same condition or are different from familial ET is unclear, and studies have varied with respect to inclusion of patients without a positive family history of tremor. These difficulties in diagnosis are reflected in the differences between diagnostic criteria that have been employed in epidemiologic studies and the great variability of the results of these studies. Louis et al demonstrated that the use of different diagnostic criteria results in widely varying prevalence rates (110). Standardization of diagnostic criteria such as the criteria of the Tremor Research Investigation Group (TIRG) will increase the consistency of findings, but their validity will only become evident when a biologic marker becomes available. Taking into account the limitations of comparability of studies using different ascertainment and diagnostic methods, the prevalence rates ranged from 0.01% to 22% (111). In an analysis of only those studies that provided diagnostic criteria for ET, defined ET as an action tremor, and used community-based rather than service-based designs, Louis et al. (111) reported a narrower range of prevalence rates from 0.4% to 3.9% in the overall population and from 1.3% to 5% in those over the age of 60 years. Incidence data are far fewer than prevalence rates, ranging from 8 per 100,000 per year (15) to 23.7 per 100,000 in a longitudinal study in Rochester, Minnesota (112). This study also showed an increase in annual age- and sex-adjusted incidence rate from 5.8 in 1935–1949 to 23.7 in 1964–1979, most likely resulting from underdiagnosis of ET in earlier years. Despite the differences in diagnosis and case ascertainment, which make it difficult to compare incidence and prevalence rates, it is clear that the prevalence of ET increases with age. In one study, the age at onset showed bimodal distribution with peaks in the second and sixth decades (103). In a Finnish study (113), the peak prevalence of ET was 12.6% in the age group 70–79 years, and in a study in Mississippi, there was a tenfold higher prevalence in those aged 70–79 compared with those aged 40–69 (114). In an incidence study from Rochester, Minnesota, incidence rates continuously increased up to the oldest age group with a sharp increase after age 49 (112). However, in a study by Bain et al., which restricted the analysis to family members of index cases with familial ET, all affected family members were symptomatic by the age of 50 with a bimodal age of tremor onset and a median onset age of 15 years (115). Tremor severity and disability, on the other hand, increased with advancing age and tremor duration, possibly in part accounting for the finding of increasing prevalence in cross-sectional studies. Life expectancy of patients with ET is similar to that of the general population, although ET has also been claimed to increase longevity (106,116). Apart from a few studies that found a higher prevalence in women (114) or men (117), ET is largely found to be equally common in women and men. Although few comparative data across different ethnic populations are available, two studies have reported a slightly higher prevalence of ET in white than black Americans (114,117).

ET is generally thought to be an autosomal dominantly inherited condition with high but age-dependent penetrance (115). However, the reported percentage of patients with ET with a family history ranges from 17.4% to 100%. This wide range may partly be artifactual and the result of different inclusion criteria as well as underreporting of a family history, but may also reflect the heterogeneity of this condition. The phenotype of pure autosomal dominantly

inherited essential tremor has been well described (115), but it is possible that other phenotypes also exist. Further description of the clinical phenotype will also provide better understanding about the heterogeneity of the condition. Linkage of familial cases of ET with the *DYT 1* gene for childhood-onset generalized dystonia has been excluded (118), but in isolated families linkage of ET to different chromosomes was established. In Iceland a locus on chromosome 3q13 was linked to 16 kindreds with ET fulfilling the TIRG criteria, named *FET1* (119), and linkage has also been reported to a locus on chromosome 2p22-25 (120,121) named *ETM* or *ET2*, but in other families with ET linkage to these loci has been excluded (122). Some studies have reported anticipation in successive generations of families with ET (120), but others could not confirm these findings (115,123), which may have resulted from heightened awareness in the families of such patients. To my knowledge, only one case-control study to assess the influence of nongenetic factors on the occurrence of ET has been reported. Exposure to agricultural chemicals and domestic animals were suggested as potential risk factors for the occurrence of ET, but this association was not statistically significant in this small study (28 controls and age-matched controls) (124).

DYSTONIA

Data on the prevalence of dystonia are likely to underestimate the true prevalence of the disorder, as dystonia is commonly underdiagnosed or underreported. In addition to the problems of all epidemiologic studies of movement disorders (lack of a pathologic substrate, reliance on a clinical diagnosis, and a high rate of underdiagnosis), there are also difficulties in the classification (e.g., primary vs. secondary dystonia, generalized vs. focal dystonia) that limit comparability of studies (125). However, since the early descriptions of primary torsion dystonia (PTD) (126), it has been recognized that dystonia is relatively common in Jewish populations, particularly in Jews of Eastern European ancestry (Ashkenazi) (127–130). The initial prevalence rate reported for PTD in Ashkenazi Jews in Israel was 10.8 per million (129), but this was later recognized to be an underestimate due to incomplete case ascertainment in this early survey, and subsequent reassessment of the population resulted in a higher prevalence rate of 4.3 per 100,000 for generalized dystonia (130). Dystonia has also been reported in many other ethnic groups, albeit with varying frequency (12,131–134). A review of hospital records at the Mayo Clinic in Rochester, Minnesota, over three decades (125) yielded prevalence rates of 3.4 per 100,000 for generalized dystonia and 29.5 for focal dystonia. A similarly high prevalence of focal dystonia was also reported in an abstract from Spain (134), where prevalence of focal dystonia was 27.9 per 100,000. A combined approach of case record review, inclusion of members of the Dystonia Society, and recruitment from the population through advertising and raising of awareness was used to determine the prevalence of dystonia in a study in northern England (135). The prevalence rates were slightly lower than in Rochester with 1.42 per 100,000 for generalized dystonia and 13 per 100,000 for focal dystonia. In a recent multinational European study (Epidemiologic Study of Dystonia in Europe, ESDE), the overall prevalence rate of focal dystonia based on diagnosed cases similarly was found to be 11.7 per 100,000 (136). There were considerable differences of prevalence rates across study centers but the authors attributed these mainly to differences in methodology. As the authors remarked, these data must be regarded as conservative estimates of a probably considerable higher population prevalence as these rates were based on already diagnosed cases. Prevalence data from a record review are also available from Japan, where the rates in the Tottori prefecture were reported as 0.2 for generalized and 6.1 for focal dystonia (137). This considerably lower prevalence figure than that from Minnesota may be due to genetic differences, as suggested by the authors, but may partly reflect differences in the rate of underdiagnosis in these hospital-based surveys. Therefore, population-based studies are of particular relevance, though few have been conducted (12,138). The prevalence rates reported from China (12) and Egypt (138) were comparatively low, with 5 cases of generalized and 3 cases of cervical dystonia per 100,000 in China, and 10 cases of focal dystonia per 100,000 in Egypt. In both studies the only focal dystonia seen was cervical dystonia, and in Egypt no cases with generalized dystonia were found. It has therefore been suggested (135) that case ascertainment was incomplete. A different approach was taken by Risch et al., who calculated the prevalence of early limb-onset generalized dystonia in Ashkenazim in New York from the number of affected individuals on the database from the Dystonia Medical Research Center at the Columbia Presbyterian Medical Center using the number of Ashkenazi Jews from the *American Jewish Yearbook* as the reference population. This resulted in a crude prevalence rate of 4.98 per 100,000. Assuming a rate of undiagnosed cases of approximately 50% and accounting for those younger than the median age of onset, the prevalence of early limb-onset dystonia was estimated to be as high as high as 11 per 100,000 (139). Although it is likely that the prevalence rate of early limb-onset dystonia in the Ashkenazi population is higher than previously reported, these data need to be interpreted with caution as they are derived indirectly and are based on a number of assumptions.

Among the different types of focal dystonia, the most common type in one study (135) was cervical dystonia (43%) followed by blepharospasm (32%), whereas writer's cramp and spasmodic dysphonia were relatively uncommon (5% and 6%, respectively), which contrasted with the findings from a clinic-based sample (140) in which writer's cramp occurred in 19%. In the European collaborative study (136), writer's cramp similarly represented 9% of the sample whereas cervical dystonia and blepharospasm accounted for 38% and 24% of primary dystonia, respectively.

Age-adjusted annual incidence rates in the early epidemiologic study in Israel population were 0.43 per million in the total Jewish population, 0.98 in European Jews, and 0.11 in Afro-Asians Jews (129). In Rochester, Minnesota, in the years 1950 to 1982, the annual incidence rate of all focal dystonias was reported as 2.4 per 100,000 and of generalized dystonia with 0.2 per 100,000 (125). An incidence study in Britain, relying on referral of all neurologic cases by a number of primary care physicians, obtained an incidence rate of 1 per 100,000 for focal dystonia, but it is likely that underdiagnosis may have affected the results of this study (15).

With the exception of writer's cramp, focal and segmental dystonia has mostly been reported to be more common in females than males (135,136,140–142).

A gene for generalized PTD with childhood onset, which contains a three-nucleotide (GAG) deletion and codes for the previously unknown protein torsin A, has been identified on chromosome 9q34 *(DYT1)* (143). It is responsible for most cases of early limb-onset PTD in both Jewish and non-Jewish kindreds (144,145). Transmission mostly follows an autosomal dominant pattern of inheritance with low penetrance. Although there is considerable phenotypic heterogeneity within and between kindreds, the typical clinical features of *DYT1*-associated dystonia are limb onset and spread to the trunk but rare involvement of craniofacial muscles. In contrast, late-onset PTD tends to begin in craniocervical muscles or an arm and rarely becomes generalized. In a minority of cases, late-onset dystonia is associated with a positive family history (146), but it is not usually associated with the *DYT1* gene (147). However, other loci causing PTD have recently been mapped on chromosome 18p *(DYT7)* in a large German pedigree (148) and chromosome 8 *(DYT6)* in two Mennonite families (149). Recently, a locus on chromosome 1p *(DYT13)* has been mapped in an Italian family (150), and other loci are likely to be identified in adult-onset focal dystonias. The D5 receptor gene has also been implicated in cervical dystonia (151). These findings provide evidence for the genetic heterogeneity of dystonia. The report of a family, including a pair of monozygotic twins, with variable phenotype (152) also provides evidence for *phenotypic* heterogeneity in adult onset focal dystonia. It is therefore likely that environmental factors have a role in the expression of genetic predisposition to develop adult-onset PTD. Patients often report trauma or significant viral infection preceding the onset of symptoms (128,141), but epidemiologic evidence regarding the role of such factors is controversial. Fletcher et al. (153) found in a case-control study that a family history of tremor or stuttering was significantly more common among patients with PTD than control subjects, whereas trauma was not more common in patients with PTD. The authors suggested that if trauma was important in the development of dystonia, it is likely that this is in combination with a preexisting susceptibility. Defazio et al. performed a large case-control study on risk factors for the development of primary adult-onset dystonia in Italy (154). In 202 patients with adult-onset dystonia and 202 age- and sex-matched controls, head or face trauma with loss of consciousness and family history of tremor or dystonia were associated with an increased risk of adult-onset dystonia, whereas hypertension and cigarette smoking exerted a protective effect. There was also a positive association between local injury to a body part and dystonia of that body part. The same group also reported that previous head or face trauma with loss of consciousness, age of onset, and female sex increased the risk of spread in patients with blepharospasm (155).

Age of onset is generally older in patients with blepharospasm and oromandibular dystonia than in patients with other focal dystonias, and younger for generalized dystonia (125,135). However, Nutt et al. reported that any of the focal dystonias could occur later in life (125). Progression of dystonia is more likely in cases with early-onset dystonia, whereas in most cases of adult-onset primary dystonia there is no or minimal spread to contiguous body parts (128). In a study of 115 patients with PTD with onset before age 22 and 472 with onset after age 21, Greene et al. reported that patients with onset in the lower extremities tended to be younger at onset than those with onset in the upper extremities, to have rapid spread of symptoms to other body parts, and to develop generalized dystonia. Patients with onset in the upper extremities were more likely to experience spread of symptoms many years after the disease began. In less than 20% of those with onset before age 22, symptoms began with torticollis and in 67% of them there was no spread to other body parts. In adults, dystonic symptoms remained focal in the majority (156). Similarly, in 51 PTD cases identified in Israel the most rapid deterioration occurred in patients with juvenile onset in the lower limbs, particularly in the first 2 years following onset. The rate of evolution was not influenced by gender or familial inheritance, but was more rapid in non-Ashkenazi Jews (157). Remissions of dystonia occur in a minority of patients (128,141).

TOURETTE'S SYNDROME

Tourette's syndrome (TS) is a disorder of multiple motor tics and one or more vocal (phonic) tics, which are typically waxing and waning. This variability in symptoms and lack of awareness in many subjects, in addition to the absence of a biologic marker and controversies on diagnostic criteria, pose difficult problems for the conduct of epidemiologic studies. Furthermore, studies in populations of different age groups and different sex distribution are difficult to compare because TS is more common in the male population and symptoms decrease with age (see below). Most epidemiologic studies in adults have yielded prevalence rates of 30 to 50 per 100,000 (158–163). However, surveys in schoolchildren have yielded higher rates. The more recent epidemiologic studies have found that TS affects between 0.1 and 3.0 percent of schoolchildren (158,164–168), and an even higher percentage have tics not fulfilling *DSM-IV* criteria for TS (which, among other things, require that the tics cause impairment or are distressing to the individual). It is unclear whether these milder tic disorders represent forme fruste of TS or a separate disorder, and this difficulty in delineation of the phenotype complicates epidemiologic and genetic research. In addition, there is an association and considerable overlap with a number of other disorders, such as attention deficit hyperactivity disorder, obsessive-compulsive disorder, depression, or self-injurious behavior (168,169). The exact relationship of these to TS is unclear as they may reflect the variable expression of a single disorder, a shared underlying etiology, selection bias, or a consequence of the social and personal impact of the disorder. Comorbidity with these disorders appears to be more common in males with the exception of obsessive-compulsive behaviors (170–175) and is associated with higher levels of behavioral problems and functional impairment (160,176). The prevalence of TS in children with special educational needs is with 7.5% and 8.6%, considerably higher than in regular schoolchildren, and other tic disorders occur in almost 30% of these children (158,177,178). In one study, 65% of children with emotional and behavioral difficulties, 24% of children with learning difficulties, and 6% of "problem children" had tics, most of whom fulfilled criteria for TS, whereas none of the normal children did. Conversely, 46% of 138 children with TS were found to have experienced school-related problems, whereby the presence of attention deficit hyperactivity disorder was a significant predictor of these (179). Children with autism have also been reported to have an increased rate of TS, with 4.3% fulfilling criteria for TS and an additional 2.2% having probable TS (180). Although many patients with TS even without comorbidity underachieve socially, the condition is found in all socioeconomic groups. TS has been described worldwide, and its characteristics are very similar across cultures (181,182), supporting a common genetic basis. Males are probably about four times more commonly affected than females, but the male-to-female ratio ranges from 1.6 to 10.1 (160,161,163,181,183–185).

It has been suggested that there has been an increase in the prevalence of TS over the last decade (186), but this may have been the result of greater recognition of this disorder and higher referral to hospitals (187) because very few of all patients in the community (16%) consult a doctor (188). The incidence of TS has been reported from a study in Rochester, Minnesota (187), which identified individuals seeking medical advice in over a 12-year period. Only 3 male individuals were identified, yielding an annual incidence rate of 0.46 per 100,000. However, since many subjects are unaware of their tics or insufficiently disabled to seek medical advice, and since physicians often do not correctly diagnose the disorder, the true incidence is likely to be much higher.

The natural history of TS is relatively well studied. The average onset age of motor tics in TS is 7 years but ranges from 2 to 21 years. Phonic tics usually occur later, with a mean age of onset of 11 years. Tic frequency or severity improve in the majority of TS patients in late adolescence or early adulthood (189,190). In a birth cohort study, Leckman et al. (191) found progressive worsening of tics until the age of 10, with a subsequent improvement of tic severity in the majority of cases. By the age of 18, half of the cohort were virtually tic free.

There is no doubt that genetic factors play an important role in the etiology of TS (192,193). The inheritance mostly follows an autosomal dominant inheritance pattern with variable expression and penetrance (170,171,194), and several areas have been implicated to be associated with TS (195). There is also growing evidence for bilineal transmission, with the father typically affected by childhood tics and the mother by symptoms of obsessive-compulsive disorder (196–198). Despite enormous research efforts, a gene responsible for TS has not yet been found. A number of reasons for this difficulty have been suggested. The assumed model for inheritance may be wrong; the phenotype may not be accurately delineated or the condition may be genetically heterogeneous; multiple genes may interact to produce TS (199); or environmental factors, such as infection or birth injury, in addition to a genetic vulnerability may determine the manifestation of TS (165,200–203). Particularly the recent description of the PANDAS syndrome (pediatric autoimmune neuropsychiatric disorders associated with streptococcal infections) (204), which links the occurrence of obsessive-compulsive disorder and/or tic disorder with prepubertal symptom onset to streptococcal infections and neuropsychiatric symptoms, has strengthened the argument for the relevance of infectious factors in the pathogenesis of TS.

HUNTINGTON'S DISEASE

Huntington's disease (HD), an autosomal dominantly inherited disorder with complete penetrance, is caused by an expanded sequence of CAG repeats in a gene on chromosome 4p16.3, which codes for the huntingtin protein (205). Nongenetic factors do not appear to influence the disease expression (206). HD occurs worldwide with prevalence rates between 2 and 12 per 100,000 (207), but lower prevalence rates have been reported in black populations, as well as in Finland, Japan, and China. Lower frequency of HD has been associated with smaller CAG repeat lengths

and different distribution of CCG alleles in these populations compared with Western European populations, suggesting that, in addition to European emigration, new mutations make a contribution to geographic variation of prevalence rates (208,209). The investigation of clusters, such as in Venezuela (210), has significantly advanced genetic research in HD. The incidence rate of HD is approximately 0.02 to 0.65 per 100,000 (211,212). Although it has been suggested that prevalence rates have declined through genetic counseling (213), such a decline in incidence and prevalence rates has not been confirmed by others. Age at onset is mostly in the mid-40s, but ranges from 2 years to more than 80 years. Younger onset is associated with more common presentation of rigidity, tremor, myoclonus, and epilepsy (Westphal variant), but many older patients also become akinetic-rigid and dystonic in the advanced stages. Onset age has been shown to inversely correlate with the length of the CAG repeat segment, particularly if onset is before age 30 years. In addition, paternal transmission is associated with earlier onset, leading to anticipation over several generations when the gene is inherited through the father (214). Median survival has been reported as long as 16.2 years (215), and many patients survive for more than 20 years, probably depending on the quality of care during the advanced stages. The main cause of death are pneumonia and cardiovascular disease (216), but the risk of suicide is also increased in patients with HD as well as unaffected siblings at risk for HD (216,217).

TARDIVE DYSKINESIA

Prolonged treatment with a variety of agents, particularly dopamine receptor–blocking drugs, can cause involuntary hyperkinetic movements or tardive dyskinesia (TD). TD comprises the whole range of abnormal involuntary movements, including chorea, tics, myoclonus, tremor, stereotypies, and dystonia, although tardive dystonia differs from TD with respect to risk factors and prognosis (218). Particularly characteristic are buccolinguomasticatory dyskinesias and involuntary movements of axial muscles, such as body rocking, but TD may involve also any other body part, often with a bizarre appearance. TD is frequently also associated with drug-induced parkinsonism and tardive motor restlessness (akathisia). Few data are available on the frequency of TD in the general population as the frequency and severity correlates with exposure to TD-inducing medication (219) and therefore depends on treatment practices. However, in a prospective community-based study in people over the age of 65, the community prevalence of TD over a 6-year follow-up was low (0.22%) (220) and was not associated with antipsychotic medication. In contrast, a review of 56 prevalence surveys of TD in neuroleptic-treated patients and 19 samples of untreated individuals yielded an average prevalence of 20%

in neuroleptic-treated patients and a 5% prevalence of "spontaneous" dyskinesia (221). Another meta-analysis of studies in patients with untreated schizophrenia estimated the prevalence of TD in this patient group from 4% in first-episode schizophrenia to 12% for chronically ill patients younger than 30, 25% for those between 30 and 50, and to 40% for those older than 60 (222). However, the authors acknowledged the limited precision of this estimate because only data from the preneuroleptic era, evaluations of first-episode patients before neuroleptic treatment, and assessment of drug-naive patients in developing countries could be used. The reported prevalence of TD among patients on long-term treatment with dopamine receptor–blocking agents is highly variable between 1.5 and 62% (218), reflecting differences in sample characteristics, duration of exposure, and type of medication (223–227). Prospective studies, which are likely to more accurately reflect risk than retrospective studies, have yielded a risk of TD after 5 years of treatment with neuroleptics between 20% (219) and 35% (228), with similar rates of 22.3% reported in Japan (223). The annual incidence rate was reported to be much higher in adults older than 45 with 30% than in younger adults with 4% to 5% (224). Overall, increased risk for the development of TD has been found in patients with older age (229), dementia (229), affective disorder (230), or diabetes mellitus (231), and in women (232,233). However, it is unclear whether these risk factors are merely a reflection of populations more likely to have greater exposure to dopamine receptor–blocking drugs or indicate greater susceptibility in these populations. In addition, it has been reported that those with other extrapyramidal side effects of neuroleptics, such as acute dystonic reaction or drug-induced parkinsonism, are more likely to develop TD, suggesting that an underlying susceptibility to extrapyramidal side effects exists that predisposes some patients to the development of TD on dopamine receptor antagonists. Comparisons across different ethnic groups are hampered by differences in study populations and exposure to dopamine receptor–blocking drugs. Nevertheless, it has been suggested that the risk may be lower in some Asian populations (232,234,235), whereas others have found a higher risk of TD in nonwhite populations (219).

The prognosis of TD is controversial and depends on a number of factors, including age, cumulative dose, and duration of exposure to the provoking drug. After discontinuation of neuroleptics, many patients improve during the months following withdrawal, especially if they are younger than 60 years. However, cessation of neuroleptic treatment may also be followed by the onset or worsening of TD (in about 40% of previously asymptomatic patients), so-called withdrawal dyskinesia (236), which usually but not always resolves. Other patients will exhibit irreversible dyskinesias even after cessation of treatment. Reports of improvement or cessation have varied in the time of follow-up, cumulative dose, and type of treatment, and studies involving consistent drug exposure are difficult to conduct

as treatment usually is dependent on individual patients' requirements of treatment for their underlying disorder. The range of reported partial or complete remission rates has therefore varied widely from 2% (237) to 100% (238). In patients with ongoing neuroleptic treatment, TD tends to plateau, although TD increases in severity in some patients and improves in others (224,228,239,240). Yassa et al. (241) reported that after a 10-year follow-up of 44 patients with TD, 50% had no change in their TD severity, 20% experienced improvement, and 30% experienced a worsening of their TD. In a study from Japan (234), the severity of TD was unchanged in 39%, improved in 18%, fluctuated in 21%, and worsened in only 21%. Fernandez et al. (242) reported resolution of TD symptoms in 62%, improvement in 4%, no change in 15%, and deterioration in 19%. In this study, parkinsonism worsened in 81% despite falling daily drug burden. Reported predictors of improvement have been younger age and affective disorder (243), but not all studies have confirmed this (234).

RESTLESS LEGS SYNDROME

Restless legs syndrome (RLS), also known as Ekbom's syndrome, is characterized by sleep-disrupting unpleasant leg sensations, often accompanied by daytime behavioral problems. Most cases of RLS remain undiagnosed in the community, and reported prevalence rates in studies using varying criteria have ranged from 4% to 15% (245–249). In a study reporting interviews with 2,018 Canadians, 15% reported leg restlessness at bedtime and 10% unpleasant leg sensations associated with awakening at night and the irresistible need to move (244). In a population-based survey using the minimal symptoms criteria published by the International Restless Legs Syndrome Study Group, the prevalence of RLS in persons aged 65 to 83 was found to be 9.8% (245). In this elderly sample, there was no association with age in women, but an inverse relationship in men. Another recent population-based postal survey followed up by telephone interviews revealed RLS symptoms during 5 or more nights per month in 10% of the population with no difference between genders. However, while it was uncommon (3%) in those between 18 and 29 years, it affected 19% of those 80 years and older (246). Associated with RLS were increased age and body mass index, lower income, smoking, lack of exercise, low alcohol consumption, and diabetes. In a study from Sweden, 11.4% of 200 randomly selected women between 18 and 64 years fulfilled criteria for RSL. Women with RLS had a higher prevalence of sleep-related complaints and daytime headache than those without (247). On the other hand, a postal survey on disturbances of sleep in the clerks of the Berne main post office revealed symptoms of RLS in only 4% of this working adult sample (248). Although prevalence increases with age, about one third of patients reported that their first symptoms started before age 10 (249). Remissions of at least a month occurred in 15% in one study, but severity generally also increases with age (249,250). Severity of RLS appears to be higher in women, and some studies have found a female preponderance of RLS (245) (13.9% vs. 6.1%), whereas others did not find a gender difference (246). RLS has been reported in European and American populations, but few data are available from other ethnic populations. In Singapore, a study based on interviews found a low prevalence of RSL of 0.6% in people older than 55 and 0.1% in subjects 21 or older (251). There is no doubt the genetic factors are important in RLS, with approximately 50% of affected individuals reporting a positive family history (249), and autosomal dominant inheritance with possible anticipation has been implicated in such families (250). On the other hand, RLS is more common in patients with uremia than in controls (25.9% vs. 13%) (252), and has been found to be associated with pregnancy, diabetes mellitus, iron deficiency with or without anemia, neuropathy and radiculopathy, rheumatoid arthritis, folate and magnesium deficiencies. Therefore, a distinction between hereditary and nonhereditary RLS has been made, and hereditary cases have been found to be associated with earlier symptom onset and slower progression (253). In order to assess the validity of this differentiation, Winkelmann et al. assessed the risk factors in 300 patients diagnosed with RLS. In 23%, RLS was associated with uremia (254). Forty-two percent of those with idiopathic RLS and 12% of those with uremic RLS had a definite family history of RLS confirmed by interview with the affected family member. Another 13% and 6%, respectively, had a possible family history of RLS. Age of onset was younger in those with hereditary RLS. However, apart from worsening during pregnancy in those with hereditary RLS, there were no differences in the phenotype between those with hereditary and nonhereditary RLS, indicating that both subgroups of RLS present with a very similar phenotype.

PSYCHOGENIC MOVEMENT DISORDERS

The diagnosis of psychogenic movement disorder (PMD) is conspicuously difficult. As no laboratory test is available to diagnose this condition, the diagnosis depends on clinical judgment and the neurologist's clinical experience with movement disorders. Diagnostic criteria, which are based on the degree of diagnostic certainty, have been developed (255). Factor et al. reported that 3.3% of patients in a movement disorder clinic fulfilled the categories of "documented" and "clinically established" PMD (summarized as "clinically definite") based on those criteria (256). Earlier studies from other movement disorder clinics have also reported similar rates (257,258). Population-based data on the prevalence of PMD are not available, but PMDs are among the most common medically unexplained symp-

toms; according to some estimates, 25% to 60% of symptoms investigated in primary care do not have a physical explanation (259). As the majority of patients with mild or transient form of medically unexplained symptoms are not referred to tertiary referral centers, probably only the more persistent or severe forms of PMD are seen in movement disorder clinics. Few data on the prognosis of PMD are available. In the study by Factor et al., tremor was the most common PMD (256), followed by dystonia, myoclonus, and parkinsonism. In other centers, psychogenic dystonia was the most common psychogenic movement disorder. Williams and Fahn reported that the majority of patients suffered from multiple types of movement disorders and only 21% had a single type of movement disorder that remained stable over time (255). In a study that followed patients with PMD seen in a movement disorder clinic for a mean of 3.2 years, outcome was poor, with persistence in abnormal movements in more than 90% of subjects. There was also a high prevalence of mental illness, especially anxiety, depression, and other somatic complaints. Poor outcome was associated with long duration of symptoms, insidious onset of movements, and psychiatric comorbidity (260). This relatively poor outcome was consistent with that reported for somatoform disorders in general (261).

Epidemiologic studies give important clues to the etiology of disease, provide the basis for health policy and planning, and guide the clinicians in giving prognostic advice. Although advances in diagnostic measures, progress in genetic research, and effective treatments that improve the prognosis have become available for many movement disorders, diagnostic difficulties still impede epidemiologic research and comparability among studies. Improved and more standardized diagnostic criteria and ascertainment methods, as well as collaborative cross-cultural and interdisciplinary efforts incorporating genetic, epidemiologic, and diagnostic methods, are required for future studies to advance our knowledge of the epidemiology of movement disorders.

REFERENCES

1. de Rijk MC, Launer LJ, Berger K, et al. Prevalence of Parkinson's disease in Europe: a collaborative study of population-based cohorts—Neurologic Diseases in the Elderly Research Group. *Neurology* 2000;54:S21–S23.
2. Zhang ZX, Roman GC. Worldwide occurrence of Parkinson's disease: an updated review. *Neuroepidemiology* 1993;12:195–208.
3. Wermuth L, Joensen P, Bunger N, et al. High prevalence of Parkinson's disease in the Faroe Islands. *Neurology* 1997;49:426–432.
4. Bharucha NE, Bharucha EP, Bharucha AE, et al. Prevalence of Parkinson's disease in the Parsi community of Bombay, India. *Arch Neurol* 1988;45:1321–1323.
5. Morgante L, Salemi G, Meneghini F, et al. Parkinson disease survival: a population-based study. *Arch Neurol* 2000;57:507–512.

6. Milanov I, Kmetski TS, Lyons KE, et al. Prevalence of Parkinson's disease in Bulgarian gypsies. *Neuroepidemiology* 2000;19:206–209.
7. Ashok PP, Radhakrishnan K, Sridharan R, et al. Epidemiology of Parkinson's disease in Benghazi, North-East Libya. *Clin Neurol Neurosurg* 1986;88:109–113.
8. Mayeux R, Marder K, Cote LJ, et al. The frequency of idiopathic Parkinson's disease by age, ethnic group, and sex in northern Manhattan, 1988–1993. *Am J Epidemiol* 1995;142:820–827.
9. Giroud Benitez JL, Collado-Mesa F, Esteban EM. Prevalence of Parkinson disease in an urban area of the Ciudad de La Habana province, Cuba: door-to-door population study. *Neurologia* 2000;15:269–273.
10. Schoenberg BS, Anderson DW, Haerer AF. Prevalence of Parkinson's disease in the biracial population of Copiah County, Mississippi. *Neurology* 1985;35:841–845.
11. Schoenberg BS, Osuntokun BO, Adeuja AO, et al. Comparison of the prevalence of Parkinson's disease in black populations in the rural United States and in rural Nigeria: door-to-door community studies. *Neurology* 1988;38:645–646.
12. Li SC, Schoenberg BS, Wang CC, et al. A prevalence survey of Parkinson's disease and other movement disorders in the People's Republic of China. *Arch Neurol* 1985;42:655–657.
13. Wang SJ, Fuh JL, Teng EL, et al. A door-to-door survey of Parkinson's disease in a Chinese population in Kinmen. *Arch Neurol* 1996;53:66–71.
14. Wang YS, Shi YM, Wu ZY, et al. Parkinson's disease in China. Coordinational Group of Neuroepidemiology, PLA. *Chin Med J (Engl)* 1991;104:960–964.
15. MacDonald BK, Cockerell OC, Sander JW, et al. The incidence and lifetime prevalence of neurological disorders in a prospective community-based study in the UK. *Brain* 2000;123(Pt 4):665–676.
16. Rajput AH, Offord KP, Beard CM, et al. Epidemiology of parkinsonism: incidence, classification, and mortality. *Ann Neurol* 1984;16:278–282.
17. Bower JH, Maraganore DM, McDonnell SK, et al. Incidence and distribution of parkinsonism in Olmsted County, Minnesota, 1976–1990. *Neurology* 1999;52:1214–1220.
18. Kuopio AM, Marttila RJ, Helenius H, et al. Changing epidemiology of Parkinson's disease in southwestern Finland. *Neurology* 1999;52:302–308.
19. Marttila RJ, Rinne UK. Epidemiology of Parkinson's disease in Finland. *Acta Neurol Scand* 1976;53:81–102.
20. Baldereschi M, Di Carlo A, Rocca WA, et al. Parkinson's disease and parkinsonism in a longitudinal study: two-fold higher incidence in men. ILSA Working Group. Italian Longitudinal Study on Aging. *Neurology* 2000;55:1358–1363.
21. de Rijk MC, Tzourio C, Breteler MM, et al. Prevalence of parkinsonism and Parkinson's disease in Europe: the Europarkinson Collaborative Study. European Community Concerted Action on the Epidemiology of Parkinson's disease. *J Neurol Neurosurg Psychiatry* 1997;62:10–15.
22. Ben Shlomo Y. How far are we in understanding the cause of Parkinson's disease? *J Neurol Neurosurg Psychiatry* 1996;61:4–16.
23. Tison F, Dartigues JF, Dubes L, et al. Prevalence of Parkinson's disease in the elderly: a population study in Gironde, France. *Acta Neurol Scand* 1994;90:111–115.
24. Maraganore DM, Anderson DW, Bower JH, et al. Autopsy patterns for Parkinson's disease and related disorders in Olmsted County, Minnesota. *Neurology* 1999;53:1342–1344.
25. Bennett DA, Beckett LA, Murray AM, et al. Prevalence of parkinsonian signs and associated mortality in a community population of older people. *N Engl J Med* 1996;334:71–76.
26. Tanner CM, Aston DA. Epidemiology of Parkinson's disease and akinetic syndromes. *Curr Opin Neurol* 2000;13:427–430.
27. Ben Shlomo Y. The epidemiology of Parkinson's disease. *Baillieres Clin Neurol* 1997;6:55–68.
28. Rocca WA, Bower JH, McDonnell SK, et al. Time trends in the incidence of parkinsonism in Olmsted County, Minnesota. *Neurology* 2001;57:462–467.
29. Tanner CM, Goldman SM. Epidemiology of Parkinson's disease. *Neurol Clin* 1996;14:317–335.
30. Taylor CA, Saint-Hilaire MH, Cupples LA, et al. Environmental, medical, and family history risk factors for Parkinson's disease: a New England–based case control study. *Am J Med Genet* 1999;88:742–749.
31. Rybicki BA, Johnson CC, Peterson EL, et al. A family history of Parkinson's disease and its effect on other PD risk factors. *Neuroepidemiology* 1999;18:270–278.
32. Duvoisin RC, Eldridge R, Williams A, et al. Twin study of Parkinson disease. *Neurology* 1981;31:77–80.
33. Marttila RJ, Kaprio J, Koskenvuo M, et al. Parkinson's disease in a nationwide twin cohort. *Neurology* 1988;38:1217–1219.
34. Tanner CM, Ottman R, Goldman SM, et al. Parkinson disease in twins: an etiologic study. *JAMA* 1999;281:341–346.
35. Vieregge P, Hagenah J, Heberlein I, et al. Parkinson's disease in twins: a follow-up study. *Neurology* 1999;53:566–572.
36. Piccini P, Burn DJ, Ceravolo R, et al. The role of inheritance in sporadic Parkinson's disease: evidence from a longitudinal study of dopaminergic function in twins. *Ann Neurol* 1999;45:577–582.
37. Chan DK, Mellick G, Cai H, et al. The alpha-synuclein gene and Parkinson disease in a Chinese population. *Arch Neurol* 2000;57:501–503.
38. Lucking CB, Durr A, Bonifati V, et al. Association between early-onset Parkinson's disease and mutations in the *parkin* gene. French Parkinson's Disease Genetics Study Group. *N Engl J Med* 2000;342:1560–1567.
39. Klein C, Pramstaller PP, Kis B, et al. Parkin deletions in a family with adult-onset, tremor-dominant parkinsonism: expanding the phenotype. *Ann Neurol* 2000;48:65–71.
40. Gorell JM, Rybicki BA, Johnson CC, et al. Smoking and Parkinson's disease: a dose-response relationship. *Neurology* 1999;52:115–119.
41. Hellenbrand W, Seidler A, Robra BP, et al. Smoking and Parkinson's disease: a case-control study in Germany. *Int J Epidemiol* 1997;26:328–339.
42. Seidler A, Hellenbrand W, Robra BP, et al. Possible environmental, occupational, and other etiologic factors for Parkinson's disease: a case-control study in Germany. *Neurology* 1996;46:1275–1284.
43. Kuopio AM, Marttila RJ, Helenius H, et al. Environmental risk factors in Parkinson's disease. *Mov Disord* 1999;14:928–939.
44. Ross GW, Abbott RD, Petrovitch H, et al. Association of coffee and caffeine intake with the risk of Parkinson disease. *JAMA* 2000;283:2674–2679.
45. Hellenbrand W, Seidler A, Boeing H, et al. Diet and Parkinson's disease. I: A possible role for the past intake of specific foods and food groups—results from a self-administered food-frequency questionnaire in a case-control study. *Neurology* 1996;47:636–643.
46. Hellenbrand W, Boeing H, Robra BP, et al. Diet and Parkinson's disease. II: A possible role for the past intake of specific nutrients—results from a self-administered food-frequency questionnaire in a case-control study. *Neurology* 1996;47:644–650.
47. Benedetti MD, Bower JH, Maraganore DM, et al. Smoking, alcohol, and coffee consumption preceding Parkinson's disease: a case-control study. *Neurology* 2000;55:1350–1358.
48. Paganini-Hill A. Risk factors for Parkinson's disease: the leisure world cohort study. *Neuroepidemiology* 2001;20:118–124.

49. Tsui JK, Calne DB, Wang Y, et al. Occupational risk factors in Parkinson's disease. *Can J Public Health* 1999;90:334–337.

50. Marion SA. The epidemiology of Parkinson's disease—current issues. *Adv Neurol* 2001;86:163–172.

51. Elbaz A, Grigoletto F, Baldereschi M, et al. Familial aggregation of Parkinson's disease: a population-based case-control study in Europe. Europarkinson Study Group. *Neurology* 1999;52:1876–1882.

52. Jankovic J, Kapadia AS. Functional decline in Parkinson disease. *Arch Neurol* 2001;58:1611–1615.

53. Hely MA, Morris JG, Reid WG, et al. Age at onset: the major determinant of outcome in Parkinson's disease. *Acta Neurol Scand* 1995;92:455–463.

54. Goetz CG, Tanner CM, Stebbins GT, et al. Risk factors for progression in Parkinson's disease. *Neurology* 1988;38:1841–1844.

55. Schrag A, Ben Shlomo Y, Brown R, et al. Young-onset Parkinson's disease revisited—clinical features, natural history, and mortality. *Mov Disord* 1998;13:885–894.

56. Denny AP, Behari M. Motor fluctuations in Parkinson's disease. *J Neurol Sci* 1999;165:18–23.

57. Hely MA, Morris JG, Traficante R, et al. The Sydney multicentre study of Parkinson's disease: progression and mortality at 10 years. *J Neurol Neurosurg Psychiatry* 1999;67:300–307.

58. Montastruc JL, Desboeuf K, Lapeyre-Mestre M, et al. Long-term mortality results of the randomized controlled study comparing bromocriptine to which levodopa was later added with levodopa alone in previously untreated patients with Parkinson's disease. *Mov Disord* 2001;16:511–514.

59. Uitti RJ, Ahlskog JE, Maraganore DM, et al. Levodopa therapy and survival in idiopathic Parkinson's disease: Olmsted County project. *Neurology* 1993;43:1918–1926.

60. Poewe W. The Sydney multicentre study of Parkinson's disease. *J Neurol Neurosurg Psychiatry* 1999;67:280–281.

61. Wermuth L, Stenager EN, Stenager E, et al. Mortality in patients with Parkinson's disease. *Acta Neurol Scand* 1995;92:55–58.

62. Hughes AJ, Daniel SE, Lees AJ. Improved accuracy of clinical diagnosis of Lewy body Parkinson's disease. *Neurology* 2001;57:1497–1499.

63. Hughes AJ, Daniel SE, Kilford L, et al. Accuracy of clinical diagnosis of idiopathic Parkinson's disease: a clinico-pathological study of 100 cases. *J Neurol Neurosurg Psychiatry* 1992;55:181–184.

64. Rajput AH, Rozdilsky B, Rajput A. Accuracy of clinical diagnosis in parkinsonism—a prospective study. *Can J Neurol Sci* 1991;18:275–278.

65. Schrag A, Ben Shlomo Y, Quinn NP. Prevalence of progressive supranuclear palsy and multiple system atrophy: a cross-sectional study. *Lancet* 1999;354:1771–1775.

66. Nath U, Ben Shlomo Y, Thomson RG, et al. The prevalence of progressive supranuclear palsy (Steele-Richardson-Olszewski syndrome) in the UK. *Brain* 2001;124:1438–1449.

67. Trenkwalder C, Schwarz J, Gebhard J, et al. Starnberg trial on epidemiology of Parkinsonism and hypertension in the elderly: prevalence of Parkinson's disease and related disorders assessed by a door-to-door survey of inhabitants older than 65 years. *Arch Neurol* 1995;52:1017–1022.

68. Tison F, Yekhlef F, Chrysostome V, et al. Prevalence of multiple system atrophy. *Lancet* 2000;355:495–496.

69. Vanacore N, Bonifati V, Fabbrini G, et al. Epidemiology of multiple system atrophy. ESGAP Consortium. European Study Group on Atypical Parkinsonisms. *Neurol Sci* 2001;22:97–99.

70. Golbe LI, Davis PH, Schoenberg BS, et al. Prevalence and natural history of progressive supranuclear palsy. *Neurology* 1988;38:1031–1034.

71. Vanacore N, Bonifati V, Colosimo C, et al. Epidemiology of progressive supranuclear palsy. ESGAP Consortium. European Study Group on Atypical Parkinsonisms. *Neurol Sci* 2001;22:101–103.

72. Bower JH, Maraganore DM, McDonnell SK, et al. Incidence of progressive supranuclear palsy and multiple system atrophy in Olmsted County, Minnesota, 1976 to 1990. *Neurology* 1997;49:1284–1288.

73. Iwatsubo T. [Japanese clinical statistical data of progressive supranuclear palsy.] *Nippon Rinsho* 1992;50[Suppl]:134–138.

74. Scrimgeour EM. Progressive supranuclear palsy in a Zimbabwean man. *West Afr J Med* 1993;12:175–176.

75. Radhakrishnan K, Thacker AK, Maloo JC, et al. Descriptive epidemiology of some rare neurological diseases in Benghazi, Libya. *Neuroepidemiology* 1988;7:159–164.

76. Caparros-Lefebvre D, Elbaz A. Possible relation of atypical parkinsonism in the French West Indies with consumption of tropical plants: a case-control study. Caribbean Parkinsonism Study Group. *Lancet* 1999;354:281–286.

77. Chaudhuri KR, Hu MT, Brooks DJ. Atypical parkinsonism in Afro-Caribbean and Indian origin immigrants to the UK. *Mov Disord* 2000;15:18–23.

78. Santacruz P, Uttl B, Litvan I, et al. Progressive supranuclear palsy: a survey of the disease course. *Neurology* 1998;50:1637–1647.

79. Litvan I, Mangone CA, McKee A, et al. Natural history of progressive supranuclear palsy (Steele-Richardson-Olszewski syndrome) and clinical predictors of survival: a clinicopathological study. *J Neurol Neurosurg Psychiatry* 1996;60:615–620.

80. de Yebenes JG, Sarasa JL, Daniel SE, et al. Familial progressive supranuclear palsy: description of a pedigree and review of the literature. *Brain* 1995;118(Pt 5):1095–1103.

81. Golbe LI. The epidemiology of progressive supranuclear palsy. *Adv Neurol* 1996;69:25–31.

82. Maher ER, Lees AJ. The clinical features and natural history of the Steele-Richardson-Olszewski syndrome (progressive supranuclear palsy). *Neurology* 1986;36:1005–1008.

83. Frasca J, Blumbergs PC, Henschke P, et al. A clinical and pathological study of progressive supranuclear palsy. *Clin Exp Neurol* 1991;28:79–89.

84. Litvan I, Baker M, Hutton M. Tau genotype: no effect on onset, symptom severity, or survival in progressive supranuclear palsy. *Neurology* 2001;57:138–140.

85. Morris HR, Schrag A, Nath U, et al. Effect of ApoE and tau on age of onset of progressive supranuclear palsy and multiple system atrophy. *Neurosci Lett* 2001;312:118–120.

86. Molinuevo JL, Valldeoriola F, Alegret M, et al. Progressive supranuclear palsy: earlier age of onset in patients with the tau protein A0/A0 genotype. *J Neurol* 2000;247:206–208.

87. Davis PH, Golbe LI, Duvoisin RC, et al. Risk factors for progressive supranuclear palsy. *Neurology* 1988;38:1546–1552.

88. Golbe LI, Rubin RS, Cody RP, et al. Follow-up study of risk factors in progressive supranuclear palsy. *Neurology* 1996;47:148–154.

89. Ben Shlomo Y, Wenning GK, Tison F, et al. Survival of patients with pathologically proven multiple system atrophy: a meta-analysis. *Neurology* 1997;48:384–393.

90. Wenning GK, Ben Shlomo Y, Magalhaes M, et al. Clinical features and natural history of multiple system atrophy: an analysis of 100 cases. *Brain* 1994;117(Pt 4):835–845.

91. Saito Y, Matsuoka Y, Takahashi A, et al. Survival of patients with multiple system atrophy. *Intern Med* 1994;33:321–325.

92. Testa D, Filippini G, Farinotti M, et al. Survival in multiple system atrophy: a study of prognostic factors in 59 cases. *J Neurol* 1996;243:401–404.

93. Kurisaki H. [Prognosis of multiple system atrophy—survival time with or without tracheostomy.] *Rinsho Shinkeigaku* 1999;39:503–507.

94. Nee LE, Gomez MR, Dambrosia J, et al. Environmental-occupational risk factors and familial associations in multiple system atrophy: a preliminary investigation. *Clin Auton Res* 1991;1: 9–13.

95. Iwahashi K, Miyatake R, Tsuneoka Y, et al. A novel cytochrome P-450IID6 (CYPIID6) mutant gene associated with multiple system atrophy. *J Neurol Neurosurg Psychiatry* 1995;58: 263–264.

96. Vanacore N, Bonifati V, Fabbrini G, et al. Smoking habits in multiple system atrophy and progressive supranuclear palsy. European Study Group on Atypical Parkinsonisms. *Neurology* 2000;54:114–119.

97. Schrag A, Ben Shlomo Y, Quinn NP. Cross sectional prevalence survey of idiopathic Parkinson's disease and parkinsonism in London. *BMJ* 2000;321:21–22.

98. Munchau A, Schrag A, Chuang C, et al. Arm tremor in cervical dystonia differs from essential tremor and can be classified by onset age and spread of symptoms. *Brain* 2001;124: 1765–1776.

99. Louis ED, Ford B, Barnes LF. Clinical subtypes of essential tremor. *Arch Neurol* 2000;57:1194–1198.

100. Dubinsky RM, Gray CS, Koller WC. Essential tremor and dystonia. *Neurology* 1993;43:2382–2384.

101. Singer MS, Wissel JW, Mueller JM, et al. Prevalence of tremor syndromes in focal and segmental dystonia: a service based epidemiological study in the adult population of Tyrol, Austria. *Mov Disord* 2000;15[Suppl 3]:155.

102. Koller WC, Busenbark K, Miner K. The relationship of essential tremor to other movement disorders: report on 678 patients. Essential Tremor Study Group. *Ann Neurol* 1994;35: 717–723.

103. Lou JS, Jankovic J. Essential tremor: clinical correlates in 350 patients. *Neurology* 1991;41:234–238.

104. Jedynak CP, Bonnet AM, Agid Y. Tremor and idiopathic dystonia. *Mov Disord* 1991;6:230–236.

105. Elble RJ, Moody C, Higgins C. Primary writing tremor: a form of focal dystonia? *Mov Disord* 1990;5:118–126.

106. Jankovic J, Beach J, Schwartz K, et al. Tremor and longevity in relatives of patients with Parkinson's disease, essential tremor, and control subjects. *Neurology* 1995;45:645–648.

107. Pahwa R, Koller WC. Is there a relationship between Parkinson's disease and essential tremor? *Clin Neuropharmacol* 1993; 16:30–35.

108. Cardoso FE, Jankovic J. Hereditary motor-sensory neuropathy and movement disorders. *Muscle Nerve* 1993;16:904–910.

109. Baloh RW, Foster CA, Yue Q, et al. Familial migraine with vertigo and essential tremor. *Neurology* 1996;46:458–460.

110. Louis ED, Ford B, Lee H, et al. Diagnostic criteria for essential tremor: a population perspective. *Arch Neurol* 1998;55: 823–828.

111. Louis ED, Ottman R, Hauser WA. How common is the most common adult movement disorder? Estimates of the prevalence of essential tremor throughout the world. *Mov Disord* 1998;13:5–10.

112. Rajput AH, Offord KP, Beard CM, et al. Essential tremor in Rochester, Minnesota: a 45-year study. *J Neurol Neurosurg Psychiatry* 1984;47:466–470.

113. Rautakorpi I, Takala J, Marttila RJ, et al. Essential tremor in a Finnish population. *Acta Neurol Scand* 1982;66:58–67.

114. Haerer AF, Anderson DW, Schoenberg BS. Prevalence of essential tremor: results from the Copiah County study. *Arch Neurol* 1982;39:750–751.

115. Bain PG, Findley LJ, Thompson PD, et al. A study of hereditary essential tremor. *Brain* 1994;117(Pt 4):805–824.

116. Herskovits E, Figueroa E, Mangone C. Hereditary essential tremor in Buenos Aires (Argentina). *Arq Neuropsiquiatr* 1988; 46:238–247.

117. Louis ED, Marder K, Cote L, et al. Differences in the prevalence of essential tremor among elderly African Americans, whites, and Hispanics in northern Manhattan, NY. *Arch Neurol* 1995;52:1201–1205.

118. Conway D, Bain PG, Warner TT, et al. Linkage analysis with chromosome 9 markers in hereditary essential tremor. *Mov Disord* 1993;8:374–376.

119. Gulcher JR, Jonsson P, Kong A, et al. Mapping of a familial essential tremor gene, *FET1*, to chromosome 3q13. *Nat Genet* 1997;17:84–87.

120. Higgins JJ, Pho LT, Nee LE. A gene *(ETM)* for essential tremor maps to chromosome 2p22-p25. *Mov Disord* 1997;12: 859–864.

121. Higgins JJ, Loveless JM, Jankovic J, et al. Evidence that a gene for essential tremor maps to chromosome 2p in four families. *Mov Disord* 1998;13:972–977.

122. Kovach MJ, Ruiz J, Kimonis K, et al. Genetic heterogeneity in autosomal dominant essential tremor. *Genet Med* 2001;3: 197–199.

123. Mengano A, Di Maio L, Maggio MA, et al. Benign essential tremor: a clinical survey of 82 patients from Campania, a region of southern Italy. *Acta Neurol (Napoli)* 1989;11: 239–246.

124. Salemi G, Aridon P, Calagna G, et al. Population-based case-control study of essential tremor. *Ital J Neurol Sci* 1998;19: 301–305.

125. Nutt JG, Muenter MD, Aronson A, et al. Epidemiology of focal and generalized dystonia in Rochester, Minnesota. *Mov Disord* 1988;3:188–194.

126. Schwalbe W. *Eine eigentuemliche tonische Krampfform mit hysterischen Symptomen.* Berlin: Universitaets-Buchdruckerei von Gustav Schade, 1980.

127. Alter M, Kahana E, Feldman S. Differences in torsion dystonia among Israeli ethnic groups. *Adv Neurol* 1976;14:115–120.

128. Cooper IS, Cullinan T, Riklan M. The natural history of dystonia. *Adv Neurol* 1976;14:157–169.

129. Korczyn AD, Kahana E, Zilber N, et al. Torsion dystonia in Israel. *Ann Neurol* 1980;8:387–391.

130. Zilber N, Korczyn AD, Kahana E, et al. Inheritance of idiopathic torsion dystonia among Jews. *J Med Genet* 1984;21:13–20.

131. Lee LV, Pascasio FM, Fuentes FD, et al. Torsion dystonia in Panay, Philippines. *Adv Neurol* 1976;14:137–151.

132. Gimenez-Roldan S, Lopez-Fraile IP, Esteban A. Dystonia in Spain: study of a Gypsy family and general survey. *Adv Neurol* 1976;14:125–136.

133. Golden GS. Dystonia in the black and Puerto Rican population. *Adv Neurol* 1976;14:121–124.

134. Sempere AP, Duarte C, Coria F, et al. Prevalence of idiopathic focal dystonias in the province of Segovia, Spain. *J Neurol* 1994; 241:S124.

135. Duffey PO, Butler AG, Hawthorne MR, et al. The epidemiology of the primary dystonias in the north of England. *Adv Neurol* 1998;78:121–125.

136. The Epidemiological Study of Dystonia in Europe (ESDE) Collaborative Group. A prevalence study of primary dystonia in eight European countries. *J Neurol* 2000;247:787–792.

137. Nakashima K, Kusumi M, Inoue Y, et al. Prevalence of focal dystonias in the western area of Tottori Prefecture in Japan. *Mov Disord* 1995;10:440–443.

138. Kandil MR, Tohamy SA, Fattah MA, et al. Prevalence of chorea, dystonia, and athetosis in Assiut, Egypt: a clinical and epidemiological study. *Neuroepidemiology* 1994;13:202–210.

139. Risch N, de Leon D, Ozelius L, et al. Genetic analysis of idiopathic torsion dystonia in Ashkenazi Jews and their recent descent from a small founder population. *Nat Genet* 1995;9: 152–159.

140. Soland VL, Bhatia KP, Marsden CD. Sex prevalence of focal dystonias. *J Neurol Neurosurg Psychiatry* 1996;60:204–205.

141. Claypool DW, Duane DD, Ilstrup DM, et al. Epidemiology and outcome of cervical dystonia (spasmodic torticollis) in Rochester, Minnesota. *Mov Disord* 1995;10:608–614.

142. Castelon Konkiewitz ECK, Trender I, Kamm CK, et al. The epidemiology of dystonia in Munich. *Mov Disord* 2000;15 [Suppl 3]:145.

143. Ozelius LJ, Page CE, Klein C, et al. The *TOR1A (DYT1)* gene family and its role in early onset torsion dystonia. *Genomics* 1999;62:377–384.

144. Klein C, Brin MF, de Leon D, et al. De novo mutations (GAG deletion) in the *DYT1* gene in two non-Jewish patients with early-onset dystonia. *Hum Mol Genet* 1998;7:1133–1136.

145. Warner TT, Fletcher NA, Davis MB, et al. Linkage analysis in British and French families with idiopathic torsion dystonia. *Brain* 1993;116(Pt 3):739–744.

146. Stojanovic M, Cvetkovic D, Kostic VS. A genetic study of idiopathic focal dystonias. *J Neurol* 1995;242:508–511.

147. Bressman SB, Heiman GA, Nygaard TG, et al. A study of idiopathic torsion dystonia in a non-Jewish family: evidence for genetic heterogeneity. *Neurology* 1994;44:283–287.

148. Leube B, Kessler KR, Goecke T, et al. Frequency of familial inheritance among 488 index patients with idiopathic focal dystonia and clinical variability in a large family. *Mov Disord* 1997;12:1000–1006.

149. Almasy L, Bressman SB, Raymond D, et al. Idiopathic torsion dystonia linked to chromosome 8 in two Mennonite families. *Ann Neurol* 1997;42:670–673.

150. Valente EM, Bentivoglio AR, Cassetta E, et al. DYT13, a novel primary torsion dystonia locus, maps to chromosome 1p36.13-36.32 in an Italian family with cranial-cervical or upper limb onset. *Ann Neurol* 2001;49:362–366.

151. Placzek MR, Misbahuddin A, Chaudhuri KR, et al. Cervical dystonia is associated with a polymorphism in the dopamine (D5) receptor gene. *J Neurol Neurosurg Psychiatry* 2001;71:262–264.

152. Uitti RJ, Maraganore DM. Adult onset familial cervical dystonia: report of a family including monozygotic twins. *Mov Disord* 1993;8:489–494.

153. Fletcher NA, Harding AE, Marsden CD. A case-control study of idiopathic torsion dystonia. *Mov Disord* 1991;6:304–309.

154. Defazio G, Berardelli A, Abbruzzese G, et al. Possible risk factors for primary adult onset dystonia: a case-control investigation by the Italian Movement Disorders Study Group. *J Neurol Neurosurg Psychiatry* 1998;64:25–32.

155. Defazio G, Berardelli A, Abbruzzese G, et al. Risk factors for spread of primary adult onset blepharospasm: a multicentre investigation of the Italian Movement Disorders Study Group. *J Neurol Neurosurg Psychiatry* 1999;67:613–619.

156. Greene P, Kang UJ, Fahn S. Spread of symptoms in idiopathic torsion dystonia. *Mov Disord* 1995;10:143–152.

157. Zilber N, Inzelberg R, Kahana E, et al. Natural course of idiopathic torsion dystonia among Jews. *Neuroepidemiology* 1994;13:195–201.

158. Comings DE, Himes JA, Comings BG. An epidemiologic study of Tourette's syndrome in a single school district. *J Clin Psychiatry* 1990;51:463–469.

159. Bruun RD. Gilles de la Tourette's syndrome: an overview of clinical experience. *J Am Acad Child Psychiatry* 1984;23:126–133.

160. Caine ED, McBride MC, Chiverton P, et al. Tourette's syndrome in Monroe County school children. *Neurology* 1988;38:472–475.

161. Burd L, Kerbeshian J, Wikenheiser M, et al. Prevalence of Gilles de la Tourette's syndrome in North Dakota adults. *Am J Psychiatry* 1986;143:787–788.

162. Apter A, Pauls DL, Bleich A, et al. A population-based epidemiological study of Tourette syndrome among adolescents in Israel. *Adv Neurol* 1992;58:61–65.

163. Apter A, Pauls DL, Bleich A, et al. An epidemiologic study of Gilles de la Tourette's syndrome in Israel. *Arch Gen Psychiatry* 1993;50:734–738.

164. Wong CK, Lau JT. Psychiatric morbidity in a Chinese primary school in Hong Kong. *Aust N Z J Psychiatry* 1992;26:459–466.

165. Mason A, Banerjee S, Eapen V, et al. The prevalence of Tourette syndrome in a mainstream school population. *Dev Med Child Neurol* 1998;40:292–296.

166. Zohar AH, Ratzoni G, Pauls DL, et al. An epidemiological study of obsessive-compulsive disorder and related disorders in Israeli adolescents. *J Am Acad Child Adolesc Psychiatry* 1992;31:1057–1061.

167. Nomoto F, Machiyama Y. An epidemiological study of tics. *Jpn J Psychiatry Neurol* 1990;44:649–655.

168. Kadesjo B, Gillberg C. Tourette's disorder: epidemiology and comorbidity in primary school children. *J Am Acad Child Adolesc Psychiatry* 2000;39:548–555.

169. Robertson MM. Tourette syndrome: associated conditions and the complexities of treatment. *Brain* 2000;123(Pt 3):425–462.

170. Curtis D, Robertson MM, Gurling HM. Autosomal dominant gene transmission in a large kindred with Gilles de la Tourette syndrome. *Br J Psychiatry* 1992;160:845–849.

171. Eapen V, Pauls DL, Robertson MM. Evidence for autosomal dominant transmission in Tourette's syndrome: United Kingdom cohort study. *Br J Psychiatry* 1993;162:593–596.

172. Noshirvani HF, Kasvikis Y, Marks IM, et al. Gender-divergent aetiological factors in obsessive-compulsive disorder. *Br J Psychiatry* 1991;158:260–263.

173. Pauls DL, Raymond CL, Stevenson JM, et al. A family study of Gilles de la Tourette syndrome. *Am J Hum Genet* 1991;48:154–163.

174. Grados MA, Riddle MA, Samuels JF, et al. The familial phenotype of obsessive-compulsive disorder in relation to tic disorders: the Hopkins OCD family study. *Biol Psychiatry* 2001;50:559–565.

175. Santangelo SL, Pauls DL, Goldstein JM, et al. Tourette's syndrome: what are the influences of gender and comorbid obsessive-compulsive disorder? *J Am Acad Child Adolesc Psychiatry* 1994;33:795–804.

176. Freeman RD, Fast DK, Burd L, et al. An international perspective on Tourette syndrome: selected findings from 3,500 individuals in 22 countries. *Dev Med Child Neurol* 2000;42:436–447.

177. Kurlan R, Whitmore D, Irvine C, et al. Tourette's syndrome in a special education population: a pilot study involving a single school district. *Neurology* 1994;44:699–702.

178. Kurlan R, McDermott MP, Deeley C, et al. Prevalence of tics in schoolchildren and association with placement in special education. *Neurology* 2001;57:1383–1388.

179. Eapen V, Robertson MM, Zeitlin H, et al. Gilles de la Tourette's syndrome in special education schools: a United Kingdom study. *J Neurol* 1997;244:378–382.

180. Burd L, Severud R, Klug MG, et al. Prenatal and perinatal risk factors for Tourette disorder. *J Perinat Med* 1999;27:295–302.

181. Staley D, Wand R, Shady G. Tourette disorder: a cross-cultural review. *Compr Psychiatry* 1997;38:6–16.

182. Robertson MM, Trimble MR. Gilles de la Tourette syndrome in the Middle East: report of a cohort and a multiply affected large pedigree. *Br J Psychiatry* 1991;158:416–419.

183. Baron-Cohen S, Scahill VL, Izaguirre J, et al. The prevalence of Gilles de la Tourette syndrome in children and adolescents with autism: a large scale study. *Psychol Med* 1999;29:1151–1159.

184. Robertson MM. The Gilles de la Tourette syndrome: the current status. *Br J Psychiatry* 1989;154:147–169.

185. Tanner CM, Goldman SM. Epidemiology of Tourette syndrome. *Neurol Clin* 1997;15:395–402.

186. Traverse L. Prevalence of Tourette syndrome in a mainstream school population. *Dev Med Child Neurol* 1998;40:847–848.

187. Lucas AR, Beard CM, Rajput AH, et al. Tourette syndrome in Rochester, Minnesota, 1968–1979. *Adv Neurol* 1982;35: 267–269.

188. Baron-Cohen S, Mortimore C, Moriarty J, et al. The prevalence of Gilles de la Tourette's syndrome in children and adolescents with autism. *J Child Psychol Psychiatry* 1999;40:213–218.

189. Bruun RD, Shapiro AK, Shapiro E, et al. A follow-up of 78 patients with Gilles de la Tourette's syndrome. *Am J Psychiatry* 1976;133:944–947.

190. Erenberg G, Cruse RP, Rothner AD. The natural history of Tourette syndrome: a follow-up study. *Ann Neurol* 1987;22:383–385.

191. Leckman JF, Zhang H, Vitale A, et al. Course of tic severity in Tourette syndrome: the first two decades. *Pediatrics* 1998;102: 14–19.

192. Abe K, Oda N. Incidence of tics in the offspring of childhood tiquers: a controlled follow-up study. *Dev Med Child Neurol* 1980;22:649–653.

193. Pauls DL. Update on the genetics of Tourette syndrome. *Adv Neurol* 2001;85:281–293.

194. Pauls DL, Leckman JF. The inheritance of Gilles de la Tourette's syndrome and associated behaviors: evidence for autosomal dominant transmission. *N Engl J Med* 1986;315:993–997.

195. Simonic I, Nyholt DR, Gericke GS, et al. Further evidence for linkage of Gilles de la Tourette syndrome (GTS) susceptibility loci on chromosomes 2p11, 8q22, and 11q23-24 in South African Afrikaners. *Am J Med Genet* 2001;105:163–167.

196. Kurlan R, Eapen V, Stern J, et al. Bilineal transmission in Tourette's syndrome families. *Neurology* 1994;44:2336–2342.

197. McMahon WM, van de Wetering BJ, Filloux F, et al. Bilineal transmission and phenotypic variation of Tourette's disorder in a large pedigree. *J Am Acad Child Adolesc Psychiatry* 1996;35: 672–680.

198. Hanna PA, Janjua FN, Contant CF, et al. Bilineal transmission in Tourette syndrome. *Neurology* 1999;53:813–818.

199. Comings DE, Wu S, Chiu C, et al. Polygenic inheritance of Tourette syndrome, stuttering, attention deficit hyperactivity, conduct, and oppositional defiant disorder: the additive and subtractive effect of the three dopaminergic genes—*DRD2, D beta H*, and *DAT1*. *Am J Med Genet* 1996;67:264–288.

200. Hasstedt SJ, Leppert M, Filloux F, et al. Intermediate inheritance of Tourette syndrome, assuming assortative mating. *Am J Hum Genet* 1995;57:682–689.

201. Walkup JT, LaBuda MC, Singer HS, et al. Family study and segregation analysis of Tourette syndrome: evidence for a mixed model of inheritance. *Am J Hum Genet* 1996;59:684–693.

202. Lougee L, Perlmutter SJ, Nicolson R, et al. Psychiatric disorders in first-degree relatives of children with pediatric autoimmune neuropsychiatric disorders associated with streptococcal infections (PANDAS). *J Am Acad Child Adolesc Psychiatry* 2000;39: 1120–1126.

203. Leckman JF, Dolnansky ES, Hardin MT, et al. Perinatal factors in the expression of Tourette's syndrome: an exploratory study. *J Am Acad Child Adolesc Psychiatry* 1990;29:220–226.

204. Swedo SE, Leonard HL, Mittleman BB, et al. Identification of children with pediatric autoimmune neuropsychiatric disorders associated with streptococcal infections by a marker associated with rheumatic fever. *Am J Psychiatry* 1997;154:110–112.

205. A novel gene containing a trinucleotide repeat that is expanded and unstable on Huntington's disease chromosomes. The Huntington's Disease Collaborative Research Group. *Cell* 1993;72: 971–983.

206. Di Maio L, Squitieri F, Napolitano G, et al. Onset symptoms in 510 patients with Huntington's disease. *J Med Genet* 1993;30: 289–292.

207. Tanner CM, Goldman SM. Epidemiology of movement disorders. *Curr Opin Neurol* 1994;7:340–345.

208. Squitieri F, Andrew SE, Goldberg YP, et al. DNA haplotype analysis of Huntington disease reveals clues to the origins and mechanisms of CAG expansion and reasons for geographic variations of prevalence. *Hum Mol Genet* 1994;3:2103–2114.

209. Andrew SE, Hayden MR. Origins and evolution of Huntington disease chromosomes. *Neurodegeneration* 1995;4:239–244.

210. Penney JB Jr, Young AB, Shoulson I, et al. Huntington's disease in Venezuela: 7 years of follow-up on symptomatic and asymptomatic individuals. *Mov Disord* 1990;5:93–99.

211. Morrison PJ, Nevin NC. Huntington disease in County Donegal: epidemiological trends over four decades. *Ulster Med J* 1993;62:141–144.

212. Pavoni M, Granieri E, Govoni V, et al. Epidemiologic approach to Huntington's disease in northern Italy (Ferrara area). *Neuroepidemiology* 1990;9:306–314.

213. Harper PS, Tyler A, Smith S, et al. Decline in the predicted incidence of Huntington's chorea associated with systematic genetic counselling and family support. *Lancet* 1981;2:411–413.

214. Brackenridge CJ. Factors affecting the age at onset of Huntington's disease. *Med J Aust* 1980;1:261–263.

215. Roos RA, Hermans J, Vegter-van der Vlis M, et al. Duration of illness in Huntington's disease is not related to age at onset. *J Neurol Neurosurg Psychiatry* 1993;56:98–100.

216. Sorensen SA, Fenger K. Causes of death in patients with Huntington's disease and in unaffected first degree relatives. *J Med Genet* 1992;29:911–914.

217. Di Maio L, Squitieri F, Napolitano G, et al. Suicide risk in Huntington's disease. *J Med Genet* 1993;30:293–295.

218. Gimenez-Roldan S, Mateo D, Bartolome P. Tardive dystonia and severe tardive dyskinesia: a comparison of risk factors and prognosis. *Acta Psychiatr Scand* 1985;71:488–494.

219. Morgenstern H, Glazer WM. Identifying risk factors for tardive dyskinesia among long-term outpatients maintained with neuroleptic medications: results of the Yale Tardive Dyskinesia Study. *Arch Gen Psychiatry* 1993;50:723–733.

220. Caligiuri MP, Lacro JP, Rockwell E, et al. Incidence and risk factors for severe tardive dyskinesia in older patients. *Br J Psychiatry* 1997;171:148–153.

221. Kane JM, Smith JM. Tardive dyskinesia: prevalence and risk factors, 1959 to 1979. *Arch Gen Psychiatry* 1982;39:473–481.

222. Fenton WS. Prevalence of spontaneous dyskinesia in schizophrenia. *J Clin Psychiatry* 2000;61[Suppl 4]:10–14.

223. Koshino Y, Madokoro S, Ito T, et al. A survey of tardive dyskinesia in psychiatric inpatients in Japan. *Clin Neuropharmacol* 1992;15:34–43.

224. Jeste DV, Caligiuri MP. Tardive dyskinesia. *Schizophr Bull* 1993;19:303–315.

225. McCreadie RG, Robertson LJ, Wiles DH. The Nithsdale schizophrenia surveys. IX: Akathisia, parkinsonism, tardive dyskinesia and plasma neuroleptic levels. *Br J Psychiatry* 1992;160: 793–799.

226. Wojcik JD, Falk WE, Fink JS, et al. A review of 32 cases of tardive dystonia. *Am J Psychiatry* 1991;148:1055–1059.

227. McDermid SA, Hood J, Bockus S, et al. Adolescents on neuroleptic medication: is this population at risk for tardive dyskinesia? *Can J Psychiatry* 1998;43:629–631.

228. Yassa R, Nastase C, Dupont D, et al. Tardive dyskinesia in elderly psychiatric patients: a 5-year study. *Am J Psychiatry* 1992;149:1206–1211.

229. Krabbendam L, van Harten PN, Picus I, et al. Tardive dyskinesia is associated with impaired retrieval from long-term mem-

ory: the Curacao Extrapyramidal Syndromes Study: IV. *Schizophr Res* 2000;42:41–46.

230. O'Hara P, Brugha TS, Lesage A, et al. New findings on tardive dyskinesia in a community sample. *Psychol Med* 1993;23: 453–465.

231. Woerner MG, Saltz BL, Kane JM, et al. Diabetes and development of tardive dyskinesia. *Am J Psychiatry* 1993;150:966–968.

232. Yassa R, Jeste DV. Gender differences in tardive dyskinesia: a critical review of the literature. *Schizophr Bull* 1992;18:701–715.

233. Muscettola G, Pampallona S, Barbato G, et al. Persistent tardive dyskinesia: demographic and pharmacological risk factors. *Acta Psychiatr Scand* 1993;87:29–36.

234. Koshino Y, Wada Y, Isaki K, et al. A long-term outcome study of tardive dyskinesia in patients on antipsychotic medication. *Clin Neuropharmacol* 1991;14:537–546.

235. Pi EH, Gutierrez MA, Gray GE. Cross-cultural studies in tardive dyskinesia. *Am J Psychiatry* 1993;150:991.

236. Gardos G, Cole JO, Tarsy D. Withdrawal syndromes associated with antipsychotic drugs. *Am J Psychiatry* 1978;135:1321–1324.

237. Glazer WM, Morgenstern H, Schooler N, et al. Predictors of improvement in tardive dyskinesia following discontinuation of neuroleptic medication. *Br J Psychiatry* 1990;157:585–592.

238. Chiu HF, Leung JY, Lee S. Tardive dystonia in Chinese. *Singapore Med J* 1989;30:441–443.

239. Glazer WM, Morgenstern H. Predictors of occurrence, severity, and course of tardive dyskinesia in an outpatient population. *J Clin Psychopharmacol* 1988;8:10S–16S.

240. Gardos G, Casey DE, Cole JO, et al. Ten-year outcome of tardive dyskinesia. *Am J Psychiatry* 1994;151:836–841.

241. Yassa R, Nair NP. A 10-year follow-up study of tardive dyskinesia. *Acta Psychiatr Scand* 1992;86:262–266.

242. Fernandez HH, Krupp B, Friedman JH. The course of tardive dyskinesia and parkinsonism in psychiatric inpatients: 14-year follow-up. *Neurology* 2001;56:805–807.

243. Glazer WM, Morgenstern H, Doucette JT. Predicting the long-term risk of tardive dyskinesia in outpatients maintained on neuroleptic medications. *J Clin Psychiatry* 1993;54:133–139.

244. Lavigne GJ, Montplaisir JY. Restless legs syndrome and sleep bruxism: prevalence and association among Canadians. *Sleep* 1994;17:739–743.

245. Rothdach AJ, Trenkwalder C, Haberstock J, et al. Prevalence and risk factors of RLS in an elderly population: the MEMO study. Memory and Morbidity in Augsburg Elderly. *Neurology* 2000;54:1064–1068.

246. Phillips B, Young T, Finn L, et al. Epidemiology of restless legs symptoms in adults. *Arch Intern Med* 2000;160:2137–2141.

247. Ulfberg J, Nystrom B, Carter N, et al. Restless legs syndrome among working-aged women. *Eur Neurol* 2001;46:17–19.

248. Schmitt BE, Gugger M, Augustiny K, et al. [Prevalence of sleep disorders in an employed Swiss population: results of a questionnaire survey.] *Schweiz Med Wochenschr* 2000;130:772–778.

249. Walters AS, Hickey K, Maltzman J, et al. A questionnaire study of 138 patients with restless legs syndrome: the "Night-Walkers" survey. *Neurology* 1996;46:92–95.

250. Trenkwalder C, Seidel VC, Gasser T, et al. Clinical symptoms and possible anticipation in a large kindred of familial restless legs syndrome. *Mov Disord* 1996;11:389–394.

251. Tan EK, Seah A, See SJ, et al. Restless legs syndrome in an Asian population: a study in Singapore. *Mov Disord* 2001;16: 577–579.

252. Miranda M, Araya F, Castillo JL, et al. [Restless legs syndrome: a clinical study in adult general population and in uremic patients.] *Rev Med Chil* 2001;129:179–186.

253. Ondo W, Jankovic J. Restless legs syndrome: clinico-etiologic correlates. *Neurology* 1996;47:1435–1441.

254. Winkelmann J, Wetter TC, Collado-Seidel V, et al. Clinical characteristics and frequency of the hereditary restless legs syndrome in a population of 300 patients. *Sleep* 2000;23:597–602.

255. Fahn S, Williams DT. Psychogenic dystonia. *Adv Neurol* 1988;50:431–455.

256. Factor SA, Podskalny GD, Molho ES. Psychogenic movement disorders: frequency, clinical profile, and characteristics. *J Neurol Neurosurg Psychiatry* 1995;59:406–412.

257. Marsden CD. Hysteria—a neurologist's view. *Psychol Med* 1986;16:277–288.

258. Lempert T, Dieterich M, Huppert D, et al. Psychogenic disorders in neurology: frequency and clinical spectrum. *Acta Neurol Scand* 1990;82:335–340.

259. Kirkwood CR, Clure HR, Brodsky R, et al. The diagnostic content of family practice: 50 most common diagnoses recorded in the WAMI community practices. *J Fam Pract* 1982;15: 485–492.

260. Feinstein A, Stergiopoulos V, Fine J, et al. Psychiatric outcome in patients with a psychogenic movement disorder: a prospective study. *Neuropsychiatry Neuropsychol Behav Neurol* 2001;14: 169–176.

261. Hiller W, Rief W, Fichter MM. How disabled are patients with somatoform disorders? *Gen Hosp Psychiatry* 1997;19:432–438.

ETIOLOGY OF PARKINSON'S DISEASE

CAROLINE M. TANNER
SAMUEL M. GOLDMAN
G. WEBSTER ROSS

Parkinson's disease (PD) is one of the most common late-life neurodegenerative disorders. Because its incidence increases with age, its prevalence in the United States is expected to triple over the next 50 years with the aging of the population. Despite intensive research during the past several decades, the cause or causes of PD remain unknown. Since described in 1817, the proposed cause of PD has shifted from heredity to infection to toxin to pure genetics to multifactorial theories of gene—environment interaction. Although a handful of genetic and environmental factors have been associated with PD, few of these associations have been consistently observed. Nonetheless, significant progress is being made in elucidating genetic and environmental risk factors and neurodegenerative processes contributing to PD. This chapter reviews current evidence and research directions for identifying the cause of PD.

DEFINITION AND DIAGNOSTIC CONSIDERATIONS

Defining PD is essential to launching any investigation. Failure to identify all persons with PD and to exclude those with other disorders will complicate etiologic studies. However, this task is difficult. There is no biomarker for PD. Diagnosis during life is based on clinical findings and, ideally, confirmed by postmortem examination. The characteristic clinical features of PD are bradykinesia, resting tremor, cogwheel rigidity, and postural reflex impairment. Loss of pigmented neurons, most prominently in the substantia nigra, and associated α-synuclein-positive cytoplasmic inclusion bodies (Lewy bodies), are the chief pathologic features. Secondary parkinsonism (e.g., due to drugs or stroke) is excluded. Neurodegenerative syndromes associated with signs of more extensive neurologic injuries, and those that are pathologically not typical of PD, are also excluded (e.g., progressive supranuclear palsy, multiple system atrophy).

Earlier studies used other criteria, often grouping parkinsonism of any cause. Even when strict clinical criteria are applied, early PD may be missed. Since approximately 50% of substantia nigra pars compacta cells are lost before clinical signs appear, the underlying pathologic process likely precedes diagnosis for years, and persons who have clinically presymptomatic PD may remain undiagnosed at death. Moreover, as few as 80% of patients with clinical PD had typical neuropathology at postmortem exam (1,2). Recently, distinct genetic forms of parkinsonism with features similar to sporadic PD have been identified, leading to speculation that PD is actually a constellation of neurodegenerative disorders culminating in overlapping clinical and pathologic findings.

The uncertainty of clinical diagnosis is an important factor in the design and critical analysis of studies of causation of PD. Inclusion of case subjects who do not have typical disease results in overestimation of disease frequency; excluding recently symptomatic cases with incomplete clinical features results in underestimation. In either case–control studies or family studies, including case subjects who do not actually have PD can obscure a causative association or even result in associations with factors determining a different form of parkinsonsim. In families, the mode of inheritance of a genetic defect could also be misinterpreted. Some of these diagnostic dilemmas may be improved by new imaging techniques, careful exclusion of cases with known genetic forms of parkinsonism, and, ultimately, development of sensitive and specific biomarkers of disease.

ETIOLOGIC THEORIES

Current theories of the mechanisms underlying PD stem from both epidemiologic observations and basic research. Although the search for clues to causation often reduces to a discussion of genes versus environment, this argument presupposes that a single or, at most, a few genes or environmental factors are sufficient to cause PD in most individuals. This is not necessarily the case, however, and although this chapter reviews studies of both genetic and environmental risk as though they were operating independently, the actual situation is undoubtedly more complex, involving interaction of multiple risk factors. Regardless of triggering factors, the final mechanisms of neuronal injury and death are probably similar. For this reason we will begin with an overview of epidemiologic data and conclude with a brief review of mechanistic observations, which likely reflect final common pathways of genetic and environmental causes of PD.

EPIDEMIOLOGIC EVIDENCE

Epidemiology is the study of disease frequencies and determinants at a population level. By comparing disease frequencies between populations with differing characteristics, putative risk factors can be identified. PD epidemiology has been systematically studied in a wide variety of populations, providing a number of clues to causation.

Age

Increasing age is unequivocally associated with increasing risk for PD. This is true in all community-based studies, with annual incidence increasing dramatically from fewer than 10 per 100,000 at age 50 to at least 200 per 100,000 at age 80 (3). Although PD is intimately related to aging, it has been well documented that its underlying process is distinct from natural aging. There is a marked microglial reaction to neuronal damage in PD that is not seen in normal aging (4), and although there is an aging-related decline in the number of nigral neurons, the distribution of cell loss in PD is significantly different (5,6).

Several causative processes could explain the nearly exponential increase with age. Potentially important aging-related mechanisms include chronic or repetitive exposure to endogenous or exogenous neurotoxicants, acute neural insult on a background of normal aging-related nigral neuron attrition, a decrease in functional neural repair mechanisms, and a decrease in detoxifying mechanisms with age. Retrospective studies of personality traits (7) suggest that a preclinical dopaminergic deficit precedes clinically evident PD by many years. ^{18}F-dopa positron emission tomography (PET) studies (8), β-CIT single photon emission computed tomography (SPECT) studies (9), and autopsy series (10) suggest a 5- to 10-year preclinical period. Yet evidence that dopaminergic neuronal loss in PD is ongoing at the time of death (4) suggests that although an event or a process ultimately resulting in disease may occur or begin in youth, PD involves a progressive loss of neurons.

Temporal Variation

Has PD incidence changed over time? Periodic fluctuation in incidence could result from any episodic exposure, such

as an infectious process. In contrast, a steady increase over the past several decades could implicate exposures increasingly present, such as those due to industrialization or lifestyle practices. Conversely, if PD incidence has remained stable over time, recent environmental factors are likely relatively unimportant causes of PD.

Reviews of the Mayo Clinic database from Olmstead County, Minnesota, disclosed no change in age-specific PD incidence between 1935 and 1990 (11,12). A large Finnish study similarly found stable disease incidence between 1971 and 1992; however, a dramatic demographic shift emerged in 1992, with a strong male and rural predominance not previously observed (13).

Variation in disease frequency over even these relatively short periods is difficult to measure reliably. Changes in incidence may reflect improved diagnosis or record keeping, or possibly relative changes in mortality from competing diseases (14). In addition, there may be a long latency between exposure to causative factors and any consequent change in the rate of clinically detectable disease. If this is true, observation over a few decades may not be adequate to identify a change.

It is even less clear whether the incidence of PD has changed over longer periods, such as centuries or even millennia. Because PD is a late-life disorder, its frequency is a function of population life span. In ancient times the average life span was decades shorter, so population prevalence was likely lower even if the incidence rate among the aged was unchanged. Several historic references describe symptoms such as shaking, slowness, and stooped posture as afflictions of aging, and these are often presented as evidence that PD was present in ancient times (15,16). However, the full syndrome of PD, with the characteristic propulsive gait, hesitation of movement initiation, and tremor at rest, was not described until 1817. Whether PD, some other parkinsonian syndrome, essential tremor, or normal aging was described in the ancient texts will remain a matter for opinionated discussion, particularly since the controversy can never be resolved.

Geography

Few incidence studies have been performed worldwide. Estimates of disease *prevalence* vary widely around the world, from 31 per 100,000 persons in Libya to 657 per 100,000 in Buenos Aires, Argentina (17). Although differences in the age distributions in these populations, diagnostic criteria, ascertainment methods, access to health care, or disease survival rates may explain much of this variation, international variation in PD frequency is seen even after adjustment for many of these inconsistencies has been carried out (18). Risk factors that might vary geographically include both genetic differences in disease susceptibility and exposure to causative and protective environmental factors.

Sex

PD is nearly twice as common in men than in similarly aged women. This male preponderance is observed irrespective of geographic location or race (19,20), and is seen in both prevalence and incidence studies. In one large, multiethnic, community-based study, American women of African, Hispanic, or Caucasian descent all had a lower incidence than men of the corresponding ethnic group (21). Whether the increased risk in men is a biologic phenomenon, such as may result, for example, from the influence of sex hormones, or a cultural phenomenon, reflecting male-related occupational exposures or other behavioral factors, is not clear. The latter hypothesis is supported by a large Finnish study showing a dramatic increase in the male-to-female relative risk from 0.9 in 1971 to 1.9 in 1992 (13).

Race

PD may be more common in nations with primarily white populations, although the evidence is far from clear. Lower prevalence has been reported in nonwhites (20), but whether these differences were real or related to shorter survival or diagnostic differences is not clear. Recent studies found similar *incidence* in African-Americans (21), Asian Americans (22), and white Americans. Whether this reflects a true race-associated difference or greater similarity in environmental exposures will need to be clarified by comparing other populations.

GENETIC FACTORS

Since proposed by Gowers in 1888 and supported by many anecdotal reports, hereditary risk factors for PD have been actively sought. Modern molecular methods have led to exciting discoveries of genetic mutations that cause parkinsonism, although these are rare.

Autosomal Dominant Parkinsonism

The largest described family with pathologically typical PD—the Contursi kindred—was reported by Golbe et al. (23). The inheritance pattern is autosomal dominant with high penetrance. Mean age at disease onset is 45.6 years, compared with 60 years in the community. Disease course is also unusual, with death following onset within a mean interval of 9.2 years versus an expected mean course (assuming onset at age 45) of approximately 20 years for typical PD (2). Clinically atypical features include fluent aphasia and palilalia.

The mutation in this pedigree was identified in the α-synuclein gene on the long arm of chromosome 4 (PARK1) (24). Although the same mutation has been identified in several Greek families (25), current evidence suggests that the mutation is extremely rare (26). A second mutation of the same gene has been identified in a German family, also with an autosomal dominant pattern of inheritance associated with a similar phenotype (27).

At least two other chromosomal loci have been identified in families with an autosomal dominant pattern of inheritance for parkinsonism. In a study of six different families from northern Germany and southern Denmark, parkinsonism was linked to a locus on chromosome 2p13, but with only 40% penetrance (PARK3) (28). In addition, a parkinsonian syndrome with young age at onset, early dementia, and a rapid clinical course has been identified in a family known as the Iowa kindred (PARK4). The locus has been mapped to chromosome 4p14-16.3 (29).

Autosomal Recessive Parkinsonism

A form of juvenile parkinsonism which is responsive to levodopa has been described in Japanese patients with onset before age 40 years and a positive family history. There is also a high incidence of foot dystonia, and early development of L-dopa-induced dyskinesias and motor fluctuations, but otherwise their disease is quite similar to typical PD (30). Exon deletion mutations in a gene on chromosome 6, called *parkin*, have now been identified in several of these families (PARK2) (31).

Homozygous deletions and point mutations in *parkin* have also been associated with early onset of parkinsonism in European and North African families (32). The clinical features of these European cases are quite similar to those reported in Japanese patients.

Recent studies suggest that *parkin* mutations are among the most common causes of young-onset familial PD throughout the world (32); however, since at least 95% of parkinsonism in the community has onset after age 50 (20), PARK2 remains a rare cause of parkinsonism.

A mutation in the ubiquitin carboxy-terminal hydrolase L1 (UCH-L1) gene located on chromosome 4p has been tentatively associated with a form of young-onset autosomal recessive parkinsonism, although clinical characterization is limited (33). The significance of this mutation in terms of PD awaits verification of the neuropathology and the identification of additional affected families.

Mitochondrial Inheritance

Mitochondrial dysfunction has been proposed to underlie the pathogenesis of nerve cell death in PD. Because mitochondrial DNA is maternally inherited, a familial pattern of maternal preponderance is expected in disorders caused by defects in the mitochondrial genome. Swerdlow et al. (34) described one such family and demonstrated abnormal mitochondrial function. Two other families with apparent maternal preponderance have also been described (35). However, matrilineal inheritance has not consistently been shown by other investigations (36). One study has shown that age at onset of PD is lower in patients born to older mothers but not fathers, implicating long exposure of the ovum to an environmental factor (37).

Other Family Aggregation Studies

A positive family history for PD is more frequently reported by PD subjects than control subjects, with odds ratios ranging from 2.7 to 14.6 (38,39). When family composition (age, number of relatives) is taken into account, PD is reported to occur from 1.4 to 3.5 times more often in relatives of PD patients than in those of control subjects (40–42). This risk factor appears to be stronger in those with younger onset of disease. In one study, PD subjects with age of onset under 70 years were 8.8 times as likely as controls to report a positive family history, while those older than 70 years were only 2.8 times as likely (38). Since families share behaviors and environments, familial occurrence cannot necessarily be attributed to an underlying genetic mechanism.

Another method of addressing the role of inheritance in PD is through the assessment of the degree of relatedness of PD cases compared with that of unaffected control subjects in a population. A recent study from Iceland identified 772 cases of parkinsonism over the preceding 50 years. Using geneologic information over 11 centuries, it was found that patients with parkinsonism, including those with onset after age 50, were significantly more related to each other than were subjects in control groups (43). The risk ratio was higher for siblings (6.7) than for children (3.2), suggesting a common early environmental factor or recessively inherited modifying genes. Interestingly, in Iceland PD frequency does not increase with increasing age as is seen in other populations worldwide. These unusual demographics may be explained by a preponderance of inherited forms of parkinsonism in Iceland since these forms typically have earlier age of onset.

Recently, two groups have reported the results of genome-wide screens in familial parkinsonism (44,45). Each found *parkin* mutations in the early age at onset group. One found an association between parkinsonism and several single nucleotide polymorphisms (SNPs) in the gene encoding tau protein (46). Whether these represent PD or another form of parkinsonism will require further investigation as familial frontotemporal dementia with parkinsonism (FTDP) and progressive supranuclear palsy (PSP) both have been associated with abnormalities in this gene (FTDP) or with the SNPs tested (PSP). As cognitive testing was not performed in the subjects studied, the meaning of this association awaits clarification of the clinical features of the population. The difference in distribution of SNPs between affected and unaffected family members was small (82% vs. 79%). Because the difference is so small, this finding is not likely to be a useful way to identify persons "at risk" for familial parkinsonism. Interestingly, this finding was not replicated in the other screen. In fact, apart from *parkin*, none of the suggestive loci identified in one screen were found in the other. Extrapolation of these findings to nonfamilial parkinsonism will require further studies in the majority of PD cases not reporting an affected family member.

Twin Studies

Twin studies have also been used to test the hypothesis of a genetic contribution to PD. Intrapair concordance rates should be much higher in monozygotic (MZ) twins than in dizygotic (DZ) twins if a genetic factor is an important causative component of PD, yet similar rates of concordance in MZ and DZ twin pairs have been demonstrated in several twin studies. A recent large population-based twin study found 163 pairs with PD in at least one twin. Concordance rates were similar in MZ and DZ pairs overall (47). However, in pairs with onset in at least one twin before age 51, concordance was six times as high in MZ as in DZ, whereas in those with onset after age 50 MZ and DZ concordance rates were identical. This suggests that early-onset PD, which is rare, may have a strong genetic component. This is not unexpected given that most of the known genetic mutations related to PD produce early-onset disease.

It follows that the vastly more common later onset disease appears not to have a genetic cause. However, a limitation to studies of concordance in twins is the possibility that one twin dies or is lost to follow-up before symptoms are evident, giving the appearance of discordance in concordant twins. In a recent PET study of twin pairs clinically discordant for PD at baseline, concordance for decreased putaminal ^{18}F-dopa uptake was higher in some of the MZ but not in any of the DZ twin pairs after several years of follow-up (48). Only about half of the pairs studied at baseline were evaluated at a second time point. The relationship between this radiographic finding and subsequent clinically or pathologically diagnosed PD is unknown, and the population prevalence of decreased putaminal ^{18}F-dopa uptake is not well understood. Prospective observation of additional twin pairs will be useful in determining the significance of these interesting findings.

ENVIRONMENTAL FACTORS

Environmental causes of PD have been suspected for many years. As recently as 40 years ago, some argued that most cases of PD result from encephalitis (49), although postencephalitic parkinsonism is now recognized to be a pathologically and clinically distinct entity. A variety of toxic agents, including carbon disulfide, manganese, and hydrocarbon solvents, had also been recognized to cause parkinsonian syndromes, but their clinical and pathologic features were distinct from typical PD (50). A break occurred in 1983, when 1-methyl-4-phenyl-1,2,3,6-tetrahydropyridine (MPTP), a simple pyridine analog, was identified as the cause of a parkinsonian syndrome in a group of narcotics addicts (51). The striking similarity of MPTP parkinsonism and idiopathic PD rekindled the idea that exposure to an exogenous agent might cause PD and spurred the search for related environmental factors using both epidemiologic and laboratory research methods.

Xenobiotics

MPTP has been used as a paradigm to narrow the search for toxicants etiologically related to PD, with research focusing on toxicologically similar compounds. MPTP toxicology is well characterized (52). The compound readily crosses the blood–brain barrier because of its lipophilicity, where it is oxidized by monoamine oxidase B (MAO-B) into 1-methyl-4-phenylpyridinium (MPP$^+$). MPP$^+$ is actively taken up into nerve terminals by the dopamine transporter (DAT) and is concentrated in mitochondria. In mitochondria it binds and inhibits NADH complex I, blocking oxidative phosphorylation and ATP production, and increasing free radicals and nitric oxide, and leads to rapid apoptotic cell death.

Pesticides

A wide range of compounds are known to act as mitochondrial poisons. Pesticides are of particular interest because of an observed association between PD and farming or rural living (see below). Mitochondrial electron transport complexes and ATP synthesis are inhibited by diphenylether herbicides, DDT and other organochlorine insecticides, thiadiazole herbicides, pyrethroid insecticides, and benzimidazole fungicides, among others. Recently, Betarbet et al. (53) described an animal model of PD caused by chronic administration of the insecticide rotenone to rats. This model is remarkable for several reasons. First, pathologically, it may mimic PD even more closely than does the MPTP model. Highly specific nigrostriatal dopaminergic degeneration with corresponding Lewy body–like inclusions is accompanied by hypokinesia and rigidity. Second, the syndrome develops only after chronic administration. Third, like MPTP, rotenone is a potent inhibitor of mitochondrial complex I, which in fact is designated "the rotenone-sensitive site." Paraquat, a dipyridyl herbicide structurally similar to MPTP, and combined paraquat and maneb (manganese ethylenebisdithiocarbamate) (54) have also been shown to induce destruction of nigral dopaminergic neurons with a consequent neurobehavioral syndrome in mice.

In addition to their direct effect on mitochondrial respiration, other mechanisms could underlie pesticide toxicity. Uversky et al. (55) recently reported that several common pesticides, including rotenone, paraquat, and dieldrin, accelerate the rate of α-synuclein fibril formation. Fibril formation leads to the formation of α-synuclein protein aggregates as are found in Lewy bodies. Whether these aggregates are causative or protective remains uncertain. However, the ability of pesticides to mimic in vitro a characteristic pathologic feature of PD provides a potential important clue to the neurodegenerative process in PD.

Case-control studies also implicate pesticides. Two autopsy studies detected increased levels of the organochlorine insecticide dieldrin in PD brain (56,57), while numerous studies have reported an increased frequency of pesticide exposure (Table 7.1). A meta-analysis of 19 published studies found a combined odds ratio (OR) of 1.94 (95% CI 1.49–2.53) for pesticide exposure (58). However, specific compounds or compound classes have only rarely been identified. Liou et al. (59) reported increased risk of PD in association with paraquat (OR = 3.22) in Taiwan. Exposure to herbicides, insecticides, alkylated phosphates, organochlorines, and wood preservatives have all been reported to be associated with increased risk of PD (59–63).

TABLE 7.1. CASE-CONTROL STUDIES TESTING ASSOCIATIONS BETWEEN RURAL HOME, FARMING, PESTICIDES, AND WELL WATER DRINKING

Location	Number of Cases/Controls	Rural Home	Farming, Gardening	Pesticides	Well Water
Michigan, USA (60)	144/464	–	OR = 2.8*	+	–
Australia (175)	224/310	+	–	–	–
USA (176)	149/149	+*	NA	–	–
New York, USA (177)	89/188	+[a]	+[a]	NA	+[a]
Spain (178)	74/148	+	–	+	+
Calgary, Canada (62)	130/260	–	+	+*	NA
China (179)	100/200	–	–	+	–
Hong Kong (180)	35/105	+*	+*	+*	NA
Meta-analysis (181)	Variable	OR = 1.56*	OR = 1.42*	OR = 1.85*	OR = 1.26

[a]Only in African-Americans.
*$p < 0.05$.
NA, not applicable; OR, odds ratio.

Rural Living and Farming

Case-control studies conducted throughout the world have identified rural living, farming, gardening, and well water drinking as risk factors for PD. Some of these are summarized in Table 7.1. Although the precise nature of the association with putative rural risk factors varies across studies, the consistency of these findings is remarkable considering the different methods and locations. It is unclear how rural factors other than pesticide exposure may be related to PD.

Occupation

In addition to the association with agricultural occupations, a higher incidence of PD has been reported among carpenters and cleaners (64), teachers (65,66), health care workers (65,66), and workers chronically exposed to metals (67). In one study, welding appeared to be associated with an earlier age of PD onset; however, the effect of occupation on age at onset was only studied for welders (68) and is therefore difficult to interpret. Despite these sporadic associations, the vast majority of studies have failed to identify any occupational risk factors for PD other than agricultural work. Future research on occupational risk factors must employ more rigorous exposure assessment methodologies.

Infection

Since the observation that encephalitis preceded parkinsonism during the influenza pandemic of the early 1900s, many studies have sought to identify an infectious agent in typical PD. Although a handful of sporadic associations have been published, these have rarely been confirmed (20). Exposure to influenza virus in utero has been proposed to damage fetal substantia nigra, predisposing to PD in adulthood. Childhood diphtheria and croup have been directly associated, and childhood measles inversely associated with subsequent PD. Single studies reported increased *Helicobacter pylori* seropositivity and increased cerebrospinal fluid coronavirus titers in PD.

Nocardia asteroides has a specific affinity for substantia nigra neurons in mouse and primate, and has been shown to cause a dopa-responsive movement disorder in mice (69–71). Elevated *Nocardia* antibody titers have been observed in some studies of PD patients, but this has not been consistent.

Monoclonal antibodies against Epstein-Barr virus were recently shown to cross-react with α-synuclein in Lewy bodies in human brain (72), implicating autoimmune-mediated mechanisms. This possibility is supported by a prior observation that IgG from patients with PD induces a specific inflammatory destruction of dopaminergic neurons in rodent substantia nigra (73).

Although an infectious process could explain the familial nature of PD, the lack of clustering within generations or geographic regions and the inability to identify a specific infectious agent argues against the importance of infection as a primary etiologic factor.

Diet

Differences in diet may help to explain the geographic variability in PD prevalence or the clustering of the disease within families. The possible role of diet as a causative or protective factor in PD has been investigated in numerous case-control studies, providing several associations for further evaluation.

Due to the potential neuroprotective role of antioxidant containing foods and vitamin supplements, several studies have examined the association of these with PD. Results have been disappointingly mixed (20). To date, there are few data to support a protective role for tocopherol. No consistent association with intake of other antioxidant vitamins has been found, although this has not been thoroughly studied. Other inconsistent observations include an inverse association between niacin intake and PD risk (74), and an inverse association with consumption of nuts, legumes (75–77), and potatoes (78). Consumption of foods high in animal fat has been positively associated in several case-control studies (79–81), as has total caloric intake (74,80). Both lipid consumption and higher caloric intake are thought to increase oxidative stress, one mechanism proposed to cause neuronal degeneration in PD (see discussion on mechanisms). Dietary restriction has been found to ameliorate loss of dopaminergic neurons in rats given the neurotoxin MPTP (82).

Caffeine

An inverse association of both coffee and caffeine consumption and PD has been reported in case control and cohort studies (64,83–86). In men, the more coffee or caffeine consumed at midlife, the lower the risk of subsequently developing PD. In women, this effect is less certain although fewer women have been studied (83,84). The stimulant effect of caffeine is thought to be mediated through its antagonist action on the adenosine A2A receptor. A possible neuroprotective role for caffeine and other adenosine A2A receptor antagonists has been demonstrated in experiments where preadministration of caffeine and other adenosine A2A receptor antagonists attenuate the striatal dopamine loss in mice given MPTP (87).

Alcohol

Consumption of alcohol has been found by some to be inversely associated with PD even after controlling for possible confounding by smoking (64,74,86). One study found that fewer subjects with PD had a diagnosis of alcoholism than controls (85). Putative biological mechanisms of ethanol protection are not well understood, and the low consumption of alcohol in PD has commonly been attributed to the reserved premorbid personality previously described (7).

Head Trauma

Prior head trauma has been associated with PD in some case control studies with the injury occurring an average of more than 35 years prior to the diagnosis of PD (39,61,88). The significance of these finding is uncertain owing to the small number of studies and the likelihood that subjects are more inclined to recall past injuries (recall bias).

Depression and Stress

Major depression occurs commonly in patients with PD and is independent of the degree of functional impairment. Some studies have shown that depression may predate the motor symptoms (89); however, it is not clear whether depression is a risk factor for the future development of PD or an early manifestation of the disease. One case-control study associated depression with PD diagnosed an average of 22 years after the depressive episode (39).

Other forms of physical and psychological stress have been linked to an increased risk of PD. These physiologic states may be associated with increased turnover in catecholamines leading to neuronal oxidative stress. In two groups of ex–Far East prisoners of war, the incidence of PD was greater than expected in later life (90,91). However, follow-up in one of these populations reported no increased mortality from PD (92).

Smoking

The most consistently observed risk factor for PD is non-smoking. An inverse association between cigarette smoking and PD has been observed in diverse populations in studies spanning more than 30 years, including several large prospective investigations (85,93–95). The risk of PD in smokers appears to be about half that of nonsmokers (96), and is inversely related to lifetime "dose," suggesting a true protective effect. This hypothesis is strengthened by experimental observations that nicotine protects against age (97), transection (98), MPTP (99), and 6-hydroxydopamine-induced (100) neuronal damage in rodent substantia nigra. Furthermore, nicotine has antioxidant properties (101) and increases striatal trophic factors (102). Alternatively, smoking might afford indirect protection by inducing peripheral detoxifying enzymes or by reducing bioactivation of protoxins. This latter hypothesis is supported by the observation that cigarette smoking reduces MAO-B activity in humans (103).

Others have argued that decreased smoking in PD could be a manifestation of the conservative personality that has been observed in PD patients prior to their diagnosis. Both smoking and personality are associated with dopaminergic functions (103–105). Despite these arguments, the consistency and strength of the inverse association, the dose–response relationship, and mechanistic plausibility support a true protective effect of smoking.

SINGLE-GENE ASSOCIATIONS AND GENE–ENVIRONMENT INTERACTIONS

The evidence for the association of genetic polymorphisms with PD has been inconclusive thus far. The search for such associations has focused on genes coding for metabolic enzymes, proteins involved in dopaminergic transmission, and free-radical detoxifying enzymes. Among the earliest and most studied in relation to PD is the cytochrome P450 isoenzyme 2D6 *(CYP2D6)*. Substrates and/or competitive inhibitors of its enzymatic product, debrisoquine hydroxylase, include tricyclic antidepressants, neuroleptics, cocaine, codeine, amphetamine, MPTP, and possibly neurotransmitters. The polymorphic alleles that code for this enzyme have variable effects on its activity and substrate affinity. *CYP2D6* allelic variants associated with the poor metabolizer phenotype have been associated with increased risk of PD. Most recently, however, the bulk of the evidence from case-control studies and meta-analyses indicates no association or a small increased risk (106–108). Although the inconsistency of these associations with PD risk may represent differences in sample size, control selection, case definition, or genetic methods, they also may result from genetic interaction with environmental exposures (109). That is, these variants may only result in an increased risk if an individual is exposed to certain environmental factors resulting in toxic effects from levels of compounds that might not otherwise be toxic. Enzymatic variability may result in decreased detoxification of toxic compounds or increased bioactivation of otherwise nontoxic compounds. Work in this area is just beginning. Thus far, one study has examined the association of exposure to pesticides, herbicides, or well water consumption with CYP2D6 genotype and found no association (108).

Glutathione transferases are a group of pesticide detoxification enzymes. Homozygosity for a null mutation in the glutathione *S*-transferase (GST) M1 gene has been inconsistently associated with PD (110,111). Interestingly, a recent case-control study, though finding no association of polymorphisms in four classes of GST with PD, found that PD cases were more likely to have GST P1 genetic variants than controls when the analysis was restricted to only those who reported exposure to pesticides (112).

A well-known environmental factor associated with reduced risk of PD is cigarette smoking. One of the proposed mechanisms for this relationship is that chemicals contained in smoke reduce the activity of MAO-B. While studies examining the association of MAO-B gene polymorphisms with PD have shown variable results, a recent case-control study found an interaction between cigarette smoking and polymorphism type where reduced PD risk related to smoking was found in cases with the G allele but there was an elevated PD risk related to smoking among those with the A allele (113).

N-Acetyltransferase-2 (NAT-2) is another detoxifying enzyme. Polymorphisms of the *NAT2* gene cause slow acetylation and, therefore, impaired inactivation of neurotoxins. Studies are divided between an association of the slow acetylator genotype with increased risk of PD (114,115) or no increased risk (106,116). Thus far no studies have examined an interaction between environmental toxin exposure and NAT-2 genotype.

Similarly inconsistent results have been reported for polymorphisms of the dopamine transporter gene and the dopamine receptor genes *DRD2* and *DRD4* (114,117,118).

The genes coding for the free-radical–detoxifying enzymes superoxide dismutase (SOD) and catalase have also been investigated with no apparent associations (119,120).

Future success in the search for gene–environment interactions for PD will depend on assessment of multiple candidate genetic polymorphisms in defined populations with well-characterized exposure data.

MECHANISMS OF DISEASE

Is PD a genetic or an environmental disease? Familial clusters of parkinsonism exist, but these are rare, and their equivalence to PD is not completely clear. Twin studies argue against a major genetic basis, but PD is more common in families of patients than in control families. The MPTP cluster and the recent rotenone animal model demonstrate that environmental factors are capable of inducing very specific nigral damage similar to that seen in idiopathic PD. Yet although general environmental associations with PD are consistently observed, few specific agents have been identified, and clusters of idiopathic PD are unknown.

Irrespective of the strengths and weaknesses of the genetic and environmental hypotheses, each has contributed to our understanding of disease mechanisms. Although the long latency between disease onset and diagnosis makes it difficult to distinguish between phenomena that are consequences of the disease process and those that are causal, we have made great strides in delineating the pathophysiologic mechanisms underlying PD.

Mitochondrial Dysfunction

The recognition that the neurotoxin MPP$^+$ impairs mitochondrial oxidative phosphorylation by inhibiting complex I of the electron transport chain suggested that an inborn or acquired mitochondrial defect might underlie idiopathic PD and prompted a search for abnormalities in patients. Consistent with this hypothesis, impaired mitochondrial function has been detected in a variety of tissues from PD patients, including substantia nigra (121), platelet (122), and possibly muscle (123). Within brain the 20% to 40% decrease in complex I activity is isolated to substantia nigra and is not observed in other neurodegenerative diseases, such as PSP (124) or multiple system atrophy (121). Deficiencies of complexes II to IV have rarely been reported.

Changes in mitochondrial function could be secondary to the disease process rather than causal. In support of this possibility, Przedborski et al. (125) found that complex I activity is inhibited by levodopa and dopamine in a dose-dependent manner, suggesting that observed changes may be a consequence of drug treatment or of increased dopamine turnover in surviving cell populations. However, the lack of similar decreases in respiratory chain activity in other neurodegenerative disorders and the observation that these changes are present in early untreated PD (122,126) lend support to the hypothesis that impaired mitochondrial function is etiologically significant.

Elucidation of the causes of mitochondrial dysfunction is difficult for several reasons. First, mitochondrial defects may be inherited or acquired. If acquired, toxicants may be exogenous, as in the case of MPTP or rotenone, or endogenous, as exemplified by the tetraisoquinolines (127) or cysteinyldopamines and dihydrobenzothiazines (128). Second, mitochondrial proteins are encoded by both mitochondrial and nuclear genomes, obscuring hereditary patterns. For example, complex I is composed of 43 protein subunits, 7 of which are encoded by mitochondrial DNA (mtDNA), and 36 by the nuclear genome (129). Third, assays of mitochondrial "activity" are not standardized, may be insensitive, and may measure functional attributes of questionable relevance to PD.

Although there is minimal epidemiologic evidence supporting a maternal inheritance pattern (34,35), mtDNA deletions and mutations are sometimes associated with PD. Hattori et al. (130) found a significantly increased frequency of a complex I polymorphism in PD patients, with an odds ratio of 2.4 for homozygotes. Other investigators have observed specific mutations or an increased frequency of mtDNA mutations in PD (131,132), but this is not consistently reported (133,134). One interesting research method involves the transfer of platelet mtDNA from PD patients into cell lines devoid of mtDNA, creating so-called cybrids. Using this methodology several investigators have shown that a complex I deficit is transferrable via PD mtDNA, strongly suggesting that the complex I deficit in some cases of PD derives at least in part from mtDNA (135,136).

Could a mild impairment of mitochondrial function cause the highly localized neuropathology of PD? Animal models of PD argue in favor of this possibility. In the rotenone model, complex I is inhibited in all tissues yet pathology is limited to dopaminergic nigral neurons. A possible explanation for this selective vulnerability is high metabolic demand on a background of oxidative stress (see below). Energetically compromised mitochondria, for example, are 30-fold more sensitive to apoptosis induced by dopamine metabolites than are fully energized mitochondria (137). They are also much more vulnerable to oxidative stress (138). In the MPTP model, selective vulnerability is due to specific regional accumulation of the complex I toxin. Either or both of these vulnerability mechanisms could operate in typical idiopathic PD.

Oxidative Stress

Oxidative stress has been proposed as a contributing factor in many systemic and neurodegenerative diseases, and several lines of evidence implicate its role in PD pathogenesis. Hydrogen peroxide and free-radical byproducts of oxygen-based metabolic processes react with and can damage all cellular components, including DNA, proteins, and membranes. Their production is in balance with protective reductive and repair mechanisms, the most important of which are vitamins A and related carotenoids, E (α-tocopherol) and C (ascorbate), and the enzymes SOD, catalase, and glutathione peroxidase. Other compounds and nutrients, such as uric acid, polyunsaturated fatty acids, and estrogen, may also confer oxidant resistance. If the capacity of local antioxidant defenses is exceeded, cell death or carcinogenesis may result.

The high metabolic demands and limited replicative potential of neurons make them especially vulnerable to the effects of oxidative processes, and a large body of evidence suggests that oxidative damage contributes to PD. Two characteristics of the substantia nigra place it at particular risk for oxidant damage. First, dopamine and its metabolic byproducts are directly toxic to neurons. Second, the neuromelanin found in pigmented neurons, which itself is formed by dopamine autoxidation, acts as a repository for iron and other reactive metals (139). In human postmortem studies, the neurons containing the highest amount of neuromelanin are those that degenerate in PD (140).

The enzymatic catabolism of dopamine by MAO generates hydrogen peroxide and superoxide radical (O_2) at a rate proportional to dopamine turnover, whereas nonenzymatic metabolism generates dopamine quinone and cysteinyl conjugates. Each of these compounds is toxic to dopaminergic cells in vitro (141) and in vivo (142). Dopamine-derived hydrogen peroxide can react with the reduced (ferric) iron of neuromelanin through the Fenton reaction, generating highly toxic hydroxyl radical ($\cdot OH$) (143). Consistent with this hypothesis, intranigral iron injection induces lipid peroxidation, a large selective decrease in dopamine, and a parkinsonian syndrome in rats (144). Sim-

ilarly, PD patients appear to have increased levels of nonferritin iron in substantia nigra relative to controls (145,146), as well as increased lipid peroxidation products (147,148). Whether these changes are primary or secondary disease phenomena is unclear.

Oxidant defenses also appear to be reduced in PD. Levels of reduced glutathione (GSH) are consistently found to be lower in PD substantia nigra than in normal controls or subjects with other neurodegenerative diseases also affecting nigral cell populations (148,149). This suggests that the depletion of GSH in PD is not simply a consequence of cell death. GSH depletion increases the neuronal toxicity of many compounds including MPTP (150), sulfite and peroxynitrite (151), and, perhaps most importantly, dopamine (152). Increased dopamine turnover itself may deplete GSH through MAO-catalyzed generation of H_2O_2 (153). Furthermore, the depletion of GSH appears to cause mitochondrial complex I inhibition due to increased thiol oxidation (154) and may therefore create a vicious cycle of increasing oxidative stress with decreasing defenses (Fig. 7.1).

Other affected antioxidant systems include SOD, which is enhanced in parkinsonian nigra, perhaps in response to increased levels of dopamine-derived superoxide radical (155), and catalase, which may have diminished activity (156), resulting in increased production and decreased clearance of H_2O_2. Toxic tyrosyl radical and reactive nitrogen species such as peroxynitrite have also been found at increased levels in parkinsonian brain (157). Furthermore, the activity of nitric oxide synthase, the enzyme that produces reactive nitric oxide, is increased in parkinsonian nigra (158) and is directly involved in MPTP toxicity (159). Finally, both nigral (160) and serum (161) uric acid levels are reduced in PD, the latter found many years prior to disease onset, suggesting that this is not a consequence of neurodegeneration or of treatment.

Although many of the oxidative phenomena observed in PD may not precipitate the neurodegenerative cascade, there is a broad and convincing body of evidence to support at least a contributory role for oxidative stress in the etiology of PD.

ABNORMAL PROTEIN AGGREGATION

The discoveries that rare mutations of the α-synuclein gene can cause parkinsonism coupled with the finding that antibodies to α-synuclein detect Lewy bodies in sporadic PD have focused attention on abnormal protein metabolism and accumulation of insoluble aggregates of α-synuclein as contributing to the mechanisms underlying the dopaminergic neuronal loss of PD (162–165). In fact, α-synuclein aggregates are also found in the cortical Lewy bodies of dementia with Lewy bodies and in the glial cytoplasmic inclusions found in multiple system atrophy, prompting reference to these conditions collectively as α-synucle-inopathies (166).

The function of α-synuclein is unknown but it is normally abundant in nerve terminals. In vitro, it has been shown that wild-type α-synuclein and both mutant types linked to PD form fibrillar aggregates and that aggregation is accelerated by both mutants (167,168). Furthermore, the expression of normal or mutant forms of α-synuclein in fruit flies that normally have no α-synuclein produces mobility disturbances, dopamine neuron loss, and Lewy-like inclusions in adult flies (169).

Normally, the ubiquitin-proteasome system is responsible for the degradation of abnormal proteins before they can aggregate. This process occurs in several steps, beginning with the activation of the protein ubiquitin and the ligation of ubiquitin to protein substrates by ubiquitin ligases (169,170). Ubiquitinization marks the protein for degradation by the proteasome. Interestingly, parkin has been discovered to act as a ubiquitin protein ligase. Parkin gene mutations may result in absent or ineffective ubiquitin ligase activity resulting in abnormal protein processing (171,172). Evidence that the proteins α-synuclein and parkin may be linked in a common process comes from a study demonstrating similar patterns of expression of α-synuclein and parkin mRNA in limited areas of normal human brains (173).

Many questions remain regarding the role of abnormal protein aggregation in PD. First, the processes that trigger fibrillogenesis of α-synuclein in PD are unknown. In addition to genetic mutations, it is speculated that environmental toxins may promote aggregation either directly or through a cascade of events beginning, for example, with mitochondrial toxicity leading to free-radical accumulation and the creation of an environment conducive to accelerated synuclein aggregation (165,174). In addition, it is not known whether abnormal synuclein aggregation is responsible for dopaminergic neuronal degeneration or is merely an end result of some other process that damages neurons.

SUMMARY

Recent advances in epidemiologic, genetic, and basic science research are generating plausible hypotheses regarding the cause of PD. These advances, rather than narrowing the focus to a single genetic or environmental cause, have led to an understanding of PD as a very complex disorder with multiple causes. In fact, the very definition of PD is undergoing reappraisal because the familial forms of the disease often have atypical clinical and pathologic features. Although rare, genetic mutations causing PD have led to improved understanding of mechanisms that are likely important in sporadic disease. α-Synuclein is an important constituent in Lewy bodies, and environmental as well as genetic influences may lead to abnormal aggregation of this protein that, in turn, could cause neuronal dysfunction and death. The role of parkin in the ubiquitin-proteasomal system suggests that impaired regulation of protein degradation may play a role in PD. Exposure to environmental toxins may interrupt energy production in the mitochondria or cause increased levels of oxidative stress that, in turn, might lead directly to cell injury or death. An individual's ability to respond to these insults may be determined by genetic polymorphisms that code for metabolic enzymes with reduced or increased ability to metabolize environmental toxins. Alternatively, other environmental factors, such as dietary antioxidants, caffeine, or nicotine-like substances, may protect neurons from these injuries.

Although the numerous potential causes of dopaminergic neuronal degeneration and clinical PD are complex and daunting, they also provide the opportunity for intervention at multiple steps. The development of successful future therapies and preventive measures depends on a sound understanding of the interaction of environmental, molecular, and genetic factors involved in PD.

REFERENCES

1. Rajput AH, Rozdilsky B. Accuracy of clinical diagnosis in parkinsonism—a prospective study. *Can J Neurol Sci* 1991;18:275–278.
2. Hughes AJ, Daniel SE, Blankson S, et al. A clinicopathologic study of 100 cases of Parkinson's disease. *Arch Neurol* 1993;50: 140–148.
3. Tanner CM, Aston DA. Epidemiology of Parkinson's disease and akinetic syndromes. *Curr Opin Neurol* 2000;13:427–430.
4. McGeer P, Itagaki S, Akiyama H, et al. Rate of cell death in parkinsonism indicates active neuropathological process. *Ann Neurol* 1988;24:574–576.
5. Fearnley JM, Lees AJ. Ageing and Parkinson's disease: substantia nigra regional selectivity. *Brain* 1991;114:2283–2301.
6. Gibb WR, Lees AJ. Anatomy, pigmentation, ventral and dorsal subpopulations of the substantia nigra, and differential cell death in Parkinson's disease. *J Neurol Neurosurg Psychiatry* 1991; 54:388–396.
7. Menza M. The personality associated with Parkinson's disease. *Curr Psychiatry Rep* 2000;2:421–426.
8. Morrish PK, Rakshi JS, Bailey DL, et al. Measuring the rate of progression and estimating the preclinical period of Parkinson's disease with [18F]dopa PET. *J Neurol Neurosurg Psychiatry* 1998;64:314–319.
9. Brucke T, Djamshidian S, Bencsits G, et al. SPECT and PET imaging of the dopaminergic system in Parkinson's disease. *J Neurol* 2000;247[Suppl 4]:IV/2–7.
10. Gibb WRG, Lees AJ. The relevance of the Lewy body to the pathogenesis of idiopathic Parkinson's disease. *J Neurol Neurosurg Psychiatry* 1988;51:745–752.
11. Rajput AH, Offord KP, Beard CM, et al. Epidemiology of parkinsonism: incidence, classification, and mortality. *Ann Neurol* 1984;16:278–282.
12. Rocca WA, Bower JH, McDonnell SK, et al. Time trends in the incidence of parkinsonism in Olmsted County, Minnesota. *Neurology* 2001;57:462–467.
13. Kuopio AM, Marttila RJ, Helenius H, et al. Changing epidemiology of Parkinson's disease in southwestern Finland. *Neurology* 1999;52:302–308.

14. Riggs JE. The nonenvironmental basis for rising mortality from Parkinson's disease. *Arch Neurol* 1993;50:653–656.

15. Parkinson J. *An essay on the shaking palsy.* London: Sherwood, Neeley, and Jones, 1817.

16. Manyam BV. Paralysis agitans and levodopa in "Ayurveda": ancient Indian medical treatise. *Mov Disord* 1990;5:47–48.

17. Tanner CM, Ben-Shlomo Y. Epidemiology of Parkinson's disease. *Adv Neurol* 1999;80:153–159.

18. Zhang Z, Roman G. Worldwide occurrence of Parkinson's disease: an updated review. *Neuroepidemiology* 1993;12:195–208.

19. Baldereschi M, Di Carlo A, Rocca WA, et al. Parkinson's disease and parkinsonism in a longitudinal study: two-fold higher incidence in men. ILSA Working Group. Italian Longitudinal Study on Aging. *Neurology* 2000;55:1358–1363.

20. Tanner C, Goldman S. Epidemiology of Parkinson's disease. *Neurol Clin* 1996;14:317–335.

21. Mayeux R, Marder K, Cote LJ, et al. The frequency of idiopathic Parkinson's disease by age, ethnic group, and sex in northern Manhattan, 1988–1993. *Am J Epidemiol* 1995;142:820–827.

22. Morens DM, Davis JW, Grandinetti A, et al. Epidemiologic observations on Parkinson's disease: incidence and mortality in a prospective study of middle-aged men. *Neurology* 1996;46:1044–1050.

23. Golbe LI, Di Iorio G, Sanges G, et al. Clinical genetic analysis of Parkinson's disease in the Contursi kindred. *Ann Neurol* 1996;40:767–775.

24. Polymeropoulos M, Lavedan C, Leroy E, et al. Mutation in the α-synuclein gene identified in families with Parkinson's disease. *Science* 1997:2045–2047.

25. Papadimitriou A, Veletza V, Hadjigeorgiou GM, et al. Mutated α-synuclein gene in two Greek kindreds with familial PD: incomplete penetrance? *Neurology* 1999;52:651–654.

26. Chan P, Tanner CM, Jiang X, et al. Failure to find the α-synuclein gene missense mutation (G209A) in 100 patients with younger onset Parkinson's disease. *Neurology* 1998;50:513–514.

27. Kruger R, Kuhn W, Muller T, et al. Ala30Pro mutation in the gene encoding α-synuclein in Parkinson's disease. *Nat Genet* 1998;18:106–108.

28. Gasser T, Muller-Myhsok B, Wszolek ZK, et al. A susceptibility locus for Parkinson's disease maps to chromosome 2p13. *Nat Genet* 1998;18:262–265.

29. Farrer M, Gwinn-Hardy K, Muenter M, et al. A chromosome 4p haplotype segregating with Parkinson's disease and postural tremor. *Hum Mol Genet* 1999;8:81–85.

30. Yokochi M, Narabayashi H, Iizuka R, et al. Juvenile parkinsonism—some clinical, pharmacological, and neuropathological aspects. In: Hassler RG, Christ JF, eds. *Advances in neurology, vol 40.* New York: Raven Press, 1984:407–413.

31. Kitada T, Asakawa S, Hattori N, et al. Mutations in the *parkin* gene cause autosomal recessive juvenile parkinsonism. *Nature* 1998;392:605–608.

32. Lucking CB, Durr A, Bonifati V, et al. Association between early-onset Parkinson's disease and mutations in the *parkin* gene. French Parkinson's Disease Genetics Study Group. *N Engl J Med* 2000;342:1560–1567.

33. Leroy E, Anastasopoulos D, Konitsiotis S, et al. Deletions in the *parkin* gene and genetic heterogeneity in a Greek family with early onset Parkinson's disease. *Hum Genet* 1998;103:424–427.

34. Swerdlow RH, Parks JK, Davis JN Jr, et al. Matrilineal inheritance of complex I dysfunction in a multigenerational Parkinson's disease family. *Ann Neurol* 1998;44:873–881.

35. Wooten GF, Currie LJ, Bennett JP, et al. Maternal inheritance in Parkinson's disease. *Ann Neurol* 1997;41:265–268.

36. Zweig RM, Singh A, Cardillo JE, et al. The familial occurrence of Parkinson's disease: lack of evidence for maternal inheritance. *Arch Neurol* 1992;49:1205–1207.

37. de la Fuente-Fernandez R. Maternal effect on Parkinson's disease. *Ann Neurol* 2000;48:782–787.

38. Rybicki BA, Johnson CC, Peterson EL, et al. A family history of Parkinson's disease and its effect on other PD risk factors. *Neuroepidemiology* 1999;18:270–278.

39. Taylor CA, Saint-Hilaire MH, Cupples LA, et al. Environmental, medical, and family history risk factors for Parkinson's disease: a New England–based case control study. *Am J Med Genet* 1999;88:742–749.

40. Payami H, Larsen K, Bernard S, et al. Increased risk of Parkinson's disease in parents and siblings of patients. *Ann Neurol* 1994;36:659–661.

41. Autere JM, Moilanen JS, Myllyla VV, et al. Familial aggregation of Parkinson's disease in a Finnish population. *J Neurol Neurosurg Psychiatry* 2000;69:107–109.

42. Kuopio A, Marttila RJ, Helenius H, et al. Familial occurrence of Parkinson's disease in a community-based case-control study. *Parkinsonism Relat Disord* 2001;7:297–303.

43. Sveinbjornsdottir S, Hicks AA, Jonsson T, et al. Familial aggregation of Parkinson's disease in Iceland. *N Engl J Med* 2000;343:1765–1770.

44. Scott WK, Nance MA, Watts RL, et al. Complete genomic screen in Parkinson disease: evidence for multiple genes. *JAMA* 2001;286:2239–2244.

45. DeStefano AL, Golbe LI, Mark MH, et al. Genome-wide scan for Parkinson's disease: the Gene PD Study. *Neurology* 2001;57:1124–1126.

46. Martin ER, Scott WK, Nance MA, et al. Association of single-nucleotide polymorphisms of the tau gene with late-onset Parkinson disease. *JAMA* 2001;286:2245–2250.

47. Tanner CM, Ottman R, Goldman SM, et al. Parkinson disease in twins: an etiologic study. *JAMA* 1999;281:341–346.

48. Piccini P, Burn DJ, Ceravolo R, et al. The role of inheritance in sporadic Parkinson's disease: evidence from a longitudinal study of dopaminergic function in twins. *Ann Neurol* 1999;45:577–582.

49. Poskanzer DC, Schwab RS. Cohort analysis of Parkinson's syndrome: evidence for a single etiology related to subclinical infection about 1920. *J Chronic Diseases* 1963;16:961–973.

50. Goetz C. *Neurotoxins in clinical practice.* New York: Medical and Scientific Books, 1985.

51. Langston JW, Ballard PA, Tetrud JW, et al. Chronic parkinsonism in humans due to a product of meperidine analog synthesis. *Science* 1983;219:979–980.

52. Langston JW. The etiology of Parkinson's disease with emphasis on the MPTP story. *Neurology* 1996;47:S153–S160.

53. Betarbet R, Sherer TB, MacKenzie G, et al. Chronic systemic pesticide exposure reproduces features of Parkinson's disease. *Nat Neurosci* 2000;3:1301–1306.

54. Thiruchelvam M, Brockel BJ, Richfield EK, et al. Potentiated and preferential effects of combined paraquat and maneb on nigrostriatal dopamine systems: environmental risk factors for Parkinson's disease? *Brain Res* 2000;873:225–234.

55. Uversky VN, Li J, Fink AL. Pesticides directly accelerate the rate of α-synuclein fibril formation: a possible factor in Parkinson's disease. *FEBS Lett* 2001;500:105–108.

56. Fleming L, Mann JB, Bean J, et al. Parkinson's disease and brain levels of organochlorine pesticides. *Ann Neurol* 1994;36:100–103.

57. Corrigan FM, Wienburg CL, Shore RF, et al. Organochlorine insecticides in substantia nigra in Parkinson's disease. *J Toxicol Environ Health A* 2000;59:229–234.

58. Priyadarshi A, Khuder SA, Schaub EA, et al. A meta-analysis of Parkinson's disease and exposure to pesticides. *Neurotoxicology* 2000;21:435–440.

59. Liou HH, Tsai MC, Chen CJ, et al. Environmental risk factors

and Parkinson's disease: a case-control study in Taiwan. *Neurology* 1997;48:1583–1588.

60. Gorell JM, Johnson CC, Rybicki BA, et al. The risk of Parkinson's disease with exposure to pesticides, farming, well water, and rural living. *Neurology* 1998;50:1346–1350.

61. Seidler A, Hellenbrand W, Robra BP, et al. Possible environmental, occupational, and other etiologic factors for Parkinson's disease: a case-control study in Germany. *Neurology* 1996;46:1275–1284.

62. Semchuk KM, Love EJ, Lee RG. Parkinson's disease and exposure to agricultural work and pesticide chemicals. *Neurology* 1992;42:1328–1335.

63. Butterfield PG, Valanis BG, Spencer PS, et al. Environmental antecedents of young-onset Parkinson's disease. *Neurology* 1993;43:1150–1158.

64. Fall PA, Fredrikson M, Axelson O, et al. Nutritional and occupational factors influencing the risk of Parkinson's disease: a case-control study in southeastern Sweden. *Mov Disord* 1999;14:28–37.

65. Schulte PA, Burnett CA, Boeniger MF, et al. Neurodegenerative diseases: occupational occurrence and potential risk factors, 1982 through 1991. *Am J Public Health* 1996;86:1281–1288.

66. Tsui JK, Calne DB, Wang Y, et al. Occupational risk factors in Parkinson's disease. *Can J Public Health* 1999;90:334–337.

67. Gorell JM, Johnson CC, Rybicki BA, et al. Occupational exposure to manganese, copper, lead, iron, mercury, and zinc and the risk of Parkinson's disease. *Neurotoxicology* 1999;20:239–247.

68. Racette BA, McGee-Minnich L, Moerlein SM, et al. Welding-related parkinsonism: clinical features, treatment, and pathophysiology. *Neurology* 2001;56:8–13.

69. Beaman BL, Canfield D, Anderson J, et al. Site-specific invasion of the basal ganglia by *Nocardia asteroides* GUH-2. *Med Microbiol Immunol (Berl)* 2000;188:161–168.

70. Kohbata S, Beaman BL. L-dopa-responsive movement disorder caused by *Nocardia asteroides* localized in the brains of mice. *Infect Immun* 1991;59:181–191.

71. Beaman BL. *Nocardia* as a pathogen of the brain: mechanisms of interactions in the murine brain—a review. *Gene* 1992;115:213–217.

72. Woulfe J, Hoogendoorn H, Tarnopolsky M, et al. Monoclonal antibodies against Epstein-Barr virus cross-react with α-synuclein in human brain. *Neurology* 2000;55:1398–1401.

73. Chen S, Le WD, Xie WJ, et al. Experimental destruction of substantia nigra initiated by Parkinson disease immunoglobulins. *Arch Neurol* 1998;55:1075–1080.

74. Hellenbrand W, Boeing H, Robra BP, et al. Diet and Parkinson's disease. II: A possible role for the past intake of specific nutrients—results from a self-administered food-frequency questionnaire in a case-control study. *Neurology* 1996;47:644–650.

75. Morens DM, Grandinetti A, Waslien CI, et al. Case-control study of idiopathic Parkinson's disease and dietary vitamin E intake. *Neurology* 1996;46:1270–1274.

76. Golbe LI, Farrell TM, Davis PH. Follow-up study of early-life protective and risk factors in Parkinson's disease. *Mov Disord* 1990;5:66–70.

77. Golbe LI, Farrell TM, Davis PH. Case-control study of early life dietary factors in Parkinson's disease. *Arch Neurol* 1988;45:1350–1353.

78. Hellenbrand W, Seidler A, Boeing H, et al. Diet and Parkinson's disease. I: A possible role for the past intake of specific foods and food groups—results from a self-administered food-frequency questionnaire in a case-control study. *Neurology* 1996;47:636–643.

79. Anderson C, Checkoway H, Franklin GM, et al. Dietary factors in Parkinson's disease: the role of food groups and specific foods. *Mov Disord* 1999;14:21–27.

80. Logroscino G, Marder K, Cote L, et al. Dietary lipids and antioxidants in Parkinson's disease: a population-based, case-control study. *Ann Neurol* 1996;39:89–94.

81. Gorell J, Johnson C, Rybicki B, Peterson E. A population-based case-control study of nutrient intake in Parkinson's disease. *Neurology* 1997;48:A298.

82. Duan W, Mattson MP. Dietary restriction and 2-deoxyglucose administration improve behavioral outcome and reduce degeneration of dopaminergic neurons in models of Parkinson's disease. *J Neurosci Res* 1999;57:195–206.

83. Ross GW, Abbott RD, Petrovitch H, et al. Association of coffee and caffeine intake with the risk of Parkinson disease. *JAMA* 2000;283:2674–2679.

84. Ascherio A, Zhang SM, Hernan MA, et al. Prospective study of caffeine consumption and risk of Parkinson's disease in men and women. *Ann Neurol* 2001;50:56–63.

85. Benedetti MD, Bower JH, Maraganore DM, et al. Smoking, alcohol, and coffee consumption preceding Parkinson's disease: a case-control study. *Neurology* 2000;55:1350–1358.

86. Paganini-Hill A. Risk factors for Parkinson's disease: the leisure world cohort study. *Neuroepidemiology* 2001;20:118–124.

87. Chen JF, Xu K, Petzer JP, et al. Neuroprotection by caffeine and A(2A) adenosine receptor inactivation in a model of Parkinson's disease. *J Neurosci* 2001;21:RC143.

88. Factor SA, Weiner WJ. Prior history of head trauma in Parkinson's disease. *Mov Disord* 1991;6(3):225–229.

89. Santamaria J, Tolosa E, Valles A. Parkinson's disease with depression: a possible subgroup of idiopathic parkinsonism. *Neurology* 1986;36:1130–1133.

90. Gibberd FB, Simmonds JP. Neurological disease in ex-Far-East prisoners of war. *Lancet* 1980;2:135–137.

91. Page WF, Tanner CM. Parkinson's disease and motor-neuron disease in former prisoners-of-war. *Lancet* 2000;355:843.

92. Gale CR, Braidwood EA, Winter PD, et al. Mortality from Parkinson's disease and other causes in men who were prisoners of war in the Far East. *Lancet* 1999;354:2116–2118.

93. Grandinetti A, Morens DM, Reed D, et al. Prospective study of cigarette smoking and the risk of developing idiopathic Parkinson's disease. *Am J Epidemiol* 1994;139:1129–1138.

94. Willems-Giesbergen P, de Rijk M, van Swieten J, et al. Smoking, alcohol, and coffee consumption and the risk of PD: results from the Rotterdam study. *Neurology* 2000;54:A347.

95. Doll R, Peto R, Wheatley K, et al. Mortality in relation to smoking: 40 years' observations on male British doctors. *BMJ* 1994;309:901–911.

96. Sugita M, Izuno T, Tatemichi M, et al. Meta-analysis for epidemiologic studies on the relationship between smoking and Parkinson's disease. *J Epidemiol* 2001;11:87–94.

97. Prasad C, Ikegami H, Shimizu I, et al. Chronic nicotine intake decelerates aging of nigrostriatal dopaminergic neurons. *Life Sci* 1994;54:1169–1184.

98. Janson AM, Moller A. Chronic nicotine treatment counteracts nigral cell loss induced by a partial mesodiencephalic hemitransection: an analysis of the total number and mean volume of neurons and glia in substantia nigra of the male rat. *Neuroscience* 1993;57:931–941.

99. Carr LA, Rowell PP. Attenuation of 1-methyl-4-phenyl-1,2,3,6-tetrahydropyridine-induced neurotoxicity by tobacco smoke. *Neuropharmacology* 1990;29:311–314.

100. Costa G, Abin-Carriquiry JA, Dajas F. Nicotine prevents striatal dopamine loss produced by 6-hydroxydopamine lesion in the substantia nigra. *Brain Res* 2001;888:336–342.

101. Ferger B, Spratt C, Earl CD, et al. Effects of nicotine on hydroxyl free radical formation in vitro and on MPTP-induced neurotoxicity in vivo. *Naunyn Schmiedebergs Arch Pharmacol* 1998;358:351–359.

102. Maggio R, Riva M, Vaglini F, et al. Striatal increase of neurotrophic factors as a mechanism of nicotine protection in experimental parkinsonism. *J Neural Transm* 1997;104: 1113–1123.

103. Fowler J, Volkow N, Wang G, et al. Inhibition of monoamine oxidase B in the brains of smokers. *Nature* 1996;379:733–736.

104. Compton P, Anglin M, Khalsa-Denison M, et al. The D2 dopamine receptor gene, addiction, and personality: clinical correlates in cocaine abusers. *Biol Psychiatry* 1996;39:302–304.

105. Benjamin J, Li L, Patterson C, et al. Population and familial association between the D4 dopamine receptor gene and measures of novelty seeking. *Nat Genet* 1996;12:81–84.

106. Nicholl DJ, Bennett P, Hiller L, et al. A study of five candidate genes in Parkinson's disease and related neurodegenerative disorders: European Study Group on Atypical Parkinsonism. *Neurology* 1999;53:1415–1421.

107. Sabbagh N, Brice A, Marez D, et al. CYP2D6 polymorphism and Parkinson's disease susceptibility. *Mov Disord* 1999;14: 230–236.

108. Joost O, Taylor CA, Thomas CA, et al. Absence of effect of seven functional mutations in the *CYP2D6* gene in Parkinson's disease. *Mov Disord* 1999;14:590–595.

109. Landi MT, Ceroni M, Martignoni E, et al. Gene–environment interaction in Parkinson's disease—the case of *CYP2D6* gene polymorphisms. *Adv Neurol* 1996;69:61–72.

110. Bandmann O, Marsden CD, Wood NW. Genetic polymorphisms of three detoxification enzymes in familial and sporadic Parkinson's disease. *Neurology* 1997;48:A182–A183.

111. Stroombergen MCMJ, Waring RH, Bennett P, et al. Determination of the *GSTM1* gene deletion frequency in Parkinson's disease by allele specific PCR. *Parkinsonism Rel Disord* 1996;2 (3):151–154.

112. Menegon A, Board PG, Blackburn AC, et al. Parkinson's disease, pesticides, and glutathione transferase polymorphisms. *Lancet* 1998;352:1344–1346.

113. Checkoway H, Franklin GM, Costa-Mallen P, et al. A genetic polymorphism of MAO-B modifies the association of cigarette smoking and Parkinson's disease. *Neurology* 1998;50: 1458–1461.

114. Tan EK, Khajavi M, Thornby JI, et al. Variability and validity of polymorphism association studies in Parkinson's disease. *Neurology* 2000;55:533–538.

115. Bandmann O, Vaughan J, Holmans P, et al. Association of slow acetylator genotype for N-acetyltransferase 2 with familial Parkinson's disease. *Lancet* 1997;350:1136–1139.

116. Maraganore DM, Farrer MJ, Hardy JA, et al. Case-control study of debrisoquine 4-hydroxylase, *N*-acetyltransferase 2, and apolipoprotein E gene polymorphisms in Parkinson's disease. *Mov Disord* 2000;15:714–719.

117. Kimura M, Matsushita S, Arai H, et al. No evidence of association between a dopamine transporter gene polymorphism (1215A/G) and Parkinson's disease. *Ann Neurol* 2001;49: 276–277.

118. Morino H, Kawarai T, Izumi Y, et al. A single nucleotide polymorphism of dopamine transporter gene is associated with Parkinson's disease. *Ann Neurol* 2000;47:528–531.

119. Gasser T, Wszolek ZK, Trofatter J, et al. Genetic linkage studies in autosomal dominant parkinsonism: evaluation of seven candidate genes. *Ann Neurol* 1994;36:387–396.

120. Farin FM, Hitosis Y, Hallagan SE, et al. Genetic polymorphisms of superoxide dismutase in Parkinson's disease. *Mov Disord* 2001;16:705–707.

121. Schapira AH, Mann VM, Cooper JM, et al. Anatomic and disease specificity of NADH CoQ1 reductase (complex I) deficiency in Parkinson's disease. *J Neurochem* 1990;55:2142–2145.

122. Haas RH, Nasirian F, Nakano K, et al. Low platelet mitochondrial complex I and complex II/III activity in early untreated Parkinson's disease. *Ann Neurol* 1995;37:714–722.

123. Bindoff LA, Birch-Machin MA, Cartlidge NE, et al. Respiratory chain abnormalities in skeletal muscle from patients with Parkinson's disease. *J Neurol Sci* 1991;104:203–208.

124. Albers DS, Augood SJ, Park LC, et al. Frontal lobe dysfunction in progressive supranuclear palsy: evidence for oxidative stress and mitochondrial impairment. *J Neurochem* 2000;74: 878–881.

125. Przedborski S, Jackson-Lewis V, Muthane U, et al. Chronic levodopa administration alters cerebral mitochondrial respiratory chain activity. *Ann Neurol* 1993;34:715–723.

126. Dexter DT, Sian J, Rose S, et al. Indices of oxidative stress and mitochondrial function in individuals with incidental Lewy body disease. *Ann Neurol* 1994;35:38–44.

127. Naoi M, Maruyama W, Dostert P, et al. N-Methyl-(R)salsolinol as a dopaminergic neurotoxin: from an animal model to an early marker of Parkinson's disease. *J Neural Transm Suppl* 1997; 50:89–105.

128. Li H, Dryhurst G. Irreversible inhibition of mitochondrial complex I by 7-(2-aminoethyl)-3,4-dihydro-5-hydroxy-2H-1,4-benzothiazine-3-carboxylic acid (DHBT-1): a putative nigral endotoxin of relevance to Parkinson's disease. *J Neurochem* 1997;69:1530–1541.

129. Hatefi Y. The mitochondrial electron transport and oxidative phosphorylation system. *Annu Rev Biochem* 1985;54: 1015–1069.

130. Hattori N, Yoshino H, Tanaka M, et al. Genotype in the 24-kDa subunit gene *(NDUFV2)* of mitochondrial complex I and susceptibility to Parkinson disease. *Genomics* 1998;49:52–58.

131. Tanaka M, Kovalenko SA, Gong JS, et al. Accumulation of deletions and point mutations in mitochondrial genome in degenerative diseases. *Ann NY Acad Sci* 1996;786:102–111.

132. Ikebe S, Tanaka M, Ozawa T. Point mutations of mitochondrial genome in Parkinson's disease. *Mol Brain Res* 1995;28: 281–295.

133. Simon DK, Mayeux R, Marder K, et al. Mitochondrial DNA mutations in complex I and tRNA genes in Parkinson's disease. *Neurology* 2000;54:703–709.

134. Lestienne P, Nelson I, Riederer P, et al. Mitochondrial DNA in postmortem brain from patients with Parkinson's disease. *J Neurochem* 1991;56:1819.

135. Swerdlow RH, Parks JK, Miller SW, et al. Origin and functional consequences of the complex I defect in Parkinson's disease. *Ann Neurol* 1996;40:663–671.

136. Schapira AH, Gu M, Taanman JW, et al. Mitochondria in the etiology and pathogenesis of Parkinson's disease. *Ann Neurol* 1998;44:S89–S98.

137. Kristal BS, Conway AD, Brown AM, et al. Selective dopaminergic vulnerability: 3,4-dihydroxyphenylacetaldehyde targets mitochondria. *Free Radic Biol Med* 2001;30:924–931.

138. Chinopoulos C, Adam-Vizi V. Mitochondria deficient in complex I activity are depolarized by hydrogen peroxide in nerve terminals: relevance to Parkinson's disease. *J Neurochem* 2001; 76:302–306.

139. Zecca L, Pietra R, Goj C, et al. Iron and other metals in neuromelanin, substantia nigra, and putamen of human brain. *J Neurochem* 1994;62:1097–1101.

140. Hirsch E, Graybiel AM, Agid YA. Melanized dopaminergic neurons are differentially susceptible to degeneration in Parkinson's disease. *Nature* 1988;334:345–348.

141. Berman SB, Hastings TG. Dopamine oxidation alters mitochondrial respiration and induces permeability transition in brain mitochondria: implications for Parkinson's disease. *J Neurochem* 1999;73:1127–1137.

142. Rabinovic AD, Lewis DA, Hastings TG. Role of oxidative

changes in the degeneration of dopamine terminals after injection of neurotoxic levels of dopamine. *Neuroscience* 2000;101: 67–76.

143. Youdim MB, Ben-Shachar D, Eshel G, et al. The neurotoxicity of iron and nitric oxide: relevance to the etiology of Parkinson's disease. *Adv Neurol* 1993;60:259–266.

144. Ben-Shachar D, Youdim MBH. Intranigral iron injection induces behavioural and biochemical "parkinsonism" in rats. *J Neurochem* 1991;57:2133–2135.

145. Mann VM, Cooper JM, Daniel SE, et al. Complex I, iron, and ferritin in Parkinson's disease substantia nigra. *Ann Neurol* 1994;36:876–881.

146. Hirsch EC, Brandel J-P, Galle P, et al. Iron and aluminum increase in the substantia nigra of patients with Parkinson's disease: an x-ray microanalysis. *J Neurochem* 1991;56:446–451.

147. Dexter DT, Carter CJ, Wells FR, et al. Basal lipid peroxidation in substantia nigra is increased in Parkinson's disease. *J Neurochem* 1989;52:381–389.

148. Jenner P, Dexter DT, Sian J, et al. Oxidative stress as a cause of nigral cell death in Parkinson's disease and incidental Lewy body disease. *Ann Neurol* 1992;32[Suppl]:S82–S87.

149. Sian J, Dexter DT, Lees AJ, et al. Alterations in glutathione levels in Parkinson's disease and other neurodegenerative disorders affecting basal ganglia. *Ann Neurol* 1994;36:348–355.

150. Klivenyi P, Andreassen OA, Ferrante RJ, et al. Mice deficient in cellular glutathione peroxidase show increased vulnerability to malonate, 3-nitropropionic acid, and 1-methyl-4-phenyl-1,2,5, 6-tetrahydropyridine. *J Neurosci* 2000;20:1–7.

151. Marshall KA, Reist M, Jenner P, et al. The neuronal toxicity of sulfite plus peroxynitrite is enhanced by glutathione depletion: implications for Parkinson's disease. *Free Radical Biol Med* 1999; 27:515–520.

152. Hastings TG, Lewis DA, Zigmond MJ. Role of oxidation in the neurotoxic effects of intrastriatal dopamine injections. *Proc Natl Acad Sci USA* 1996;93:1956–1961.

153. Spina M, Cohen G. Dopamine turnover and glutathione oxidation: implications for Parkinson's disease. *Proc Natl Acad Sci USA* 1989;86:1398–1400.

154. Jha N, Jurma O, Lalli G, et al. Glutathione depletion in PC12 results in selective inhibition of mitochondrial complex I activity: implications for Parkinson's disease. *J Biol Chem* 2000; 275:26096–26101.

155. Saggu H, Cooksey J, Dexter DT, et al. A selective increase in particulate superoxide dismutase activity in parkinsonian substantia nigra. *J Neurochem* 1989;53:692–697.

156. Riederer P, Sofic E, Rausch WD, et al. Transition metals, ferritin, glutathione, and ascorbic acid in parkinsonian brains. *J Neurochem* 1989;52:515–520.

157. Good PF, Hsu A, Werner P, et al. Protein nitration in Parkinson's disease. *J Neuropathol Exp Neurol* 1998;57:338–342.

158. Knott C, Stern G, Wilkin GP. Inflammatory regulators in Parkinson's disease: iNOS, lipocortin-1, and cyclooxygenases-1 and -2. *Mol Cell Neurosci* 2000;16:724–739.

159. Liberatore GT, Jackson-Lewis V, Vukosavic S, et al. Inducible nitric oxide synthase stimulates dopaminergic neurodegeneration in the MPTP model of Parkinson disease. *Nat Med* 1999; 5:1403–1409.

160. Church WH, Ward VL. Uric acid is reduced in the substantia nigra in Parkinson's disease: effect on dopamine oxidation. *Brain Res Bull* 1994;33:419–425.

161. Davis JW, Grandinetti A, Waslien CI, et al. Observations on serum uric acid levels and the risk of idiopathic Parkinson's disease. *Am J Epidem* 1996;144:480–484.

162. Spillantini M, Schmidt M, Lee V, et al. α-Synuclein in Lewy bodies. *Nature* 1997;388:839–840.

163. Baba M, Nakajo S, Tu PH, et al. Aggregation of α-synuclein in Lewy bodies of sporadic Parkinson's disease and dementia with Lewy bodies. *Am J Pathol* 1998;152:879–884.

164. Mezey E, Dehejia AM, Harta G, et al. α-Synuclein is present in Lewy bodies in sporadic Parkinson's disease. *Mol Psychiatry* 1998;3:493–499.

165. Trojanowski JQ, Lee VM. Parkinson's disease and related neurodegenerative synucleinopathies linked to progressive accumulations of synuclein aggregates in brain. *Parkinsonism Relat Disord* 2001;7:247–251.

166. Spillantini MG, Goedert M. The α-synucleinopathies: Parkinson's disease, dementia with Lewy bodies, and multiple system atrophy. *Ann NY Acad Sci* 2000;920:16–27.

167. Narhi L, Wood SJ, Steavenson S, et al. Both familial Parkinson's disease mutations accelerate α-synuclein aggregation. *J Biol Chem* 1999;274:9843–9846.

168. Conway KA, Harper JD, Lansbury PT. Accelerated in vitro fibril formation by a mutant α-synuclein linked to early-onset Parkinson disease. *Nat Med* 1998;4:1318–1320.

169. Feany MB, Bender WW. A *Drosophila* model of Parkinson's disease. *Nature* 2000;404:394–398.

170. Alves-Rodrigues A, Gregori L, Figueiredo-Pereira ME. Ubiquitin, cellular inclusions, and their role in neurodegeneration. *Trends Neurosci* 1998;21:516–520.

171. Shimura H, Hattori N, Kubo S, et al. Familial Parkinson disease gene product, parkin, is a ubiquitin-protein ligase. *Nat Genet* 2000;25:302–305.

172. Mizuno Y, Hattori N, Mori H, et al. Parkin and Parkinson's disease. *Curr Opin Neurol* 2001;14:477–482.

173. Solano SM, Miller DW, Augood SJ, et al. Expression of α-synuclein, parkin, and ubiquitin carboxy-terminal hydrolase L1 mRNA in human brain: genes associated with familial Parkinson's disease. *Ann Neurol* 2000;47:201–210.

174. Golbe LI. α-Synuclein and Parkinson's disease. *Mov Disord* 1999;14:6–9.

175. McCann SJ, LeCouteur DG, Green AC, et al. The epidemiology of Parkinson's disease in an Australian population. *Neuroepidemiology* 1998;17:310–317.

176. Stern M, Dulaney E, Gruber SB, et al. The epidemiology of Parkinson's disease: a case-control study of young-onset and old-onset patients. *Arch Neurol* 1991;48:903–907.

177. Marder K, Logroscino G, Alfaro B, et al. Environmental risk factors for Parkinson's disease in an urban multiethnic community. *Neurology* 1998;50:279–281.

178. Morano A, Jimenez-Jimenez FJ, Molina JA, et al. Risk-factors for Parkinson's disease: case-control study in the province of Caceres, Spain. *Acta Neurol Scand* 1994;89:164–170.

179. Tanner CM, Chen B, Wang W, et al. Environmental factors and Parkinson's disease: a case-control study in China. *Neurology* 1989;39:660–664.

180. Ho SC, Woo J, Lee CM. Epidemiologic study of Parkinson's disease in Hong Kong. *Neurology* 1989;39:1314–1318.

181. Priyadarshi A, Khuder SA, Schaub EA, et al. Environmental risk factors and Parkinson's disease: a meta-analysis. *Environ Res* 2001;86:122–127.

LEVODOPA IN PARKINSON'S DISEASE: MECHANISMS OF ACTION AND PATHOPHYSIOLOGY OF LATE FAILURE

WERNER POEWE
GREGOR WENNING

Until we are better informed respecting the nature of the disease, the employment of internal medicine is scarcely warrantable.—J. Parkinson, 1817 (1).

In contrast to poorly understood empirical approaches to the management of Parkinson's disease (PD), such as the use of belladonna alkaloids in the 1860s, the introduction of levodopa in the 1960s was firmly based on major advances in the understanding of the neurochemical abnormalities underlying the disease. Levodopa was first given to PD patients after Carlsson et al. (2,3) showed that cerebral dopamine (DA) was concentrated in the striatum and that levodopa could reverse the akinetic effects of reserpine in experimental animals, and after Ehringer and Hornykiewicz (4) demonstrated striatal DA depletion as a key neurochemical finding in parkinsonian brains.

Following early reports by Birkmayer and Hornykiewicz (5) and Barbeau et al. (6) about the antiparkinsonian efficacy of small doses (50 to 100 mg) of levodopa administered to patients intravenously, Cotzias et al. (7) eventually demonstrated the dramatic clinical effects of high-dose oral levodopa substitution in idiopathic Parkinson's disease (IPD). Until now, oral levodopa has remained the single most effective treatment for IPD, and none of the orally active DA agonists studied in comparative clinical trials have so far matched levodopa's effect size on parkinsonian motor symptoms (8–10).

However, two major areas of uncertainty still surround this type of antiparkinsonian treatment. One concerns the precise mechanism by which oral levodopa works so well in the early stages of IPD that responsiveness has become a differential diagnostic criterion for this disease (11). The other is the opposite, namely, why long-term levodopa substitution in IPD eventually fails in a majority of patients by producing increasingly capricious response oscillations and abnormal involuntary movements. Both aspects are the focus of the clinical and pathophysiologic considerations in this chapter.

MECHANISMS OF ACTION

The basic rationale behind the introduction of levodopa into antiparkinsonian drug treatment was that it would be converted to DA, thus correcting the striatal DA depletion. In trying to understand how oral levodopa eventually can restore striatal DA deficiency, a number of pharmacokinetic and pharmacodynamic mechanisms must be considered. However, even after more than 30 years of successful clinical application, the exact central mode of action of levodopa is still not fully understood.

Pharmacokinetics

The peripheral pharmacokinetics of levodopa have been analyzed in human studies in healthy and parkinsonian subjects. No significant differences in the main pharmacokinetic parameters (Table 8.1) have been found. However, there is some variation among the data of the different studies. They most often fit a two-compartment model with a rapid α phase that has a half-life of approximately 5 to 10 minutes and a slower terminal β phase that has a half-life of 50 to 120 minutes. The apparent volume of distribution is large, and skeletal muscle is one of the candidate compartments where levodopa can be pooled. The other is 3-*o*-methyldopa (3-OMD), formed in large quantities after blockade of aromatic amino acid decarboxylase (AAAD) by decarboxylase inhibitors (DCI). 3-OMD has a long half-life of more than 12 hours (12), and theoretically can act as a reservoir for levodopa, since the enzymatic reaction catalyzed by AAAD is reversible (13). However, 3-OMD has never been exploitable as a clinically relevant levodopa donor, and it is capable of competing with levodopa blood–brain barrier transport (14–16).

Coadministration of peripherally active DCIs prevents premature and excessive decarboxylation to DA by the

TABLE 8.1. LEVODOPA PHARMACOKINETIC PARAMETERS: SUMMARY OF HUMAN STUDIES

Study	V_d	Cl_p	$t\frac{1}{2}\ \alpha$	$t\frac{1}{2}\ \beta$
Hardie et al., 1986	83.1 L	36.2 L/hr^{-1}	5.5 min	1.6 hr
Sasahara et al., 1980	87.8 L	96.6 L/hr^{-1}	—	0.6 hr
Fabbrini et al., 1987	0.26 L/kg^{-1}	0.13 L/kg^{-1} hr^{-1}	—	1.4 hr
Nutt et al., 1985	0.67 L/kg^{-1}	0.3 L/kg^{-1} hr^{-1}	—	1.4 hr
Poewe et al. (unpublished data)	3.0 L/kg^{-1}	1.4 L/kg^{-1} hr^{-1}	5.4 min	1.5 hr

^{a}V_d, apparent volume of distribution; Cl_p, plasma clearance; $t\frac{1}{2}$, half-life.

AAAD that is amply present in the gastrointestinal mucosa and liver, and thus it is essential for the reduction of peripheral side effects and enhancement of central efficacy of oral levodopa. The main change in levodopa pharmacokinetics induced by decarboxylase inhibition is a 50% decrease in the elimination rate and a corresponding increase in bioavailability without major effect on half-life (17).

The normal enzymatic handling of oral levodopa primarily entails peripheral conversion to DA by AAAD, which is followed by the action of catechol-*O*-methyltransferase (COMT) and monoamine oxidase (MAO) to produce 3,4-dioxyphenylacetic acid (DOPAC) and homovanillic acid (HVA) as the major metabolites. Following decarboxylase inhibition, this metabolic pathway shifts toward excessive production of 3-OMD via the action of COMT (Fig. 8.1). Inhibition of COMT in the periphery therefore results in a longer plasma half-life of levodopa, giving rise to an increase of the area under the levodopa plasma concentration/time curve (AUC) approximately doubling its bioavailability. However, the average levodopa maximal plasma concentration (C_{max}) and the time to C_{max} (t_{max}) are generally unaffected (18,19).

From Gut to Brain: Transport

Orally ingested levodopa is rapidly taken up from resorption sites of the duodenum and proximal jejunum. Standard formulations of levodopa typically achieve C_{max} between 15 and 45 minutes after oral intake. Erratic gastric emptying may influence the onset of clinical effects from individual levodopa doses, and factors that may alter gastric motility have particular relevance. They include meals, antacids, and anticholinergics, which may delay gastric emptying rate, and antiemetics, which may enhance it (20). Delayed gastric emptying or enteral absorption failure of various reasons are associated with "delayed-on" or "no-on" phenomena in fluctuating Parkinson's disease (see above; 21).

Mucosal transport of levodopa across the gut wall is an active energy-dependent carrier-mediated process. The carriers involved with mucosal transport of amino acids exhibit limited stereospecificity, such that levodopa shares a saturable transport system with a group of other large neutral amino acids (LNAAs) (22). Competitive inhibition of levodopa absorption thus occurs with rising concentrations of neutral amino acids from the diet, which explains part of the negative effects of oral protein intake on the clinical efficacy of individual oral doses of the drug (Fig. 8.2).

The blood–brain barrier for levodopa is essentially enzymatic and is represented by AAAD in endothelial cells. This is another target of coadministration of DCIs with levodopa. Blood–brain barrier transport of levodopa also depends on the same active carrier systems as its transport across gut mucosa, so that similar competitive interactions occur with other LNAAs (23–25). Striatal influx of levodopa, the presumed crucial prerequisite for its clinical action, is thus a function not only of levodopa plasma con-

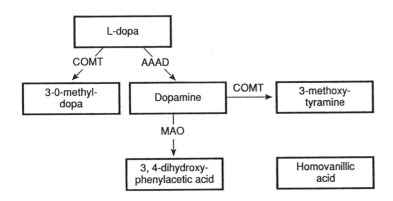

FIG. 8.1. Two major avenues of enzymatic handling of levodopa. Conversion to 3-*O*-methyldopa (3-OMD) by catechol-*O*-methyltransferase (COMT) becomes important when aromatic amino acid decarboxylase (AAAD) is blocked by coadministration of decarboxylase inhibitors (DCIs).

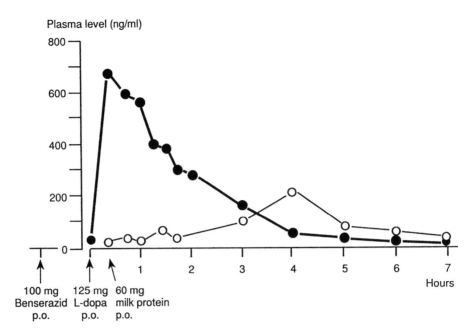

FIG. 8.2. Levodopa plasma levels following a standard oral dose of 125 mg given on an empty stomach *(dark symbols)* or with a 60-mg milk protein drink *(open symbols)*. Note delayed plasma peak and reduced area under the curve when the drug was taken with protein.

centration but also of the ratio of that concentration to the levels of the sum of competing LNAAs (26).

Presynaptic Central Handling

When clinical symptoms of IPD first become apparent, about 40% to 50% of dopaminergic nigrostriatal projection neurons still survive (27). The classic hypothesis about levodopa's central mechanisms of action thus assumes that the drug is taken up into surviving nigrostriatal nerve terminals, decarboxylated by sufficient residual amounts of AAAD in these neurons, stored as DA, and finally released presynaptically. This synaptic release of DA formed from exogenous sources may very well be regulated in the same way as that from normal DA neurons, although there seems to be a compensatory increase in DA turnover in surviving nigral neurons in IPD. With this type of presynaptic handling, the efficacy of oral levodopa replacement should decline as disease progresses because of progressive loss of striatal DA nerve terminals. However, a closer look reveals that this clearly is not the case, and this is just one of several inconsistencies in the theory of levodopa's mechanism of action outlined earlier. The major uncertainties concern the following:

■ At what exact location is exogenous levodopa decarboxylated to DA?
■ Is there presynaptic storage of DA derived from exogenous sources?

■ Does physiologically regulated neuronal synaptic release of such DA occur, and is this release pulsatile or tonic?

Presynaptic Storage and Release of Levodopa-derived Dopamine

Levodopa administration increases striatal DA concentrations in parkinsonian brains (28,29). According to a classic hypothesis, exogenous levodopa, once it has reached the striatum, is handled in a way qualitatively similar to that of its endogenous counterpart formed from L-tyrosine after conversion by tyrosine hydroxylase (TH). Under physiologic conditions, enhanced firing rates of DA neurons lead to increases in DA synthesis and release, and it was postulated that under conditions of partial denervation both the use and turnover of both endogenous (from tyrosine hydroxylation) and exogenous levodopa are enhanced. Such hyperactivity of surviving dopaminergic neurons would compensate for the state of partial striatal denervation by synthesizing and releasing sufficient amounts of DA to restore normal or nearly normal striatal dopaminergic neurotransmission (30).

However, several lines of evidence from animal experiments argue against parts of this postulated sequence of events. A number of studies have shown that in unilaterally DA-depleted rats, behavioral activation induced by levodopa administration outlasts the elevation in DA observed in the denervated striatum (31,32). Furthermore, the increase in extracellular DA in the DA-depleted striatum following a single administration of levodopa has been shown to remain constant during a course of repeated treatments, even though the behavorial effects were observed to increase with successive doses of the drug (33). Therefore, the effects of levodopa-induced changes on DA levels within the striatum appear to be insufficient to account for the therapeutic actions of this drug. Melamed et al. (34) have demonstrated that experimental destruction of dopaminergic vesicles with reserpine in rats had little effect on the elevations of striatal DA concentrations observed after levodopa administration. Since DA pooling in dopaminergic neurons includes vesicular storage plus extravesicular cytosolic compartmenting, the authors concluded that it was mainly in the extravesicular cystolic form that DA from exogenous levodopa occurred in surviving nigrostriatal nerve terminals in IPD. Such findings also imply that levodopa-derived DA is not subject to firing-coupled vesicular release, since the cytosolic DA compartment is thought to be a nonreleasable reserve pool (35). Indeed, it has been shown in animal studies that modifying the firing rate of dopaminergic neurons by administration of DA agonists or by direct electrical neuronal stimulation does not affect the synthesis and release rates of DA from exogenous levodopa (36,37). Extrapolating such experiments to the mechanism of action of levodopa in patients, one may assume that there is extravesicular presynaptic pooling of DA derived from the drug with concentration-dependent unregulated leaking of DA into the synaptic cleft. This is not compatible with pulsatile, firing-coupled DA release but rather would produce tonic bathing of striatal neurons in a DA-containing environment.

This assumption would have important implications for how the nigrostriatal DA projection works physiologically. The fact that oral levodopa substitution exerts a dramatic effect on the symptoms of IPD patients and virtually brings their motor functioning back to normal hardly is compatible with a tightly firing, single-motor action–coupled physiologic mode of action of striatal DA cells, since such actions in all likelihood are not at all reproduced by administering oral levodopa to patients. If, however, there is a physiologic tonic DA release onto striatal neurons, this may be restored in a similar way by administering exogenous levodopa or DA agonists.

However, recent experimental findings suggest that motor behavior may depend on phasic DA release rather than on tonic DA receptor stimulation. Using microelectrode recording of DA cells in 6-hydroxydopamine-lesioned rats subjected to chronic intermittent levodopa treatment, Harden and Grace (38) reported a substantial increase in the proportion of DA neurons exhibiting spontaneous spike firing suggestive of phasic DA release into the synaptic cleft. In contrast, the extrasynaptic DA levels showed tonic elevations (steady-state increases) following chronic intermittent levodopa administration. The investigators speculated that the rapid restoration of tonic DA levels might underlie its

immediate antirigidity action, whereas the delayed increase in DA cell spike activity may be required for control of bradykinesia. These and other experimental findings illustrate that the exact mode of presynaptic storage and release of DA remains a matter of controversy.

SITE OF CEREBRAL LEVODOPA DECARBOXYLATION

Exclusive conversion of exogenous levodopa neurons to DA in surviving nigrostriatal neurons (30) should lead to progressive decline in the effectiveness of the drug as nigrostriatal denervation proceeds. However, this is not observed in patients who in cases of pure IPD continue to respond dramatically to oral levodopa even after many years of advancing disease (39). More importantly, such patients regularly have a better clinical response to individual levodopa doses than to postsynaptically active DA agonists. All of this is difficult to reconcile with exclusive decarboxylation of levodopa in nigrostriatal terminals. Correspondingly, striatal decarboxylase activity cannot be annihilated by extensive destruction of the rat's nigrostriatal projection, indicating AAAD activity in nondopaminergic compartments (40,41). Melamed et al. (42) have performed a number of experiments to define striatal nondopaminergic sites of levodopa decarboxylation and have failed to detect evidence for such transformation in serotonergic or adrenergic neurons, endothelial cells, or glia. These authors suggested that decarboxylation may occur in nonaminergic striatal interneurons with subsequent leakage of DA from the cytosol of these cells into the environment, where the transmitter would tonically activate DA receptors. In support of this hypothesis, Tashiro et al. (43) reported the presence of sparse medium-sized spiny neurons that show intensive immunoreactivity similar to that of aromatic amino acid decarboxylase (AADC) in the rat striatum and that increase in number after dopaminergic denervation. However, these observations were not confirmed subsequently (44). That levodopa metabolism can occur independently of dopaminergic neuronal activity has been recently reported by Mizoguchi et al. (45). These investigators observed that DA formation after levodopa administration occurred both in the rat striatum and the hippocampus, although the latter is practically devoid of dopaminergic innervation. An important finding was that the outflow of newly synthesized DA was not coupled to neuronal activity. Tison et al. (46) have described nonmonoaminergic neuronal cells within rat brainstem that decarboxylate exogenous levodopa into DA; however, the presence of striatal projections has yet to be demonstrated. Finally, recent evidence that other neural cells, as well as glial cells, can express AADC ought to be taken into consideration (47).

These findings suggest that our knowledge of the site of levodopa action is far from complete, and the common belief that striatal AADC is associated exclusively with dopaminergic nigrostriatal neurons should be critically examined.

POSTSYNAPTIC CENTRAL HANDLING OF LEVODOPA

As with the presynaptic handling of exogenous levodopa by the parkinsonian striatum, many details of levodopa's post-synaptic mode of action remain obscure. Although there is little doubt that levodopa therapy for IPD leads to increased striatal activation of postsynaptic DA receptors, less is known about the alterations in the pharmacodynamic state of these receptors induced by the denervating disease and its pharmacologic treatment. The following questions have been only partially resolved:

- Are striatal DA receptors supersensitive in de novo patients with IPD, and does such supersensitivity affect all DA subtypes?
- Does levodopa treatment lead to down-regulation of primarily supersensitive receptors?
- Does pulsatile stimulation of DA receptors by exogenous levodopa have different effects on receptor pharmacodynamics than continuous stimulation?
- Are clinical effects coupled with receptor occupancy?

DISEASE- AND TREATMENT-DEPENDENT ALTERATIONS IN STRIATAL DOPAMINERGIC RECEPTOR SENSITIVITY

It has been suggested that loss of dopaminergic nigrostriatal afferents leads to a denervation type of supersensitivity of postsynaptic DA receptors (30). Such up-regulation of receptor sensitivity was also postulated to explain the striking effectiveness of levodopa substitution, and subsequent treatment-induced down-regulation was suggested as a possible explanation for increased dose demand and/or reduced efficacy in the course of therapy.

Accordingly, animal experiments showed increases in the density of striatal *N*-propylnorapomorphine binding sites after 6-hydroxydopamine lesions of the nigrostriatal tract in rats (48), with subsequent declines below baseline within 1 year. Positron emission tomography (PET) studies in a monkey using the D2 receptor ligand raclopride also showed a 50% increase in striatal tracer binding ipsilateral to unilateral carotid injection of 1-methyl-4-phenyl-1,2,3,6-tetrahydropyridine (MPTP) (49). Again, this up-regulation subsequently normalized. These preliminary findings have been confirmed by a more recent monkey study showing that striatal D2 receptor binding was increased by 32% following acute MPTP intoxication, decreasing to 18% several years following the intoxication

(50). Postmortem studies of drug-naive PD patients have yielded inconsistent results, showing both normal (51–53) and increased (54,55) striatal D2 densities. Similarly, Rinne et al. (56) found both lowered and raised striatal spiroperi-dole binding among 15 untreated PD patients.

Human PET studies of putaminal D2 receptor binding in untreated PD patients using raclopride as a tracer generally are consistent with modest up-regulation of putaminal D2 binding sites, showing increases of tracer uptake between 10% and 15%, either globally or contralaterally to the affected side in patients with unilateral disease (57–61). Such evidence as there is from human PET and single photon emission computed tomography (SPECT) studies with D2 ligands suggests that sustained treatment with levodopa or DA agonists is associated with decreases in striatal tracer uptake in the order of 20% to 30% (58,59,62–65). However, experimental work in nonhuman primates has shown a normalization of raclopride binding to the D2 receptor within months or years after MPTP exposure despite the fact that the monkeys never received any levodopa treatment (50).

After balancing all these various lines of evidence, it appears likely that nigrostriatal denervation in IPD is associated with putaminal D2 receptor up-regulation with a subsequent decline, possibly below baseline levels, which may be related to both disease and treatment. However, it remains unclear whether and to what extent such changes in dopaminergic receptor sensitivity are responsible for the clinical problems of long-term treatment with levodopa, in particular response oscillations and abnormal involuntary movements (discussed later).

Little is know about differential responses of receptor subtypes within the D2 family to levodopa. Recent evidence suggests that levodopa exposure may induce D3 receptor expression in the ventral striatum (66). In the hemiparkinsonian rat model this is associated with behavioral sensitization to levodopa, but it is unclear if this mechanism is involved in any of the long-term motor complications associated with levodopa treatment of Parkinson's disease.

Furthermore, it is unclear whether and to what extent D1 receptors are involved in such pharmacodynamic sensitivity changes.

PULSATILE VERSUS CONTINUOUS DOPAMINERGIC STIMULATION: HOW TO DELIVER LEVODOPA

Experimental work in animals suggests that under physiologic conditions nigrostriatal dopaminergic projection neurons exhibit a more or less constant firing rate that is not modified by active or passive limb movement (67). This suggests that striatal neurons are under tonic dopaminergic—possibly modulatory—influence, with little physiologic variation of striatal DA concentrations. At the same time ample experimental data show different behavioral effects of intermittent pulsatile versus tonic continuous dopaminergic striatal stimulation (68,69). Intermittent stimulation generally has been found to be associated with behavioral sensitization, but this does not seem to be the case with continuous modes of DA receptor activation.

Human experience with continuous intravenous or intrajejunal infusions of levodopa or subcutaneous infusions of apomorphine in fluctuating PD also indicates that such continuous treatment strategies lead to adaptive pharmacodynamic receptor changes with increased dyskinesia thresholds (discussed later). With respect to oral levodopa replacement therapy this may mean that the initial use of sustained-release preparations or combinations of levodopa with COMT inhibitors may have long-term benefits over standard formulations by reducing the risk of motor complications. Unfortunately, randomized controlled trials comparing standard versus slow-release levodopa in de novo patients have failed to demonstrate such benefits (70,71) and similar trials with COMT inhibitors have not been performed.

DURATION OF ACTION: IS IT DETERMINED BY POSTRECEPTOR EVENTS?

Muenter and Tyce (72) were the first to distinguish between a short-duration response, measured in hours, and a long-duration response, measured in days, following oral doses of levodopa. The mechanisms underlying both types of response are poorly understood. The long-duration response to levodopa, which is defined as gradual reemergence of parkinsonian disability over days following withdrawal of levodopa, is believed to depend on exogenous levodopa that enters the remaining dopamine nerve terminals to supplement the endogenous levodopa (73,74). In contrast, the short-duration response may be a nonphysiologic response that relates to a number of factors, such as DA synthesis in nondopaminergic terminals, lack of normal feedback control, and absence of DA reuptake mechanisms (74).

With respect to the short-duration response, there is usually some lag between attainment of peak plasma levels and the emergence of clinical benefit (72,75,76), and clinical effects generally persist during the declining phase of plasma levels. One possible interpretation of this dissociation between time courses of levodopa blood levels and clinical effects is that the initial lag is the time needed for levodopa to become equilibrated with the striatal compartment, decarboxylated, and released as DA into the vicinity of postsynaptic DA receptors. Persisting motor benefit after the decline of blood levels may indicate storage in and continuing release from nerve terminals. Such persistence of motor effects is illustrated by counterclockwise hysteresis curves plotted in sequential plasma concentration effects (77).

As outlined earlier, there is some doubt as to whether presynaptic storage of levodopa-derived DA actually occurs. Persisting motor effects beyond the period of suprathreshold blood levels may equally well be postreceptor events outlasting the period of receptor occupancy. Gancher et al. (77) presented evidence for the latter using subcutaneous, apomorphine challenges and levodopa short infusions. Plasma concentration effect curves were similar for both types of dopaminergic stimulation, although apomorphine is rapidly equilibrated with the central compartment, has short receptor occupancy in the range of minutes, and has no intraneuronal storage. Further elucidating such postsynaptic events thus may offer important clues for understanding the pathogenesis of and possible treatment strategies for levodopa response fluctuations.

DOES LEVODOPA ACT EXCLUSIVELY THROUGH CENTRAL CONVERSION TO DOPAMINE?

Levodopa is widely believed to be an inert amino acid that acts as a substrate for catecholamine synthesis in brain. However, there is growing evidence that levodopa has multiple roles within the central nervous system. The idea that levodopa is a neurotransmitter is supported in several reports concerning the existence of levodopa neurons in the rat (78) and human brain (79). Such neurons seem to produce levodopa as their end product. However, specific levodopa receptors have yet to be identified. Direct effects of levodopa on striatal DA receptors have recently been observed in vivo in experimental animals. It has been demonstrated using PET that acute levodopa treatment leads to increased binding of the D2 receptor ligand raclopride in rat striatum. This action was unaltered by AADC inhibition (80). This finding appears to be supported by the report that bolus levodopa administration produces an increase in the number of D2 binding sites in rat striatum. The effect of such treatment on D1 binding was even more pronounced, and it was preceded by a significant increase in D1 messenger RNA (mRNA). The mechanism of DA receptor supersensitivity after acute levodopa administration is not understood at present. However, it is interesting that these acute effects habituated after chronic treatment (81), indicating tolerance to levodopa that may well contribute to the wearing-off fluctuations in advanced IPD.

LATE LEVODOPA FAILURE

Although a marked to excellent initial response to oral levodopa replacement is one of the clinical hallmarks of IPD, up to 50% of all patients treated for 5 years or more develop instability of their motor response (8,71,82). Initially this consists of dose-related periods of improvement followed by

TABLE 8.2. LATE LEVODOPA FAILURE

Drug-related motor complications
  Response fluctuations
    Wearing-off
    On-off
  Drug-induced dyskinesias
    Interdose chorea
    Diphasic dyskinesia
    Off-period dystonia
Disease-related motor complications
  Postural imbalance
  Freezing
  Dysarthria
  Dysphagia
Nonmotor complications
  Depression
  Dementia
  Drug-induced psychosis
  Sleep disorders
  Autonomic dysfunction

TABLE 8.3. PATHOPHYSIOLOGIC MECHANISMS OF LEVODOPA RESPONSE FLUCTUATIONS

Peripheral mechanisms
  Levodopa pharmacokinetics (short $t\frac{1}{2}$; conversion to 3-OMD)
  Gastric emptying
  Intestinal absorption (levodopa vs. LNAA)
  Blood–brain barrier transport (levodopa vs. LNAA)
Central mechanisms
  Loss of presynaptic storage capacity
  Pharmacodynamic receptor changes

3-OMD, 3-O-methyldopa; LNAA, large neutral amino acid.

the wearing off of clinical effects some 3 to 4 hours after dosing. However, with progressing disease these fluctuations in motor performance become increasingly capricious and unpredictable (Table 8.2), while the magnitude of the motor response amplitude to levodopa administration is maintained or even enlarged until late in the course of disease (83). As a result of wearing-off fluctuations patients must cope with several episodes of failing symptomatic relief each day despite optimal oral dosing regimes of levodopa, resulting in many hours of cumulative daily off time. In rough parallel to such response oscillations, most of those affected also exhibit various types and degrees of levodopa-induced abnormal involuntary movements, which in them may cause significant motor disability. The underlying mechanisms of these aspects of late failure of oral levodopa treatment are incompletely understood, and they are a major challenge in the drug therapy of advanced stages of IPD.

PATHOPHYSIOLOGIC MECHANISMS OF LEVODOPA-RELATED RESPONSE FLUCTUATIONS

Several mechanisms clearly contribute to a short-lived and unpredictable clinical response to oral levodopa. They can be divided into aspects of peripheral pharmacokinetic handling of the drug and central pharmacokinetic and pharmacodynamic factors (Table 8.3).

Peripheral Pharmacokinetic Mechanisms

As outlined earlier in the chapter, the half-life of levodopa is short and therefore predisposes to short-lived clinical effects. Absorption following oral ingestion may vary as a

result of erratic gastric emptying and/or competition with dietary amino acids for mucosal transport. Indeed, a radionuclide study demonstrated prolonged gastric emptying in fluctuating PD patients with delayed-on and no-on episodes (21). Delayed-on may account for up to 50% of off-time in fluctuating PD patients. Similarly, blood–brain barrier transport of plasma levodopa may be compromised by competing plasma amino acids. That such transport competition can indeed contribute to clinical response oscillations in patients has long been recognized for gastrointestinal absorption, in which negative effects of oral protein on the effectiveness of levodopa were first observed by Mena and Cotzias (84).

Moreover, it was recognized recently that oral protein or amino acid loading can induce off time in fluctuating patients who were stabilized by continuous intravenous infusions of levodopa despite constant levodopa plasma levels (24), indicating blood–brain barrier transport inhibition. Direct human evidence for this effect of LNAA on brain influx of levodopa was obtained by ^{18}F-dopa PET scanning (85). These studies illustrate that it is the influx of levodopa into the brain that is critical for clinical effects and that this not only is a function of levodopa plasma levels but is also correlated inversely with the concentration of the sum of all competing LNAAs (26). In clinical practice inhibition of blood–brain barrier transport by amino acids seems to be more relevant for possible induction of off time than the variation in intestinal absorption produced by protein meals (86). The latter probably exert most of their negative effects on the action of levodopa by delaying gastric emptying.

Although the mechanisms outlined here certainly contribute to clinical fluctuations in patients, clearly they are operative from the very beginning of treatment and thus do not readily explain the late occurrence of on–off oscillations.

Central Pathophysiologic Mechanisms

One popular hypothesis to explain the late occurrence of levodopa-related response fluctuations was based on the original assumption that exogenous levodopa would act through conversion to DA within surviving nigrostriatal nerve terminals, where it would be stored presynaptically and released in a more or less physiologic manner. Such presynaptic storage would be responsible for the long-duration, seemingly dose-independent initial response, and progressive nigrostriatal degeneration would diminish such storage capacity and make a patient more and more dependent on continuous influx of levodopa from exogenous sources, resulting in dose-related response swings. This hypothesis is attractive not only because it helps to explain the different temporary response characteristics to individual levodopa doses in early and later phases of the disease, but also because it has gained some additional support from ^{18}F-dopa PET studies showing less striatal accumulation of the tracer in fluctuating than in stable responders (86). However, ^{18}F-dopa uptake is critically dependent on availability of striatal AADC activity; therefore, results of such studies may overestimate dopaminergic activity in PD and mask the real disease status because reduced striatal DA levels seem to trigger a relative up-regulation of AADC. This observation indicates that AADC activity marks neuronal survival but not dopaminergic integrity (41). In addition, two studies found only poor correlations between the duration of action of individual doses of levodopa and duration of the disease (87,88). However, Sohn et al. (89) demonstrated a significant correlation between levodopa peak response time and symptom duration that was not observed for apomorphine peak response time. The investigators concluded that peak response time to levodopa may provide an index of the degree of DA neuron degeneration in parkinsonian patients.

The second major hypothesis about the pathogenesis of levodopa response fluctuations therefore assumes delayed development of alterations in the pharmacodynamics of postsynaptic DA receptors. Such pharmacodynamic receptor changes have been implicated in progressive steepening of motor effect decay curves assessed after cessation of short levodopa infusions in patients progressing from stable response to wearing off and finally on–off patterns of clinical response: while efficacy half-life paralleled plasma half-life in wearing-off patients, it was shorter than that in on–off oscillators (90). Similarly, dyskinetic threshold doses of intravenous levodopa declined progressively between groups of drug-naive patients and those with a stable response, wearing-off, or on–off fluctuations, with no change in threshold of antiparkinsonism. This led to progressive narrowing of the therapeutic window between antiparkinsonian and dyskinetic threshold doses (91). Although the initial appearance of wearing-off phenomena probably reflects to some extent the degeneration of presynaptic dopaminergic neurons, recent experiments suggest that secondary changes at the postsynaptic level ultimately contribute substantially to this complication. In rats rendered parkinsonian by a unilateral 6-hydroxydopamine-induced lesion of the nigrostriatal system, twice-daily

administration of levodopa for 3 weeks led to progressive shortening in the rotational response to each injection (92). Since the number of DA neurons remained unchanged during this period, the shorter duration of response presumably reflects alterations at the postsynaptic level. In IPD patients the plasma half-life of apomorphine was unaffected by disease progression, but the rate of antiparkinsonian response decline following withdrawal of a steady-state optimal dose infusion became significantly faster. Since the motor effects of this DA agonist are mediated postsynaptically, wearing-off phenomena must in part reflect modifications at the postjunctional level (93). Indeed, recent postmortem studies of human parkinsonian brains revealed increased preproenkephalin mRNA but unchanged preprotachykinin mRNA. The failure of intermittent levodopa therapy, which was administered to all patients in the study, to fully reverse up-regulation of the indirect striatal output pathway while completely reversing the down-regulation of the direct pathway may result in an imbalance that can affect the pathogenesis of fluctuations seen in levodopa-treated patients (94). Chase et al. (95) estimated that approximately two thirds of the shortening of levodopa's response duration in patients with advanced IPD is attributable to postsynaptic changes.

Interestingly, evidence suggests that such changes may be related to pulsatile stimulation of DA receptors as achieved by periodic oral dosing of levodopa, leading to short sequences of peaks and troughs of plasma and presumably striatal levels. Such chronic pulsatile stimulation of dopamine receptors activates a cascade of molecular and biochemical events, including defective regulation of Fos proteins belonging to the FosB family, increased expression of neuropeptides, and impaired GABA- and glutamate-mediated neurotransmission in the basal ganglia output structures (96,97). Continuous intrajejunal infusions of levodopa are associated with decreases of dose requirement and lessened degrees of preexisting dyskinesias over time (98,99). Response characteristics to single-dose challenges may change toward increased dyskinetic thresholds following as little as 1 week of continuous intravenous infusions of levodopa (100).

NOVEL PHARMACOKINETIC APPROACHES TO L-DOPA THERAPY

Although the exact mechanism underlying the development of levodopa-related motor complications are incompletely understood, the pharmacokinetics of levodopa and its gastrointestinal absorption mechanisms are important contributing factors to the erratic absorption of levodopa and fluctuating plasma levels. Whereas levodopa slow-release preparations and add-on treatment with COMT inhibitors are aimed at increasing half-life and bioavailability of levodopa, a number of strategies have been used to improve gastrointestinal absorption of levodopa. These modifications are aiming at improvement of delayed "on" or "no-on" phenomena due to absorption failure as well as providing more constant gastrointestinal delivery. Such formulations and delivery routes include dispersible levodopa preparations or levodopa prodrugs with high water solubility like levodopa methyl ester and levodopa ethyl ester, all aimed at achieving faster peak plasma levels after oral ingestion as well as dual release formulations of levodopa designed to overcome the delay in C_{max} of sustained-release preparations (21,101–105).

Enteral infusions of levodopa bypass the stomach and thus avoid gastric emptying as a factor for delayed and erratic levodopa absorption. Using infusion pumps they also provide a means of constant levodopa delivery with similar plasma level profiles to intravenous levodopa infusions (106).

IS LEVODOPA TOXIC?

A number of studies have provided evidence for oxidative stress as a pathogenetic factor involved in the progressive loss of nigral DA neurons in Parkinson's disease (107,108). Brain DA undergoes oxidative metabolism associated with generation of reactive free-radical species as well as the formation of potentially toxic quinones via autoxidation. Therefore, there is theoretical concern that enhancing DA production by exogenous levodopa in a failing nigrostriatal system that has lost part of its radical buffering capacity (108) might contribute to increased oxidative stress and accelerated neuronal fallout (109). A number of in vitro experiments in neuroblastoma or pheochromocytoma cell cultures as well as in cultures of chick sympathetic neurons have shown that the addition of high concentrations of levodopa can induce cytotoxic effects via generation of free radicals and mitochondrial energy failure (for review, see 109). However, there have also been in vitro studies showing neurotrophic effects of low concentrations of levodopa, particularly when cell cultures were cocultivated with glial cells (110,111). Similarly contradictory results have been observed regarding levodopa toxicity in experimental in vivo systems. Levodopa was observed to both increase and reduce dopaminergic cell loss in 6-hydroxydopamine-lesioned rats in different experiments (111–113). Therefore, experimental data regarding potential levodopa toxicity in in vitro and in vivo systems are inconsistent and do not provide conclusive evidence for neurotoxic effects of levodopa (114).

Postmortem studies of human brains of patients exposed to levodopa (with or without Parkinson's disease) have also failed to provide any evidence for harmful levodopa effects (115). Clinically levodopa treatment is associated with reduced progression of disability and mortality in Parkinson's disease (116).

More recently, randomized controlled clinical trials have used β-CIT SPECT or fluorodopa PET sequential scans as surrogate markers for progression of nigrostriatal denervation in de novo Parkinson's disease patients exposed to either levodopa or DA agonists, such as pramipexole, ropinirole, or pergolide, in order to assess the differential effects of these drugs on disease progression. All of these trials have shown trends for reduced rates of decline of nigrostriatal function indices in favor of DA agonists versus levodopa, but these differences were not statistically significant (9,117). Follow-up studies are ongoing. However, due to the lack of placebo-controlled arms, these approaches are not suitable to support a conclusion regarding the detrimental effects of either drug on progression of nigral cell loss.

CONCLUSION

After more than 25 years of routine use of levodopa for Parkinson's disease important aspects of its basic mechanisms of action remain incompletely understood. This is also true for the underlying sequence of late development of response oscillations and drug-induced dyskinesias. Advances in the understanding of both types of mechanisms are likely to be interdependent. Such progress is needed for improvement of the long-term success of oral levodopa therapy of IPD.

REFERENCES

1. Parkinson J. *An essay on the shaking palsy.* Parkinson J, ed. London: Whittingham and Rowland, 1817.
2. Carlsson A, Lindqvist M, Magnusson T. 3,4-Dihydroxyphenylalanine and 5-hydroxytryptophan as reserpine antagonists. *Nature (Lond)* 1957;180:1200.
3. Carlsson A, Lindqvist M, Magnusson T, et al. On the presence of 3-hydroxytyramine in brain. *Science* 1958;127:471.
4. Ehringer H, Hornykiewicz O. Verteilung von Noradrenalin und Dopamin (3-Hydroxytyramin) im Gehirn des Menschen und ihr Verhalten bei Erkrankungen des extrapyramidalen Systems. *Klin Wochenschr* 1960;38:1236–1239.
5. Birkmayer W, Hornykiewicz O. Der L-Dioxyphenylalanin (= L-DOPA) Effekt beim Parkinson-Syndrom des Menschen: Zur Pathogenese und Behandlung der Parkinson-Akinese. *Arch Psychiatr Nervenkr* 1962;203:560–574.
6. Barbeau A, Sourkes TL, Murphy CF. Les catecholamines de la maladie de Parkinson. In: Ajuriaguerra J, ed. *Monoamines et systeeme nerveux central.* Geneve: George; Paris: Masson, 1962: 247–262.
7. Cotzias CG, Van Woert MH, Schiffer LM. Aromatic amino acids and modification of Parkinsonism. *N Engl J Med* 1967; 276:374–379.
8. Rascol O, Brooks DJ, Korczyn AD, et al. A five-year study of the incidence of dyskinesias in patients with early Parkinson's disease who were treated with ropinirole or levodopa. 056 Study Group. *N Engl J Med* 2000;342:1484–1491.
9. Parkinson Study Group. Pramipexole vs. levodopa as initial treatment for Parkinson's disease. *JAMA* 2000;284: 1931–1938.

10. Rinne UK, Bracco F, Chouza C, et al. Cabergoline in the treatment of early Parkinson's disease: results of the first year of treatment in a double-blind comparison of cabergoline and levodopa—the PKDS009 Collaborative Study Group. *Neurology* 1997;48:363–368.

11. Gibb WRG, Lees AJ. The relevance of the Lewy body to the pathogenesis of idiopathic Parkinson's disease. *N Neurol Neurosurg Psychiatry* 1988;51:745–752.

12. Kuruma I, Bartholini G, Tissot R, et al. The metabolism of L-3-O-methyldopa, a precursor of dopa in man. *Clin Pharmacol Ther* 1971;12:678–682.

13. Bartholini G, Kuruma I, Pletscher A. 3-O-Methyldopa, a new precursor of dopamine. *Nature* 1971;230:533–534.

14. Muenter MD, Dinapoli RP, Sharpless NS, et al. 3-O-Methyldopa, L-dopa, and trihexyphenidyl in the treatment of Parkinson's disease. *Mayo Clin Proc* 1973;48:173–183.

15. Nutt JG, Woodward WR, Cancher STT, et al. 3-O-Methyldopa and the response to levodopa in Parkinson's disease. *Ann Neurol* 1987;21:584–588.

16. Wade LA, Katzman R. 3-O-Methyldopa uptake and inhibition of L-dopa at the blood-brain barrier. *Life Sci* 1975;17:131–136.

17. Nutt JG, Woodward WR, Anderson JL. Effect of carbidopa on pharmacokinetics of intravenously administered levodopa: implications for mechanism of action of carbidopa in the treatment of parkinsonism. *Ann Neurol* 1985;13:537–544.

18. Merello M, Lees AJ, Webster R, et al. Effect of entacapone, a peripherally acting catechol-O-methyltransferase inhibitor, on the motor response to acute treatment with levodopa in patients with Parkinson's disease. *J Neurol Neurosurg Psychiatry* 1994;57:186–189.

19. Kaakkola S, Teravainen H, Ahtila S, et al. Effect of entacapone, a COMT inhibitor, on clinical disability and levodopa metabolism in parkinsonian patients. *Neurology* 1994;44(1):77–80.

20. Nutt JG, Fellman JH. Pharmacokinetics of levodopa. *Clin Neuropharmacol* 1984;7:35–49.

21. Djaldetti R, Baron J, Ziv I, et al. Gastric emptying in Parkinson's disease: patients with and without response fluctuations. *Neurology* 1996;46:1051–1054.

22. Wade DN, Mearrick PT, Morris JL. Active transport of L-DOPA in the intestine. *Nature* 1973;242:463–465.

23. Daniel PM, Moorhouse SR, Pratt OE. Do changes in blood levels of other aromatic amino acids influence levodopa therapy? *Lancet* 1976;1:95.

24. Nutt JG, Woodward WR, Hammerstad JP, et al. The "on-off" phenomenon in Parkinson's disease: relation to levodopa absorption and transport. *N Engl J Med* 1984;310:483–488.

25. Leenders KL, Poewe WH, Palmer AJ, et al. Inhibition of [18F]fluorodopa uptake into human brain by amino acids demonstrated by positron emission tomography. *Ann Neurol* 1986;20:258–262.

26. Nutt JG, Woodward WR, Carter JH, et al. Influence of fluctuations of plasma large neutral amino acids with normal diets on the clinical response to levodopa. *J Neurol Neurosurg Psychiatry* 1989;52:481–487.

27. Fearnley JU, Lees AJ. Ageing and Parkinson's disease: substantia nigra regional selectivity. *Brain* 1991;114:2283–2301.

28. Bernheimer H, Birkmayer W, Hornykiewicz O, et al. Brain dopamine and syndromes of Parkinson and Huntington. *J Neurol Sci* 1975;30:415–455.

29. Lloyd KG, Davidson L, Hornykiewicz O. The neurochemistry of Parkinson's disease: effect of L-dopa therapy. *J Pharmacol Exp Ther* 1975;195:453–464.

30. Hornykiewicz O. The mechanisms of action of L-dopa in Parkinson's disease. *Life Sci* 1974;15:1249–1259.

31. Spencer SE, Wooten GF. Pharmacologic effects of L-dopa are not closely linked temporally to striatal dopamine concentration. *Neurology* 1984;34:1609–1611.

32. Robertson GS, Robertson HA. Evidence that L-dopa induced rotational behaviour is dependent on both striatal and nigral mechanisms. *J Neurosci* 1989;9:3326–3331.

33. Wachtel SR, Abercrombie ED. Long-term L-dopa administration to rats with 6-OHDA lesions: behaviour and striatal neurochemistry. *Soc Neurosci Abstr* 1993;19:1370.

34. Melamed E, Globus M, Uzzan A, et al. Is dopamine formed from exogenous L-dopa stored within vesicles in striatal dopaminergic nerve terminals: implications for L-dopa's mechanism of action in Parkinson's disease. *Neurology* 1985;35[Suppl 1]:118.

35. Glowinski J. Properties and functions of intraneuronal monoamine compartments in central aminergic neurons. In: Iversen LL, Iversen SD, Snyder SH, eds. *Handbook of clinical psychopharmacology, vol 3. Biochemistry of biogenic amines.* New York: Plenum Press, 1975:139–167.

36. Hefti F, Melamed E. Dopamine release in rat striatum after administration of L-dopa as studied with in vivo electrochemistry. *Brain Res* 1981;295:333–346.

37. Melamed E, Dafni N. Effect of electrical stimulation of nigrostriatal dopaminergic neurons on utilization of exogenous L-dopa in rat corpus striatum. *J Pharm Pharmacol* 1982;34:820–822.

38. Harden DG, Grace AA. Activation of dopamine cell firing by repeated L-dopa administration to dopamine-depleted rats: its potential role in mediating the therapeutic response to L-dopa treatment. *J Neurosci* 1995;15:6157–6166.

39. Poewe WH, Wenning GK. The natural history of Parkinson's disease. *Neurology* 1996;47[Suppl 3]:146–152.

40. Hefti F, Melamed E, Wurtman RJ. The site of dopamine formation in rat striatum after L-dopa administration. *J Pharmacol Exp Ther* 1981;217(1):189–197.

41. Opacka-Juffry J, Brooks DJ. L-dihydroxyphenylalanine and its decarboxylase: new ideas on their neuroregulatory roles. *Mov Disord* 1995;10:241–249.

42. Melamed E, Hefti F, Wurtman RJ. Nonaminergic striatal neurons convert exogenous L-dopa to dopamine in parkinsonism. *Ann Neurol* 1980;8:559–563.

43. Tashiro Y, Kaneko T, Sugimoto T, et al. Striatal neurons with aromatic L-amino acid decarboxylase-like immunoreactivity in the rat. *Neurosci Lett* 1989;100:29–34.

44. Kang UJ, Park DH, Wessel T, et al. DOPA-decarboxylation in the striata of rats with unilateral substantia nigra lesions. *Neurosci Lett* 1992;147:53–57.

45. Mizoguchi K, Yokoo H, Yoshida M, et al. Dopamine formation from L-dopa administered exogenously is independent of dopaminergic neuronal activity: studies with in vivo microdialysis. *Brain Res* 1993;611:152–154.

46. Tison F, Normand E, Jaber M, et al. Aromatic L-amino-acid decarboxylase (DOPA decarboxylase) gene expression in dopaminergic and serotonergic cells of the rat brainstem. *Neurosci Lett* 1991;127:203–206.

47. Li XM, Juorio AV, Paterson IA, et al. Gene expression of aromatic L-amino acid decarboxylation in rat cultured glial cells. *J Neurochem* 1992;59:1172–1175.

48. Fuxe K, Agnati LF, et al. Characterisation of normal and supersensitive dopamine receptors: effects of ergot drugs and neuropeptides. *J Neural Transm* 1981;51:3–37.

49. Leenders KL, Aquilonius SM, Bergström K, et al. Unilateral MPTP lesion in a rhesus monkey: effects on the striatal dopaminergic systems measured in vivo with PET using various novel tracers. *Brain Res* 1988;445:61–67.

50. Doudet DJ, Holden JE, Jivan S, et al. In-vivo PET studies of the dopamine D2 receptors in rhesus monkeys with long-term MPTP-induced parkinsonism. *Synapse* 2000;38:105–113.

51. Quik M, Spokes E, MacKay A, et al. Alterations in [3H]spiperone binding in human caudate nucleus, substantia nigra, and frontal cortex in the Shy-Drager syndrome and Parkinson's disease. *J Neurol Sci* 1979;43:429–437.

52. Bokobza B, Ruber M, Scatton B, et al. [3H]spiperone binding, dopamine and HVA concentrations in Parkinson's disease and supranuclear palsy. *Eur J Pharmacol* 1984;99:167–175.

53. Cortes R, Camps M, Gueye B, et al. Dopamine receptors in the human brain: autoradiographic distribution of D1 and D2 sites in Parkinson syndrome of different etiology. *Brain Res* 1989; 483:30–38.

54. Lee T, Seeman P, Rajput A, et al. Receptor basis for dopaminergic supersensitivity in Parkinson's disease. *Nature* 1978;273: 59–61.

55. Guttman M, Seeman P. Dopamine D2 receptor density in parkinsonian brain is constant for duration of disease, age, and duration of L-dopa therapy. *Adv Neurol* 1986;45:51–57.

56. Rinne UK, Lönnberg P, Koskinen V. Dopamine receptors in the parkinsonian brain. *J Neural Transm* 1981;51:97–106.

57. Rinne UK, Laihinen A, Rinne JO, et al. Positron emission tomography demonstrates dopamine D2 receptor supersensitivity in the striatum of patients with early Parkinson's disease. *Mov Disord* 1990;5:55–59.

58. Brooks DJ, Ibanez V, Sawle GV, et al. Striatal D2 receptor status in patients with Parkinson's disease, striatonigra degeneration, and progressive supranuclear palsy, measured with ^{11}C-raclopride and positron emission tomography. *Ann Neurol* 1992;31:184–192.

59. Antonini A, Schwarz J, Oertel WH, et al. Long-term changes of striatal dopamine D2 receptors in patients with Parkinson's disease: a study with positron emission tomography and ^{11}C-raclopride. *Mov Disord* 1997;12:33–38.

60. Wenning GK, Donnemiller E, Granata R, et al. ^{123}I-beta CIT and ^{123}I-IBZM-SPECT scanning in levodopa-naive Parkinson's disease. *Mov Disord* 1998;13:438–445.

61. Ichise M, Kim YJ, Ballinger JR, et al. SPECT imaging of pre- and postsynaptic dopaminergic alterations in L-dopa-untreated PD. *Neurology* 1999;52:1206–1214.

62. Leenders KL, Herold S, Palmer AJ, et al. Human cerebral dopamine system measured in vivo using PET. *J Cereb Blood Flow Metab* 1985;5:157–158.

63. Wienhard K, Coenen HH, Pawlik G, et al. PET studies of dopamine receptor distribution using (^{18}F-)fluorethylspiperone: findings in disorders related to the dopaminergic system. *J Neural Transm* 1990;81:195–213.

64. Brücke T, Podreka I, Angelberger P, et al. Dopamine D2 receptor imaging with SPECT: studies in different neuropsychiatric disorders. *J Cereb Blood Flow Metab* 1991;11:220–228.

65. Turjanski N, Lees AJ, Brooks DJ. In-vivo studies on striatal dopamine D1 and D2 site binding in L-dopa treated Parkinson's disease with and without dyskinesias. *Neurology* 1997;49:717–723.

66. Bordet R, Ridray S, Carboni S, et al. Induction of dopamine D3 receptor expression as a mechanism of behavioural sensitization to levodopa. *Proc Natl Acad Sci USA* 1997;94:3363–3367.

67. Bunny BS, Walter JR, Roth RH, et al. Dopaminergic neurons: effects of antipsychotic drugs and amphetamine on single cell activity. *J Pharmacol Exp Ther* 1973;85:560–571.

68. Costall B, Domency AM, Naylor RJ. A comparison of the behavioral consequences of chronic stimulation of dopamine receptors in the nucleus accumbens of rat brain affected by continuous infusion or by single daily injections. *Naunyn Schmiedebergs Arch Pharmacol* 1984;324:27–33.

69. Juncos JL, Engber TM, Raisman R, et al. Continuous and intermittent levodopa differentially affect basal ganglia function. *Ann Neurol* 1989;25:437–478.

70. Dupont E, Anderson A, Boqs J, et al. Sustained-release Madopar HBS compared with standard Madopar in the long-term treatment of de novo parkinsonian patients. *Acta Neurol Scand* 1996;93:14–20.

71. Koller WC, Hutton JT, Tolosa E, et al., Carbidopa/Levodopa Study Group. Immediate-release and controlled-release carbidopa/levodopa in PD: a 5-year randomized multicenter study. *Neurology* 1999;53:1012–1019.

72. Muenter MD, Tyce GM. L-Dopa therapy of Parkinson's disease: plasma L-dopa concentration, therapeutic response, and side effects. *Mayo Clin Proc* 1971;46:231–239.

73. Nutt JG, Carter JH, Woodward WR. Long-duration response to levodopa. *Neurology* 1995;45:1613–1616.

74. Nutt JG, Holford NHG. The response to levodopa in Parkinson's disease: imposing pharmacological law and order. *Neurology* 1996;39:561–573.

75. Shoulson I, Glaubiger GA, Chase TN. On–off response: clinical and biochemical correlation during oral and intravenous levodopa administration in parkinsonian patients. *Neurology* 1975; 25:1144–1148.

76. Nutt JG, Woodward WR. Levodopa pharmacokinetics and pharmacodynamics in fluctuating parkinsonian patients. *Neurology* 1986;36:739–744.

77. Gancher ST, Woodward WR, Gliessman P, et al. The short-duration response to apomorphine: implications for the mechanism of dopaminergic effects in parkinsonism. *Ann Neurol* 1990;27:660–665.

78. Tison F, Mons N, Rouet-Karama S, et al. Endogenous L-DOPA in the rat dorsal vagal complex: an immunocytochemical study by light and electron microscopy. *Brain Res* 1989;497:260–270.

79. Komori K, Uesaka S, Yamaoka H, et al. Identification of L-dopa immunoreactivity in some neurons in the human mesencephalic region: a novel dopa neuron group? *Neurosci Lett* 1993;157:13–16.

80. Hume SP, Myers R, Opacka-Juffry J, et al. Effect of L-dopa and 6-OHDA lesioning on ^{11}C-raclopride binding in rat striatum quantified using PET. *J Cereb Blood Flow Metab* 1993;13 [Suppl]:295.

81. Murata M, Kanazawa I. Repeated L-dopa administration reduces the ability of dopamine storage and abolishes the supersensitivity of dopamine receptors in the striatum of intact rats. *Neurosci Res* 1993;16:15–23.

82. Schrag A, Quinn N. Dyskinesias and motor fluctuations in Parkinson's disease: a community-based study. *Brain* 2000;123: 2297–2305.

83. Hughes AJ, Frankel JP, Kempster PA, et al. Motor response to levodopa in patients with parkinsonian motor fluctuations: a follow-up study over three years. *J Neurol Neurosurg Psychiatry* 1994;57:430–434.

84. Mena MA, Cotzias GC. Protein intake and treatment of Parkinson's disease with levodopa. *N Engl J Med* 1975;292:131–134.

85. Leenders KL, Palmer AJ, Quinn N, et al. Brain dopamine metabolism in patients with Parkinson's disease measured with positron emission tomography. *J Neurol Neurosurg Psychiatry* 1986;49:853–860.

86. Frankel JP, Kempster PA, Bovingdon M, et al. The effects of oral protein on the absorption of intraduodenal levodopa and motor performance. *J Neurol Neurosurg Psychiatry* 1989;52: 1063–1067.

87. Gancher ST, Nutt JG, Woodward W. Response to brief levodopa infusions in parkinsonian patients with and without motor fluctuations. *Neurology* 1988;38:712–716.

88. Kempster PA, Frankel JP, Bovingdon M, et al. Levodopa peripheral pharmacokinetics and duration of motor response in Parkinson's disease. *J Neurol Neurosurg Psychiatry* 1989;52: 718–723.

89. Sohn YH, Verhagen Metman L, et al. Levodopa peak response time reflects severity of dopamine neuron loss in Parkinson's disease. *Neurology* 1994;44:755–757.

90. Fabbrini G, Mouradian MM, Juncos JL, et al. Motor fluctuations in Parkinson's disease: central pathophysiological mechanisms: Part I. *Ann Neurol* 1987;24:366–371.

91. Mouradian MM, Juncos JL, Fabbrini G, et al. Motor fluctuations in Parkinson's disease: central pathophysiological mechanisms, part II. *Ann Neurol* 1988;24:372–378.

92. Pappa SM, Engber TM, Chase TN. Motor response variations produced by chronic levodopa treatment in 6-hydroxydopamine lesioned rats. *Neurology* 1993;43:A152.

93. Bravi D, Mouradian MM, Roberts JW, et al. "Wearing-off" fluctuations in Parkinson's disease: contribution of postsynaptic mechanisms. *Ann Neurol* 1994;36:27–31.

94. Nisbet AP, Foster OJF, Kingsbury A, et al. Preproenkephalin and preprotachykinin messenger RNA expression in normal human basal ganglia and in Parkinson's disease. *Neuroscience* 1995;66:361–376.

95. Chase TN, Engber T, Mouradian MM. Palliative and prophylactic benefits of continuously administered dopaminomimetics in Parkinson's disease. *Neurology* 1994;44[Suppl 6]:15–18.

96. Calon F, Hadj Tahar A, Blanchet PJ, et al. Dopamine-receptor stimulation: biobehavioral and biochemical consequences. *Trends Neurosci* 2000;23[Suppl 10]:92–100.

97. Chase TN, Oh JD. Striatal dopamine- and glutamate-mediated dysregulation in experimental parkinsonism. *Trends Neurosci* 2000;23[Suppl 10]:86–91.

98. Sage JI, Trooskin S, Sonsalla PK, et al. Long-term duodenal infusion of levodopa for motor fluctuations in parkinsonism. *Ann Neurol* 1988;24:87–89.

99. Nutt JG, Carter JH. Apomorphine can sustain the long-duration response to L-dopa in fluctuating PD. *Neurology* 2000;54:247–250.

100. Mouradian MM, Heuser IJE, Baronti F, et al. Modification of central dopaminergic mechanisms by continuous levodopa therapy for advanced Parkinson's disease. *Ann Neurol* 1990;27:18–23.

101. Cooper DR, Marrel C, van de Waterbeemd H, et al. L-Dopa esters as potential prodrugs: behavioural activity in experimental models of Parkinson's disease. *J Pharm Pharmacol* 1987;39;627–635.

102. Juncos JL, Fabbrini G, Mouradian MM, et al. Controlled release levodopa-carbidopa (CR-5) in the management of parkinsonian motor fluctuations. *Arch Neurol* 1987;44:1010–1012.

103. Ruggieri S, Stocci F, Carta A, et al. Jejunal delivery of levodopa methyl ester. *Lancet* 1989;2(8653):45–46.

104. Contin M, Riva R, Martinelli P, et al. Concentration–effect relationship of levodopa-benserazide dispersible formulation versus standard form in the treatment of complicated motor response fluctuations in Parkinson's disease. *Clin Neuropharmacol* 1999;22:351–355.

105. Descombes S, Bonnet AM, Gasser UE, et al. Dual-release formulation, a novel principle in L-dopa treatment of Parkinson's disease. *Neurology* 2001;56:1239–1242.

106. Nilsson D, Hansson LE, Johansson K, et al. Long-term intraduodenal infusion of a water based levodopa-carbidopa dispersion in very advanced Parkinson's disease. *Acta Neurol Scand* 1998;97:175–183.

107. Jenner P, Olanow W. Understanding cell death in Parkinson's disease. *Ann Neurol* 1998;44:72–84.

108. Dexter DT, Sian J, Rose S, et al. Indices of oxidative stress and mitochondrial function in individuals with incidental Lewy body disease. *Ann Neurol* 1994;35:38–44.

109. Fahn S. Is levodopa toxic? *Neurology* 1996;47:184–195.

110. Mena MA, Casarejos MJ, Carazo A, et al. Glia conditioned medium protects fetal rat midbrain neurones in culture from L-dopa toxicity. *Neuroreport* 1996;7:441–415.

111. Dziewczapolski G, Murer G, Agid Y, et al. Absence of neurotoxicity of chronic L-dopa treatment in 6-hydroxydopamine lesioned rats. *Neuroreport* 1997;8:975–979.

112. Blunt SB, Jenner P, Marsden CD. Suppressive effect of L-dopa on dopamine cells remaining in the ventral tegmental area of rats previously exposed to the neurotoxin 6-hydroxydopamine. *Mov Disord* 1993;8:129–133.

113. Datla KP, Blunt SB, Dexter DT. Chronic L-DOPA administration is not toxic to the remaining dopaminergic nigrostriatal neurons, but instead may promote their functional recovery, in rats with partial 6-OHDA or FeCl₃ nigrostriatal lesion. *Mov Disord* 2001;16:424–434.

114. Agid Y. Levodopa: is toxicity a myth? *Neurology* 1998;50:858–863.

115. Rajput AH, Fenton M, Birdi S, et al. Is levodopa toxic to human substantia nigra? *Mov Disord* 1997;12:634–638. Parkinson's disease. *Ann Neurol* 1998;44:1–9.

116. Poewe WH, Wenning GK. The natural history of Parkinson's disease. Ann Neurol 1998;44:1–9.

117. Oertel WH. Pergolide versus L-dopa (PELMOPET). *Mov Disord* 2000;15[Suppl 3]:4.

9

THERAPEUTIC STRATEGIES IN PARKINSON'S DISEASE

JOSEPH J. JANKOVIC

Few neurologic disorders have received more attention from the medical and lay communities in the recent past than Parkinson's disease (PD). The growing interest in this neurodegenerative disease has been generated largely as a result of better understanding of the circuitry of the basal ganglia and how its function is altered in a diseased state, improved knowledge about the mechanisms of cell death, the introduction of novel therapeutic strategies, and the disclosure of the diagnosis by many important public figures (1). This extraordinary progress has been fueled by scientific discoveries that are providing new insights into the etiology and pathogenesis of PD. These advances in basic research are now being translated into clinical practice.

Although much progress has been made since James Parkinson's first description of the disease in 1817, at which time he suggested that blood letting and iatrogenic pus formation constituted the best treatments, PD continues to be one of the most common causes of disability among the elderly. The disorder affects about 1% of the population 60 years of age or older, and it has been estimated that 1 person in 40 will develop parkinsonian symptoms during a normal lifetime. While the longevity of patients with PD has increased, largely as a result of advances in medical and surgical therapies, the cost of PD has been escalating (2). According to a 1997 study sponsored by the Parkinson's Disease Foundation, the annual cost has been estimated to be $24,041 per patient and the aggregate annual cost has been estimated to be $24 billion for the entire country (3).

The various therapeutic options in PD can be divided into the following approaches: (a) Dopaminergic—enhances dopaminergic transmission by (i) increasing synaptic dopamine (DA) concentration (levodopa), (ii) administering DA agonists, (iii) enhancing DA release, (iv) blocking DA reuptake, and (v) inhibiting DA degradation; (b) Nondopaminergic—manipulates nondopaminergic neurotransmitters by anticholinergic drugs, and other drugs modulating nondopaminergic systems; (c) Symptomatic—treats specific parkinsonian symptoms; (d) Neuroprotective—attempts to slow disease progression by protecting or

rescuing surviving neurons; (e) Surgery—(i) ablative (e.g., thalamotomy, pallidotomy), (ii) deep brain stimulation, (iii) brain grafting (attempts to repair or reverse underlying pathology); and (f) Preventive (will require finding the cause of PD).

Experimental therapeutics of PD is a rapidly evolving field. In order to assess the efficacy of novel therapeutic interventions it is essential that the motor and other impairments be measured as objectively as possible. Although a variety of neurophysiologic and computer-based methods have been proposed, such as the Bradykinesia Akinesia Incoordination Test (BRAIN, a simple computer keyboard test; www.anaesthetist.com/software/brain.htm) (4), most studies still rely on clinical rating scales, particularly the Unified Parkinson's Disease Rating Scale (UPDRS) (5–10). Rating scales for levodopa-induced dyskinesias (11–14) and diaries (15) are also being developed and increasingly utilized in studies of dopaminergic therapy of PD. In addition, portable devices based on a triaxial accelerometer, worn on the shoulder, have been reported to provide valid data that correlate well with various dyskinesia scales (16,17). Finally, there are ongoing attempts to develop instruments that not only can measure specific motor functions in PD but that can assess quality of life as well (18).

Besides utilizing the most appropriate measures to quantitate the response it is also imperative that the methodology and the design of the clinical trial considers as many potential confounding variables as possible, including a placebo effect, which may persist for 6 months or longer (19,20). In one provocative study using positron emission tomography (PET) scan to image ^{11}C-raclopride binding to D2 DA receptors, placebo administration (subcutaneous injection of saline) was associated with marked reduction in D2 binding indicating that a release of endogenous DA mediates the placebo effect (21). This suggests that the observed placebo response is mediated by or results in actual physiologic and neurotransmitter changes.

In addition to improvements in motor function, the therapeutic advances have had a positive impact on the quality of life of PD patients. When levodopa was introduced in late 1960s, the mortality rate of PD initially improved, probably because of improved mobility of severely disabled PD patients. However, more recent studies have shown that the life expectancy of PD patients is still shorter than that of age-matched controls (22,23). However, in a prospective study of 800 patients followed longitudinally from early stages of their disease for an average of 8.2 years, the overall death rate (2.1% per year) was similar to that of an age- and gender-matched U.S. population without PD (24).

DOPAMINERGIC THERAPY

Levodopa

While levodopa remains the most effective drug for management of the symptoms of PD, side effects, particularly motor fluctuations and dyskinesias, limit its usefulness (25) (Tables 9.1–9.5; Fig. 9.1). Because of the levodopa-related complications and the theoretical consideration that levodopa increases oxidative stress and may thus accelerate neuronal degeneration, there is an ongoing debate as to when in the course of PD it is most appropriate to initiate levodopa therapy (26–28). Several algorithms and decision trees have been offered as treatment

TABLE 9.1. THERAPEUTIC STRATEGIES IN PARKINSON'S DISEASE

Enhance Dopaminergic Transmission
A. Increase DA synthesis
   1. Stimulate tyrosine hydroxylase (tetrahydrobiopterin, oxyferris-corbone)
   2. DA precursors (tyrosine, levodopa)
   3. Modify levodopa pharmacokinetics
     a. Dietary modification (minimize AA intake, administer antacids)
     b. Block peripheral dopa decarboxylase (carbidopa, benserazide)
     c. Slow-release levodopa (Sinemet CR, Madopar HBS)
     d. Improve delivery of drugs with infusions (intravenous, intraduodenal, intraventricular)
     e. Subcutaneous and brain implants of levodopa in polymer matrix
B. Enhance DA release
   1. Methylphenidate
   2. Dextroamphetamine
   3. Pemoline
   4. Amantadine
   5. Nicotine
   6. Electroconvulsive therapy
C. Block DA reuptake
   1. Tricyclics
   2. Bupropion
   3. Mazindol
   4. Benztropine
D. Inhibit DA catabolism (degradation)
   1. COMT inhibitors
   2. MAO-B inhibitors (deprenyl, lazabemide)
E. Administer DA agonists
   1. Bromocriptine
   2. Pergolide
   3. Lisuride
   4. Apomorphine
   5. Pramipexole
   6. Ropinirole
   7. Cabergoline
Manipulating Nondopaminergic Neurotransmitters
A. ACh (anticholinergics, tricyclics, amantadine)

B. NE (L-threodihydroxyphenylserine or DOPS)
C. 5-HT (5-hydroxytryptamine, clonazepam, lisuride)
D. GABA (progabide)
E. Block glutamate receptors (NMDA and AMPA antagonists)
F. Block glutamate release (riluzole)
Neurosurgical Approaches to Parkinson's Disease
A. Thalamotomy (VIM)
B. Pallidotomy (posteroventral)
C. Deep Brain Stimulation
   1. Thalamus (VIM)
   2. Globus pallidus
   3. Subthalamic nucleus
D. Implantation (subcutaneous, brain)
   1. Levodopa polymer matrix
   2. Levodopa-containing biodegradable microspheres
   3. Polymer-encapsulated dopaminergic cell lines
   4. Autologous adrenal medulla
   5. Fetal (human, porcine) mesencephalon
   6. Vectors (fibroblasts, astrocytes, viruses), genetically modified to produce DA, trophic factors
Slowing Progression by Protecting Surviving Neurons
A. Levodopa-sparing strategies
B. Antioxidants
C. Free radical trappers
D. Iron chelators
E. Glutamate antagonists
F. Trophic factors (GDNF)
G. GM1 gangliosides
Repairing or Reversing Pathology
A. Brain implants
   1. Autologous adrenal medulla (with cografts)
   2. Fetal substantia nigra
   3. Cell suspensions or cultured tissue
   4. Genetically engineered cells or vectors
B. Gene replacement therapy
C. Trophic factors
Prevention
A. Avoid drugs/toxins and other known causes of parkinsonism
B. Find a population at risk for Parkinson's disease and then design a specific preventive program

DA, dopamine; AA, amino acids; COMT, catecholamine *O*-methyltransferase; MAO-B, monoamine oxidase B; ACh, acetylcholine; NE, norepinephrine; DOPS, L-threodihydroxyphenylserine; 5-HT, 5-hydroxytryptamine; GABA, gamma aminobutyric acid; NMDA, *N*-methyl-D-aspartate; AMPA, α-amino-3-hydroxy-5-methyl-4-isoxazolepropionate; VIM, ventralis intermedius; GDNF, glial-derived neurotrophic factor.

TABLE 9.2. PRIMARY DRUGS USED IN THE MANAGEMENT OF PARKINSON'S DISEASE

Generic Name	Dosage Unit	Daily Dose (mg)	Mechanism of Action
Deprenyl	Tabs (5 mg)	10	MAO-B (Selegiline) inhibitor
Trihexyphenidyl	Tabs (2 and 5 mg)	4–8	Anticholinergic
Benztropine	Tabs (0.5, 1, and 2 mg)	0.5–8	Anticholinergic
	Ampules 2 mL (1 mg/mL)		
Amantadine	Caps (100 mg)	100–300	Release of DA, anticholinergic, NMDA antagonist
Levodopa	Tabs and caps (100, 250, 500 mg)	3,000–8,000	DA precursor
Carbidopa/levodopa	Tabs (10/100, 30/300–25/100 and 200/2,000 25/250 mg)		Dopa decarboxylase inhibitor/DA precursor
Carbidopa/levodopa CR	Tabs (25/100, 50/200 mg)	50/200–250/2,000	Dopa decarboxylase inhibitor/DA precursor
Bromocriptine	Tabs (2.5 mg)	7.5–40	DA agonist
	Caps (5 mg)		
Pergolide	Tabs (0.05, 0.25, and 1 mg)	0.5–6	DA agonist
Ropinirole	Tabs (0.25, 0.5, 1.0, 2.0, 5.0)	0.5–24	DA agonist
Pramipexole	Tabs (0.125, 0.25, 1.0, 1.5 mg)	0.1–15	DA agonist
Cabergoline	Tabs (0.5 mg)	2–10	DA agonist
Entacapone	N/A	200–400	COMT inhibitor
Tolcapone	N/A	300–1,200	COMT inhibitor

DA, dopamine; MAO-B, monoamine oxidase B; NMDA, *N*-methyl-D-asparate; COMT, catecholamine *O*-methyltransferase.

TABLE 9.3. LEVODOPA SIDE EFFECTS

System	Management
Peripheral (and Medullary Emetic Center)	
Nausea, vomiting, anorexia	A. Carbidopa
	B. Diphenidol, hydroxyzine, cyclizine
	C. Ondansetron
	D. Domperidone
Orthostatic hypotension	A. Carbidopa
	B. Fluorinef, NaCl
	C. Midodrine
	D. Elastic stockings
Central	
Chorea, stereotypy, punding	A. Reduce levodopa
	B. Reduce anticholinergic
	C. Amantadine
	D. Yohimbine
	E. Glutamate antagonists
	F. Surgery
Dystonia[a]	A. Reduce levodopa (in D-I-D increase dose)
	B. Sinemet CR, Madopar HBS
	C. Anticholinergics
	D. Tricyclics
	E. Baclofen, tizanidine, mexilitine
	F. DA agonists
	G. Lithium
	H. Botulinum toxin
	I. Surgery
Myoclonus[a]	A. Reduce levodopa
	B. Clonazepam
	C. Valproate
Akathisia[a]	A. Anxiolytics
	B. Propranolol
	C. Naltrexone
Hallucinations[a]	A. Reduce levodopa
	B. Clozapine
	C. Ondasetron
	D. Olanzapine
	E. "Drug holiday"

[a]May not be related to levodopa therapy.

TABLE 9.4. FLUCTUATIONS IN PARKINSON'S DISEASE

Fluctuation	Management
End-of-dose deterioration ("wearing-off")	A. Increase frequency of levodopa doses B. Sinemet CR C. DA agonists D. MAO inhibitors E. COMT inhibitors F. Apomorphine rescue G. Surgery
Delayed onset of response	A. Give before meals B. Reduce protein C. Antacids D. Liquid levodopa E. Apomorphine
Drug-resistant "offs"	A. Increase levodopa dose and frequency B. Give before meals C. Liquid levodopa D. Apomorphine
Random oscillation ("on-off")	A. DA agonists B. Infusions (levodopa, apomorphine) C. "Drug holiday"
Freezing[a]	A. Increase dose B. DA agonists C. MAO inhibitors D. Desipramine (?) E. DOPS (?) F. Gait training G. Botulinum toxin injections (?) H. Surgery (?)
Fluctuations in blood pressure, mood, sensory symptoms, sleep pattern, etc.[a]	

[a]May not be related to levodopa therapy.
DA, dopamine; MAO, monoamine oxidase; COMT, catecholamine *O*-methyltransferase; DOPS, L-threodihydroxyphenylserine.

guidelines (29). In this section we will review the pharmacology of levodopa and discuss the rationale for delaying the introduction of levodopa until the PD symptoms become troublesome or interfere with a patient's functioning at home or at work.

Levodopa is almost entirely absorbed at the level of the small intestine, but only 30% of the administered dose

TABLE 9.5. DYSKINESIAS IN PARKINSON'S DISEASE

Dyskinesia	Management
Peak dose dyskinesia (I-D-I)	A. Reduce each dose of levodopa B. DA agonists C. Amantadine D. Clozapine, olanzapine E. Glutamate antagonists F. Yohimbine G. Botulinum toxin H. Surgery (pallidotomy, DBS)
Diphasic dyskinesia (D-I-D)	A. Increase each dose of levodopa (?) B. DA agonists C. Botulinum toxin D. Surgery (pallidotomy, DBS)

DA, dopamine; DBS, deep brain stimulation.

remains as the parent compound in the periphery; the rest is metabolized in the liver, kidneys, and the blood. Only 1% of the ingested levodopa dose enters the brain (30). Levodopa is transported across the duodenum wall by a saturable, facilitated carrier system (the aromatic and branched chain L-amino acid system). Amino acids contained in protein meals may, therefore, compete with levodopa transport across the intestinal mucosa and at the blood–brain barrier. Levodopa absorption, both at the gut and at the blood–brain barrier, can therefore be optimized by regulating dietary protein intake, and many clinicians advise their patients, particularly those who have developed motor complications, to take levodopa with small meals containing minimal amounts of protein (31).

The therapeutic benefits of levodopa have been markedly enhanced by the addition of carbidopa or benserazide, peripheral dopa decarboxylase inhibitors (32). Since the medullary vomiting center is not protected by the blood–brain barrier, the "peripheral" dopa decarboxylase inhibitor (carbidopa) is effective in blocking the conversion of levodopa to DA in this region, thus reducing levodopa-related anorexia, nausea, and vomiting. When combined with carbidopa, the total levodopa dosage can be reduced by 75% to 80%. Although earlier studies indicated that 75

Motor Fluctuations and Dyskinesias Related to Levodopa Therapy

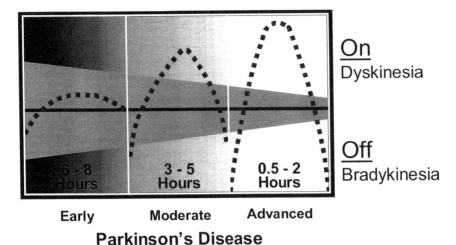

FIG. 9.1. Diagrammatic representation of the occurrence of motor fluctuations and dyskinesias with narrowing of the therapeutic window related to duration of levodopa treatment.

mg of carbidopa is sufficient to inhibit peripheral dopa decarboxylase, subsequent data suggested that a higher dose of carbidopa is needed to completely block peripheral dopa decarboxylase (33). However, when the dosage of carbidopa exceeds 150 mg, it may partially enter the brain where it could block the conversion of levodopa to DA. Therefore, dosages above 150 mg/day are not advisable. In the United States and many other countries, Sinemet (*sin,* without; *emet,* emesis) and generic preparations of levodopa combined with carbidopa are the conventional forms of levodopa used in clinical practice (Table 9.4). Madopar, a combination of levodopa and benserazide, is used in some European and other countries. In this chapter, levodopa/carbidopa combination will be referred to as *Sinemet,* but it should be noted that there are many generic formulations of levodopa/carbidopa. Carbidopa alone (Lodosyn) can be prescribed to patients who experience nausea, particularly when Sinemet is introduced and the dosage of carbidopa in Sinemet is not sufficient to prevent this side effect. In addition to the commercial preparations of levodopa, some patients, particularly in the Middle East, have reported beneficial effects from a natural source of levodopa in the cooked broad bean (*Vicia faba* seedlings and pods) (34).

The surviving striatal dopaminergic terminals are primarily responsible for conversion of levodopa to DA, but nonneuronal cells (e.g., glia) may also participate in this process. However, with progression of the disease and accompanying cellular loss, the capacity for conversion of levodopa to DA is reduced. This leads to a shortening of the striatal half-life and the development of motor fluctuations, dyskinesias, and symptomatic deterioration. Poor response to levodopa should suggest the following possibilities: (a) wrong diagnosis (e.g., one of the postsynaptic forms of

parkinsonism such as the "parkinsonism plus" syndromes), (b) adverse drug interaction (e.g., certain antipsychotic and antiemetic drugs, which act by blocking DA receptors), and (c) pharmacokinetic effects (e.g., insufficient dosage, slow stomach emptying, competition for absorption at small intestine and blood–brain barrier by amino acids in protein meals). The three most important reasons why PD patients lose their response to levodopa are (a) natural progression of the disease with gradual loss of dopaminergic neurons and terminals, (b) development of complications as a result of chronic levodopa therapy, and (c) emergence of symptoms not directly related to dopaminergic deficiency, such as cognitive decline, depression, freezing, and dysautonomia.

One of the most challenging problems in the management of PD is the treatment of levodopa complications (36–39) (Tables 9.2–9.5). Side effects caused by peripheral DA (and DA stimulation of the medullary vomiting center, which is not protected by the blood–brain barrier) include gastrointestinal symptoms, tachycardia, and orthostatic hypotension. Common central side effects of levodopa therapy include motor fluctuations, dyskinesias, and psychiatric problems. In a large prospective study of 352 patients originally enrolled in the DATATOP study (see below), the following complications occurred after 20.5 ± 8.8 months of levodopa therapy: wearing off in about half, dyskinesia in one third, and severe on–off in about one tenth of subjects (40). This is consistent with some previous studies (41), but in a study of 618 patients enrolled in the CR First Study, in which standard and CR Sinemet were compared, only 22% of the patients developed fluctuations or dyskinesias during a 5-year prospective follow-up (42). The difference may be explained in part by the more stringent criteria for the detection of the time to onset of motor fluctuations in the CR First Study: when more than 20% of the waking day was spent in the "off" state or when more than 10% of the waking day was spent in the "on with dyskinesia" state. Nutt et al. (43) showed that when patients are carefully observed, a majority of patients develop motor fluctuations and dyskinesias even during the first year of levodopa therapy. In a review of 74 publications with adequate data related to frequency of levodopa-induced fluctuations and dyskinesias, Ahlskog and Muenter (44) concluded that after 5 years of levodopa therapy about 40% of patients experience fluctuations and the same number experience dyskinesias. The limitations of such a survey, including marked heterogeneity of diagnostic criteria, doses, duration of follow-up, and other problems, must be carefully considered when interpreting this data.

The most common form of clinical fluctuation, the wearing-off effect, is characterized by end-of-dose deterioration and recurrence of parkinsonian symptoms as a result of shorter (sometimes only 1 to 2 hours) duration of benefit after a given dose of levodopa. Besides motor deterioration many patients experience a variety of cognitive, behavioral (depression), autonomic, sensory, and other nonmotor symptoms during their off periods (45). Some patients even exhibit an addictive behavior ("hedonistic homeostatic dysregulation") similar to substance abuse (46). In addition to this short-duration response lasting several hours, many PD patients also experience a long-duration response, which usually lasts several days and gradually diminishes with the progression of the disease (47). In their subsequent study, Zappia et al. (48) found that a multiple daily intake of small single doses of levodopa, as is currently done in clinical practice, was not adequate to provide a sustained long-duration response but that full doses once or three times a day ensured sustained long-duration response. Although they suggest that these findings may be relevant to the treatment of PD, the studies were done in patients with early PD who are not taking DA agonists, in whom frequent, small-dose administration is usually not used. Nutt (49) in an accompanying editorial concluded that these studies do not provide sufficient evidence for clinicians to change their practice.

There are several different types of levodopa-induced dyskinesias, such as peak-dose, diphasic, and wearing-off dyskinesias (50–53). The phenomenology of the dyskinesias also varies from one individual to another. Even within the same patient the dyskinesias vary from minute to minute or from one anatomic location to another. Besides chorea, other levodopa-related dyskinesias include various stereotypies, dystonia, and myoclonus. Although these involuntary movements can be quite violent and disabling, many patients prefer being "on" with dyskinesia than being "off" without dyskinesia. The most common type, peak-dose dyskinesia, usually consists of choreiform or stereotypic movements involving the head, trunk, and limbs, and, occasionally, the respiratory muscles (54,55). One relatively

rare form of stereotypic motor behavior related to levodopa is "punding," characterized by intense fascination with repetitive handling, examining, sorting, and arranging of objects (56). Another form of levodopa-related dyskinesia, occurring in about 15% to 20% of patients chronically treated with levodopa, is so-called diphasic dyskinesia. In contrast to the more common peak-dose dyskinesias, manifested by the sequence of parkinsonism-*i*mprovement-*d*yskinesia- *i*mprovement-parkinsonism (I-D-I), the diphasic response is characterized by parkinsonism-*d*yskinesia-*i*mprovement- *d*yskinesia-parkinsonism (D-I-D). Dystonia tends to occur when plasma, and presumably brain, levels either rise or fall, and is usually manifested by painful flexion or extension of the toes and other dystonic movements or postures. The most common form of dystonia in levodopa-treated PD patients consists of early morning or nocturnal dystonia, such as painful foot cramps (57,58). Careful studies of patients during periods of dyskinesia suggest that levodopa-induced dyskinesias usually start in the foot, ipsilateral to the side most affected by PD (59,60). This is consistent with early loss of dopaminergic innervation in the dorsolateral striatum, which corresponds somatotopically to the foot area.

Whether motor fluctuations and dyskinesias are more related to duration of levodopa treatment or to duration of disease has been debated since these adverse effects first became recognized. Whatever the mechanism, there is a growing body of evidence suggesting that the shortening of response to levodopa and the wearing-off effect are related to shortening of levodopa's half-life in the striatum, without a measurable change in the peripheral pharmacokinetics. Thus, as a result of loss of striatal dopaminergic terminals, the brain's ability to store and buffer the shifts in striatal concentration of levodopa is lost (38,61). Dopaminergic transmission in the nigrostriatal system is converted from the normal tonic firing rate (nigral neurons normally fire at a constant rate of 5 Hz) to a phasic response. Although there is no direct clinical evidence for this theory, there are some experimental models, such as 6-hydroxydopamine (6-OHDA)–lesioned rats, that provide support for the notion that intermittent (pulsatile) dosing of levodopa is more likely associated with shortening of response to each dose of levodopa than continuous administration (62).

In addition to the presynaptic mechanisms, there is increasing evidence supporting the role of postsynaptic mechanisms in the development of wearing-off and on–off phenomenon. The postsynaptic mechanisms for motor fluctuations is supported by the observation that the response to apomorphine is shortest and steepest in patients with the most severe motor fluctuations (63) and that apomorphine is capable of sustaining a long-duration response similar to that produced by oral levodopa (64). In 28 patients with various degrees of motor fluctuations, the duration of antiparkinsonian response was 43% shorter in the group of patients with the most severe (on–off) fluctuation as compared to the patients in early stage of the disease never treated with levodopa (63). Furthermore, the slope of dose–response curve was the steepest and the therapeutic window narrowest for the most fluctuating patients. Because apomorphine acts directly at postsynaptic receptors the observed differences in response were thought to represent changes "within, or downstream from, striatal dopaminoceptive neurons" (63). The authors suggested that "chronic nonphysiologic intermittent stimulation of dopaminergic receptors on medium-sized GABAergic efferent neurons may activate signal transduction mechanisms that elicit long-term potentiation of *N*-methyl-D-aspartate (NMDA)–mediated responses." The role of glutamate and its receptors in motor fluctuation and dyskinesias is supported by the observation that NMDA receptor blockers, such as amantadine, ameliorate these motor responses in parkinsonian animals and patients (65,66). Whether NMDA antagonists primarily affect the interaction of DA and NMDA receptors at dendritic spines of striatal GABAergic neurons or at the level of the pallidum is not known. The NMDA receptor blocker MK-801 has been shown to reduce apomorphine-induced excitation of pallidal neurons in rats (67). Furthermore, globus pallidus has been found to be hyperactive in monkeys made parkinsonian by infusion of the toxin 1-methyl-4-phenyl-1,2,3,6-tetrahydropyridine (MPTP) with dyskinesias induced by DA agonists (68) and pallidotomy clearly ameliorates levodopa-induced dyskinesias in PD patients (see below) (1). The mechanism by which pallidotomy improves levodopa-induced dyskinesia is not known, but single-cell recordings in the internal globus pallidus (GPi) of parkinsonian monkeys show a marked reduction in firing rates only when dyskinesias were present (69). The average firing rate decreased from 46 Hz during "off" state, to 26 Hz during "on" state, and to 7.6 Hz during dyskinesia. It has been hypothesized that either overactive GPi (in a parkinsonian state) or low GPi activity (during dyskinesias) results in an abnormal ("noisy") input to the thalamocortical circuit. Dopaminergic drugs (70) as well as pallidotomy and high frequency pallidal stimulation tend to reduce or eliminate the "noise" and "normalize" the output (71).

The mechanisms of levodopa-induced dyskinesias and how they contribute to the broad spectrum of phenomenology are poorly understood (51,61,72). Many studies support the notion that levodopa-induced dyskinesias involve overactivity of the direct striatal output pathway and GPe, but dystonic dyskinesia additionally involves the motor component of the subthalamic nucleus (STN) (61). Although levodopa may induce dyskinesias even in normal squirrel monkeys, suggesting that preexisting striatal degeneration is not necessary for levodopa-induced dyskinesias (73), many studies have shown that motor fluctuations and dyskinesias are primarily related to dose and duration of levodopa treatment (74). Besides dose and duration of levodopa therapy, there are other risk factors that should be

considered when initiating treatment with levodopa. Young-onset PD patients seem to be particularly likely to develop levodopa-induced dyskinesias early in the course of therapy (75,76). Since levodopa-induced dyskinesias usually do not occur in patients with atypical postsynaptic parkinsonism, it has been proposed that this complication is mediated in PD patients by intact or supersensitive postsynaptic receptors (77,78). In a case-control study of 136 patients with PD and 224 controls, Oliveri et al. (79) found that certain alleles of the short tandem repeat polymorphism of the D2 receptor gene reduce the risk of developing levodopa-induced dyskinesias. In another study, *DRD2Taq1A* polymorphism was associated with increased risk for developing motor fluctuations (80).

The neural mechanisms underlying levodopa-induced dyskinesias are not fully understood, but recent studies suggest that pulsatile stimulation of DA receptors and downstream changes in proteins and genes result in alterations in the firing patterns from the basal ganglia to the cortex. Bezard et al. (61) have proposed that in addition to external globus pallidus (GPe) overactivity and STN inhibition, the direct striatum-GPi pathway is responsible for the underactivity and altered firing pattern of the basal ganglia outputs in levodopa-induced dyskinesias. Disinhibition (overactivity) of the primary and associated motor cortex secondary to increased activity of the outflow pallidothalamocortical motor pathway has been suggested as a mechanism of levodopa-induced dyskinesias (81). This is supported by studies utilizing intravenous ^{133}Xe single photon emission computed tomography (SPECT) to measure regional cerebral blood flow, which show that dyskinetic parkinsonian patients have a significant overactivation in the supplementary motor area and ipsi- and contralateral primary motor areas induced by simple motor tasks. A reduction in the striatal uptake of ^{18}F-dopa has been demonstrated by PET scans in fluctuating but not in stable parkinsonian patients (82). However, there is no difference in the DA receptor density as measured by PET scans between patients with or without dyskinesias (83). Using [^{11}C]dopa and PET, Ekesbo et al. (84) concluded that DA autoreceptor function is lost in advanced PD. Progressive shortening of the response to levodopa during long-term therapy may be also explained in part by the development of tolerance. This is supported by the observation that a 2- to 4-day levodopa withdrawal ("drug holiday") results in prolongation of the response to levodopa infusion (85). One 3-year follow-up study using PET and [^{11}C]raclopride as D2 receptor ligand, found that patients who later developed wearing-off fluctuations had estimated levels of synaptic DA 3 times higher at 1 hour in response to oral levodopa than patients who had a stable response to levodopa treatment (86). The [^{11}C]raclopride reduction returned to baseline in 4 hours in the fluctuating group but was maintained for 4 hours in the nonfluctuating group. Although the authors attribute the observed differences in different concentrations of synaptic

DA, the exaggerated levodopa effect could have been due to more severe baseline depletion of DA or altered D2 receptors in the fluctuating group of patients.

There is a growing body of evidence to support the notion that intermittent dopaminergic stimulation activates signal transduction pathways in the striatum (particularly the medium spiny neurons) facilitating the development of motor fluctuations and dyskinesias (38). Studies of mRNA expression of enkephalin (preproenkephalin) and of substance P (preprotachykinin) as markers for the indirect and direct striatopallidal pathways, respectively, may provide insights into the pathogenesis of levodopa-induced dyskinesia (72). In animals made parkinsonian by 6-OHDA or MPTP, the striatal enkephalin mRNA as well as Fos-related antigens are increased whereas the mRNA for substance P is decreased (72,87). Treatment with levodopa increases the substance P mRNA, but it fails to correct the elevated levels of enkephalin mRNA. In another study involving 6-OHDA rats, levels of expression of FosB-related proteins were correlated with severity of abnormal movements and with increased prodynorphin mRNA in the striatum (88). In addition, there is growing evidence that the opioid system is also involved in dyskinesias. Levodopa-induced dyskinesia is associated with marked decrease in κ-receptor binding, suggesting that enhanced stimulation of κ-receptor in levodopa-induced dyskinesia is accompanied by down-regulation in receptor number as a result of elevation of endogenous opioids (61). These and other studies suggest that levodopa-induced dyskinesias are partly related to pulsatile activation of the D2-mediated indirect striatopallidal pathway but also involve overactivity of the direct pathway, as well as increased opioid levels. Therefore, opioid antagonists may be useful in the treatment of levodopa-induced dyskinesias.

Despite previous notions that levodopa does not cause dyskinesia in normal animals or humans, levodopa in high doses has been demonstrated to produce dyskinesias in normal monkeys. This phenomenon is associated with increased preproenkephalin, again providing support for the importance of the D2-mediated indirect pathway in levodopa-induced dyskinesia (89). In addition, studies in MPTP monkeys have demonstrated a striking association between induction of dyskinesias and Fos-related antigens, particularly when the drugs (levodopa or D1 or D2 agonists) were administered in a pulsatile manner (72). While DA receptor binding and mRNA studies have not demonstrated a consistent correlation with levodopa-induced dyskinesias, increased preproenkephalin in the striatum and GABA$_A$ binding in the GPi were consistently related to dyskinesias. In addition, pulsatile dopaminergic treatment increases Fos-related antigens, JunD and CREB phosphorylation resulting in increased AP-1 binding in the striatum. These changes may represent "a form of pathological learning that results from deficient gating of glutamatergic inputs to the striatum by dopamine" (72). Thus, there is growing evidence to support the concept that pulsatile

stimulation of DA receptors causes dysregulation of "downstream" genes and proteins resulting in altered neuronal firing patterns in GPe-STN-GPi (36,62,90–92). The alteration in signal transduction pathways in the striatum may also lead to enhanced phosphorylation of NMDA subunits, causing increased sensitivity of these receptors to glutamatergic corticostriatal input. It has been hypothesized that this change in the NMDA receptors eventually translates clinically into motor fluctuations and dyskinesias (38). Levodopa-induced dyskinesias may be associated with abnormalities in the phosphorylation status and subsequent subcellular localization of NMDA receptors (61).

Postmortem ligand studies as well as in vivo PET studies have provided support for the notion that denervation supersensitivity is the most likely mechanism for levodopa-induced dyskinesias. Using PET and the opioid receptor ligand [^{11}C]diprenorphine, Piccini et al. (93) found that opioid receptor binding is decreased in the striatum, thalamus, and in cingulate and prefrontal areas of patients with levodopa-induced dyskinesia, but not in patients without dyskinesia. It has been hypothesized that increased endogenous levels of opioids produced by levodopa results in down-regulation of the opioid receptors and disinhibition of the GPi and dyskinesias. In animals, the synthesis of dynorphin is enhanced by an intermittent stimulation of D1 receptors. Levodopa not only increases levels of opioids, but also induces redistribution of D1 receptors from plasma membrane of medium-sized spiny neurons to the cytoplasm of these neurons (94). The altered localization of D1 receptors may contribute to the development of levodopa-related motor complications. Furthermore, abnormal expression of striatal D3 receptors may also contribute to levodopa-induced complications (95). These receptors are normally found in the striatum and limbic areas (particularly the nucleus accumbens), but the density of these receptors is low in the striatum. However, the D3 receptors are markedly increased in the putamen of animals exhibiting behavioral sensitization to levodopa (96). In contrast to the striatal D2 receptors that are usually increased in PD, the D3 receptors are decreased in ventral striatum, particularly in patients with advanced PD (95,97). The role of D3 receptors in mediating antiparkinsonian effect of DA agonists is not known, but D3 activation decreases locomotor activity in the experimental animals (98).

Strategies designed to prolong and smooth out the therapeutic concentrations of levodopa are most helpful in patients with motor fluctuations (99). Slow-release preparations of levodopa, such as Sinemet CR, offer the possibility of "smoothing out" clinical fluctuations by slowly releasing the levodopa from a special matrix. Sinemet CR prolongs the plasma (and presumably brain) levels and, has been found useful in the treatment, and possibly prevention, of motor fluctuations, particularly the wearing-off effect (100). Once the decision is made to start levodopa therapy, Sinemet CR may be the preferable formulation. This recommendation is based on the theory that more constant activation of DA receptors may cause less receptor alterations, and more predictable and longer response, than pulsatile or intermittent dopaminergic stimulation (101–103). Sinemet CR consists of a mixture of 200 mg of levodopa and 50 mg of carbidopa (Sinemet CR 50/200) or 100 mg of levodopa and 25 mg of carbidopa (Sinemet CR 25/100); and, in contrast to standard Sinemet (25/100 or 25/250), which dissolves within 30 minutes, Sinemet CR may take up to 3 hours to fully dissolve. Although Sinemet CR can be taken less frequently, the total daily dosage of levodopa is about 30% higher as compared with standard Sinemet. In addition to prolonging the "on" time, smoothing out the wearing-off response, and reducing the total number of doses and tablets taken per day, Sinemet CR also seems helpful in alleviating troublesome nighttime rigidity, thus allowing patients to have more restful nights and better nighttime mobility. Potential disadvantages of Sinemet CR over the standard preparations include delayed or poor response after the morning dose (absence of the "the morning kick") and an exacerbation and prolongation of peak-dose dyskinesias. These problems, however, can be alleviated by proper dosing and timing and by combining Sinemet CR with standard Sinemet. For example, Sinemet 25/100 can be used in the morning to provide a rapid relief of parkinsonian symptoms, and Sinemet CR can be used during the rest of the day. As the individual patient's needs increase, the 25/250 Sinemet preparation may be required to maintain adequate therapeutic response. The goal of levodopa therapy is not to completely eliminate all the symptoms, but to satisfactorily improve patient's functioning at the lowest daily dosage. In a study of 618 patients followed for 5 years from the initiation of levodopa, in a form of Sinemet 25/100 or Sinemet CR 50/200, there was no difference in the frequency of motor fluctuations or dyskinesias, but patients randomized to Sinemet CR had slightly better ADL (activities of daily living) scores (42,104). Approximately 60% of each group remained in the study, and the end-of-study doses were 426 mg/day IR and 510 mg/day "bioequivalent" CR.

Other methods currently investigated in an attempt to provide more continuous dopaminergic stimulation include duodenal infusions of levodopa (105–108), oral solutions of levodopa made by dissolving it with ascorbic acid in water (109,110), subcutaneous or intramuscular injections of levodopa ethyl ester (111), intravenous (and intraventricular) administration of levodopa methyl ester (112, 113), the use of catechol-*O*-methyltransferase (COMT) inhibitors (114–116), monoamine oxidase (MAO) inhibitors (117), and the use of DA agonists (see below). In one double-blind, placebo-controlled study, liquid levodopa/carbidopa significantly improved motor function without exacerbating dyskinesia (110). The mechanism of this observation is not clear because this method of administration achieved this effect without diminishing the number of fluctuations. The authors recommend the use of liquid levodopa/carbidopa in "patients with poor overall motor function, instead of those specifically plagued with frequent

oscillations." Although all of their patients apparently elected to continue taking liquid levodopa/carbidopa, many of our patients prefer simply dissolving the levodopa/carbidopa in carbonated beverage to reduce latency and improve motor response.

Levodopa-related motor fluctuations usually improve by increasing the frequency of administration of levodopa and by the methods outlined above. Recent clinical pharmacologic studies have demonstrated that, contrary to the commonly advised practice of giving smaller, more frequent levodopa doses in order to ameliorate dyskinesias, higher doses of levodopa may be more beneficial since this will not shorten the motor response or necessarily increase dyskinesias (118). However, the observation that, due to an all-or-nothing response, suprathreshold doses of levodopa may not necessarily increase dyskinesias may not be easily translated into practice. Some patients are bothered by their dyskinesias; therefore, the levodopa dosage has to be adjusted accordingly. Furthermore, the nonmotor side effects of levodopa, such as hallucinations and orthostatic hypotension, are dose related, and these adverse effects could offset the potential benefits of prolonged motor response. In addition to adjusting levodopa dosing, reductions of anticholinergic drugs may also ameliorate dyskinesias. Dystonia often improves with the administration of baclofen, anticholinergic drugs, DA agonists, lithium, and local injections of botulinum toxin (58,119). Although rarely a disabling symptom, myoclonus often responds to clonazepam and methysergide.

There are several drugs that have been reported to improve levodopa-induced dyskinesias without necessitating a reduction in levodopa dosage (120,121). In a double-blind, placebo-controlled study of 18 patients with advanced PD, Verhagen Metman et al. (122) showed that amantadine reduced dyskinesia severity by 60% compared with placebo. They suggested that this antidyskinetic effect was mediated by the inhibition of NMDA receptors and that the beneficial effects are maintained for at least a year (66). Clozapine (Clozaril), an atypical neuroleptic, may improve dyskinesias without exacerbating parkinsonian symptoms (123). Clozapine has been reported to also help PD tremor (124,125). Fluoxetine, a classic selective serotonin reuptake inhibitor (SSRI), has been also reported to have beneficial effects on levodopa-induced dyskinesia (126). Administration of propranolol to a small group of patients improved choreic and ballistic, but not dystonic, levodopa-induced dyskinesias (127). The cannabinoid receptor agonist nabilone has been demonstrated to reduce levodopa-induced dyskinesias possibly by stimulating cannabinoid receptors in the lateral segment of GPi by reducing γ-aminobutyric acid (GABA) reuptake and enhancing GABA transmission (128). The novel adenosine A2a receptor antagonist KW-6002 has been shown to reverse parkinsonian symptoms in experimental parkinsonian models without causing dyskinesias (129,130). Strategies designed to prevent pulsatile dopaminergic stimulation and the consequent downstream effects may prevent the development of levodopa-induced dyskinesias (131).

Novel delivery methods for levodopa are currently being explored in experimental animals and in pilot human trials. Levodopa- or DA-secreting tissue cell lines, encapsulated in slow-release polymer systems or biodegradable microspheres and implanted subcutaneously or directly in the striatum, have been shown in experimental models to prolong dopaminergic transmission by providing a continuous delivery of DA in the striatum (132–134).

In addition to motor side effects related to levodopa therapy, many PD patients experience a variety of psychiatric reactions, particularly agitation, visual hallucinations, psychosis, paranoia, and hypersexuality (135,136). These symptoms can be controlled by reducing the dosage of dopaminergic drugs (levodopa, DA agonists) and eliminating all other drugs that are not absolutely essential, such as deprenyl, anticholinergics, and amantadine. In addition, propranolol and other beta blockers and benzodiazepines may provide anxiolytic effect in some patients. Naltrexone and other opioid agonists may be useful in the treatment of some patients with troublesome akathisia (137). In general, typical antipsychotic drugs should be avoided in PD because they may exacerbate parkinsonian symptoms by blocking central DA receptors. Atypical antipsychotics offer the best strategy for controlling drug-induced psychosis without the need to adjust the dosage of dopaminergic drugs (138). In contrast to the traditional (typical) antipsychotics, the new atypical antipsychotics usually control hallucinations and other psychiatric side effects without exacerbating the underlying parkinsonism. Clozapine, an atypical neuroleptic and a relatively specific D4 receptor antagonist, has been shown to effectively control levodopa-induced hallucinations and psychosis without exacerbating parkinsonian symptoms (123,139–141). Because of its potential for causing agranulocytosis, close hematologic monitoring is required. Clozapine may also cause myotoxicity (142). Ondansetron (Zofran), a 5-hydroxytryptophan type 3 (5-HT$_3$) receptor antagonist used primarily in the management of nausea associated with cancer chemotherapy, has been found to have a potent antipsychotic effect, similar to that seen with clozapine. Although this drug does not have the potentially life-threatening side effects of clozapine, its use is limited by high cost (143). Olanzapine (Zyprexa), another atypical neuroleptic, has been reported to exert an antipsychotic effect similar to that of clozapine but without the risk of agranulocytosis (144). However, in several studies olanzapine was associated with exacerbation of parkinsonian motor disability (145–147). Quetiapine fumarate (Seroquel), a dibenzothiazepine that blocks not only D1 and D2 receptors but also 5-HT$_{1A}$ and 5-HT$_2$ receptors, has been also found to have a beneficial effect in PD patients with hallucinations described previously with the other atypical neuroleptics (148). Indeed, quetiapine is our drug of choice for psychosis in patients with PD, followed by clozapine and olanzapine.

Treatment of cognitive deficit in association with PD is as challenging as the treatment of Alzheimer's disease and other dementias. With the introduction of cholinesterase inhibitors such as donepezil (Aricept) and rivastigmine (Exelon), it is possible that cognition, orientation, and language function will improve, and that such improvement will lead to a meaningful improvement in function. Rivastigmine inhibits not only acetylcholinesterase but also butyrylcholinesterase, which in contrast to its relative absence in normal brain, accounts for 40% of cholinergic activity in the cortex and 60% in the hippocampus in AD brains. In a small, open-label trial in 11 patients with probable dementia with Lewy bodies, McKeith et al. (149) found rivastigmine to be safe and to effectively ameliorate delusions, apathy, agitation, and hallucinations.

Gastrointestinal side effects of levodopa are usually brought under control by carbidopa (Lodosyn) or diphenidol, cyclizine, hydroxyzine, or domperidone, a peripheral D2 receptor blocker that is not yet available in the United States. Ondansetron may also be helpful in the management of levodopa-induced nausea (150). Granisetron (Kytril), another selective 5-HT$_3$ receptor antagonist, may be used as a safe and effective antinauseant and antiemetic agent. Cardiac dysrhythmias, including sinus and atrial tachycardia and premature ventricular contractions, can be treated with β-adrenergic receptor blocking agents. Orthostatic hypotension usually improves with the addition of salt to patient's diet and the use of fludrocortisone (Florinef) and midodrine (ProAmatine) (151,152).

Temporary levodopa withdrawal ("drug holiday") has been suggested as a useful strategy to restore levodopa's efficacy, but its long-term benefits are debatable (85,153,154). When managed by skilled nursing staff in the hospital, complications such as aspiration pneumonia and other infections, as well as other complications potentially associated with levodopa withdrawal, such as neuroleptic malignant syndrome (155), can be prevented or effectively managed. Although this procedure often improves gastrointestinal and psychiatric side effects and it may restore the efficacy of levodopa, the benefit is only temporary, lasting about 6 months (153). Therefore, the procedure should be performed only in selected patients in whom all other therapeutic maneuvers have failed. A less radical strategy than complete levodopa withdrawal is partial reduction in daily levodopa dosage (50% reduction for 6 days). Alternatively, patients in whom symptoms are relatively well controlled with a low maintenance dose may benefit from a complete levodopa withdrawal on a selected day each week or on weekends. However, the potential protective effect of this latter strategy has not been assessed. A subgroup of patients experience definite sleep benefit, responding better to levodopa after a night's sleep, but the mechanism of this phenomenon is unknown (156,157).

In addition to the well-recognized complications associated with levodopa therapy, there are some theoretical, but yet unproven, concerns about the potential neurotoxic effects of levodopa (158,159). In the process of enzymatic and nonenzymatic oxidation of DA, toxic compounds, such as hydrogen peroxide and quinones, are produced (160). Levodopa, by increasing the brain levels of DA, may therefore exert potentially neurotoxic effects. This concern is supported by studies demonstrating levodopa's toxicity on a catecholamine-rich neuroblastoma cell line. There is, however, no direct evidence that levodopa is neurotoxic in vivo (161), and the in vitro studies have been challenged, partly because the culture media employed in these studies had either a reduced number or absence of potentially neuroprotective glial cells (162–165). Non-PD patients exposed chronically to high doses of levodopa have not developed parkinsonian features (161). A 6-month oral levodopa treatment of rats, made parkinsonian by 6-OHDA, actually promoted the recovery of striatal innervation (165). In another study in rats with partial 6-OHDA or $FeCl_3$ nigrostriatal lesions, Datla et al. (166) found no detrimental effects of chronic (i.e., 24 weeks) levodopa therapy on the remaining dopaminergic neurons. In fact, long-term levodopa administration was associated with an increase in the number of tyrosine hydroxylase (TH–expressing neurons. In this study, oral levodopa treatment began 7 days after the chemical lesion and continued for 6 months. Number of dopaminergic neurons remaining was determined by TH immunocytochemistry. DA neurons decreased in both vehicle-treated and levodopa-treated animals for 12 weeks, with no significant difference between the groups. Between 12 and 24 weeks, DA neurons increased significantly in the levodopa group but not in the vehicle-treated group. $FeCl_3$ also produced no excess DA cell death versus vehicle, but no increase was seen over time in this group. The mechanism of this finding is not known, but levodopa has been shown to increase the expression of brain-derived neurotrophic factor (BDNF) mRNA in the mouse striatum (167). Furthermore, the "oxidative stress" produced by levodopa may stimulate certain antioxidant mechanisms, such as reduced glutathione (GSH) (168). Although one controlled, prospective study showed higher mortality in patients receiving levodopa as compared with the group treated with bromocriptine (169), additional studies are needed to answer the question of whether levodopa is neurotoxic in patients with PD. A large, multicenter study, the ELLDOPA trial, which is evaluating the effects of levodopa on progression of PD is currently being conducted in multiple centers in North America (26). The debate about whether levodopa is toxic or not will probably continue until the results of this or other studies become available (170,171).

COMT Inhibitors

Another strategy to enhance and prolong DA response utilizes the inhibition of COMT by drugs such as entacapone (Comtan) (172,173) and tolcapone (Tasmar) (174,175). Although tolcapone has both central and peripheral effects, as compared with entacapone (which inhibits only peripheral

COMT), it is not clear whether this difference produces different clinical pharmacologic effects. Tolcapone has a longer half-life than entacapone (2 hours vs. 1 hour) and can be administered 3 times per day (e.g., 100–400 mg TID), whereas entacapone, because of its shorter half-life, requires more frequent administration (200 mg, up to 8 times per day). Most patients take entacapone with each dose of levodopa. Because of its relatively short half-life, the clinical effects disappear within a few hours of discontinuation of the drug. It is not yet known whether COMT inhibitors offer any advantages over other strategies, such as Sinemet CR and DA agonists, designed to prolong the "on" time in PD patients who fluctuate. Theoretically, the COMT inhibitors have an advantage over Sinemet CR in that they do not delay the absorption of levodopa and, although they increase the levodopa plasma concentration area under the curve (AUC) by about 50%, they do not increase the time to reach the peak concentration (T_{max}) or the maximal concentration (C_{max}) of levodopa (176). This pharmacologic action of the COMT inhibitors may prolong the "on" time without markedly increasing dyskinesias (114,177), but most studies do report higher frequency of levodopa-induced dyskinesia in patients treated with COMT inhibitors (116,161,178). In one study of 12 patients, entacapone increased "on" time by 30 minutes when added to standard Sinemet ($p = 0.03$) and by 48 minutes when added to Sinemet CR ($p = 0.05$) without increasing the severity or duration of dyskinesias (179). In comparison with bromocriptine, tolcapone was clinically more effective and better tolerated (175,180); however, additional studies are needed to determine the relative roles of COMT inhibitors and DA agonists.

Both tolcapone (released in 1998) and entacapone (released in 1999) have been previously shown to prolong the "on" time in patients with motor fluctuations. In a multicenter, placebo-controlled study of 205 PD patients with motor fluctuations, entacapone (200 mg with each dose of levodopa, up to 10 doses per day) increased the percent "on" time by 5%, which represented about 1 extra hour of "on" time, reduced UPDRS score by about 10%, and reduced daily levodopa dosage by 100 mg (181). Although this benefit was associated with mild increase in dyskinesia and nausea, the drug was otherwise well tolerated. Other studies have demonstrated more robust improvement in "on" time as well as a substantial decrease in levodopa dosage. For example, Rinne et al. (172) showed that compared with placebo, entacapone increased "on" time by 1.2 hours (13%) and decreased "off" time by 1.3 hours (22%). Furthermore, the average daily dose of levodopa was reduced by 50% in the entacapone group as compared with only 10% in the placebo group. In another multicenter study involving 151 patients, tolcapone decreased "off" time by up to 47% (at 400 mg TID) and increased "on" time by about 25% as compared to a placebo (116). Although there was no significant reduction in UPDRS, the enhancement of levodopa's effect allowed a significant reduction in levodopa dosage. Similar reduction in daily levodopa dose was demonstrated in another study involving 298 patients with PD and without motor fluctuations treated with tolcapone (182). However, one should not be seduced into thinking that COMT inhibitors produce levodopa-sparing effect; they merely make levodopa more effective. In the study of Kurth et al. (116), dyskinesia was significantly more common in the tolcapone group (50%) as compared with the placebo group (21.4%). Other side effects included nausea and postural hypotension, but diarrhea, noted in prior studies (182), was not significantly more common in this study. Both COMT inhibitors cause "orange" discoloration of urine.

The two COMT inhibitors have not been directly compared, but their clinical effects seem similar. Tolcapone has the theoretical advantage over entacapone in that it inhibits both peripheral and central COMT; it also has a longer duration of action and, therefore, can be administered 3 times per day. On the other hand, it can cause explosive diarrhea (in about 5% of patients) and abnormal results of liver function test (LFT), reported in up to 5% of patients treated with tolcapone. Acute fulminant liver failure has been rarely associated with tolcapone (183), but this risk has prompted the Food and Drug Administration (FDA) and the manufacturer to recommend obtaining a consent form and frequent monitoring of LFTs. Although it is not known whether frequent laboratory monitoring prevents the occurrence of liver failure, it is considered a prudent practice to obtain alanine aminotransferase (ALT) and aspartate aminotransferase (AST) levels at baseline and every 2 weeks for the first year of therapy, every 4 weeks for the next 6 months, and every 8 weeks thereafter. If the patient exhibits laboratory or clinical evidence of liver disease (or if no observable symptomatic benefit is seen within 3 weeks of initiation therapy), the drug should be withdrawn. Less rigorous monitoring was recommended by the Tasmar Advisory Panel (184). Rat toxicology studies have shown that tolcapone, but not entacapone, causes hepatotoxicity (185). Entacapone usually does not cause diarrhea or abnormal LFTs, and can be administered with each dose of levodopa up to 8 times per day. It is likely that combination tablets containing both dopa decarboxylase and COMT inhibitors will be used in the future in combination with levodopa.

Dopamine Agonists

DA agonists exert their pharmacologic effect by directly activating DA receptors, bypassing the presynaptic synthesis of DA. DA receptors have been traditionally divided into two types: the D1 class of receptors (composed of subtypes D1 and D5), linked to the enzyme adenylate cyclase, and the D2 class of receptors (composed of subtypes D2, D3, and D4), which are coupled to inhibitory G proteins and inhibit adenylate cyclase (186–189). A wealth of information about the anatomic distribution and pharmacologic properties of these five receptor subtypes has accumulated since their discovery. D1 receptors are preferentially distributed in the striatum giving rise to the direct pathway projecting to the GPi and D2 receptors are primarily localized in the indirect pathway projecting from the striatum to the GPe. Furthermore, D1-, D2-, and D3-receptor mutant mice have been characterized behaviorally and neurochemically (187). In addition to the classic D1 and D2 receptors, three additional receptors have been characterized and cloned (Table 9.6). The rapidly expanding knowledge about anatomic distribution and functional specificity of different DA receptors should yield new compounds that not only are more potent but are more selective in their pharmacologic and clinical action (187, 190).

Experimental and clinical studies have provided evidence that activation of the D2 receptors is important in mediating the beneficial antiparkinsonian effects of DA agonists, but concurrent D1 and D2 stimulation is required to produce optimal physiologic and behavioral effects (191,192). Bromocriptine has served as the prototype for other ergot derivatives, including pergolide; these two are the only DA agonists clinically used in the United States until 1997 (193). At that time two additional DA agonists, ropinirole and pramipexole, became available in the United States. In contrast to bromocriptine, pergolide does not require endogenous DA for its pharmacologic effect, possibly because it activates both D1 and D2 receptors, whereas bromocriptine stimulates D2 and inhibits D1 receptors. Pergolide is 20 times more potent than bromocriptine in inhibiting pro-

TABLE 9.6. DOPAMINE RECEPTORS AND AGONISTS

	D1	D2	D3	D4	D5
Receptor Type					
Human chromosome	5	11	3	11	4
Agonist					
Dopamine	+	++	+++	++	+++
Bromocriptine	−	++	+	+	+
Pergolide	+	+++	+++	+++	+
Pramipexole	−	+++	++++	++	−
Ropinirole	−	+++	+++	−	−

lactin secretion, and its half-life is three times longer. Although an earlier study comparing the two currently available DA agonists showed that they have similar efficacy in PD patients (194), more recent studies suggest that pergolide may be more effective than bromocriptine (195). Despite similar efficacy of the two DA agonists, some patients obtain new benefit when they are switched from one agonist to another. The starting dosage should be very low (bromocriptine at 1.25 mg twice a day and pergolide at 0.05 mg/day) and increased slowly so as to prevent orthostatic hypotension, gastrointestinal, cardiac, and other potential side effects. Cabergoline, a potent D2 agonist with a half-life of about 65 hours, can be administered as a once-a-day agonist (196–198). In one double-blind controlled study of de novo PD patients, cabergoline at a mean dose of 2.8 mg/day was found to be nearly as effective as levodopa when used as monotherapy during the first year of treatment (198). Cabergoline, probably because of its long duration of action, is very effective in reducing levodopa-induced dyskinesias in MPTP monkeys (199). Cabergoline (Dostinex) is available as a 0.5-mg tablet in the United States, but is indicated only for the treatment of hyperprolactinemic disorders.

In contrast to the traditional DA agonists, pramipexole and ropinirole are nonergolines and therefore are expected to have a lower risk of such complications as peptic ulcer disease, vasoconstrictive effects, erythromelalgia, and pulmonary and retroperitoneal fibrosis (200). While pramipexole has been promoted as a D3 agonist (201), other dopamine agonists have been found to be also active at the D3 receptor. Perachon et al. (202) measured the affinities of bromocriptine, pramipexole, pergolide, and ropinirole at human recombinant dopamine D1, D2, and D3 receptors in binding and functional tests. All four compounds were found to bind with high affinity at the dopamine D3 receptor; bromocriptine and pergolide also had high affinity for the dopamine D2 receptor, whereas only pergolide had significant, though moderate, affinity for the dopamine D1 receptor. Pramipexole has little effect on D1, 5-HT, or muscarinic or adrenergic receptors. In the striatum, the D3 receptor is colocalized with D1 receptors on substance P/dynorphin-containing GABA neurons (203). The observation that D3 receptors are primarily located in the mesolimbic system may explain the putative antidepressant effect of pramipexole and ropinirole (204,205). D3 activation may be also responsible for the occurrence of hallucinations noted particularly with higher dosages of dopamine agonists. In a long-term study, pramipexole was found to be well tolerated for up to 4 years, with the following side effects encountered in more than 10% of patients: dyskinesias, orthostatic hypotension, dizziness, insomnia, and hallucinations (206). Pramipexole has been also reported to cause dose-dependent and idiosyncratic peripheral edema (207). Although counterintuitive, activation of D3 receptors has been associated with a reduction in locomotor activity in experimental animals (98).

Pramipexole has been shown to be a safe and effective drug when used as monotherapy in early stages of PD

(208,209) and in mild to moderate PD (206,210). A study of 301 patients in early stages of PD, followed in a double-blinded fashion for a mean of 2 years, after randomization to pramipexole or levodopa (CALM-PD), found marked reduction in the risk of motor complications in the pramipexole group (211,212). Open-label supplementation with levodopa was permitted. The difference in the frequency of wearing-off was 24% versus 38% ($p = 0.009$), dyskinesias 10% versus 31% ($p = 0.0002$), on–off effects 1% versus 5% ($p = 0.07$). However, the magnitude of the symptomatic improvement was greater in the levodopa group; there was a mean reduction of 9.2 points in total UPDRS score from baseline in the levodopa group and 4.4 in the pramipexole group ($p = 0.0002$). In addition, hallucinations, somnolence, and edema were more common in the pramipexole group as compared with patients treated with levodopa alone. Furthermore, sequential β-CIT SPECT scans show that the rate of loss of dopamine transporters, as measured by the decline in β-CIT over the 46-month period of follow-up, was significantly lower in the group initially treated with pramipexole (16%) as compared with the levodopa group (25.5%) ($p=0.01$) (211). Ropinirole has been also demonstrated to be effective in early PD (213,214). In one study, 268 patients with early PD were randomized to either ropinirole ($N = 179$) or levodopa ($N = 89$) and followed for more than 5 years (215). After 5 years, approximately half of patients remained in the study (47% in the ropinirole group and 51% in the levodopa group) and 34% of those randomized to ropinirole remained on monotherapy (16.5 mg/day). The mean levodopa dose was 750 mg/day. Prior to the addition of levodopa only 5% of the ropinirole-treated patients developed dyskinesia in contrast to 36% of those treated with levodopa. After 5 years, only 20% of patients on ropinirole or ropinirole/levodopa exhibited dyskinesias, versus 46% of those on levodopa had dyskinesia. No significant differences were seen among groups for wearing-off, freezing, or dopaminergic side effects, except hallucinations, which were more common in the ropinirole group. This study showed that the risk for developing dyskinesias was substantially less with ropinirole monotherapy or with ropinirole plus levodopa supplementation. A follow-up study utilizing F-dopa-PET (REAL-PET) showed significantly slower decline in F-dopa uptake in patients on ropinirole versus on levodopa. In this double-blind, multinational 2-year follow-up study, 1,186 de novo patients (not previously treated with dopaminergic drugs) were randomized to ropinirole or Sinemet (Whone et al., 2002). The primary endpont was a change in putamen ^{18}F-dopa uptake measured with 3-D positron emission tomography (PET) and secondary endpoints included incidence of dyskinesias. Although changes in UPDRS motor score on medication favored the L-dopa group by six points ($p=NS$), there was significantly less dyskinesia with ropinirole. Various statistical analyses of the PET data showed significantly slower (30%–35%) loss of dopamine terminal function in early PD patients treated with ropinirole compared with L-dopa (215a).

While a number of studies have confirmed the efficacy of monotherapy with DA agonists in early stages of the disease, in more advanced stages of disease DA agonists must be combined with levodopa to achieve optimal therapeutic effect (216). Furthermore, pramipexole has been shown to smooth out clinical fluctuations in patients with advanced PD and its use facilitates the reduction in levodopa dosage (217). This is possibly due to the effect of pramipexole on the pharmacokinetics of levodopa, with earlier time to reach maximum plasma concentration (T_{max}) and a greater maximum plasma concentration (C_{max}). In one study, pramipexole up to 3.4 mg/day was found to be more effective than bromocriptine up to 22.6 mg/day in reducing parkinsonian motor score (218). Since pramipexole is excreted largely unchanged and it does not interact with the cytochrome P450 enzymes, inhibitors of this enzyme system would not be expected to have an effect on the pharmacokinetics of the drug (219). In addition to its beneficial effects on the PD clinical symptoms and levodopa sparing (about 25% reduction in daily levodopa dosage), pramipexole has been demonstrated to possibly exert neuroprotective effect and to enhance neurotrophic activity in mesencephalic dopaminergic cultures (220–222). In contrast to pramipexole, which in addition to its D2 receptor activity has a strong affinity for the D3 receptor, ropinirole is a relatively pure D2 receptor agonist (223). Similar to pramipexole, ropinirole, when added to levodopa, reduced the daily "off" time and allows for a substantial reduction in the daily dose of levodopa (35% of ropinirole patients reduced their levodopa by 20%) (224). In contrast to pramipexole, ropinirole is metabolized by CYP1A2; therefore, ciprofloxacin, estrogens, and other drugs may significantly reduce its clearance. Thus, pramipexole may be safer particularly in elderly patients who take multiple medications. Pramipexole (and even more so levodopa) down-regulates striatal DAT (dopamine transporter), which could further increase dopaminergic neurotransmission (225).

There have been few head-to-head comparisons to determine the relative efficacy and safety of the various dopamine agonists (226). When patients treated with pergolide were switched to pramipexole (mean dose ratio of 3.2 mg to 2.1 mg), there was no statistically significant difference in efficacy (227). There are no specific guidelines on conversion from one DA agonist to another, but rapid conversion to the full converted dose the day after stopping the previous DA agonist seems safe (16,228). Comparing seven placebo-controlled studies involving 1,756 patients treated with pergolide, pramipexole, ropinirole, entacapone, or tolcapone, Inzelberg et al. (229) concluded that although all drugs caused more dyskinesias than placebo, pramipexole and entacapone had the best efficacy and tolerability profile.

Both pramipexole and ropinirole (and possibly other DA agonists) have been associated with irresistible sleep attacks leading to motor vehicle mishaps (230,231). Initially described in only 8 patients (7 taking pramipexole, 1 taking ropinirole) (230), subsequent study of 37 patients taking pramipexole showed that 57% experienced somnolence and 7 of 14 (50%) reported falling asleep while driving (231). Although excessive daytime drowsiness appears to occur in about 15% of patients with PD as compared with 1% of healthy elderly people (232–235), this problem is not unique to pramipexole or ropinirole and occurs with other anti-PD drugs including levodopa (236) and other anti-PD medications (237). It may correlate with increased age, advanced disease, and higher doses (233). The mechanisms of irresistible sleepiness in PD are not well understood, but it may represent sedative effects of dopaminergic agents "superimposed on the background of sleep disruption" (238). Although clearly not specific for the D3 dopamine agonists, it is interesting to note that microdialysis of the D3 agonist quinpirole into the diencephalon (D11) of narcoleptic Dobermans aggravates cataplexy (239).

The risk of accidents can be prevented by discussing this potential side effect with the patient and their family, by warning them not to drive if they feel drowsy, and by encouraging them to take short naps on the side of the road as needed (240). Modafinil (Provigil) at 100 to 200 mg twice a day is effective in reversing the excessive daytime drowsiness and the sedative effects of anti-PD medications (241,242). More recent studies suggest that modafinil may exert an entirely different benefit to patients with PD because of its neuroprotective properties (243).

Apomorphine is water soluble and, therefore, suitable for intravenous, subcutaneous, sublingual, or intranasal administration (63,244–251). In one study of 19 patients with severe motor fluctuations and disabling levodopa dyskinesias, subcutaneous apomorphine therapy (at a mean daily dose of 90.6 mg) for an average of 2.7 years resulted in a 65% reduction in dyskinesia and the waking time "off" decreased from 35% to only 10% (245). Furthermore, 9 (47%) were able to discontinue levodopa completely and the others substantially decreased their daily levodopa dosage. Subcutaneous injections or continuous infusions have been found useful even in advanced PD by reducing the "off" time to half without necessarily increasing dyskinesias (246). In one study, 95% of apomorphine versus 23% of placebo subcutaneous injections resulted in a successful abortion of the "off" state (248). Apomorphine administered intravenously via a long-term indwelling venous catheter significantly improved "off" time, dyskinesias, and quality of life in six patients (251). However, the complication rate was "unacceptably high," chiefly related to crystal aggregation and thrombus formation. Another mode of administration, found to be effective as a rescue therapy, is the intranasal spray (247). In our study of a novel preparation of sublingual apomorphine in patients with advanced PD, we found a marked reduction in the UPDRS score, an increase in "on" time, an increase in tapping speed, and a significant reduction in levodopa dosage (252). More recently, several reports have suggested that apomorphine may exert a neuroprotective effect in MPTP animals and other models (253).

Rotigotine CDS (constant-delivery system), also referred to as N-0923 and SPM 962, a new 5-hydroxy-2-aminotetralin derivative, is a highly selective, lipid-soluble, D2 agonist that is currently undergoing clinical trials (254–256). In addition to its effects on the D2 receptor, this nonergoline dopamine agonist also activates D3 and D1 receptors. Administration via a transdermal patch bypasses metabolism by liver and as a result of sustained delivery more steady plasma and brain levels can be achieved. Although the half-life is only 5.5 hours, the CDS system promises to result in smoother response and less severe motor complications. Rotigotine CDS, in a silicone-based transdermal system (4.5 to 18 mg per patch) is currently undergoing clinical trials in the United States and abroad. Preliminary results suggest that the drug is well tolerated at plasma levels that produce clinical improvement at doses of 8.4 to 67 mg, except for some side effects usually associated with DA agonists, such as somnolence, nausea, vomiting, and occasional skin irritation. Furthermore, the dosage of levodopa could be substantially reduced when rotigotine CDS was added. In another study of 85 patients with PD treated with transdermal N-0923 (Rotigotine CDS), Hutton et al. (255) showed 26% to 28% reduction in levodopa dosage in patients randomized to the active drug group in comparison with only a 7% reduction in the placebo group. In addition to the transdermal route, N-0923 has been also found to be effective when given as a continuous infusion (257). Another DA agonist currently being evaluated is α-dihydroergocryptine (α-DHEC). This D2 agonist (and partial D1 agonist) has been found to be more efficacious and safer than lisuride (258), and safe and effective in improving symptoms in previously untreated patients with PD (259). Piribedil, a D2 agonist, administered in a 50-mg transdermal patch formulation, was found to be ineffective in a randomized, double-blind study involving 27 PD patients (260). PNU 95666, a selective D2 receptor agonist with some 5-HT_{1D} activity, is currently being investigated in patients with PD and, because of its selectivity for the D2 receptor subtype, is predicted to have increased efficacy and relatively few side effects (261). SLV 308 (Solvay) is a D2 partial agonist and 5-HT_{1A} agonist that is currently being studied as a potential antiparkinsonian, antidepressant, and anxiolytic agent (262).

The possibility that levodopa is neurotoxic and that the onset of levodopa-induced complications may be related to the duration of treatment are the two most important reasons why many experts recommend delaying levodopa therapy until parkinsonian symptoms clearly begin to interfere with patients' functioning and normal lifestyle. In order to delay or prevent levodopa-induced complications many parkinsonologists recommend using DA agonists as the initial or early form of dopaminergic therapy (1). When used as monotherapy, DA agonists provide only modest improvement in parkinsonian symptoms, but the improvement may be sufficient to delay the introduction of levodopa by several months or years.

Several studies have demonstrated that when used early in the course of treatment, DA agonists can delay the development of dyskinesias and possibly motor fluctuations (263). Furthermore, DA agonists when used alone (monotherapy) produce little or no clinical fluctuations and dyskinesias

(191). This is particularly true with long-acting DA agonists, such as cabergoline (264), or with continuous administration of short-acting DA agonists (265). In one study with a 5-year follow-up, monotherapy with bromocriptine followed by levodopa therapy significantly delayed complications usually associated with levodopa therapy (266). In a 3-month, double-blind, randomized trial, pergolide monotherapy at a mean dose of 2.1 mg/day produced significantly greater reduction in UPDRS score than placebo (267). In a multicenter study of 241 patients with early PD, ropinirole at doses up to 8 mg 3 times per day was associated with a 24% reduction in the total UPDRS score, whereas the placebo group had a 3% increase in the score ($p < 0.001$) (268). Twice as many patients with early PD treated with ropinirole completed a 12-month study as compared with those treated with placebo (44% vs. 22%) (269). In another study of 335 patients with early PD, pramipexole, at doses of 3.8 to 4.0 mg administered over a 6-month period, reduced UPDRS part II ADL and motor examination scores by 25% and 30%, respectively (210).

Although DA agonists provide some symptomatic benefit when used as monotherapy, these drugs are most frequently used as adjunctive therapy in patients with levodopa-induced fluctuations and levodopa failures. In a double-blind, parallel, multicenter trial of 376 patients with PD treated with pergolide plus levodopa or placebo plus levodopa for up to 24 weeks, 48% noted 25% improvement in the pergolide group ($N = 189$) and 20% noted similar degree of improvement in the placebo group ($N = 187$; $p < 0.001$) (270). Furthermore, total daily dose of levodopa was reduced by 27% in the pergolide group and by 6% in the placebo group ($p < 0.001$). Whereas some patients experience sustained improvement with pergolide over several years, other lose the benefit after 2 years of therapy. The beneficial effects of DA agonists in "smoothing out" clinical fluctuations partly relates to their relatively long plasma half-life and even longer behavioral effect. In contrast to levodopa, DA agonists do not induce dyskinesias in naive MPTP parkinsonian animals. However, DA agonists do induce dyskinesias if the animals have been previously exposed to levodopa (even with only a single dose). This finding that levodopa primes for the development of dyskinesia provides rationale for using DA agonists in early stages of therapy, before the introduction of levodopa.

Besides D2 receptor activation, there is a growing interest in D1 agonists as therapeutic agents in PD (271). Activation of D1 receptors has been associated not only with antiparkinsonian effect but also with improvement in bladder function, presumably by suppression of detrusor hyperreflexia, in MPTP monkeys (272). SKF-38393, the first selective D1 agonist, as well as other D1 agonists (SKF-89626, SKF-8298, CY-208243) have been shown to be ineffective in parkinsonian animals or patients with PD (273). Other D1 agonists, such as ABT-431 and dihydrexidine, have been thought to have a relative advantage over D2 agonists in that they are less likely to cause dyskinesia and may even reverse it (274,275). Unfortunately, dihydrexidine was discontinued from clinical trials and ABT-431 is currently available experimentally only in a parenteral form. In one study, 1-hour intravenous infusions of ABT-431 were associated with antiparkinsonian efficacy with reduction in dyskinesias in 14 patients with levodopa-responsive PD (275). In another study, intravenous ABT-431 was found to produce antiparkinsonian response and dyskinesia similar to levodopa (215). Dinapsoline (DAR-201), a full D1 agonist, has been shown to have good oral availability and significant antiparkinsonian effects in MPTP marmosets (273,276). This potent D1 agonist, with only limited effect on D2 receptors, has been shown to produce contralateral rotation in 6-OHDA rat that can be blocked by the D1 receptor antagonist SCH-23390 but not by the D2 receptor antagonist raclopride (276). No selective D1 agonists are currently clinically available, but apomorphine and pergolide activate both D1 and D2 receptors. Blockade of D1 receptors improves levodopa-induced dyskinesia but exacerbates parkinsonism in MPTP monkeys (277).

There is increasing support from various experimental studies of the notion that DA agonists not only provide a meaningful symptomatic effect but also may exert a neuroprotective effect and, therefore, should be introduced early in antiparkinsonian therapy (278–280). To the extent that levodopa may be neurotoxic (at least in in vitro studies) and that it produces motor complications, delaying levodopa therapy and levodopa-sparing strategies would seem to be desirable strategy. However, DA agonists may have a neuroprotective role not only because of their levodopa-sparing effect but also for a number of other reasons. By stimulating DA autoreceptors, DA agonists decrease DA turnover, thus reducing oxidative stress (281). DA agonists have been demonstrated to scavenge the hydroxyl, superoxide, and nitric oxide radicals (282–285) and induce up-regulation of the free-radical scavenging enzyme superoxide dismutase (SOD) and other proteins that scavenge free radicals (286,287). In vitro studies have shown that certain DA agonists enhance growth and survival of cultured dopaminergic neurons (222,288). In one study, preincubation with bromocriptine provided neuroprotection against glutamate-induced neuronal death in cultured rat mesencephalic neurons (287). Zou et al. (222) showed that pretreatment with pramipexole in a concentration of 4 to 100 μM significantly attenuates DA and levodopa-induced cytotoxicity and apoptosis. This effect appears to be independent of its receptor agonist action because it is not blocked by D3 or D2 receptor antagonists. The investigators also showed that pramipexole protects dopaminergic cell lines from hydrogen peroxide induced cytotoxicity, perhaps by scavenging hydrogen peroxide. Furthermore, in a cell-free system pramipexole inhibits the formation of melanin, an end product of DA and levodopa oxidation. In another study, pramipexole was found to reduce levels of oxygen radicals produced by MPP^+ and it inhibits the opening of mitochondrial permeability transition pores (PTP) induced by calcium and phosphate or MPP^+ (289). Tanaka et al. (290) concluded that ropinirole suppresses autoxidation by increasing GSH synthesis. Felten et al. (291) showed that pergolide, when administered in the diet (0.5 mg/kg per day) to male rats from age 3 months to age 26 months, prevented age-related losses of fluorescent DA cell bodies in the substantia nigra (SN) and fluorescent DA terminals in the striatum. The mechanism of this apparent anti-aging effect of pergolide is unknown, but it is possible that the activation of presynaptic DA receptors reduces baseline release of DA and slows the formation of toxic oxidative metabolites.

Although most clinicians advocate the use of DA agonists early in the treatment of PD, not all agree with this strategy. A 10-year follow-up study showed that starting with DA agonist bromocriptine did not reduce mortality, and although there was a slightly lower incidence of motor fluctuations, this occurred at the expense of more severe disability during the early years of therapy (292). Prospective longitudinal studies with the newer DA agonists are currently in progress.

DA agonists are not without side effects. In addition to nausea, vomiting, anorexia, malaise, orthostatic hypotension, and psychiatric reactions, they may also produce acroparesthesias due to digital vasospasm, and may exacerbate peptic ulcer disease and angina. Erythromelalgia, a painful reddish discoloration of the skin, though occasionally seen with levodopa therapy is more typically observed in patients treated with ergot DA agonists. Finally, pulmonary and retroperitonal fibrosis occasionally complicate chronic therapy with bromocriptine and, rarely, with pergolide. The full potential of these and other new DA agonists has yet to be fully explored in order to determine whether their advantages outweigh their disadvantages (Table 9.7).

TABLE 9.7. POSSIBLE ADVANTAGES AND DISADVANTAGES OF DOPAMINE AGONISTS

Advantages

Pharmacologic advantages
1. Directly stimulate DA receptors, bypassing degenerating nigrostriatal neurons
2. Do not require enzymatic conversion
3. Longer striatal half-life than levodopa
4. Do not compete for transport in the gut or at the blood–brain barrier
5. Selective receptor activation may be possible
6. Alternate routes of administration may be possible (lisuride, apomorphine, N-0923)

Possible protective effects (reduce oxidative stress)
1. Do not generate free radicals or potentially toxic products
2. May decrease presynaptic DA turnover
3. Delay levodopa initiation and side effects

Disadvantages

1. Less effective than levodopa in reducing Parkinson's symptoms
2. More adverse effects (psychiatric phenomena, orthostatic hypotension, peptic ulcer, vasoconstrictive effects, erythromelalgia, pulmonary effects, and retroperitoneal fibrosis)
3. More down-regulation of receptors
4. Higher cost

DA, dopamine.

OTHER SYMPTOMATIC AND SUPPORTIVE THERAPY

Although it is generally desirable to use as few medications as possible, "polypharmacy" is often necessary in the treatment of PD, particularly in the advanced stages. It is important to point out that many parkinsonian symptoms do not respond to dopaminergic therapy (Table 9.8). These symptoms may be mediated by nondopaminergic mechanisms or may represent manifestations of a different parkinsonian disorder, such as progressive supranuclear palsy, multiple system atrophy, and other atypical disorders (293). Selected motor and nonmotor symptoms of PD may require specific symptomatic therapy (Table 9.9).

In some cases, motor features other than the cardinal signs (e.g., painful rigidity or dystonia) and nonmotor symptoms precede the onset of other parkinsonian signs, which may considerably delay the correct diagnosis. For example, many patients exhibit neurobehavioral disturbances, such as depression, dementia, tip-of-the-tongue phenomenon, various psychiatric symptoms, and sleep disorders (294–296). The tricyclic antidepressants, such as amitriptyline or nortriptyline, may be helpful in the management of depression and in addition may improve sialorrhea because of their anticholinergic side effects. However, these drugs must be used with caution in patients with cognitive compromise. Mirtazepine, in addition to its antidepressant effects, has been reported to also have an antitremor effect (297). While the SSRIs may be helpful in the management of depression and anxiety associated with PD, these drugs may exacerbate tremor. Rapid eye movement (REM) sleep behavior disorder (RBD), which may be the initial manifestations of parkinsonism (298), may respond to nighttime clonazepam. Drooling (sialorrhea), one of the most embarrassing symptoms of PD caused by impaired swallowing, has been successfully managed with botulinum toxin injections (299–301). Dysphagia (302) and constipation (303) represent the most common gastrointestinal manifestations of PD. Seborrhea, a common manifestation

TABLE 9.8. SYMPTOMS REFRACTORY TO LEVODOPA

Postural instability
Freezing
Speech abnormalities
Mental changes
    Dementia
    Depression
Sleep disturbance
Dysautonomia
    Constipation
    Sexual dysfunction
    Bladder dysfunction
    Sweating
Sensory phenomena

TABLE 9.9. MANAGEMENT OF SPECIFIC PARKINSON'S SYMPTOMS

Symptom	Management
Depression	A. Tricyclics and other antidepressants
	B. Electroconvulsive therapy
Dysarthria	A. Clonazepam
Sialorrhea	A. Anticholinergics
	B. Bethanechol
	C. Tympanic neurectomy
	D. Salivary duct ligation
	E. Botulinum toxin
Action tremor	A. Beta blockers
	B. Primidone
	C. Clonazepam
Pain	A. Methylphenidate
	B. Nonsteroidals
Painful rigidity	A. Muscle relaxants (cyclobenzaprine, orphenadrine)
	B. Pallidotomy
Disabling unilateral tremor–rigidity	A. Anticholinergics
	B. Dopaminergic drugs
	C. Clozapine
	D. Pallidotomy or STN/VIM DBS
Paroxysmal drenching sweats	A. Beta blockers
	B. Anticholinergics
	C. Botulinum toxin
REM sleep behavior disorder	A. Clonazepam
Urinary frequency	A. Oxybutynin
	B. Tolterodine
Constipation	A. Cisapride

STN, subthalamic nucleus; VIM, ventralis intermedius; DBS, deep brain stimulation.

in PD, and evidence of peripheral involvement, may occasionally require topical application of steroids. Sensory complaints, such as paresthesias, akathisia, and oral and genital pain (304), are difficult to manage but may respond to tricyclic antidepressants, carbamazepine, or gabapentin.

Dysautonomia, such as orthostatic hypotension, sphincter dysfunction, and sexual impotence, also requires specific treatments. For example, orthostatic hypotension can be treated with salt, fludrocortisone and midodrine (151,152). Increased urinary frequency due to overactive bladder often improves with antimuscarinic oxybutynin (Ditropan), 5 mg 3 to 4 times per day, and tolterodine (Detrol), 2 mg 3 times per day. The latter drug may be better tolerated because it has 8 times less affinity for the salivary gland, thus having much lower frequency of dry mouth. The alpha blocker tamsulosin (Flomax), 0.4 twice a day, may be effective if the urinary frequency is associated with benign prostatic hypertrophy; this condition must be excluded prior to the use of antimuscarinic agents. Urinary incontinence is rarely a complication of PD, although it is a common manifestation of multiple system atrophy (305). Sildenafil citrate (Viagra) has been found to be safe and effective in the management of erectile dysfunction associated with PD, but it may

Pharmacologic Treatment in PD

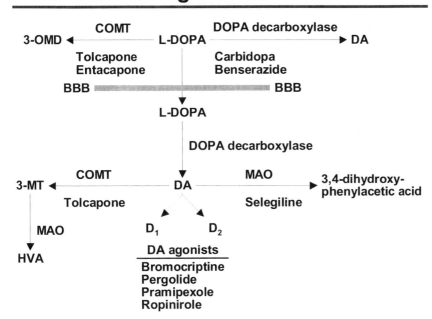

FIG. 9.2. Pharmacologic therapy for Parkinson's disease.

unmask orthostatic hypotension in patients with multiple system atrophy (306,307).

The most important principle designed to optimize the management of PD is to individualize therapy and to target the most disabling symptoms (1) (Figs. 9.2 and 9.3). The selected therapy should be based on scientific rationale and designed not only to control symptoms but to slow the progression of the disease. Since younger patients are likely to require dopaminergic therapy for longer time and are at increased risk for the development of levodopa complications, levodopa-sparing strategies, such as the use of MAO inhibitors and DA agonists, is even more critical in this population. It is very likely that with better understanding of the mechanisms of neurodegeneration novel and more effective therapeutic strategies will be available in the near future.

Before leaving the topic of symptomatic pharmacologic therapy of PD, it is worth commenting on some special cir-

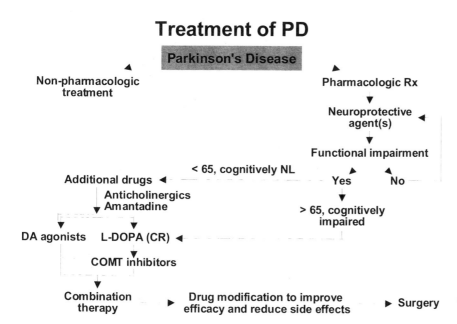

FIG. 9.3. Decision tree for the management of Parkinson's disease.

cumstances that may influence the selection of a particular drug or drugs. For example, there are few or no data on the use of various anti-PD medications in pregnant women. Although the majority of studies in animals have not shown any teratogenicity, malformations of the skeletal and circulatory system and other teratogenic effects have been reported with amantadine and selegiline (308). Levodopa has not been found to produce teratogenic effects in mice, rats, or rabbits except in a single report. Fetal complications have been rarely reported in cases of human PD managed with levodopa. Another circumstance when levodopa and other dopaminergic drugs are sometimes withheld is in a setting of malignant melanoma. In the early 1970s, levodopa therapy was considered contraindicated in malignant melanoma because of its apparent carcinogenic effects. However, subsequent studies failed to provide any evidence that levodopa accelerates malignant melanoma (309,310). Finally, it is important to reemphasize that certain symptoms of PD, such as dysarthria, dysphagia, freezing, and other "axial" symptoms, usually do not respond to dopaminergic therapy and may be mediated by non-dopaminergic systems (311,312).

Neuroprotective Therapy

Neuroprotective therapies can be defined as such medical or surgical interventions that favorably alter the underlying etiology or pathogenesis and therefore delay the onset or slow, or even halt, the progression of the neurodegenerative process. In contrast to symptomatic therapy, which is designed to merely ameliorate the clinical features of the illness, the goal of neuroprotective therapy is to protect or rescue neurons that are vulnerable to the neurodegenerative process. To the extent that such neuroprotective strategies may prevent the neurodegenerative process, it is essential that they be implemented early in the course of the disease. There are many agents that have been reported to exert such a protective effect, such as antioxidants, antiexcitatory drugs, and dopamine agonists. These drugs and their symptomatic and putative neuroprotective effects are reviewed below; in this section we will focus on the MAO inhibitors because these drugs have been tested first as predominantly neuroprotective agents (313).

Deprenyl (Selegiline)

The metabolism and deactivation of DA is mediated via the DA reuptake system (DA transporter) and the DA-degrading enzymes (MAO and COMT). Deprenyl, the L isomer of *N*-propynylmethamphetamine, acts as a "suicide substrate" for MAO-B, irreversibly inhibiting this enzyme (314). Intracellular recordings from midbrain dopaminergic neurons show that MAO inhibitors prolong the electrophysiologic effects of DA (315). Restoration of MAO activity after inhibition by deprenyl requires de novo synthesis of

MAO. The rate of MAO-B regeneration may take several weeks, possibly months. In contrast to MAO-A, which preferentially deaminates tyramine, 5-HT, and norepinephrine (NE), deprenyl inhibits only MAO-B and is, therefore, devoid of the pressor "cheese" effect. This complication of MAO-A inhibition consists of sympathomimetic crisis (hypertension, tachycardia, headache) and it is due to ingestion of foods rich in tyramine and other monoamines normally metabolized in the gut and liver by MAO-A. When MAO-A is inhibited this results in excess absorption of these monoamines and displacement of NE from nerve terminals. Certain MAO-A inhibitors, such as moclobemide, do not seem to produce the "cheese effect" because they selectively inhibit MAO-A, so that the remaining MAO-B is capable of deaminating tyramine. Furthermore, high concentrations of tyramine (more than 150 mg) competitively interact with MAO-A, displacing the drug from the enzyme's active site (most meals contain less than 40 mg of tyramine) (316).

Deprenyl is readily absorbed, reaching maximal plasma levels within 0.5 to 2 hours. The major metabolite of deprenyl, L-desmethyldeprenyl, has a mean half-life of 2 hours; the other metabolites, L-amphetamine and L-methamphetamine, have a considerably longer mean half-life (17.7 and 20.5 hours, respectively). Nearly half of the administered deprenyl is excreted in the urine in the form of these metabolites within 48 hours. Although less biologically active than their D isomers, these amphetamine metabolites may exert some CNS stimulatory effect and may therefore be responsible for some of the symptomatic improvement. Deprenyl is well tolerated at the usual doses (5 mg after breakfast and 5 mg after lunch), but it occasionally causes nausea, insomnia, and hallucinations, and when combined with levodopa, it enhances levodopa-related dyskinesias. Since 5 mg/day may be as effective as 10 mg/day, we prescribe one tablet daily (317).

The finding that deprenyl (selegiline) prevents MPTP-induced parkinsonism has stimulated interest in antioxidative therapy as a means of retarding progression of PD and other neurodegenerative diseases (313). The largest clinical trial designed to address the potential protective effects of deprenyl, "Deprenyl and Tocopherol Antioxidative Therapy of Parkinsonism" (DATATOP), was carried out by the Parkinson Study Group in 800 patients with early, untreated PD in 28 North American centers (313,318, 319). Using a 2×2 factorial design, the study aimed to assess the outcomes of treatments with deprenyl 10 mg/day, α-tocopherol (vitamin E) 2,000 IU/day, and a combination of these putative antioxidants in comparison with a placebo. The results showed that after a mean follow-up of 14 ± 6 months after randomization, 154 of 399 deprenyl-treated subjects reached the end point, as compared with 222 of 401 subjects who were not receiving deprenyl (319). The projected median length of time to reach the end point was 9 months longer in the deprenyl-treated group than in the group treated with placebo or tocopherol. The waning of the effects of deprenyl on delaying end point after the first year, coupled with slight but significant improvement in motor performance after initiation of deprenyl (a reduction of mean of 1.9 points on the UPDRS scale after 4 weeks) and worsening after 2-month washout, has been used as an argument in favor of a predominantly symptomatic rather than a protective effect. However, in another study, no deterioration after washout was demonstrated in de novo patients initially treated with deprenyl (320). However, the fact that survival rates appear to be the same whether end-pointed subjects did or did not have detectable symptomatic antiparkinsonian effects at the start of deprenyl treatment suggests that symptomatic effects alone cannot entirely explain the delay in reaching the end point in deprenyl-treated patients (319). Some studies have concluded that while deprenyl can delay the need for levodopa therapy this does not necessarily translate into meaningful long-term therapeutic benefits (321). Furthermore, although deprenyl appears to delay disability and the need for levodopa, this initial benefit is not sustained (322, and the drug does not appear to prevent the development of levodopa-related motor fluctuations and dyskinesias (40).

There is a growing body of evidence to support the notion that deprenyl may exert its neuroprotective effects through mechanisms other than MAO inhibition (222,323). MPTP-exposed striatal neurons were partially "rescued" from eventual death by deprenyl even when given after MPTP is completely converted to 1-methyl-4-phenylpyridinium ion (MPP^+). In the original study, a 5-day course of deprenyl (or saline) treatment was administered to mice 3 days after the last dose of MPTP. There was a 37% to 42% loss of TH immunoreactive neurons with MPTP; this loss was reduced to 14% to 16% with deprenyl. Further support for the rescue effect of deprenyl is provided by the demonstration of enhanced survival of axotomized facial neurons in animals treated with the drug (324). Since the rescue effects of deprenyl in various experimental studies occurred at doses much lower than those required for inhibition of MAO-B, Tatton (325) has estimated that dosages of 0.4 to 1.0 mg/day should be sufficient to provide similar effect in patients with PD. The drug increases SOD and catalase activity in the striatum of rats in low doses, but it inhibits these neuroprotective enzymes in higher doses (326). Deprenyl has been shown to stimulate the production of interleukin-6 (327). It has been postulated that this cytokine may have a neuroprotective effect. Deprenyl increases reactive astrogliosis during the first 3 days after facial nerve transection (and decreases the gliosis thereafter) (328). Deprenyl also activates astrocytes immediately after striatal injury as demonstrated by increased glial fibrillary acidic protein (GFAP) immunoreactivity (329). It has been postulated that the drug somehow augments the production of or sensitivity to ciliary neutrophilic factor (CNTF), neurotensin-3 (NT-3), and possibly other trophic factors

(330) and that L-deprenyl (but not D-deprenyl) prevents apoptosis in PC-12 cells deprived of serum and nerve growth factor (331).

Before discussing the possible anti-apoptotic effects of deprenyl, it is useful to briefly review the presumed mechanisms of apoptosis. The following cascade of intracellular events has been postulated as a mechanism of neurodegeneration: (a) increased cytosolic calcium (possibly as a result of excitotoxicity) and oxidative radicals, coupled with impaired mitochondrial complexes, results in (b) decreased mitochondrial membrane potential ($\Delta\Psi_M$), which in turn (c) opens the mitochondrial PTP, (d) releases apoptosis initiating factors (e.g., cytochrome *c*), and ultimately leads to (e) apoptosis (332,333). We documented that (–)-deprenyl at concentrations of 0.1 to 10 μM significantly reduced MPP^+-induced apoptosis in MES 23.5, a dopaminergic cell line that does not contain MAO-B (221). Deprenyl prevents reduction in mitochondrial membrane potential in pre-apoptotic neurons and induces expression of certain anti-apoptotic genes, including those for SOD, nitric oxide synthase (NOS), c-Jun, and bcl-2 (323,334).

The hypothesis that deprenyl may exert a protective effect is supported by several studies showing a delay in disability in patients with early PD treated with deprenyl (318, 319,335,336) and by retrospective analyses (337). One such study (336) showed that patients treated with deprenyl experienced significantly less deterioration as compared with those on placebo, but this study has been challenged because of possible methodologic flaws (338). In addition to delaying disability and the need for levodopa therapy, deprenyl clearly has a moderate, albeit transient, beneficial symptomatic effect on parkinsonian symptoms (339). Deprenyl is also associated with a smaller need for levodopa dosage as compared with placebo, suggesting that the drug has a levodopa-sparing effect (340). Finally, deprenyl clearly prolongs the effects of levodopa and smooths out levodopa-related motor fluctuations, possibly by prolonging dopamine-induced responses in midbrain dopaminergic neurons (315).

Whether deprenyl actually retards the progression of neuronal degeneration (protective effect) or whether the slower rate of disability can be explained by its symptomatic effect has been debated since the original reports (341,342). Although there is a theoretical consideration that deprenyl could exert neuroprotective actions, this notion has been challenged by the observation from the Parkinson's Study Group of the United Kingdom of 520 patients with early PD showing a 60% higher mortality in patients treated with deprenyl in contrast to levodopa alone (44/249 or 17.7% vs. 76/271 or 28.0%, respectively) after 5.6 years of follow-up (343–345). However, this study has been criticized because of methodologic and other problems (346,347). Furthermore, there was no excess mortality attributable to deprenyl treatment during the first 5 years of the DATATOP study (24) and a meta-analysis of other deprenyl studies also failed to demonstrate an increase in mortality associated with deprenyl (348). In another study, deprenyl reduced mortality of 97 PD patients to the level of age-matched controls (349). Additional studies are necessary before the controversy as to whether the delay in need for levodopa is due to deprenyl's neuroprotective, symptomatic, or combined effect can be resolved.

Various new formulations of deprenyl are being developed. For example, Zydis, a fast-dissolving deprenyl, may be useful for patients who have difficulties swallowing. The pregastric absorption avoids extensive first-pass metabolism in the liver and, therefore, the concentration of amphetamine-like metabolites is much lower. Although the manufacturer has cautioned about the use of deprenyl in combination with either tricyclic antidepressants or SSRIs, a survey of experienced parkinsonologists showed that serious adverse experiences, including the "serotonin syndrome," related to the use of this combination is extremely rare (350).

Compounds structurally related to deprenyl, such as CGP 3466 or TCH 346, but without MAO-A or MAO-B activity, have been shown to bind to glyceride-3-phosphate dehydrogenase (GAPDH). This glycolytic enzyme with multiple functions has been shown to have an anti-apoptotic effect, which is 100-fold more potent than deprenyl in both in vitro and in vivo models (351). TCH 346 is currently undergoing preclinical and early clinical trials.

Other MAO Inhibitors

Besides deprenyl, other MAO inhibitors have been investigated as potential neuroprotective agents. Lazabemide (Ro19-6327), a short-acting, reversible MAO-B inhibitor, has been found to delay the need for levodopa and mildly improved PD symptoms in one study (352). Despite its excellent tolerance, it is unlikely that this drug will be developed for clinical use in the future. Fahn and Chouinard (353) advocate the use of tranylcypromine (Parnate), an irreversible inhibitor of MAO-A and B, but patients have to be on a low-tyramine diet in order to prevent the cheese effect. In their study, 37 patients with early PD not requiring symptomatic therapy were treated with tranylcypromine for up to 33 months. In addition to erectile dysfunction and insomnia, this drug may cause hypertensive crises and hemorrhagic strokes. Its long-term safety and efficacy have not been established, but the drug must be discontinued once the patient requires treatment with levodopa.

Rasagiline, coded TVP 1012, is a selective, irreversible MAO-B inhibitor that is five times more potent than selegiline in preventing MPTP-induced parkinsonism (354). Its major metabolite, 1-(R)-aminoindan, is devoid of amphetamine-like properties, which is in contrast to deprenyl. Although the drug appears to be well tolerated, long-term

clinical data are lacking. However, experimental studies indicate that rasagiline rescues dying neurons and, in addition to its neuroprotective action, has a symptomatic, dopaminergic effect (355,356). In clinical studies, rasagiline provides a modest benefit as an adjunctive therapy in PD patients experiencing levodopa-related motor fluctuations (357). Despite the sound scientific rationale for the use of antioxidants in PD, the preliminary clinical trials have been thus far disappointing, possibly because the appropriate dosage has not been determined, the therapy is instituted too late, and the end points for determining progression of disease are not sensitive enough to show the difference between the antioxidant and placebo (358).

Antiglutamatergic Drugs

Interactions between dopamine and glutamate in striatal medium spiny neurons have been found to play an increasingly important role in PD (359). Furthermore, there is considerable theoretical and experimental support for the use of glutamate antagonists, such as NBQX (2,3-dihydroxy-6-nitro-7-sulfamoylbenzo(f)quinoxaline), remacemide, and other antiglutamate agents, as potential neuroprotective drugs (360, 361). Several studies have demonstrated that the neuronal activity is increased in the STN and GPi of parkinsonian animals and humans (36,362). Since STN provides excitatory, glutamatergic input to GPi, glutamate inhibition would be expected to improve parkinsonism. Some studies indeed have shown that NMDA antagonists prevent the selective toxicity of MPP^+ and, therefore, may have a protective effect (363). Furthermore, ablation of STN attenuates the loss of DA neurons in rats exposed to the mitochondrial toxin 3-nitropropionic acid (3-NP) or the catecholamine toxin 6-OHDA (364). In naive monoamine-depleted rats MK-801, an NMDA antagonist, increased locomotor activity and potentiated the anti-akinetic effects of levodopa. Certain anticholinergic drugs and amantadine possess NMDA-blocking properties (360,365). Amantadine has been shown to not only ameliorate parkinsonian symptoms, but also to improve motor fluctuations and levodopa-induced dyskinesias (66,366). Furthermore, amantadine has been reported to improve survival of PD patients (367). The noncompetitive NMDA antagonist memantine, an antispasticity drug not yet available in the United States, has been also shown to have some antiparkinsonian effects (368). Budipine is another NMDA antagonist with demonstrated antiparkinsonian effects (369). Remacemide, an anticonvulsant with anti-NMDA effects, has been shown to enhance the effects of levodopa in parkinsonian rats and monkeys (363). In a randomized, controlled trial of remacemide in 279 patients with PD and levodopa-related motor fluctuations, "trends" toward improvement in the percent "on" time were noted, but the study failed to show clinically meaningful benefit (361). The selective NMDA antagonist LY 235959, administered subcutaneously to MPTP monkeys, has been shown to improve levodopa-induced dyskinesias (65). At 3.0 mg/kg the drug abolished oral dyskinesias and reduced limb chorea by 68%, but it had no effect on levodopa-induced dystonia and actually produced dystonia at higher doses (5 mg/kg). The drug did not reduce the antiparkinsonian effects of levodopa and had no effect on motor function when given alone. Similarly, the NMDA antagonist ifenprodil, which selectively inhibits the NR2B subunit of the NMDA receptor, has been found to have an antiparkinsonian effect without causing dyskinesias in MPTP primates (370). Dextromethorphan, another antiglutamatergic agent, has been found to reduce the severity of levodopa-induced dyskinesias by 50% (365).

Although there is no evidence that the antiexcitatoxic drugs slow the progression of PD, there is a growing support for the use of antiglutamate agents as a neuroprotective strategy in amyotrophic lateral sclerosis (ALS) (371,372). Riluzole, amino-2-trifluoromethoxy-6-benzothiazole (RP-54274), acts primarily by inhibiting glutamic acid release and by noncompetitively blocking NMDA receptors. As such it should exert antiexcitotoxic, and potentially neuroprotective, effects. This drug has been demonstrated to delay disability in some patients with ALS and preserves motor function in a transgenic model of familial ALS (373). The neuroprotective effects of riluzole have also been demonstrated in studies of 6-OHDA- and MPTP-induced parkinsonism in rodents (374) and rhesus monkeys (375). When riluzole was administered before the injection of MPTP, parkinsonian symptoms, particularly bradykinesia and rigidity, were prevented. The preliminary results of this study suggest that riluzole could possess neuroprotective and palliative effects in a primate model of PD. There are no published data on the effects of riluzole in patients with PD except for a small series of patients with levodopa-induced dyskinesia apparently benefitting from riluzole (376). A study of riluzole in early stages of PD recently completed at Baylor's Parkinson's Disease Center indicates that the drug is well tolerated in patients with PD but does not appear to provide a significant symptomatic benefit (377). A large, multicenter study of riluzole in early and more advanced stages of PD has been discontinued because of lack of benefit based in an interim data analysis. Lamotrigine, another glutamate release inhibitor, failed to provide any symptomatic benefit in patients with PD in one controlled trial (378). Additional studies are needed to answer the question of whether glutamate antagonists and glutatame depleters exert symptomatic or neuroprotective effect.

Trophic Factors

One particularly promising therapeutic and potentially neuroprotective approach involves the use of neurotrophic factors, particularly the glial-derived neurotrophic factor (GDNF) (379,380). This trophic factor has been reported to enhance the survival of midbrain dopaminergic neurons in vitro and to rescue degenerating neurons in vivo. Tseng et al. (381) showed that GDNF continuously released from polymer-encapsulated, genetically engineered cells prevented the loss of TH immunoreactivity in rats subjected to unilateral medial forebrain bundle (MFB) axotomy. In addition, GDNF reduced the abnormal turning response to amphetamine. Since this behavioral improvement occurred despite the loss of striatal DA, it was attributed to GDNF-induced dendritic sprouting in the SN. Another strategy to deliver GDNF to or near the SN involves the use of a replication-defective adenoviral vectors encoding human GDNF (382). Intraventricular administration of GDNF in monkeys resulted in amelioration of parkinsonian findings, an increase in midbrain and globus pallidus levels, and a 20% enlargement of nigral neurons accompanied by increased fiber density (383). GDNF-levodopa combination reportedly reduces the levodopa-induced side effects in experimental monkeys (384). These encouraging observations have led to a pilot human trial in patients with moderately advanced PD conducted in several centers in North America. However, because of lack of observed efficacy and frequent occurrence of nausea, anorexia, tingling (L'hermitte's sign), hallucinations, and depression, these trials were suspended in April 1999 (385). In one postmortem case, there was no evidence of significant trophic effect on nigrostriatal neurons (386). Using lentiviral vector as a means of delivery of GDNF to the striatum and SN of monkeys made parkinsonian with MPTP, Kordower et al. (387) demonstrated reversal of functional deficit, extensive and long-term (8 months) GDNF expression, augmentation of dopaminergic function, and prevention of nigrostriatal degeneration. This exciting report suggests that this novel delivery system of atrophic factor may provide a new therapeutic strategy for management of PD.

Immunomodulators

The growing interest in immunologic mechanisms of cell death in PD has some obvious therapeutic implications (388). First, dopaminergic drugs have been shown to antagonize the normal age-related decline in interferon-γ. Furthermore, immunomodulating agents, such as anti-inflammatory drugs including nonsteroidal anti-inflammatory drugs (389), cyclooxygenase isoenzymes COX-1 and COX-2 (390), thalidomide (which blocks tumor necrosis factor-α) (391,392), and α-melanocyte-stimulating hormone inhibitors (393), may exert neuroprotective effects.

Another evidence that the immune system may have a role in cell survival is the observation that immunophilin-binding proteins are 10- to 50-fold more abundant in the brain than in the immune system and certain immunosuppressive drugs that bind to immunophilin-binding proteins can produce nerve growth in vitro and in vivo (394,395). Immunophilins are intracellular receptor proteins that bind to the immunosuppressive drugs cyclosporin A, FK506, and rapamycin. The immunophilin ligands combine with immunophilins and cause suppression of the immune system by inhibiting the calcium-activated phosphatase calcineurin. Certain synthetic immunophilin ligands, such GPI 1046 (Guilford Pharmaceuticals) and AMG-474-00 or NIL-A (Amgen), have been shown to promote neuronal outgrowth even more potently than trophic factors without exhibiting any immunosuppressive activity (396,397). These agents have been found to promote growth of nigrostriatal dopaminergic neurons spared after MPTP-induced damage to the SN. In contrast to trophic factors, they exert their effects after oral administration. Although subsequent studies failed to confirm the initially observed robust effects of GPI 1046 (398) and AMG-474-00 (NIL-A), a more potent immunophilin ligand, clinical trials with the latter drug have been suspended, even though possible benefits have been suggested in a double-blind, placebo-controlled study of 300 patients with mild or moderate PD. In this study, NIL-A at 1,000 mg 4 times per day was apparently associated with a 21% reduction in Hoehn and Yahr score, as compared with 11% reduction with placebo ($p = 0.028$) (press release, July 26, 2001, Guilford Pharmaceuticals). Additional studies are needed to determine whether these or other immunophilin ligands will have utility in slowing or reversing PD.

Caspase inhibition is increasingly studied as a potential neuroprotective strategy in PD because caspase-1 and caspase-3 are increased in the SN of brains of patients with PD (399), and caspase-3 has been shown to be increased in the presence of neuronal apoptosis in PD (400). Minocycline, an antibiotic used for treatment of infections and dermatologic problems, has been shown to delay disease progression in various animal models of Huntington's disease, presumably by inhibiting caspase-1 and caspase-3 mRNA up-regulation and decreasing inducible NOS activity (401–403). Furthermore, an injection of minocycline into 6-OHDA mouse model of parkinsonism has been shown to inhibit microglial activation by 47% and protects TH-positive (dopaminergic) neurons by 27% at 7 days and 38% at 14 days after injection (404). Clinical studies that are currently underway were designed to determine the long-term safety and efficacy of minocycline in PD and other neurodegenerative diseases.

Other Neuroprotective Strategies

Other potentially promising neuroprotective strategies currently tested in preclinical and clinical trials include (a) MAO-A inhibitors such as brofaromide and moclobemide (405); (b) other antioxidants and free-radical trappers or scavengers, such as thioctic (lipoic) acid, dihydrolipoic acid, SOD, 21-amino steroids (lazaroids), OPC-14117, deferoxamine (406), aspirin and salicylate (407,408), coenzyme Q_{10} (409,410), thiolic antioxidants such as *N*-acetylcysteine (411), and certain dopamine agonists (222, 253); (c) DA transport inhibitors such as mazindol (412); (d) anti-apop-

totic agents such as certain dopamine agonists (222,289), inhibitors of the JNK signaling pathway (e.g., CEP-1347) (413,414); (e) GABA agonists, such as zolpidem (415); (f) trophic factors such as GDNF, BDNF, insulin-like growth factor, fibroblast growth factor, epidermal growth factor, and G_{M1} ganglioside (383,416); (g) non-adenine-based purines, such as AIT-082 (neotrofin) (417); (h) caspase inhibitors such as minocycline; (i) neural implants, including human nigral grafts, xenotransplants, and engineered stem cells (418,419); and (j) efforts to control potential risk factors.

Besides drugs already discussed, other strategies have been suggested to have a neuroprotective effect, including the stimulant modafinil (92) and green tea, which contains polyphenol (−)-epigallocatechin-3-gallate and has been reported to block the uptake of MPP$^+$ (420).

FUTURE STUDIES

Prevention of parkinsonism induced by animals with the neurotoxin MPTP is often used to study putative neuroprotective effects of certain drugs or other therapies. It is not known whether rotenone, a lipophilic pesticide and a potent inhibitor of mitochondrial complex I, found to produce parkinsonism in rats, will be a useful model for the study of neuroprotection (421). We have developed a selective nigral dopaminergic neuron degeneration animal model by knockout *Nurr1* gene (in human called *NOT*) in mouse (422). Nurr1 is a member of the nuclear receptor superfamily and is highly expressed in midbrain dopaminergic neurons beginning in embryonic stages and continuing into adulthood. Disruption of the gene induces massive apoptosis of dopaminergic precursor neurons in SN. The homozygous *Nurr1* gene knockout (Nurr1−/−) mice display a selective and complete loss of dopaminergic neurons in SN and DA levels in the striatum and die in 24 hours, whereas the heterozygous *Nurr1* gene knockout (Nurr1+/−) mice that have minimal alteration of dopaminergic neurons and DA levels in the nigrostriatal system confer increased vulnerability to dopaminergic neurotoxin MPTP compared with wild-type (Nurr1+/+) mice. Furthermore, the heterozygous Nurr1+/− mice exhibit age-related, accelerated dopaminergic deficiency and other biochemical and behavioral features of parkinsonism. Manifested by progressive, rather than acute (toxin-induced), parkinsonism, this model may be particularly suitable for the study of neuroprotection.

Future studies of neuroprotective agents should utilize not only clinical ratings but also ancillary techniques such as ^{18}F-dopa PET and ^{123}I β-CIT SPECT to measure longitudinally the progression of nigrostriatal degeneration. Assuming a 9% annual change in the baseline putamen ^{18}F-dopa uptake (K_i), Morrish et al. (423) estimated that 130 patients in early stages of PD would have to be enrolled to demonstrate 50% protection. In their study, they found that the mean change was 8 points in total UPDRS points per year. This is in contrast to the 1.4 to 1.5 units annual rate of decline in the total UPDRS scores in longitudinally followed patients (424,425). Future research will undoubtedly find a therapeutic intervention that will favorably alter the natural course of the disease by promoting survival and growth of degenerating neurons.

NEUROSURGERY

It is beyond the scope of this chapter to comprehensively review the advances in neurosurgical treatment of PD. The reader is referred to other chapters in this book as well as other reviews of this topic (71,426,427).

OTHER THERAPEUTIC APPROACHES

Besides pharmacologic and surgical treatments, there are many other strategies currently being explored in the treatment of some PD symptoms (1). For example, electroconvulsive therapy (ECT) and pre-frontal rapid-rate, repetitive transcranial magnetic stimulation (rTCMS), may be helpful not only in the management of depression, but also in the treatment of other parkinsonian symptoms (428,429). However, a more comprehensive study of rTCMS could not demonstrate any beneficial effect in patients with PD (430). Nevertheless, encouraged by the initial reports of rTCMS on PD, some investigators have tried extradural motor cortex simulation using a quadripolar electrostimulator and reported bilateral benefits in PD motor signs and in dyskinesias (431). The results of these preliminary studies, however, must be confirmed by a larger study before this procedure can be considered as a potential treatment in PD.

Any discussion of the management of PD would not be complete without emphasizing the importance of physical therapy and improved conditioning of patients with PD (432–434). In one long-term study, 16 patients with early PD underwent 14 weeks of an intensive exercise program, including gait, balance, strength, and coordination exercises (434). Significant improvements were seen on all various clinical scales, with small losses between 14 weeks and 20 weeks. In one study, the incorporation of external sensory cues in the rehabilitation protocol extended the short-term benefits of physical therapy (435). While benefits of physical therapy are intuitive, rehabilitation in PD has not been evaluated by well-designed trials using appropriate outcome measures (436). Speech therapy designed to stimulate increased vocal fold adduction with instructions to "increase loudness," the so-called Lee Silverman Voice Treatment (LSVT) (437,438), using various verbal cues to regulate speech volume (439), and percutaneous collagen augmentation of the vocal folds (440) have been used successfully to treat the hypophonic, hypokinetic dysarthria associated with PD. Finally, psychological support on the part of family members, friends, and physicians is essential for patients to maintain as much independence as physically possible. Patients should be encouraged to learn about their disease (perhaps by reading educational material provided by the national and local support organizations) and to be physically and socially active.

EXPERIMENTAL THERAPEUTICS

There are many therapeutic agents in the classes of the drugs we previously described, but some novel therapies do not fit the traditional classification and will be briefly reviewed here.

In contrast to anticholinergic drugs, which tend to improve some symptoms of PD, the cholinergic drugs would be expected to increase parkinsonian motor deficits. However, the novel nicotinic acetylcholine receptor agonist SIB-1508Y has been found to have a potentially beneficial effects not only on motor deficits but on cognitive deficits associated with PD as well, particularly when combined with levodopa (441). Furthermore, cognitive and motor benefits have been observed in patients with PD managed with intravenous or transdermal (patch) nicotine (442). Interestingly, nicotine has been found to initially activate midbrain dopamine neurons, but after longer exposure to nicotine these neurons become desensitized (443). Despite some evidence of possible protective effects of smoking, particularly in young patients with PD (444), and antioxidant effects of nicotine (445), transdermal nicotine administration has been associated with no effect (446) or worsening (447) of motor performance in patients with PD.

Another promising strategy in the treatment of PD is the use of adenosine antagonists. Adenosine A2a receptors are colocalized with striatal dopamine D2 receptors on GABAergic medium spiny neurons that project via the "indirect" striatopallidal pathway to the GPe (448). The novel adenosine A2a receptor antagonist KW-6002, synthesized at the Pharmaceutical Research Institute at Kyowa Hakko Kogyo Company, has been shown to reverse parkinsonian symptoms in 6-OHDA rats and MPTP marmosets without causing dyskinesias (129,130). These results were later confirmed by Grondin et al. (449) in MPTP cynomolgus monkeys. The elimination half-life of KW-6002 is about 30 hours. Phase I studies have demonstrated that KW-6002 can cause nausea, vomiting, abdominal pain, fever, sleep disorder, and mild elevation in white cell count and possibly in liver enzymes. A multicenter study evaluating the safety and efficacy of a once-a-day administration of 5 to 40 mg of KW-6002 in patients with moderately advanced PD is currently underway. Theophylline acts as an adenosine A2 antagonist, and the drug has been shown to increase "on" time and smooth out motor fluctuations in some patients with moderately advanced PD (450,451).

As our knowledge about mechanisms of neurodegeneration grows, novel therapeutic strategies will become available for investigation. For example, it is possible that caspase inhibitors will have a role in the treatment and even prevention of neurodegeneration in PD and related disorders (452,453). Another potential approach is immunization for PD, similar to the vaccination approach using injection or nasal administration of amyloid-β peptide, currently investigated in Alzheimer's disease (454,455).

The encouraging results of fetal grafting in the management of experimental as well as human parkinsonism has stimulated the research in gene therapy of PD (456,457). This approach has received a great deal of publicity, but until recently the results in experimental animals have been disappointing. Viral vectors are currently being used to deliver genes to the animal brain in an attempt to restore dopaminergic transmission or promote survival of dying neurons. For example, the TH gene and a gene encoding GTP-cyclohydrolase-1 have been used to enhance the activity of TH. Leff et al. (458) have shown that gene therapy with a recombinant amino acid decarboxylase (AADC) gene can provide long-term AADC expression in 6-OHDA-lesioned rats. Furthermore, a replication-defective adenoviral vectors encoding human GDNF has been used to deliver this trophic factor into the brain (382). There are many methodologic challenges that have to be solved before gene therapy can be considered for clinical trials.

Observations that cell division can occur in an adult brain have led to speculations that stem cell technology may be applied to neurodegenerative diseases, including PD (418, 419,459–465). One of the most exciting areas of current research is the potential use of cultured, well-characterized stem cells, with the ability to generate neurons and glia, for therapeutic applications in PD. This interest has been fueled by the encouraging findings from clinical trials utilizing fetal grafts into brains of PD patients (see below). It has become possible to generate CNS cells that express neuronal and glial properties by manipulating the tissue cultures with various cytokines and growth factors. When these progenitor cells are injected into an intact striatum they acquire the characteristics of striatal cells (but when injected into a lesioned brain they differentiate into glia). In one experiment, neuronal progenitor cells from a neonatal anterior subventricular zone were implanted in an adult rat with unilateral nigrostriatal denervation by 6-OHDA and were found to differentiate into neuronal phenotype as long as 5 months postimplantation (466). In another study, embryonic stem cells derived from somatic cells via nuclear transfer differentiated into dopaminergic and serotonergic neurons in vitro and germ cells in vivo, demonstrating the full pluripotency of cloned cells and their potential usefulness in the management of PD (419). Rietz et al. (467) found that a population of neuronal stem cells located in both ependymal and subventricular zones acts as functional stem cells in vivo and has a potential to differentiate not only neuronal but also nonneuronal cells. These studies suggest the possibility that in PD the progenitor or stem cells can eventually be used to replace lost or degenerated cells.

ALGORITHM AND THERAPEUTICS GUIDELINES

Although a cure is not yet in sight, tremendous strides have been made in the treatment of patients with PD (1,99,468). Levodopa is the most potent antiparkinsonian agent, but its use is associated with the development of motor complications. Furthermore, there is a growing body of evidence that levodopa primes for the development of motor complications and may be neurotoxic. For these reasons, most parkinsonologists prefer to delay the introduction of levodopa and recommend a variety of levodopa-sparing strategies. Deprenyl not only inhibits MAO-B but may also exert rescuing and trophic effects on dopaminergic neurons, independent of its antioxidant properties. Since it also delays the need for levodopa, deprenyl should be used soon after the diagnosis of PD is made. DA agonists not only reduce the need for levodopa but may also have an independent neuroprotective effect. It is, therefore, reasonable to consider using DA agonists early in the course of PD therapy. Although they are not as effective as levodopa, they often provide satisfactory relief in patients with mild symptoms. In patients whose symptoms are severe enough to interfere with their social or occupational activities, early symptomatic treatment with levodopa, later combined with a DA agonist, may be necessary. In addition, the anticholinergic drugs and amantadine may provide some symptomatic relief in early phases of anti-PD therapy. However, these drugs can cause undesirable side effects, particularly in the elderly, and therefore we prefer to use these drugs only in younger individuals. Surgery, such as thalamotomy, pallidotomy, and STN or GPi deep brain stimulation, should be reserved only for patients whose PD symptoms or levodopa-induced dyskinesias are so troublesome as to cause disability at home or at work. We understand that many of the issues raised in this chapter are controversial. We offer these practical treatment guidelines in the hope that they will be useful to practitioners involved in the management of PD and related disorders. The recommendations are based on our interpretation of the available basic and clinical information, coupled with our own clinical experience. The decision tree presented here seems quite sensible, although it should be continuously reevaluated and modified as relevant information becomes available.

REFERENCES

1. Jankovic J. New and emerging therapies for Parkinson disease. *Arch Neurol* 1999;56:785–790.

2. Siderowf AD, Holloway RG, Stern MB. Cost-effectiveness analysis in Parkinson's disease: determining the value of interventions. *Mov Disord* 2000;15:439–445.

3. Whetten-Gladstone K, et al. The burden of Parkinson's disease on society, family, and the individual. *J Am Geriatric Soc* 1997; 45:844–849.

4. Homann CN, Suppan K, Wenzel K, et al. The bradykinesia akinesia incoordination test (BRAIN[c]), an objective and user-friendly means to evaluate patients with parkinsonism. *Mov Disord* 2000;15:641–647.

5. Fahn S, Elton RL, members of the UPDRS Development Committee. The Unified Parkinson's Disease Rating Scale. In Fahn S, Marsden CD, Calne DB, et al., eds. *Recent developments in Parkinson's disease,* vol 2. Florham Park, NJ: Macmillan Healthcare Information, 1987:153–163, 293–304.

6. Goetz CG, Stebbins GT, Shale HM, et al. Utility of an objective dyskinesia rating scale for Parkinson's disease: inter- and intrareliability assessment. *Mov Disord* 1994;9:390–394.

7. Goetz CG, Stebbins GT, Chmura TA, et al. Teaching tape for the motor section of the Unified Parkinson's Disease Rating Scale. *Mov Disord* 1995;10:263–266.

8. Goetz CG, Stebins GT, Blasucci LM, et al. Efficacy of a patient-training videotape on motor fluctuations for on–off diaries in Parkinson's disease. *Mov Disord* 1997;12:1039–1041.

9. Martinez-Martin P, Gil-Nagel A, Garcia LM, et al. Unified Parkinson's Disease Rating Scale characteristics and structure. *Mov Disord* 1994;9:76–83.

10. Bennett DA, Shannon KM, Beckett LA, et al. Metric properties of nurses' ratings of parkinsonian signs with a modified Unified Parkinson's Disease Rating Scale. *Neurology* 1997;49: 1580–1587.

11. Burkhard PR, Shale H, Langston JW, et al. Quantitation of dyskinesia in Parkinson's disease: validation of a novel instrumental method. *Mov Disord* 1999;14:754–763.

12. Goetz CG. Rating scales for dyskinesias in Parkinson's disease. *Mov Disord* 1999;14[Suppl 1]:48–53.

13. Hoff JI, van Hilten BJ, Roos RA. A review of the assessment of dyskinesias. *Mov Disord* 1999;14:737–743.

14. Parkinson Study Group. Evaluation of dyskinesias in a pilot, randomized, placebo-controlled trial of remacemide in advanced Parkinson disease. *Arch Neurol* 2001;58:1660–1668a.

15. Hauser RA, Friedlander J, Zesiewicz TA, et al. A home diary to assess functional status in patients with Parkinson's disease with motor fluctuations and dyskinesia. *Clin Neuropharmacol* 2000; 2:75–81.

16. Goetz CG, Blasucci L, Stebbins GT. Switching dopamine agonists in advanced Parkinson's disease: is rapid titration preferable to slow? *Neurology* 1999;52:1227–1229.

17. Manson AJ, Brown P, O'Sullivan JD, et al. An ambulatory dyskinesia monitor. *J Neurol Neurosurg Psychiatry* 2000;68: 196–201.

18. Schrag A, Selai C, Jahanshahi M, et al. He Q-5D—generic quality of life measure—is a useful instrument to measure quality of life in patients with Parkinson's disease. *J Neurol Neurosurg Psychiatry* 2000;69:67–73.

19. Shetty N, Friedman JH, Kieburtz K, et al. The placebo response in Parkinson's disease. *Clin Neuropharmacol* 1999;22:207–212.

20. Goetz CG, Leurgans S, Raman R, et al. Objective changes in motor function during placebo treatment in PD. *Neurology* 2000;54:710–714.

21. De la Fuente-Fernandez R, Ruth TJ, Sossi V, et al. Expectation and dopamine release: mechanism of the placebo effect in Parkinson's disease. *Science* 2001;293:1164–1166a.

22. Lilienfeld DE, Chan E, Ehland J, et al. Two decades of increasing mortality from Parkinson's disease among the U.S. elderly. *Arch Neurol* 1990;47:731–734.

23. Clarke CE. Does levodopa therapy delay death in Parkinson's disease? A review of the evidence. *Mov Disord* 1995;10: 250–256.

24. Parkinson Study Group. Mortality in DATATOP: a multicenter trial in early Parkinson's disease. *Ann Neurol* 1998;43: 318–325.

25. Jankovic J. Complications and limitations of drug therapy for movement disorders. *Neurology Suppl* 2000;55[Suppl 6]:S2–S6.

26. Fahn S. Parkinson's disease, the effect of levodopa, and the ELLDOPA trial. *Arch Neurol* 1999;56:529–535.

27. Weiner WJ. The initial treatment of Parkinson's disease should begin with levodopa. *Mov Disord* 1999;14:716–724.

28. Montastruc JL, Rascol O, Senard J-M. Treatment of Parkinson's disease should begin with a dopamine agonist. *Mov Disord* 1999;14:725–730.

29. Olanow CW, Watts RL, Koller WC. An algorithm (decision tree) for the management of Parkinson's disease (2001): treatment guidelines. *Neurology* 2001;56[Suppl 5]:S1–S88.

30. Männistö PT, Kaakola S. Rationale for selective COMT inhibitors as adjuvants in the drug treatment of Parkinson's disease. *Pharmacol Toxicol* 1990;66:317–323

31. Karstaedt PJ, Pincus JH. Protein redistribution diet remains effective in patients with fluctuating parkinsonism. *Arch Neurol* 1992;49:149–151.

32. Opacka-Juffrey J, Brooks DJ. L-Dihydroxyphenylalanine and its decarboxylase: new ideas on the neuroregulatory roles. *Mov Disord* 1995;10:241–249.

33. Cedarbaum JM, Kutt H, Dhar AK, et al. Effect of supplemental carbidopa on bioavailability of L-dopa. *Clin Neuropharmacol* 1986;9:153–159.

34. Apaydin H, Ertan S, Özekmerci S. Broad bean *(Vicia faba)*—a natural source of L-dopa—prolongs "on" periods in patients with Parkinson's disease who have "on–off" fluctuations. *Mov Disord* 2000;15:164–166.

35. Nutt JG, Holford NHG. The response to levodopa in Parkinson's disease: imposing pharmacological law and order. *Ann Neurol* 1996;39:561–573.

36. Obeso JA, Rodriguez-Oroz MAC, Rodriguez M, et al. Pathophysiology of levodopa-induced dyskinesias in Parkinson's disease: problems with the current model. *Ann Neurol* 2000;47 [Suppl 1]:S22–S34b.

37. Obeo JA, Olanow CW, Nutt JG. Levodopa motor complications in Parkinson's disease. *TINS* 2000;23[Suppl]:S2–S7c.

38. Verhagen Metman L, Konitsiotis S, Chase TN. Pathophysiology of motor response complications in Parkinson's disease: hypotheses on the why, where, and what. *Mov Disord* 2000; 15:3–8.

39. Waters CH. Managing the late complications of Parkinson's disease. *Neurology* 1997;49[Suppl 1]:S49–S57.

40. Parkinson Study Group. Impact of deprenyl and tocopherol treatment on Parkinson's disease in DATATOP patients requiring levodopa. *Ann Neurol* 1996;39:37–45b.

41. Poewe WH, Lees AJ, Stern GM. Low-dose L-dopa therapy in Parkinson's disease: a 6-year follow-up study. *Neurology* 1986;36:1528–1530.

42. Block G, Liss C, Reines S, et al. Comparison of immediate-release and controlled release carbidopa/levodopa in Parkinson's disease: a multicenter 5-year study. *Eur Neurol* 1997;37:23–27.

43. Nutt JG, Carter JH, Van Houten L, et al. Short- and long-duration responses to levodopa during the first year of levodopa therapy. *Ann Neurol* 1997;42:349–355.

44. Ahlskog JE, Muenter MD. Frequency of levodopa-related dyskinesias and motor fluctuations as estimated from the cumulative literature. *Mov Disord* 2001;16:448–458.

45. Raudino F. Non-motor off in Parkinson's disease. *Acta Neurol Scand* 2001;104:312–315.

46. Giovannoni G, O'Sullivan JD, Turner K, et al. Hedonistic homeostatic dysregulation in patients with Parkinson's disease on dopamine replacement therapies. *J Neurol Neurosurg Psychiatry* 2000;68:423–428.

47. Zappia M, Oliveri RL, Montesanti R, et al. Loss of long-duration response to levodopa over time in PD: implications for wearing off. *Neurology* 1999;52:763–767.

48. Zappia M, Oliveri RL, Bosco D, et al. The long-duration response to L-dopa in the treatment of early PD. *Neurology* 2000;54:1910–1915.

49. Nutt JG. Response to L-dopa in PD: the long and short of it. *Neurology* 2000;54:1884–1885.

50. Luquin MR, Scipioni O, Vaamonde J, et al. Levodopa-induced dyskinesias in Parkinson's disease: clinical and pharmacological classification. *Mov Disord* 1992;7:117–124a.

51. Riley DE, Lang AE. The spectrum of levodopa-related fluctuations in Parkinson's disease. *Neurology* 1993;43:1459–1464.

52. Vidailhet M, Bonnet AM, Marconi N. The phenomenology of L-dopa–induced dyskinesias in Parkinson's disease. *Mov Disord* 1999;14[Suppl 1]:13–18.

53. Fahn S. The spectrum of levodopa-induced dyskinesias. *Ann Neurol* 2000;47[Suppl 1]:S2–S11.

54. Jankovic J, Nour F. Respiratory dyskinesia in Parkinson's disease. *Neurology* 1986;36:303–304.

55. Rascol O. L-Dopa–induced peak-dose dyskinesias in patients with Parkinson's disease: a clinical pharmacologic approach. *Mov Disord* 1999;14[Suppl 1]:19–32.

56. Fernandez HH, Friedman JH. Punding on L-dopa. *Mov Disord* 1999;14:836–838.

57. Cubo E, Gracies J-M, Benabou R, et al. Early morning off-medication dyskinesias, dystonia, and choreic subtypes. *Arch Neurol* 2001;58:1379–1382.

58. Jankovic J, Tintner R. Dystonia and parkinsonism. *Parkinsonism Relat Disord* 2001;8:109–121.

59. Marconi R, Lefebvre-Caparros D, Bonnet A-M, et al. Levodopa-induced dyskinesia in Parkinson's disease: phenomenology and pathophysiology. *Mov Disord* 1994;9:2–12.

60. Vidailhet M, Bonnet AM, Marconi N, et al. Do parkinsonian symptoms and levodopa-induced dyskinesias start in the foot? *Neurology* 1994;44:1613–1616.

61. Bezard E, Brotchie JM, Gross CE. Pathophysiology of levodopa-induced dyskinesia: potential for new therapies. *Nat Rev Neurosci* 2001;2:577–588.

62. Olanow CW, Schapira AHV, Rascol O. Continuous dopamine-receptor stimulation in early Parkinson's disease. *TINS* 2000;23[Suppl]:S117–S126.

63. Verhagen Metman L, Locatelli ER, Bravi D, et al. Apomorphine responses in Parkinson's disease and the pathogenesis of motor complications. *Neurology* 1997;48:369–372.

64. Nutt JG, Carter JH. Apomorphine can sustain the long-duration response to L-DOPA in fluctuating PD. *Neurology* 2000;54:247–250.

65. Papa SM, Chase TN. Levodopa-induced dyskinesias improved by a glutamate antagonist in parkinsonian monkeys. *Ann Neurol* 1996;39:574–578.

66. Verhagen Metman L, Dotto PD, LePoole K, et al. Amantadine for levodopa-induced dyskinesias: a 1-year follow-up study. *Arch Neurol* 1999;56:1383–1386.

67. Kelland MD, Walters JR. Apomorphine-induced changes in striatal and pallidal neuronal activity are modified by NMDA and muscarinic receptor blockade. *Life Sci* 1992;50:PL179–PL184.

68. Filion M, Tremblay L, Bedard PJ. Effects of dopamine agonists on the spontaneous activity of globus pallidus neurons in monkeys with MPTP-induced parkinsonism. *Brain Res* 1991;547:152–161.

69. Papa SM, Desimone R, Fiorani M, et al. Internal globus pallidus discharge is nearly suppressed during levodopa-induced dyskinesias. *Ann Neurol* 1999;46:732–738.

70. Boraud T, Bezard E, Bioulac B, et al. Dopamine agonist-induced dyskinesias are correlated to both firing pattern and frequency alterations of pallidal neurons in the MPTP-treated monkey. *Brain* 2001;124:546–557.

71. Lang AE. Surgery for levodopa-induced dyskinesias. *Ann Neurol* 2000;47[Suppl 1]:S193–S202.

72. Bedard PJ, Blanchet PJ, Levesque D, et al. Pathophysiology of L-dopa–induced dyskinesias. *Mov Disord* 1999;14[Suppl 1]:4–8.

73. Togasaki DM, Tan L, Protell P, et al. Levodopa induces dyskinesias in normal squirrel monkeys. *Ann Neurol* 2001;50:254–257.

74. Schrag AS, Quinn N. Dyskinesias and moto fluctuations in Parkinson's disease: a community-based study. *Brain* 2000;123:2297–2305.

75. Quinn NP, Critchely P, Marsden CD. Young-onset parkinsonism. *Mov Disord* 1987;2:73–91.

76. Jankovic J, Linfante I, Dawson LE, et al. Young-onset versus late-onset Parkinson's disease: clinical features and disease progression. *Ann Neurol* 1997;42:448.

77. Boyce S, Rupniak NMJ, Steventon MJ, et al. Differential effects of D1 and D2 agonists in MPTP-treated primates: functional implications for Parkinson's disease. *Neurology* 1990;40:927–933.

78. Luquin MR, Laguna J, Obeso JA. Selective D2 receptor stimulation induces dyskinesia in parkinsonian monkeys. *Ann Neurol* 1992;31:551–554b.

79. Oliveri RL, Annesi G, Zappia M, et al. Dopamine D2 receptor gene polymorphism and the risk of levodopa-induced dyskinesias in PD. *Neurology* 1999;53:1425–1430.

80. Wang J, Liu Z-L, Chen B. Association study of dopamine D2, D3 receptor gene polymorphisms with motor fluctuations in PD. *Neurology* 2001;56:1757–1759.

81. Rascol O, Sabatini U, Brefel C, et al. Cortical and motor over-activation in parkinsonian patients with L-dopa–induced peak-dose dyskinesia. *Brain* 1998;121:527–533.

82. Leenders KL, Poweve WH, Palmer AJ, et al. Inhibition of [18F]fluorodopa uptake into human brain by amino acids demonstrated by positron emission tomography. *Ann Neurol* 1986;20:258–262.

83. Turjanski N, Lees AJ, Brooks DJ. In vivo studies on striatal dopamine D_1 and D_2 site binding in L-dopa–treated Parkinson's disease patients with and without dyskinesias. *Neurology* 1997;49:717–723.

84. Ekesbo A, Rydin E, Torstenson R, et al. Dopamine autoreceptor function is lost in advanced Parkinson's disease. *Neurology* 1999;52:120–125.

85. Nutt JG, Carter JH, Woodward WR. Effect of brief levodopa holidays on the short-duration response to levodopa: evidence for tolerance to the antiparkinsonian effects. *Neurology* 1994;44:1617–1622.

86. De la Fuente-Fernandez R, Lu J-Q L, Sossi V, et al. Biochemical variations in the synaptic level of dopamine precede motor fluctuations in Parkinson's disease: PET evidence of increased dopamine turnover. *Ann Neurol* 2001;49:298–303b.

87. Jolkkonen J, Jenner P, Marsden CD. L-DOPA reverses altered gene expression of substance P but not enkephalin in the caudate-putamen of common marmosets treated with MPTP. *Mol Brain Res* 1995;32:297–307.

88. Andersson M, Hilbertson A, Cenci MA. Striatal fosB expression is causally linked with L-dopa–induced abnormal involuntary movements and the associated upregulation of striatal prodynorphin mRNA in a rat model of Parkinson's disease. *Neurobiol Dis* 2000;6:461–474.

89. Pearce RKB, Jackson M, Smith L, et al. Chronic L-DOPA administration induces dyskinesias in the 1-methyl-4-phenyl-1,2,3,6-tetrahydropyridine-treated common marmoset *(Callithrix jacchus)*. *Mov Disord* 1995;10:731–740.

90. Canales JJ, Graybiel AM. Patterns of gene expression and behavior induced by chronic dopamine treatments. *Ann Neurol* 2000;47[Suppl 1]:S53–S59.

91. Calon F, Grondin R Morissette M, et al. Molecular basis of levodopa-induced dyskinesias. *Ann Neurol* 2000;47[Suppl 1]:S70–S78.

92. Jenner P. Factors influencing the onset and persistence of dyskinesia in MPTP-treated primates. *Ann Neurol* 2000;47[Suppl 1]:S90–S104.

93. Piccini P, Weeks RA, Brooks DJ. Alterations in opioid receptor binding in Parkinson's disease with levodopa-induced dyskinesias. *Ann Neurol* 1997;42:720–726.

94. Muriel M-P, Bernard V, Levey AI, et al. Levodopa induced cytoplasmic localization of D1 dopamine receptors in striatal neurons in Parkinson's disease. *Ann Neurol* 1999;46:103–111.

95. Gurevich EV, Joyce JN. Distribution of dopamine D3 receptor expressing neurons in the human forebrain: comparison with D2 receptor expressing neurons. *Neuropsychopharmacology* 1999;1:60–80.

96. Bordet R, Ridray S, Carboni S, et al. Induction of dopamine D3 receptor expression as a mechanism of behavioral sensitization to levodopa. *Proc Natl Acad Sci USA* 1997;94:3363–3367.

97. Ryoo HL, Pierrotti D, Joyce JN. Dopamine D3 receptor is decreased and D2 receptor is elevated in the striatum of Parkinson's disease. *Mov Disord* 1998;13:788–797.

98. Svensonn KA, Carlsson A, Huff RM, et al. Behavioral and biochemical data suggest functional differences between dopamine D2 and D3 receptors. *Eur J Pharmacol* 1994;263(3):235–243.

99. Ahlskog JE. Medical treatment of later-stage motor problems of Parkinson disease. *Mayo Clin Proc* 1999;74:1239–1254.

100. Jankovic J, Schwartz K, Van der Linden C. Comparison of Sinemet CR4 and standard Sinemet: double-blind and long-term open trial in parkinsonian patients with fluctuations. *Mov Disord* 1989;4:303–309.

101. Davis TL, Brughitta G, Baronti F, et al. Acute effects of pulsatile levodopa administration on central dopamine pharmacodynamics. *Neurology* 1991;41:630–633.

102. Sage JI, Mark MH. The rationale for continuous dopaminergic stimulation in patients with Parkinson's disease. *Neurology* 1992;42[Suppl 1]:23–28.

103. Hammerstad JP, Woodward WR, Nutt JG, et al. Controlled release levodopa/carbidopa 25/100 (Sinemet CR 25/100): pharmacokinetics and clinical efficacy in untreated parkinsonian patients. *Clin Neuropharmacol* 1994;17:429–434.

104. Koller WC, Hutton JT, Tolosa E, et al., and the Carbidopa/Levodopa Study Group. Immediate-release and controlled-release carbidopa/levodopa in PD. *Neurology* 1999;53:1012–1019.

105. Nilsson D, Hansson L-E, Johansson K, et al. Long-term intraduodenal infusion of a water based levodopa-carbidopa dispersion in very advanced Parkinson's disease. *Acta Neurol Scand* 1998;97:175–183.

106. Syed N, Zimmerman T, Mark MH, et al. Ten years' experience with enteral levodopa infusions for motor fluctuations in Parkinson's disease. *Mov Disord* 1998;13:336–338.

107. Hanson ND, Johansson L-E, Nystrom A, et al. Long-term intraduodenal infusion of a water based levodopa-carbidopa dispersion in very advanced Parkinson's disease. *Acta Neurol Scand* 1998;97:175–183.

108. Nilsson D, Nyholm ND, Aquilonius S-M. Dudodenal levodopa infusion in Parkinson's disease—long-term experience. *Acta Neurol Scand* 2001;104:343–348.

109. Verhagen Metman L, Hoff J, Mouradian MM, et al. Fluctua-

tions in plasma levodopa and motor responses with liquid and tablet levodopa/carbidopa. *Mov Disord* 1994;9:463–465.

110. Pappert EJ, Goetz CG, Niederman F, et al. Liquid levodopa/carbidopa produces significant improvement in motor function without dyskinesia exacerbation. *Neurology* 1996;47:1493–1495.

111. Djaldetti R, Melamed E. Levodopa ethylester: a novel rescue therapy for response fluctuations in Parkinson's disease. *Ann Neurol* 1996;39:400–404.

112. Stocci F, Ruggieri S, Carta A, et al. Intravenous boluses and continuous infusions of L-DOPA methyl ester in fluctuating patients with Parkinson's disease. *Mov Disord* 1992;7:249–256.

113. Schu LA, Bennett JP. Suppression of dyskinesias in advanced Parkinson's disease. I. Continuous intravenous levodopa shifts dose response for production of dyskinesias but not for relief of parkinsonism in patients with advanced Parkinson's disease. *Neurology* 1993;43:1545–1550.

114. Merello M, Lees AJ, Webster R, et al. Effect of entacapone, a peripherally acting catechol-*O*-methyltransferase inhibitor, on the motor response to acute treatment with levodopa in patients with Parkinson's disease. *J Neurol Neurosurg* 1994;57:186–189.

115. Nutt JG, Woodward WR, Beckner RM, et al. Effect of peripheral catechol-*O*-methyltransferase on the pharmacokinetics and pharmacodynamics of levodopa in parkinsonian patients. *Neurology* 1994;44:913–919b.

116. Kurth MC, Adler CH, Hilaire M St, et al. Tolcapone improves motor function and reduces levodopa requirement in patients with Parkinson's disease experiencing motor fluctuations: a multicenter, double-blind, randomized, placebo-controlled trial. *Neurology* 1997;48:81–87.

117. Parkinson Study Group. A controlled trial of lazabemide (Ro 19-6327) in levodopa-treated Parkinson's disease. *Arch Neurol* 1994;51:342–347.

118. Verhagen Metman L, va den Munckhof, Klaassen AAG, et al. Effects of supra-threshold levodopa doses on dyskinesias in advanced Parkinson's disease. *Neurology* 1997;49:711–713.

119. Jankovic J. Dystonia: medical therapy and botulinum toxin in dystonia. In: Fahn S, Marsden CD, DeLong DR, eds. *Dystonia 3.* Advances in neurology, vol 78. Philadelphia: Lippincott–Raven Publishers, 1998:169–184.

120. Rascol O, on behalf of the 056 Study Group. Ropinirole reduces risk of dyskinesia when used in early PD. *Parkinsonism Rel Disord* 1999;5:S83–S84.

121. Rascol O. Medical treatment of levodopa-induced dyskinesias. *Ann Neurol* 2000;47[Suppl 1]:S179–S188.

122. Verhagen Metman L, Del Dotto P, va den Munckhof P, et al. Amantadine as treatment for dyskinesias and motor fluctuations in Parkinson's disease. *Neurology* 1998;50:1323–1326.

123. Bennett JP, Landow ER, Dietrich S, et al. Suppression of dyskinesias in advanced Parkinson's disease: moderate daily clozapine doses provide long-term dyskinesia reduction. *Mov Disord* 1994;9:409–414.

124. Friedman JH, Koller WC, Lannon MC, et al. Benztropine versus clozapine for the treatment of tremor in Parkinson's disease. *Neurology* 1997;48:1077–1081.

125. Bonucceli U, Ceravolo R, Salvetti S, et al. Clozapine in Parkinson's disease tremor: effects of acute and chronic administration. *Neurology* 1997;49:1587–1590.

126. Durif F, Vidailhet M, Bonnet AM, et al. Levodopa-induced dyskinesias are improved by fluoxetine. *Neurology* 1995;45:1855–1858.

127. Carpentier AF, Bonnet AM, Vidailhet M, et al. Improvement of levodopa-induced dyskinesia by propranolol in Parkinson's disease. *Neurology* 1996;46:1548–1551.

128. Sieradzan KA, Fox SH, Hill M, et al. Cannabinoids reduce lev-

odopa-induced dyskinesia in Parkinson's disease: a pilot study. *Neurology* 2001;57:2108–2111.

129. Kanda T, Jacson MJ, Smith LA, et al. Adenosine A$_{2A}$ antagonist: a novel antiparkinsonian agent that does not provoke dyskinesia in parkinsonian monkeys. *Ann Neurol* 1998;43:507–513.

130. Kanda T, Jackson MJ, Smith LA, et al. Combined use of the adenosine A$_{2A}$ antagonist KW-6002 with L-DOPA or with selective D1 or D2 dopamine agonists: increases antiparkinsonian activity but not dyskinesia in MPTP-treated monkeys. *Exp Neurol* 2000;162:321–327.

131. Olanow CW, Obeso JA. Preventing levodopa-induced dyskinesias. *Ann Neurol* 2000;479[Suppl 1]:S167–S178.

132. Sabel BA, Dominiak P, Hauser W, et al. Levodopa delivery from controlled-release polymer matrix: delivery of more than 600 days in vitro and 225 days of elevated plasma levels after subcutaneous implantation in rats. *J Pharmacol Exp Ther* 1990;255:914–922.

133. Aebischer P, Tresco PA, Sagen J, et al. Transplantation of microencapsulated bovine chromaffin cells reduces lesion-induced rational asymmetry in rats. *Brain Res* 1991;560:43–49.

134. McRae A, Ling EA, Hjorth S, et al. Catecholamine-containing biodegradable microsphere implants as a novel approach in the treatment of CNS neurodegenerative disease: a review of experimental studies in DA-lesioned rats. *Mol Neurobiol* 1994;9:191–205.

135. Fénelon G, Mahieux F, Huon R, et al. Hallucinations in Parkinson's disease: prevalence, phenomenology, and risk factors. *Brain* 2000;123:733–745.

136. Goetz CG, Leurgans S, Pappert EJ, et al. Prospective longitudinal assessment of hallucinations in Parkinson's disease. *Neurology* 2001;57:2078–2082.

137. Lang AE. Akathisia and the restless legs syndrome. In: Jankovic J, Tolosa E, eds. *Parkinson's disease and movement disorders,* 2nd ed. Baltimore: Williams & Wilkins, 1993:399–418.

138. Friedman JH, Factor SA. Atypical antipsychotics in the treatment of drug-induced psychosis in Parkinson's disease. *Mov Disord* 2000;15:201–211.

139. Factor SA, Brown D. Clozapine prevents recurrence of psychosis in Parkinson's disease. *Mov Disord* 1992;7:125–131.

140. Rabey JM, Treves TA, Neufeld MY, et al. Low-dose clozapine in the treatment of levodopa-induced mental disturbances in Parkinson's disease. *Neurology* 1995; 45:432–434.

141. Parkinson Study Group. Low dose clozapine for the treatment of drug-induced psychosis in Parkinson's disease. *N Engl J Med* 1999;340:757–763.

142. Scelsa SN, Simpson DM, McQuistion et al. Clozapine-induced myotoxicity in patients with chronic psychotic disorders. *Neurology* 1996;47:1518–1523.

143. Zoldan J, Friedberg G, Livneh M, et al. Psychosis in advanced Parkinson's disease: treatment with ondansetron, 5-HT3 receptor antagonist. *Neurology* 1995;45:1305–1308.

144. Wolters EC, Jansen ENH, Tuynman-Qua, et al. Olanzapine in the treatment of dopaminomimetic psychosis in patients with Parkinson's disease. *Neurology* 1996;47:1085–1087.

145. Graham JM, Kay JD, Ford K, et al. Olanzapine in the treatment of hallucinosis in idiopathic Parkinson's disease: a cautionary note. *J Neurol Neurosurg Psychiatry* 1998;65:774–777.

146. Manson AJ, Schrag A, Lees AJ. Low-dose olanzapine for levodopa-induced dyskinesias. *Neurology* 2000;55:795–799.

147. Ondo WG, Hunter C, Vuong KD, et al. Olanzapine treatment for hallucinations induced by dopaminergic drugs. *Mov Disord* 2002 (in press).

148. Fernandez HH, Friedman JH, Jacques C, et al. Quetiapine for the treatment of drug-induced psychosis in Parkinson's disease. *Mov Disord* 1999;14:484–487.

149. McKeith IG, Grace JB, Walker Z, et al. Rivastigmine in the treatment of dementia with lewy bodies: preliminary findings from an open trial. *Int J Geriatr Psychiatry* 2000;15:387–392.

150. Wilde MI, Markham A. Ondansetron: a review of its pharmacology and preliminary clinical findings in novel applications. *Drugs* 1996;52:773–794.

151. Jankovic J, Gilden JL, Hiner BC, et al. Neurogenic orthostatic hypotension: a double-blind placebo-controlled study with midodrine. *Am J Med* 1993;95:38–48.

152. Low PA, Gilden JL, Freeman R, et al. Efficacy of midodrine vs. placebo in neurogenic orthostatic hypotension: a randomized, double-blind multicenter study. *JAMA* 1997;277:1046–1051.

153. Kurlan R, Tanner CM, Goetz C, et al. Levodopa drug holiday versus drug dosage reduction in Parkinson's disease. *Clin Neuropharmacol* 1994;17:117–127.

154. Corona T, Rivera C, Otero E, et al. A longitudinal study of the effects of an L-dopa drug holiday on the course of Parkinson's disease. *Clin Neuropharmacol* 1995;18:325–332.

155. Ueda M, Hamamoto M, Nagayama H, et al. Susceptibility to neuroleptic malignant syndrome in Parkinson's disease. *Neurology* 1999;52:777–781.

156. Currie LJ, Bennett JP, Harrison MB, et al. Clinical correlates of sleep benefit in Parkinson's disease. *Neurology* 1997;48:1115–1117.

157. Högl BE, Gómez-Arévalo G, García S, et al. A clinical, pharmacologic, and polysomnographic study of sleep benefit in Parkinson's disease. *Neurology* 1998;50:1323–1339.

158. Fahn S. Levodopa-induced neurotoxicity: does it represent a problem for the treatment of Parkinson's disease? *CNS Drugs* 1997;8:376–393.

159. Fahn S. Welcome news about levodopa, but uncertainty remains. *Ann Neurol* 1998;43:551–554.

160. Olanow CW. A rationale for dopamine agonists as primary therapy for Parkinson's disease. *Can J Neurol Sci* 1992;19:108–112a.

161. Rajput AH, Fenton ME, Birdi S, et al. Is levodopa toxic to human substantia nigra? *Mov Disord* 1997;12:634–638.

162. Desagher S, Glowinski J, Premont J. Astrocytes protect neurons from hydrogen peroxide toxicity. *J Neurosci* 1996;16:2553–2562.

163. Agid Y. Levodopa: is toxicity a myth? *Neurology* 1998;50:858–863.

164. Mena MA, Casarejos MJ, Carazo A, et al. Glia conditioned medium protect fetal rat midbrain neurons in culture from L-dopa toxicity. *Neuroreport* 1996;7:441–445.

165. Murer MG, Dziewczapolski G, Menalled LB, et al. Chronic levodopa is not toxic for remaining dopamine neurons, but instead promotes their recovery, in rats with moderate nigrostriatal lesions. *Ann Neurol* 1998;43:561–575.

166. Datla KP, Blunt SB, Dexter DT. Chronic L-DOPA administration is not toxic to the remaining dopaminergic nigrostriatal neurons, but instead may promote their functional recovery, in rats with partial 6-OHDA or FeCl$_3$ nigrostrial lesions. *Mov Disord* 2001;16:424–434.

167. Okazawa H, Murata M, Watanabe M, et al. Dopaminergic stimulation upregulates in vivo expression of brain derived neurotrophic factor (BDNF) in the striatum. *FEBS Lett* 1992;313:138–142.

168. Han SK, Mytilineou C, Cohen G. L-DOPA upregulated glutathione and protects mesencephalic structures against oxidative stress. *J Neurochem* 1996;66:501–510.

169. Przuntek H, Welzel D, Blumner E, et al. Bromocriptine lessens the incidence of mortality in L-dopa-treated parkinsonian patients: PRADO study discontinued. *Eur J Clin Pharmacol* 1992;43:357–363.

170. Shulman LM. Levodopa toxicity in Parkinson disease: reality or myth? Reality—practice patterns should change. *Arch Neurol* 2000;57:406–410.

171. Weiner WJ. Is levodopa toxic? *Arch Neurol* 2000;57:408–409.

172. Rinne UK, Larsen JP, Siden A, et al. Entacapone enhances the response to levodopa in parkinsonian patients with motor fluctuations. *Neurology* 1998;51:1309–1314.

173. Holm KJ, Spencer CM. Entacapone: a review fits us in Parkinson's disease. *Drugs* 1999;58:159–177.

174. Kurth MC, Adler CH. COMT inhibition: a new treatment strategy for Parkinson's disease. *Neurology* 1998;50[Suppl 5]:S3–S14.

175. Tolcapone Study Group. Efficacy and tolerability of tolcapone compare with bromocriptine in levodopa-treated parkinsonian patients. *Mov Disord* 1999;14:38–44.

176. Ruottine HM, Rinne UK. COMT inhibition in the treatment of Parkinson's disease. *J Neurol* 1998;245[Suppl 3]:25–34.

177. Roberts JW, Cora-Locatelli G, Bravi D, et al. Catechol-*O*-methyltransferase inhibitor tolcapone prolongs levodopa/carbidopa action in parkinsonian patients. *Neurology* 1993;43:2685–2688.

178. Baas H, Beiske AG, Ghika J, et al. Catechol-*O*-methyltransferase inhibition with tolcapone reduces the "wearing off" phenomenon and levodopa requirements in fluctuating parkinsonian patients. *J Neurol Neurosurg Psychiatry* 1997;63:421–428.

179. Piccini P, Brooks DJ, Korpela K, et al. The catechol-*O*-methyltransferase (COMT) inhibitor entacapone enhances the pharmacokinetic and clinical response to Sinemet CR in Parkinson's disease. *J Neurol Neurosurg Psychiatry* 2000;68:589–594.

180. Agid Y, Destée A, Durif F, et al. Tolcapone, bromocriptine, and Parkinson's disease. *Lancet* 1997;350:712–713.

181. Parkinson Study Group. Entacapone improves motor fluctuations in levodopa-treated Parkinson's disease patients. *Ann Neurol* 1997;42:747–755.

182. Waters CH, Kurth M, Bailey P, et al. Tolcapone in stable Parkinson's disease: efficacy and safety of long-term treatment. *Neurology* 1997;49:665–671.

183. Assal F, Spahr L, Hadengue A, et al. Tolcapone and fulminant hepatitis. *Lancet* 1998;352:958.

184. Olanow CW, and the Tasmar Advisory Panel. Tolcapone and hepatotoxic effects. *Arch Neurol* 2000;57:263–267.

185. Haasio K, Sopanen L, Vaalavirta L, et al. Comparative toxicological study n the hepatic safety of entacapone and tolcapanoe in the rat. *J Neural Transm* 2001;108:79–91.

186. Missale C, Nash SR, Robinson SW, et al. Dopamine receptors: from structure to function. *Physiol Rev* 1998;78:189–225.

187. Schmauss C. Dopamine receptors: novel insights from biochemical and genetic studies. *Neuroscientist* 2000;6:127–138.

188. Sealfon SC, Olanow CW. Dopamine receptors: from structure to behavior. *TINS* 2000;23[Suppl]:S34–S40.

189. Gerfen CR. Molecular effects of dopamine on striatal-projection pathways. *TINS* 2000;23[Suppl]:S64–S70.

190. Sealfon SC. Dopamine receptors and locomotor responses: molecular aspects. *Ann Neurol* 2000;47[Suppl 1]:S12–S21.

191. Jenner P. Is stimulation of D-1 and D-2 dopamine receptors important for optimal motor functioning in Parkinson's disease? *Eur J Neurol* 1997;4[Suppl 3]:S3–S11.

192. Brooks DJ. Dopamine agonists: their role in the treatment of Parkinson's disease. *J Neurol Neurosurg Psychiatry* 2000;68:685–690.

193. Jankovic J. Long-term study of pergolide in Parkinson's disease. *Neurology* 1985;35:296–299.

194. LeWitt PA, Ward CD, Larsen TA, et al. Comparison of pergolide and bromocriptine therapy in parkinsonism. *Neurology* 1983;33:1009–1014.

195. Pezzoli G, Martigoni E, Pacchetti C, et al. Pergolide compared with bromocriptine in Parkinson's disease: a multicenter, crossover, controlled study. *Mov Disord* 1994;9:431–436.

196. Hutton JT, Koller WC, Ahlskog JE, et al. Multicenter, placebo-controlled trial of cabergoline taken once daily in the treatment of Parkinson's disease. *Neurology* 1996;46:1062–1065.

197. Inzelberg R, Nisipeanu P, Rabey JM, et al. Double-blind comparison of cabergoline and bromocriptine in Parkinson's disease patients with motor fluctuations. *Neurology* 1996;47:785–788.

198. Rinne UK, Bracco F, Chouza C, et al. Cabergoline in the treatment of early Parkinson's disease: results of the first year of treatment in a double-blind comparison of cabergoline and levodopa. *Neurology* 1997;48:363–368.

199. Tahar HA, Gregoire L, Bangassoro E, et al. Sustained cabergoline treatment reverses levodopa-induced dyskinesias in parkinsonian monkeys. *Clin Neuropharmacol* 2000;23:195–202.

200. Shaunak S, Wilkins A, Pilling JB, et al. Pericardial, retroperitoneal, and pleural fibrosis induced by pergolide. *J Neurol Neurosurg Psychiatry* 1999;66:79–81.

201. Bennett JP, Piercey MF. Pramipexole—new dopamine agonist for the treatment of Parkinson's disease. *J Neurol Sci* 1999;163:25–31.

202. Perachon S, Schwartz JC, Sokoloff P. Functional potencies of new antiparkinsonian drugs at recombinant human dopamine D1, D2, and D3 receptors. *Eur J Pharmacol* 1999;5:293–300.

203. Surmeir DJ, Song WJ, Yan Z. Coordinated expression of dopamine receptors in neostriatal medium spiny neurons. *J Neurosci* 1996;16:6569–6591.

204. Corrigan MH, Denahan AQ, Wright CE, et al. Comparison of pramipexole, fluoxetine, and placebo in patients with major depression. *Depression and Anxiety* 2000;11:58–65.

205. Perugi G, Toni C, Ruffolo G, et al. Adjunctive dopamine agonists in treatment-resistant bipolar II depression: an open case series. *Pharmacopsychiatry* 2001;34:137–141.

206. Weiner WJ, Factor SA, Jankovic J, et al. The long-term safety and efficacy of pramipexole in advanced Parkinson's disease. *Parkinsonism Relat Disord* 2001;7:115–120.

207. Tan EK, Ondo W. Clinical characteristics of pramipexole-induced peripheral edema. *Arch Neurol* 2000;57:729–732.

208. Parkinson Study Group. Safety and efficacy of pramipexole in early Parkinson disease: a randomized dose-ranging study. *JAMA* 1997;278:125–130.

209. Parkinson Study Group. Pramipexole vs. levodopa as initial treatment for Parkinson's disease: a randomized controlled trial. *JAMA* 2000;284:1931–1938.

210. Shannon KM, Bennett JP, Friedman JH, et al. Efficacy of pramipexole, a novel dopamine agonist, as monotherapy in mild to moderate Parkinson's disease. *Neurology* 1997;49:724–728.

211. Parkinson Study Group. Dopamine transporter brain imaging to assess the effects of pramipexole vs. levodopa on Parkinson disease progression. *JAMA* 2002;287:1653–1661.

212. Tanner CM. Dopamine agonists in early therapy for Parkinson disease: promise and problems. *JAMA* 2000;284:1971–1973.

213. Rascol O, Brooks DJ, Brunt ER, et al. Ropinirole in the treatment of early Parkinson's disease: a 6-month interim report of a 5-year levodopa-controlled study. *Mov Disord* 1998;13:39–45.

214. Korczyn AD, Brunt ER, Larsen JP, et al. A 3-year randomized trial of ropinirole and bromocriptine in early Parkinson's disease. *Neurology* 1999;53:364–370.

215. Rascol O, Nutt JG, Blin O, et al. Induction by dopamine Da receptor agonist ABT-431 of dyskinesia similar to levodopa in patients with Parkinson disease. *Arch Neurol* 2001;58:249–254.

215a. Whone AL, Remy P, Davis MR, et al. The REAL-PET study: slower progression in early Parkinson's disease treated with ropinirole compared to L-dopa. *Neurology* 2002;58(Suppl 3):A82–A83.

216. Pinter MM, Pogarell O, Oertel WH. Efficacy, safety, and tolerance of the non-ergoline dopamine agonist pramipexole in the treatment of advanced Parkinson's disease: a double-blind, pacebo-controlled, randomised, multicentre study. *J Neurol Neurosurg Psychiatry* 1999;66:436–441.

217. Lieberman A, Ranhosky A, Korts D. Clinical evaluation of pramipexole in advanced Parkinson's disease: results of a dou-

ble-blind, placebo-controlled, parallel-group study. *Neurology* 1997;49:162–168.

218. Guttman M, and the International Pramipexole-Bromocriptine Study Group. Double-blind comparison of pramipexole and bromocriptine treatment with placebo in advanced Parkinson's disease. *Neurology* 1997;49:1060–1065.

219. Wynalda MA, Wienkers LC. Assessment of potential interactions between dopamine receptor agonists and various human cytochrome P450 enzymes using a simple in vitro inhibition screen. *Drug Metabolism and Disposition* 1997;25:1211–1214.

220. Hall ED, Andrus PK, Oostveen JA, et al. Neuroprotective effects of the dopamine D2/D3 agonist pramipexole against postischemic or methamphetamine-induced degeneration of nigrostriatal neurons. *Brain Res* 1996;742:80–88.

221. Le W, Jankovic J, Xie W, et al. (-)-Deprenyl protection of 1-methyl-4 phenyl-pyridium ion (MPP+)-induced apoptosis independent of MAO-B inhibition. *Neurosci Letters* 1997;224: 197–200.

222. Zou L, Jankovic J, Rowe DB, et al. Neuroprotection by pramipexole against dopamine- and levodopa-induced cytotoxicity. *Life Sci* 1999;64:1275–1285.

223. Tulloch IF. Pharmacologic profile of ropinirole: a nonergoline dopamine agonist. *Neurology* 1997;49[Suppl 1]:S58–S62.

224. Lieberman A, Olanow CW, Sethi K, et al. A multicenter trial of ropinirole as adjunct treatment for Parkinson's disease. *Neurology* 1998;51:1057–1062.

225. Guttman M, Stewart D, Hussey D, et al. Influence of L-dopa and pramipexole on striatal dopamine transporter in early PD. *Neurology* 2001;56:1559–1564.

226. Tan EK, Jankovic J. Choosing dopamine agonists in Parkinson's disease. *Clin Neuropharmacol* 2001;24:247–253.

227. Hanna PA, Ratkos L, Ondo WG, et al. Switching from pergolide to pramipexole in patients with Parkinson's disease. *J Neural Transm* 2001;108:63–70.

228. Caesi M, Antonini A, Mariani CB, et al. An overnight switch to ropinirole therapy in patients with Parkinson's disease. *J Neural Transmission* 1999;106:925–929.

229. Inzelberg R, Carasso RL, Schechtman E, et al. A comparison of dopamine agonists and catechol-*O*-methyltransferase inhibitors in Parkinson's disease. *Clin Neuropharmacol* 2000;5:262–266.

230. Frucht S, Rogers JD, Greene PE, et al. Falling asleep at the wheel: motor vehicle mishaps in persons taking pramipexole and ropinirole. *Neurology* 1999;52:1908–1910.

231. Hauser RA, Gauger L, Anderson WM, et al. Pramipexole-induced somnolence and episodes of daytime sleep. *Mov Disord* 2000;15:658–663.

232. Ferreira JJ, Galitzky M, Montastruc JL, et al. Sleep attacks and Parkinson's disease treatment. *Lancet* 2000;355:1333–1334.

233. Ondo WG, Vuong KV, Khan H, et al. Sleep disorders in patients with Parkinson's disease. *Neurology* 2001;57: 1392–1396.

234. Pal S, Bhattacharya KF, Agapito C, et al. A study of excessive daytime sleepiness and its clinical significance in three groups of Parkinson's disease patients taking pramipexole, cabergoline and levodopa mono and combination therapy. *J Neural Transm* 2001;108:71–77.

235. Larsen JP, Tandberg E. Sleep disorders in patients with Parkinson's disease: epidemiology and management. *CNS Drugs* 2001; 15:267–275.

236. Andreu N, Chale JJ, Senard JM, et al. L-Dopa-induced sedation: a double-blind cross-over controlled study versus triazolam and placebo in healthy volunteers. *Clin Neuropharmacol* 1999;22:15–23.

237. Tandberg E, Larsen JP, Karlsen K. Excessive daytime sleepiness and sleep benefit in Parkinson's disease: a community-based study. *Mov Disord* 1999;14:922–927.

238. Olanow CW, Schapira AHV, Roth T. Waking up to sleep episodes in Parkinson's disease. *Mov Disord* 2000;15:212–215.

239. Okura M, Honda K, Riehl J, et al. Roles of diencephalic dopaminergic cell groups in regulation of cataplexy in canine narcolepsy. *Sleep* 1999;22:S1.

240. Reyner LA, Horne JA. Falling asleep whilst driving: are drivers aware of prior sleepiness? *Int J Legal Med* 1998;111:120–123.

241. U.S. Modafinil in Narcolepsy Multicenter Study Group. Randomized trial of modafinil as a treatment for the excessive daytime somnolence of narcolepsy. *Neurology* 2000;54:1166–1175.

242. Hauser RA, Wahba MN, Anderson WM. Modafinil treatment of pramipexole-associated somnolence. *Mov Disord* 2000;15: 1269–1271.

243. Jenner P, Zeng BY, Smith LA, et al. Antiparkinsonian and neuroprotective effects of modafinil in the MPTP-treated common marmoset. *Exp Brain Res* 2000;133:178–188.

244. Van Laar T, Neef C, Danhof M, et al. A new sublingual formulation of apomorphine in the treatment of patients with Parkinson's disease. *Mov Disord* 1996;11:633–638.

245. Colzi A, Turner K, Lees AJ. Continuous subcutaneous waking day apomorphine in the long-term treatment of levodopa induced intredose dyskinesias in Parkinson's disease. *J Neurol Neurosurg Psychiatry* 1998;64:573–576.

246. Pietz K, Hagell P, Odin P. Subcutaneous apomorphine in late stage Parkinson's disease: a long-term follow-up. *J Neurol Neurosurg Psychiatry* 1998;65:709–716.

247. Dewey RB, Maraganore DM, Ahklskog JE, et al. A double-blind, placebo-controlled study of intranasal apomorphine spray as a rescue agent for "off" states in Parkinson's disease. *Mov Disord* 1998;13:782–787.

248. Dewey RB, Hutton JT, LeWitt PA, et al. A randomized, double-blind, placebo-controlled trial of subcutaneously injected apomrophine for parkinsonian off-state events. *Arch Neurol* 2001;58:1385–1392.

249. Poewe W, Wenning GK. Apomorphine: an underutilized therapy for Parkinson's disease. *Mov Disord* 2000;15:789–794.

250. Ondo W, Hunter C, Almaguer M, et al. Efficacy and tolerability of a novel sublingual apomorphine preparation in patients with fluctuating Parkinson's disease. *Clin Neuropharmacol* 1999; 22:1–4a.

251. Manson AJ, Hanagasi H, Turner K, et al. Intravenous apomorphine therapy in Parkinson's disease: clinical and pharmacokinetic observations. *Brain* 2001;124:331–340.

252. Ondo W, Hunter C, Almaguer M, et al. Sublingual apomorphine in patients with fluctuating Parkinson's disease. *Mov Disord* 1999;14:664–668b.

253. Grünblatt E, Mandel S, Berkuzki T, et al. Apomorphine protects against MPTP-induced neurotoxicity in mice. *Mov Disord* 1999;14:612–618.

254. Belluzi JD, Domino EF, May JM, et al. N-0923, a selective dopamine D2 receptor agonist, is efficacious in rat and monkey models of Parkinson's disease. *Mov Disord* 1994;9:147–154.

255. Hutton JT, Metman LV, Chase TN, et al. Transdermal dopaminergic D2 receptor agonist in Parkinson's disease with N-0923 TDS: a double-blind, placebo-controlled study. *Mov Disord* 2001;16:459–463.

256. Verhagen Metman L, Gillespie M, Farmer C, et al. Continuous transdermal dopaminergic stimulation in advanced Parkinson's disease. *Clin Neuropharmacol* 2001;24:163–169.

257. Calabrese VP, Lloyd KA, Brancazio P, et al. N-0923, a novel soluble dopamine D2 in the treatment of parkinsonism. *Mov Disord* 1998;13:768–774.

258. Battistin L, Bardin PG, Ferro-Milone F, et al. Alpha-dihydroergocryptine in Parkinson's disease: a multicenter randomized double parallel group study. *Acta Neurol Scand* 1999;99:36–42.

259. Bergamasco B, Frattola L, Muratorio A, et al. Alpha-dihydroer-

gocryptine in the treatment of de novo parkinsonian patients: results of a multicentre, randomized, double-blind, placebo-controlled study. *Acta Neurol Scand* 2000;101:372–380.

260. Montastruc JL, Ziegler M, Rascol O, et al. A randomized, double-blind study of a skin patch of a dopaminergic agonist, Piribedil, in Parkinson's disease. *Mov Disord* 1999;14:336–341.

261. Durham RA, Eaton MJ, Moore KE, et al. Effects of selective activation of dopamine D2 and D3 receptors on prolactin secretion and the activity of tuberoinfundibular dopamine neurons. *Eur J Pharmacol* 1997;17;335:37–42.

262. Feenstra R, Ronken E, Koopman T, et al. SLV308. *Drugs and Future* 2001;26:128–132.

263. Hely MA, Morris JGL, Reid WGJ, et al. The Sydney multicenter study of Parkinson's disease: a randomized, prospective five-year study comparing low dose bromocriptine with low dose levodopa-carbidopa. *J Neurol Neurosurg Psychiatry* 1994;57:903–910.

264. Grondin C, Goulet M, Di Paolo T, et al. Cabergoline, a long-acting D2 receptor agonist, produces a sustained antiparkinsonian effect with transient dyskinesias. *Brain Res* 1996;735:298–306.

265. Blanchet PJ, Calon F, Martel JC, et al. Continuous administration decreases and pulsatile administration increases behavioural sensitivity to a novel D-2 agonist (U-91356A) in MPTP monkeys. *J Pharmacol Exp Ther* 1995;272:854–859.

266. Montastruc JL, Rascol O, Senard JM, et al. A randomised controlled study comparing bromocriptine to which levodopa was later added, with levodopa alone in previously untreated patients with Parkinson's disease: a five-year follow-up. *J Neurol Neurosurg Psychiatry* 1994;57:1034–1038.

267. Barone P, Bravi D, Bernejo-Pareja F, et al. Pergolide monotherapy in the treatment of early PD: a randomized, controlled study. *Neurology* 1999;53:573–579.

268. Adler CH, Sethi KD, Hauser RA, et al. Ropinirole for the treatment of early Parkinson's disease. *Neurology* 1997;49:393–399.

269. Sethi KD, O'Brien CF, Hammerstad JP, et al. Ropinirole for the treatment of early Parkinson disease: a 12-month experience. *Arch Neurol* 1998;55:1211–1216.

270. Olanow CW, Fahn S, Muenter M, et al. A multicenter double-blind placebo-controlled trial of pergolide as an adjunct to Sinemet in Parkinson's disease. *Mov Disord* 1994;9:40–47.

271. Huang X, Lawler CP, Lewis MM, et al. D1 dopamine receptors. *Int Rev Neurobiology* 2001;48:65–139.

272. Yoshimura N, Mizuta E, Kuno S, et al. The dopamine D-1 receptor agonist SKF 38303 suppresses detrusor hyperreflexia in the monkey with parkinsonism induced by 1-methyl-4-phenyl-1,2,3,6-tetrahydropyridine (MPTP). *Neuropharmacology* 1993;32:315–321.

273. Mailman R, Huang X, Nichols DE. Parkinson's disease and D1 dopamine receptors. *Curr Opin Invest Drugs* 2001;2:1582–1591.

274. Shiosaki K, Jenner P, Asin KE, et al. ABT-431: the diacetyl prodrug of A-86929, a potent and selective dopamine D1 receptor agonist—in vitro characterization and effects in animal models of Parkinson's disease. *J Pharmacol Exp Ther* 1996;276:150–160.

275. Rascol O, Blin O, Thalamas C, et al. ABT-431, a D1 receptor agonist has efficacy in Parkinson's disease. *Ann Neurol* 1999;45:736–741.

276. Gulwadi AG, Korpinen CD, Mailman RB, et al. Dinapsoline: characterization of a D1 dopamine receptor agonist in a rat model of Parkinson's disease. *J Pharmacol Exp Ther* 2001;296:338–344.

277. Grondin R, Doan VD, Gregoire L, et al. D1 receptor blockade improves L-dopa-induced dyskinesia but worsens parkinsonism in MPTP monkeys. *Neurology* 1999;52:771–776.

278. Bravi D, Nohria V, Megas LF. Dopamine agonists in the clini-

cal management of Parkinson's disease: symptomatic or neuroprotective treatment? *Eur J Neurol* 1996;3[Suppl 1]:13–18.

279. Olanow CW. Dopamine agonists as initial symptomatic treatment for Parkinson's disease. *Eur J Neurol* 1997;4[Suppl 3]:S13–S18.

280. Le W-D, Jankovic J. Are dopamine receptor agonists neuroprotective in Parkinson's disease? *Drugs Aging* 2001;18:389–396.

281. Ogawa N, Tanaka K, Asanuma M, et al. Bromocriptine protects mice against 6-hydroxy-dopamine and scavenges hydroxyl free radical in vitro. *Brain Res* 1994;657:207–213.

282. Yoshikawa T, Minamiyama Y, Naito Y, et al. Antioxidant properties of bromocriptine, a dopamine agonist. *J Neurochem* 1994;62:1034–1038.

283. Nishibayashi S, Asanuma M, Kohno M, et al. Scavenging effects of dopamine agonists on nitric oxide radicals. *J Neurochem* 1996;67:2208–2211.

284. Gassen M, Gross A, Youdim MBH. Apomorphine enantiomers protect cultured pheochromocytoma (PC12) cells from oxidative stress induced by H_2O_2 and 6-hydroxydopamine. *Mov Disord* 1998;13:242–248.

285. Gomez-Vargas M, Nishibayashi-Asanuma S, Asanuma S, et al. Pergolide scavenges both hydroxyl and nitric oxide free radicals in vitro and inhibits lipid peroxidation in different regions of the rat brain. *Brain Res* 1998;790:202–208.

286. Clow A, Freestone C, Lewis E, et al. The effect of pergolide and MDL 72974 on rat brain CuZn superoxide dismutase. *Neurosci Lett* 1993;164:41–43.

287. Sawada H, Ibi M, Kihara T, et al. Dopamine D2-type agonists protect mesencephalic neurons from glutamate neurotoxicity: mechanisms of neuroprotective treatment against oxidative stress. *Ann Neurol* 1998;44:110–119.

288. Carvey PM, Pieri S, Ling ZD. Attenuation of levodopa-induced toxicity in mesencephalic cultures by pramipexole. *J Neural Transm* 1997;104:209–228.

289. Cassarino DS, Fall CP, Smith TS, et al. Pramipexole reduces reactive oxygen species production in vivo and in vitro and inhibits the mitochondrial permeability transition produced by the parkinsonian neurotoxin methylpyridinium ion. *J Neurochem* 1998;71:295–301.

290. Tanak K, Miyazaki I, Fujita N, et al. Molecular mechanism in activation of glutathione system by ropinirole, a selective dopamine D2 agonist. *Neurochem Res* 2001;26:31–36.

291. Felten DL, Felten SY, Fuller RW, et al. Chronic dietary pergolide preserves nigrostriatal neuronal integrity in aged-Fischer-344 rats. *J Biol Aging* 1992;13:339–351.

292. Lees AJ, Katzenschlager R, Head J, et al. Ten-year follow-up of three different initial treatments in de-novo PD: a randomized trial. *Neurology* 2001;57:1687–1694.

293. Jankovic J. Parkinsonian syndromes. In: Kurlan R, ed. *Treatment of movement disorders.* Philadelphia: JB Lippincott, 1995:95–114.

294. Pal PK, Calne S, Samii A, et al. A review of normal sleep and its disturbances in Parkinson's disease. *Parkinsonism Relat Disord* 1999;5:1–17.

295. Aarsland D, Larsen JP, Lim NG, et al. Range of neuropsychiatric disturbances in patients with Parkinson's disease. *J Neurol Neurosurg Psychiatry* 1999;67:492–496.

296. Friedman JH, Fernandez HH. The nonmotor problems of Parkinson's disease. *Neurologist* 2000;6:18–27.

297. Pact V, Giduz T. Mirtazapine treats resting tremor, essential tremor, and levodopa-induced dyskinesias. *Neurology* 1999;53:1154.

298. Comella CL, Nardine TM, Diederich NJ, et al. Sleep-related violence, injury, and REM sleep behavior disorder in Parkinson's disease. *Neurology* 1998;51:526–529.

299. Bushara KA. Sialorrhea in amyotrophic lateral sclerosis: a

hypothesis of a new treatment—botulinum toxin A injections of the parotid glands. *Med Hypotheses* 1997;48:337–339.

300. Pal PK, Calne DB, Calne S, et al. Botulinum—a toxin in the treatment of sialorrhea in patients with Parkinson's disease. *Parkinsonism Relat Disord* 1999;5:S82.

301. Bhatia KP, Münchau A, Brown P. Botulinum toxin is a useful treatment in excessive drooling of saliva. *J Neurol Neurosurg Psychiatry* 1999;67:697.

302. Hunter PC, Crameri J, Austin S, et al. Response of parkinsonian swallowing dysfunction to dopaminergic stimulation. *J Neurol Neurosurg Psychiatry* 1997;63:579–583.

303. Ashraf W, Pfeiffer RF, Park F, et al. Constipation in Parkinson's disease: objective assessment and response to psyllium. *Mov Disord* 1997;12:946–951.

304. Ford B, Louis ED, Greene P, et al. Oral and genital pain syndromes in Parkinson's disease. *Mov Disord* 1996;11:421–426.

305. Scientific Committee of the First International Consultation on Incontinence. Assessment and treatment of urinary incontinence. *Lancet* 2000;355:2153–2158.

306. Zesiewicz TA, Helal M, Hauser RA. Sildenafil citrate (Viagra) for the treatment of erectile dysfunction in men with Parkinson's disease. *Mov Disord* 2000;15:305–308.

307. Hussain IF, Brady CM, Swinn MJ, et al. Treatment of erectile dysfunction with sildenafil citrate (Viagra) in parkinsonism due to Parkinson's disease or multiple system atrophy with observations on orthostatic hypotension. *J Neurol Neurosurg Psychiatry* 2001;71:371–374.

308. Hagell P, Odin P, Vinge E. Pregnancy in Parkinson's disease: a review of the literature and a case report. *Mov Disord* 1998;13:34–38.

309. Woofter MJ, Manyam BV. Safety of long-term levodopa therapy in malignant melanoma. *Clin Neuropharmacol* 1994;17:315–319.

310. Pfutzner W, Przybilla B. Malignant melanoma and levodopa: is there a relationship? Two new cases and a review of the literature. *J Am Acad Dermatol* 1997;37:332–336.

311. Bonnet A-M. Involvement of non-dopaminergic pathways in Parkinson's disease: pathophysiology and therapeutic implications. *CNS Drugs* 2000;13:351–364.

312. Kompoliti K, Wang QE, Goetz CG, et al. Effects of central dopaminergic stimulation by apomorphine on speech in Parkinson's disease. *Neurology* 2000;54:458–462.

313. Shoulson I, and the Parkinson Study Group. DATATOP: a decade of neuroprotective inquiry. *Ann Neurol* 1998;44[Suppl 1]:S160–S166.

314. Knoll J. The pharmacological profile of (-) deprenyl (Selegiline) and its relevance for humans: a personal view. *Pharmacol Toxicol* 1992;70:317–321.

315. Mercuri NB, Scarponi M, Bonci A, et al. Monoamine oxidase inhibition causes a long-term prolongation of the dopamine-induced responses in rat midbrain dopaminergic cells. *J Neurosci* 1997;17:2267–2272.

316. Freeman H. Moclobemide. *Lancet* 1993;342:1528–1532.

317. Hubble JP, Koller WC, Waters C. Effects of selegiline dosing on motor fluctuations in Parkinson's disease. *Clin Neuropharmacol* 1993;16:83–87.

318. Parkinson Study Group. Effect of deprenyl on the progression of disability in early Parkinson's disease. *N Engl J Med* 1989;321:1364–1371.

319. Parkinson Study Group. Effects of tocopherol and deprenyl on the progression of disability in early Parkinson's disease. *N Engl J Med* 1993;328:176–183a.

320. Palhagen S, Heinonen EH, Hagglund J, et al. Selegiline delays the onset of disability in de novo parkinsonian patients. *Neurology* 1998;51:520–525.

321. Brannan T, Yahr MD. Comparative study of selegiline plus L-dopa-carbidopa versus L-dopa-carbidopa alone in the treatment of Parkinson's disease. *Ann Neurol* 1995;37:95–98.

322. Parkinson Study Group. Impact of deprenyl and tocopherol treatment on Parkinson's disease in DATATOP patients not requiring levodopa. *Ann Neurol* 1996;39:29–36a.

323. Tatton WG, Chalmers-Redman RME. Mitochondria in neurodegenerative apoptosis: an opportunity for therapy? *Ann Neurol* 1998;44[Suppl 1]:S134–S141.

324. Ansari KS, Yu PH, Kruck TP, et al. Rescue of axotomized immature rat facial motoneurons by R(-)-deprenyl: stereospecificity and independence from monoamine oxidase inhibition. *J Neurosci* 1993;13:4042–4053.

325. Tatton WG. Selegiline can mediate neuronal rescue rather than neuronal protection. *Mov Disord* 1993;8:S20–S30.

326. Carrillo MC, Kanai S, Sato Y, et al. The optimal dosage of (-) deprenyl for increasing superoxide dismutase activities in several brain regions decreases with age in male Fischer 344 rats. *Life Sci* 1993;52:1925–1934b.

327. Kuhn W, Müller Th, Krüger R, et al. Selegiline stimulates biosynthesis of cytokines interleukin-1 beta and interleukin-6. *Neuroreport* 1996;7:2847–2848.

328. Ju WYH, Hollan DP, Tatton WG. (-)Deprenyl alters the time course of death of axotomized facial motoneurons and the hypertrophy of neighboring astrocytes in immature rats. *Exp Neurol* 1994;126:1–14.

329. Biagini G, Zoli M, Fuxe K, et al. L-deprenyl increases GFAP immunoreactivity selectively in activated astrocytes in rat brain. *Neuroreport* 1993;4:955–958.

330. Lindsay RM, Wiegand SJ, Altar CA, et al. Neurotrophic factors: from molecule to man. *TINS* 1994;17:182–190.

331. Tatton WG, Holland DP, Ju WYL, et al. Blockade of PC12 cell apoptosis by (-)-deprenyl requires new protein synthesis. *J Neurochem* 1994;63:1572–1575.

332. Olanow CW, Myllylä VV, Sotaniemi KA, et al. Effect of selegiline on mortality in patients with Parkinson's disease: a meta-analysis. *Neurology* 1998;1998;51:825–830.

333. Miller RJ. Mitochondrial—the Kraken wakes! *TINS* 1998;21:95–97.

334. Reed JC. Double identity for proteins of the Bcl-2 family. *Nature* 1997;387:773–776.

335. McDermott MP, Jankovic J, Carter J, et al. Factors predictive of the need for levodopa therapy in early, untreated Parkinson's disease. *Arch Neurol* 1995;52:565–570.

336. Olanow CW, Hauser RA, Gauger L, et al. The effect of deprenyl and levodopa on the progression of Parkinson's disease. *Ann Neurol* 1995;38:771–777.

337. Rinne JO, Roytta M, Paljarvi L, et al. Selegiline (deprenyl) treatment and death of nigral neurons in Parkinson's disease. *Neurology* 1991;41:859–861.

338. Van Hilten JJ, Bloem BR, Klaassen AAG. Deprenyl's neuroprotective action remains unresolved. *Ann Neurol* 1996;40:266.

339. Elizan TS, Moros DA, Yahr MD. Early combination of selegiline and low-dose levodopa as initial symptomatic therapy in Parkinson's disease. *Arch Neurol* 1991;48:31–34.

340. Myllylä VV, Sotaniemi KA, Hakulinen P, et al. Selegiline as the primary treatment of Parkinson's disease: a long-term double-blind study. *Acta Neurol Scand* 1997;95:211–288.

341. Jankovic J. Neuroprotection: a reachable therapeutic goal? In: Stern MB, ed. *Beyond the decade of the brain.* Kent, UK: Wells Medical Ltd, 1994:109–130.

342. Ward CD. Does selegiline delay progression of Parkinson's disease? A critical reevaluation of the DATATOP study. *J Neurol Neurosurg Psychiatry* 1994;57:217–220.

343. Lees AJ, and the Parkinson's Disease Research Group of the United Kingdom. Comparison of therapeutic effects and mortality data of levodopa and levodopa combined with selegeline

in patients with early, mild Parkinson's disease. *BMJ* 1995;311: 1602–1607.

344. Calne DB. Selegiline in Parkinson's disease. *BMJ* 1995;311: 1583–1584.

345. Lees AJ, Head J, Ben-Shlomo Y. Selegiline and mortality in Parkinson's disease: another view. *Ann Neurol* 1997;41: 282–283.

346. Olanow CW, Godbold JH, Koller W. Patients taking selegiline may have received more levodopa than necessary. *BMJ* 1996; 312:702–703.

347. Olanow CW, Fahn S, Langston JW, et al. Selegiline and mortality in Parkinson's disease. *Ann Neurol* 1996;40:841–845.

348. Olanow CW, Jenner P, Tatton NA, et al. Neurodegeneration and Parkinson's disease. In: Jankovic J, Tolosa E, eds. *Parkinson's disease and movement disorders,* 3rd ed. Baltimore: Williams & Wilkins, 1998:67–104.

349. Donnan PT, Steinke DT, Stubbings C, et al. Selegiline and mortality in subjects with PD: a longitudinal community study. *Neurology* 2000;55:1785–1788.

350. Richard IH, Kurlan R, Tanner C, et al. Serotonin syndrome and the combined use of deprenyl and an antidepressant in Parkinson's disease. *Neurology* 1997;48:1070.

351. Waldmeier PC, Boulton AA, Cools AR, et al. Neurorescuing effects of the GAPDH ligand CGP 3466B. *J Neural Transm* 2000;[Suppl]60:197–214.

352. Parkinson Study Group. A controlled trial of lazabemide (Ro19-6327) in untreated Parkinson's disease. *Ann Neurol* 1993;33:350–356b.

353. Fahn S, Chouinard S. Experience with tranylcypromine in early Parkinson's disease. *J Neural Transm* 1998;[Suppl]52:49–61.

354. Lamensdorf I, Youdim MBH, Finberg JPM. Effect of long-term treatment with selective monoamine oxidase A and B inhibitors on dopamine release from rat striatum in vivo. *J Neurochem* 1996;67:1532–1539.

355. Finberg JP, Lamensdorf I, Commissiong JW, et al. Pharmacology and neuroprotective properties of rasagiline. *J Neural Transmission* 1996;[Suppl 48]:95–101.

356. Finberg JPM, Takeshima T, Johnston JM, et al. Increased survival of dopaminergic neurons by rasagiline, a monoamine oxidase B inhibitor. *Neuroreport* 1998;9:703–707.

357. Rabey JM, Sagi I, Huberman M, et al. for the Rasagiline Study Group. Rasagiline mesylate, a new MAO-B inhibitor for the treatment of Parkinson's disease: a double-blind study as adjunctive therapy to levodopa. *Clin Neuropharmacol* 2000;23: 324–330.

358. Delanty N, Dichter MA. Antioxidant therapy in neurologic disease. *Arch Neurol* 2000;57:1265–1270.

359. Chase TN, Oh JD. Striatal dopamine- and glutamate-mediated dysregulation in experimental parkinsonism. *TINS* 2000;23 [Suppl]:S86–S91.

360. Greenamyre JT. Pharmacologic pallidotomy with glutamate antagonists. *Ann Neurol* 1996;39:537–538.

361. Parkinson Study Group. A randomized, controlled trial of remacemide for motor complication in Parkinson's disease. *Neurology* 2001;56:455–462b.

362. Bergman H, Wichmann T, DeLong MR. Reversal of experimental parkinsonism by lesions of the subthalamic nucleus. *Science* 1990;249:1436–1438.

363. Greenamyre JT, Eller RV, Zhang Z, et al. Antiparkinsonian effects of remacemide hydrochloride, a glutamate antagonist, in rodent and primate models of Parkinson's disease. *Ann Neurol* 1994;35:655–661.

364. Nakao N, Nakai E, Nakai K, et al. Ablation of the subthalamic nucleus supports the survival of nigral dopaminergic neurons after nigrostriatal lesions induced by the mitochondrial toxin 3-nitropropionic acid. *Ann Neurol* 1999;45:640–651.

365. Verhagen Metman LV, Dotto Del P, Natte R, et al. Dextromethorphan improved levodopa-induced dyskinesias in Parkinson's disease. *Neurology* 1998;51:203–206.

366. Luginger E, Wenning GK, Bösch S, et al. Beneficial effects of amantadine on L-Dopa–induced dyskinesias in Parkinson's disease. *Mov Disord* 2000;15:873–878.

367. Uitti RJ, Rajput AH, Ahlskog JE, et al. Amantadine treatment is an independent predictor of improved survival in Parkinson's disease. *Neurology* 1996;46:1551–1556.

368. Rabey JM, Nissipeanu P, Korczyn AD. Efficacy of memantine, an NMDA receptor antagonist, in the treatment of Parkinson's disease. *J Neurol Transm Park Dis Dement Sect* 1992;4:277–282.

369. Klockgether T, Jacobsen P, Löschmann PA, et al. The antiparkinsonian agent budipine as an N-methyl-D-aspartate antagonist. *J Neurol Transm Park Dis Dement Sect* 1993;5: 101–106.

370. Fox SH, Nash JE, Hill MP, et al. A novel therapeutic approach to the treatment of Parkinson's disease based on blockade of NR2B containing NMDA receptors in the striatum. *J Neurol Neurosurg Psychiatry* 1998;65:416(abst).

371. Brown RH. Superoxide dismutase and familial amyotrophic lateral sclerosis: new insights into mechanisms and treatments. *Ann Neurol* 1996;39:145–146.

372. Gurney ME, Cutting FB, Zhai P, et al. Benefit of vitamin E, riluzole, and gabapentin in transgenic model of familial amyotrophic lateral sclerosis. *Ann Neurol* 1996;39:147–157.

373. Gurney ME, Fleck TJ, Hines S, et al. Riluzole preserves motor function in a trangenic model of familial amyotrophic lateral sclerosis. *Neurology* 1998;50:62–66.

374. Barnéoud P, Mazadier M, Miquet J-M, et al. Neuroprotective effects of riluzole on a model of Parkinson's disease in the rat. *Neuroscience* 1996;74:971–983.

375. Benazzouz A, Boraud T, Dubedat P, et al. Riluzole prevents MPTP-induced parkinsonism in the rhesus monkey: a pilot study. *Eur J Pharmacol* 1995;284:299–307.

376. Merims D, Ziv I, Djaldetti R, et al. Riluzole for levodopa-induced dyskinesias in advanced Parkinson's disease. *Lancet* 1999;353:1764–1765.

377. Jankovic J, Hunter C. A double-blind, placebo-controlled and longitudinal study to assess safety and efficacy of riluzole in early Parkinson's disease. *Parkinsonism Rel Disord* 2002;8: 271–277.

378. Shimotoh H, Vingerhoets FJG, Lee CS, et al. Lamotrigine trial in idiopathic parkinsonism: a double-blind, placebo-controlled crossover study. *Neurology* 1997;48:1282–1285.

379. Lapchak PA. A preclinical development strategy designed to optimize the use of glial cell line–derived neurotrophic factor in the treatment of Parkinson's disease. *Mov Disord* 1998;13[Suppl 1]:49–54.

380. Gash DM, Zhang Z, Gerhardt G. Neuroprotective and neurorestorative properties of GDNF. *Ann Neurol* 1998;44[Suppl 1]:S121–S125.

381. Tseng JL, Baetge EE, Zurn AD, et al. GDNF reduces drug-induced rotational behavior after medial forebrain bundle transection by a mechanism not involving striatal dopamine. *J Neurosci* 1997;17:325–333.

382. Choi-Lundberg DL, Lin Q, Chang Y-N, et al. Dopaminergic neurons protected from degeneration by GDNF gene therapy. *Science* 1997;275:838–841.

383. Gash DM, Zhang Z, Ovadia A, et al. Functional recovery in parkinsonian monkeys treated with GDNF. *Nature* 1996;380: 252–255.

384. Miyoshi Y, Zhang Z, Ovadia A, et al. Glial cell line-derived neurotrophic factor–levodopa interactions and reduction of side effects in parkinsonian monkeys. *Ann Neurol* 1997;42: 208–214.

385. Nutt JG, Comella C, Jankovic J, et al. Intraventricular administration of GDNF in the treatment of Parkinson's disease. *Neurology* 2002 (in press).

386. Kordower JH, Palfi S, Chen E-Y, et al. Clinicopathological findings following intraventricular glial-derived neurotrophic factor treatment in a patient with Parkinson's disease. *Ann Neurol* 1999;46:419–424.

387. Kordower JH, Emborg ME, Bloch J, et al. Neurodegeneration prevented by lentiviral vector delivery of GDNF in primate models of Parkinson's disease. *Science* 2000;290:767–773.

388. Kuhn W, Müller T, Nstos I, et al. The neuroimmune hypothesis in Parkinson's disease. *Rev Neurosci* 1997;8:29–34.

389. Bas A, Veld I, Ruitenberg A, et al. Nonsteroidal anti-inflammatory drugs and the risk of Alzheimer's disease. *N Engl J Med* 2001;345:1515–1521.

390. Teismann P, Ferger B. Inhibition of the cyclooxygenase isoenzymes COX-1 and COX-2 provide neuroprotection in the MPTP-mouse model of Parkinson's disease. *Synapse* 2001;39:167–174.

391. Klausner JD, Freedman VH, Kaplan G. Thalidomide as an anti-TNF-α inhibitor: implications for clinical use. *J Immunol Immunopathol* 1996;81:219–223.

392. Zwingenberger K, Wnendt S. Immunomodulation by thalidomide: systematic review of the literature and of unpublished observations. *J Inflam* 1996;46:177–211.

393. Rajora N, Boccoli G, Burns D, et al. α-MSH modulates local and circulating tumor necrosis factor-α in experimental brain inflammation. *J Neurosci* 1997;17:2181–2186.

394. Snyder SH, Sabatini DM, Lai MM, et al. Neural actions of immunophilin ligands. *Trends Pharmacol Sci* 1998;19:21–26.

395. Guo X, Dillman JF, Dawson VL, et al. Neuroimmunophilins: novel neuroprotective and neurodegenerative targets. *Ann Neurol* 2001;50:6–16.

396. Steiner JP, Hamilton GS, Ross DT, et al. Neurotrophic immunophilin ligands stimulate structural and functional recovery in neurodegenerative animal models. *Proc Natl Acad Sci USA* 1997;94:2019–2024.

397. Gold BG, Zeleny-Pooley M, Chaturverdi P, et al. Oral administration of a nonimmunosuppressant FKBP-12 ligand speeds nerve regeneration. *Neuroreport* 1998;9:553–558.

398. Harper S, Bilsland J, Young L, et al. Analysis of the neurotrophic effects of GPI-1046 on neuron survival and regeneration in culture and in vivo. *Neuroscience* 1999;88:257–267.

399. Mogi M, Togari A, Kondo T, et al. Caspase activities and tumor necrosis factor receptor R1 (p55) level are elevated in the substantia nigra from parkinsonian brain. *J Neural Transm* 2000;107:335–341.

400. Tatton NA. Increased caspase 3 and Bax immunoreactivity accompany nuclear GAPDH translocation and neuronal apoptosis in Parkinson's disease. *Exp Neurol* 2000;166:29–43.

401. Chen M, Ona VO, Li M, et al. Minocycline inhibits caspase-1 and caspase-3 expression and delays mortality in a transgenic mouse model of Huntington disease. *Nat Med* 2000;6:797–801.

402. Yamamoto A, Lucas JJ, Hen R. Reversal of neuropathology and motor dysfunction in a conditional model of Huntington's disease. *Cell* 2000;101:57–66.

403. Tikka T, Fiebich BL, Goldsteins G, et al. Minocycline, a tetracycline derivative, is neuroprotective against excitotoxicity by inhibiting and proliferation of microglia. *J Neuroscience* 2001;21:2580–2588.

404. He Y, Appel S, Le W. Minocycline inhibits microglial activation and protects nigral cells after 6-hydroxydopamine injection into mouse striatum. *Brain Res* 2001;909(1–2):187–193.

405. Gleiter CH, Nilsson E, Muhlbauer B, et al. Effective selective MAO-A inhibitors brofaromine, clorgyline and moclobenide on human platelet MAO-B activity. *J Neural Transm* 1992;89:129–133.

406. Hall ED. Lazaroids: mechanisms of action and implications for disorders of the CNS. *Neuroscientist* 1997;2:42–51.

407. Aubin N, Curet O, Deffois A, et al. Aspirin and salicylate protect against MPTP-induced dopamine depletion in mice. *J Neurochem* 1998;71:1635–1642.

408. Ferger B, Teisman P, Earl CD, et al. Salicylate protects against MPTP-induced impairments in dopaminergic transmission at the striatal and nigral level in mice. *Naunyn-Schmiedeberg's Arch Pharmacol* 1999;360:256–261.

409. Matthews RT, Yang L, Browne S, et al. Coenzyme Q10 administration increases brain mitochondrial concentrations and exerts neuroprotective effects. *Proc Natl Acad Sci USA* 1998;95:8892–8897.

410. Shults CW, Beal FM, Fontaine D, et al. Absorption, tolerability, and effects on mitochondrial activity of oral coenzyme Q10 in parkinsonian patients. *Neurology* 1998;50:793–795.

411. Martinez M, Marinez N, Hernandez AI, et al. Can N-acetylcysteine be beneficial in Parkinson's disease? *Life Sci* 1999;64:1253–1257.

412. Uhl G. Neurotransmitter transporters (plus): a promising new gene family. *Trends Neurosci* 1992;15:265–271.

413. Maroney AC, Glicksman MA, Basma AN, et al. Motoneuron apoptosis is blocked by CEP-1347 (KT 7515), a novel inhibitor of the JNK signaling pathway. *J Neurosci* 1998;18:104–111.

414. Saporito MS, Brown EM, Miller MS, et al. CEP-1347/KT-7515, an inhibitor of c-jun N-terminal kinase activation, attenuates the 1-methyl-4-phenyl tetrahydropyridine-mediated loss of nigrostriatal dopaminergic neurons in vivo. *J Pharmacol Exp Ther* 1999;288:421–427.

415. Daniele A, Albanese A, Gainotti G, et al. Zolpidem in Parkinson's disease. *Lancet* 1997;349:1222–1223.

416. Schneider JS, Roeltgen DP, Mancall EL, et al. Parkinson's disease: improved function with GM1 ganglioside treatment in a randomized placebo-controlled study. *Neurology* 1998;50:1630–1636.

417. Rathbone MP, Middlesmiss PJ, Gysbers J, et al. Physiology and pharmacology of natural and synthetic nonadenine-based purines in the nervous system. *Drug Develop Research* 1998;45:356–372.

418. Vescovi AL, Snyder EY. Establishment and properties of neural stem cell clones: plasticity in vitro and in vivo. *Brain Pathology* 1999;9:569–598.

419. Wakayama T, Tabar V, Rodriguez I, et al. Differentiation of embryonic stem cell lines generated from adult somatic cells by nuclear transfer. *Science* 2001;292:740–743.

420. Levites Y, Weinreb O, Maor G, et al. Green tea polyphenol (-)-epigallocatechin-3-gallate prevents N-methyl-4-phenyl-1,2,3,6-tetrahydropyridine-induced dopaminergic neurodegeneration. *J Neurochem* 2001;78:1073–1082.

421. Betarbet R, Sherer TB, MacKenzie G, et al. Chronic systemic pesticide exposure reproduces features of Parkinson's disease. *Nat Neurosci* 2002;3:1301–1306.

422. Le WD, Conneely OM, He Y, et al. Reduced Nurr1 expression increases the vulnerability of mesencephalic dopamine neurons to MPTP-induced injury. *J Neurochem* 1999;73:2218–2221.

423. Morrish PK, Rakshi JS, Brooks DJ. Can the neuroprotective efficacy of an agent ever be conclusively proven? *E J Neurol* 1997;4[Suppl 3]:S19–S24.

424. Louis ED, Tang MX, Cote L, et al. Progression of parkinsonian signs in Parkinson disease. *Arch Neurol* 1999;56:334–337.

425. Jankovic J, Kapadia AS. Functional decline in Parkinson's disease. *Arch Neurol* 2001;58:1611–1615.

426. Jankovic J. Surgery for Parkinson's disease and other movement disorders: benefits and limitations of ablation, stimulation, restoration, and radiation. *Arch Neurol* 2001;58:1970–1972.

427. Krauss JK, Jankovic J, Grossman RG, eds. *Surgery for movement disorders.* Philadelphia: Lippincott Williams & Wilkins, 2001.

428. Pascual-Leone A, Rubio B, Pallardo F, Catala MD. Rapid-rate transcranial magnetic stimulation of left dorsolateral prefrontal cortex in drug-resistant depression. *Lancet* 1996;347:233–237.

429. Lance JW, Hickie I, Wakefiled D, et al. An akinetic-rigid syndrome, depression, and stereotypies in a young man. *Mov Disord* 1998;13:835–844.

430. Ghabra MB, Hallett M, Wassermann EM. Simultaneous repetitive transcranial magnetic stimulation does not speed fine movement in PD. *Neurology* 1999;52:768–770.

431. Canavero S, Paolotti R. Extradural motor cortex stimulation for advanced Parkinson's disease: a case report. *Mov Disord* 2000; 15:169–171.

432. Comella CL, Stebbins GT, Brown-Toms N, et al. Physical therapy and Parkinson's disease: a controlled clinical trial. *Neurology* 1994;44:376–378.

433. Protas EJ, Stanley R, Jankovic J, MacNeill B. Cardiovascular and metabolic responses to upper and lower extremity exercise in men with idiopathic Parkinson's disease. *Phys Ther* 1996;76:34–40.

434. Reuter I, Engelhardt M, Stecker K, et al. Therapeutic value of exercise training in Parkinson's disease. *Med Sci Sports Exerc* 1999;31:1544–1549

435. Marchese R, Diverio M, Zucchi F, et al. The role of sensory cues in the rehabilitation of parkinsonian patients: a comparison of two physical therapy protocols. *Mov Disord* 2001;15:879–883.

436. Thompson AJ, Playford ED. Rehabilitation for patients with Parkinson's disease. *Lancet* 2001;357:410–411.

437. Ramig LO, Countryman S, O'Brien C, et al. Intensive speech treatment for patients with Parkinson's disease: short- and long-term comparison of two techniques. *Neurology* 1996;47: 1496–1504.

438. Ramig LO, Sapir S, Fox C, et al. Changes in vocal loudness following intensive voice treatment (LSVT®) in individuals with Parkinson's disease: a comparison with untreated patients and normal age-matched controls. *Mov Disord* 2001;16:79–83.

439. Ho AK, Bradshaw JL, Iansek R, et al. Speech volume regulation in Parkinson's disease: effects of implicit cues and explicit instructions. *Neuropsychologia* 1999;37:1453–1460

440. Berke GS, Gerrast B, Kreiman J, et al. Treatment of parkinson hypothonia with percutaneous collagen augmentation. *Laryngoscope* 1999;109:1295–1299.

441. Schneider JS, Van Velson M, Menzaghi F, et al. Effects of the nicotinic acetylcholine receptor agonist SIB-1508Y on object retrieval performance in MPTP-treated monkeys: comparison with levodopa treatment. *Ann Neurol* 1998;43:311–317.

442. Newhouse PA, Potter A, Levin ED. Nicotinic system involvement in Alzheimer's and Parkinson's diseases: implications for therapeutics. *Drugs Aging* 1997;11:206–228.

443. Pidoplichko VI, DeBiasi M, Williams JT, et al. Nicotine activates and desensitizes midbrain dopamine neurons. *Nature* 1997;390:401–404.

444. Tzourio C, Rocca WA, Breteler MM, et al. Smoking and Parkinson's disease: an age-dependent risk effect. *Neurology* 1997;49:1267–1272.

445. Linert W, Bridge MH, Huber M, et al. In vitro and in vivo studies investigating possible antioxidant actions of nicotine: relevance to Parkinson's and Alzheimer's diseases. *Biochim Biophys Acta* 1999;1454:143–152.

446. Vieregge A, Sieberer M, Jacobs H, et al. Transdermal nicotine in PD: a randomized, double-blind, placebo-controlled study. *Neurology* 2001;57:1032–1035.

447. Ebersbach G, Stock M, Muller J, et al. Worsening of motor performance in patients with Parkinson's disease following transdermal nicotine administration. *Mov Disord* 1999;14: 1011–1013.

448. Richardson PJ, Kase H, Jenner PG. Adenosine A$_{2A}$ receptor antagonists as new agents for the treatment of Parkinson's disease. *TIPS* 1997;18:338–344.

449. Grondin R, Bédard PJ, Tahar H, et al. Antiparkinsonian effect of a new selective adenosine A$_{2A}$ receptor antagonist in MPTP-treated monkeys. *Neurology* 1999;52:1673–1677.

450. Svetel M, Sternic N, Kostic V, et al. Antiparkinsonian effects of adenosine antagonist in de novo and advanced Parkinson's patients. *Ann Neurol* 1998;44:501(abst.).

451. Kostic VS, Svetel M, Sternic N, et al. Theophyllin increases "on" time in advanced parkinsonian patients. *Neurology* 1999; 52:1916.

452. Li M, Ona VO, Guegan C, et al. Functional role of caspase-1 and caspase-3 in ALS transgenic mouse model. *Science* 2000; 288:335–339.

453. Friedlander RM. Role of caspase 1 in neurologic disease. *Arch Neurol* 2000;57:1273–1276.

454. Levey AI. Immunization for Alzheimer's disease: a shot in the arm or a whiff? *Ann Neurol* 2000;48:553–555.

455. Weiner HL, Lemere C, Maron R, et al. Nasal administration of amyloid-β peptide decreases cerebral amyloid burden in a mouse model of Alzheimer's disease. *Ann Neurol* 2000;48: 567–579.

456. Latchman DS, Coffin RS. Viral vectors in the treatment of Parkinson's disease. *Mov Disord* 2000;15:9–17.

457. Kang UJ, Isacson O. The potentials of gene therapy for treatment of Parkinson's disease. In: Krauss JK, Jankovic J, Grossman RG, eds. *Surgery for movement disorders.* Philadelphia: Lippincott Williams & Wilkins, 2000.

458. Leff SE, Spratt SK, Snyder RO, et al. Long-term restoration of striatal L-aromatic amino acid decarboxylase activity using recombinant adeno-associated vector gene transfer in a rodent model of Parkinson's disease. *Neuroscience* 1999;92:185–196.

459. Studer L, Tabar V, McKay RDG. Transplantation of expanded mesencephalic precursor leads to recovery in parkinsonian rats. *Nature Neurosci* 1998;1:290–295.

460. Shihabuddin LA, Ray J, Gage FH. Stem cell technology for basic science and clinical applications. *Arch Neurol* 1999;56: 29–32.

461. Dunnett S, Björklund A. Prospects for new restorative and neuroprotective treatments in Parkinson's disease. *Nature* 1999;399[Suppl]:A32–A39.

462. Mehler MF, Kessler JA. Progenitor cell biology: implications for neural regeneration. *Arch Neurol* 1999;56:780–784.

463. Svendsen CN, Smith AG. New prospects for human stem-cell therapy in the nervous system. *TINS* 1999;22:357–364.

464. Lee S-H, Lumelsky N, Studer L, et al. Efficient generation of midbrain and hindbrain neurons from mouse embryonic stem cells. *Nature Biotechnol* 2000;18:675–679.

465. Deng H-X, Siddique T. Transgenic mouse models and human neurodegenerative disorders. *Arch Neurol* 2000;57:1695–1702.

466. Zigova T, Pencea V, Betarbet R, et al. Neuronal progenitor cells of the neonatal suventricular zone differentiate and disperse following transplantation into the adult rat striatum. *Cell Transplantation* 1998;7:137–156.

467. Rietze RL, Valcanis H, Brooker GF, et al. Purification of a pluripotent neural stem cell from the adult mouse brain. *Nature* 2001;412:736–739.

468. Lang AE, Lozano AM. Parkinson's disease. *N Engl J Med* 1998; 339:1044–1053, 1130–1143.

PROGRESSIVE SUPRANUCLEAR PALSY

EDUARDO TOLOSA
FRANCESC VALLDEORIOLA
PAU PASTOR

Progressive supranuclear palsy (PSP) is a prominent member of a group of several chronic progressive neurodegenerative disorders in which extrapyramidal features, chiefly bradykinesia and rigidity, dominate the clinical picture. It is frequently referred to as a form of atypical Parkinson's disease (PD). The first clinicopathologic descriptions were published in 1963 and 1964 and have proved to be remarkably accurate. Only in the past 10 years has the interest of neurologists and basic scientists again focused on this disorder. As a consequence, following an initial conference solely devoted to PSP that took place in Barcelona in 1991, similar meetings have taken place. Two lay societies for PSP, a North American and a European one, are actively assisting patients, and notable advances in defining the basic epidemiologic and clinical features of the disorder have taken place. New advances in the neurobiology, neurophysiology, and neuroimaging have provided remarkable insight into the pathophysiology of PSP, a disorder now classified as a tauopathy since, as it occurs in other degenerative disorders of the nervous system, neurofibrillary tangles (NFTs) that are aggregates of tau are present in the degenerating neurons. Finally, genetic factors linked to the *tau* gene in chromosome 17q21 have been shown to be necessary to cause PSP, although additional, exogenous or genetic factors seem to be required for the disease to develop.

EPIDEMIOLOGY AND ETIOLOGY

Sex Distribution and Natural History

Published cases of PSP reveal a slightly higher prevalence of male cases, with sex ratios (M/F) of 2:1. As with idiopathic Parkinson's disease (IPD), first symptoms of PSP occur in the late 50s or early 60s. Mean age at onset has ranged in published series from 60 to 63 years (1).

Median survival from onset of symptoms, actuarially adjusted, was estimated as 5.9 (2) and 9.7 (1) years. The interval from initial symptom to the need for a cane, walker, or constant assistance when walking is 3.1 years. The interval to confinement to a chair or bed is 8.2 years (1). The

most common causes of death are pulmonary emboli, pneumonia, and renal infection (3).

Prevalence and Incidence

Prevalence data derived from tertiary centers suggest that PSP affects 4% to 6% of patients with parkinsonism (4). However, population-based studies, such as the one by Golbe et al. (1) in two New Jersey counties, found a prevalence ratio of 1.4 per 100,000, suggesting that this disorder is approximately 1% as common as IPD. A recent population-based study conducted in the United Kingdom analyzing both neurologists' and nonneurologists' clinics found an age-adjusted prevalence of PSP of 3.1 and 2.4 per 100,000, respectively (5). In another recent population study in the United Kingdom, Schrag et al. (6) reported an age-adjusted prevalence for PSP of 6.4 per 100,000. Since PSP is frequently misdiagnosed or diagnosis is made several years after onset of symptoms, these figures probably underestimate the prevalence of PSP.

Incidence has been assessed in Rochester, Minnesota (7), and Perth, Australia (8), giving crude incidence rates of 3 to 4 per million per year, approximately 5% of that of Parkinson's disease.

Causation, Risk Factors, and Genetics

The cause of PSP is unknown. Davis et al. (9) investigated the risk factors for PSP in a cohort of 41 patients and 82 healthy controls. Their findings suggested a more frequent rural residence for patients with PSP as the only significant risk factor. In a follow-up study the same investigators (10) found that patients with PSP were less likely to have completed at least 12 years of school. The authors hypothesized that this finding may be a result of poor early-life nutrition or occupational or residential exposure to an unidentified toxin. Infection has been considered as a cause because the NFTs in PSP resemble those found in brains of patients with postencephalitic parkinsonism and with Guam parkinsonism-dementia complex. A slow virus seems unlikely, since after a mean observation of 9.8 years, 29 chimpanzees given intracerebral inoculations of brain tissue from 10 patients with PSP yielded negative results. Furthermore, Jendroska et al. (11) were unable to identify pathologic prion proteins in patients with PSP, suggesting that a causative role for prions is not likely.

Recently, a cluster of patients with the syndrome of PSP has been identified in the French West Indies. In the isle of Guadaloupe a series of 83 cases of parkinsonism have been studied during a 2-year period in the island's only neurology clinic. Of these cases, only 22 involved PD and 30 fulfilled criteria for probable PSP. In this population statistically significant associations have been observed between consumption of tropical fruit or herbal tea and risk of PSP and atypical parkinsonisms in comparison with controls. It is therefore thought that this cluster of Caribbean PSP could be related to the exposure to environmental neurotoxins such as the benzyltetrahydroisoquinolines, found in both tropical fruits and herbal teas (12).

PSP is considered a sporadic disorder, but in the past few years there have appeared reports of five families with at least two members suspected to have PSP and pathologic confirmation in one or more individuals (13–18). Recent studies show that a small proportion of cases are inherited in an autosomal dominant fashion. The genetic abnormality associated with familial PSP is not yet known. No evidence of linkage has been reported between PSP and the α-synuclein gene (19). Because of tau pathology and the known association of the allele 4 of the *APOE* gene as a risk factor for Alzheimer's disease (AD), PSP patients have been genotyped for *APOE* in search for a correlation, but no association was found (20). A recent case-control study showed a significant association between the *tau* gene AO/AO genotype and PSP not found in other neurodegenerative diseases, suggesting that the disease may be associated with a genetically determined alter-

ation in the *tau* gene (21). We (22) and others (19,23) have also found a highly significant overrepresentation in homozygous AO/AO individuals for the *tau* gene dinucleotide polymorphism compared with a control group.

The A0, A1, and A2 alleles of the intronic tau polymorphism are linked to other alleles of additional polymorphisms located along the *tau* gene, defining a new extended *tau* gene haplotype (H1) of approximately 100 kb (24). The association of the H1 haplotype in its homozygous form with PSP is even stronger than the association with the A0/A0 genotype alone (24). An extended 5′-tau haplotype, HapA, corresponding to four contiguous single-nucleotide polymorphisms (SNPs) in exons 1, 4A, and 8 has been identified in 98% of PSP cases. HapA appears to be the most sensitive marker for PSP, but HapA was also found in 33% of controls, pointing that the specificity of the HapA is low (25). These results indicate that mutations contained in the haplotype associated with PSP could behave at least as a risk factor to develop PSP.

Also a statistically significant overrepresentation of the H1 haplotype frequency, extended up to the promoter of the *tau* gene, has been reported in PSP patients in comparison with controls (26). This extension has been confirmed in another study (27). These authors have found allelic variants in two consensus binding sequences for the transcriptional factors c-myc and AP-2 (26), suggesting that PSP may in part be due to an increased amount of *tau* transcripts (27).

Recent study analyzing some microsatellites and SNPs located in the common region of linkage (D17S800-D17S791) associated with FTDP-17 has shown that the D17S810 2 and 3 alleles, the SNP rs1816 A allele, and the SNP rs937 delG allele formed a new haplotype named H1E (Fig. 10.1). The H1E haplotype, which has an approximate

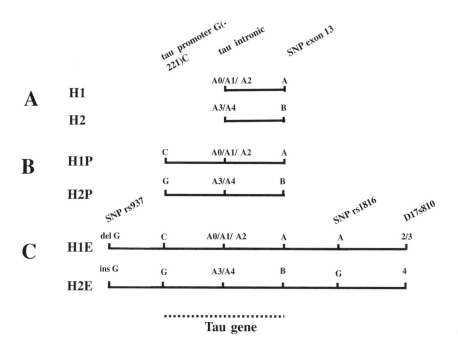

FIG. 10.1. Haplotypes formed through the analysis of the markers that are overrepresented in progressive supranuclear palsy. **A:** Haplotypes initially described by Baker et al. (24) indicating the most distal markers. **B:** Haplotypes that included the G(–221)C polymorphism of the tau promoter gene described previously (26). **C:** Extended haplotypes most recently described (28).

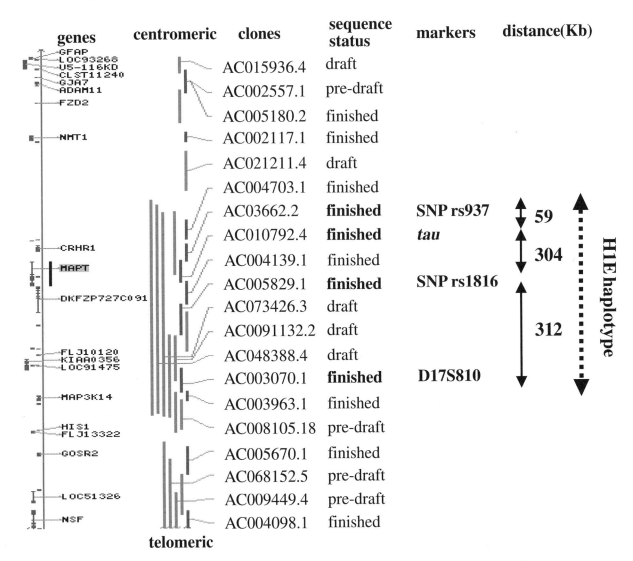

FIG. 10.2. Current location of the tau gene and the markers linked to progressive supranuclear palsy (PSP). The clones, markers, and gene locations have been obtained from NCBI database (updated on August 23, 2001). The broken line indicates the extension of the region associated to PSP. Approximate distances among markers are shown.

extension of 670 kb, in its homozygote state has been shown to be overrepresented in PSP (84.4% PSP vs. 33.3% controls; *p* < 0.001) (28). These data support the hypothesis that a change either in the 5′ or in the 3′ flanking regions of the *tau* gene or even other genes contained in the H1E haplotype could be related to the etiology of the disease. Several genes and transcripts have been mapped in the region associated with PSP (Fig. 10.2). Identification of its precise site, probably linked to H1E haplotype, seems critical.

Genetically Determined Tauopathies Resembling PSP

Frontotemporal dementia linked to chromosome 17 mutations (FTDP-17) is a hereditary form of tauopathy

due to heterozygous mutations in the *tau* gene (29–31). In familial multisystem tauopathy with presenile dementia, a heterozygous splice–donor site mutation of *tau* gene has been identified leading to a clinical phenotype and brain tau pathology reminiscent of PSP and corticobasal degeneration (CBD) (31). Also, other missense heterozygous tau mutations have been described associated to kindreds with clinical and pathologic phenotypes closely resembling PSP (32,33).

Recently, a homozygous tau mutation (del296N) has been described in one of two affected brothers (VI:23 and VI:25) born from a third-degree consanguineous marriage (Fig. 10.3). The phenotype of the two brothers resembled mostly PSP. Also the two patients exhibited variably cortical signs, such as apraxia, sensory cortical

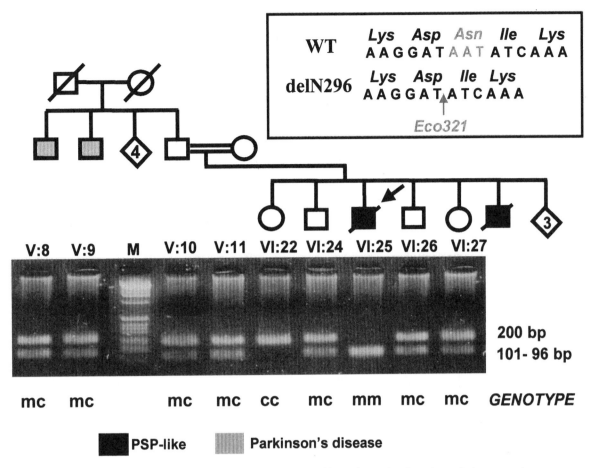

FIG. 10.3. *Pedigree of the family in which two siblings have developed atypical progressive supranuclear palsy (PSP), one of them being delN296 homozygous. An arrowhead indicates the proband of this family. mm, homozygous for the delN296 mutant allele; mc, heterozygous for the delN296 mutant allele; cc, homozygous for the common allele. Roman numbers to the left of the pedigree denote generations. The mutation delN296 creates a new Eco321 restriction site. The mutant product containing homozygous delN296 (mm) generates two 101- and 96-base pair (bp) fragments after endonuclease digestion that are superimposed in the gel. When the delN296 mutation was heterozygous (mc), an additional fragment of 200 bp appears corresponding to normal allele, whereas the nonmutated polymerase chain reaction products (cc) were not digested and only one fragment appears (200 bp) (24).*

signs, and language difficulties (34). The neuropathologic study of the patient carrying the del296N mutation in homozygous state (VI:25) (data not published) revealed severe neuronal loss in the brainstem and moderate in the frontal gray matter, globose tau-immunoreactive NFTs in a large number of neurons in the brainstem and in a smaller number in frontal cortex, and a great number of tau-positive inclusions, mainly in oligodendrocytes, in precentral frontal cortex and brainstem. Thus, the clinical and neuropathologic phenotype of the patient carrying the homozygous delN296 *tau* mutation resembles some of the clinical and pathologic features characteristic of PSP.

These data lead to hypothesize that underlying abnormalities in the *tau* gene may be responsible for the etiology of sporadic cases of PSP. In fact, several mutational studies

in a series of PSP patients have discovered new genetic variants in the *tau* gene associated with PSP (24,25,35). However, these *tau* variations are either not clearly pathogenic or are absent in the transcripts from the adult human brain. This could indicate that probably these changes are uncommon polymorphisms in disequilibrium with another mutation unknown to date.

Up to now, no clear pathogenic mutations in the *tau* gene have been found in several series of patients with familial and sporadic PSP (24,25,35,36).

Oxidative Damage

In the last years several studies have been focused on the role of free-radical-induced oxidative stress in several neurodegenerative diseases. Free radicals such as hydroxyl

(OH), superoxide (O^{2-}) and peroxynitrite ($ONOO^-$) extract electrons from neighboring molecules, thus leading to the oxidation of proteins, DNA, RNA, and membrane lipids. Particularly, membrane lipid peroxidation can render tau resistant to dephosphorylation in PSP (37). The levels of several markers of lipid peroxidation, such as malondialdehyde (MDA) and 4-hydroxynonenal, have been reported to be increased in PSP brains (39,40). Also, inducible nitric oxide synthetase is increased in tufted astrocytes, suggesting a possible role of the glial cells in the oxidative damage of PSP (41).

Also supporting a role for oxidative stress in the pathogenesis of PSP is the finding of increased levels of superoxide dismutase (SOD), glutathione, and matrix metalloproteinases 2 and 9 (MMP-2 and MMP-9). Such changes could represent compensatory mechanisms against oxidative stress (42–44). Recently, PSP-designed cytoplasmic cybrids have revealed specific defects in complex I activity (45), impaired oxygen consumption, significantly decreased levels of ATP, and loss of the activity of the iron-sulfur enzyme aconitase (46,47). The aged-related incidence and progressive nature of PSP might be caused by interactions between oxidative damage and defects in energy metabolism. Mitochondrial dysfunction in PSP, in combination with genetic and environmental factors, might lead to the instability of microtubules and hyperphosphorylation of specific tau isoforms (mostly 4R tau isoforms), resulting in the formation of NFTs and neuronal loss seen in PSP (47).

NEUROPATHOLOGY

Macroscopic Findings

On gross examination the brain shows only minor abnormalities or may even appear normal, but mild atrophy of the frontal lobes may be seen in some cases. The brain weight is usually normal or slightly reduced. Examining the cerebral cortex reveals no evident abnormalities. The globus pallidus and the thalamus are usually somewhat shrunken, but there are no changes in the caudate nucleus or in the putamen (48). The lateral ventricles, the third ventricle, and the cerebral aqueduct are usually enlarged. The midbrain is shrunken, the substantia nigra is pale, and the red nucleus discolored. The pontine tegmentum shows a remarkable atrophy, and the locus ceruleus is also discolored, as are the subthalamic regions and the globus pallidus.

Microscopic Findings

Histopathologically PSP is characterized by neuronal loss and gliosis variably affecting mostly subcortical structures.

Consistently the globus pallidus, the subthalamic nucleus, and the substantia nigra show marked neuronal loss. With appropriate stains and inmunostaining for tau, NFTs, and a variety of other inclusions can be detected, including pretangles (neurons with nonfilamentous granular cytoplasmic tau inmunoreactivity), neuropil threads (tau-positive fibers), and tau-positive tufts of abnormal fibers (tufted astrocytes) most common in motor cortex and striatum.

A specific distribution is generally observed. The most affected sites are substantia nigra, globus pallidus, and subthalamic nucleus. The globus pallidus shows neuronal loss, gliosis, and NFTs as well as iron pigment deposits and granular neuraxonal spheroids. By contrast the nucleus basalis of Meynert has moderate neuronal loss but extensive pretangle pathology. The brainstem nuclei are extensively affected and the cerebellar peduncle may show grumose degeneration (49). Spinal cord is often affected but it is not usually examined (50).

NFTs are the single most important neuropathologic hallmark of PSP. Electron microscopy reveals that they consist of bundles of straight 15- to 18-nm-diameter filaments and many fewer common paired helical filaments as seen in AD. NFTs can also be distinguished from those in AD by the paucity of ubiquitin inmunoreactivity and because they have far less fluorescence to thioflavin S stains.

Neuropil threads are short, thin, randomly oriented neurites scattered through the neuropil of the subcortical gray matter structures. They can be stained by silver impregnation method of Gallyas, and by inmunolabeling with tau filaments and isolated paired filaments (51,52). The presence of abundant neuropil threads has been related to dementia in PSP, but not all studies have replicated this observation (53). Neuropil treads have been found extensively in the subcortical gray matter, neocortex, and hippocampus of PSP cases colocalizing with NFTs (51). Thus, the presence of neuropil threads in subcortical gray matter has become for some authors one of the main pathologic criteria for diagnosis of the disease (54).

Cortical pathology in PSP is less pronounced than in other tauopathies, but NFT and tufted astrocytes are concentrated in the motor and premotor cortices (55,56). Neuronal fibrillar degeneration in the hippocampus is variable in PSP; apparently it is not intrinsic to the disease but rather more consistent with concurrent age-related pathology or coincidental pathologic states such as AD (57). The exception is the involvement of dentate granule hippocampal cells in PSP (58). When this occurs, the number of NFTs may correlate with the degree of mental deterioration (59) as in aging and AD (60). Areas of pathologic involvement in PSP and the suggested clinical correlate are summarized in Table 10.1.

TABLE 10.1. CLINICOPATHOLOGIC CORRELATES IN PROGRESSIVE SUPRANUCLEAR PALSY

Lesion Topography	Clinical Correlate
Frontal cortex, nucleus basalis of Meynert, groping, pedunculopontine nucleus	Poor verbal fluency, grasping, imitation behavior, echolalia, palilalia
Substantia nigra, striatum, medial pallidum, subthalamic nucleus	Bradykinesia, limb rigidity
Rostral interstitial nucleus of the medial longitudinal fasciculus, interstitial nucleus of Cajal, n. of Darkshewitsch	Impairment of vertical saccades
Pontine nuclei	Impaired horizontal smooth-pursuit eye movements
Paramedian pontine reticular formation	Altered rapid horizontal eye movements
Interstitial nucleus of Cajal	Nuchal dystonia
Nucleus of Edinger-Westphall	Pupillary abnormalities
Superior colliculus	Increased axial tone
Pedunculopontine nucleus, raphe nuclei, locus ceruleus	Sleep disorders
Raphe nuclei	Mood disorders
Dentate and pedunculopontine nucleus	Postural instability

Morphologic Diagnostic Criteria

Although the neuropathologic findings of PSP are relatively stereotyped (61), it has become evident in recent years that PSP may have a wide neuropathologic spectrum. Table 10.2 lists the inclusionary and exclusionary features included in the NINDS adopted neuropathologic criteria (54). Several neuropathologists from a total of 62 histologic cases have tested the validity of these criteria recently. This study demonstrates that NINDS criteria were not accurate enough to distinguish corticobasal ganglionic degeneration and Pick's disease from PSP (62). The separation into typical and atypical cases has the virtue of drawing attention to the fact that topography of the lesions is quite variable but has only limited interest for the clinician.

Some authors have pointed out that pathologic changes in PSP can be associated with those typical of AD or of IPD (63). In addition, the recently described syndrome of dementia with argyrophilic grains (64,65) at least sometimes is associated with subcortical tangles and neuropil threads. When associated with neuropil threads, it has been considered as a possible variant of PSP (66). According to preliminary National Institute of Neurological Disorders and Stroke (NINDS) criteria (54), the morphologic diagnosis of PSP cannot be considered when pathologic changes indicating PSP are associated with pathologic features characteristic of AD, multiple system atrophy (MSA), or Creutzfeldt-Jakob disease or when associated with Lewy bodies, Pick bodies, or basophilic, argyrophilic, and tau-positive inclusions.

To these cases with characteristic PSP changes plus additional neuropathologic findings we proposed (67) that a more descriptive term, such as "PSP-plus," be applied to avoid use of the word "combined," which is suggestive of the coexistence of two different diseases. Litvan et al. (68) restricted the use of the term "combined-PSP" to the coexistence of neuropathologically typical PSP and vascular lesions in the brainstem. Otherwise, when vascular lesions are found in areas distinct from those characteristically affected in PSP or when other disorders of the central nervous system occur, the diagnosis should be typical PSP plus the associated disease.

Tau Brain Immunochemistry

Tau protein is the major component of fibrillar lesions described in several neurodegenerative disorders referred to

TABLE 10.2. NINDS NEUROPATHOLOGIC CRITERIA FOR TYPICAL PSP

Inclusion Criteria	Exclusion Criteria
A high density of neurofibrillary tangles and neuropil threads in at least three of the following areas: pallidum, subthalamic nucleus, substantia nigra, or pons; and a low to high density of neurofibrillary tangles or neuropil threads in at least three of the following areas: striatum, oculomotor complex, medulla, or dentate nucleus and clinical history compatible with PSP.	Large or numerous infarcts; marked diffuse or focal atrophy; Lewy bodies; changes diagnostic of Alzheimer's disease, oligodendroglial argyrophilic Inclusions; Pick bodies; diffuse spongiosis; prion P-positive amyloid plaques

NINDS, National Institute of Neurological Disorders and Stroke; PSP, progressive supranuclear palsy.

as tauopathies (69,70). Tau is a microtubule-associated protein that is involved in tubulin assembly and stabilization. In adult human brain, six mRNA tau isoforms are derived from a single gene. They differ from each other by the presence or absence of 29- or 58-amino-acid inserts located in the amino-terminal and 31-amino-acid repeat located in the carboxy-terminal half, which correspond at the DNA genomic level to exons 2, 3, and 10, respectively. Inclusion (or not) of the region codified by exon 10 gives rise to the four (or three) tau isoforms, which each have four (or three) repeats (4R or 3R). These repeats and the surrounding sequences constitute the microtubule-binding domain of tau to tubulin (71).

In normal cerebral cortex, there is a slight preponderance of 3R over 4R tau mRNA isoforms (69). Moreover, tau isoforms are variably phosphorylated at specific serine and threonine residues (72–77). Pathologic accumulation of hyperphosphorylated tau isoforms comprises the abnormal inclusions in neurons and glia seen in tauopathies. Immunochemical and electrophoretic studies of cerebral cortex and basal ganglia confirm that the glial and neuronal inclusions in each tauopathy are composed of a specific set of hyperphosphorylated tau (72–81). Two-dimensional gel electrophoresis and phospho-specific tau antibodies in PSP and CBD brains reveal the presence of the 64- and 68-kd hyperphosphorylated tau isoforms. The detergent-insoluble tau in PSP is mostly composed of tau with 4R. A similar situation exists in CBD. However, the use of antibodies to exon 3 tau-specific epitopes confirms that, in contrast to PSP, inclusions in CBD lack exon 3 sequences (82).

Recently, tau and amyloid burdens, and the ratio of 4R to 3R detergent-insoluble tau, were measured in the basal ganglia from brains with PSP and AD (83). The insoluble tau from PSP was not composed exclusively of 4R tau. All brains had a mixture of 4R and 3R tau but, in PSP there was less 3R than 4R tau, whereas the ratio was reversed in AD. In PSP cases with concurrent Alzheimer-type pathology, the ratio of 4R to 3R was intermediate between AD and PSP. The H1 tau haplotype had no effect on the 4R to 3R ratio or on tau and amyloid burdens of the brains examined (83).

The electrophoretic pattern of tau in other tauopathies, such as Pick's disease, is characterized by a 60- and 64-kd doublet, composed of 3-repeat tau isoforms, while the Western blots of detergent-insoluble tau from AD brains reveal three bands 60, 64, and 68 kd, composed of both 3- and 4-repeat tau isoforms.

Thus, biochemical studies in PSP and other tauopathies provide a potential helpful instrument to improve the neuropathologic characterization of these disorders. Differences in the morphology and distribution of brain tau immunoreactivity suggest that the different tau isoforms could be involved in the diverse neuropathologic expression of the tauopathies.

CLINICAL DIAGNOSIS

Clinical Manifestations

The clinical picture of PSP is characteristic and has been outlined in detail by several authors (1,2,84–88). The cardinal manifestations include supranuclear ophthalmoplegia (SNO), pseudobulbar palsy, prominent neck dystonia, behavioral and cognitive disturbances, parkinsonism, gait disturbances, poor equilibrium, and falls. When these clinical features are encountered in an adult patient with a gradual progressive course, the clinical diagnosis of PSP is almost always certain. SNO, initially affecting saccadic eye movements on downward direction, is the hallmark of the disease. Other clinical features, sometimes considered atypical, at times are prominent. For example, focal or segmental dystonia in the form of limb dystonia or blepharospasm is not uncommon (89–91), and a variety of neuro-ophthalmologic features other than SNO can be present (Table 10.3). Likewise, asymmetric apraxia resembling CBD can occur (92). Sleep disturbances, such as insomnia, frequent nocturnal awakenings, and sleep-related behavioral disturbances, can also be an important cause of morbidity (93) not sufficiently emphasized. Micturition disturbances, including urinary incontinence, are not uncommon (94,95) except in the early stages.

More unusual symptoms and signs include schizophreniform psychoses, chorea, rest tremor, muscle atrophy, and paroxysmal kinesigenic dystonia, among others (96). Hardly ever encountered are some clinical signs such as aphasia, visual agnosia, prominent cerebellar dysfunction, polyneuropathy, focal sensory deficits, and unilateral limb apraxia. Asymmetric onset is also uncommon. The presence of one or more of these signs makes the diagnosis of PSP quite improbable (97). Onset before age 40 and disease duration of more than 20 years are also features that do not support the diagnosis of PSP.

Difficulties in the Clinical Diagnosis

The clinical features of PSP are so characteristic that seemingly diagnostic errors should be uncommon in patients with the full clinical syndrome. Recent clinicopathologic studies (98,99) indicate that a significant proportion of patients are erroneously diagnosed during life, some because they have unusual symptoms and signs, others because of lack of typical manifestations, such as supranuclear gaze palsy. However, in a recent review of the literature (100) involving 90 pathologically proven cases, only 69% of cases met standard diagnostic criteria for PSP.

Problems in the clinical diagnosis of PSP arise mostly in three circumstances. First, the disorder is difficult to diagnose in the early stages, before the characteristic gaze palsy

TABLE 10.3. NEURO-OPHTHALMOLOGIC FEATURES OF PROGRESSIVE SUPRANUCLEAR PALSY

Ocular Abnormalities Preceding Gaze Palsy
Defective visual suppression of the vestibuloocular reflex
Loss of the fast component of the optokinetic nystagmus
Ocular fixation instability with square-wave jerks
Impersistence of gaze
Hesitancy when initiating an eye movement to command, usually to look down
Slow and hipometric saccades (first on the vertical plane)
Supranuclear gaze palsy
Vertical supranuclear gaze palsy: saccadic movements affected before smooth-pursuit system; downgaze more disturbed than upgaze; oculocephalic movements preserved
Limitation or absence of convergence
Global supranuclear ophthalmoplegia in advanced phases of the illness

Other, Less Common Oculomotor Disturbances
Internuclear ophthalmoplegia
Loss of Bell's phenomenon
Loss of oculocephalic movements
Eyelid disturbances in progressive supranuclear palsy
Eyelid retractions (Cowper's sign) with wide-eyed staring look
Blepharospasm (eyebrow elevation usually associated)
Palpebral ptosis due to levator inhibition
Apraxia of lid opening and closure
Blink rate diminution (may result in exposure keratitis)

and neck dystonia have occurred. Even more problematic is the diagnosis of PSP when some cardinal features, such as gaze palsy, do not occur or unusual manifestations, such as dementia, dominate the clinical course. Finally, a number of well-defined neurologic conditions may mimic the clinical features of PSP (101) and cause the clinician to erroneously diagnose PSP (Table 10.4).

Early Diagnosis

The diagnosis of PSP in the early stages, when most of the characteristic signs are yet to manifest, is difficult if not impossible, and description of pathologically proven cases frequently indicates early misdiagnosis. The mean duration of symptoms before diagnosis in Kristensen's review of 325 cases collected from the literature (88) was 3.9 years. Other authors, including Pfaffenbach et al. (102), report an even longer average delay in the diagnosis after symptom onset. These difficulties in diagnosis are undoubtedly in part due to the variable clinical presentation of the disorder and to the fact that its most characteristic manifestation, the supranuclear gaze palsy, frequently appears months or years after onset of symptoms. Brusa et al. (87), in their review of 75 reported cases with neuropathologic confirmation, found that in half of the cases slowness and limitation of

TABLE 10.4. NEUROLOGIC DISORDERS THAT MAY RESEMBLE PROGRESSIVE SUPRANUCLEAR PALSY

Disorders Associated with Parkinsonism	Dementing Processes	Other Diseases
Idiopathic Parkinson's disease	Alzheimer's disease	Amyotrophic lateral sclerosis
Postencephalitic parkinsonism	Punch-drunk syndrome	Multi-infarct state
Guam parkinsonism-dementia complex	Progressive subcortical gliosis	Brain tumors
Multiple system atrophy (especially striatonigral type)	Diffuse Lewy body disease	Progressive external ophthalmoplegia
Corticobasal ganglionic degeneration	Pick's disease	Myasthenia gravis
Rigid form of Huntington's disease	Normal-pressure hydrocephalus	Whipple's disease
Machado-Joseph Azorean disease	Creutzfeldt-Jakob disease	
Hallervorden-Spatz disease		
Rare forms of neurometabolic disorders (e.g., Gaucher's disease)		
Wilson's disease		
Acquired hepatocerebral degeneration		
Pallidoluysian degeneration		

both conjugate voluntary and vergence movements occurred 2 to 4 years after the onset of any other symptoms.

The onset of PSP is insidious, and there is often a prolonged phase of vague, nonspecific symptoms such as fatigue, dizziness, headaches, arthralgias, and depression. These symptoms frequently bring the patient to medical attention before abnormal clinical signs are recognized. The family may note subtle personality changes, with the patient becoming introverted and withdrawn from social activities. Other frequent complaints at onset are memory loss, gait instability, slowness of movements as in PD, diplopia, and other visual and pseudobulbar symptoms. In a neuropathologic study (3) the most common symptoms at disease onset were postural instability and falls (63%), dysarthria (35%), bradykinesia (13%), and visual disturbances such as diplopia, blurred vision, burning eyes, and light sensitivity (13%). It is therefore not surprising that several alternative diagnoses are considered before the appearance of the typical gaze palsy. When behavioral changes or motor symptoms occur early, disorders such as IPD; MSA; CBD; the sporadic ataxias; AD and other dementing disorders, such as the frontal lobe dementias, Creutzfeldt-Jakob disease, Pick's disease, normopressure hydrocephalus, and multi-infarct encephalopathy; and psychiatric conditions, such as depression, can be entertained (103). Early prominent bulbar findings suggest the bulbar forms of motor neuron disease and can also resemble a multi-infarct state. The early ocular manifestations can lead to an erroneous diagnosis of progressive external ophthalmoplegia on a myopathic basis or to myasthenia gravis, particularly if the manifestation is atypical, as with internuclear ophthalmoplegia. In the early stages, before SNO sets in, certain clinical signs that are uncommon in PSP or are not well recognized as part of the syndrome can also create diagnostic problems. Examples of such abnormalities are early apraxia of lid opening and prominent limb dystonia.

In summary, there is a substantial period during which patients with PSP are symptomatic and under medical care but are not yet correctly diagnosed. As Duvoisin (97) suggested, perhaps about twice as many PSP patients are in this category as have been diagnosed.

Clinical Variants

Particularly difficult from a diagnostic point of view are cases in which the clinical presentation is unusual or the cardinal features appear late or not at all. Examples such circumstances would be those in which patients never develop the characteristic ophthalmoparesis (104–106). Sometimes a gaze abnormality is suspected but difficult to confirm. This can be due to the changing characteristics of the gaze disorder, which can vary from one day to another. Occasionally severe cervical dystonia, particularly during flexion, makes proper evaluation impossible.

In a study of four pathologically proven cases of PSP (105), the clinical manifestations developed before age 34 in mentally subnormal individuals. These patients presented with a prominent neuropsychiatric disorder that included violent behavior, bursts of irritability, aggressiveness, restlessness, and disorientation, resulting in early admission to psychiatric hospitals. Other similar cases have not been reported.

PSP has been diagnosed at autopsy in patients in whom progressive dementia was the dominant clinical manifestation throughout the course of the illness. Such patients with prominent dementia are frequently misdiagnosed as having AD or other dementing disorder. In 5 of 13 patients with pathologically proven PSP reported by Gearing et al. (63), the clinical diagnosis during life was AD. Correct diagnosis of the dementing form of PSP can be made in life only if the cardinal features of the illness appear in conjunction with the dementing state (63,66,107).

Another clinical variant of PSP is the akinetic-rigid form with poor or no response to levodopa. These cases can be confused with Parkinson's disease and other parkinsonian syndromes, such as those encountered in MSA with predominantly parkinsonian features (MSA-P; striatonigral degeneration). It is unclear how many patients with PSP go through the entire course of the illness believed to have an isolated parkinsonian syndrome with transient or poor response to levodopa. In a recent prevalence investigation in the United Kingdom (5), 17 individuals with PSP were identified in a community study via diagnostic and therapeutic registers. Seven of the 17 individuals identified had an alternative diagnosis prior to the study, the most common misdiagnosis being Parkinson's disease (3 cases) and cerebrovascular disease (3 cases). In a clinicopathologic study by the Parkinson's Disease Society Brain Bank in the United Kingdom, 6 of 17 patients pathologically diagnosed as having PSP in life carried the diagnosis of IPD. An additional one had been diagnosed as having nonidiopathic Parkinson's syndrome. However, in none of the 12 pathologically proven cases reported by Collins et al. (98) was IPD the clinical diagnosis during life. In this series, one case was classified as Parkinson's-plus and another as undetermined extrapyramidal disease. Helpful features in differentiating IPD from the akinetic-rigid syndrome that can occur in PSP are shown in Table 10.5. Probably disturbances in ocular and eyelid motility provide the greatest help in differentiating the akinetic rigid form of PSP from the parkinsonian variant of MSA, as discussed by Duvoisin (97), but the two disorders can be confused even by experienced clinicians.

Pure akinesia is a recently described syndrome (108,109) characterized by gait initiation failure, dysarthria, and micrography without other parkinsonian features, such as bradykinesia, postural instability, rigidity, or tremor. Some authors have pointed out that this clinical presentation may

TABLE 10.5. CLINICAL DIFFERENCES BETWEEN PROGRESSIVE SUPRANUCLEAR PALSY AND IDIOPATHIC PARKINSON'S DISEASE

PSP	IPD
Symmetric parkinsonian symptoms	Asymmetric at onset
Gait impaired early in course	Early impairment rare
Falls early in course	Falls late in the course
Early impairment of postural reflexes	Normal in early stages
Stiff gait, legs extended at the knee	Marché à petit pas
Trunk posture in extension	Body flexion when walking
Arm swing when walking may be present	Early loss of arm swing
"Astonished" facial expression	Facial hypokimia
Blink rate 3–5 per minute	Blink rate 10–14 per minute
Rest tremor uncommon	Rest tremor frequent
More common axial than limb dystonia	Limb dystonia more common
Axial rigidity more common	Limb rigidity more common
Absence of hand deformity	Characteristic hand deformity
Absent or poor response to levodopa	Good response to levodopa
Levodopa-induced dyskinesias rare	Dyskinesias common
Wearing-off, on–off phenomena unusual	Wearing-off, on–off phenomena common

PSP, progressive supranuclear palsy; IPD, idiopathic Parkinson's disease.

be a variant of PSP and that the recognition of this syndrome may suggest PSP before the development of abnormalities of ocular movement (110).

Disorders That May Mimic Progressive Supranuclear Palsy

Rarely other neurologic disorders mimic the clinical picture of PSP, manifesting several of the characteristic clinical features of this disorder. Such reported conditions include diffuse Lewy body disease, AD, progressive subcortical gliosis, CBD, and MSA in both its parkinsonian and cerebellar variant. Multi-infarct states can also reproduce the syndrome of PSP (111), and diagnostic difficulties can arise with disorders in which a supranuclear gaze palsy accompanies an extrapyramidal syndrome such as normopressure hydrocephalus (112), rigid forms of Huntington's disease, Creutzfeldt-Jakob disease (113), Whipple's disease, and Guam parkinsonism-dementia complex (114,115). Differential diagnosis must be occasionally established with other disorders, such as Wilson's disease, Machado-Joseph disease (116), juvenile dystonic lipoidosis (117), Gaucher's disease (118), Pick's disease, punch-drunk syndrome (119), and postencephalitic parkinsonism (120). These various case descriptions clearly show that various neurologic disorders can manifest some of the main clinical features of PSP. However, in the majority of these cases misdiagnosed as PSP the clinical picture was in other respects different from that of typical PSP, and if standard clinical diagnostic criteria had been applied to these cases, the diagnosis before death generally would not have been PSP. Judging from the clinical diagnoses in life reported in recent clinicopathologic studies (99), cerebrovascular disease, AD, and

IPD are the three disorders most commonly mistaken for PSP during life. The use of appropriate clinical diagnostic criteria should minimize the frequency with which clinicians misdiagnose PSP, but until we have more accurate diagnostic markers for the disorder, false-positive diagnoses will be unavoidable.

CLINICAL DIAGNOSTIC CRITERIA

In an attempt to improve diagnostic accuracy, to provide appropriate prognosis to patients and their families, and to select appropriate cases for epidemiologic studies, drug studies, and so on, several clinical diagnostic criteria for PSP have been developed. Criteria frequently used are those of Jackson et al. (4), Lees (96), Blin et al. (121), Golbe and Davis (122), Tolosa et al. (103), and Collins et al. (98). Understandably, these criteria differ considerably. Some, such as those proposed by Lees and by Tolosa's group, require SNO for the diagnosis of PSP, either probable or possible. Others accept the diagnosis of possible PSP without SNO. Some consider the presence of bradykinesia to be a necessary requirement; others do not. These sets of criteria also use different items to complement the necessary criteria. NINDS and Society for PSP (SPSP) (68) have formulated clinical research criteria for the diagnosis of PSP based on an extensive review of the literature, comparison with published sets of criteria, and the consensus of experts and validated on a clinical dataset from autopsy-confirmed cases of PSP. The criteria specify three degrees of diagnostic certainty: possible, probable, and definite PSP. The criteria for probable PSP are highly specific (100%) and are therefore suitable for clinical drug trials and other studies for which it is essential to exclude subjects with illnesses other

TABLE 10.6. CRITERIA FOR CLINICAL DIAGNOSIS OF PROGRESSIVE SUPRANUCLEAR PALSY

Major criteria:
    Onset after age 40
    Progressive course
    Supranuclear gaze palsy with involvement of downward gaze
Plus the following manifestations (probable PSP if three or more are present; possible PSP if
    two are present)
Early postural instability, falls
Bradykinesia
Early dysphagia or dysarthria
Prominent frontal lobe syndrome (e.g., bradyphrenia, apathy, perseveration, grasping)
Prominent axial dystonia (neck or trunk hyperextended)
Plus absence of all of the following
Prominent cerebellar signs
Unexplained polyneuropathy
Unexplained dysautonomic symptoms (early incontinence or symptomatic postural hypotension)
Focal sensory deficits, primary or cortical
Unilateral limb apraxia or alien-hand syndrome
Parkinsonism with full and persistent response to levodopa

From Tolosa E, Valldeoriola F, Cruz-Sanchez F. Progressive supranuclear palsy: clinical and pathological diagnosis. *Eur J Neurol* 1995;2:258–273.

than PSP. Criteria for possible PSP, with a sensitivity of 83%, are more suitable for descriptive epidemiologic studies and clinical care, when it is important to identify all cases of PSP even at the cost of including a few false-positive cases. The clinical criteria we use in our movement disorder unit (67) (Table 10.6) differ fundamentally from those of NINDS and SPSP. For the diagnosis of probable PSP we require downgaze supranuclear palsy, but we do not require prominent postural instability with falls in the first year of disease. Since only few neurologic disorders other than PSP have the characteristic combination of supranuclear gaze palsy, pseudobulbar palsy, parkinsonism, disequilibrium, falls, bradyphrenia, frontal lobe signs, and neck dystonia, the use of the criteria we propose or similar criteria excludes the conditions most commonly misdiagnosed as PSP. Our criteria yield only a small rate of false-positive diagnosis when patients with the full-blown syndrome are evaluated. We leave undiagnosed those patients without ophthalmoplegia as well as those with clinical variants such as a pure akinesia syndrome or dementia without ophthalmoplegia.

The validity of the various proposed criteria remains to be tested in prospective clinicopathologic studies. At this time we recommend using the NINDS and SPSP diagnostic criteria for all research studies in PSP.

DIAGNOSTIC INVESTIGATIONS

Magnetic Resonance

Magnetic resonance (MR) studies of patients with PSP demonstrate midbrain atrophy, thinning of the quadrigeminal plate, enlargement of the third ventricle, pontine tegmental atrophy, increased signal intensity in the periaqueductal gray, and frontal and temporal lobe atrophy (123–126). None of these abnormalities is a constant finding. The size of some brainstem diameters and structures might help to differentiate between PSP from other parkinsonian syndromes. In PSP patients the midbrain tegmentum diameter is reduced below the lower limit of normal range but the pontine diameter is within normal range; by contrast, patients with MSA present a normal brainstem tegmentum diameter but a reduced pontine diameter (127). Lower midbrain diameters have also been described in patients with PSP as opposed to Parkinson's disease (128). However, in the latter study, midbrain and pontine diameter measurement did not help to distinguish between PSP and MSA.

Magnetic resonance (^{1}H) spectroscopic studies in PSP have shown reduced *N*-acetylaspartate/creatine-phosphocreatine ratio in the brainstem, centrum semiovale, frontal and precentral cortex, and reduced *N*-acetylaspartate/choline ratio in the lentiform nucleus (129). Other MR (^{1}H) spectroscopic studies have disclosed a significant reduction in the median concentration from *N*-acetyl groups in the pallidum in comparison with control subjects (130), probably reflecting the predominant neuronal loss taking place in the pallidum.

In summary, it is now generally accepted that the presence of a reduced midbrain diameter, signal increase in the midbrain, dilatation of the third ventricle, atrophy or signal increase of the red nucleus, and frontal or temporal atrophy are typical radiologic manifestations of PSP not usually found in other parkinsonian syndromes. MSA, the most frequently confounding disease, typically presents putaminal hyperintensity or putaminal rim; dilatation of the fourth ventricle; and signal increase in the cerebellum, middle cerebellar peduncles, and pons. The radiologic analysis of these brain areas has proved helpful in the differentiation between PSP and other parkinsonian syndromes, with a sensitivity up to 70% (131). However, these studies are of little help in establishing the diagnosis of the disease in early stages. MR studies are also of interest to rule out the existence of nondegenerative pathology, such as vascular or tumoral lesions.

Positron Emission Tomography and Single Photon Emission Computed Tomography

Positron emission tomography (PET) studies in PSP have shown global cerebral hypometabolism with frontal areas particularly targeted (132–134). This finding is not specific for PSP. Basal ganglia, cerebellar, and thalamic glucose metabolism is also depressed in PSP, thus distinguishing it from PD were metabolism is preserved. Studies with fluorodopa PET have shown a reduction in the ^{18}F-dopa influx in the caudate and putamen, in line with the known degeneration of the nigrostriatal pathway that takes place in this disorder. This finding has also been documented in four asymptomatic relatives of patients with familial PSP (135), suggesting that ^{F}18-dopa and deoxydopa PET could detect subclinical cases of PSP. These findings contrasts with those in PD where caudate is less severely affected (136). Caudate and putamen D2 binding has also been evaluated in PSP with both PET and single photon emission computed tomography (SPECT) (137). Overall D2 receptor density is reduced in PSP but, again, this alteration is not specific to PSP. Differences between PSP and PD have also been found in the patterns of dopamine transporter loss in a study using the radiotracer [^{11}C]-WIN 35,428 and PET (138). In this study, patients with PD showed the most important abnormality in the posterior putamen, with a less marked presence in the anterior putamen and caudate. By contrast, PSP patients showed a relatively uniform degree of involvement in these areas. SPECT studies using ^{123}I-β-CIT, which binds to the dopamine transporter, have also shown reduction in transporter density in both caudate and putamen, similar to what is encountered in MSA (139). It is not yet possible to differentiate among different types of parkinsonian syndromes with this technique because the overall reduction of the striatal binding is similar in PSP, PD, MSA, and CBD (140,141).

Recent studies have measured levels of acetylcholinesterase activity using *N*-methyl-4-[^{11}C]piperidyl acetate and PET in PSP and PD. In one study, PD patients showed a reduction of 17% of cerebral cortical acetylcholinesterase activity, whereas there was only a slight reduction of cortical activity in PSP patients. By contrast, there was a prominent reduction (38%) of thalamic activity in PSP patients, whereas only a minimal reduction of thalamic activity occurred in PD patients (142). Another study

obtained similar findings with nondemented Parkinson's disease patients and demented PSP patients. These studies suggest that there is a different loss of the ascending cholinergic systems in Parkinson's disease and PSP, with a preferential loss of cholinergic innervation to the thalamus in PSP, and that the cerebral cortical cholinergic system may not have a major role in cognitive dysfunction in PSP.

Evoked Potentials

Brainstem evoked potentials are near normal in this entity (143). However, event-related potentials show delayed P2 and P300 components (144,145). Enlarged cortical responses have been found in somatosensory evoked potentials studies in 13 of 14 patients with PSP (146). In the same study, motor evoked potentials were normal in all cases.

Electro-oculography

An excess of square-wave jerks on eye movement recording has been reported as a common finding in PSP but it is not a specific finding (147,148). Recording eye movements may also be of help in diagnosis in the initial phases of the disease (149,150). A recent longitudinal ocular motor study of visually guided saccades and antisaccades in patients with PSP and CBD has shown (151) that PSP patients had decreased saccade velocity throughout the disease course, whereas patients with CBD showed preserved saccade velocity but an important increase in saccade latency ipsilateral to the apractic side.

Polisomnography

Although daytime somnolence is not a typical feature in PSP patients, sleep architecture and sleep efficiency is severely distorted in PSP. Polisomnographic studies have shown a diminished total sleep time, lower sleep efficiency, increased awakenings, reduction in sleep spindles, atonic slow-wave sleep, and a lower percentage of REM sleep (152–157). REM efficiency and latency seem to be no different from that in control subjects (157). These disturbances can be understood on the basis of the alteration of the brainstem structures crucial to generate normal sleep patterns.

Other Brainstem Reflexes

The acoustic startle response, in which brainstem circuits are implicated, has been found to be abnormal in PSP (150), whereas it is generally normal in PD and MSA (158,159). The startle circuit is mediated by reticulospinal pathways. The absence of startle responses as well as the lack of reaction time shortening after a startling stimulus (160) or after transcranial magnetic stimulation (161) suggests a massive derangement of the reticular system in PSP.

Blink reflex excitability-recovery curve to paired stimuli is enhanced in PSP as well as in other parkinsonian syndromes (162). However, the orbicularis oculi response to median nerve stimulation is absent in patients with PSP in which the response of the mentalis muscle to the same stimulus is preserved. This fact can be helpful in distinguishing PSP patients from those with other parkinsonian syndromes (163).

Anal Sphincter Electromyography and Urodynamic Studies

Although not common, some PSP patients present fecal or urinary incontinence, which could be attributed to a neuronal loss in the Onuf's nuclei of the S2-S4 segments of the anterior horn of the spinal cord (164). Problems of micturition are less common than in MSA but more common than in PD (94,165). Anal sphincter EMG has proved its interest in the diagnosis of MSA (166) but we and others have shown that anal sphincter EMG is also abnormal in PSP (42% of patients), rendering this test of little value in distinguishing PSP from MSA (94,167). Urodynamic studies in PSP patients have shown detrusor hyperreflexia or dyssynergia (94).

TREATMENT

There is no effective pharmacologic or surgical treatment for PSP. Unlike in Parkinson's disease, neurotransmitter replacement is of little help, probably because the widespread pathologic derangement that occurs in PSP implies the alteration in many neurochemical systems.

Dopaminergic therapy is rarely of help in the control of PSP symptoms, and its benefit is almost always brief or absent. This minimal response refers only to bradykinesia and rigidity but not to other symptoms of the disease. A retrospective study confirmed this clinical impression, demonstrating a minimal response to levodopa in only 38% of patients with PSP, close to the accepted placebo response in PD drug trials (30%) (168). Similarly, 75% of 16 pathologically proven cases of PSP showed no response to levodopa treatment during life in a comparative retrospective study of different parkinsonian syndromes (169). Other postmortem studies have also shown the lack of efficacy of dopaminergic and other neurotransmitter replacement therapies (170). Dopamine agonists (e.g., pramipexole 4.5 mg daily) have also been ineffective in controlling the symptoms of the disease (170–172) and cause frequent side effects.

Despite the widespread degeneration of cholinergic systems in PSP, trials with cholinergic drugs have also been disappointing (173,174). A recent trial with donepezil, a centrally acting cholinesterase inhibitor, did not show any significant change in motor, cognitive, and activities of daily living performance in PSP patients (175). Another study with this drug showed mild improvement of cognitive function, but activities of daily living and motor scores significantly worsened (176).

Serotonin replacement has also been ineffective. There is controversial experimental information demonstrating the alteration of serotonergic system in patients with PSP in the brainstem (105,177,178), but pharmacologic trials with serotonin reuptake blockers have been not favorable (168). There is a case report showing amelioration in rigidity and nuchal dystonia with the serotonin reuptake blocker trazodone (179). In a double-blind trial, the efficacy of amitriptyline was tested in four PSP patients with slight improvement of gait disorders and rigidity (180). Other study has shown improvement of bradykinesia, dysphagia, and dysarthria with low-dose amitriptyline (181). None of these results has been reproduced in a larger group of patients.

N-Methyl-D-aspartate receptor antagonists, such as amantadine, have been used in a study of patients with gait disorders (182). The results showed minor improvement of certain aspects of gait, such as start hesitation and freezing, but studies showing efficacy in PSP are lacking.

α_2-Receptor noradrenergic antagonists such as idazoxan (183) or the newer, more potent efaroxan have been tested in PSP in an attempt to increase central noradrenaline levels, also without success.

Reduced neurotransmission of γ-aminobutyric acid (GABA) in the striatum and globus pallidus (184) could contribute to the symptoms of PSP; consequently, drugs that act specifically on the GABAergic systems in the basal ganglia might be helpful in management of the disorder. A trial with valproic acid produced no clinical benefit (168). More recently, improvement in saccadic eye movements and motor performance in ten patients with PSP has been reported with zolpidem (185), which is a short-acting, hypnotic, GABAergic drug. Zolpidem is a selective agonist of the benzodiazepine subtype receptor BZ1, with the highest density of this receptor being in the ventral globus pallidus and substantia nigra pars reticulata.

In addition to neurotransmission replacement therapy, other palliative treatments should be considered. Physical therapy may teach patients how to rise from and descend to chairs safely. The use of walkers should be considered in patients suffering falls. Swallowing should be regularly evaluated to avoid aspiration pneumonia. Dysphagia can be managed by using straws, food thickeners, or soft processed food. Placement of percutaneous endoscopic gastroscopy may help with oral feedings in patients who have had major episodes of aspiration pneumonia or significant weight loss related to poor intake.

Botulinum toxin A has been found useful in the treatment of rigidity and the dystonic phenomena such as blepharospasm or focal limb dystonia (186) and in the so-called eye-opening apraxia where the best results seem to be obtained with injections directed toward the junction of the preseptal and pretarsal parts of the palpebral orbicularis oculi (187).

REFERENCES

1. Golbe LI, Davis PH, Schoenberg BS, et al. Prevalence and natural history of progressive supranuclear palsy. *Neurology* 1988; 38:1031–1034.
2. Maher ER, Lees AJ. The clinical features and the natural history of the Steele-Richardson-Olszewski syndrome (progressive supranuclear palsy). *Neurology* 1986;1005–1008.
3. Litvan I, Mangone CA, McKee A, et al. Natural history of progressive supranuclear palsy (Steele-Richardson-Olszewski syndrome) and clinical predictors of survival: a clinicopathological study. *J Neurol Neurosurg Psychiatry* 1996;61:615–620.
4. Jackson JA, Jankovic J, Ford J. Progressive supranuclear palsy: clinical features and response to treatment in 16 patients. *Ann Neurol* 1983;13:273–278.
5. Nath U, Ben-Shlomo Y, Thomson RG, et al. The prevalence of progressive supranuclear palsy (Steele-Richardson-Olszewski syndrome) in the U.K. *Brain* 2001;124:1438–1449.
6. Schrag A, Ben-Shlomo Y, Quinn NP. Prevalence of progressive supranuclear palsy and multiple system atrophy: a cross-sectional study. *Lancet* 1999;354:1771–1775.
7. Rajput AH, Offord KP, Beard CM, et al. Epidemiology of parkinsonism: incidence, classification, and mortality. *Ann Neurol* 1984;16:278–282.
8. Mastaglia FL, Grainger K, Kee F, et al. Progressive supranuclear palsy (the Steele-Richardson-Olszewski syndrome): clinical and electrophysiological observations in eleven cases. *Proc Aust Assoc Neurol* 1973;10:35–44.
9. Davis PH, Golbe LI, Duvoisin RC, et al. Risk factors for progressive supranuclear palsy. *Neurology* 1988;38:1546–1552.
10. Golbe LI, Rubin RS, Cody RP, et al. Follow-up study of risk factors in progressive supranuclear palsy. *Neurology* 1996;47: 148–154.
11. Jendroska K, Hoffmann O, Schelosky L, et al. Absence of disease related prion protein in neurodegenerative disorders presenting with Parkinson's syndrome. *J Neurol Neurosurg Psychiatry* 1994;57:1249–1251.
12. Caparros-Lefebvre D, Elbaz A. Possible relation of atypical parkinsonism in the French West Indies with consumption of tropical plants: a case-control study. Caribbean Parkinsonism Study Group. *Lancet* 1999;354:281–286.
13. Brown J, Lantos P, Stratton M, et al. Familial progressive supranuclear palsy. *J Neurol Neurosurg Psychiatry* 1993;56: 473–476.
14. Ohara S, Kondo K, Morita H, et al. Progressive supranuclear palsy-like syndrome in two siblings of a consanguineous marriage. *Neurology* 1992;42:1009–1014.
15. Golbe LI, Dickson DW. Familial autopsy-proven progressive supranuclear palsy. *Neurology* 1995;45[Suppl 4]:A255.
16. Tetrud JW, Golbe LI, Farmer PM, et al. Autopsy proven progressive supranuclear palsy in two siblings. *Neurology* 1996;46: 931–934.
17. Gazely S, Maguire J. Familial progressive supranuclear palsy. *Brain Pathol* 1994;4:534.
18. Garcia de Yébenes J, Sarasa JL, Daniel SE, et al. Familial progressive supranuclear palsy: description of a pedigree and review of the literature. *Brain* 1995;118:1094–1103.
19. Higgins JJ, Litvan I, Pho LT, et al. Progressive supranuclear gaze palsy is in linkage disequilibrium with the tau and not the alpha-synuclein gene. *Neurology* 1998;50:270–273.
20. Tabaton M, Rolleri M, Masturzo P, et al. Apolipoprotein E-4 allele frequency is not increased in progressive supranuclear palsy. *Neurology* 1995;45:1764–1765.
21. Conrad C, Andreadis A, Trojanowski JQ, et al. Genetic evidence for the involvement of τ (tau) in progressive supranuclear palsy. *Ann Neurol* 1997;41:277–281.
22. Oliva R, Tolosa E, Ezquerra M, et al. Significant changes in the tau A0 and A3 alleles in progressive supranuclear palsy and improved genotyping by silver detection. *Arch Neurol* 1998;55: 1122–1124.
23. Bennett P, Bonifati V, Bonuccelli U, et al. Direct genetic evidence for involvement of tau in progressive supranuclear palsy. European Study Group on Atypical Parkinsonism Consortium. *Neurology* 1998;51:982–985.
24. Baker M, Litvan I, Houlden H, et al. Association of an extended haplotype in the tau gene with progressive supranuclear palsy. *Hum Mol Genet* 1999;8:711–715.
25. Higgins JJ, Golbe LI, De Biase A, et al. An extended 5′-tau susceptibility haplotype in progressive supranuclear palsy. *Neurology* 2000;55:1364–1367.
26. Ezquerra M, Pastor P, Valldeoriola F, et al. Identification of a novel polymorphism in the promoter region of the tau gene highly associated to progressive supranuclear palsy in humans. *Neurosci Lett* 1999;275:183–186.
27. de Silva R, Weiler M, Morris HR, et al. Strong association of a novel Tau promoter haplotype in progressive supranuclear palsy. *Neurosci Lett* 2001;311:145–148.
28. Pastor P, Ezquerra M, Tolosa E, et al. Further extension of the H1 haplotype associated with progressive supranuclear palsy. *Mov Dis* 2002;17:550–556.
29. Dumanchin C, Camuzat A, Campion D, et al. Segregation of a missense mutation in the microtubule-associated protein tau gene with familial frontotemporal dementia and parkinsonism. *Hum Mol Genet* 1998;7:1825–1829.
30. Hutton M, Lendon CL, Rizzu P, et al. Association of missense and 5′-splice-site mutations in tau with the inherited dementia FTDP-17. *Nature* 1998;393:702–705.
31. Spillantini MG, Murrell JR, Goedert M, et al. Mutation in the tau gene in familial multiple system tauopathy with presenile dementia. *Proc Natl Acad Sci USA* 1998;95:7737–7741.
32. Stanford PM, Halliday GM, Brooks WS, et al. Progressive supranuclear palsy pathology caused by a novel silent mutation in exon 10 of the tau gene: expansion of the disease phenotype caused by tau gene mutations. *Brain* 2000;123:880–893.
33. Delisle MB, Murrell JR, Richardson R, et al. A mutation at codon 279 (N279K) in exon 10 of the Tau gene causes a tauopathy with dementia and supranuclear palsy. *Acta Neuropathol* 1999;98:62–77.
34. Pastor P, Pastor E, Carnero C, et al. Familial atypical progressive supranuclear palsy associated with homozygosity for the delN296 mutation in the tau gene. *Ann Neurol* 2001;49: 263–267.
35. Bonifati V, Joosse M, Nicholl DJ, et al. The tau gene in progressive supranuclear palsy: exclusion of mutations in coding exons and exon 10 splice sites, and identification of a new intronic variant of the disease-associated H1 haplotype in Italian cases. *Neurosci Lett* 1999;274:61–65.
36. Hoenicka J, Perez M, Perez-Tur J, et al. The tau gene A0 allele and progressive supranuclear palsy. *Neurology* 1999;53:1219–1225.
37. Mattson MP, Pedersen WA. Effects of amyloid precursor protein derivatives and oxidative stress on basal forebrain cholinergic systems in Alzheimer's disease. *Int J Dev Neurosci* 1998;16: 737–753.
38. Albers DS, Augood SJ, Martin DM, et al. Evidence for oxidative stress in the subthalamic nucleus in progressive supranuclear palsy. *J Neurochem* 1999;73:881–884.

39. Albers DS, Augood SJ, Park LC, et al. Frontal lobe dysfunction in progressive supranuclear palsy: evidence for oxidative stress and mitochondrial impairment. *J Neurochem* 2000;74:878–881.

40. Odetti P, Garibaldi S, Norese R, et al. Lipoperoxidation is selectively involved in progressive supranuclear palsy. *J Neuropathol Exp Neurol* 2000;59:393–397.

41. Komori T, Shibata N, Kobayashi M, et al. Inducible nitric oxide synthase (iNOS)–like immunoreactivity in argyrophilic, tau-positive astrocytes in progressive supranuclear palsy. *Acta Neuropathol* 1998;95:338–344.

42. Perry TL, Hansen S, Jones K. Brain amino acids and glutathione in progressive supranuclear palsy. *Neurology* 1988;38:943–946.

43. Yong VW, Krekoski CA, Forsyth PA, et al. Matrix metalloproteinases and diseases of the CNS. *Trends Neurosci* 1998;21:75–80.

44. Albers DS, Beal MF. Mitochondrial dysfunction and oxidative stress in aging and neurodegenerative disease. *J Neural Transm* 2000;59:[Suppl]133–154.

45. Swerdlow RH, Golbe LI, Parks JK, et al. Mitochondrial dysfunction in cybrid lines expressing mitochondrial genes from patients with progressive supranuclear palsy. *J Neurochem* 2000;75:1681–1684.

46. Albers DS, Swerdlow RH, Manfredi G, et al. Further evidence for mitochondrial dysfunction in progressive supranuclear palsy. *Exp Neurol* 2001;168:196–198.

47. Albers DS, Augood SJ. New insights into progressive supranuclear palsy. *Trends Neurosci* 2001;24:347–353.

48. Mann DMA, Oliver R, Snowden JS. The topographic distribution of brain atrophy in Huntington's disease and progressive supranuclear palsy. *Acta Neuropathol* 1993;85:553–559.

49. Arai N. "Grumose degeneration" of the dentate nucleus: a light and electron microscopic study in progressive supranuclear palsy and dentatorubropallidoluysial atrophy. *J Neurol Sci* 1989;90:131–145.

50. Litvan I, Grafman J, Gomez C, et al. Memory impairment in patients with progressive supranuclear palsy. *Arch Neurol* 1989;46:765–767.

51. Probst A, Langui D, Lautenschlager C, et al. Progressive supranuclear palsy: extensive neuropil threads in addition to neurofibrillary tangles: very similar antigenicity of subcortical neuronal pathology in progressive supranuclear palsy and Alzheimer's disease. *Acta Neuropathol* 1988;77:61–68.

52. Yamada T, McGeer PLI, McGeer EG. Appearance of paired nucleated, tau-positive glia in patients with progressive supranuclear palsy. *Neurosci Lett* 1992;135:99–102.

53. Davis DG, Wang HZ, Markesbery WR. Image analysis of neuropil threads in Alzheimer's, Pick's, diffuse Lewy body disease, and in progressive supranuclear palsy. *J Neuropathol Exp Neurol* 1992;51:594–600.

54. Hauw JJ, Daniel SE, Dickson D, et al. Preliminary NINDS neuropathologic criteria for Steele-Richardson-Olszewski syndrome (progressive supranuclear palsy). *Neurology* 1994;44:2015–2019.

55. Hauw JJ, Verny M, Cervera P, et al. Constant neurofibrillary changes in the neocortex in progressive supranuclear palsy: basic differences with Alzheimer's disease and aging. *Neurosci Lett* 1990;119:182–186.

56. Hof PR, Delacourte A, Bouras C. Distribution of cortical neurofibrillary tangles in progressive supranuclear palsy: a quantitative analysis of six cases. *Acta Neuropathol* 1992;84:45–51.

57. Braak H, Braak E. Argyrophilic grains: characteristic pathology of cerebral cortex in cases of adult onset dementia without Alzheimer changes. *Neurosci Lett* 1987;76:124–127.

58. Hof PR, Bouras C, Buee L, et al. Differential distribution of neurofibrillary tangles in the cerebral cortex of dementia pugilistica and Alzheimer's disease cases. *Acta Neuropathol* 1992;85:23–30.

59. Dickson DW. Neuropathologic differentiation of progressive supranuclear palsy and corticobasal degeneration. *J Neurol* 1999;246:116.

60. Braak H, Braak E. Neuropathological staging of Alzheimer-related changes. *Acta Neuropathol* 1991;82:239–259.

61. Kleinschmidt-DeMasters BK. Early progressive supranuclear palsy: pathology and clinical presentation. *Clin Neuropathol* 1989;8:79–84.

62. Litvan I, Mangone CA, McKee A, et al. Natural history of progressive supranuclear palsy (Steele-Richardson-Olszewski syndrome) and clinical predictors of survival: a clinicopathological study. *J Neurol Neurosurg Psychiatry* 1996;60:615–620.

63. Gearing M, Olson DA, Watts RL, et al. Progressive supranuclear palsy: neuropathologic and clinical heterogeneity. *Neurology* 1994;44:1015–1024.

64. Braak H, Braak E. Argyrophilic grains: characteristic pathology of cerebral cortex in cases of adult onset dementia without Alzheimer changes. *Neurosci Lett* 1987;76:124–127.

65. Braak H, Braak E. Cortical and subcortical argyrophilic grains characterize a disease associated with adult onset dementia. *Neuropathol Appl Neurobiol* 1989;15:13–26.

66. Masliah E, Hansen LA, Quijada S, et al. Late onset dementia with argyrophilic grains and subcortical tangles or atypical progressive supranuclear palsy? *Ann Neurol* 1991;29:389–396.

67. Tolosa E, Valldeoriola F, Cruz-Sanchez F. Progressive supranuclear palsy: clinical and pathological diagnosis. *Eur J Neurol* 1995;2:259–273.

68. Litvan I, Agid Y, Calne D, et al. Clinical research criteria for the diagnosis of progressive supranuclear palsy (Steele-Richardson-Olszewski syndrome): report of the NINDS-SPSP International Workshop. *Neurology* 1996;47:1–9.

69. Spillantini MG, Goedert M. Tau protein pathology in neurodegenerative diseases. *Trends Neurosci* 1998;21:428–433.

70. Vermersch P, Robitaille Y, Bernier L, et al. Biochemical mapping of neurofibrillary degeneration in a case of progressive supranuclear palsy: evidence for general cortical involvement. *Acta Neuropathol* 1994;87:572–577.

71. Goedert M, Spillantini MG, Jakes R, et al. Multiple isoforms of human microtubule-associated protein tau: sequences and localization in neurofibrillary tangles of Alzheimer's disease. *Neuron* 1989;3:519–526.

72. Goedert M, Jakes R. Expression of separate isoforms of human tau protein: correlation with the tau pattern in brain and effects on tubulin polymerization. *EMBO J* 1990;9:4225–4230.

73. Iqbal K, Grundke-Iqbal I. Ubiquitination and abnormal phosphorylation of paired helical filaments in Alzheimer's disease. *Mol Neurobiol* 1991;5:399–410.

74. Ksiezak-Reding H, Binder LI, Yen SH. Alzheimer disease proteins (A68) share epitopes with tau but show distinct biochemical properties. *J Neurosci Res* 1990;25:420–430.

75. Ksiezak-Reding H, Dickson DW, Davies P, et al. Recognition of tau epitopes by anti-neurofilament antibodies that bind to Alzheimer neurofibrillary tangles. *Proc Natl Acad Sci USA* 1987;84:3410–3414.

76. Ksiezak-Reding H, Liu WK, Yen SH. Phosphate analysis and dephosphorylation of modified tau associated with paired helical filaments. *Brain Res* 1992;597:209–219.

77. Lichtenberg-Kraag B, Mandelkow EM, Biernat J, et al. Phosphorylation-dependent epitopes of neurofilament antibodies on tau protein and relationship with Alzheimer tau. *Proc Natl Acad Sci USA* 1992;89:5384–5388.

78. Delacourte A, Robitaille Y, Sergeant N, et al. Specific pathological Tau protein variants characterize Pick's disease. *J Neuropathol Exp Neurol* 1996;55:159–168.

79. Flament S, Delacourte A, Verny M, et al. Abnormal Tau proteins in progressive supranuclear palsy: similarities and differences with the neurofibrillary degeneration of the Alzheimer type. *Acta Neuropathol* 1991;81:591–596.

80. Greenberg SG, Davies P. A preparation of Alzheimer-paired helical filaments that displays distinct tau proteins by polyacrylamide gel electrophoresis. *Proc Natl Acad Sci USA* 1990;87:5827–5831.

81. Ksiezak-Reding H, Morgan K, Dickson DW. Tau immunoreactivity and SDS solubility of two populations of paired helical filaments that differ in morphology. *Brain Res* 1994;649:185–196.

82. Feany MB, Ksiezak-Reding H, Liu WK, et al. Epitope expression and hyperphosphorylation of tau protein in corticobasal degeneration: differentiation from progressive supranuclear palsy. *Acta Neuropathol* 1995;90:37–43.

83. Liu WK, Le TV, Adamson J, et al. Relationship of the extended tau haplotype to tau biochemistry and neuropathology in progressive supranuclear palsy. *Ann Neurol* 2001;50:494–502.

84. Steele JC, Richardson JC, Olszewski J. Progressive supranuclear palsy: a heterogeneous degeneration involving the brainstem, basal ganglia and cerebellum with vertical gaze and pseudobulbar palsy, nuchal dystonia, and dementia. *Arch Neurol* 1964;10:333–358.

85. Steele JC. Progressive supranuclear palsy. *Brain* 1972;95:693–704.

86. Steele JC. Progressive supranuclear palsy. In: Vinken PJ, Bruyn GW, dejong JMB, eds. *Handbook of clinical neurology: system disorders and atrophies,* Part 2. Amsterdam: North-Holland, 1975:217–219.

87. Brusa A, Mancardi GL, Bugiani O. Progressive supranuclear palsy 1979: an overview. *Ital J Neurol Sci* 1979;1:205–222.

88. Kristensen MO. Progressive supranuclear palsy 20 years later. *Acta Neurol Scand* 1985;71:177–189.

89. Rafal R, Friedman J. Limb dystonia in progressive supranuclear palsy. *Neurology* 1987;37:1546–1549.

90. Rivest J, Quinn N, Marsden CD. Dystonia in Parkinson's disease, multiple system atrophy, and progressive supranuclear palsy. *Neurology* 1990;40:1571–1578.

91. Barclay GL, Lang AE. Dystonia in progressive supranuclear palsy. *J Neurol Neurosurg Psychiatry* 1997;62:352–356.

92. Gibb WRG, Luthert PJ, Marsden CD. Corticobasal degeneration. *Brain* 1989;112:1171–1192.

93. De Bruin VS, Machado C, Howard RS, et al. Nocturnal and respiratory disturbances in Steele-Richardson-Olszewski syndrome (progressive supranuclear palsy). *Postgrad Med J* 1996;72:293–296.

94. Sakakibara R, Hattori T, Tojo M, et al. Micturitional disturbance in progressive supranuclear palsy. *J Auton Nerv Syst* 1993;45:101–106.

95. Tolosa E, Espuña M, Valls J, et al. Bladder dysfunction in progressive supranuclear palsy and other parkinsonian disorders. *Mov Disord* 1997;12:272.

96. Lees AJ. The Steele-Richardson-Olszewski syndrome (progressive supranuclear palsy). In: Marsden DC, Fahn S, eds. *Movement disorders.* London: Butterworth, 1987;2:272–287.

97. Duvoisin RC. Differential diagnosis of PSP. *J Neural Transm Suppl* 1994;42:51–67.

98. Collins SJ, Ahlskog JE, Parisi JE, et al. Progressive supranuclear palsy: neuropathologically based diagnostic clinical criteria. *J Neurol Neurosurg Psychiatry* 1995;58:167–173.

99. Daniel SE, de Bruin VMS, Lees AJ. The clinical and pathological spectrum of Steele-Richardson-Olszewski syndrome: progressive supranuclear palsy—a reappraisal. *Brain* 1995;118:759–770.

100. De Bruin VMS, Lees AJ. Subcortical neurofibrillary degenera-tion presenting as Steele-Richardson-Olszewski and other related syndromes: a review of 90 pathologically verified cases. *Mov Disord* 1994;9:381–389.

101. Barr AN. Progressive supranuclear palsy. In: Vinken PJ, Bruyn GW, Klawans HL, eds. *Handbook of clinical neurology.* Amsterdam: North Holland, 1979;49:233–256.

102. Pfaffenbach DD, Layton OD, Kearns TP. Ocular manifestations in progressive supranuclear palsy. *Am J Ophthalmol* 1972;74:1174–1184.

103. Tolosa E, Valldeoriola F, Marti Mi. Clinical diagnosis and diagnostic criteria of progressive supranuclear palsy (Steele-Richardson-Olszewski syndrome). *J Neural Transm Suppl* 1994;42:15–31.

104. Dubas F, Gray F, Escourelle R. Maladie de Steele-Richardson-Olszewski sans ophtalmoplegie: six cas anatomo-cliniques. *Rev Neurol (Paris)* 1983;139:407–416.

105. Jellinger K, Riederer P, Tomonaga M. Progressive supranuclear palsy: clinico-pathological and biochemical studies. *J Neural Transm Suppl* 1980;16:111–128.

106. Probst A. Dégénérescence neurofibrillaire sous-corticale sénile avec présence de tubules contournés et de filaments droits: form atypique de la paralysie supranucléaire progressive. *Rev Neurol (Paris)* 1977;133:417–428.

107. Davis PH, Bergeron C, McLachlan R. Atypical presentation of progressive supranuclear palsy. *Ann Neurol* 1985;17:337–343.

108. Matsuo H, Takashima H, Jishinawa M, et al. Pure akinesia: an atypical manifestation of progressive supranuclear palsy. *J Neurol Neurosurg Psychiatry* 1991;54:397–400.

109. Yamamoto T, Kawamura J, Hashimoto S, et al. Pallidonigroluysian atrophy, progressive supranuclear palsy and adult onset Hallervorden-Spatz disease: a case of akinesia as a predominant feature of parkinsonism. *J Neurol Sci* 1990;101:98–106.

110. Riley DE, Fogt N, Leigh RJ. The syndrome of "pure akinesia" and its relationship to progressive supranuclear palsy. *Neurology* 1994;44:1025–1029.

111. Winikates J, Jankovic J. Vascular progressive supranuclear palsy. *J Neural Transm Suppl* 1994;42:189–204.

112. Morariu MA. Progressive supranuclear palsy and normal-pressure hydrocephalus. *Neurology* 1979;29:1544–1546.

113. Ross-Russell R. Supranuclear palsy of eyelid closure. *Brain* 1980;103:71–82.

114. Steele JC, Guzmán T. Observations about amyotrophic lateral sclerosis and the parkinsonism-dementia complex of Guam with regard to epidemiology and etiology. *Can J Neurol Sci* 1987;14:358–362.

115. Tanner CM, Steele JC, Perl DP, et al. Parkinsonism, dementia, and gaze paresis in Chamorros on Guam: a progressive supranuclear palsy-like syndrome. *Ann Neurol* 1987;22:174.

116. Rosenberg B, Hyhan WL, Day C, et al. Autosomal dominant strionigral degeneration. *Neurology* 1976;26:703–714.

117. Neville BRG, Lake BD, Stephens R, et al. A neurovisceral storage disease with vertical supranuclear ophthalmoplegia, and its relation with Niemann-Pick disease. *Brain* 1973;96:97–120.

118. Tripp JH, Lake BD, Young E, et al. Juvenile Gaucher's disease with horizontal gaze palsy in 3 siblings. *J Neurol Neurosurg Psychiatry* 1977;40:470–478.

119. Ross RJ, Cole M, Thompson JS, et al. Boxers: computed tomography, EEG, and neurological evaluation. *JAMA* 1983;249:211–213.

120. Perkin GD, Lees AJ, Stern GM, et al. Problems in the diagnosis of progressive supranuclear palsy. *Can J Neurol Sci* 1978;5:167–173.

121. Blin J, Baron JC, Dubois B, et al. Positron emission tomography study in progressive supranuclear palsy: brain hypometabolic pattern and clinico-metabolic correlations. *Arch Neurol* 1990;47:747–752.

122. Golbe LI, Davis PH. Progressive supranuclear palsy. In: Jankovic J, Tolosa E, eds. *Parkinson's disease and movement disorders,* 2nd ed. Baltimore: William & Wilkins, 1993:145–161.

123. Drayer BP, Olanow W, Burger P, et al. Parkinson plus syndrome: diagnosis using high field MR imaging of brain iron. *Radiology* 1986;159:493–498.

124. Schonfeld SM, Golbe LI, Safer J. et al. Computed tomographic findings in progressive supranuclear palsy: correlation with clinical grade. *Mov Disord* 1987;2:263–278.

125. Stem MB, Braffman BH, Skolnick BE, et al. Magnetic resonance imaging in Parkinson's disease and parkinsonian syndromes. *Neurology* 1989;39:1524–1526.

126. Savoiardo M, Girotti F, Strada L, et al. Magnetic resonance imaging in progressive supranuclear palsy and other parkinsonian disorders. *J Neural Transm Suppl* 1994;42:93–110.

127. Asato R, Akiguchi I, Masunaga S, et al. Magnetic resonance imaging distinguishes progressive supranuclear palsy from multiple system atrophy. *J Neural Transm* 2000;107:1427–1436.

128. Warmuth-Metz M, Naumann M, Csoti I, et al. Measurement of the midbrain diameter on routine magnetic resonance imaging: a simple and accurate method of differentiating between Parkinson disease and progressive supranuclear palsy. *Arch Neurol* 2001;58:1076–1079.

129. Tedeschi G, Litvan I, Bonavita S, et al. Proton magnetic resonance spectroscopic imaging in progressive supranuclear palsy, Parkinson's disease, and corticobasal degeneration. *Brain* 1997; 120:1541–1552.

130. Davie CA, Barker GJ, Machado C, et al. 1H Magnetic resonance spectroscopy in Steele-Richardson-Olszewski syndrome. *Mov Disord* 1997;12(abst.):270.

131. Schrag A, Good CD, Miszkiel K, et al. Differentiation of atypical parkinsonian syndromes with routine MRI. *Neurology* 2000;54:697–702.

132. Foster NL, Gilman S, Berent S, et al. Cerebral hypometabolism in progressive supranuclear palsy studied with positron emission tomography. *Ann Neurol* 1988;24:399–406.

133. Blin J, Baron JC, Dubois B, et al. Positron emission tomography study in progressive supranuclear palsy: brain hypometabolic pattern and clinico-metabolic correlations. *Arch Neurol* 1990;47:747–752.

134. Foster NL, Gilman S, Berent S, et al. Progressive subcortical gliosis and progressive supranuclear palsy can have similar clinical and PET abnormalities. *J Neurol Neurosurg Psychiatry* 1992; 55:707–713.

135. Piccini P, de Yébenes J, Lees AJ, et al. Familial progressive supranuclear palsy: detection of subclinical cases using 18F-dopa and 18fluorodeoxyglucose positron emission tomography. *Arch Neurol* 2001;58:1846–1851.

136. Brooks DJ, Ibáñez V, Sawle GV, et al. Differing patterns of striatal [18F]-dopa uptake in Parkinson's disease, multiple system atrophy, and progressive supranuclear palsy. *Ann Neurol* 1990; 28:547–555.

137. van Royen E, Verhoeff NF, Speelman JD, et al. Multiple system atrophy and progressive supranuclear palsy: diminished striatal D2 dopamine receptor activity demonstrated by 123I-IBZM single photon emission computed tomography. *Arch Neurol* 1993;50:513–516.

138. Ilgin N, Zubieta J, Reich SG, et al. PET imaging of the dopamine transporter in progressive supranuclear palsy and Parkinson's disease. *Neurology* 1999;52:1221–1226.

139. Messa C, Volonte MA, Fazio F, et al. Differential distribution of striatal [123I]beta-CIT in Parkinson's disease and progressive supranuclear palsy, evaluated with single-photon emission tomography. *Eur J Nucl Med* 1998;25:1270–1276.

140. Brucke T, Asenbaum S, Pirker W, et al. Measurement of the dopaminergic degeneration in Parkinson's disease with [123I]

beta-CIT and SPECT: correlation with clinical findings and comparison with multiple system atrophy and progressive supranuclear palsy. *J Neural Transm Suppl* 1997;50:9–24.

141. Pirker W, Asenbaum S, Bencsits G, et al. [123I]beta-CIT SPECT in multiple system atrophy, progressive supranuclear palsy, and corticobasal degeneration. *Mov Disord* 2000;15: 1158–1167.

142. Shinotoh H, Namba H, Yamaguchi M, et al. Positron emission tomographic measurement of acetylcholinesterase activity reveals differential loss of ascending cholinergic systems in Parkinson's disease and progressive supranuclear palsy. *Ann Neurol* 1999;46:62–69.

143. Tolosa E, Zeese JA. Brainstem auditory evoked responses in progressive supranuclear palsy. *Ann Neurol* 1979;6:639.

144. Pierrot-Deseilligny C, Turell E, Penet C, et al. Increased wave P300 latency in progressive supranuclear palsy. *J Neurol Neurosurg Psychiatry* 1989;52:656–658.

145. Johnson RJ, Litvan I, Grafman J. Progressive supranuclear palsy: altered sensory processing leads to degraded cognition. *Neurology* 1991;41:1257–1262.

146. Kofler M, Muller J, Reggiani L, et al. Somatosensory evoked potentials in progressive supranuclear palsy. *J Neurol Sci* 2000; 179(S 1-2):85–91.

147. Lepore FE. Disorders of ocular motility in the olivopontocerebellar atrophies. In: Duvoisin RC, Plaitakis A, eds. *The olivopontocerebellar atrophies.* New York: Raven Press, 1984:97–103.

148. Rascol O, Sabatini U, Simonetta-Moreau M, et al. Square wave jerks in parkinsonian syndromes. *J Neurol Neurosurg Psychiatry* 1991;54:599–602.

149. Troost B. Neuro-ophthalmological aspects. In: Litvan Y, Agid Y, eds. *Progressive supranuclear palsy: clinical and research approaches.* New York: Oxford University Press, 1992:44–88.

150. Vidailhet M, Rivaud S, Gouider-Khouja N, et al. Eye movements in parkinsonian syndromes. *Ann Neurol* 1994;35: 420–426.

151. Rivaud-Pechoux S, Vidailhet M, Gallouedec G, et al. Longitudinal ocular motor study in corticobasal degeneration and progressive supranuclear palsy. *Neurology* 2000;54:1029–1032.

152. Gross RA, Spehlmann R, Daniels JC. Sleep disturbances in progressive supranuclear palsy. *Clin Neurophysiol* 1978;48: 16–25.

153. Laffont F, Autret A, Minz M, et al. Etude polygraphique du sommeil dans 9 cas de maladie de Steele-Richardson. *Rev Neurol (Paris)* 1979;135:127–142.

154. Aldrich MS, Foster NL, White RF, et al. Sleep abnormalities in progressive supranuclear palsy. *Ann Neurol* 1989;49:323–329.

155. Santamaría J, Cardozo A, Martí MJ, et al. Alteraciones del sueño en la parálisis supranuclear progresiva. *Neurología* 1992;7: 292.

156. Santamaría J, Iranzo A. Alteraciones del sueño en los trastornos del movimiento. *Neurologia* 1997;12[Suppl 3]:35–47.

157. Montplaisir J, Petit D, Decary A, et al. Sleep and quantitative EEG in patients with progressive supranuclear palsy. *Neurology* 1997;49:999–1003.

158. Valldeoriola F, Valls-Solé J, Tolosa E, et al. The acoustic startle response is normal in patients with multiple system atrophy. *Mov Disord* 1997;12:697–700.

159. Kofler M, Müller J, Wenning GK, et al. The auditory startle reaction in parkinsonian disorders. *Mov Disord* 2001;16:62–71.

160. Valldeoriola F, Valls-Solé J, Tolosa E, et al. The effect of a startling acoustic stimulus on reaction time in patients with different parkinsonian syndromes. *Neurology* 1998;51: 1315–1320.

161. Molinuevo JL, Valls-Solé J, Valldeoriola F. The effect of transcranial magnetic stimulation on reaction time in progressive supranuclear palsy. *Clin Neurophysiol* 2000;111:2008–2013.

162. Valls-Solé J. Neurophysiological characterization of parkinsonian syndromes. *Clin Neurophysiol* 2000;30:352–367.

163. Valls Solé J, Valldeoriola F, Tolosa E, et al. Distinctive abnormalities of facial reflexes in patients with progressive supranuclear palsy. *Brain* 1997;120:1877–1883.

164. Scaravilli T, Pramstaller PP, Salerno A, et al. Neuronal loss in Onuf's nucleus in three patients with progressive supranuclear palsy. *Ann Neurol* 2000;48:97–101.

165. Wenning GK, Scherfler C, Granata R, et al. Time course of symptomatic orthostatic hypotension and urinary incontinence in patients with postmortem confirmed parkinsonian syndromes: a clinicopathological study. *J Neurol Neurosurg Psychiatry* 1999;67:620–623.

166. Eardley I, Quinn NP, Fowler CJ, et al. The values of urethral sphincter electromyography in the differential diagnosis of parkinsonism. *Br J Urol* 1989;64:360–362.

167. Valldeoriola F, Valls-Solé J, Tolosa ES, et al. Striated anal sphincter denervation in patients with progressive supranuclear palsy. *Mov Disord* 1995;10:550–555.

168. Nieforth KA, Golbe LI. Retrospective study of drug response in 87 patients with progressive supranuclear palsy. *Clin Neuropharmacol* 1993;16:338–346.

169. Colosimo C, Albanese A, Hughes AJ, et al. Some specific clinical features differentiate multiple system atrophy (striatonigral variety) from Parkinson's disease. *Arch Neurol* 1995;52:294–298.

170. Kompoliti K, Goetz CG, Litvan I, et al. Pharmacological therapy in progressive supranuclear palsy. *Arch Neurol* 1998;55:1099–1102.

171. Weiner WJ, Minagar A, Shulman LM. Pramipexole in progressive supranuclear palsy. *Neurology* 1999;52:873–874.

172. Goetz CG, Kompoliti K, Litvan Y, et al. Pharmacological therapy in progressive supranuclear palsy (PSP). *Mov Disord* 1997;12(abst.):273.

173. Litvan I, Blesa R, Clark K, et al. Pharmacological evaluation of the cholinergic system in progressive supranuclear palsy. *Ann Neurol* 1994;36:55–61.

174. Frattali CM, Sonies BC, Chi-Fishman G, et al. Effects of physostigmine on swallowing and oral motor functions in patients with progressive supranuclear palsy: a pilot study. *Dysphagia* 1999;14:165–168.

175. Fabbrini G, Barbanti P, Bonifati V, et al. Donepezil in the treatment of progressive supranuclear palsy. *Acta Neurol Scand* 2001;103:123–125.

176. Litvan I, Phipps M, Pharr VL, et al. Randomized placebo-controlled trial of donepezil in patients with progressive supranuclear palsy. *Neurology* 2001;57:467–473.

177. Chinaglia G, Landwehrmeyer B, Probst A, et al. Serotoninergic terminal transporters are differentially affected in Parkinson's disease and progressive supranuclear palsy: an autoradiographic study with [3H]citalopram. *Neurosci* 1993;54:691–699.

178. Hornykiewicz O, Shannak KJ. Brain monoamines in progressive supranuclear palsy—comparison with idiopathic Parkinson's disease. *Neural Trans Suppl* 1994;42:219–227.

179. Kato E, Takahashi S, Abe T, et al. A case of progressive supranuclear palsy showing improvement of rigidity, nuchal dystonia, and autonomic failure with trazodone. *Rinsho Shinkeigaku* 1994;34:1013–1017.

180. Newman GC. Treatment of progressive supranuclear palsy with tryciclic antidepressants. *Neurology* 1985;35:1189–1193.

181. Engel PA. Treatment of progressive supranuclear palsy with amitriptyline: therapeutic and toxic effects. *J Am Geriatr Soc* 1996;44:1072–1074.

182. Cohen S, Oster M, Hennerici M. Amantadin improves gait disorders in patients with age related gait abnormalities. *J Neurol* 1995;242[Suppl 2]:13.

183. Ghika J, Tennis M, Hoffman E, et al. Idazoxan treatment in progressive supranuclear palsy. *Neurology* 1991;41:986–991.

184. Levy R, Ruberg M, Herrero MT, et al. Alterations of GABAergic neurons in the basal ganglia of patients with progressive supranuclear palsy: an in situ hybridization study of GAD67 messenger RNA. *Neurology* 1995;45:127–134.

185. Daniele A, Moro E, Bentivoglio AR. Zolpidem in progressive supranuclear palsy. *N Engl J Med* 1999;12;341:543–544.

186. Polo KB, Jabbari B. Botulinum toxin-A improves the rigidity of progressive supranuclear palsy. *Ann Neurol* 1994;35:237–239.

187. Krack P, Marion MH. "Apraxia of lid opening," a focal eyelid dystonia: clinical study of 32 patients. *Mov Disord* 1994;9:610–615.

11

MULTIPLE SYSTEM ATROPHY

SID GILMAN

Multiple system atrophy (MSA) is a neurodegenerative disease occurring sporadically and characterized by parkinsonism, cerebellar dysfunction, and autonomic insufficiency in any combination. When parkinsonism dominates the clinical picture, the disorder is termed MSA-P (i.e., MSA with predominantly parkinsonian features). When cerebellar ataxia is the dominant clinical disorder, the disease is termed MSA-C. The disease affects both sexes, usually beginning in middle age and progressing continuously. The extrapyramidal disorders appear similar to those in Parkinson's disease, including bradykinesia with rigidity, postural instability, hypokinetic speech, and occasionally tremor, usually with a poor or unsustained response to chronic levodopa therapy. The signs of cerebellar dysfunction include disorders of extraocular movements (Table 11.1), ataxia of speech, and ataxia of limb movements and gait resulting in postural instability and frequent falls. Autonomic insufficiency results in orthostatic hypotension, urinary retention or incontinence, and impotence, often accompanied by constipation and decreased sweating (Table 11.2). According to a consensus committee decision, the definition of orthostatic hypotension is a reduction of systolic blood pressure of at least 20 mm Hg or a diastolic blood pressure of at least 10 mm Hg within 3 minutes of rising from the recumbent position (1). For the diagnosis of MSA, however, a subsequent consensus committee utilized a reduction of systolic blood pressure by 30 mm Hg systolic or 15 mm Hg diastolic as a criterion (2). Confounding variables include food ingestion, time of day, state of hydration, ambient temperature, recent recumbency, postural deconditioning, hypertension, medications, gender, and age.

TABLE 11.1. COMMON DISORDERS OF EXTRAOCULAR MOVEMENTS IN MULTIPLE SYSTEM ATROPHY

Square-wave jerks
Saccadic pursuit movements
Nystagmus in primary gaze or upon lateral gaze
Overshoot or undershoot dysmetria
Slowness of pursuit movements

TABLE 11.2. AUTONOMIC DYSFUNCTION IN MULTIPLE SYSTEM ATROPHY

Common Features
Orthostatic hypotension (reduction of systolic blood pressure of at least 20 mm Hg or diastolic blood pressure of at least 10 mm Hg within 3 min of standing from the recumbent position) unexplained by medication
Impotence (in males)
Urinary incontinence or retention
Less Common Features
Impaired sweating
Constipation
Iris atrophy

Extrapyramidal, cerebellar, and autonomic features often occur in combination in MSA, but one or in some patients two features may predominate. The neuropathologic changes consist of neuronal cell loss with reactive gliosis in some or all of the following structures: putamen, caudate nucleus, globus pallidus, substantia nigra, inferior olives, pontine nuclei, cerebellar Purkinje cells, autonomic nuclei of the brainstem, and the intermediolateral cell columns and Onuf's nucleus in the spinal cord. Glial and neuronal cytoplasmic inclusions are found in multiple structures of the central nervous system. α-Synuclein is a major component of these inclusions (3), and currently MSA can be viewed as a synucleinopathy. Although it has many clinical variations, MSA is a distinct entity that should be differentiated from both the sporadic multiple system degenerations, such as progressive supranuclear palsy (PSP) and corticobasal ganglionic degeneration, and the hereditary multiple system degenerations, such as Machado-Joseph disease and some families with the *SCA1* gene disorder (4).

TERMINOLOGY

The terms *striatonigral degeneration, Shy-Drager syndrome,* and, at least in some cases, *sporadic olivopontocerebellar atrophy* refer to various manifestations of MSA. Striatonigral degeneration is a neurologic disorder characterized pathologically by neuronal degeneration with reactive gliosis in the striatum and substantia nigra and clinically by parkinsonian features of bradykinesia, rigidity, postural instability, and hypokinetic speech (5), all poorly responsive or unresponsive to levodopa medication. This disorder is now recognized as a form of MSA and is best placed in the category of possible MSA, as described below. The term *Shy-Drager syndrome* (6) as currently used refers to a combination of striatonigral degeneration and autonomic insufficiency manifested by orthostatic hypotension, impotence, and urinary retention or incontinence. Sporadic olivopontocerebellar atrophy (sOPCA) is characterized neuropathologically by neuronal degeneration with reactive gliosis in the inferior olives, pons, and cerebellar vermis and hemispheres, and clinically by progressive ataxia of extraocular movements, speech, gait, and limb movements. This disorder is best considered as a form

of possible MSA; however, it is not clear whether all patients with sOPCA progress to develop MSA (7).

LEVELS OF DIAGNOSTIC CERTAINTY

MSA is a complex disorder, and several efforts have been made to develop diagnostic criteria. A consensus committee recently published a set of diagnostic criteria that provide guidelines for categorizing patients based on their clinical findings (2) (Table 11.3). The guidelines took into account the complex nature of the disorder and the level of certainty that a particular patient might have MSA. Accordingly, three levels of diagnostic certainty were described: possible, probable, and definite (Table 11.4). With these guidelines, sOPCA patients would qualify for the diagnosis of possible MSA if they had one parkinsonian feature plus one auto-

TABLE 11.3. MULTIPLE SYSTEM ATROPHY: CONSENSUS CRITERIA

These criteria utilize clinical domains, features and criteria for the diagnosis of MSA. Clinical domains refer to autonomic and urinary dysfunction, parkinsonism, and cerebellar ataxia.
Features (a) are defined as characteristics of the disease and criteria (b) consist of defining features or composites of features required for diagnosis. For tests of orthostatic hypotension, the clinician measures the blood pressure after the patient has been in the recumbent position for 2 min and then in the standing position for 2 min.

Clinical Domains
I. Autonomic and urinary dysfunction
  A. Autonomic and urinary features
    1. Orthostatic hypotension (a decline of 20 mm Hg systolic or 10 mm Hg diastolic)
    2. Urinary incontinence or incomplete bladder emptying
  B. Criterion for autonomic failure or urinary dysfunction in MSA
    1. Orthostatic fall in blood pressure (by 30 mm Hg systolic or 15 mm Hg diastolic) or
    2. Urinary incontinence (persistent, involuntary partial or total bladder emptying, accompanied by erectile dysfunction in men) or both
II. Parkinsonism
  A. Parkinsonian features
    1. Bradykinesia (slowness of voluntary movement with a progressive reduction of speed and amplitude)
    2. Rigidity
    3. Postural instability (not due to primary visual, vestibular, cerebellar, or proprioceptive dysfunction)
    4. Tremor (postural, resting or both)
  B. Criterion for parkinsonism in MSA
    Bradykinesia plus at least one of items 2–4
III. Cerebellar dysfunction
  A. Cerebellar features
    1. Gait ataxia (wide based stance with steps irregular in length and direction)
    2. Ataxic dysarthria
    3. Limb ataxia
    4. Sustained gaze-evoked nystagmus
  B. Criterion for cerebellar dysfunction in MSA
    Gait ataxia plus at least one of items 2–4
IV. Corticospinal tract dysfunction
  A. Corticospinal tract features
    Extensor plantar responses with hyperreflexia
  B. Criterion for corticospinal tract dysfunction
    Corticospinal dysfunction is not considered in the diagnosis

Based on Gilman et al., 1999.

TABLE 11.4. DIAGNOSTIC CATEGORIES OF MULTIPLE SYSTEM ATROPHY

Possible MSA: One criterion plus two features from separate other domains. When the criterion is parkinsonism, a poor levodopa response qualifies as one feature (hence only one additional feature is required);

Probable MSA: Criterion for autonomic failure/urinary dysfunction plus poorly levodopa responsive parkinsonism or cerebellar dysfunction;

Definite MSA: Pathologically confirmed by the presence of a high density of glial cytoplasmic inclusions in association with a combination of degenerative changes in the nigrostriatal and olivopontocerebellar pathways

Based on Gilman et al., 1999 (2).

nomic feature, either urinary incontinence or orthostatic hypotension (at the level of a 20 mm Hg decline systolic or 10 mm Hg decline diastolic). Similarly, striatonigral patients would qualify for the diagnosis of possible MSA if they had one cerebellar feature plus one autonomic feature. Striatonigral patients would also qualify for the diagnosis of possible MSA if they had a poor response to levodopa plus either one cerebellar feature or one autonomic feature. The diagnosis of probable MSA requires the presence of autonomic failure or urinary dysfunction plus poorly levodopa-responsive parkinsonism or cerebellar dysfunction (Table 11.4). The diagnosis of definite MSA requires neuropathologic confirmation of the disease. The consensus conference developed exclusion criteria for the diagnosis of MSA (Table 11.5).

TABLE 11.5. EXCLUSION CRITERIA FOR THE DIAGNOSIS OF MULTIPLE SYSTEM ATROPHY

I. History
  A. Symptomatic onset under age 30 years
  B. Family history of a similar disorder
  C. Systemic diseases or other identifiable causes for features listed in Table 11.1
  D. Hallucinations unrelated to medication
II. Physical Examination
  A. DSM–IV criteria for dementia
  B. Prominent slowing of vertical saccades or vertical supranuclear gaze palsy[a]
  C. Evidence of focal cortical dysfunction such as aphasia, alien-limb syndrome, and parietal dysfunction
III. Laboratory Investigation
  Metabolic, molecular genetic, and imaging evidence of an alternative cause of features listed in Table 11.3

[a]In practice, MSA is most frequently confused with Parkinson's disease or PSP. Mild limitation of upward gaze alone is nonspecific, whereas a prominent (>50%) limitation of upward gaze or any limitation of downward gaze suggests PSP. Before the onset of vertical gaze limitation, a clinically obvious slowing of voluntary vertical saccades is usually easily detectable in PSP and assists in the early differentiation of these two disorders.
DSM–IV, Diagnostic and Statistical Manual of Mental Disorders; PSP, progressive supranuclear palsy.
Based on Gilman et al., 1999–IV (2).

HISTORICAL NOTES

Dejerine and Thomas (8) first described olivopontocerebellar atrophy in two patients without a family history of similar disorders. Clinically these patients had cerebellar, parkinsonian, and autonomic disorders, and neuropathologic examination revealed neuronal loss and gliosis in the inferior olives, pons, and cerebellum. The authors did not mention the basal ganglia in their description of neuropathologic changes. Subsequently, Bradbury and Eggleston (9) reported three patients with postural hypotension, including one with impotence and constipation and another with brisk muscle stretch reflexes and extensor plantar responses. In retrospect, these patients probably had MSA.

Shy and Drager (6) described two patients with orthostatic hypotension, impotence, an atonic bladder resulting in urinary incontinence, loss of rectal sphincter tone with fecal incontinence, loss of sweating, iris atrophy, external ocular palsies, rigidity, tremor, loss of associated movements, fasciculations, and wasting of distal muscles. Neuropathologic examination in one of the patients revealed neuronal loss and gliosis in the substantia nigra, striatum, olives, pons, cerebellum, and intermediolateral cells of the spinal cord. Even though the patients described by Shy and Drager had clinical symptoms indicating widespread neurologic disease and one of them showed extensive neuropathologic changes, many clinicians now use the term Shy-Drager syndrome to designate patients with the combination of autonomic insufficiency and parkinsonism poorly responsive to levodopa. Quinn et al. (10) have commented appropriately that the entity described by Shy and Drager does not correspond to the disorder currently designated with their names, and thus the term "Shy-Drager syndrome" should not be used.

Adams et al. (5) described the clinical and neuropathologic findings of an entity that they termed striatonigral degeneration, although the patients clinically manifested cerebellar, pyramidal tract, and autonomic dysfunction and neuropathologically showed neuronal and gliosis in the striatum, substantia nigra, inferior olives, pons, and cerebellum.

In a classic paper presenting one new patient studied clinically and neuropathologically, Graham and Oppenheimer (11) pulled together the entities described previously and recommended designating these disorders as "multiple system atrophy," a term they coined. The patient they described had shown autonomic failure, cerebellar ataxia, and probably signs of corticospinal tract disease, but not parkinsonism during life, and neuropathologic examination disclosed neuronal cell loss and gliosis in the substantia nigra, putamen, inferior olives, pons, cerebellum, and intermediolateral columns of the spinal cord. This paper established MSA as a clinical entity and demonstrated the features that are seen in common in striatonigral degeneration, Shy-Drager syndrome, and sOPCA.

Lantos and Papp (12) identified glial cytoplasmic inclusions in the oligodendrocytes of MSA patients, thereby establishing a neuropathologic basis for considering striatonigral degeneration, Shy-Drager syndrome, and at least some cases of sOPCA as manifestations of MSA. Subsequently, several investigators determined that α-synuclein is a key component of glial cytoplasmic inclusions and that MSA is a synucleinopathy (3).

INCIDENCE AND PREVALENCE

Determining the incidence and prevalence of MSA is difficult, as only a few epidemiologic studies have been reported. Estimates of the prevalence of MSA (per 100,000 in the population) in four studies were 2.3 (13), 4.4 (14), 4.9 (15), and 310 (16). In a single study, the annual incidence of MSA was estimated to be 3.0/100,000 people over the age of 50 years (17).

CLINICAL PRESENTATION

Onset

MSA is a disease of adult life that commonly causes clinical symptoms beginning in the sixth decade, although occasionally symptoms commence as early as the fourth decade (18). In a series of 100 cases of MSA reported by Wenning et al. (19), the median age of onset was 53 and the range was 33 to 76 years.

Initial Symptomatology

In the series of Wenning et al. (19), almost half of patients with MSA developed symptoms of autonomic dysfunction as their initial feature, and 97% experienced these symptoms at latest follow-up. The most common symptoms of autonomic insufficiency were impotence in men and urinary incontinence in women. Symptomatic orthostatic hypotension, although present in 68% of cases, was severe in only 15%. Extrapyramidal disorders of the parkinsonian type were the initial feature in 46%, but these disturbances subsequently developed in 91% of subjects. Although akinesia and rigidity were the predominant clinical abnormalities, tremor at rest was found in 29% of patients. The response to levodopa was good to excellent in 29% of patients at some stage of the disease, but only 13% maintained this response over time. Patients with onset before the age of 49 years tended to have a better levodopa response than patients with later onset. Signs of cerebellar disorder were the only initial features in 5% of cases, but 47% later developed these disturbances. A cerebellar syndrome was the only motor disorder in 9% of patients and the predominant motor disturbance in another 9%. MSA-

C presented most commonly with ataxia of gait and cerebellar tremor. Signs of pyramidal dysfunction and myoclonus were more common in MSA-P than in MSA-C. Signs of cerebellar disorder were present in 42% of patients with the MSA-P, and parkinsonian signs were found in 50% of patients with MSA-C.

The predominance of parkinsonian symptomatology in the series of Wenning et al. (19) may result in part from a sampling bias, reflecting the investigators' interest in parkinsonian syndromes and the identification of these patients in a clinic specializing in Parkinson's disease. A recent study suggests that a substantial proportion of patients with sOPCA will progress to develop MSA. This study followed the clinical course of 51 sOPCA patients age 20 years or older initially evaluated in an ataxia clinic over 14 years and followed at 3- to 6-month intervals for 3 months to 10 years (7). Seventeen evolved to develop MSA, whereas the remaining 34 manifested only progressively worsening cerebellar ataxia. The features of the MSA cases included autonomic failure and parkinsonism in 10, autonomic failure without parkinsonism in 6, and parkinsonism without autonomic failure in 1. A survival analysis demonstrated that 24% of subjects in this population would evolve to MSA within 5 years of the onset of sOPCA symptoms. An older age of onset of symptoms and a shorter time from onset of symptoms to first presentation in a neurology specialty clinic were both highly predictive of evolution to MSA. The estimated median survival time from time of transition to death was 3.5 years.

Progression

MSA is a chronically progressive disease characterized by the gradual onset of symptoms of autonomic insufficiency, extrapyramidal disorder, or cerebellar ataxia followed by worsening of these symptoms and accumulation of symptoms reflecting involvement of the systems initially unaffected. Thus, patients who present initially with extrapyramidal features commonly progress to develop autonomic disturbances, cerebellar disorders, or both. Conversely, patients who begin with symptoms of cerebellar dysfunction often progress to develop extrapyramidal or autonomic disorders, or both. Patients whose symptoms initially are autonomic may later develop cerebellar, extrapyramidal, or both types of disorders.

ASSOCIATED CLINICAL FEATURES

Peripheral Neuropathy

Patients with MSA frequently have a mild and often subclinical peripheral neuropathy. In a study of 74 patients with the clinical diagnosis of MSA, 90% had an abnormal sphincter electromyographic examination, indicating denervation and reinnervation owing to loss of anterior horn cells in Onuf's nucleus (20). In the same study, however, only 40% had abnormal peripheral nerve conduction and electromyographic studies. These abnormal studies included a mixed sensory and motor axonal neuropathy in 17.5% of patients and an abnormal skeletal muscle electromyogram, suggesting partial denervation in 22.5%. These findings indicate that MSA affects both motor and sensory nerve fibers to some extent, and that the anterior horn cells of Onuf's nucleus innervating the external sphincter muscles are particularly vulnerable.

Sleep Disorders

MSA patients have multiple sleep-related symptoms, including excessive daytime sleepiness, insomnia, arrhythmic respiration, sleep apnea, rapid eye movement sleep behavior disorder (RBD), and sleep-related stridor from vocal cord paresis. REM sleep and slow-wave sleep are reduced, and RBD affects at least two thirds of MSA patients, at times preceding the onset of other clinical features. Obstructive sleep apnea (OSA) and central sleep apnea (CSA) frequently occur in MSA and may cause sudden death (21). This is clinically important, as OSA can be treated effectively with continuous positive airway pressure (CPAP) or with various surgical procedures (21).

Cognitive Function

Patients with MSA usually retain normal intelligence levels, but abnormalities of neuropsychological function have been described (22). In one study, a distinctive pattern of cognitive defects was found suggesting normal intelligence but disorders of frontal lobe function (23). These included difficulties with attentional set shifting when extradimensional shifting was required, impairment in subject-ordered tests of spatial working memory, and deficits in speed of thinking (rather than of accuracy) in the Tower of London task. Another study in patients with striatonigral degeneration demonstrated impairment on category and phonemic fluency, frontal behaviors, trail making tests A and B, and free recall in the Grober and Buschke test (24). These patients were normal on the revised Wechsler Adult Intelligence Scale verbal scale, Wechsler memory scale, Raven 47 colored progressive matrices, California Verbal Learning Test, Wisconsin Card Sorting Test, and the Stroop interference condition. In the same study, a group of patients with Parkinson's disease had similar disorders. In a third study, deficits in attention tasks, particularly the Stroop test, were significantly greater in MSA-P than in patients with Parkinson's disease (22).

Other Disorders

Patients with MSA commonly experience emotional disorders, most frequently depression but also emotional liability. Signs of pyramidal tract disease occur frequently and include spasticity and hyperreflexia with extensor plantar responses. MSA patients can show antecollis, myoclonus, and Raynaud's phenomenon, and a supranuclear ophthalmoplegia resembling the findings in PSP can occur. Pain has been reported in up to 50% of MSA patients, classified as rheumatic in 64%, sensory in 28%, dystonic in 21%, and levodopa related in 16% (25). Pain in association with levodopa administration was related to off-periods or diphasic dystonias. Olfactory function is impaired in MSA, though the impairment is not as great as in idiopathic Parkinson's disease (19). Abnormal vestibulo-ocular reflex cancellation has been found in MSA as well as in PSP, but not in Parkinson's disease (26).

NEUROPATHOLOGIC CHANGES

Neuronal Cell Loss and Gliosis

The neurodegenerative changes in MSA consist of neuronal loss with reactive gliosis in the substantia nigra, locus ceruleus, putamen, lateral segment of the globus pallidus, inferior olivary nucleus, pons, cerebellar cortex, autonomic nuclei of the brainstem, and intermediolateral columns of the spinal cord (12). Degenerative changes occur more consistently in the inferior olives, pons, and cerebellum than in the basal ganglia. The caudate nucleus and medial segment of the globus pallidus usually become less affected than the putamen and lateral segment of the globus pallidus, and can be spared. A clinical pathologic study of 35 cases of MSA revealed pronounced loss of neurons in the putamen in 61% of cases and moderate to mild loss in 11% (27). The caudate nucleus showed severe neuronal loss in only 6% of cases and only mild to moderate gliosis in 60%. Degenerative changes of the inferior olives, pons, and cerebellum were observed in 85% of 34 cases studied. The changes in the cerebellar cortex consisted of pronounced Purkinje cell depletion in the cerebellar cortex in 35% of the cases and moderate changes in 50%. When present, cell loss was more severe in the cerebellar vermis than in the hemispheres in 70% of the 17 cases in which comparisons were made. The dentate nuclei were only mildly affected, showing gliosis without neuronal loss.

Glial and Neuronal Cytoplasmic Inclusions

Lantos and Papp (12) found cytoplasmic inclusions in cells of the central nervous system in patients with MSA, initially in glia and later in neurons. They concluded that these inclusions are both pathognomonic of the disorder and important in the clinical symptomatology (Fig. 11.1). Many investigators have confirmed these findings. These inclusions appear in several locations, including oligodendrocyte cytoplasm, oligodendrocyte nuclei, neuronal cyto-

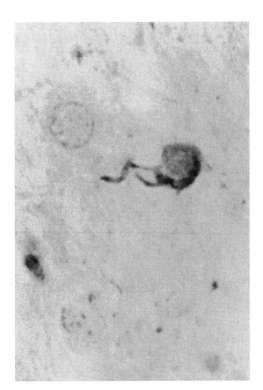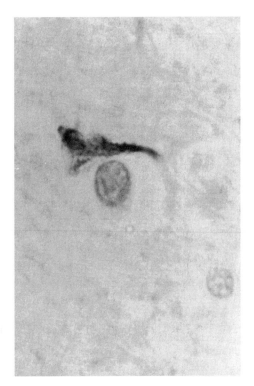

FIG. 11.1. Intracytoplasmic oligodendroglial inclusions immunostained with tau *(left)* and ubiquitin *(right)* (×2,240). (Courtesy of Dr. A.A.F. Sima and Ms. C. D'Amato, Pathology Department, University of Michigan.)

plasm, neuronal nuclei, and axons. Glial cytoplasmic inclusions (GCIs) are found predominantly in the motor and autonomic system, including cortical motor regions, putamen, caudate, pallidum, reticular formation of the brainstem, basis pontis, and intermediate zone of the spinal cord. The density of GCIs exceeds the degree of neuronal degeneration, as demonstrated by neuronal cytoplasmic and nuclear inclusions, degenerated neurons, and loss of nerve cells. This suggests that GCIs may precede neuronal loss and that they constitute the primary pathologic change in MSA. Current evidence indicates that, although glial and neuronal cytoplasmic inclusions appear in most and probably all cases of MSA, they can also be found in patients with other neurodegenerative disorders. These include PSP (28), corticobasal ganglionic degeneration (28), and dominantly inherited multiple system degeneration resulting from the *SCA1* gene (4). Thus, these inclusions are not specific for MSA and they are not diagnostic for this disorder. Nevertheless, they appear to be highly important in the pathophysiology of the disorder.

α-Synuclein in Multiple System Atrophy

α-Synuclein constitutes a major component of both glial and neuronal cytoplasmic inclusions (3). Degenerating neurites also contain α-synuclein. GCIs also contain β-crystallin, tubulins, and ubiquitin. α-Synuclein is one

component of a family that now includes β-synuclein (also designated phosphoneuronoprotein 14 or PNP14) and γ-synuclein (also called breast cancer–specific gene 1 or *BCSG1* and persyn) (29). Separate genes on chromosome 4q21.3-q22, 5q35, and 10q23 encode α, β, and γ-synuclein, respectively. All of these synucleins can be found in brain, primarily in axon terminals and presynaptic sites. Other tissues also express these proteins, notably breast, ovary, skin, and retina. Two mutations in the gene encoding α-synuclein are associated with autosomal dominantly inherited parkinsonism (30). Moreover, aggregates of α-synuclein appear not only in GCIs of MSA cases, but also in glia and neurons in PD and related Lewy body disorders (31). The finding of selective nitration of α-synuclein in GCIs of MSA and other α-synuclein lesions in related α-synucleinopathies implicates nitrative and perhaps oxidative damage in mechanisms of brain degeneration in these neurodegenerative disorders (32). Because MSA is a sporadic disorder, nongenetic (e.g., environmental) causes of MSA have been sought. While there is currently no evidence that most cases of MSA are caused by a specific environmental cause, rarely autopsy-proven cases of MSA have been attributed to exposure to certain toxins known to cause neuronal cell death, such as formaldehyde, malathion, diazinon, *n*-hexane, benzene, methylisobutylketone, and pesticides (32a).

DIFFERENTIAL DIAGNOSIS

Parkinsonian Features

Many patients with MSA develop striatonigral degeneration and experience as their earliest symptoms the parkinsonian features of bradykinesia, rigidity, and postural instability. In these patients, the differential diagnosis includes the many disorders that comprise parkinsonian symptoms and signs, including idiopathic Parkinson's disease and many parkinsonian syndromes (Table 11.6). An excellent response to levodopa in the absence of significant autonomic failure is the best means of differentiating Parkinson's disease from MSA-P (Table 11.7). A poor response to levodopa, symptomatic autonomic dysfunction, and clinical evidence of a cerebellar disorder suggests a diagnosis other than idiopathic Parkinson's disease

TABLE 11.6. PARKINSONIAN SYNDROMES

Neurodegenerative disorders
  Idiopathic Parkinson's disease
  Diffuse Lewy body disease
  Striatonigral degeneration (multiple system atrophy)
  Shy-Drager syndrome (multiple system atrophy)
  Progressive supranuclear palsy
  Alzheimer's disease with extrapyramidal features
  Corticobasal ganglionic degeneration
  Guam parkinsonism-dementia-amyotrophic lateral sclerosis
    complex
Cerebrovascular disease
  Infarctions of the substantia nigra and basal ganglia
Disorders of cerebrospinal fluid circulation
  Normal pressure hydrocephalus
Infectious diseases
  Encephalitis
  Postencephalitic parkinsonism (encephalitis lethargica)
  Creutzfeldt-Jakob disease
Craniocerebral trauma
Brain tumors
Drugs
  Neuroleptics: dopamine receptor blockers, dopamine
    storage depleters
Toxins
  (1-Methyl-4-phenyl-1,2,3,6-tetrahydropyridine) (MPTP)
  Carbon monoxide
  Manganese
  Cobalt
  Cyanide
Inherited disorders
  Wilson's disease
  Huntington's disease
  Hallervorden-Spatz disease
  Neuroacanthosis
  Frontotemporal dementia and parkinsonism linked to
    chromosome 17
Metabolic disorders
  Hypoparathyroidism with basal ganglia calcification
  Hepatocerebral degeneration

TABLE 11.7. FINDINGS COMPATIBLE WITH THE DIAGNOSIS OF PARKINSON'S DISEASE

Bradykinesia and rigidity with postural instability
Distal limb tremor at rest
Unilateral onset and persistent asymmetry affecting the side of symptom onset
Excellent response to levodopa
Levodopa-induced chorea
Levodopa response for 5 years or more
Clinical course for 10 years or more without dementia or autonomic features

(Table 11.8). Moreover, symptom onset after neuroleptic medication, the finding of an alien arm, and dementia preceding or at the onset of parkinsonian symptoms make the diagnosis of idiopathic Parkinson's disease unlikely (Table 11.9). Although difficult at the onset of symptoms in some patients, PSP can be differentiated from MSA by demonstration of a supranuclear downgaze or upgaze palsy, marked nuchal and trunk rigidity, and severe postural instability with a poor or absent response to levodopa. A prion disorder such as Creutzfeldt-Jakob disease can present with the rapid onset and progression of parkinsonian features accompanied by ataxia leading to motor disability within several months, even without myoclonus or a severe dementia initially. Dementia preceding or occurring at the onset of a parkinsonian syndrome suggests the possibility of diffuse Lewy body disease or Alzheimer's disease with extrapyramidal features, and the addition of an alien arm leads to consideration of corticobasal ganglionic degeneration. The combination of a behavioral disorder with dementia and parkinsonism and a family history of a similar disorder raises the possibility of a chromosome 17–linked dementia.

Autonomic Insufficiency

Patients with MSA often develop autonomic insufficiency before other symptoms appear, but people are prone to accept these symptoms as a consequence of normal aging. Thus, impotence in men and urinary disorders in both men and women may begin 5 or 10 years prior to the onset of parkinsonian or cerebellar symptoms. Orthostatic hypotension usually occurs later and may be symptomatic or asymp-

TABLE 11.8. UNUSUAL CLINICAL FINDINGS IN IDIOPATHIC PARKINSON'S DISEASE

Poor response to levodopa
Moderate or severe autonomic dysfunction
Cerebellar disorder
Peripheral neuropathy
Supranuclear gaze palsy
Several affected relatives

TABLE 11.9. FEATURES THAT MAKE THE DIAGNOSIS OF IDIOPATHIC PARKINSON'S DISEASE UNLIKELY

Symptom onset after administration of neuroleptic medication
Dementia preceding or at onset of parkinsonian symptoms
Supranuclear gaze palsy
Alien arm
Poor response to levodopa

tomatic. Symptomatic orthostatic hypotension usually occurs with standing from the recumbent position and usually resolves with return to the recumbent position. The symptoms may include light-headedness, dizziness, blurred vision, weakness, fatigue, cognitive impairment, nausea, palpitations, tremulousness, headache, and neck ache. In idiopathic Parkinson's disease, postural faintness can occur, particularly when the patient is receiving dopaminergic drugs, and urinary frequency and urgency can be missed unless the clinician is alert to the possibility of MSA, even in patients showing a good response to levodopa. Physicians evaluating patients with parkinsonian or cerebellar disorders should make specific inquiries about urinary and sexual functions. Examination of these patients should include determination of the systolic and diastolic blood pressure and the pulse initially with the patient recumbent and then 3 minutes after standing. The diagnosis of orthostatic hypotension requires the demonstration of a decline of systolic blood pressure of 20 mm Hg or more and of diastolic blood pressure of 10 mm Hg or more, usually with a change of pulse rate no more than 10 per minute. Mitigating factors include medications (particularly beta blockers and agents containing levodopa), the patient's state of hydration, and the recent ingestion of a large meal, all of which can promote postural hypotension.

Cerebellar Disorders

The differential diagnosis of a patient with a nonhereditary progressive ataxia of gait, speech, and limb coordination includes a long list of disorders (Table 11.10). In most

TABLE 11.10. DIFFERENTIAL DIAGNOSIS OF NONHEREDITARY PROGRESSIVE ATAXIA

Neoplasms, both primary and metastatic
Paraneoplastic syndromes
Infections
Cerebrovascular diseases, including infarction and hemorrhage
Demyelinative disorders
Deficiency diseases
Craniocerebral trauma
Metabolic diseases
Endocrinologic disorders
Malformations
Neurodegenerative disorders

cases, systematic laboratory investigations are needed for definitive diagnosis, including blood counts; screening tests of hepatic, renal, and thyroid function; a serologic test for syphilis; and levels of vitamin B_{12}, folate, and vitamin E. Neuroimaging studies are important, and magnetic resonance imaging (MRI), including T2-weighted images to detect demyelinative disease, is the preferred type of anatomic imaging. Demonstration of cerebellar and brainstem atrophy in MR images is helpful in the diagnosis of sOPCA, but may not be found early or, in some cases, even late in the disease process. In many patients with clinically symptomatic sOPCA, MR images demonstrate cerebellar but not brainstem atrophy, particularly early in the course. In these patients, differentiation of cerebellar cortical atrophy from sOPCA can be difficult. In patients who, after full evaluation are thought to have sOPCA, the history should be probed for symptoms relevant to autonomic and extrapyramidal function. Next the examining physician should measure the blood pressure and pulse in the recumbent and upright positions, and examine resistance to passive manipulation of the limbs to detect cogwheel rigidity. Positive findings lead to consideration of the possibility that the patient's disorder is evolving into MSA.

SPECIAL LABORATORY INVESTIGATIONS

Sphincter Electromyographic Examination

Initial reports suggested that the most specific single test for diagnosis of MSA is external urethral or anal sphincter electromyography (20). This shows pathologic increases of amplitude duration and polyphasic potentials indicating denervation and renervation secondary to anterior horn cell loss in Onuf's nucleus in the S2 and S3 segments of the sacral spinal cord. Subsequent reports indicated that these abnormalities would identify patients with MSA with good sensitivity and specificity (33). Recently, however, abnormal sphincter EMGs have been found in patients with advanced PD and PSP, indicating that this test may not be specific for MSA (34).

Studies of Autonomic Function

Although the clinical history, detection of orthostatic hypotension during clinical examination, and urologic evaluation of bladder function usually suffice for diagnosis, quantitative evaluation of autonomic function can be helpful in differentiating MSA from both Parkinson's disease and primary autonomic failure. The tests helpful in differentiating MSA from Parkinson's disease include evaluation of orthostatic blood pressure regulation, percentage of anhidrosis on thermal regulatory sweat testing, quantitative pseudomotor axon reflex testing, and heart rate response to deep breathing. For differentiating MSA from primary autonomic failure, the effect of upright tilt on circulating vasopressin can be helpful. In primary autonomic failure, upright tilt induces hypotension and a pronounced increase in the plasma concentration of vasopressin, and in MSA hypotension occurs with little or no change in circulating levels of vasopressin.

Cardiac Imaging

The ligand [^{123}I]metaiodobenzylguanidine (MIBG), which is structurally similar to norepinephrine, can be utilized with single photon emission computed tomography (SPECT) to visualize the autonomic innervation of the heart, as it labels postganglionic adrenergic neurons. Studies with this ligand have compared patients with Parkinson's disease (PD) and autonomic failure with MSA patients (35). The studies were based on the notion that in PD autonomic failure results from degeneration of postganglionic neurons, whereas in MSA preganglionic neurons degenerate and postganglionic neurons remain preserved. The investigation revealed that in all PD patients with autonomic failure studied, the heart to mediastinum ratio of MIBG was pathologically impaired whereas this ratio was normal in the MSA patients. In a subsequent study comparing early-stage PD patients with MSA patients, the median cardiac [^{123}I]MIBG uptake was significantly decreased in both groups of patients compared with controls (36). In the PD group, uptake was significantly lower than in MSA, but the two groups overlapped. Even the PD patients without clinical evidence of autonomic failure had significantly lower uptake than the MSA patients. These studies suggest that [^{123}I]MIBG with SPECT may be helpful in differentiating MSA from PD, even in early stages of the diseases.

Anatomical Imaging

Computed tomography (CT) scanning can be helpful diagnostically by demonstrating cerebellar atrophy in MSA. Hardening artifacts in the posterior fossa in CT scans limit their utility in evaluating the brainstem for atrophy. MRI is usually more helpful because visualization of the posterior fossa allows detection of both cerebellar and brainstem atrophy (Fig. 11.2). In 1.5-tesla MR images, T2-weighted images may show putaminal hypointensity relative to the globus pallidus. These scans also may show slit-like hyperintensity in the outer margin of the putamen (Fig. 11.3). However, changes in the putamen are not specific because they can be found not only in persons with MSA, but also in those with PSP and even in 30% of elderly normal subjects (37). In patients with possible MSA-P (those who do not have signs of cerebel-

lar degeneration or autonomic insufficiency), MRI can be helpful by showing atrophy of cerebellar and brainstem structures. As a group, these patients show a significant decrease in the size of the cerebellum and brainstem, though patients with possible MSA-C show greater atrophy.

Several studies have examined the utility of these findings in differentiating MSA from PD, PSP, and corticobasal degeneration (CBD). In the first study, two neuroradiologists blindly rated axial T2-weighted and proton density MRI of probable MSA patients with idiopathic PD and age-matched control subjects (38). Putaminal atrophy, a hyperintense putaminal rim, and infratentorial signal change had high specificity but low sensitivity for MSA. The infratentorial changes included atrophy of the cerebellum, middle cerebellar peduncles, and midbrain and signal change in the pons ("hot cross bun") and the cerebellar peduncles. For MSA in comparison with idiopathic PD, the overall sensitivity was 88%; the specificity of these findings for MSA in comparison with idiopathic PD was 93% and for MSA in comparison with controls was 91%. Putaminal isointensity or hypointensity relative to globus pallidus, absolute putaminal hypointensity, and altered size of olives were not useful discriminators. In a similar investigation comparing MSA with PD and PSP, the combination of hypointense regions within the dorsolateral putamen and a hyperintense rim proved a highly specific (100%) but only moderately sensitive (60%) sign of MSA (39). The finding of hypointensity alone was a sensitive but nonspecific sign of MSA (39). Another investigation evaluated the sensitivity of MRI in the diagnosis of MSA, PSP, and CBD (40). Findings indicating the diagnosis of MSA-P were hyperintense putaminal rim, putaminal atrophy and hyperintensity, atrophy and signal decrease of the globus pallidus, thinning or smudging of the substantia nigra, and increased infratentorial signal and atrophy. All MSA-C cases showed increased infratentorial signal and atrophy. None of the CBD cases showed increased infratentorial signal, putaminal hyperintense rim, or globus pallidus atrophy. Signs typical of PSP included midbrain diameter below 17 mm, increased midbrain signal, dilatation of the third ventricle, frontal or temporal atrophy, increased globus pallidus signal and atrophy, and increased red nucleus signal. More than 70% patients with PSP and more than 80% of patients with MSA-C could be classified correctly, and no patient in these groups was misclassified. The remaining could not be differentiated clearly. Moreover, only about half of patients with MSA-P could be classified correctly, and almost 20% of them were misclassified. The conclusion is that a hyperintense rim lateral to the putamen with hypointensity or atrophy in the putamen is relatively specific for MSA. These findings can differentiate MSA from PD. Increased infratentorial signal and atrophy can help to distinguish MSA from PD and other forms of atypical parkinsonism, such as PSP and CBD.

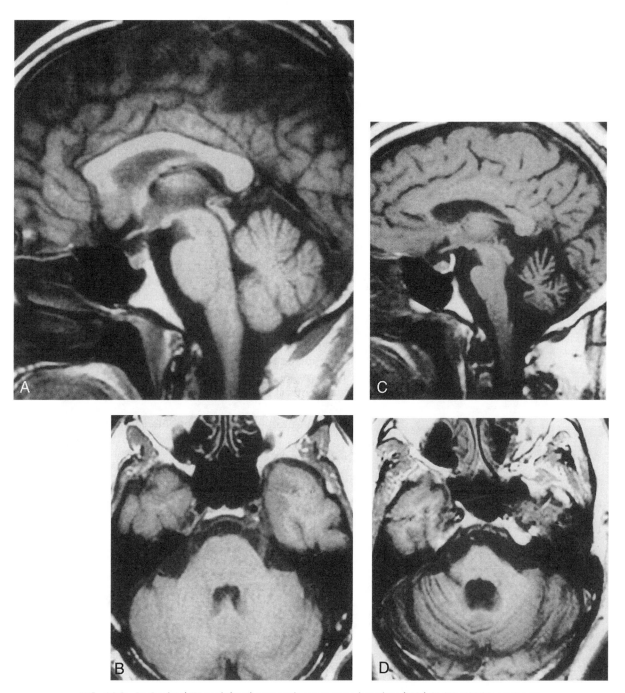

FIG. 11.2. A: Sagittal T1-weighted magnetic resonance imaging (MRI) TR/TE 500/20 ms 5 mm thick in a 57-year-old male normal control subject. **B:** Axial T1-weighted MRI TR/TE 500/20 in the same normal control subject. **C:** Sagittal T1-weighted MRI TR/TE 500/20 ms 5 mm thick in a 50-year-old man with probable multiple system atrophy of the olivopontocerebellar atrophy type showing decreased volume of the caudal portion of the pons, enlargement of the fourth ventricle, and decreased volume of the cerebellar vermis. **D:** Axial T1-weighted MRI TR/TE 500/20 ms in a 50-year-old man with probable multiple system atrophy of the olivopontocerebellar atrophy type showing enlargement of the fourth ventricle, decreased size of the middle cerebellar peduncle, and mild volume loss of the cerebellar hemispheres. (Courtesy of Dr. J. Brunberg, Radiology Department, University of Michigan.)

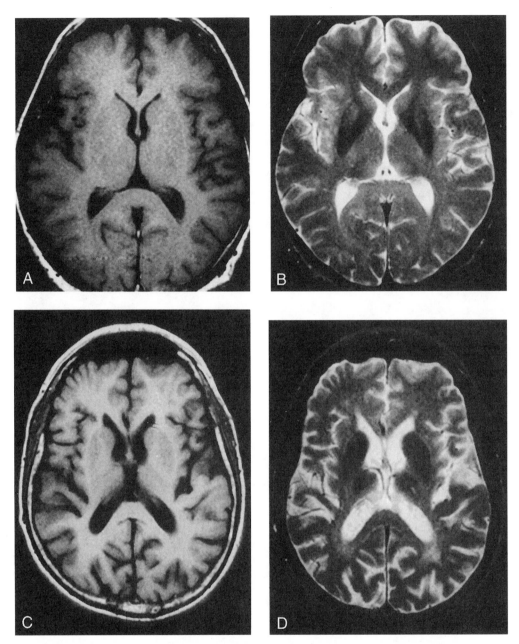

FIG. 11.3. A: Axial T1-weighted magnetic resonance imaging (MRI) TR/TE 500/20 ms 5 mm thick in a 57-year-old male normal control subject. **B:** Axial T2-weighted MRI 3500/90 (TR/TE) in the same normal control subject. **C:** Axial T1-weighted MRI TR/TE 600/20 ms 5 mm thick in a 59-year-old man with probable multiple system atrophy (MSA) of the subthalamic nucleus (striatonigral degeneration) type showing decreased volume of the putamen bilaterally, slightly increased size of the lateral ventricles, and volume loss in the cerebral cortex with increased size of the sulci. **D:** Axial T2-weighted MRI 3500/90 (TR/TE) in a 59-year-old man with probable MSA of the striato–nigral degeneration type showing decreased signal intensity of the putamen and caudate nucleus bilaterally, slit-like hyperintensity along the outer margin of the putamen, slightly increased size of the lateral ventricles, and volume loss in the cerebral cortex with increased size of the sulci. (Courtesy of Dr. J. Brunberg, Radiology Department, University of Michigan.)

Functional Imaging

Positron emission tomography (PET) studies with [18F]fluorodeoxyglucose have contributed useful information about the diagnosis of MSA. These investigations demonstrate widespread central nervous system hypometabolism in both MSA and sOPCA as compared with normal controls, including brainstem, cerebellum, putamen, thalamus, and cerebral cortex (41) (Fig. 11.4). However, some overlap between normal controls and MSA patients has been reported (42). In MSA patients with predominantly unilateral parkinsonian signs, hypometabolism is more conspicuous in the putamen on the side contralateral to the symptomatic limbs than on the ipsilateral side (43). The finding of hypometabolism in the cerebellum and putamen constitute the most helpful aid to diagnosis and assists in distinguishing MSA from Parkinson's disease.

Several other ligands have been used with PET in studies of MSA patients. Scans with [18F]fluorodopa have shown decreased uptake in striatal dopaminergic terminals, suggesting degeneration of nigrostriatal projections (44). Studies with [11C]dihydrotetrabenazine and PET also have demonstrated decreased striatal monoaminergic terminals in MSA patients (45). This new ligand appears to be advantageous because regulatory changes from medication do not influence its binding. PET scans with [11C]raclopride (46) and SPECT scans with [123I]iodobenzamine (47) have indicated that striatal D2 receptor activity is decreased. SPECT with [123I]iodobenzamine was used prospectively in an attempt to differentiate PD from "Parkinson-plus" patients (the latter presumably were developing MSA) (48). The Parkinson-plus group had significantly lower binding than the PD group at both the beginning and the end of a study over 11 to 53 months. Also, binding declined over the course of the study in the Parkinson-plus cases but not in the PD cases. Studies with PET and [11C]SCH-23390 suggest that striatal D1 receptor activity is also diminished (49). PET

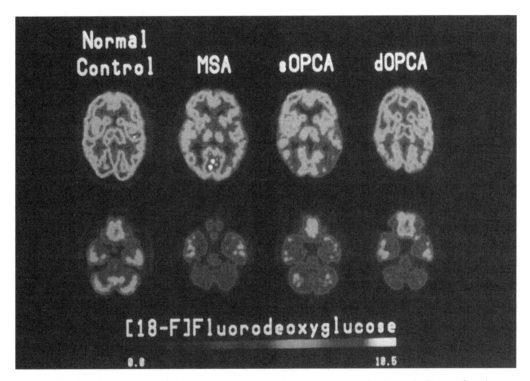

FIG. 11.4. PET scan with [18F]-fluorodeoxyglucose showing local cerebral metabolic rate for glucose (lCMR$_{glc}$) in a 52-year-old male normal control subject *(left upper and lower images)*, a 61-year-old man with probable multiple system atrophy (MSA) of the olivopontocerebellar type (MSA, *upper and lower images second from left*), a 46-year-old man with sporadic olivopontocerebellar ataxia (sOPCA) *(upper and lower images third from left),* and a 37-year-old man with dominantly inherited olivopontocerebellar atrophy (dOPCA, *right upper and lower images*). Scans in the upper row show axial sections at the level of the cerebral cortex, basal ganglia, and thalamus. Scans in the lower row show axial sections at the level of the cerebellum and the base of the temporal and frontal lobes. The color bar indicated the rate of cerebral glucose use for all scans expressed as milligrams per 100 grams per minute extending from 0.0 to 10.5. The scans show decreased lCMR$_{glc}$ in the brainstem and cerebellum of all three patients in comparison with the normal control subject but decreased lCMR$_{glc}$ in the cerebral cortex, basal ganglia, and thalamus of the patients with MSA and sOPCA but not dOPCA. (Reprinted with permission from Gilman et al., 1994 [41].)

studies with [^{11}C]diprenorphine indicate that striatal opioid binding is diminished in MSA (50).

PET with a combination of [^{18}F]fluorodeoxyglucose, [^{18}F]fluorodopa, and [^{11}C]raclopride has been used to differentiate PD from MSA and normal controls (51). The binding of [^{18}F]fluorodopa distinguished the PD patients from normal controls. Binding of [^{11}C]raclopride separated MSA patients from PD patients and normal controls. The data obtained with [^{18}F]fluorodeoxyglucose also differentiated MSA from both PD and normal controls.

A general conclusion is that PET with [^{18}F]fluorodeoxyglucose can differentiate MSA patients from PD patients and normal controls. It is not yet clear whether [^{18}F]fluorodeoxyglucose studies can differentiate MSA from PSP and CBD patients. Studies with markers of presynaptic dopaminergic terminals cannot differentiate among PD, MSA, and PSP cases but may be able to predict the sOPCA patients destined to develop MSA. Ligands for the D2 receptor can distinguish MSA from PD patients, but may not be able to differentiate between MSA and PSP or CBD patients.

MANAGEMENT

Extrapyramidal Features

In MSA patients with bradykinesia, rigidity, and tremor, levodopa may be helpful, but usually the magnitude of the effect is small and not well sustained (52). Nevertheless, treatment should be initiated with carbidopa/levodopa 25/100 three times daily, with an increase in dose every other day as tolerated to a total dose of eight tablets per day. The principal side effects are nausea, involuntary movements of the choreiform or dystonic type, postural hypotension, and psychological disturbances such as depression, paranoid ideation, and hallucinations. Some patients with MSA require and tolerate larger doses than most patients with Parkinson's disease. If levodopa/carbidopa is ineffective, other dopaminergic agonist agents usually do not help. Nevertheless, it is worthwhile instituting a trial of anticholinergics such as trihexyphenidyl 1 mg once daily with an increase in dose by 2 mg every 3 to 5 days to a total daily dose of 10 to 12 mg in three divided doses daily as tolerated. The principal side effects are dry mouth, blurred vision, and nausea. Amantadine 100 mg twice daily can also be tried if both dopaminergic and anticholinergic agents fail. The effects of tricyclic antidepressants and monoamine oxidase inhibitors have not been ascertained in MSA.

Autonomic Disorder

It is extremely important to monitor and manage symptomatic orthostatic hypotension. Patients should be cautioned to sit down or lie down as soon as symptoms appear, which is usually upon rising from the recumbent or seated position. Patients should be advised to avoid extreme heat because of reflex peripheral vasodilatation and also to avoid acts that increase vagal activity, such as overeating and straining at stool. Medical treatment begins with attempting to increase blood volume by increasing sodium intake unless the patient is at risk for congestive heart failure or has renal insufficiency. Pressure stockings should be prescribed and worn constantly to increase central venous volume. The head of the patient's bed should be elevated 6 inches to increase renin secretion. If symptomatic orthostatic hypotension persists despite simpler measures, fludrocortisone should be instituted at 0.1 mg daily and increased to a maximum of 0.4 mg/day in two divided doses. If this measure is not helpful, administration of indomethacin 25 mg three times daily with meals increasing to 50 mg three times daily may be helpful by inhibition of prostaglandin synthesis, which has vasodilator effects. An alternative to this is to administer the α-adrenergic agonist clonidine 0.1 mg twice daily increasing to 0.3 mg twice daily. Ephedrine administered at 25 mg three times daily can be helpful through its peripheral vasoconstrictor effects.

MSA results in three fundamental abnormalities of lower urinary tract function. (a) Involuntary detrusor contraction occurs in response to bladder filling, perhaps due to loss of inhibitory influences from the corpus striatum and substantia nigra. (b) MSA patients lose the ability to initiate a voluntary micturition reflex, probably reflecting degeneration of neurons in pontine and medullary nuclei and in sacral intermediolateral columns of the sacral spinal cord and a reduction in the density of acetylcholinesterase-containing nerves innervating the bladder musculature. (c) Severe urethral dysfunction occurs, partly due to dysfunction of the striated component of the urethral sphincter musculature, resulting in bladder neck incompetence. Urinary symptoms, including frequency and incontinence, often respond to a peripherally acting anticholinergic agent such as oxybutynin 5 to 10 mg at bedtime. An alternative therapy is propantheline 15 to 30 mg at bedtime, which is useful for detrusor hyperreflexia. Anticholinergic treatment of the urinary dysfunction can worsen the constipation that frequently occurs in MSA.

Constipation should be treated with a high-fiber diet, including daily administration of one to three doses of psyllium, a high-fiber cereal at breakfast, an apple, and at least one serving of broccoli or similar high-fiber vegetable. Stool softening is readily accomplished with one 8-ounce glass of prune juice and additional servings of other fruit juices as needed.

Treatment of ataxia in MSA has not been effective. The only agent that is worth using for a therapeutic trial is clonazepam, 0.05 mg (1/2 tablet) at bedtime, increasing to 0.1 mg.

PROGNOSIS

MSA is a progressive disorder associated with a shortened life span, with death occurring on average within about 10 years of symptom onset. In one clinical study, the median survival from onset of symptoms was 9.5 years (19), and in another 7.5 years (53). Similar average survivals were reported in two autopsy-verified series of MSA patients, 8.7 years in one (27) and 8.0 years in another (52).

REFERENCES

1. Consensus Committee of the American Autonomic Society and the American Academy of Neurology. Consensus statement on the definition of orthostatic hypotension, pure autonomic failure, and multiple system atrophy. *Neurology* 1996;46:1470.
2. Gilman S, Low PA, Quinn N, et al. Consensus statement on the diagnosis of multiple system atrophy. *J Neurol Sci* 1999;163:94–98.
3. Gai WP, Power JH, Blumbergs PC, et al. Multiple-system atrophy: a new α-synuclein disease? *Lancet* 1998;352:547–548.
4. Gilman S, Sima AF, Junck L, et al. Spinocerebellar ataxia type 1 with multiple system degeneration and glial cytoplasmic inclusions. *Ann Neurol* 1996;39:241–255.
5. Adams RD, van Bogaert L, van der Eecken H. Dégénérescences nigro-striées et cérébello-nigro-striées. *Psychiatry Neurol* 1961;142:219–259.
6. Shy GM, Drager GA. A neurologic syndrome associated with orthostatic hypotension. *Arch Neurol* 1960;2:511–527.
7. Gilman S, Little R, Johanns J, et al. Evolution of sporadic olivopontocerebellar atrophy into multiple system atrophy. *Neurology* 2000;55:527–532.
8. Dejerine J, Thomas AA. L'atrophie olivo-ponto-cérébelleuse. *Nouv Iconog de la Salpêtrière* 1900;13:330–370.
9. Bradbury S, Eggleston C. Postural hypotension: a report of three cases. *Am Heart J* 1925;1:73–86.
10. Quinn NP, Wenning G, Marsden GD. The Shy-Drager syndrome: what did Shy and Drager really describe? *Arch Neurol* 1995;52:656–657.
11. Graham JG, Oppenheimer DR. Orthostatic hypotension and nicotine sensitivity in a case of multiple system atrophy. *J Neurol Neurosurg Psychiatry* 1969;32:28–34.
12. Lantos PL, Papp MI. Cellular pathology of multiple system atrophy: a review. *J Neurol Neurosurg Psychiatry* 1994;57:129–133.
13. Wermuth L, Joensen P, Bunger N, et al. High prevalence of Parkinson's disease in the Faroe Islands. *Neurology* 1997;49:426–432.
14. Schrag A, Ben-Shlomo Y, Quinn NP. Prevalence of progressive supranuclear palsy and multiple system atrophy: a cross-sectional study. *Lancet* 1999;354:1771–1775.
15. Chio A, Magnani C, Schiffer D. Prevalence of Parkinson's disease in northwestern Italy: comparison of tracer methodology and clinical ascertainment of cases. *Mov Disord* 1998;13:400–405.
16. Trenkwalder C, Schwarz J, Gebhard J, et al. Starnberg trial on epidemiology of Parkinsonism and hypertension in the elderly: prevalence of Parkinson's disease and related disorders assessed by a door-to-door survey of inhabitants older than 65 years. *Arch Neurol* 1995;52:1017–1022.
17. Bower JH, Maraganore DM, McDonnell SK, et al. Incidence of progressive supranuclear palsy and multiple system atrophy in Olmsted County, Minnesota, 1976 to 1990. *Neurology* 1997;49:1284–1288.
18. Sima AAF, Caplan M, D'Amato CJ, et al. Fulminant multiple system atrophy in a young adult presenting as motor neuron disease. *Neurology* 1993;43:2031–2035.
19. Wenning GK, Ben-Shlomo Y, Magalhães M, et al. Clinical features and natural history of multiple system atrophy: an analysis of 100 cases. *Brain* 1994;117:835–845.
20. Pramstaller PP, Wenning GK, Smith SJM, et al. Nerve conduction studies, skeletal muscle EMG, and sphincter EMG in multiple system atrophy. *J Neurol Neurosurg Psychiatry* 1995;58:618–621.
21. Harcourt J, Spraggs P, Mathias C, et al. Sleep-related breathing disorders in the Shy-Drager syndrome: observations on investigation and management. *Eur J Neurol* 1996;3:186–190.
22. Meco G, Gasparini M, Doricchi F. Attentional functions in multiple system atrophy and Parkinson's disease. *J Neurol Neurosurg Psychiatry* 1996;60:393–398.
23. Robbins TW, James M, Lange KW, et al. Cognitive performance in multiple system atrophy. *Brain* 1992;115:271–291.
24. Pillon B, Gouider-Khouja N, Deweer B, et al. Neuropsychological pattern of striatonigral degeneration: comparison with Parkinson's disease and progressive supranuclear palsy. *J Neurol Neurosurg Psychiatry* 1995;58:174–179.
25. Tison F, Wenning GK, Volonte MA, et al. Pain in multiple system atrophy. *Neurology* 1996;243:153–156.
26. Rascol O, Sabatini U, Fabre N, et al. Abnormal vestibuloocular reflex cancellation in multiple system atrophy and progressive supranuclear palsy but not in Parkinson's disease. *Mov Disord* 1995;10:163–170.
27. Wenning GK, Ben-Shlomo Y, Magalhães M, et al. Clinicopathological study of 35 cases of multiple system atrophy. *J Neurol Neurosurg Psychiatry* 1995;58:160–166.
28. Daniel SE, Geddes JF, Revesz T. Glial cytoplasmic inclusions are not exclusive to multiple system atrophy (letter). *J Neurol Neurosurg Psychiatry* 1995;58:262.
29. Souza JM, Giasson BI, Lee VM, et al. Chaperone-like activity of α-synucleins. *FEBS Lett* 2000;474:116–119.
30. Kruger R, Kuhn W, Muller T, et al. Ala30Pro mutation in the gene encoding α-synuclein in Parkinson's disease. *Nature Genetics* 1998;18:106–108.
31. Dickson DW. α-Synuclein and the Lewy body disorders. *Curr Opin Neurology* 2001;14:423–432.
32. Giasson BI, Duda JE, Murray IV, et al. Oxidative damage linked to neurodegeneration by selective α-Synuclein nitration in synucleinopathy lesions. *Science* 2000;290:985–989.
32a. Hanna P, Jankovic J, Kilkpatrick J. Multiple system atrophy: the putative causative role of environmental toxins. *Arch Neurol* 1999;56:90–94.
33. Tison F, Arne P, Sourgen C, et al. The value of external anal sphincter electromyography for the diagnosis of multiple system atrophy. *Mov Disord* 2000;15:1148–1157.
34. Giladi N, Simon ES, Korczyn AD, et al. Anal sphincter EMG does not distinguish between multiple system atrophy and Parkinson's disease. *Muscle Nerve* 2000;23:731–734.
35. Braune S, Reinhardt M, Schnitzer R, et al. Cardiac uptake of [123I]MIBG separates Parkinson's disease from multiple system atrophy. *Neurology* 1999;53:1020–1025.
36. Druschky A. Hilz MJ. Platsch G. et al. Differentiation of Parkinson's disease and multiple system atrophy in early disease stages by means of I-123-MIBG-SPECT. *J Neurol Sci* 2000;175:3–12.
37. Brooks DJ. Reply to the diagnosis of multiple system atrophy by T. caraceni. *Ann Neurol* 1991;29:690.
38. Schrag A, Kingsley D, Phatouros C, et al. Clinical usefulness of magnetic resonance imaging in multiple system atrophy. *J Neurol Neurosurg Psychiatry* 1998;65:65–71.
39. Kraft E, Schwarz J, Trenkwalder C, et al. The combination of

hypointense and hyperintense signal changes on T2-weighted magnetic resonance imaging sequences: a specific marker of multiple system atrophy? *Arch Neurol* 1999;56:225–228.

40. Schrag A, Good CD, Miszkiel K, et al. Differentiation of atypical parkinsonian syndromes with routine MRI. *Neurology* 2000; 54:697–702.

41. Gilman S, Koeppe RA, Junck L, et al. Patterns of cerebral glucose metabolism detected with PET differ in multiple system atrophy and olivopontocerebellar atrophy. *Ann Neurol* 1994;36: 166–175.

42. Otsuka M, Kuwabara Y, Ichiya Y, et al. Differentiating between multiple system atrophy and Parkinson's disease by positron emission tomography with 18F-dopa and 18F-FDG. *Ann Nucl Med* 1997;11:251–257.

43. Kume A, Shiratori M, Takahashi A, et al. Hemi-parkinsonism in multiple system atrophy: a PET and MRI study. *J Neurol Sci* 1992;110:37–45.

44. Burn DJ, Sawle GV, Brooks DJ. Differential diagnosis of Parkinson's disease, multiple system atrophy, and Steele-Richardson-Olszewski syndrome: discriminant analysis of striatal ^{18}F-dopa PET data. *J Neurol Neurosurg Psychiatry* 1994;57:278–284.

45. Gilman S, Koeppe RA, Junck L, et al. Decreased striatal monoaminergic terminals in multiple system atrophy detected with PET. *Ann Neurol* 1999;45:769–777.

46. Brooks DJ, Ibanez V, Sawle GV, e al. Striatal D_2 receptor status in patients with Parkinson's disease, striatonigral degeneration, and progressive supranuclear palsy, measured with ^{11}C-raclopride

and positron emission tomography. *Ann Neurol* 1992;31: 184–192.

47. Schulz JB, Klockgether T, Petersen D, et al. Multiple system atrophy: natural history, MRI morphology, and dopamine receptor imaging with ^{123}IBZM-SPECT. *J Neurol Neurosurg Psychiatry* 1994;57:1047–1056.

48. Hierholzer J, Cordes M, Venz S, et al. Loss of dopamine-D2 receptor binding sites in parkinsonian plus syndromes. *J Nuclear Med* 1998;39:954–960.

49. Shinotoh H, Inoue O, Hirayama K, et al. Dopamine D1 receptors in Parkinson's disease and striatonigral degeneration: a positron emission tomography study. *J Neurol Neurosurg Psychiatry* 1993;56:467–472.

50. Rinne JO, Burn DJ, Mathias CJ, et al. Positron emission tomography studies on the dopaminergic system and striatal opioid binding in the olivopontocerebellar atrophy variant of multiple system atrophy. *Ann Neurol* 1995;37:568–573.

51. Antonini A, Leenders KL, Vontobel P, et al. Complementary PET studies of striatal neuronal function in the differential diagnosis between multiple system atrophy and Parkinson's disease. *Brain* 1997;120:2187–2195.

52. Hughes AJ, Colosimo C, Kleedorfer B, et al. The dopaminergic response in multiple system atrophy. *J Neurol Neurosurg Psychiatry* 1992;55:1009–1013.

53. Testa D, Filippini G, Farinotti M, et al. Survival in multiple system atrophy: a study of prognostic factors in 59 cases. *Neurology* 1996;243:401–404.

CORTICOBASAL DEGENERATION

RAJEEV KUMAR
CATHERINE BERGERON
ANTHONY E. LANG

Corticobasal degeneration (CBD) was first described by Rebeiz et al. in their 1968 paper entitled "Corticodentatonigral Degeneration with Neuronal Achromasia" (1). More than 100 cases have since been described in the literature, often under such essentially synonymous terms as "cortical-basal ganglionic degeneration" and "corticonigral degeneration with neuronal achromasia" (1–4). Although originally described as a late-adult-onset, progressive, neurodegenerative disorder presenting as a distinctive asymmetric akinetic-rigid syndrome with associated involuntary movements and signs of cortical dysfunction, a wider spectrum of clinical phenotypes has been recently recognized, including presentations with dementia, dysphasia, and altered behavior dependent on the topography of the predominant lesion. Furthermore, a variety of alternative pathologies (or "mimickers") have been reported to occasionally cause the prototypical syndrome (Fig. 12.1). Comparative studies with other neurodegenerative diseases utilizing new immunochemical techniques and electron microscopy have lead to the recognition of substantial similarities—particularly with progressive supranuclear palsy (PSP), Pick's disease, and frontotemporal dementia and parkinsonism linked to chromosome 17 (FTDP-17)—and possibly unique morphologic and biochemical features. The

hypothesis that fundamental abnormalities in tau processing may underlie these disorders has been supported by genetic linkage studies. Each of these issues in the clinical and pathologic diagnosis of CBD and its overlap with other neurodegenerative diseases will be emphasized.

CLASSICAL CLINICAL FEATURES AND NATURAL HISTORY

Classically, CBD presents in the sixth, seventh, or eighth decade of life with a varied combination of symptoms including stiffness, clumsiness, jerking, and sensory impairment affecting an arm or, less frequently, a leg (Table 12.1) (4,5). Over the next 2 to 7 years, symptoms and accompanying disability progress as additional limbs are affected—usually the unaffected ipsilateral limb before the contralateral limbs. Mean survival is 7 years after symptom onset with death secondary to a complication of generalized immobility (6,7). Early bilateral bradykinesia or a frontal syndrome (including early dementia, memory or attention disturbances) is predictive of a shorter survival (7). Recent clinicopathologic correlation has cast considerable doubt on the specificity of the classical clinical syndrome for the

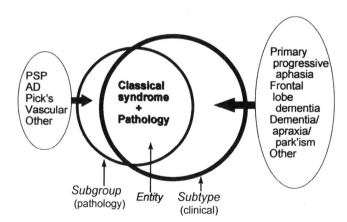

FIG. 12.1. The spectrum of corticobasal degeneration.

TABLE 12.1. NATURAL HISTORY OF THE CLASSICAL SYNDROME OF CORTICOBASAL DEGENERATION IN COMPARISON TO PROGRESSIVE SUPRANUCLEAR PALSY AND STRIATONIGRAL DEGENERATION

Clinical Features	CBD	PSP	SND
Movement disorders			
Akinesia, rigidity	At presentation—frequent; develops universally	Universal	Universal
Limb dystonia	At presentation—uncommon; develops in ~60–70%	At presentation—rare; develops occasionally (~25%); may be levodopa induced	Uncommon, but develops commonly with levodopa therapy (facial dystonia may be an early clue to diagnosis)
Focal reflex myoclonus[a]	At presentation—occasional; develops in ~60–70%	Uncommon	Frequent
Postural and action tremor	At presentation—occasional; develops in ~50%	Rare	At presentation—occasional; develops frequently
Postural instability, falls, or dysequilibrium	Rare at presentation (though abnormal gait is common in those with leg onset symptoms); develops late in course frequently (~70–80%)	At presentation—frequent; develops universally	At presentation—occasional; develops frequently
Other dyskinesias (especially athetosis or pseudoathetosis	At presentation—rare; develops occasionally	Rare	Rare
Cerebrocortical features			
Cortical sensory loss	At presentation—uncommon; develops in ~50%	Rare	Rare
Apraxia	At presentation—frequent; develops universally	At presentation—uncommon; develops commonly	Rare
Alien limb	At presentation—rare; develops in ~50%	Rare, though levitation may occur in the presence of marked cortical degeneration	Rare
Frontal release signs, including grasp	At presentation—uncommon; develops in ~50%	At presentation—common; develops frequently	At presentation—rare; develops occasionally
Dementia	At presentation—rare; develops in ~25%[b]	At presentation—uncommon; develops frequently	Rare
Dysphasia	At presentation—rare; develops uncommonly (~15%)[b]	Rare	At presentation—rare; develops occasionally
Corticospinal tract signs	At presentation—occasional; develops frequently (~70%)	At presentation—uncommon; develops frequently	At presentation—uncommon; develops frequently
Oculomotor dysfunction	At presentation—occasional (predominantly saccadic pursuit and hypometric saccades); develops frequently (~60–70%) (true supranuclear gaze palsy remains uncommon throughout course)	At presentation—frequent (may just be impairment of saccades and generation of opticokinetic nystagmus); vertical supranuclear gaze palsy develops in almost all patients (>90%)	At presentation—rare; develops ataxic eye movements occasionally
Eyelid motor dysfunction	At presentation—uncommon (usually only decreased blink rate or speed); develops frequently with apraxia of lid opening (~20%) or blepharospasm occasionally	At presentation—uncommon; develops frequently with apraxia of lid opening or blepharospasm	At presentation—rare; develops uncommonly
Dysarthria	At presentation—rare; develops frequently (~50–60%) (often pseudobulbar in character)	At presentation—common; develops frequently (often pseudobulbar in character)	At presentation—uncommon; develops frequently
Dysphagia	At presentation—rare; develops frequently	At presentation—rare; develops frequently	At presentation—rare; develops frequently
Autonomic failure	At presentation—rare; incontinence develops frequently	At presentation—rare; incontinence develops frequently	At presentation—occasional (often impotence is first symptom, incontinence or orthostasis may also be present); severe orthostasis and incontinence develops frequently
Cerebellar signs	Rare	Rare	At presentation—uncommon; develops frequently

[a]See text for discussion of unique physiologic characteristics of myoclonus in corticobasal ganglionic degeneration.
[b]These features, especially dementia, may be much more common than generally appreciated in patients who do no present with the "classical" CBD phenotype (see text for details).
Note: Approximate percentage frequencies provided in addition to descriptors where adequate data exists. Rare = <10%; uncommon = 10–20%; occasional = 20–30%; common = 30–50%; frequent = >50%; universal = >90%.
CBD, corticobasal degeneration; PSP, progressive supranuclear palsy; SND, striatonigral degeneration.
Adapted in part from data by Rinne et al. (5), Wenning et al. (14,50), and Litvan et al. (51), with modifications based on our personal experience.

pathologic diagnosis of CBD (8–10). Despite several reports of such patients with alternative pathologic findings at postmortem [including PSP, Pick's disease, FTDP-17, nonspecific cortical degeneration with status spongiosus, Alzheimer's disease (AD), vascular disease, Creutzfeldt-Jakob disease (CJD), sudanophilic leukodystrophy], the typical pathologic features of CBD seem to most commonly accompany this constellation of clinical features (11).

On examination at presentation, most patients demonstrate rigidity, bradykinesia, and apraxia of the affected limbs without significant global intellectual impairment or dysphasia. Little or no levodopa response of parkinsonism is noted. Pronounced asymmetry of limb involvement is a hallmark of the classical disorder. In our experience, buccofacial apraxia at presentation is uncommon (but when present can significantly impair speech) (12). Although it has been said that limb-kinetic apraxia is the commonest form of apraxia seen in CBD, it is difficult to distinguish this from the clumsiness caused by accompanying bradykinesia, rigidity, and dystonia. It is important not to "overdiagnose" the presence of apraxia when these motor disturbances are prominent; this has been a common source of misdiagnosis in our experience. Ideomotor limb apraxia is almost universal during the course of CBD (5). Heilman et al. have proposed that the dominant parietal lobe stores representations of learned skilled movements (known as praxicons), which are converted into motor programs by anterior premotor regions [especially the supplementary motor area (SMA)] upon verbal command or other external or internal signal (13). Two forms of ideomotor apraxia may result: (a) lesions of the dominant parietal lobe damage the praxicons and result in a bilateral deficit in the performance of skilled movements in addition to difficulty comprehending and discriminating between well- and poorly pantomimed actions; (b) dominant SMA lesions (or subcortical lesions that disconnect the dominant parietal lobe from the SMA) cause a contralateral performance deficit without a discrimination deficit. Leiguarda and colleagues found ideomotor apraxia without a discrimination deficit to be most common in patients with clinically diagnosed CBD lacking ideational apraxia and significant cognitive impairment, thus suggesting predominant SMA cortical pathology early in the course of classical CBD, with recent fluorodeoxyglucose (FDG) positron emission tomography (PET) findings congruent with this pathologic localization (14). The presence of ideational apraxia in three patients correlated with more severe global cognitive impairment, and all such patients had ideomotor apraxia with a discrimination deficit. This is consistent with dominant parietal, and possibly, more diffuse cortical involvement developing with disease progression.

A rigid, dystonically postured arm with some fingers extended and others forcibly flexed into the palm causing skin maceration characteristically develops early in the course of the illness in a substantial minority (4,5). Jerking of the affected limb due to action-induced and stimulus-sensitive focal reflex myoclonus commonly precedes or accompanies the development of such dystonic postures and, if rhythmic, may mimic tremor (15). However, classical parkinsonian resting tremor is not a feature of CBD. Application of light touch or pinprick stimuli usually elicits multiple flexion jerks, which although initially distal, with disease progression may affect the entire limb almost synchronously. Spontaneous myoclonus may also occur but is always superimposed on a background of muscle activity (15). With time, combinations of apraxia, dystonia, rigidity, akinesia, and myoclonus make a limb functionally useless. In those with initial leg involvement, the early development of apraxia may interfere with walking, resulting in a frontal gait disorder with shuffling, start hesitation, and freezing (5). However, isolated gait ignition failure is not a feature of CBD. With disease progression, dysequilibrium becomes a common feature in all patients, and postural instability with falls becomes common.

At presentation, oculomotor function may be normal or, alternatively, may be abnormal with saccadic pursuit and increased latency of pursuit onset, as well as increased saccade latency and difficulty initiating voluntary saccades to command when spontaneous saccades in the same directions are successfully performed (sometimes referred to as apraxia of eye movement) (16). Patients may use head thrusts to improve horizontal saccades (head–eye synergy). Although a true supranuclear gaze palsy may develop later in the clinical course once marked generalized disability is present, an early vertical supranuclear gaze palsy raises the diagnostic possibility of PSP with "atypical" features due to accompanying cortical degeneration (to be discussed below) (5,16,17). Furthermore, in CBD there is usually equally severe vertical and horizontal gaze palsy.

New clinical features develop and preexisting symptoms and signs worsen as the disease progresses with pathologic involvement of additional cortical and subcortical areas. Alien-limb phenomenon (ALP) develops in approximately 50% of patients (18). Classification schemes and definitions for ALP have been proposed. Feinberg et al. have proposed that ALP be divided into frontal and callosal types (19). Frontal ALP occurs in the dominant hand, is characterized by a strong grasp reflex and an uncontrollable tendency to reach for and manipulate objects, and is due to a lesion involving the dominant medial prefrontal cortex, SMA, anterior cingulate gyrus, and anterior corpus callosum. Callosal ALP results from an anterior or midbody corpus callosum lesion, with the nondominant hand demonstrating intermanual conflict and diagonistic dyspraxia (acting at cross-purposes in tasks requiring both hands). In CBD patients with ALP, transcranial magnetic stimulation studies indicate an enhanced excitability, or reduced inhibition, of the motor area of the hemisphere contralateral to the ALP, and ipsilateral responses are noted compatible with a disinhibited transcallosal input (20). *Levitation* consists of relatively simple and nonpurposeful movements of a limb caused by a contralateral parietal lobe lesion, is much less specific for CBD, and may result in misdiagnosis. We would agree with other authorities in requiring more complex behavior to fulfill criteria for true ALP. In our experience the most common semipurposeful movement found in CBD that could be characterized as an ALP is utilization behavior with groping and manipulation. It should be borne in mind that among neurodegenerations, ALP is not specific for CBD, and complex forms of ALP may be present in AD and CJD (18).

Cortical sensory deficits, such as sensory extinction, astereognosis, agraphesthesia, and impaired two-point discrimination, account for some patients' complaints of numbness or paresthesias, but are initially present in only a minority of patients. Later, severe sensory dysfunction may result in pseudoathetotic movements or wandering of the limb without patient awareness. Visual inattentiveness may also develop. Similarly, frontal release signs (e.g., grasp), signs of corticospinal tract dysfunction (including extensor plantar responses and exaggerated deep tendon reflexes), and bulbar dysfunction are uncommon at presentation but become very common later in the disease course. Pseudobulbar palsy with emotional lability or inappropriate jocularity may also be observed (21). Hypokinetic and mixed-type dysarthria frequently impairs communication, and dysphagia with resulting aspiration pneumonia becomes a common source of morbidity and mortality (22). In contrast, severe dysphasia and global dementia remain uncommon (in the classical CBD phenotype) even when mobility is severely compromised probably due to the topographically restricted predisposition for frontoparietal/pericentral cortical involvement. Extensive neuropsychological testing has revealed mild to moderate global deficits and some specific similarities to PSP (and differences from AD), including a frontal dysexecutive syndrome, explicit learning deficits without retention difficulties easily compensated for by the use of semantic cues for encoding and retrieval, and disorders of dynamic motor execution (temporal organization, bimanual coordination, control, and inhibition) (23). However, as in the case of AD, patients with CBD display prominent deficits on tests of sustained attention/mental control and verbal fluency, and mild deficits on confrontation naming (24). Psychomotor depression is more common and severe than in AD possibly because of underlying basal ganglia pathology or psychological reaction to debilitating motor deficits with greater preservation of insight (24). Similarly, both depression and irritability are more common than in PSP in which apathy predominates (25). Unlike both AD and PSP, patients with CBD have asymmetric praxis disorders (23). Evidence for cognitive asymmetry corresponding to the patients' motor asymmetry is typically lacking. For example, in patients presenting with the classical syndrome dysphasia does not appear to be associated with initial involvement of the dominant hemisphere

but is more likely to occur in the presence of cognitive impairment late in the course of the disease. In reviewing the results of these neuropsychological reports it is important to emphasize that the patients studied presented with the classical disorder. It is likely that other neuropsychological patterns would be found in those presenting with alternative features (see below).

DIFFERENTIAL DIAGNOSIS

CBD may at times be difficult to differentiate from other parkinsonian syndromes such as multiple system atrophy (MSA) and PSP (Table 12.1). Misdiagnosis has resulted from misinterpretation of poor performance on manual tasks as due to apraxia when in fact severe bradykinesia, rigidity, or dystonia was causative. Stimulus-sensitive myoclonus in MSA and PSP may also encourage a misdiagnosis of CBD. PSP may share clinical features more commonly associated with CBD, including apraxia, asymmetric dystonia, and arm levitation. When supranuclear gaze palsy is mild or absent, as it can sometimes be early on, and these features are present, the differentiation between PSP and CBD becomes most difficult. Leiguarda et al. also found bilateral ideomotor apraxia for transitive and intransitive movements in 67% and 33%, respectively, of patients with PSP (26). Severity of apraxia correlated with cognitive deficit measured by Mini-Mental State Examination. Although 2 of 12 patients performed abnormally on multiple-step tasks, no patient with PSP failed to comprehend pantomimed tasks or to discriminate between well and poorly performed pantomimes. Although blepharospasm has been well recognized in PSP, the presence of other forms of dystonia has not been emphasized. Barclay and Lang found that 45% of PSP patients seen at our center manifested some form of dystonia (27). Limb dystonia was common; it developed spontaneously in 20 (24%) patients and was L-dopa induced in 2 patients. We have also observed arm levitation in pathologically proven PSP (17). These "unusual" clinical features may be more common in the presence of coexistent cortical degeneration. Severe autonomic dysfunction or delusions or hallucinations unrelated to levodopa therapy have never been reported in pathologically confirmed CBD. MSA may cause the former, and dementia with Lewy bodies (DLB) may cause both of these problems. AD and nonspecific cortical degeneration (which more often presents as a frontal lobe dementia) may present with an asymmetric motor syndrome (especially progressive apraxia) that is initially indistinguishable from CBD (8,11). Nevertheless, clues that CBD is not the causative pathology include the absence of limb dystonia, milder parkinsonism, and usually more severe cognitive dysfunction. Parietal-predominant Pick's disease may be clinically indistinguishable from CBD. Nevertheless, multiple infarcts and CJD may mimic CBD. A stepwise or rapid progression, respectively, should be the important clue to these alternative diagnoses. Lastly, FTDP-17 should also be considered in patients with any family history or parkinsonism or dementia. The role of functional neuroimaging and electrophysiologic studies (see below) in distinguishing these disorders from CBD remains uncertain (with the exception of imaging for multiple infarcts). The above comments apply to the differential diagnosis of the classical syndrome of CBD outlined in the previous section. However, as will be emphasized below, the fact that the pathology of CBD may result in alternative clinical presentations broadens the differential diagnosis problem considerably.

ALTERNATIVE CLINICAL PRESENTATIONS

It has recently become increasingly clear that CBD may present with any of a variety of asymmetric cortical degeneration syndromes more commonly associated with other neurodegenerative diseases (Table 12.2) (28). These syndromes include primary progressive aphasia, frontal lobe dementia, posterior cortical atrophy (parieto-occipital degeneration), progressive hemiparesis, progressive apraxia, etc. (10,11,28). From pathologic studies, it is apparent that CBD commonly presents with a frontal lobe dementia syndrome, especially when the cortical degeneration predominantly involves the frontal lobes (29,30). CBD should be suspected when patients present with a dementia phenotype characterized by severe cognitive disturbances (especially frontal lobe disturbances, such as severe executive dysfunction and poor attentiveness), dysphasia, and later development of bilateral motor signs (including non-levodopa-

responsive parkinsonism and pyramidal signs) and urinary incontinence (29). Similarly, when the superior temporal gyrus is the site of early cortical degeneration presentation with the syndrome of primary progressive aphasia may result (10). When the lateral dominant frontal lobe is affected early the rare syndrome of pure orofacial apraxia and speech impairment may present long before other features develop (12). The broad clinical phenotype of asymmetric cortical degeneration syndromes seems to reflect the predominant area of pathological cortical degeneration and is not specific for any one disease. This situation makes accurate antemortem diagnosis in the absence of a sensitive and specific clinical or laboratory marker very difficult.

Attempts have been made to assess the accuracy of neurologists' clinical diagnosis of CBD. Litvan et al. have assessed the accuracy of neurologists' clinical diagnoses of CBD: mean sensitivity for CBD was low (35%) but specificity was near perfect (99.6%) (9). Boeve et al. developed diagnostic criteria based on previously published pathologically proven cases and then prospectively applied these criteria (8). At postmortem, only 7 in 13 cases defined as clinically definite, probable, or possible using their criteria had the classical pathology of CBD whereas the remainder demonstrated alternative findings. These studies mandate the development of validated diagnostic criteria. Given that the classical syndrome seems to correlate best with the pathology of CBD, we propose the research diagnostic criteria outlined in Table 12.3, acknowledging that these rigid clinical criteria are likely to exclude large numbers of patients, especially those with "atypical" or alternative presentations. However, using these criteria, a homogeneous patient population or registry might be gathered for future research studies.

TABLE 12.2. COMMON ALTERNATIVE CLINICAL PRESENTATIONS OF CORTICOBASAL DEGENERATION

Clinical Syndrome	Main Clinical Features[a]	Other Common Pathologies
Primary progressive aphasia	Progressive nonfluent and/or fluent aphasia without global dementia or significant anterograde amnesia often presenting initially with anomia, frequent paraphasic errors, and loss of speech fluency. Occasionally orofacial apraxia.	Pick's disease FTDP-17 Nonspecific cortical degeneration Alzheimer's disease Motor neuron disease with aphasic dementia Creutzfeldt-Jakob disease
Frontal lobe dementia	Progressive loss of judgment with disinhibition (including distractibility, impulsiveness, compulsiveness, or perseveration), social misconduct, or social withdrawal out of proportion to the degree of anterograde amnesia. Psychometric testing abnormalities on trailmaking, verbal fluency, mazes, or categorization. Affective symptoms including depression, anxiety, emotional unconcern, or abulia. Early primitive reflexes and incontinence.	Pick's disease FTDP-17 Nonspecific cortical degeneration Alzheimer's disease Motor neuron disease with frontal dementia

[a]Predominant clinical features at presentation and in the early clinical course; thereafter, additional signs commonly develop.
FTDP-17, frontotemporal dementia and parkinsonism linked to chromosome 17.

TABLE 12.3. PROPOSED RESEARCH CRITERIA FOR THE DIAGNOSIS OF THE CLINICAL SYNDROME USUALLY ACCOMPANIED BY THE PATHOLOGY OF CORTICOBASAL DEGENERATION

I. Chronic progressive course
II. Asymmetric at onset (includes speech dyspraxia, dysphasia)
III. Presence of:
    A. Higher cortical dysfunction
      and
    B. Movement disorders
      1. Higher cortical dysfunction
        a. Apraxia
          or
        b. Cortical sensory loss
          or
        c. Alien limb
      2. Movement Disorder
        a. *Rigid*/akinetic syndrome resistant to L-dopa
          and
          i) Dystonic limb posturing
          ii) Spontaneous and reflex focal myoclonus

Qualifications of Clinical Features

- Rigidity: must be easily detectable without reinforcement.
- Apraxia: must be more than simple use of limb as object; absence of cognitive/motor abnormalities sufficient to account for the disturbance must be clear.
- Cortical sensory loss: must be able to demonstrate preserved primary sensation and be highly asymmetric to verify that the patient understands the test assignment.
- Alien-limb phenomenon: must be more than simple *levitation.*
- Dystonia: must affect a limb and be present at rest from the outset (i.e., not purely action induced).
- Myoclonus: must spread beyond the digits when provoked by external stimuli.

Exclusion Criteria

- Presentation with cognitive disturbances other than apraxias or speech or language disorders.[a]
- Presence of moderate to severe global dementia while the patient remains ambulatory.[a]
- Presence of levodopa responsivity (other than mild worsening on withdrawal).
- Presence of downgaze palsy (including absence of fast component of optokinetic nystagmus) while patient is still ambulatory.[a]
- Presence of typical parkinsonian rest tremor.
- Presence of severe autonomic disturbances, including symptomatic postural hypotension, urinary or bowel incontinence, and constipation to the point of repeated impaction.
- Presence of sufficient and appropriately located lesions on imaging studies to account for the clinical disturbances.

[a]May exclude cases of classical pathology but more often excludes alternative pathologies (i.e., reduces sensitivity but increases specificity even more).
Adapted from Lang AE, Riley DE, Bergeron C. Cortical-basal ganglionic degeneration. In: Calne DB, ed. *Neurodegeneration diseases.* Philadelphia: WB Saunders, 1994:877–894.

EPIDEMIOLOGY

Although CBD has become a more widely recognized entity, it remains a rare disease of unknown incidence and prevalence. Furthermore, it is not clear what proportion of all patients harboring CBD pathology present in the classical fashion as opposed to an alternative asymmetric cortical degeneration syndrome because current data are largely based on biased samples derived from small autopsy series with cases originating from movement disorder or dementia clinics rather than from more widely dispersed or population-based sources. It is seen considerably less commonly than PSP, which accounts for approximately 5% of cases of parkinsonism seen in specialized movement disorder clinics. CBD was present in 0.9% of patients seen in one large movement disorders clinic. Based on this estimate and corrections for underdiagnosis, Togasaki et al. estimated that the total number of people who will develop CBD in the population is about 4% to 6% of the number of those with parkinsonism (31). Based on the incidence of Parkinson's disease, they estimated that the CBD incidence rate would be 0.62–0.92/100,000 per year. Based on a mean survival of 7.9 years, they estimated a prevalence rate of 4.9–7.3/100,000. In considering these estimates, one must keep in mind that overestimation is likely because patients with CBD are more likely to be referred to specialized clinics; however, these estimates may be low because they consider only the classic lateralized movement disorder presentation and not the dementia phenotype. The cause and risk factors for the development of CBD are currently unknown.

NEUROIMAGING AND NEUROPHYSIOLOGY

Structural and functional imaging and electrophysiologic techniques have been used in an attempt to provide useful adjunctive information in the diagnosis of CBD and information about the pathophysiology of various clinical signs. For the most part, systematic studies have been carried out only in patients diagnosed with the classical clinical syndrome. Recognizing the clinical heterogeneity of CBD and variability of pathologic conditions causing the clinical syndrome, it must be acknowledged that it is uncertain how sensitive and specific the defined imaging and physiologic abnormalities are for the pathology of CBD as opposed to a specific topographic distribution that may be affected by multiple pathologic entities.

Magnetic resonance imaging (MRI) may demonstrate asymmetric pericentral cortical atrophy in approximately 50% to 96% of cases (32). However, Caselli et al. have suggested that three-dimensional surface-rendered MRI may be considerably more sensitive in detecting subtle cortical atrophy (28). Computerized quantitation and detection of accelerated regional or generalized cerebral atrophy using serial MRI images as in patients with AD might also be applicable in CBD and other asymmetric cortical degeneration syndromes. Hyperintensity of the atrophic cortex and the underlying white matter may be seen on fluid-attenuated reversion recovery (FLAIR) images in some cases (32). Hypointensity in the putamina and globus pallidi may also be evident on T2-weighted images, although we have not been impressed with the presence of these abnormalities, and they certainly do not reach the degree seen in striatonigral degeneration or neurodegeneration with brain iron accumulation type 1 (Hallervorden–Spatz syndrome) (32). Compared with controls, proton magnetic resonance spectroscopic imaging demonstrates significantly reduced *N*-acetylaspartate/creatine-phosphocreatine ratio in the centrum semiovale and reduced *N*-acetylaspartate/choline ratio in the lentiform nucleus and parietal cortex (predominantly contralateral to the worst affected side) (33). Functional imaging studies may help differentiate between CBD and other neurodegenerative diseases (Table 12.4) especially when [^{18}F]FDG and [^{18}F]fluoro-L-dopa (F-dopa) PET are both utilized in a single patient (34). Widespread abnormalities may be revealed even when structural imaging studies appear normal or minimally abnormal. Areas of cortical hypometabolism or reduced blood flow may reflect a combination of local neuronal loss and deafferentation from adjacent cortical and subcortical regions. Typically FDG scans show asymmetric medial frontal, inferior parietal, and temporal cortical hypometabolism as well as hypometabolism in the lenticular nucleus and thalamus. Eidelberg has also suggested that the severity of apraxia and dystonia correlates with the severity of cortical and basal ganglia hypometabolism, respectively, in individual patients (34). Assessment of the presynaptic dopamine system shows severe, asymmetric reduction in striatal F-dopa uptake, which is equal in putamen and caudate. There is also reduced basal ganglia iodobenzamide (IBZM) binding on single photon emission computed tomography (SPECT) examination of postsynaptic D2 receptors. These findings are congruent with widespread substantia nigra neuron loss and similar, though less severe, striatal degeneration (34). Recent studies have also demonstrated differences between

PSP and Parkinson's disease with respect to muscarinic and opioid receptor binding; further discrimination of CBD might also be possible using these ligands (34).

Conventional electrophysiologic studies are generally nonspecifically abnormal or unrevealing (15), although upper limb somatosensory evoked potentials (SEPs) may be delayed in early CBD in an apraxic upper limb compared with the normal arm. Action and spontaneous myoclonus consists of 25- to 50-ms bursts of agonist and antagonist muscle co-contraction with a proximal-to-distal pattern of activation. Stimulus-sensitive and action myoclonus is often repetitive with 60- to 80-ms interburst intervals. Clinically apparent spontaneous myoclonus occurs on a background of ongoing muscle activity (often dystonic) and subsides if muscle relaxation (as recorded by surface electromyography) can be achieved (15). Unlike typical cortical reflex myoclonus (e.g., as seen in progressive myoclonus epilepsy/ataxia), electroencephalographic back-averaging rarely provides evidence of a preceding cortical discharge (15). Studies with magnetoencephalography may provide further insight into the nature of the cortical mechanisms of myoclonus in CBD; cortical activation on back-averaged magnetoencephalography preceding myoclonus in CBD has been detected that was not evident on electroencephalography (15). Cortical SEPs are usually not enlarged. Later components of the parietal SEPs are poorly formed and dominated by a broad positive wave with a peak latency of about 45 ms possibly due to abnormal processing in the sensory cortex (15). Cutaneous reflex latencies in CBD (mean 50 ms) are considerably shorter than in patients with MSA or dementia plus Parkinson's disease (mean 63.5 ms) (15). To the best of our knowledge, no other pathologic entity has been reported to result in myoclonus with these physiologic characteristics; therefore, this feature may help differentiate CBD from pathologic mimickers that otherwise clinically appear typical of CBD (Fig. 12.2). Further evaluation of this technique in pathologically verified cases is necessary to confirm its sensitivity and specificity. The latency of typical cortical reflex myoclonus is approximately 8 ms longer than that of CBD and is thought to involve

TABLE 12.4. FUNCTIONAL IMAGING IN NEURODEGENERATIVE DISEASES

Pathology	FDG PET or HMPAO SPECT Scanning	F-dopa PET Scanning
CBD	Asymmetric hypometabolism in striatum, thalamus, posterior frontal, inferior parietal, and lateral temporal cortex	Reduced uptake equally in caudate and putamen (may be asymmetric)
PSP	Bilateral medial frontal, thalamus, and midbrain hypometabolism	Same as CBD, but symmetric
AD	Hypometabolism in parietotemporal and frontal association cortex (occasionally asymmetric)	Usually normal
Parkinson's disease with dementia	May be same as AD	Uptake reduced in putamen much greater than caudate (usually asymmetric)

CBD, corticobasal degeneration; PSP, progressive supranuclear palsy; AD, Alzheimer's disease; FDG, fluorodeoxyglucose; PET, positron emission tomography; HMPAO, hexamethylpropyleneamine oxime; SPECT, single photon emission computed tomography.

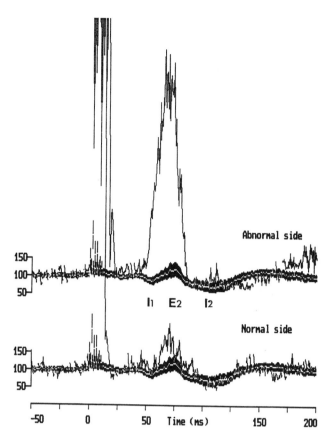

FIG. 12.2. Effect of stimulating the middle finger (5 pulses at 500 Hz at twice perception threshold given at time zero) on electromyogram (EMG) of the first dorsal interosseous muscle (FDI) during a 30% maxima contraction (50 sweeps rectified and averaged). The darkened zone represents the mean ± 2 SE from normal subjects. (From Chen et al., 1992). On the abnormal side of patient no. 2 *(top trace)* digital nerve stimulation resulted in a strong facilitation of the FDI EMG with a latency of 46 ms replacing the normal inhibitory period "I1." This was not seen on the patients "normal" side *(bottom trace).* The mean value of the prestimulus EMG has been normalized to 100%. (Courtesy of Dr. P. Ashby.)

abnormal relays through the sensory cortex to motor cortex. Thompson et al. have suggested that a direct sensory input from ventrolateral thalamic nuclei to the motor cortex (bypassing the primary sensory cortex) may be the basis for the very short latency reflex myoclonus in CBD, which is only 1 to 2 ms longer than the sum of the afferent and efferent times to and from the cortex (15). Intracortical or thalamocortical neuronal inhibition may also be reduced in CBD. This is supported by studies using transcranial magnetic stimulation, which demonstrates reduced inhibition of voluntary electromyographic activity with subthreshold stimuli, whereas single suprathreshold stimuli frequently cause repetitive muscle facilitation that has been attributed to repetitive cortical activation (17). Furthermore, a shorter silent period following use of transcranial magnetic stimulation on the affected side of the brain may be found (15).

PATHOLOGY

Recently, several advances have been made in the pathologic characterization of CBD coupled with recognition of overlapping features with other neurodegenerative diseases. As a result, controversy exists with respect to its differentiation from PSP and Pick's disease. Indeed, Kertesz and Munoz have argued for use of the term "Pick complex" to lump together a variety of diagnoses, both clinically and pathologically (10). Nevertheless, we believe that CBD is a pathologically distinct disorder with unique histologic and biochemical features. On gross examination, frontoparietal cortical atrophy is usually present but may be mild. Dementing and primary progressive aphasia presentations are associated with additional involvement of the frontal and temporal lobes. Asymmetry is often less obvious pathologically than clinically. A variable degree of ventricular dilatation may be seen. The substantia nigra is severely depigmented in most cases, but this may be much less evident in patients with severe early cognitive symptoms. Routine histologic examination of the cortex reveals neuronal loss and gliosis most prominent in the superficial layers; in the most severely involved areas, status spongiosus may be observed. These changes are most evident in grossly atrophic areas but can be seen to a milder degree in less overtly atrophic cortex. Gliosis is usually observed in the subcortical white matter and parallels the degree of cortical degeneration. Neuronal gloss, gliosis, and "corticobasal inclusions" (see below) are invariably found in the substantia nigra (2). There is variable involvement of other deep gray structures, including lateral thalamic nuclei, subthalamic nucleus, globus pallidus, striatum, amygdala, deep cerebellar nuclei, and other brainstem nuclei.

Ballooned neurons (BNs) (Fig. 12.3A) are characterized by perikaryal swelling, dispersion of Nissl substance, an eccentrically located nucleus, loss of typical cytoplasmic staining *(achromasia),* and occasional cytoplasmic vacuolation. BNs stain variably with antibodies to ubiquitin and tau, but are consistently stained with antibodies to phosphorylated neurofilament epitopes and β-crystallin (30). Among neurodegenerative diseases, the presence of BNs was previously thought to be characteristic of Pick's disease (so-called "Pick cells") and CBD. However, they have been increasingly recognized in some cases of PSP and less commonly in AD, frontotemporal dementia and parkinsonism motor neuron disease, and CJD (30). Thus, the presence of swollen neurons does not discriminate among different diseases, although their quantity and distribution is of diagnostic relevance.

The occasional presence of frank cortical degeneration predominantly confined to the premotor and motor cortex with neuronal loss, gliosis, and occasional BNs in PSP blurs its distinction from CBD (17). Unusual clinical features may be associated with such cases including limb apraxia, focal dystonia, arm levitation, and absence of supranuclear

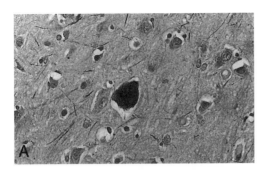

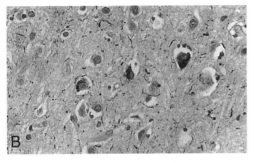

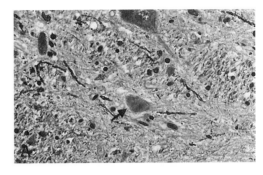

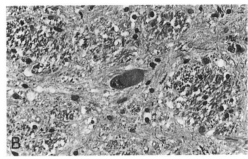

FIG. 12.3. Ballooned neuron **(A)** and tau immunoreactive neuronal deposits **(B)** in the neocortex. Thin tau immunoreactive profiles are scattered in the neuropil **(B)**. Neurofilament **(A)** and tau **(B)** immunostains, original magnification ×60.

FIG. 12.4. Corticobasal inclusions vary in their appearance. They include coarse fibrillary tangles **(A)** and more homogeneous basophilic inclusions **(B)**. Hematoxylin-eosin/luxol fast blue. Original magnification ×60.

gaze palsy. Despite these features, CBD can be differentiated on the basis of other pathologic findings as discussed below.

Feaney and Dickson have studied the cytoskeletal abnormalities and the neuropathologic overlap between CBD, Pick's disease, and PSP using sensitive immunohistochemical methods (30). All of the disorders have numerous tau-immunoreactive neuronal and glial inclusions in cortical and subcortical regions. Pathologic diagnostic separation can be achieved by identifying the characteristic *distribution* of neuronal and glial lesions. Cortical tau-positive neuronal inclusions in CBD are found in pyramidal and nonpyramidal neurons and may have a distinctive perinuclear, coiled filamentous appearance, but in general vary greatly in appearance (Fig. 12.3B). Weakly basophilic nigral neuronal inclusions were first described by Gibb et al. and were initially thought to be specific for CBD (corticobasal inclusions); however, examination of additional cases has revealed considerable morphologic heterogeneity, ranging from slightly fibrillar to frankly filamentous (Fig. 12.4) (2). As a result, these inclusions are not reliably distinguishable from tau-positive neurofibrillary tangles (NFTs) commonly associated with PSP. Thus, the morphology of neuronal tau-positive inclusions is often not sufficiently distinctive to allow differentiation between different diseases. Cortical tau-positive neuronal inclusions are considerably more common in CBD than in PSP; in contrast, in PSP the neuronal inclusions in the deep gray matter and brainstem are more abundant than in CBD.

Diagnostic confusion between Pick's disease and CBD has resulted from old classifications describing three subtypes of Pick's disease, recognition that CBD may present with a frontal lobe dementia syndrome, and recent studies describing cytoskeletal abnormalities similar to those seen in CBD and other conditions. Pick bodies (PBs) are spherical cortical intraneuronal inclusions seen predominantly in the hippocampal dentate gyrus and frontotemporal cortex that are argyrophilic and ubiquitin and tau immunoreactive. The light microscopic appearance of an individual PB is nonspecific, and both PSP and CBD may contain tau-positive structures that appear similar to PBs (30). Nevertheless, when present in sufficient quantity and appropriate distribution they confirm the diagnosis of Pick's disease. Furthermore, PBs and the "Pick-like" bodies of CBD have distinct staining characteristics. PBs are strongly argentophilic with Bodian's and Bielschowsky's stains, but negative with Gallyas's stain. The converse is true in CBD. The tau immunoreactivity is also different: typical PBs fail to stain with the anti-tau antibody 12E8, which detects phosphorylation at SER 262/356, whereas the CBD inclusions are recognized by 12E8 (35,36).

Astrocytic plaques are distinctive annular clusters of thick, short, tau-positive deposits within distal processes of cortical astrocytes specific for CBD (37) (Fig. 12.5A). These plaques are not associated with β-amyloid. Astrocytic plaques must be distinguished from thorn-shaped astrocytes, which are not disease specific, and tufted astrocytes most commonly seen in PSP (30). Thorn-shaped astrocytes

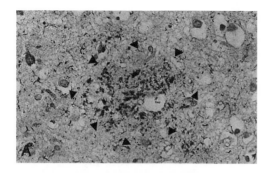

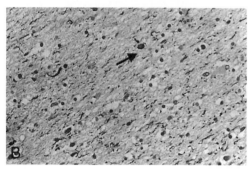

FIG. 12.5. Tau immunoreactive astrocytic plaque in the neocortex **(A)**. In the white matter, tau immunoreactive profiles and coils *(arrow)* are common **(B)**. Tau immunostain, original magnification ×60.

have their tau immunoreactivity mainly localized to perikaryal cytoplasm with extension into the proximal portions of cell processes, whereas the abnormal inclusions of tufted astrocytes are mainly in distal and proximal processes and radiate from the periphery of the astrocytic perikaryon. In CBD, astrocytic inclusions are more common in cortex than in deep gray matter or the brainstem. In each disease, abnormal tau accumulates preferentially in specific subcellular regions of astrocytes. This differential distribution may reflect distinctive pathogenetic mechanisms.

Coiled bodies are oligodendroglial inclusions that appear as a fine bundle of filaments coiled around a nucleus and

extend to the proximal part of the cell process (Fig. 12.5B). These ubiquitin-negative, tau-immunoreactive inclusions are morphologically and antigenically distinct from glial cytoplasmic inclusions seen in MSA and, though nonspecific, are most common in cortical and subcortical regions of CBD (30). Thin tau-immunoreactive threads of neuronal and glial origin are seen throughout the gray and white matter (Figs. 12.3B and 12.5B). Although also found in Pick's disease, they are particularly numerous in CBD and PSP.

MOLECULAR NEUROPATHOLOGY

Unique antigenic, biochemical, and ultrastructural characteristics serve to differentiate CBD from other neurodegenerative diseases. Aberrant phosphatase activity has been implicated in the production of abnormal tau protein, and pathologic accumulation of hyperphosphorylated tau comprises the abnormal inclusions in neurons and glia. The *tau* gene is localized to chromosome 17 and has 13 exons. Variable splicing of exons 2, 3, and 10 results in six tau isoforms, which are variably phosphorylated at specific serine and threonine residues (30,37). Three of these isoforms carry the segment specified by exon 10 and four repeats of a microtubule-binding domain (4R tau); the other three isoforms lack this fourth domain (3R tau). Normally, 3R and 4R tau are in equal concentration. Phosphorylation and differential exon splicing alter the affinity of tau binding to microtubules. Since phosphorylation decreases electrophoretic mobility, tau isoforms cannot be precisely differentiated by electrophoresis alone. Studies using antibodies to exon-specific epitopes allow further differentiation. Differences in the morphology and distribution of tau-immunoreactivity suggest that different isoforms may be implicated in different neurodegenerative diseases (Table 12.5). Immunochemical analysis of cortex in AD, CBD, and Pick's disease and basal ganglia in PSP reveals elec-

TABLE 12.5. COMPARATIVE MOLECULAR PATHOLOGY OF SELECT NEURODEGENERATIVE DISEASES

Disease	Western Blot of Predominant Insoluble Tau	Tau Exon 10 Expression (Four Repeat Tau)	Ultrastructure of Abnormal Filaments
CBD	Two bands (64 and 68 kd)	Present	15-nm straight filaments and wide twisted double-stranded form
Pick's disease	Two bands (55 and 64 kd)	Absent (three repeat tau)	15-nm straight filaments and wide twisted double-stranded form
PSP	Two bands (64 and 68 kd)	Present	15-nm straight filaments
Chromosome-17-linked dementia (select exon 10 and splice site mutations)	Two bands (64 and 68 kd)	Present (overproduction of four repeat tau)	15-nm straight filaments and wide twisted double-stranded form
Chromosome-17-linked dementia (select nonexon 10 mutations)	Three bands (55, 64, and 68 kd as in AD)	Present	22-nm paired helical filaments (AD-like)

CBD, corticobasal degeneration; PSP, progressive supranuclear palsy; AD, Alzheimer's disease.
Adapted from Dickson DW, Liu W-K, Ksiezak-Reding W, et al. Neuropathologic and molecular considerations. *Adv Neurol* 2000;82:9–28.

trophoretic patterns, confirming that the glial and neuronal inclusions in each disease are composed of a distinct complement of phosphorylated tau variants (Table 12.5) (30). There is similarity of the electrophoretic profile of tau in CBD and PSP (68- and 64-kd doublets); however, application of antibodies to exon 3 tau-specific epitopes confirms that, in contrast to PSP, inclusions in CBD lack exon 3 sequences. Immunoblot analysis in CBD and PSP shows distinctive patterns of tau fragments suggesting differing intracellular processing of aggregated tau in these two diseases despite an identical composition of tau isoforms (38). Immunoblots from AD cerebrospinal fluid (CSF) reveal a triplet identical to that found in AD brain homogenate. Increased total CSF tau protein has also been reported in patients with CBD compared with normal controls and patients with PSP (39). Therefore, an antemortem diagnostic test for CBD and other neurodegenerative diseases might be developed if disease-specific electrophoretic profiles of tau protein in CSF are the same as those from postmortem brain homogenates.

The tau in CBD forms paired helical filaments (PHFs) that differ from those in AD by being wider, unstable, more polymorphic, and having a longer periodicity of the helical twist. Using scanning transmission electron microscopy, Ksiezak-Reding et al. have shown that paired helical filaments in CBD exist in a less abundant double-stranded form (with a maximal width of 29 nm and a mass per unit length of 133 kd/nm), which may separate into more abundant single-stranded filaments (which are 15 nm wide and have a mass per unit length of 62 kd/nm) (30). Although 15-nm abnormal straight filaments are also seen in PSP and Pick's disease, paired wide-twisted ribbons are seen only in Pick's disease (Table 12.5) (30). Heterogeneity of tau isoforms, differential packing of the tau protein, phosphorylation state, and possibly other posttranslational modifications may contribute to the unique ultrastructure and instability of the abnormal filaments in CBD.

ETIOLOGY

Reports of familial cases of CBD suggest that genetic predisposition may be important. Brown et al. have described a frontal lobe dementia syndrome in multiple members of two families in a pattern consistent with autosomal dominant inheritance (40). One member of each family underwent pathologic study with findings most consistent with CBD. Furthermore, in two other pathologically proven cases a first-degree relative with dementia was noted (41). Vérin et al. have reported two brothers with clinical, radiologic, and metabolic imaging features of CBD, though pathologic confirmation was lacking (42). Caselli et al. have reported two clinically discordant monozygotic twins in which the proband had clinical and imaging evidence suggestive of CBD; neuropsychological testing in the clinically

unaffected twin suggested mild left hemispheric dysfunction, and FDG PET scanning revealed mild global hypometabolism, though MRI was normal (43). Despite the absence of pathologic confirmation, these findings suggest that the second twin might have presymptomatic CBD. The role of nongenetic factors is unclear, but might account for the interval between the twins' symptom onset. If presymptomatic detection becomes possible, trials of neuroprotective therapy might be instituted. Schneider et al. found increased $\epsilon 4$ allele frequency (0.32) of apoenzyme E (apoE) in their 11 cases of CBD and suggested that apoE genotype might be important in CBD pathophysiology (21). These results require confirmation in a larger study as three of their cases had concomitant AD, and Aβ-immunoreactive plaques were identified in five of seven cases with at least one $\epsilon 4$ allele, whereas none of the remaining four cases with a 3/3 genotype demonstrated any Aβ deposition.

The clinical and pathologic overlap of CBD with PSP (including the presence of widespread tau-immunoreactive pathology) combined with the recent identification of an association between homozygosity for the tau H1 haplotype in PSP encouraged similar studies in CBD. Using pathologically confirmed cases (to avoid diagnostic errors), an identical association with the H1 haplotype as in PSP has been demonstrated for CBD (44). This has led to speculation that underlying abnormalities in the *tau* gene (on chromosome 17q) may be responsible for both CBD and PSP. This raises an important question of the relationship between CBD and a number of disorders linked to chromosome 17q21-22 [frontotemporal dementia and parkinsonism (FTDP-17) or the so-called tauopathies]. Recent molecular genetic studies have confirmed that autosomal dominantly inherited FTDP-17 is due to a wide variety of mutations in the *tau* gene that reduce the ability of tau to bind to microtubules and promote microtubule assembly (37). Families with certain mutations located in exon 10 or the 5′ exon splice site of exon 10 have a pathologic phenotype that is similar to CBD, whereas those with tau mutations outside the microtubule-binding domain show either nonspecific pathology or Alzheimer-type pathology without plaques (30). Furthermore, Western blots of detergent-soluble tau and ultrastructural studies in these groups of mutations demonstrate additional similarities to CBD and PSP, respectively (Table 12.5). Most of the intron splice site mutations and certain exon 10 mutations result in an increase in the production of 4R tau isoforms, which may form toxic filaments and cause neuron dysfunction and death. Other exon mutations are associated with decreased microtubule binding and assembly, disrupt the neuronal cytoskeleton, and alter fast axonal transport resulting in neuronal dysfunction. Either a change in the ratio of 3R to 4R tau or mutations in tau can lead to abnormal tau deposition within neurons and glia. This concept has been validated in transgenic mice with overexpression of either wild-type 4R tau or mutant 3R/4R tau causing neurodegeneration and intracellular accumulation of fibrillar deposits of tau (45). Mutations leading to increased 4R tau cause an accumulation of straight filaments, while 3R tau accumulation leads to PHFs (like AD) (30). Straight filaments do not stain with silver, whereas PHFs are argyrophilic. Further complicating the situation is the fact that familial forms of Pick's disease with tau mutations have recently been reported (46).

FTDP-17 has an age of onset of less than 65 years (often in the fifth decade) and demonstrates selective frontotemporal and basal ganglia involvement. Clinical features are highly variable even with in a single family, which suggests that additional genetic or epigenetic factors influence the phenotypic manifestations of neurodegenerative tauopathies. The clinical overlap between CBD and FTDP-17 may be substantial. Buggiani et al. have described a family with a tau mutation in which the father presented with frontotemporal dementia and the son with the classic syndrome of CBD (47). As described above, CBD cases with predominantly frontal lobe involvement may be difficult to distinguish from classic frontotemporal dementia. Progressive parkinsonian dementia with pallidopontonigral degeneration, familial progressive subcortical gliosis, disinhibition-dementia-parkinsonism-amyotrophy complex, and in one family FTDP-17 resembling PSP have been reported, with pathologic findings including neuronal loss and gliosis, BNs, and tau-positive neuronal and glial inclusions (37). As a result, only the presence of astrocytic plaques and distinctive isoforms of tau clearly justify considering CBD a completely separate pathologic entity. Indeed, it is possible that PSP, CBD, and FTDP-17 represent the same disorder differing only in underlying additional biological and genetic factors. Additional molecular genetic studies of large numbers of patients with CBD are needed to determine if specific abnormalities in the *tau* gene or genes that control tau processing might be responsible for producing such a wide range of clinical and pathologic phenotypes.

TREATMENT

Unfortunately, there is no treatment that prevents or delays progression in CBD, and symptomatic therapy is usually ineffective. Kompoliti et al. retrospectively reviewed the open-label treatment of 147 patients with a variety of drugs at eight movement disorder centers (48). Parkinsonism was present in 100% of patients, and 24% of patients treated with dopaminergic agents (predominantly L-dopa) showed modest improvement in parkinsonian signs, but none responded dramatically. Poor response to L-dopa despite universal involvement of nigrostriatal dopaminergic neurons is probably due to the presence of pathology further "downstream" in the basal ganglia, thalamus, and SMA. Clonazepam reduced myoclonus in 23% of treated patients, and botulinum toxin injections improved limb dystonia or pain in six of nine patients. Other medications, such as baclofen, anticonvulsants, steroids, and anticholinergics, were not significantly useful, and central and peripheral side effects were common. Our experience is generally consistent with these results. We have observed "apraxia" of eyelid opening and closure and abnormal limb movements in two separate CBD patients taking L-dopa, which resolved with drug withdrawal. Therefore, an effort should be made to discontinue L-dopa, especially if a clinical response has been absent or unclear. The only drug that has resulted in some consistent benefit in our hands has been clonazepam used for myoclonus, whereas valproic acid has been ineffective. In contrast to the above results, we have had somewhat unfavorable results with botulinum toxin injections although others have found that electromyographically guided injections of the small muscles of the hand (especially the lumbricals) can be useful for the dystonic fisted posture. Nevertheless, botulinum toxin injections may play an important role in alleviating pain and discomfort associated with dystonia and rigidity in some cases (49). There are no data indicating that any form of currently available surgical therapy would be helpful. In addition to drug therapies, intervention by allied health professionals may be helpful. Physical therapists for gait training and use of weighted walkers may help prevent falls. Occupational therapists may devise strategies to accommodate for patients' specific disabilities. Speech therapy for dysarthria, dietary manipulation for dysphagia, and advice regarding the timing of the use of percutaneous endoscopic gastrostomy are all useful. Clearly, new experimental therapies are needed to halt the underlying neurodegeneration and provide symptomatic relief to patients.

FUTURE DIRECTIONS

Although considerable advances have been made in the recognition of the pathologic characteristics of CBD, additional work is necessary to define universally accepted pathologic diagnostic criteria based on the presence of specific markers (e.g., tau protein electrophoretic profile). Further studies are necessary to define the relationship between CBD, PSP, and the other tauopathies. The current difficulties with clinical diagnosis and clinicopathologic correlation mandate the establishment of a registry of patients who fulfill stringent diagnostic criteria, such as those proposed above (31). This will permit epidemiologic case-control studies allowing the identification of possible risk factors and the development of hypotheses that can be tested in the clinical or laboratory settings. However, if the pathology of CBD results in other clinical presentations (e.g., frontal lobe dementia) more often than the classical syndrome, epidemiologic studies will be greatly compromised. On the other hand, a homogeneous patient group might allow biochemical and genetic studies and the validation of an antemortem diagnostic marker (e.g., in CSF), which could then be applied to other clinical populations, permitting more definitive epidemiologic evaluations. Furthermore, establishing a homogeneous patient group with this rare disorder would allow more successful evaluation of new treatments in the form of multi-institutional pharmacologic therapeutic trials. As a result of this newly gained knowledge, we might be better able to alleviate the suffering experienced by these unfortunate patients.

ACKNOWLEDGMENTS

Supported in part by the Colorado Neurological Institute and the National Parkinson Foundation.

REFERENCES

1. Rebeiz JJ, Kolodny EH, Richardson EP. Corticodentatonigral degeneration with neuronal achromasia. *Arch Neurol* 1968;18: 20–33.
2. Gibb WRG, Luthert PJ, Marsden CD. Corticobasal degeneration. *Brain* 1989;112:1171–1192.
3. Lippa CF, Smith TW, Fontneau N. Corticonigral degeneration with neuronal achromasia. *J Neurol Sci* 1990;98:301–310.
4. Riley DE, Lang AE, Lewis A, et al. Cortical-basal ganglionic degeneration. *Neurology* 1990;40:1203–1212.
5. Rinne JO, Lee MS, Thompson PD, et al. Corticobasal degeneration: a clinical study of 36 cases. *Brain* 1994;117:1183–1196.
6. Litvan I, Grimes DA, Lang AE. Phenotypes and prognosis: clinicopathologic studies of corticobasal degeneration. In: Litvan I, Goetz CK, Lang AE, eds. *Advances in neurology, Vol. 82. Corticobasal degeneration and related disorders.* Philadelphia: Lippincott Williams & Wilkins, 2000b:183–196.
7. Wenning GK, Litvan I, Jankovic J, et al. Natural history and survival of 14 patients with corticobasal degeneration confirmed at postmortem examination. *J Neurol Neurosurg Psychiatry* 1998;64: 184–189.
8. Boeve BF, Maraganore DM, Parisi JE, et al. Pathologic heterogeneity in clinically diagnosed corticobasal degeneration. *Neurology* 1999;53:795–800.
9. Litvan I, Agid Y, Goetz C, et al. Accuracy of the clinical diagnosis of corticobasal degeneration: a clinicopathologic study. *Neurology* 1997;48:119–125.
10. Kertesz A, Martinez-Lage P, Davidson W, et al. The corticobasal degeneration syndrome overlaps progressive aphasia and frontotemporal dementia. *Neurology* 2000;55:1368–1375.
11. Bhatia KP, Lee SM, Rinne JO, et al. Corticobasal degeneration look-alikes. *Adv Neurol* 2000;82:169–182.
12. Lang AE. Cortical-basal ganglionic degeneration presenting with "progressive loss of speech output and orofacial dyspraxia." *J Neurol Neurosurg Psychiatry* 1992;55:1101.
13. Heilman KM. The apraxia of CBGD. *Mov Disord* 1996;11:348.
14. Leiguarda R, Lees AJ, Merello M, et al. The nature of apraxia in corticobasal degeneration. *J Neurol Neurosurg Psychiatry* 1994;57: 455–459.
15. Thompson PD, Shibasaki H. Myoclonus in corticobasal degeneration and other neurodegenerations. *Adv Neurol* 2000;82: 69–82.
16. Rivaud-Pechoux S, Vidailhet M, Gallouedec G, et al. Longitudinal ocular motor study in corticobasal degeneration and progressive supranuclear palsy. *Neurology* 2000;54:1029–1032.
17. Bergeron C, Weyer LP, et al. Cortical degeneration in progressive supranuclear palsy: a comparison with cortical-basal ganglionic degeneration. *J Neuropathol Exp Neurol* 1997;56:726–734.
18. Hanna PA, Doody RS. Alien limb sign. *Adv Neurol* 2000;82: 135–146.
19. Feinberg TE, Schindler RJ, Flanagan NG, et al. Two alien hand syndromes. *Neurology* 1992;42:19–24.
20. Valls-Sole J, Tolosa E, Marti MJ, et al. Examination of motor output pathways in patients with corticobasal ganglionic degeneration using transcranial magnetic stimulation. *Brain* 2001;124: 1131–1137.
21. Schneider JA, Watts RL, Gearing M, et al. Corticobasal degeneration: neuropathologic and clinical heterogeneity. *Neurology* 1997;48:959–969.
22. Frattali CM, Sonies BC. Speech and swallowing disturbances in corticobasal degeneration. *Adv Neurol* 2000;82:153–160.
23. Pillon B, Blin J, Vidailhet M, et al. The neuropsychological pattern of corticobasal degeneration: comparison with progressive supranuclear palsy and Alzheimer's disease. *Neurology* 1995;45:1477–1483.
24. Massman PJ, Kreiter KT, Jankovic J, et al. Neuropsychological functioning in cortical-basal ganglionic degeneration: differentiation from Alzheimer's disease. *Neurology* 1996;46:720–726.
25. Litvan I, Cummings JL, Mega M. Neuropsychiatric features of corticobasal degeneration. *J Neurol Neurosurg Psychiatry* 1998;65: 717–721.
26. Leiguarda RC, Pramstaller PP, Merello M, et al. Apraxia in Parkinson's disease, progressive supranuclear palsy, multiple system atrophy and neuroleptic-induced parkinsonism. *Brain* 1997; 120:75–90.
27. Barclay C, Lang AE. Dystonia in progressive supranuclear palsy. *J Neurol Neurosurg Psychiatry* 1997;62:352–356.
28. Caselli RJ, Jack CR. Asymmetric cortical degeneration syndromes—a proposed clinical classification. *Arch Neurol* 1992;49: 770–780.
29. Grimes DA, Lang AE, Bergeron C. Dementia is the most common presentation of cortical-basal ganglionic degeneration. *Neurology* 1999;53:1969–1974.
30. Dickson DW, Liu W-K, Ksiezak-Reding H, et al. Neuropathologic and molecular considerations. *Adv Neurol* 2000;82:9–28.
31. Togasaki DM, Tanner CM. Epidemiologic aspects. *Adv Neurol* 2000;82:53–59.
32. Savoiardo M, Grisoli M, Girotti F. Magnetic resonance imaging in CBD-related atypical parkinsonian disorders and dementias. *Adv Neurol* 2000;82:197–208.
33. Tedeschi G, Litvan I, Bonavita S, et al. Proton magnetic resonance spectroscopic imaging in progressive supranuclear palsy, Parkinson's disease, and corticobasal degeneration. *Brain* 1997; 120:1541–1552.
34. Brooks DJ. Functional imaging studies in corticobasal degeneration. *Adv Neurol* 2000;82:109–215.
35. Probst A, Tolnay M, Langui D, et al. Pick's disease: hyperphosphorylated tau protein segregates to the somatoaxonal compartment. *Acta Neuropathol (Berl)* 1996;92:588–596.
36. Bell K, Cairns NJ, Lantos PL, et al. Immunohistochemistry distinguishes: between Pick's disease and corticobasal degeneration. *J Neurol Neurosurg Psychiatry* 2000;69:835–836.
37. Lee VM, Goedert M, Trojanowski JQ. Neurodegenerative tauopathies. *Annu Rev Neurosci* 2001;24:1121–1159.
38. Arai T, Ikeda K, Akiyama H, et al. Intracellular processing of aggregated tau differs between corticobasal degeneration and progressive supranuclear palsy. *Neuroreport* 2001;12:935–938.
39. Urakami K, Wada K, Arai H, et al. Diagnostic significance of tau protein in cerebrospinal fluid from patients with corticobasal degeneration or progressive supranuclear palsy. *J Neurol Sci* 2001; 183:95–98.
40. Brown J, Lantos PL, Roques P, et al. Familial dementia with

swollen achromatic neurons and corticobasal inclusion bodies: a clinical and pathological study. *J Neurol Sci* 1996;135:21–30.

41. Mitsuyama Y, Masuda K, Inoue T, et al. Primary progressive dementia with swollen chromatolytic neurons. *Dementia* 1992;3: 223–231.

42. Verin M, Rancurel G, DeMarco O, et al. First familial cases of corticobasal degeneration. *Mov Disord* 1997;12:55.

43. Caselli RJ, Reiman EM, Timmann D, et al. Progressive apraxia in clinically discordant monozygotic twins. *Arch Neurol* 1995;52: 1004–1010.

44. Houlden H, Baker M, Morris HR, et al. Corticobasal degeneration and progressive supranuclear palsy share a common tau haplotype. *Neurology* 2001;56:1702–1706.

45. Lewis J, McGowan E, Rockwood J, et al. Neurofibrillary tangles, amyotrophy, and progressive motor disturbance in mice expressing mutant (P301L) tau protein. *Nat Genet* 2000;25:402–405.

46. Neumann M, Schulz-Schaeffer W, Crowther RA, et al. Pick's disease associated with the novel Tau gene mutation K369I. *Ann Neurol* 2001;50:503–513.

47. Bugiani O, Murrell JR, Giaccone G, et al. Frontotemporal dementia and corticobasal degeneration in a family with a P301S mutation in tau. *J Neuropathol Exp Neurol* 1999;58: 667–677.

48. Kompoliti K, Goetz CG, Boeve BF, et al. Clinical presentation and pharmacological therapy in corticobasal degeneration. *Arch Neurol* 1998;55:57–61.

49. Vanek Z, Jankovic J. Dystonia in corticobasal degeneration. *Mov Disord* 2001;16:252–257.

50. Wenning GK, Ben Shlomo Y, Magalhaes M, et al. Clinical features and natural history of multiple system atrophy: an analysis of 100 cases. *Brain* 1994;117:835–845.

51. Litvan I, Mangone CA, McKee A, et al. Natural history of progressive supranuclear palsy (Steele-Richardson-Olszewski syndrome) and clinical predictors of survival: a clinicopathological study. *J Neurol Neurosurg Psychiatry* 1996;60:615–620.

52. Lang AE, Riley DE, Bergeron C. Cortical-basal ganglionic degeneration. In: Calne DB, ed. *Neurodegenerative diseases*. Philadelphia: WB Saunders, 1994:877–894.

SECONDARY PARKINSONISM

DAVID E. RILEY

Since the last edition of this text, the list of diseases and conditions producing some or all of the clinical features of Parkinson's disease (PD) has continued to grow. We have also expanded and refined our knowledge concerning many of the previously described secondary causes of parkinsonism. As one might expect, much of this progress can be attributed to dramatic advances in our understanding of genetics. Consequently, the greatest changes in this field have occurred in the category of hereditary illnesses, where new disorders associated with parkinsonism have been reported and a genetic basis has been found for a number of others.

One item that remains unchanged is the importance of being able to distinguish Parkinson's disease from its imitators. Incorrect differential diagnosis of PD is still the greatest obstacle to research, resulting in misleading conclusions regarding studies of heredity, epidemiology, therapeutics, and all other aspects of this illness. Clinically, proper recognition of PD's imitators avoids repeated consultations, unnecessary investigations, and fruitless medication trials, and allows physicians to give more accurate information regarding natural history and prognosis. When specific treatment does become available for these conditions, it would be helpful to have patients correctly identified beforehand so that they can obtain prompt benefit. Whether using the classification proposed here (Table 13.1) or any other, neurologists should develop an approach to the differential diagnosis of PD and maintain a constant awareness of alternative causes.

To conserve space, only references published since the last edition of this text are given. Readers are urged to consult the last edition of this chapter (1) for information on causes of secondary parkinsonism not referenced in the tables of this chapter.

TABLE 13.1. CATEGORIES OF PARKINSONISM

Infectious or postinfectious (Table 13.2)
Drug-induced (Table 13.3)
Toxic (Table 13.4)
Metabolic (Table 13.5)
Familial (Table 13.6)
Parkinsonism diagnosable by imaging studies (Table 13.7)
Miscellaneous causes (Table 13.8)
Degenerative diseases causing parkinsonism (Table 13.9)

INFECTIOUS AND POSTINFECTIOUS PARKINSONISM

A number of infectious diseases (Table 13.2) may cause parkinsonism, acutely or as a long-term complication. However, none has done so with significant frequency since the heyday of encephalitis lethargica in the 1920s. In truth, the infectious nature of this illness remains an assumption because no causative agent has ever been identified (2). Occasionally a patient still merits a diagnosis of postencephalitic parkinson-

TABLE 13.2. INFECTIOUS OR POSTINFECTIOUS PARKINSONISM

AIDS
    HIV (15)
    Progressive multifocal leukoencephalopathy (PML)
    Toxoplasmosis
Cryptococcal meningoencephalitis
Cysticercosis
Fungal abscesses in striata
Herpes simplex encephalitis
Japanese encephalitis
Malaria
Mycoplasma infection (16)
Postencephalitic parkinsonism
    Coxsackie B
    Encephalitis lethargica (2)
    Influenza A
    Japanese encephalitis
    Measles
    Mumps
    Polio
    Western equine encephalitis
Postvaccinal parkinsonism
Prion diseases
    Creutzfeldt-Jakob disease (17)
    Gerstmann-Sträussler-Scheinker disease
    Kuru (18)
    Other prion disease
St. Louis encephalitis
Subacute sclerosing panencephalitis
Syphilis
Tuberculosis
Whipple's disease

AIDS, autoimmune deficiency syndrome; HIV, human immunodeficiency virus.

ism because of a history of encephalitis-like illness with excessive somnolence and because of additional features, such as early age of onset, oculogyric crises, ophthalmoplegia, behavioral and sleep disorders, and prominent dyskinesias such as dystonia and tics. A number of identifiable encephalitides may cause postinfectious parkinsonism (Table 13.2), albeit rarely. In most cases the parkinsonism remits spontaneously and completely in a matter of weeks to months.

Parkinsonism as an acute effect of nervous system infection is very rare. Historically one of the most important causes of secondary parkinsonism was a tuberculoma of the midbrain, which led to the discovery of the substantia nigra as the site of the pathology of PD. In children, acute infection with *Mycoplasma pneumoniae* may lead to striatal necrosis manifested by parkinsonism, dystonia, or both. In adults, Whipple's disease may produce a combination of parkinsonism and supranuclear gaze palsy, mimicking progressive supranuclear palsy (PSP). Creutzfeldt-Jakob and other prion diseases may cause parkinsonism, but new-variant Creutzfeldt-Jakob disease apparently does not. In addition to Creuzfeldt-Jakob disease, there are other prion diseases that may be manifested by parkinsonism, including Gerstmann-Sträussler-Scheinker disease (2a). The topic of prion disease has been recently reviewed by Prusiner, who received a Nobel Prize for his contributions to this field (2b). The most common infectious cause of parkinsonism in the early 21st century is AIDS, due either to central nervous system invasion by human immunodeficiency virus (HIV) itself, or to opportunistic infection (Table 13.2).

DRUG-INDUCED PARKINSONISM

One of the most important categories of secondary parkinsonism is drug-induced parkinsonism (Table 13.3). Most physicians are aware of the potential for dopamine receptor–blocking drugs used in a psychiatric or gastrointestinal context to cause parkinsonism, both as an isolated subacute complication and in the case of the rare neuroleptic malignant syndrome. It is important to question patients closely regarding symptoms that might prompt treatment with antidopaminergic drugs, rather than relying on their recollection of their medications. In some countries, antidopaminergic drugs may be used as counterfeit substitutes for other prescription drugs and cause parkinsonism (3). The presynaptic catecholamine-depleting drugs reserpine and tetrabenazine may have the same parkinsonian effect as dopamine receptor blockers. Recovery following withdrawal of offending agents may take weeks to months. Striatal lesions on magnetic resonance images may correlate with a slower rate of recovery.

A number of other drugs (Table 13.3) have mechanisms that are less well defined but that produce a similar clinical picture. From a practical standpoint it is important to remember that drug-induced parkinsonism is rare except in the case of antidopaminergic drugs and the calcium channel blockers cinnarizine and flunarizine. Nevertheless, a high index of sus-

TABLE 13.3. DRUG-INDUCED PARKINSONISM

α-Methyldopa
Amiodarone
Amoxapine
Amphotericin B
Antidopaminergic drugs
    Dopamine receptor blockers
    Presynaptic monoamine depletors: reserpine, tetrabenazine
Antineoplastic therapy
    Multiagent chemotherapy
    Plus radiation
Aprindine
Bethanechol (intraventricular)
Buformin
Calcium channel blockers
Captopril
Cephaloridine
Cimetidine
Clopamide—pindolol combination
Cyclosporine
Cytosine arabinoside
Diazepam
Disulfiram
5-Fluorouracil
Hexamethylmelamine
Interferon-α
Lithium
Meperidine
Perhexiline
Phenelzine
Phenytoin
Prenylamine
Procaine
Pyridostigmine
Serotonin-specific reuptake inhibitors
Trazodone
Valproate

picion is warranted so as not to overlook a highly treatable cause of secondary parkinsonism. The potential production or aggravation of parkinsonism by serotonin-specific reuptake inhibitors (SSRIs) has been widely reported but appears to affect only a minuscule portion of the huge numbers of patients using these medications. SSRIs are safely taken by many PD patients. Other frequently prescribed drugs, such as cimetidine, diazepam, and phenytoin, have caused parkinsonism in very few cases, suggesting a highly idiosyncratic effect. In all cases of drug-induced parkinsonism the effects are reversible if the offending agent is withdrawn.

TOXIC PARKINSONISM

Exposure to numerous toxins (Table 13.4) has been associated with parkinsonism. Some toxins are environmental, whereas other exposures result from drug abuse, or attempted suicide or homicide. Obviously a detailed occupational or drug use history may be the key to a correct diagnosis. Although none of the toxic agents listed here is a particularly common cause of parkinsonism, it can be argued that 1-methyl-4-phenyl-

TABLE 13.4. TOXINS ASSOCIATED WITH PARKINSONISM

Betel nut plus antipsychotics
Carbon disulfide
Carbon monoxide (19)
Contact herbicides
    Paraquat
    Diquat
Contrast agent for cardiac catheterization
Cyanide
Ethanol withdrawal
Glyphosate (20)
Hydrocarbons (*n*-hexane)
Hydrogen sulfide
Lacquer thinner
1-Methyl-4-phenyl-1,2,3,6-tetrahydropyridine
Maneb (manganese ethylenebisdithiocarbamate)
Manganese
Mercury
Methanol
Organophosphate insecticide
Petroleum products

TABLE 13.5. METABOLIC CAUSES OF PARKINSONISM

Acquired chronic hepatocerebral degeneration
Folate deficiency
Heatstroke
Hypothyroidism
Postanoxic parkinsonism (21)

parkinsonism may occur. This disorder may also result in pallidal abnormalities on imaging studies. Hypothyroidism does not cause parkinsonism per se, but it does cause a slowing down of activity that can be mistaken for PD.

HEREDITARY PARKINSONISM

Our understanding of hereditary parkinsonism has been and is being revolutionized by rapid developments in molecular genetics. Parkinsonism due to genetic abnormalities occurs in a variety of forms (Table 13.6). Many of these disorders have exceptional features and would not be mistaken for PD. However, several families have autosomal dominant parkinsonism clinically and pathologically typical for PD except for an early age of onset and a relatively rapid course (4). This disorder has been attributed to a mutation in the α-synuclein gene at 4q21-22. Another locus for autosomal dominant Parkinson's disease exists at 2p13 (5). A third site for monogenic, autosomal dominant PD, including Lewy body pathology, is located in the ubiquitin C-terminal hydrolase gene at 4p14-15 (6).

1,2,3,6-tetrahydropyridine (MPTP) is one of the most important. MPTP has become the tool of choice to create animal models for PD. The ability of MPTP toxicity in humans to mimic PD so closely has spurred an enormous effort to identify environmental toxins with similar properties that may be implicated in the pathogenesis of PD. MPTP is highly toxic to substantia nigra neurons, and the symptoms of MPTP parkinsonism respond well to levodopa. *n*-Hexane also exerts its effects on the substantia nigra, while methanol is mainly toxic to the striatum. A common target for toxic parkinsonism is the globus pallidus, which is the site of action of carbon monoxide, cyanide, and manganese.

Manganese is the most common known environmental cause of parkinsonism, being found in both exposed miners and industrial workers. Manganese toxicity causes akinesia and rigidity along with a peculiar plantar flexion action dystonia and a flexed upper limb posture, resulting in a characteristic cock-walk gait. Behavioral symptoms and signs, such as fatigue, irritability, and aggressiveness, often precede or accompany this form of parkinsonism, especially in miners. Contact and organophosphate insecticides are rare causes of parkinsonism, but are frequent suspects in discussions of epidemiologic studies that find a higher incidence of rural living and farming in the early-life environment of PD patients.

METABOLIC PARKINSONISM

Metabolic parkinsonism comprises unusual metabolic disorders and more common diseases of which parkinsonism is a rare complication (Table 13.5). Parkinsonism caused by anoxic encephalopathy is associated with lesions in the globus pallidus (Fig. 13.1). Cerebellar, cognitive, and other findings usually dominate the clinical picture in acquired chronic hepatocerebral degeneration, but a pure levodopa-responsive

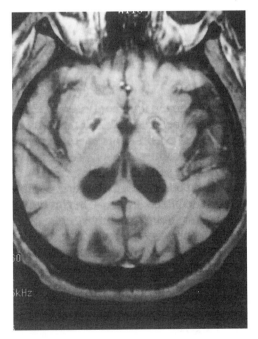

FIG. 13.1. T1-weighted magnetic resonance image of a man with postanoxic parkinsonism showing probable bilateral cavitation of the globus pallidus.

TABLE 13.6. HEREDITARY PARKINSONISM

Adult polyglucosan body disease (22)
Aromatic amino acid decarboxylase deficiency
Autosomal dominant parkinsonism linked to chromosome 2 (5)
Autosomal dominant parkinsonism with ubiquitin C–terminal hydrolase gene mutations (6)
Autosomal recessive juvenile parkinsonism (*parkin* gene mutations) (23,7)
Autosomal recessive parkinsonism due to *PARK6* mutations (8)
Autosomal recessive parkinsonism due to *PARK7* mutations (9)
Cerebrotendinous xanthomatosis (24)
Ceroid lipofuscinosis (25)
Chediak-Higashi syndrome (26)
Dentatorubropallidoluysian atrophy
Dominantly inherited early-onset parkinsonism
Dopa-responsive dystonia–parkinsonism
Familial diffuse Lewy body disease
Familial Parkinson's disease (α-synuclein gene mutations) (4)
Familial progressive subcortical gliosis
Familial progressive supranuclear palsy
Fragile X syndrome (27)
Frontotemporal dementia and parkinsonism linked to chromosome 17 (28)
G_{M1} gangliosidosis
G_{M2} gangliosidosis
Hereditary hemochromatosis
Hereditary sensorimotor neuropathy and parkinsonism
Huntington's disease (29)
Mitochondrial cytopathy (30)
Niemann-Pick disease type C
Rapid-onset dystonia–parkinsonism (31)
Spinocerebellar ataxia type 1
Spinocerebellar ataxia type 2
Spinocerebellar ataxia type 3 (Machado-Joseph disease)
Spinocerebellar ataxia type 12 (32)
Tyrosine hydroxylase deficiency (33)
Wilson's disease
X-linked dystonia–parkinsonism (Lubag)
X-linked recessive parkinsonism and mental retardation

Several types of autosomal recessive parkinsonism have been described and genetically mapped. The most common variety is autosomal recessive juvenile parkinsonism (AR-JP) (7). AR-JP characteristically develops early in life but may present at almost any age. Younger patients often experience considerable dystonia. Pathologically, AR-JP shows nigral degeneration without Lewy bodies. AR-JP is due to mutations in the *parkin* gene at 6q25.2-27. Two loci for autosomal recessive parkinsonism arising in early adulthood are near each other at chromosome 1p35-36 ("PARK6") (8) and 1p36 ("PARK7") (9). X-linked causes of parkinsonism include fragile X syndrome and lubag. Mitochondrial DNA mutations may also result in parkinsonism.

The term "frontotemporal dementia and parkinsonism linked to chromosome 17" (FTDP-17) refers to a group of autosomal dominant disorders caused by mutations in the *tau* gene at 17q21-22. Although individual kindreds express apparently distinctive clinical features, the presentation of FTDP-17 always involves either dementia or parkinsonism. If cognitive changes predominate, they are often accompanied by behavioral abnormalities, such as aggression, disinhibition, irritability, and withdrawal. If an akinetic-rigid syndrome develops first, dementia soon follows and additional features include amyotrophy, dystonia, spasticity, and ocular motor dysfunction. FTDP-17 is dealt with in greater detail elsewhere in this volume.

Although hereditary, as an autosomal recessive condition Wilson's disease (WD) often occurs without a family history. WD causes a variety of movement disorders, notably ataxia and dystonia, but parkinsonism may be the most common neurologic presentation. All parkinsonian patients younger than 40 years should undergo tests of copper metabolism and a slit-lamp examination to look for evidence of WD. Prompt induction of treatment with trien, followed by maintenance therapy with zinc, is usually lifesaving and may reverse many of the clinical manifestations.

Dopa-responsive dystonia-parkinsonism causes generalized dystonia beginning in childhood in the lower limbs, often with marked diurnal variations. The clinical spectrum includes many cases of parkinsonism with or without dystonia, mainly in older patients. Autopsy studies demonstrate a normal-appearing substantia nigra. The dominant form of dopa-responsive dystonia-parkinsonism maps to a gene defect in chromosome 14q that results in a deficiency of guanine triphosphate–cyclohydrolase I, a synthetic enzyme for tetrahydrobiopterin, the cofactor for tyrosine hydroxylase.

When the onset of Huntington's disease (HD) occurs before age 20 years, or rarely later, the principal movement disorder is often not chorea but an akinetic-rigid syndrome, often known as the Westphal variant of HD. Patients have the same expanded CAG triplet repeat sequence in the short arm of chromosome 4 as is found in the more typical choreic form. Other CAG repeat diseases show signs of parkinsonism, which may be the dominant feature in spinocerebellar ataxia (SCA) type 3 (Machado-Joseph disease). Subtle signs of parkinsonism may also form part of the clinical picture in SCA types 1, 2, and 12, typically in late stages (9a). As we identify more patients with SCA with the development of genetic tests, it becomes clear there is a great deal of overlap among SCA types, and the clinical presentation does not reliably predict the genotype. Parkinsonism is a rare feature of dentatorubropallidoluysian atrophy.

Other hereditary causes of parkinsonism may be found in Table 13.6 and among the imageable and degenerative diseases described in other sections. Characterization of familial parkinsonian disorders is somewhat hampered by variable expressions of disease in family members, and by misdiagnosis, particularly misidentification of essential tremor. Nevertheless, many families remain genetically unmapped, and more forms of hereditary parkinsonism will continue to be identified.

PARKINSONISM DIAGNOSABLE BY IMAGING STUDIES

Although diagnoses under other headings may cause imaging abnormalities, the disorders listed here (Table 13.7)

TABLE 13.7. PARKINSONISM DIAGNOSABLE BY IMAGING STUDIES

Calcification of the basal ganglia (9b)
Central pontine or striatal myelinolysis
Hydrocephalus (34)
Mass lesions
    Cyst in the cerebellar vermis
    Cyst in the mesencephalon
    Gliomatosis cerebri
    Midbrain bullet
    Neoplasms (35)
    Primary CNS lymphoma (36)
Syringomesencephalia
Vascular
    Ischemic
        Multi-infarct
        Single infarct
        Global
    Other vascular
        Midbrain bleed
        Subdural hematoma
        Cortical venous thrombosis (37)
        Giant internal carotid/middle cerebral artery aneurysm

invariably are associated with lesions visible on computed tomography (CT) or magnetic resonance imaging (MRI) studies. Indeed, imaging studies are often the only way to diagnose these conditions reliably.

Critchley popularized the concept of arteriosclerotic parkinsonism in the 1930s in a monograph that subsequently fell out of favor. In recent years, however, a variety of reports have not only solidified vascular disease as an important cause of parkinsonism but have delineated at least four pathologic types. The most common is a process of multiple lacunes similar to that underlying multi-infarct dementia, presenting acutely when lesions predominantly affect gray matter (Fig. 13.2) and insidiously when white matter is primarily involved. Also known as lower-body parkinsonism because of a propensity to produce a shuffling gait out of proportion to any other parkinsonian signs, multi-infarct parkinsonism rarely shows a positive response to dopaminergic drugs. It is also possible to develop parkinsonism contralateral to a single infarct in the striatum, thalamus, or substantia nigra. Less common vascular disorders associated with parkinsonism include Binswanger's encephalopathy (Fig. 13.3) and dilated perivascular spaces.

Parkinsonism may occur with either communicating or noncommunicating forms of hydrocephalus. Like vascular types, hydrocephalic parkinsonism (Fig. 13.4) tends to affect gait disproportionately. Hydrocephalus usually also

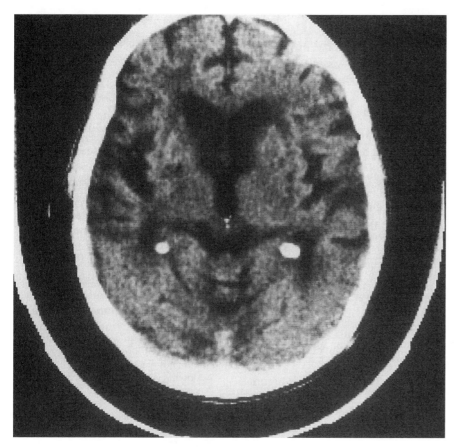

FIG. 13.2. CT scan of man with multi-infarct parkinsonism showing multiple bilateral putaminal lacunes.

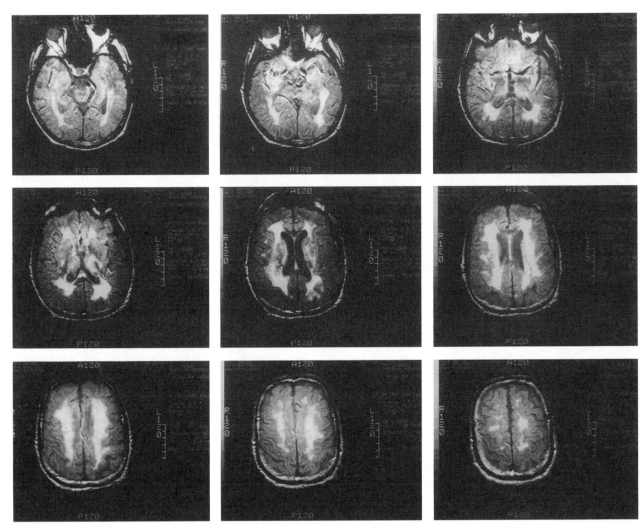

FIG. 13.3. T1-weighted magnetic resonance image of a man with lower-body parkinsonism and no dementia showing diffuse hyperintense signal in the white matter consistent with Binswanger's disease.

leads to cognitive deterioration and urinary incontinence. However, in many cases it closely mimics PD in that it causes resting tremor and responds to levodopa, occasionally with fluctuations and dyskinesias.

A small degree of calcification of the basal ganglia (CBG) involving the medial pallidum is a common incidental finding in brain imaging. Familial or idiopathic calcification of the basal ganglia associated with parkinsonism and other movement disorders, such as tremor, chorea, and dystonia, has received increased attention since the identification of a gene locus on chromosome 14q (9b). In some of these cases the calcification appears massive, affecting the entire corpus striatum and literally looking as if the patient has "rocks in the head" (Fig.

13.5). In addition to the basal ganglia, cerebral white matter and the dentate nuclei are often calcified as well. CBG may be familial, associated with a parathyroid disorder, or idiopathic. Rarely, CBG may develop rapidly after brain anoxia. A single case of calcification of the substantia nigra with parkinsonism is known.

A variety of mass lesions of different types (including hemorrhages, tumors, and abscesses) and locations have caused parkinsonism (Table 13.7). The most common neoplasm causing parkinsonism is meningioma, usually near the frontal or temporal lobes. Other lesions that can be identified on imaging studies and may cause parkinsonism include central pontine myelinolysis, striatal myelinolysis, and syringomesencephalia.

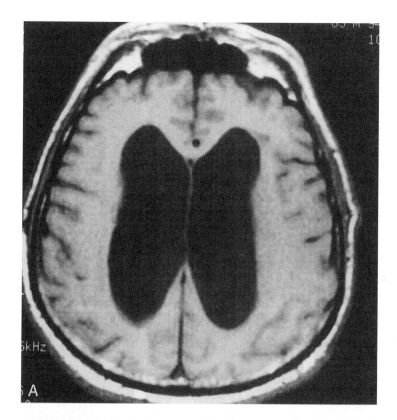

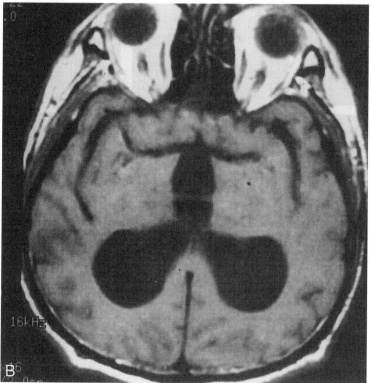

FIG. 13.4. CT scan of a man with hydrocephalic parkinsonism demonstrating enlargement of the **(A)** lateral, **(B)** third, and **(C)** fourth ventricles. *Continued on next page.*

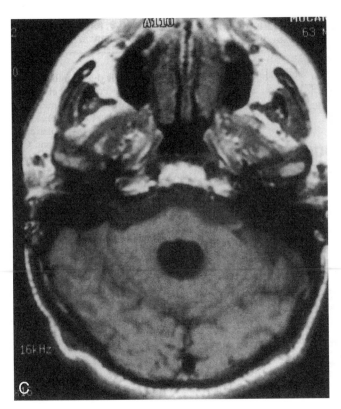

FIG. 13.4. *Continued.*

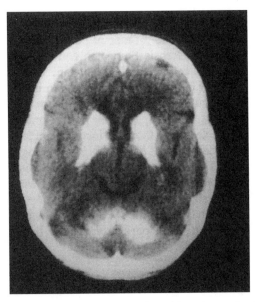

FIG. 13.5. CT scan of a woman with parkinsonism and calcification of the basal ganglia and dentate nuclei.

MISCELLANEOUS CAUSES OF PARKINSONISM

The association between trauma and parkinsonism is controversial. It is well known that a syndrome of parkinsonism may develop in boxers as a result of repeated head trauma, although dementia (punch-drunk syndrome) is a more common clinical consequence. As one might expect, the pugilists in question usually possessed inferior skills and suffered multiple knockouts. Less widely accepted is the notion that a single blow to the head can lead to parkinsonism, although there are some highly suggestive case reports. Even more controversial is the reported association of peripheral trauma with parkinsonism. These issues are obviously of great relevance to victims of motor vehicle accidents, industrial mishaps, and other causes of injury.

Another debated cause of parkinsonism is multiple sclerosis. Some contend that the relation is coincidental, but individual instances again make this difficult to accept in all cases. Psychogenic parkinsonism is suspected when there are inconsistent features or other signs of probable psychological origin. The diagnosis is difficult to establish and should be confirmed by someone with considerable experience in the study of parkinsonism. Other miscellaneous causes of parkinsonism are listed in Table 13.8.

DEGENERATIVE DISEASES

Three degenerative diseases are responsible for the majority of cases involving parkinsonism of degenerative etiology. These are dealt with in greater detail here and in other chapters.

TABLE 13.8. MISCELLANEOUS CAUSES OF PARKINSONISM

Anaphylaxis due to milk allergy (?anoxic encephalopathy)
Behçet's disease
Bone marrow transplantation
Burn
Hemiparkinsonism–hemiatrophy
Multiple sclerosis
Paraneoplastic nigral degeneration
Psychogenic parkinsonism
Rett's syndrome
Sjögren's syndrome
Trauma
    Postpugilistic parkinsonism
    Single head trauma
    Craniotomy (38)
    Peripheral trauma
Unilateral striatal necrosis

Progressive Supranuclear Palsy

Known as Steele-Richardson-Olszewski syndrome in Europe, PSP is a disease of slightly later onset than PD. The name derives from its most characteristic feature, a vertical gaze palsy affecting voluntary eye movements while sparing reflex ocular motility. This supranuclear gaze palsy is neither specific nor sensitive for PSP, and reliance on this sign frequently causes clinicians to miss the diagnosis. More common early manifestations are postural instability and falling. Other characteristic features of PSP include akinesia, axial rigidity, pseudobulbar palsy, and (usually mild) dementia. There is growing recognition of apraxia as a manifestation of PSP (10). Among the major degenerative parkinsonian syndromes, PSP is the least likely to cause tremor and other dyskinesias except dystonia.

CT or MRI may show midbrain atrophy (Fig. 13.6), but not early, when diagnostic assistance would be most useful. Patients may get vague benefit from levodopa, but it is rare to document an objective response. No other treatments show consistent results, although tricyclic antidepressants, amantadine, and other agents may help in individual cases.

Dysphagia is a common complication that often leads to death via aspiration pneumonia. Autopsy studies show degenerative changes with neurofibrillary tangle formation in remaining neurons, particularly in substantia nigra, globus pallidus, subthalamic nucleus, and midbrain nuclei. Neurofibrillary tangles contain aggregates of hyperphosphorylated microtubule-associated tau protein.

Multiple System Atrophy

The term multiple system atrophy (MSA) encompasses three entities, found in varying combinations more often than in isolation: striatonigral degeneration, olivopontocerebellar atrophy, and Shy-Drager syndrome. The three corresponding clinical syndromes are parkinsonism, cerebellar dysfunction, and autonomic failure, any of which may be prominent. The parkinsonism tends to be more symmetric, rest tremor is less common, and postural instability develops earlier, but MSA often appears identical to PD in its early stages. One feature that helps make MSA the most difficult disease to distinguish from PD is its similar

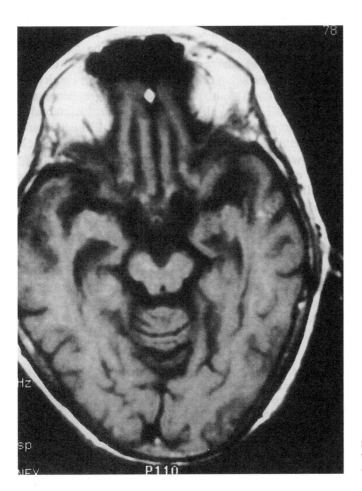

FIG. 13.6. T2-weighted magnetic resonance image of a woman with progressive supranuclear palsy demonstrating midbrain atrophy.

ability to respond to levodopa, including the production of fluctuations and dyskinesias. Clinicians depend on additional features not commonly found in PD to establish a correct diagnosis. These include orthostatic hypotension, urinary retention or incontinence, ataxia, frequent falls, stimulus-sensitive action myoclonus, facial and cervical dystonia, slurred or scanning speech, dysphonia, stridor (occasionally with laryngeal obstruction requiring tracheotomy), hand contractures, and corticospinal tract signs. Characteristic MRI abnormalities include hypointensity in the posterolateral putamen and linear hyperintensities in the lateral putamen on T2-weighted studies (Fig. 13.7), and atrophy of the cerebellum and pons. However, MRI is not a sensitive test for the diagnosis of MSA, and findings are normal in many individuals.

MSA affects a slightly younger age group than PD, but the peak onset is still in the sixth decade. Expected survival from onset is probably close to 10 years, with much variability. Pathologically there is degeneration of striatum, substantia nigra, cerebellar Purkinje cells, pontine nuclei, inferior olives, and the intermediolateral cell columns of the

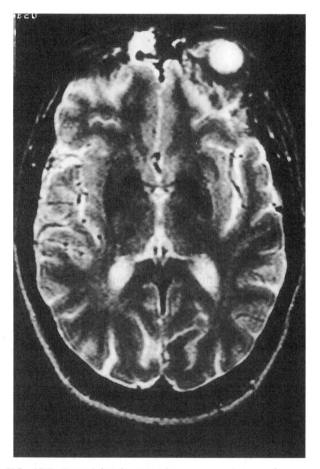

FIG. 13.7. T1-weighted magnetic resonance image of a man with multiple system atrophy showing hypointensity in the posterolateral putamen bilaterally. Note the hyperintense linear signal lateral to the left putamen.

spinal cord. Parkinsonism in MSA is associated with abnormalities in the substantia nigra, putamen, or both. Oligodendrocyte inclusion bodies known as glial cytoplasmic inclusions contain α-synuclein (11), illustrating another similarity between MSA and PD.

Treatment is symptomatic. Parkinsonism is managed much as it is in PD, although efficacy of levodopa and other medications is much less consistent. Orthostatic hypotension may respond to conservative measures, such as raising the head of the bed, compressive stockings, and liberal salt intake. Medication, such as fludrocortisone or midodrine, is commonly required. Urinary dysfunction can be managed with antispasmodics, such as oxybutynin and tolterodine, and self-catheterization.

Cortical-Basal Ganglionic Degeneration

Cortical-basal ganglionic degeneration (CBGD) produces an asymmetric akinetic-rigid picture similar to that of PD but without the resting tremor. The motor deficit is usually compounded by similarly asymmetric dystonia, apraxia, and myoclonus, all contributing to the development of the characteristic "stiff," "dystonic," "jerky," or "useless" hand. Other typical clinical findings include alien-limb phenomenon, disequilibrium with falls, and cortical sensory loss. Some patients present with other features, such as dementia, aphasia, or speech apraxia. Brain imaging studies may reveal asymmetric atrophy of the cerebral cortex, particularly in medial frontal and parietal areas (Fig. 13.8).

The major pathologic findings in CBGD are neuronal loss and formation of ballooned achromatic neurons in the cerebral cortex and degenerative changes in the substantia nigra. Surviving nigral neurons often contain cytoplasmic inclusions, nicknamed corticobasal bodies, but these are not found in every case. Immunohistochemical studies reveal cortical plaques containing abnormal tau in distal astrocytic processes as well as other abnormalities in both neurons and glia. CBGD inclusions contain the same tau isoforms as are found in PSP. There is growing evidence that CBGD and progressive supranuclear palsy share a common tau haplotype (11a).

CBGD is a source of great frustration for both patient and physician, as symptoms rarely respond to treatment to any great degree. Occasional successes are achieved with valproate or clonazepam for myoclonus or botulinum toxin for dystonia. There is no effective treatment for the cerebral cortical manifestations of CBGD.

Other Degenerative Diseases

Alzheimer's disease (AD) can produce parkinsonism and substantia nigra degeneration. Although dementia usually remains the most prominent finding, AD patients may be misdiagnosed as having PD. AD may cause the parkinsonism seen occasionally in Down's syndrome, as most brains been found to have a mutation in the *PANK-2* gene on chromosome 20p12.3-p13 coding for pantothenate kinase (14a). The term pantothenate kinase–associated neurodegeneration (PKAN) is used to describe this rare autosomal recessive neurodegenerative disorder that usually presents as a childhood-, adolescent-, or adult-onset disorder with a constellation of dystonia, rigidity, choreoathetosis, corticospinal tract dysfunction, optic nerve atrophy, and intellectual impairment. Occasionally a patient presents with a predominantly parkinsonian appearance, particularly late in life (14). MRI shows hypointense pallida on T2-weighted images (Fig. 13.9). Pallidal atrophy may occur in isolation or in any combination of degeneration of other nuclei, including subthalamic nucleus (pallidoluysian atrophy), substantia nigra, thalamus, and dentate nucleus. Cases are few and clinical manifestations are varied, so that there is no typical syndrome. However, elements of parkinsonism are often present and contribute to disability.

Other rare degenerative diseases that occasionally lead to parkinsonism are listed in Table 13.9.

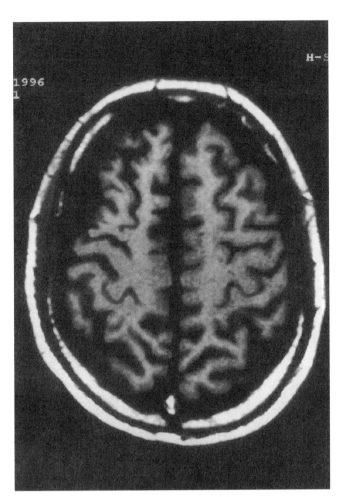

FIG. 13.8. Focal right medial frontal atrophy on T1-weighted magnetic resonance image in a man with predominantly left-sided manifestations of corticobasal ganglionic degeneration.

of Down patients show tangles rather than Lewy bodies in substantia nigra neurons. The development of parkinsonism in the setting of AD usually heralds a more rapid decline in independence. Another neurofibrillary tangle disease, the parkinsonism-dementia-amyotrophic lateral sclerosis disease complex, is endemic to three areas of the western Pacific: Guam in the Mariana Islands, where the disease is known as lytico-bodig; the Kii peninsula of Honshu Island in Japan; and western New Guinea (11b). Fortunately, the incidence of this entity has decreased dramatically, but a high incidence of atypical forms of parkinsonism has recently been noted in Caribbean (12) and Indian (13) populations.

Hallervorden-Spatz disease is a rare disorder of childhood causing dementia and a combination of pyramidal and extrapyramidal deficits. Because of Hallervorden's ethically checkered past, the disorder has been renamed neurodegeneration with brain iron accumulation type 1 (NBIA-1). Some of the patients with this syndrome have

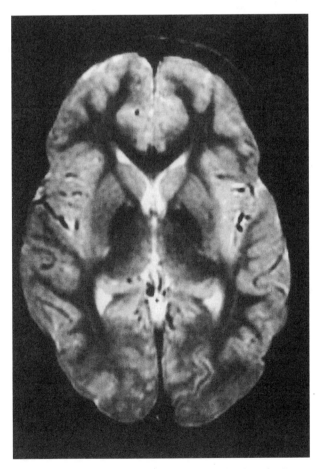

FIG. 13.9. T2-weighted magnetic resonance image of a 9-year-old girl with Hallervorden-Spatz disease showing bilateral hypointense signal in the globus pallidus.

TABLE 13.9. DEGENERATIVE DISEASES

Disorders frequently confused with PD
    Progressive supranuclear palsy
    Multiple system atrophy
    Corticobasal ganglionic degeneration
Other disorders
Alexander's disease
Alzheimer's disease (39)
Amyotrophic lateral sclerosis (40)
Caribbean atypical parkinsonism[a] (12)
Down's syndrome
Hallervorden-Spatz disease (14,14A)
Indian atypical parkinsonism[a] (13)
Neuroacanthocytosis (41)
Neurofibrillary tangle parkinsonism (?encephalitis lethargica)
Neuronal intranuclear inclusion disease (42)
Pallidal degenerations
Pallidopyramidal disease
Guam parkinsonism-dementia-amyotrophic lateral sclerosis complex
Pick's disease (43)
Substantia nigra degeneration without inclusions
Thalamo-olivary degeneration

[a]Presumed degenerative diseases. Pathology not yet defined.

PERSPECTIVE AND CONCLUSION

Despite the seemingly overwhelming number of possible causes of parkinsonism, most patients do not present much of a diagnostic puzzle. For a variety of obvious reasons, most forms of parkinsonism listed herein are not often mistaken for PD. In practice, once antidopaminergic medication has been excluded as the culprit, the majority of patients turn out to have PD. Autopsy studies indicate that the conditions that pose the greatest diagnostic challenge are MSA, PSP, AD, and multi-infarct parkinsonism, at least in part because of the lack of definitive clinical laboratory tests.

If patients have asymmetric parkinsonism with a resting tremor and are responding well to medication, no further investigations are necessary. It is the atypical features that dictate how extensive a laboratory evaluation is warranted. The most informative investigation is usually MRI, which is most useful in the case of a patient with a disproportionate gait disturbance, perhaps indicating multi-infarct parkinsonism or hydrocephalus. The most important task upon first encountering a young person with features of parkinsonism is to look for the copper metabolism disturbances associated with Wilson's disease.

In an ideal world we should be able to identify the cause of parkinsonism in all patients within a short period. However, the obstacles to full diagnostic accuracy are formidable. Patients often show too few clinical features to indicate the proper diagnosis, or combinations of features that suggest two different disorders at once. This situation is aggravated by occasional autopsy results that are inconclusive or show combinations of degenerative diseases. Further advances in genetics may improve diagnostic reliability by leading to the development of diagnostic tests.

A daunting challenge facing neurologists as we approach the 200th anniversary of the publication of James Parkinson's Essay on the Shaking Palsy is to achieve greater diagnostic accuracy as the scope of the differential diagnosis of parkinsonism widens. It is hoped that future advances in diagnostic capabilities will outstrip the growth of disorders under consideration.

REFERENCES

1. Riley DE. Secondary parkinsonism. In: Jankovic J, Tolosa E, eds. *Parkinson's disease and movement disorders,* 3rd ed. Baltimore: Williams & Wilkins, 1998:317–339.
2. Dickman MS. von Economo encephalitis. *Arch Neurol* 2001; 58:1696–1698.
2a. Panegyres PK, Toufexis K, Kakulas BA, et al. A new *PRNP* mutation (G131V) associated with Gerstmann-Sträussler-Scheinker disease. *Arch Neurol* 2001;58:1899–1902.
2b. Prusiner SB. Shattuck lecture—Neurodegenerative disease and prions. *N Engl J Med* 2001;344:1516–1551.
3. Cosentino C, Torres L, Scorticati MC, et al. Movement disorders secondary to adulterated medication. *Neurology* 2000;55:598–599.
4. Bostantjopoulou S, Katsarou Z, Papadimitriou A, et al. Clinical features of parkinsonian patients with the alpha-synuclein (G209A) mutation. *Mov Disord* 2001;16:1007–1013.
5. Gasser T, Muller-Myhsok B, Wszolek ZK, et al. A susceptibility locus for Parkinson's disease maps to chromosome 2p13. *Nat Genet* 1998;18:262–265.
6. Farrer M, Gwinn-Hardy K, Muenter M, et al. A chromosome 4p haplotype segregating with Parkinson's disease and postural tremor. *Hum Mol Genet* 1999;8:81–85.
7. Terreni L, Calabrese E, Calella AM, et al. New mutation (R42P) of the *parkin* gene in the ubiquitin-like domain associated with parkinsonism. *Neurology* 2001;56:463–466.
8. Bentivoglio AR, Cortelli P, Valente EM, et al. Phenotypic characterisation of autosomal recessive *PARK6*-linked parkinsonism in three unrelated Italian families. *Mov Disord* 2001;16: 999–1006.
9. van Duijn CM, Dekker MC, Bonifati V, et al. *Park7,* a novel locus for autosomal recessive early-onset parkinsonism, on chromosome 1p36. *Am J Hum Genet* 2001;69:629–634.
9a. Shan DE, Soong B-W, Sun C-M, et al. Spinocerebellar ataxia type 2 presenting as familial levodopa-responsive parkinsonism. *Ann Neurol* 2001;50:812–815.
9b. Manyam BV, Walters AS, Narla KR. Bilateral striopallidal calcinosis: clinical characteristics of patients seen in a registry. *Mov Disord* 2001;16:258–264.
10. Pharr V, Uttl B, Stark M, et al. Comparison of apraxia in corticobasal degeneration and progressive supranuclear palsy. *Neurology* 2001;56:957–963.
11. Galvin JE, Lee VM, Trojanowski JQ. Synucleinopathies: clinical and pathological implications. *Arch Neurol* 2001;58:186–190.
11a. Houlden H, Baker M, Morris HR, et al. Corticobasal degeneration and progressive supranuclear palsy share a common tau haplotype. *Neurology* 2001;56:1702–1705.
11b. Kuzuhara S, Kokubo Y, Sasaki R, et al. Familial amyotrophy lateral sclerosis and parkinsonism-dementia complex of the Kii peninsula of Japan: clinical and neuropathological study and tau analysis. *Ann Neurol* 2001;49:501–511.
12. Caparros-Lefebvre D, Elbaz A. Possible relation of atypical

parkinsonism in the French West Indies with consumption of tropical plants: a case-control study. Caribbean Parkinsonism Study Group. *Lancet* 1999;354:281–286.

13. Chaudhuri KR, Hu MT, Brooks DJ. Atypical parkinsonism in Afro-Caribbean and Indian origin immigrants to the UK. *Mov Disord* 2000;15:18–23.

14. Racette BA, Perry A, D'Avossa G, et al. Late-onset neurodegeneration with brain iron accumulation type 1: expanding the clinical spectrum. *Mov Disord* 2001;16:1148–1152.

14a. Zhou B, Westaway SK, Levinson B, et al. A novel pantothenate kinase gene (PANK2) is defective in Hallervorden-Spatz syndrome. *Nat Genet* 2001;28:345–349.

15. Tanaka M, Endo K, Suzuki T, et al. Parkinsonism in HIV encephalopathy. *Mov Disord* 2000;15:1032–1033.

16. Green C, Riley DE. Treatment of dystonia in striatal necrosis due to *Mycoplasma pneumoniae*. *Pediatr Neurol* 2002;26:318–320.

17. Hsiung GY, Clark AW. A 67-year-old woman with parkinsonism. *Can J Neurol Sci* 2001;28:150–154.

18. Kompoliti K, Goetz CG, Gajdusek DC, et al. Movement disorders in Kuru. *Mov Disord* 1999;14:800–804.

19. Sohn YH, Jeong Y, Kim HS, et al. The brain lesion responsible for parkinsonism after carbon monoxide poisoning. *Arch Neurol* 2000;57:1214–1218.

20. Barbosa ER, Leiros da Costa MD, Bacheschi LA, et al. Parkinsonism after glycine-derivate exposure. *Mov Disord* 2001;16:565–568.

21. Krack P, Dowsey PL, Benabid AL, et al. Ineffective subthalamic nucleus stimulation in levodopa-resistant postischemic parkinsonism. *Neurology* 2000;54:2182–2184.

22. Robertson NP, Wharton S, Anderson J, et al. Adult polyglucosan body disease associated with an extrapyramidal syndrome. *J Neurol Neurosurg Psychiatry* 1998;65:788–790.

23. Lucking CB, Durr A, Bonifati V, et al. Association between early-onset Parkinson's disease and mutations in the *parkin* gene. French Parkinson's Disease Genetics Study Group. *N Engl J Med* 2000;342:1560–1567.

24. Ohno T, Kobayashi S, Hayashi M, et al. Diphenylpyraline-responsive parkinsonism in cerebrotendinous xanthomatosis: long-term follow up of three patients. *J Neurol Sci* 2001;182:95–97.

25. Aberg LE, Rinne JO, Rajantie I, et al. A favorable response to antiparkinsonian treatment in juvenile neuronal ceroid lipofuscinosis. *Neurology* 2001;56:1236–1239.

26. Hauser RA, Friedlander J, Baker MJ, et al. Adult Chediak-Higashi parkinsonian syndrome with dystonia. *Mov Disord* 2000;15:705–708.

27. Hagerman RJ, Leehey M, Heinrichs W, et al. Intention tremor, parkinsonism, and generalized brain atrophy in male carriers of fragile X. *Neurology* 2001;57:127–130.

28. Yasuda M, Yokoyama K, Nakayasu T, et al. A Japanese patient with frontotemporal dementia and parkinsonism by a tau P301S mutation. *Neurology* 2000;55:1224–1227.

29. Reuter I, Hu MT, Andrews TC, et al. Late onset levodopa responsive Huntington's disease with minimal chorea masquerading as Parkinson plus syndrome. *J Neurol Neurosurg Psychiatry* 2000;68:238–241.

30. Casali C, Bonifati V, Santorelli FM, et al. Mitochondrial myopathy, parkinsonism, and multiple mtDNA deletions in a Sephardic Jewish family. *Neurology* 2001;56:802–805.

31. Pittock SJ, Joyce C, O'Keane V, et al. Rapid-onset dystonia-parkinsonism: a clinical and genetic analysis of a new kindred. *Neurology* 2000;55:991–995.

32. O'Hearn E, Holmes SE, Calvert PC, et al. SCA-12: tremor with cerebellar and cortical atrophy is associated with a CAG repeat expansion. *Neurology* 2001;56:299–303.

33. de Rijk-Van Andel JF, Gabreels FJ, et al. L-Dopa-responsive infantile hypokinetic rigid parkinsonism due to tyrosine hydroxylase deficiency. *Neurology* 2000;55:1926–1928.

34. Stolze H, Kuhtz-Buschbeck JP, Drucke H, et al. Comparative analysis of the gait disorder of normal pressure hydrocephalus and Parkinson's disease. *J Neurol Neurosurg Psychiatry* 2001;70:289–297.

35. Pohle T, Krauss JK. Parkinsonism in children resulting from mesencephalic tumors. *Mov Disord* 1999;14:842–846.

36. Haussermann P, Wilhelm T, Keinath S, et al. Primary central nervous system lymphoma in the SMA presenting as rapidly progressive parkinsonism. *Mov Disord* 2001;16:962–965.

37. Jenkins M, Hussain N, Lee D, et al. Reversible parkinsonism and MRI diffusion abnormalities in cortical venous thrombosis. *Neurology* 2001;57:364–366.

38. Wenning GK, Luginger E, Sailer U, et al. Postoperative parkinsonian tremor in a patient with a frontal meningioma. *Mov Disord* 1999;14:366–368.

39. Kurlan R, Richard IH, Papka M, et al. Movement disorders in Alzheimer's disease: more rigidity of definitions is needed. *Mov Disord* 2000;15:24–29.

40. Desai J, Swash M. Extrapyramidal involvement in amyotrophic lateral sclerosis: backward falls and retropulsion. *J Neurol Neurosurg Psychiatry* 1999;67:214–216.

41. Bostantjopoulou S, Katsarou Z, Kazis A, et al. Neuroacanthocytosis presenting as parkinsonism. *Mov Disord* 2000;15:1271–1273.

42. O'Sullivan JD, Hanagasi HA, Daniel SE, et al. Neuronal intranuclear inclusion disease and juvenile parkinsonism. *Mov Disord* 2000;15:990–995.

43. Hodges JR. Frontotemporal dementia (Pick's disease): clinical features and assessment. *Neurology* 2001;56[Suppl 4]:S6–S10.

HUNTINGTON'S DISEASE

KEVIN M. BIGLAN
IRA SHOULSON

Choreiform disorders have been described since the Middle Ages, and Thomas Sydenham's excellent description of chorea was published in 1686. However, it was not until the 19th century that one finds descriptions of a hereditary chorea (1). It was George Huntington's concise and eloquent description of this hereditary chorea that drew international attention and the eponymic designation. The text of his seminal lecture, "On Chorea," was published in the *Medical and Surgical Reporter* on April 13, 1872, a portion of which is cited here:

> *The hereditary chorea, as I shall call it, is confined to certain and fortunately few families and has been transmitted to them, an heirloom from generations way back in dim past... It is attended generally by all the symptoms of common chorea, only in an aggravated degree, hardly ever manifesting itself until adult or middle life, and then coming on gradually but surely, increasing by degrees and often occupying years in its development, until the hapless sufferer is but a quivering wreck of his former self... There are three marked peculiarities in this disease: 1. its hereditary nature; 2. a tendency to insanity and suicide; 3. its manifesting itself as a grave disease only in adult life* (2).

This description was based on his father's and grandfather's experience as physicians in Long Island as well as his own personal experience, and in retrospect the precision of this account is remarkable. By the turn of the 21st century it was recognized that Huntington's disease (HD) was an autosomal dominant disorder caused by an expansion of an unstable trinucleotide repeat near the telomere of chromosome 4 (3). Each offspring of an affected family member has a 50% chance of having inherited the fully penetrant mutation. Huntington also remarked on the onset of the condition in adulthood, with the average age of onset between 35 to 40 years (4)—a fact that makes HD particularly sinister because healthy individuals carrying the *HD* gene may have already passed the mutation on to their children. Huntington also commented on the psychiatric manifestations and the risk of suicide but failed to mention cognitive decline, which is now recognized as a cardinal feature of the disease.

HD represents one of the most important genetic disorders of adulthood. It was the first disease known to result from a trinucleotide expansion and detectable by presymptomatic predictive DNA testing.

EPIDEMIOLOGY

It is believed that the mutation for HD arose independently in multiple locations and does not represent a founder effect whereby all individuals with a particular disease can be traced back to a single individual or founder (5,6). However, isolated pockets of relatively increased density likely represent such an effect. The most notable of these is the population around Lake Maracaibo in Venezuela. All affected individuals can be traced back to a single woman living more than 200 years ago who has produced ten generations numbering over 13,000 individuals (6,7). This population has the highest prevalence rates worldwide, with approximately 2% of the population affected (8). This population has been incredibly important in our understanding of the clinical characteristics, natural history, and identification of the *HD* gene location and molecular mutation (7,9,10). New mutations are extraordinarily rare, accounting for a very small proportion of cases (5). It has been suggested that these "new" mutations represent expansion of the unstable trinucleotide repeat from the high-normal range in the parent to the pathologic range in the offspring (3).

HD is the most common inherited form of chorea, with a worldwide distribution that may reflect multiple introductions of the gene from European migrations (8). HD is found throughout North America, South America, and Australia in Caucasian populations. It has the highest prevalence rates in the region of Lake Maracaibo in Venezuela and the Moray Firth region of Scotland, and is relatively rare in Asian countries and among African blacks (5,11).

Throughout Europe, with the notable exception of Finland and possibly Spain, prevalence rates are relatively uniform, ranging from 2 to 8 per 100,000 (5). Finland is believed to be genetically distinct from the rest of the European population and has the lowest prevalence rates in

Europe at 0.5 per 100,000 (5). Regions of the world largely populated by individuals of European descent show a prevalence similar to that in Europe (5,12,13).

Little is known of the prevalence of HD in Africa. Hayden has carried out the only systematic survey of African populations in South Africa (11). Prevalences similar to those of European populations were found in white and mixed populations. Prevalence in populations of African origin was around ten times less than that in European populations. In American blacks of African origin, true prevalence rates are difficult to obtain; however, Folstein et al. (13) found a rate comparable to that in European studies. European origin of these cases in African-Americans could not be identified but could not be clearly excluded. It is probable that HD occurs at relatively low rates in persons of African origin.

HD has been documented in Asia, with only Japan having systematic data. Detailed studies in Japan reveal frequencies between 0.11 and 0.45 per 100,000 (5). Case reports from China, India, Turkey, and previous Soviet republics in central Asia suggest that the disease occurs in these locations; however, exact prevalence rates are not clear (5).

CLINICAL CHARACTERISTICS

HD is a progressively disabling and lethal neurodegenerative disorder characterized by the triad of a movement disorder, dementia, and behavioral disturbances. There is large variability in the clinical presentation and major clinical manifestations of the disease. Some of this variability is predictable. For example, young age at onset is associated with an akinetic-rigid phenotype, in contrast with the more typical hyperkinetic manifestations. A variety of disorders exist that may mimic HD and must be distinguished from it in order to accurately counsel patients and family members about prognosis and genetic risk.

Diagnosis

The diagnosis of HD was traditionally based solely on the adult onset of the characteristic clinical illness in the setting of a confirmatory family history (14). In 1993, the Huntington's Disease Collaborative Research Group identified the genetic mutation responsible for HD, making precise and accurate genetic diagnosis possible (3). Despite the advent of genetic testing, DNA testing for the *HD* gene is usually reserved for individuals whose family history is not clearly apparent, individuals whose clinical features are atypical, or, most commonly, healthy adults at risk for HD.

A variety of volumetric and functional neuroimaging techniques have been investigated to allow for the earlier and more accurate diagnosis of HD (15–19). Magnetic resonance imaging (MRI) and computed tomography (CT) may be useful in distinguishing secondary causes of an HD phenotype and to quantify the extent of caudate atrophy. Volumetric MRI may be more sensitive to detect early volume loss, particularly in the striatum and may correlate with motor symptoms (15,17,20). Functional imaging studies have discovered striatal abnormalities in early and presymptomatic carriers of the *HD* gene (16,18,19). These studies have revealed hypometabolism and reduced dopamine receptor binding in the striatum. Though rarely used clinically, volumetric MRI and positron emission tomography (PET) measurements may prove useful as biomarkers in future therapeutic trials in HD.

While the diagnostic approach appears relatively straightforward, the diagnosis of HD is typically only confirmed months to years after initial symptoms have appeared and individual functioning is impaired (21). The onset of disease is insidious and manifestations may be motor, behavioral, or cognitive (7,22–24), making early diagnosis challenging.

Motor Manifestations

Chorea is the prototypical motor abnormality characteristic of HD, though a wide range of other motor abnormalities have been described (25–31). Some of these motor manifestations, such as impaired ocular motility and dysdiadokinesis, may even be earlier and more sensitive markers of disease than chorea (7,9,32,33).

Chorea represents quick, arrhythmic, semipurposeful involuntary movements and is the most conspicuous feature of HD, occurring in 90% of affected patients. Although movements may be stereotyped in a single patient, they are highly variable from individual to individual and within an individual over time. The chorea begins subtly with slight movements of the fingers and toes. McCusker et al. (22) found that minimal chorea observed in the feet and toes of at-risk individuals predicted gene positivity in 86% of these subjects (positive predictive value). The chorea usually progresses with more overt movements, including facial grimacing, eyelid elevation, head bobbing, and writhing and jerking of the limbs. Parakinesia or the conversion of an involuntary movement to a seemingly voluntary one is frequently seen and may be manifested by crossing and uncrossing of the legs, smoothing of the hair, or rubbing of the chin or brow. Motor impersistence is an associated feature whereby individuals are unable to maintain tongue protrusion or eye closure.

Oculomotor abnormalities are common, with early findings in HD manifested by increased latency of response, insuppressible eye blinks or head movements associated with saccade initiation, and slowing of saccade velocity (7,9,25,32–35). Impairment is more noticeable with vertical than horizontal saccades.

The slower and more sustained postures of dystonia are also observed, especially as HD advances, and may be associated with the use of antidopaminergic therapy (7,29,36). Other movement disorders have also been reported in HD including bradykinesia, rigidity, myoclonus, tics, bruxism, and ataxia (26,27,31,37–39). Bradykinesia and rigidity, like dystonia, appear to be more common as HD progresses. Hypertonicity, representing both pyramidal (spasticity) and extrapyramidal (rigidity) tone abnormalities, may be seen, even in the same patient. Other signs of pyramidal tract dysfunction are also seen, including hyperreflexia and extensor plantar responses (39). Abnormalities in fine-motor coordination may occur early (7,9,40).

Dysarthria can occur at any stage of the illness and may become so severe as to leave individuals nearly anarthric. Despite severe dysarthria, cortical language disturbances are rare. Dysphagia tends to be most prominent in the terminal stages of the disease, and aspiration is a common cause of death (28). In fact, early reports suggest that aspiration secondary to dysphagia was the cause of death in 85% of HD patients (41).

Gait and station become impaired in HD. Superimposed chorea may give the gait a dance-like or lurching appearance. Patients will appear to be thrown off balance by sudden involuntary movements and move in a zig-zag pattern. Station is typically broad based and postural reflexes are eventually lost. Abnormalities of gait combined with dysarthria may contribute to the erroneous belief that individuals with HD are intoxicated.

Cognitive Dysfunction

Cognitive impairment occurs to a greater or lesser degree in all HD patients. As defined by global intellectual performance two standard deviations below the mean for healthy controls, dementia was seen in up to 66% of patients in one study (42), but is generally believed to be a feature of advancing illness (43). A variety of cognitive domains are involved, including memory, executive function, visuospatial abilities, cognitive speed, sensorimotor function, concentration, and the acquisition and encoding of sensory stimuli (42,44–47), but higher cortical language and gnostic operations are usually spared. Cognitive inflexibility may also be seen, whereby individuals with HD will perseverate ferociously on specific issues. This inflexibility may be extremely distressing to caregivers. It has been postulated that these deficits are the result of impairment in frontostriatal functional loops (45,48,49).

There has been considerable interest in whether cognitive difficulties antedate other manifestations of HD. Many studies evaluating cognitive measures in asymptomatic individuals who have inherited the gene have shown early cognitive impairment, frequently antedating motor symptoms (22,23,50–56). Other studies have failed to show early cognitive impairment in asymptomatic individuals (57–61).

There remains lingering uncertainty as to whether cognitive or motor manifestations represent the earliest detectable features of HD; however, motor changes appear to be more specific than cognitive changes (7,22,34).

It is clear that cognitive impairment is inevitable in HD, with the possible exception of a few individuals who have a very late onset of illness (62). Cognitive impairment typically progresses from selective deficits in psychomotor, executive, and visuospatial abilities to more global deficits, such as apraxia (43,45,47,63,64).

Behavioral Disturbances

Psychiatric difficulties have been recognized as an important aspect of HD since George Huntington's original description. Although Huntington focused on the "tendency to insanity and suicide," a wide range of psychiatric and behavioral disturbances is currently recognized in HD (65). Mood disorders, psychosis, anxiety, obsessions, compulsions, aggression, irritability, and apathy may be prominent features in the clinical manifestations of HD.

Affective disorders are an important and potentially treatable manifestation of HD. Depression is common in HD occurring in as many as half of HD patients (13,65), with manic features in 5% to 10% of HD patients (13,66). The suicide rate is fivefold that of the general population and may account for 2% of HD mortality (67). Affective disorders in HD are believed to be primarily related to the disruption of specific frontal-subcortical neural pathways regulating mood (68). Anxiety disorders seem to be important clinically, though few epidemiologic data exist on these conditions. Generalized anxiety, panic attacks, and obsessive-compulsive symptoms are seen (69).

Psychosis is also more common in HD than in the general population, occurring in up to 15% of HD patients (65,66). In addition, psychosis may be seen more commonly in earlier-onset cases (13). Paranoia is an important and underreported manifestation of psychosis in this population. Paranoid delusions may appear, but frank auditory or visual hallucinations are rare (69). The acute onset or presence of hallucinations should alert the clinician to look for other causes of the psychiatric disturbance.

Aggression in HD varies in severity from overreaction to relatively trivial issues to overt acts of violence. Aggression may represent a feature of other underlying psychopathology, such as paranoia, depression, or anxiety. Using an aggression scale, Burns et al. (70) found that nearly two thirds of HD patients had elevated levels of aggression. Closely linked to aggression is irritability, which reflects an inability to control temper or a reduced threshold for the development of anger. Irritability appears to be common in HD and may not be recognized by patients themselves (70). If left untreated, irritability may lead to aggressive behaviors and psychiatric hospitalization (71).

Apathy is a common behavioral complaint expressed by caregivers of persons with HD, and is characterized by a loss of emotion resulting in an internal feeling of disinterest or a behavioral state of inaction (70). Apathy can occur independently of depression and may be more distressing to family and friends than to the patient (72).

There has also been controversy regarding whether psychiatric disturbances predate motor manifestations in HD. Some reports suggest that psychiatric disturbances are more common in at-risk individuals who are positive for the *HD* gene in comparison with at-risk *HD* gene–negative controls (22,73). Other reports do not show such a difference (52,55). Regardless, the behavioral manifestations of HD are more variable and less specific than the motor and cognitive manifestations of illness.

Natural History

HD is a relentlessly progressive and lethal disorder. Illness may emerge at any time of life, with the highest occurrence between 35 to 40 years of age (4). Longitudinal observation of the Venezuela cohort revealed a slightly younger mean age of onset of 33 years in this population compared with a North American population (7). However, age of onset has been notoriously imprecise in this gradually developing and progressive condition. There is likely a period of time when symptoms develop until flagrant abnormalities make the diagnosis unavoidable. The average age of death in the United States is approximately 59 years (74) compared with 50 years in the Venezuelan cohort (7), perhaps reflecting differences in access to medical care. Very early age of onset seems to portend a short duration of illness, especially in juvenile-onset patients (75,76). However, others have failed to confirm the association between age of onset and disease duration (43).

The rating of total functional capacity (TFC) is a standardized measure of functional disability used extensively in HD (77). This scale ranges from a score of 13 (normal) to 0 (completely incapacitated) and assesses a patient's capacity in five relevant domains. Details of the scale can be seen in Table 14.1 (77). Numerous longitudinal studies have shown an annual decline in TFC of approximately 0.8 to 1.0 unit per year (9,36,78). This consistency across populations has made this an important tool for the evaluation of potential therapeutic interventions.

The Huntington Study Group (HSG) is an international collaboration of academic medical centers dedicated to advancing the knowledge and treatment of HD. The HSG has developed a rating scale, the Unified Huntington's Disease Rating Scale (UHDRS), to measure disease severity across four domains: motor, cognition, behavior, and functional capacity. The UHDRS has been shown to have a high degree of internal consistency and interrater reliability (79). Across time, individuals show a worsening of their motor function with increasing dystonia and stable chorea scores,

TABLE 14.1. TOTAL FUNCTIONAL CAPACITY SCALE

Occupation
0 = Unable
1 = Marginal work only
2 = Reduced capacity for usual job
3 = Normal
Finances
0 = Unable
1 = Major assistance
2 = Slight assistance
3 = Normal
Domestic Chores
0 = Unable
1 = Impaired
2 = Normal
Activities of Daily Living
0 = Total care
1 = Gross tasks only
2 = Minimal impairment
3 = Normal
Care Level
0 = Full-time skilled nursing
1 = Home or chronic care
2 = Home

worsening cognitive performance, an increased frequency of behavioral disorders, and a worsening functional status (80). The UHDRS is a useful outcome measure used extensively to evaluate the impact of experimental therapeutics on disease progression and illness severity. Details of the UHDRS, along with an accompanying instructional videotape, have been published (79).

Juvenile-onset Huntington's Disease

Juvenile-onset HD has generated interest because of its relative rareness and unique clinical phenotype. The juvenile variant of HD, where age of onset is under 20 years, is typically manifested by an akinetic-rigid phenotype in contrast with the classical hyperkinetic phenotype (76,81). In general, the earlier the age of juvenile onset the greater the likelihood of exhibiting an akinetic-rigid phenotype with prominent dystonia and occasionally even tremor (9). Seizures may occur in half of juvenile cases, and pyramidal tract dysfunction is also more prominent (81). Inheritance of the *HD* gene from an affected father is more common in juvenile-onset illness, perhaps owing to increased CAG repeat length as a consequence of spermatogenesis (6,9,75,76,81–83).

Differential Diagnosis

A variety of acquired and hereditary disorders of the central nervous system may mimic HD and may be considered in the differential diagnosis of adult-onset choreiform disorders. Differentiation from HD is important because of the major implications for treatment and genetic counseling.

Table 14.2 lists those conditions that may be difficult to distinguish clinically from HD (37,84–88).

Benign familial chorea, like HD, is inherited in an autosomal dominant fashion but is otherwise clinically distinct from HD (89). It can be distinguished clinically by the absence of dementia, behavioral disturbances, and progression. Pathologically, there is no caudate atrophy. In addition, onset usually occurs in childhood with stabilization in the second decade. Chorea tends to be abrupt, of small amplitude, and affecting the distal extremities.

Neuroacanthocytosis is a genetically heterogeneous disorder and may be clinically indistinguishable from HD (90). The presence of a sensorimotor neuropathy may be a useful clue to this diagnosis. The presence of acanthocytes on the peripheral blood smear helps to confirm the diagnosis.

Dentatorubropallidoluysian atrophy (DRPLA) is an autosomal dominant disorder with profound clinical heterogeneity (91). In Japanese populations, DRPLA is more common than HD (5). It can be clinically indistinguishable from HD, and confirmatory DNA testing may be necessary to distinguish these disorders.

The spinocerebellar ataxias (SCAs), including Machado-Joseph disease, are distinguished from HD by the prominent cerebellar dysfunction in these conditions (86). Neuroimaging may reveal cerebellar atrophy. Genetic testing is available for many of these conditions.

Creutzfeldt-Jakob disease (CJD) includes prominent myoclonus and a much more rapid course than HD. Characteristic periodic sharp and slow-wave complexes on electroencephalography may be seen (92). The 14-3-3 protein, a normal cellular constituent, is released into the cerebrospinal fluid (CSF) as a result of extensive destruction of brain tissue (93). The presence of this protein in the CSF is a sensitive and specific marker for CJD (94).

Wilson's disease rarely exhibits chorea, with dysarthria, dystonia, and tremor being more prominent features (95). Yellow–brown deposits of copper in Descemet's membrane in the cornea (Kayser-Fleischer ring) are invariably present in the setting of neurologic manifestations of Wilson's disease (96).

Sporadic disorders presenting with an HD phenotype are infrequently confused with HD. However, senile chorea deserves special mention. This disorder of isolated generalized chorea in the elderly is a controversial disorder. The etiology of this condition is unclear. However, Warren et al. (97) found that as many as half of individuals with supposed "senile chorea" actually carry the genetic mutation responsible for HD whereas an additional 25% of this cohort had other causes of chorea, such as antiphospholipid antibody syndrome. A thorough evaluation for secondary causes of chorea, particularly polycythemia and the antiphospholipid antibody syndrome (97,98), must be sought and genetic testing considered.

GENETICS

Gene Discovery

The Venezuela HD cohort, the largest known affected kinship in the world, was an ideal population in which to examine the genetic locus responsible for HD. Nancy S. Wexler and Thomas Chase surveyed the region in 1979. In 1981, a collaborative study between the U.S. National Institutes of Health and the University of Zulia in Venezuela began systematic clinical examinations and the collection of DNA blood samples from members of the affected kindred. Within 2 years of initiating this landmark field study, Gusella and his collaborators in Venezuela and North America discovered a DNA probe on the short arm of chromosome 4 that closely localized to the *HD* gene (10).

With this information in hand, a further collaborative effort was undertaken to identify and define the *HD* gene mutation. While analyzing an interesting transcript *(IT15)* on chromosome 4, the Huntington's Disease Collaborative Research Group identified an expansion of a CAG trinucleotide repeat unique to transmission of HD (3). In 98% of normal chromosomes, the CAG repeat length in both alleles ranged between 11 and 24, whereas 100% of affected individuals carried a CAG length on one allele greater than 42 repeats. This expanded repeat was also somewhat unstable, contracting or expanding in subsequent offspring. Of great importance was that in all HD families tested across ethnic and racial groups, the same CAG expansion was found, confirming a single mutation for all cases of HD. This contrasts with some predictions that multiple mutations might account for the clinical heterogeneity of HD. Figure 14.1 demonstrates the clear distinction between repeat lengths in normal controls and in 150 different HD families as initially reported by Duyao et al. (6).

TABLE 14.2. DIFFERENTIAL DIAGNOSIS OF HUNTINGTON'S DISEASE

Inherited Disorders	Sporadic Disorders
Benign familial chorea	Sydenham's chorea
Neuroacanthocytosis	Senile chorea
Dentatorubropallidoluysian atrophy	Corticobasal ganglionic degeneration
Machado-Joseph disease	Progressive supranuclear palsy
Spinocerebellar ataxias 1, 2, 6, 7	Multiple system atrophy
Hereditary Creutzfeldt-Jakob disease	Sporadic Creutzfeldt-Jakob disease
Wilson's disease	Vascular chorea
Mitochondrial disorders	Polycythemia vera
Porphyria	Systemic lupus erythematosus
	Antiphospholipid antibody syndrome
	Tardive dyskinesia

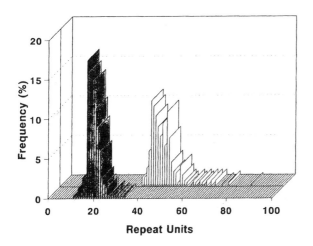

FIG. 14.1. Comparison of CAG repeat length from normal controls (*n* = 545, dark bars) and HD chromosomes (*n* = 425, open bars). (From Duyao M, Ambrose C, Myers R, et al. Trinucleotide repeat length instability and age of onset in Huntington's disease. *Nat Genet* 1993;4:387–392.)

Molecular Analysis of the Gene and Its Transcript

The *HD* gene, *IT15*, consists of 67 exons covering a genomic region of approximately 210 kb on the short arm of chromosome 4 (99). The expanded CAG repeat is found on the 5′ region of the gene. The gene encodes for a unique protein of approximately 348 kd, named huntingtin. The function of huntingtin remains unknown; however, it is believed to be critical in embryogenesis. Wild-type huntingtin is widely expressed throughout the brain but, surprisingly, is not enriched in the basal ganglia (100). In unaffected individuals the protein is found primarily in the cytoplasm of neurons, with the highest levels in the cerebellum, hippocampus, cerebral cortex, substantia nigra pars compacta, and pontine nuclei (100,101). The mutant protein also localizes to neurons, but unlike the wild type, it is found in the nucleus as well as in the cytoplasm (101–103). The expanded CAG repeat codes for an expanded polyglutamine region within the mutant protein that plays an important, but still unknown, role in HD pathogenesis.

CAG Repeat Length and Clinical Features

The Huntington's Disease Collaborative Research Group reported a generally inverse relationship between the length of the repeat and age of onset, with juvenile cases having the longest repeats (3). This observation raised the tantalizing possibility that age of onset could be accurately predicted by measuring an individual's repeat length. There was hope that even phenotypic variability might be explained by examining an individual's genes.

Since that time a number of studies have evaluated these issues (6,82,104–113). Confirmation of the association between repeat length and age of onset quickly followed identification of the gene (6,82,105). However, individuals with very early- and late-onset HD account for a large proportion of this inverse relationship. Figure 14.2 illustrates this relationship graphically.

However, despite the strong correlations demonstrated, there remained wide variability in age of onset with a 95% confidence interval of ±18 years for any given CAG repeat length (6). Others have found an increasing probability of disease onset at a given age for increasing repeat lengths (104). Table 14.3 derived from Brinkman and co-workers' (104) retrospective evaluation of 728 affected and 321 asymptomatic individuals with an expanded repeat, demonstrates the age by which 50% of individuals will be affected for a given repeat size. Much of the predictive power of these models is influenced by juvenile-onset cases with CAG repeat lengths greater than 52 (6). Therefore, CAG repeat length cannot be relied on to accurately predict age of onset for a particular individual. It is likely that other genetic or environmental modifiers have a significant role in determining age of onset (114,115).

Age of onset becomes even more difficult to predict in individuals who have fewer than 42 CAG repeats (116). Although it is generally believed that individuals with more than 40 repeats will inevitably develop symptoms of HD, some individuals with repeats lengths of 40 or 41 may not exhibit symptoms in their lifetime. This suggests reduced penetrance among carriers of such lower repeat sizes. Approximately 1% to 2% of at-risk individuals screened for HD will have repeat lengths between 36 and 39. It is difficult to predict which of these individuals will develop symptoms of HD within a normal life span. Table 14.4

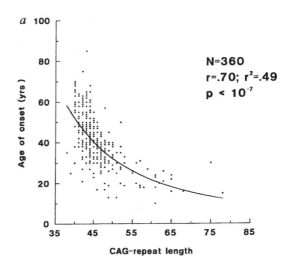

FIG. 14.2. Age of onset by length of CAG repeat. (From Andrew SE, Goldberg YP, Kremer B, et al. *Nat Genet* 1993;4:398–403.)

CAG Repeat Size	Median Age at Onset[a] (95% CI) (Yr)
39	66 (72–59)
40	59 (61–56)
41	54 (56–52)
42	49 (50–48)
43	44 (45–42)
44	42 (43–40)
45	37 (39–36)
46	36 (37–35)
47	33 (35–31)
48	32 (34–30)
49	28 (32–25)
50	27 (30–24)

[a]Age by which 50% of individuals will be affected.
From Brinkman RR, Mezei MM, Theilmann J, et al. The likelihood of being affected by Huntington disease by a particular age, for a specific CAG size. *Am J Hum Genet* 1997;60:1202–1210.

shows rough probability estimates for the development of HD for these rare intermediate repeats (116).

With the exception of juvenile-onset cases, there has been poor correlation between phenotype and CAG repeat length. Unusually long repeat lengths (i.e., >55) are characteristic of juvenile-onset patients (3). The median CAG repeat length of adult onset patients was 44, while juvenile onset patients had a median repeat length of 56.5 (82). The fact that early-onset cases are known to commonly exhibit the akinetic-rigid phenotype and may have a shorter duration of disease than midlife adult-onset cases suggests that very long repeat length may influence phenotype.

Studies evaluating the influence of CAG repeat length on the rate of illness progression have been mixed. Neuropathologic studies (109) and functional neuroimaging studies (106,111) have suggested a greater rate of clinical decline in individuals with longer repeat lengths. Some clinical studies have supported the inverse association between rate of decline and repeat length, with longer repeats progressing more rapidly (107,108). Still other studies have not revealed this correlation (110,112,113). Kieburtz et al. (113) systematically and prospectively evaluated 50 patients with manifest HD and found no relationship between the length of CAG repeats and the rate of clinical decline as measured by the TFC. Recently, the HSG confirmed that CAG repeat

TABLE 14.4. PROBABILITY OF DEVELOPING HUNTINGTON'S DISEASE FOR A GIVEN INTERMEDIATE REPEAT LENGTH

CAG Length	Probability of Disease (%)
36	25
37	50
38	75
39	90

length was not associated with functional decline in the context of a prospective therapeutic trial (117).

The association of repeat length with disease progression, functional decline, and phenotypic variability remains unclear. It is likely that other genetic, neurobiological, or environmental influences may modify phenotypic expression in HD.

CAG Repeat Length Instability

Instability of the CAG repeat length during meiosis is a genetic hallmark of HD and other trinucleotide repeat disorders (86). There exists wide variation in repeat lengths within single pedigrees, and the offspring of an affected individual usually have different repeat lengths (3,6). Duyao et al. (6) evaluated 51 parental transmissions and found alterations in repeat lengths in all 51 offspring. Increases occurred in 39 cases, whereas contractions occurred in 12.

CAG Repeat Length Variability and Parental Transmission

Of interest in Duyao and co-workers' (6) evaluation of intergenerational variability of repeat length was the propensity for paternal transmissions to result in significantly larger expansions compared with maternal transmissions, possibly owing to expansion during spermatogenesis. The largest expansions are known to occur exclusively with paternal transmission. One such expansion resulted in an increase from 42 repeats in a father to 121 in his offspring (82). This information was particularly enlightening given the relationship of age of onset to CAG repeat length and the knowledge that juvenile-onset cases were most commonly the result of paternal transmission of the *HD* gene (83).

Predictive Testing

With the discovery of the gene, it was presumed that nearly all individuals at risk for inheriting the gene would opt for presymptomatic DNA testing. However, since HD genetic testing has become available, only 3% of individuals who are at immediate risk (50:50) for HD have chosen to be tested, and only about 500 predictive DNA tests are performed in the United States annually (118). Similar low rates of testing have been observed in central Europe (119). Reasons for foregoing testing include an increased risk to offspring if the test was positive, lack of an effective treatment, potential loss of health and life insurance, costs of testing, and inability to "undo" the test results (120). Fears about testing are understandable. The relief from a negative result is offset by the grim reality of a positive one. The impact of the results may affect entire families and reach far beyond the individual tested (121).

The impact of genetic testing for HD has not been extensively evaluated. Although Wiggins et al. (122) did not find a negative psychological impact of predictive testing, others

(123) have found negative psychosocial impacts in both those who received positive and those who received negative test results. Of particular interest are studies suggesting that a significant proportion of individuals who undergo predictive genetic testing may fear or experience genetic discrimination, especially if they are refused employment or insurance based merely on genetic risk (124–127).

Clearly the decision to undergo predictive testing in HD is an exceedingly personal and complex consideration for individuals, families, and caregivers. It is essential that individuals undergo skilled genetic and psychological counseling prior to and after the administration of the test (128,129). Finally, the decision to test must be evaluated in the context of the family because of the far-reaching implications of *HD* gene test results.

NEUROPATHOLOGY

Pathologic studies demonstrate progressive and severe atrophy of the caudate and putamen (130). Grossly, the HD brain shows profound atrophy of the head of the caudate and putamen, and, to a lesser extent, of the cortex (130,131). Figure 14.3 demonstrates the gross cau-

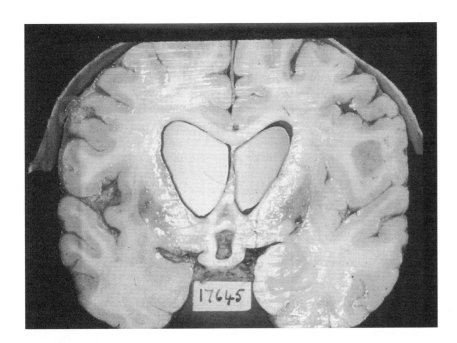

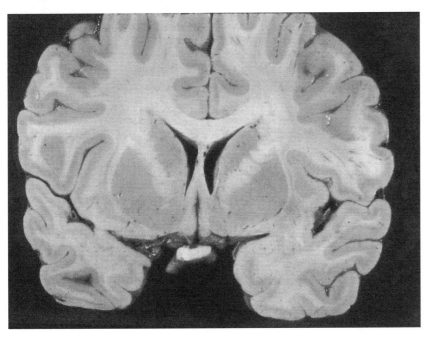

FIG. 14.3. HD brain *(top)* compared with a normal brain *(bottom)*, demonstrating caudate atrophy. (See color section.)

date atrophy of an HD brain compared with a normal brain.

Microscopically, the pathologic hallmark of the disease is the preferential loss of medium spiny neurons projecting from the striatum to the external pallidum (132). These striatal neurons contain γ-aminobutyric acid (GABA) and enkephalin as their primary neurotransmitters, which are selectively depleted, whereas neighboring neurons are unaffected (133–136).

Intraneuronal inclusions were first described by Roizin et al. (137) and have been further defined by others (138). These inclusions are seen most prominently in the nuclei and neuropil of striatal and cortical neurons and represent aggregates of the mutant huntingtin protein and ubiquitin (138,139). The presence of these inclusions seems to predate neurologic symptoms (140).

PATHOGENIC HYPOTHESES

The exact mechanisms that lead from an expansion of a CAG repeat in the *IT15* gene to selective neuronal loss and the heterogeneous clinical picture of HD are poorly understood. Hypotheses include glutamatergic excitotoxicity (141–143), mitochondrial bioenergetic dysfunction (144–146), caspase-mediated apoptosis (102,147), and transcriptional dysregulation (148–150). It is possible that all of these mechanisms participate in neuronal degeneration through a complex interaction whereby dysfunction in one area sets the stage for excitotoxic and bioenergetic vulnerabilities. For example, bioenergetic defects may predispose otherwise normal levels of glutamate to exert an excitotoxic effect (151).

Huntingtin, the mutant protein product of CAG expansion, may exert its pathogenic influence through "a gain of function" (152). The CAG expansion in the mutant *HD* gene results in translation of an expanded polyglutamine tract within the protein. In animal models, the mutant huntingtin protein appears to undergo abnormal cleavage in the cytoplasm, resulting in the translocation of the N-terminal fragment into the nucleus (153). These abnormally cleaved mutant proteins form aggregates in the nucleus, as demonstrated in in vitro and in vivo animal models (103,154). It has been debated whether these aggregates represent a byproduct of neurodegeneration or are an important component in the pathogenic process. Recent data support the latter scenario. Preventing the nuclear localization of mutant huntingtin also inhibits neurodegeneration, suggesting that the altered cleavage and subsequent nuclear translocation represent key steps in the pathogenic cascade leading to neuronal dysfunction and cell death (102). Additional support for this hypothesis comes from data demonstrating that the expression of the N-terminal fragment alone can reproduce the pathology and phenotype seen in HD (139,155,156).

The mechanism by which huntingtin aggregates induce neuronal injury is the subject of intense research. One hypothesis suggests that mutant huntingtin exerts its pathogenicity through abnormal interactions with nuclear and cytoplasmic proteins (157). Most intriguing of these abnormal interactions is the finding that the mutant huntingtin interacts with a variety of transcriptional regulatory proteins in human and animal brains (148,149). It is further postulated that huntingtin inhibits acetyltransferase activity and that the potency of this inhibition is related to polyglutamine length (i.e., CAG length) (158). The inhibition of acetyltransferases results in a reduction in histone acetylation that is reversible with histone deacetylase (HDAC) inhibitors in both in vitro and in vivo models (158). In addition, HDAC inhibitors have been shown to reverse neuronal degeneration in a *Drosophila* model of HD. Histone acetylation is an important regulator of gene transcription within the nucleus, supporting transcriptional dysregulation as an important mechanism in HD pathogenesis.

The ability of huntingtin to inhibit histone acetylation within the nucleus represents a persuasive mechanism for pathogenicity that could help unify the various pathogenic hypotheses. One can theorize that selective inhibition of histone acetylation could selectively inhibit gene expression, leading to defects in energy metabolism and increased vulnerability to oxidative and excitotoxic stress.

THERAPEUTIC STRATEGIES

There are no effective therapies to slow the progression or delay the onset of HD. Symptomatic treatments have largely focused on ameliorating the motor and psychological dysfunction of individuals affected with HD. However, scientific advances have renewed hope for the development of effective neuroprotective or preventive therapeutic strategies.

Symptomatic Treatments

Motor Impairment

The focus of therapy for motor abnormalities in HD has traditionally been on the control of chorea. However, chorea may not cause serious disability, and antichoreic therapy is beset with adverse effects. In fact, functional decline is associated with a natural reduction of chorea and emergence of dystonia (36). Dopaminergic blockade with typical antipsychotics, such as haloperidol, has been the mainstay of treatment for chorea. However, the impact of these medications on swallowing, speech, spontaneous movements, and gait may impair function out of proportion to any improvement in chorea (159). The atypical antipsychotic, clozapine, has been found to reduce chorea without the extrapyramidal side effects of the typical agents. Remacemide, an *N*-methyl-D-aspartate (NMDA) receptor antagonist, and riluzole, an inhibitor of corticostriatal glutamate release, have been shown to improve chorea, but amelioration of chorea with these antiglutamatergic agents did not result in functional improvement (117,160,161). Amantadine has also been noted to be effective in reducing chorea in a subpopulation of HD patients (162). The presynaptic monoamine–depleting agent, tetrabenazine, improves chorea; however, parkinsonism and depression are potential adverse effects (163, 164). In general, it is not recommended to treat chorea unless it is causing disabling functional or social impairment. There is limited evidence that levodopa or dopamine agonists improve the akinetic-rigid variants of HD (31, 37,165).

There are no controlled trials evaluating whether physical and occupational therapy helps motor impairment in HD or whether speech therapy improves the intelligibility of speech.

Cognitive Approaches

Pharmacologic trials to improve cognitive function in HD have been largely unsuccessful (166–169).

Behavioral Care

Antidepressants are useful in the management of depression in HD (65). The selective serotonin reuptake inhibitors (SSRIs) have become first-line agents in the treatment of depression in HD. Although there are no controlled trials of SSRIs in depressed patients with HD, these agents appeared to be well tolerated and effective. In addition, SSRIs may suppress chorea and reduce aggression in HD (170–172). Dosages should be started low and doubled every 2 to 4 weeks as necessary. The mixed serotonergic and noradrenergic reuptake inhibitor venlafaxine may also be useful; however, gastrointestinal side effects may limit its use. More traditional tricyclic antidepressants can also be effective in treating depression in HD (65,159,173). The major limitations with this class are the anticholinergic side effects. Amoxapine, a metabolite of the antipsychotic loxapine, is a novel tricyclic with some dopamine receptor blocking properties, suggesting that it may be useful in reducing chorea while improving mood (173). There are limited data suggesting that electroconvulsive therapy may be useful and safe in HD (174).

Chronic anxiety disorders may respond to SSRIs. Episodic or situational anxiety can be treated with a brief course of benzodiazepines. Obsessive-compulsive symptoms may respond to treatment with SSRIs or clomipramine (175).

Psychosis is disabling and may develop in 10% to 15% of HD patients. The mainstay of treatment is antipsychotic medication, with the newer atypical agents being preferable. The antipsychotic agents with the fewest neurologic side effects include clozapine, quetiapine, and olanzapine. More traditional neuroleptics are associated with an increased risk of tardive dyskinesia, the propensity to impair swallowing and gait, and heighten dystonia in HD (30,176,177). Clozapine can be very useful in managing psychosis and may also improve chorea (178). Its use is limited by the necessity for weekly blood monitoring and the rare risk of bone marrow suppression. As with antidepressants, antipsychotics should be initiated at low doses and titrated slowly.

In assessing aggression and irritability, secondary causes, such as paranoia, depression, and anxiety, should be sought and managed appropriately (69,179). Benzodiazepines may be used for the acute management of aggressive episodes. The anticonvulsant valproic acid may be useful in treating both aggression and irritability (180,181). Propranolol has been reported to reduce aggression in HD associated with frustration (182). The SSRIs may also be useful in management of aggression (171,172) and might be considered in the agitated depressed patient.

Apathy is a common manifestation of HD, but the treatment of apathy has not been systematically evaluated. The removal of medications, such as typical antipsychotics, that may contribute to apathy should be considered.

Surgical Approaches

Surgical approaches to the management of HD have focused on tissue transplantation strategies. This reflects results in animal models of HD, where transplanted striatal cells have been demonstrated to survive, differentiate, grow, and reverse motor and behavioral abnormalities (183–185).

Fetal neural allografts have been shown to be relatively safe in individuals with HD in preliminary, small, uncontrolled trials (186–188). Functional neuroimaging studies have shown increased metabolic activity in some patients treated with fetal tissue transplantations (189). Small improvements in motor, cognitive, and behavioral measures were seen in some patients (187–189). Caution must be used when interpreting these results, as the surgical experience is very preliminary. All studies to date have involved small numbers of patients without blinded assessments. Motor deteriorations and mood alterations also occurred in some patients (186,188). In addition, the use of fetal tissue for therapeutic uses remains controversial.

Fetal tissue transplantation for HD continues to be experimental and should only be considered within the context of a well-designed clinical trial. Large randomized controlled and potentially blinded studies are needed to further evaluate the safety and efficacy of these approaches. Guidelines for tissue transplantation in HD have been published and should be adhered to in the development of any protocol (190).

Neuroprotective Strategies and Experimental Therapeutics

Neuroprotection refers to interventions aimed at producing "enduring benefits by favorably influencing underlying etiology or pathogenesis and thereby forestalling onset of illness or clinical decline" (191). A number of neuroprotective trials have been undertaken in individuals with manifest HD, but with limited success (78,117,192–194). It may be that the failure of putative neuroprotective agents in HD is secondary to the late initiation of these therapies after irreversible pathogenic processes have developed. Ideally, neuroprotective therapy would be initiated prior to the onset of symptoms while neuronal changes are potentially reversible (140). No studies to date have evaluated potential neuroprotective agents in this presymptomatic population.

There is hope that experimental therapeutic strategies will influence both proximal and distal targets in the pathogenic cascade in order to prevent or slow the neurodegenerative process (195). Proximal targets include targeting the translation, abnormal folding, and aggregation of the mutant huntingtin protein. In addition, mutant huntingtin results in altered protein–protein interactions, caspase-mediated cleavage resulting in formation of toxic intermediates, transcriptional dysregulation, and neurotrophin depletion. These may all serve as potential proximal targets amenable to therapeutic intervention. Distal therapeutic targets represent those presumed final pathways common to neurodegenerative conditions, including excitotoxic and oxidative injury, inflammation, and apoptotic mechanisms. While less specific, distal targets may be important in slowing disease progression after a variety of molecular insults have already occurred.

The multicenter trial evaluating coenzyme Q10 and remacemide in HD illustrates attempts to target distal pathways in neurodegeneration (117). The HSG investigators working at 23 sites in the United States and Canada evaluated 347 subjects with early HD using a randomized, double-blind, placebo-controlled, parallel-group, 2×2 factorial design. Subjects were randomized to one of four treatment groups: coenzyme Q10 (an antioxidant and cofactor involved in mitochondrial electron transfer), remacemide (a noncompetitive NMDA receptor antagonist), a combination of both, or placebo. Subjects were followed for at least 30 months, with change in functional capacity as the primary outcome. Individuals treated with coenzyme Q10, 600 mg daily, showed about a 13% slowing in functional decline compared with individuals not receiving coenzyme Q10 ($p = 0.15$) and was not associated with adverse events. These results, while not statistically significant, are encouraging. Coenzyme Q10 was the first agent to show a potential neuroprotective benefit in HD. Higher dosages of coenzyme Q10 and perhaps a larger sample size may help address the value of these effects.

Other experimental compounds are currently in human clinical trials. Minocycline, a caspase inhibitor, is a second-generation tetracycline antibiotic that has a variety of anti-apoptotic, antioxidant, and anti-excitotoxic properties that may be of potential neuroprotective benefit in HD (196,197). Minocycline has been shown to be effective at delaying mortality in mouse models of HD (196). Studies are currently underway to investigate the safety, tolerability, and efficacy of minocycline in subjects with early HD. Creatine is a nutritional supplement that, like coenzyme Q10, may have neuroprotective effects in a variety of disease processes where altered bioenergetic metabolism is important in the pathogenic mechanism. Evidence from animal models suggests a neuroprotective effect of creatine (198,199). An exciting new therapeutic prospect is the potential role of HDAC inhibitors to influence transcriptional dysregulation in HD. HDAC inhibitors have been shown to be powerful tools in arresting and even reversing polyglutamine-dependent neurodegeneration in *Drosophila* (158). Importantly, HDAC inhibitors are already in use for the treatment of some types of cancer (200,201), but the risks, safety, and tolerability of these compounds in HD have not been evaluated.

OBSERVATIONAL STUDIES IN HUNTINGTON'S DISEASE: PHAROS AND PREDICT-HD

Two large prospective observational studies are currently underway to better define early and sensitive markers of disease onset in asymptomatic individuals at risk for HD. Information gleaned from these studies will form the basis for designing meaningful therapeutic or neuroprotective clinical trials in the future. The *P*rospective *H*untington *At Risk Observational Study* (PHAROS) was initiated in 1999 in an attempt to further characterize and measure the clinical onset of HD in a diverse cohort of individuals at immediate risk for HD. The aims of PHAROS include defining the earliest and most specific markers of disease onset in HD, determining the relationship of CAG repeat length and age of onset in a systematic prospective manner, and determining genetic and environmental modifiers of disease onset. Subjects and investigators remain blinded to participants *HD* gene status. Thus, individuals who do not want to know their gene status (about 95% of the at-risk population) will be examined to assess the personal beliefs, attitudes, and behaviors of individuals at direct risk for a genetic illness. In addition, PHAROS represents the first large prospective clinical research effort undertaken in an at-risk population. Neurobiological *Predict*ors of *HD* (PREDICT-HD) is a companion study of PHAROS that will prospectively assess asymptomatic individuals who have undergone presymptomatic HD DNA testing and who agree to undergo sophisticated cognitive and neuroimaging tests in an attempt to better understand the onset of illness in HD. It is believed that comprehensive neuropsychological assessment and neuroimaging data will help further define onset of illness in HD. Information gleaned from these studies will become increasingly important as more genetic illnesses are defined and presymptomatic preventive therapies become available.

FUTURE OF HUNTINGTON'S DISEASE

Novel therapeutic strategies are quickly being developed and entering clinical trials at rapidly accelerating pace. The results of the coenzyme Q10 study and the efficacy of experimental agents in animal models of HD contribute to therapeutic optimism. In the long term, understanding the complex mechanisms that occur in the pathogenic process of HD will lead to the development of more precise and effective therapeutic weapons to delay the onset or slow the progression of the disease. It is expected that successful protective and preventive strategies will be developed in the coming years. In the meantime, a rational, comprehensive, and systematic approach remains the cornerstone of therapeutics aimed at reducing the symptoms and improving the quality of life in patients and families affected by HD.

REFERENCES

1. Hayden MR. *Huntington's chorea.* New York: Springer, 1981.
2. Huntington G. On chorea. *Medical and Surgical Reporter* 1872; 26:317–321.
3. Huntington's Disease Collaborative Research Group. A novel gene containing a trinucleotide repeat that is expanded and unstable on Huntington's disease chromosomes. *Cell* 1993;72: 971–983.
4. Farrer LA, Conneally PM. A genetic model for age at onset in Huntington disease. *Am J Hum Genet* 1985;37:350–357.
5. Harper PS. The epidemiology of Huntington's disease. *Human Genetics* 1992;89:365–376.
6. Duyao M, Ambrose C, Myers R, et al. Trinucleotide repeat length instability and age of onset in Huntington's disease. *Nature Genetics* 1993;4:387–392.
7. Penney JB, Young AB, Shoulson I, et al. Huntington's disease in Venezuela: 7 years of follow up on symptomatic and asymptomatic individuals. *Mov Disord* 1990;5:93–99.
8. Giron LT Jr, Koller WC. A critical survey and update on the epidemiology of Huntington's disease. In: Gorelick PB, Alter M, eds. *Handbook of neuroepidemiology.* New York: Marcel Dekker, 1994:281–292.
9. Young AB, Shoulson I, Penney JB, et al. Huntington's disease in Venezuela: neurologic features and functional decline. *Neurology* 1986;36:244–249.
10. Gusella JF, Wexler NS, Conneally PM, et al. A polymorphic DNA marker genetically linked to Huntington's disease. *Nature* 1983;306:234–238.
11. Hayden MR, MacGregor JM, Beighton PH. The prevalence of Huntington's chorea in South Africa. *South African Medical Journal* 1980;58:193–196.
12. Kokmen E, Özekmekçi S, Beard M, et al. Incidence and prevalence of Huntington's disease in Olmsted County, Minnesota (1950 through 1989). *Arch Neurol* 1994;51:696–698.
13. Folstein SE, Chase GA, Wahl WE, et al. Huntington disease in Maryland: clinical aspects of racial variation. *Am J Hum Genet* 1987;41:168–179.
14. Folstein SE, Leigh RJ, Parhad IM, et al. The diagnosis of Huntington's disease. *Neurology* 1986;36:1279–1283.
15. Harris GJ, Codori AM, Lewis RF, et al. Reduced basal ganglia blood flow and volume in pre-symptomatic, gene-tested persons at-risk for Huntington's disease. *Brain* 1999;122: 1667–1678.
16. Young AB, Penney JB, Starosta-Rubenstein S, et al. PET scan investigations of Huntington's disease: cerebral metabolic correlates of neurological features and functional decline. *Ann Neurol* 1986;20:296–303.
17. Aylward E, Brandt J, Codori AM, et al. Reduced basal ganglia volume associated with the gene for Huntington's disease in asymptomatic at-risk person. *Neurology* 1994;44:823–828.
18. Grafton ST, Mazziotta JC, Pahl JJ, et al. A comparison of neurological, metabolic, structural, and genetic evaluations in persons at risk for Huntington's disease. *Ann Neurol* 1990;28: 614–621.
19. Andrews TC, Weeks RA, Turjanski N, et al. Huntington's disease progression PET and clinical observations. *Brain* 1999; 122:2353–2363.
20. Harris GJ, Pearlson GD, Peyser CE, et al. Putamen volume reduction on magnetic resonance imaging exceeds caudate changes in mild Huntington's disease. *Ann Neurol* 1992;31: 69–75.
21. Greenamyre JT, Shoulson I. Huntington's disease. In: Calne DB, ed. *Neurodegenerative diseases.* Philadelphia: WB Saunders, 1994:685–704.
22. McCusker E, Richards F, Sillence D, et al. Huntington's disease: neurological assessment of potential gene carriers presenting for predictive DNA testing. *J Clin Neurosci* 2000;7:38–41.
23. Hahn-Barma V, Deweer B, Durr A, et al. Are cognitive changes the first symptoms of Huntington's disease? A study of gene carriers. *Journal of Neurology, Neurosurgery & Psychiatry* 1998;62: 172–177.
24. Baxter LR Jr, Mazziotta JC, Pahl JJ, et al. Psychiatric, genetic, and positron emission tomographic evaluation of persons at risk for Huntington's disease. *Arch Gen Psychiatry* 1992;49: 148–154.
25. Tian JR, Zee D, Lasker AG, et al. Saccades in Huntington's disease: predictive tracking and interaction between release of fixation and initiation of saccades. *Neurology* 1991;41:875–881.
26. Carella F, Scaioli V, Ciano C, et al. Adult onset myoclonic Huntington's disease. *Mov Disord* 1993;8:201–205.
27. Jankovic J, Ashizawa T. Tourettism associated with Huntington's disease. *Mov Disord* 1995;10:103–105.
28. Leopold N, Kagel M. Dysphagia in Huntington's disease. *Arch Neurol* 1985;42:57–60.
29. Louis ED, Lee P, Quinn L, et al. Dystonia in Huntington's disease: prevalence and clinical characteristics. *Mov Disord* 1999;14:95–101.
30. van Vugt JP, van Hilten BJ, Roos RA. Hypokinesia in Huntington's disease. *Mov Disord* 1996;11:384–388.
31. Racette BA, Perlmutter JS. Levodopa responsive parkinsonism in an adult with Huntington's disease. *J Neurol Neurosurg Psychiatry* 1998;65:577–579.
32. Beenen N, Buttner U, Lange HW. The diagnostic value of eye movement recordings in patients with Huntington's disease and their offspring. *Electroenceph Clin Neurophysiol* 1986;63: 119–127.
33. Collewijn H, Went LN, Tamminga EP, et al. Oculomotor deficits in patients with Huntington's disease and their offspring. *J Neurol Sci* 1988;86:307–320.
34. Kirkwood SC, Siemers E, Bond C, et al. Confirmation of subtle motor changes among presymptomatic carriers of the Huntington disease gene. *Arch Neurol* 2000;57:1040–1044.
35. Oepen G, Clarenbach P, Thoden U. Disturbance of eye movements in Huntington's chorea. *Archiv Psychiatrie Nervenkrankheiten* 1981;229:205–213.
36. Feigin A, Kieburtz K, Bordwell K, et al. Functional decline in Huntington's disease. *Mov Disord* 1995;10:211–214.
37. Reuter I, Hu MT, Andrews TC, et al. Late onset levodopa responsive Huntington's disease with minimal chorea mas-

querading as Parkinson plus syndrome. *J Neurol Neurosurg Psychiatry* 2000;68:238–241.

38. Tan E, Jankovic J, Ondo W. Bruxism in Huntington's disease. *Mov Disord* 2000;15:171–173.

39. Paulson GW. Diagnosis of Huntington's disease. In: Chase TN, Wexler NS, Barbeau A, eds. *Huntington's disease.* New York: Raven Press, 1979;177–184.

40. Siemers E, Foroud T, Bill DJ, et al. Motor changes in presymptomatic Huntington disease gene carriers. *Arch Neurol* 1996; 53:487–492.

41. Edmonds C. Huntington's chorea, dysphagia, and death. *Med J Aust* 1966;2:273–274.

42. Pillon B, Dubois B, Ploska A, et al. Severity and specificity of cognitive impairment in Alzheimer's, Huntington's, and Parkinson's diseases and progressive supranuclear palsy. *Neurology* 1991;41:634–643.

43. Josiassen RC, Curry LM, Mancall EL. Development of neuropsychological deficits in Huntington's disease. *Arch Neurol* 1983;40:791–796.

44. Morris M. Dementia and cognitive changes in Huntington's disease. In: Weiner WJ, Lang AE, eds. *Behavioral neurology of movement disorderss* New York: Raven Press, 1995:187–200.

45. Bamford KA, Caine ED, Kido DK, et al. Clinical-pathologic correlation in Huntington's disease: a neuropsychological and computed tomography study. *Neurology* 1989;39:796–801.

46. Huber SJ, Paulson GW. Memory impairment associated with progression of Huntington's disease. *Cortex* 1987;23:275–283.

47. Lawrence AD, Sahakian B, Hodges JR, et al. Executive and mnemonic functions in early Huntington's disease. *Brain* 1996; 119:1633–1645.

48. Watkins L, Rogers RD, Lawrence AD, et al. Impaired planning but intact decision making in early Huntington's disease: implications for specific fronto-striatal pathology. *Neuropsychologia* 2000;38:1112–1125.

49. Lawrence AD, Weeks RA, Brooks DJ, et al. The relationship between striatal dopamine receptor binding and cognitive performance in Huntington's disease. *Brain* 1998;121:1343–1355.

50. Paulsen JS, Zhao H, Stout JC, et al. Clinical markers of early disease in persons near onset of Huntington's disease. *Neurology* 2001;57:658–662.

51. Foroud T, Siemers E, Kleindorfer D, et al. Cognitive scores in carriers of Huntington's disease gene compared to noncarriers. *Ann Neurol* 1995;37:657–664.

52. Strauss ME, Brandt J. Are there neuropsychologic manifestations of the gene for Huntington's disease in asymptomatic, at-risk individuals? *Arch Neurol* 1990;47:905–908.

53. Diamond R, White RF, Myers RH, et al. Evidence of presymptomatic cognitive decline in Huntington's disease. *J Clin Exp Neuropsychol* 1992;14:961–975.

54. Jason GW, Pajurkova EM, Suchowersky O, et al. Presymptomatic neuropsychological impairment in Huntington's disease. *Arch Neurol* 1988;45:769–773.

55. Rosenberg NK, Sorenson SA, Christensen AL. Neuropsychological characteristics of Huntington's disease carriers: a double blind study. *J Med Genet* 1995;32:600–604.

56. Lawrence AD, Hodges JR, Rosser AE, et al. Evidence for specific cognitive deficits in preclinical Huntington's disease. *Brain* 1998;121:1329–1341.

57. Giordani B, Berent S, Boivin MJ, et al. Longitudinal neuropsychological and genetic linkage analysis of persons at risk for Huntington's disease. *Arch Neurol* 1995;52:59–64.

58. de Boo GM, Tibben A, Lanser JBK, et al. Early cognitive and motor symptoms in identified carriers of the gene for Huntington disease. *Arch Neurol* 1997;54:1353–1357.

59. Blackmore L, Simpson SA, Crawford JR. Cognitive performance in UK sample of presymptomatic people carrying the gene for Huntington's disease. *J Med Genetics* 1995;32: 358–362.

60. Rothlind JC, Brandt J, Zee D, et al. Unimpaired verbal memory and oculomotor control in asymptomatic adults with the genetic marker for Huntington's disease. *Arch Neurol* 1993;50: 799–802.

61. Wexler NS. Perceptual-motor, cognitive, and emotional characteristics of persons at risk for Huntington's disease. In: Chase TN, Wexler NS, Barbeau A, eds. *Huntington's disease.* New York: Raven Press, 1979:257–271.

62. Britton JW, Uitti RJ, Ahlskog JE, et al. Hereditary late-onset chorea without significant dementia: genetic evidence for substantial phenotypic variation in Huntington's disease. *Neurology* 1995;45:443–447.

63. Wilson RS, Garron DC. Cognitive and affective aspects of Huntington's disease. In: Chase TN, Wexler NS, Barbeau A, eds. *Huntington's disease.* New York: Raven Press, 1979: 193–201.

64. Shelton PA, Knopman DS. Ideomotor apraxia in Huntington's disease. *Arch Neurol* 1991;48:35–41.

65. Caine ED, Shoulson I. Psychiatric syndromes in Huntington's disease. *Am J Psychiatry* 1983;140:728–733.

66. Mendez MF. Huntington's disease: update and review of neuropsychiatric aspects. *Int J Psychiatry Med* 1994;24:189–208.

67. Schoenfeld M, Myers RH, Cupples LA, et al. Increased rate of suicide among patients with Huntington's disease. *J Neurol Neurosurg Psychiatry* 1984;47:1283–1287.

68. Mayberg HS, Starkstein SE, Peyser CE, et al. Paralimbic frontal lobe hypometabolism in depression associated with Huntington's disease. *Neurology* 1992;42:1791–1797.

69. Guttman M, Alpay M, Chouinard S, et al. Clinical management of psychosis and mood disorders in Huntington's disease. In: Bedard MA, Agid Y, Chouinard G, et al, eds. *Mental and behavioral dysfunction in movement disorders.* Totowa, NJ: Humana Press, 2002 (in press).

70. Burns A, Folstein S, Brandt J, et al. Clinical assessment of irritability, aggression, and apathy in Huntington and Alzheimer disease. *J Nerv Ment Dis* 1990;178:20–26.

71. Dewhurst K, Oliver JE, McKnight AL. Socio-psychiatric consequences of Huntington's disease. *Br J Psychiatry* 1970;116: 255–258.

72. Levy ML, Cummings JL, Fairbanks LA, et al. Apathy is not depression. *J Neuropsychiatry Clin Neurosci* 1998;10:314–319.

73. Shiwach RS, Norbury CG. A controlled psychiatric study of individuals at risk for Huntington's disease. *Br J Psychiatry* 1994;165:500–505.

74. Lanska DJ, Lavine L, Lanska MJ, et al. Huntington's disease mortality in the United States. *Neurology* 1988;38:769–772.

75. Foroud T, Gray J, Ivashina J, et al. Differences in duration of Huntington's disease based on age at onset. *J Neurol Neurosurg Psychiatry* 1999;66:52–56.

76. van Dijk G, Van der Velde EA, Roos RA, et al. Juvenile Huntington's disease. *Hum Genet* 1986;73:235–239.

77. Shoulson I, Kurlan R, Rubin A. Assessment of functional capacity in neurodegenerative movement disorders: Huntington's disease as a prototype. In: Munsat TL, ed. *Quantification of neurologic deficit.* Boston: Butterworths, 1989:285–306.

78. Shoulson I, Odoroff C, Oakes D, et al. A controlled clinical trial of baclofen as protective therapy in early Huntington's disease. *Ann Neurol* 1989;25:252–259.

79. Huntington Study Group. Unified Huntington's disease rating scale: reliability and consistency. *Mov Disord* 1996;11:136–142.

80. Siesling S, van Vugt JP, Zwinderman AH, et al. Unified Huntington's Disease Rating Scale: a follow up. *Mov Disord* 1998;13: 915–919.

81. Rasmussen A, Macias R, Yescas P, et al. Huntington disease in

children: genotype–phenotype correlation. *Neuropediatrics* 2000;31:190–194.

82. Andrew SE, Goldberg YP, Kremer B, et al. The relationship between trinucleotide (CAG) repeat length and clinical features of Huntington's disease. *Nat Genet* 1993;4:398–403.

83. Roos RA, Vegter-Van der Vlis M, Hermans J, et al. Age at onset in Huntington's disease: effect of line of inheritance of patient's sex. *Med Genet* 1991;28:515–519.

84. Shoulson I. On chorea. *Clin Neuropharmacol* 1986;9:S85–S99.

85. Rosenblatt A, Ranen N, Rubinsztein DC, et al. Patients with features similar to Huntington's disease, without CAG expansion in huntingtin. *Neurology* 1998;51:215–220.

86. Nance M. Clinical aspects of CAG repeat diseases. *Brain Pathol* 1997;7:881–890.

87. Bateman D, Boughey AM, Scaravilli F, et al. A follow-up study of isolated cases of suspected Huntington's disease. *Ann Neurology* 1992;31:293–298.

88. Shinotoh H, Calne DB, Snow B, et al. Normal CAG repeat length in the Huntington's disease gene in senile chorea. *Neurology* 1994;44:2183–2184.

89. Fernandez M, Raskind W, Matsushita M, et al. Hereditary benign chorea: clinical and genetic features of a distinct disease. *Neurology* 2001;57:106–110.

90. Hardie RJ, Pullon HW, Harding AE, et al. Neuroacanthocytosis: a clinical, haemotological, and pathological study of 19 cases. *Brain* 1991;114:13–49.

91. Farmer TW, Wingfield MS, Lynch SA, et al. Ataxia, chorea, seizures, and dementia: pathological features of a newly defined familial disorder. *Arch Neurol* 1989;46:774–779.

92. Brown P. EEG findings in Creutzfeldt-Jakob disease. *JAMA* 1993;269:3168–3168.

93. Hsich G, Kenney K, Gibbs CJ, et al. The 14-3-3 brain protein in cerebrospinal fluid as a marker for transmissible spongiform encephalopathies. *N Engl J Med* 1996;335:924–930.

94. Lemstra AW, van Meegen MT, Vreyling JP, et al. 14-3-3 testing in diagnosing Creutzfeldt-Jakob disease: a prospective study in 112 patients. *Neurology* 2000;55:514–516.

95. LeWitt PA, Pfeiffer RF. Neurologic aspects of Wilson's disease: clinical manifestations and treatment considerations. In: Jankovic J, Tolosa E, eds. *Parkinson's disease and related movement disorders,* 3rd ed. Philadelphia: Lippincott Williams & Wilkins, 1998:377–399.

96. Scheinberg IH, Sternlieb I. *Wilson's disease.* Philadelphia: WB Saunders, 1984.

97. Warren JD, Firgaira F, Thompson EM, et al. The causes of sporadic and "senile" chorea. *Aust N Z J Med* 1998;28:429–431.

98. Bruyn GW, Padberg G. Chorea and polycythaemia. *Eur Neurol* 1984;23:26–33.

99. Goldberg YP, Telenius H, Hayden MR. The molecular genetics of Huntington's disease. *Curr Opin Neurol* 1994;7:325–332.

100. Landwehrmeyer GB, McNeil SM, Dure LS, et al. Huntington's disease gene: regional and cellular expression in brain of normal and affected individuals. *Ann Neurol* 1901;37:218–230.

101. Sapp E, Schwarz C, Chase K, et al. Huntingtin localization in brains of normal and Huntington's disease patients. *Ann Neurol* 1997;42:604–612.

102. Saudou F, Finkbeiner S, Devys D, et al. Huntingtin acts in the nucleus to induce apoptosis but death does not correlate with the formation of intranuclear inclusions. *Cell* 1998;95:55–66.

103. Jones AL. The localization and interactions of huntingtin. *Philos Trans R Soc Lond Biol Sci* 1999;354:1021–1027.

104. Brinkman RR, Mezei MM, Theilmann J, et al. The likelihood of being affected with Huntington disease by a particular age, for a specific CAG size. *Am J Hum Genet* 1997;60:1202–1210.

105. Snell RG, MacMillan JC, Cheadle JP, et al. Relationship between trinucletoided repeat expansion and phenotypic variation in Huntington's disease. *Nat Genet* 1993;4:393–397.

106. Jenkins BG, Rosas HD, Chen Y, et al. ^{1}H NMR spectroscopy studies of Huntington's disease: correlations with CAG repeat numbers. *Neurology* 1998;50:1357–1365.

107. Illarioshkin S, Igarashi S, Onodera O, et al. Trinucleotide repeat length and rate of progression of Huntington's disease. *Ann Neurol* 1994;36:630–635.

108. Brandt J, Bylsma FW, Gross BA, et al. Trinucleotide repeat length and clinical progression in Huntington's disease. *Neurology* 1996;46:527–531.

109. Furtado S, Suchowersky O, Rewcastle B, et al. Relationship between trinucleotide repeats and neuropathological changes in Huntington's disease. *Ann Neurol* 1996;39:132–136.

110. Ashizawa T, Wong L, Richards CS, et al. CAG repeat size and clinical presentation in Huntington's disease. *Neurology* 1994;44:1137–1143.

111. Antonini A, Leenders K, Eidelberg D. Raclopride-PET studies of the Huntington's disease rate of progression: relevance of the trinucleotide repeat length. *Ann Neurol* 1998;43:253–255.

112. Claes S, Van Zand K, Legius E, et al. Correlations between triplet repeat expansion and clinical features in Huntington's disease. *Arch Neurol* 1995;52:749–753.

113. Kieburtz K, MacDonald ME, Shih C, et al. Trinucleotide repeat length and progression of illness in Huntington's disease. *J Med Genetics* 1994;31:872–874.

114. MacDonald ME, Vonsattel JP, Srinidhi J, et al. Evidence for the *GluR6* gene associated with younger onset age of Huntington's disease. *Neurology* 1999;53:1330–1332.

115. Gusella JF, Persichetti F, MacDonald ME. The genetic defect causing Huntington's disease: repeated in other contexts? *Mol Med* 1997;3:238–246.

116. Myers RH, Marans K, MacDonald ME. Huntington's disease. In: Warren ST, Wells RT, eds. *Genetic instabilities and hereditary neurological diseases.* San Diego: Academic Press, 1998: 301–323.

117. Huntington Study Group. A randomized, placebo-controlled trial of coenzyme Q10 and remacemide in Huntington's disease. *Neurology* 2001;57:397–404.

118. Nance MA, Myers RH, the U.S. Huntington Disease Genetic Testing Group. Trends in predictive and prenatal testing for Huntington's disease 1993–1999. *Am J Hum Genet* 1999;65: A406.

119. Laccone F, Engel U, Holinski-Feder E, et al. DNA analysis of Huntington's disease: five years of experience in Germany, Austria, and Switzerland. *Neurology* 1999;53:801–806.

120. Quaid KA, Morris M. Reluctance to undergo predictive testing: the case of Huntington disease. *Am J Med Genet* 1993;45: 41–45.

121. Hayes C. Genetic testing for Huntington's disease—a family issue. *N Engl J Med* 1992;327:1449–1451.

122. Wiggins S, Whyte P, Huggins M, et al. The psychological consequences of predictive testing for Huntington's disease. *N Engl J Med* 1992;327:1401–1405.

123. Tibben A, Frets P, van de Kamp J, et al. On attitudes and appreciation 6 months after predictive DNA testing for Huntington disease in the Dutch program. *Am J Med Genet* 1993;48: 103–111.

124. Alper JS, Geller LN, Barash CI, et al. Genetic discrimination and screening for hemochromatosis. *J Public Health Pol* 1994; 15:345–358.

125. Low L, King S, Wilkie T. Genetic discrimination in life insurance: empirical evidence from a cross sectional survey of genetic support groups in the United Kingdom. *BMJ* 1998;317: 1632–1635.

126. Billings PR, Kohn MA, de Cuevas M, et al. Discrimination as a

consequence of genetic testing. *Am J Hum Genet* 1992;50: 476–482.

127. Lapham EV, Kozma C, Weiss JO. Genetic discrimination: perspectives of consumers. *Science* 1996;274:621–624.

128. Tibben A, Duivenvoorden H, Vegter-Van der Vlis M, et al. Presymptomatic DNA testing for Huntington disease: identifying the need for psychological intervention. *Am J Med Genet* 1993;48:137–144.

129. Quaid KA, Brandt J, Faden RR, et al. Knowledge, attitude, and the decision to be tested for Huntington's disease. *Clinical Genetics* 1989;36:431–438.

130. Vonsattel JP, Myers RH, Stevens TJ, et al. Neuropathological classification of Huntington's disease. *J Neuropathol Exp Neuro* 1985;44:559–577.

131. Sotrel A, Paskevich PA, Kiely DK, et al. Morphometric analysis of the prefrontal cortex in Huntington's disease. *Neurology* 1991;41:1117–1123.

132. Mitchell IJ, Cooper AJ, Griffiths MR. The selective vulnerability of striatopallidal neurons. *Prog Neurobiol* 1999;59:691–719.

133. Perry TL, Hansen S, Kloster M. Huntington's chorea: deficiency of gamma-aminobutyric acid in brain. *N Engl J Med* 1973;288:337–342.

134. Reiner A, Albin RL, D'Amato C, et al. Differential loss of striatal projection neurons in Huntington disease. *Proc Natl Acad Sci USA* 1988;85:5733–5737.

135. Sapp E, Ge P, Aizawa H, et al. Evidence for a preferential loss of enkephalin immunoreactivity in the external globus pallidus in low grade Huntington's disease using high resolution image analysis. *Neuroscience* 1995;64:397–404.

136. Richfield EK, Maguire-Zeiss KA, Vonkemank HE, et al. Preferential loss of preproenkephalin versus preprotachykinin neurons from the striatum of Huntington's disease patients. *Ann Neurol* 1995;38:852–861.

137. Roizin L, Stellar S, Willson N, et al. Electron microscope and enzyme studies in cerebral biopsies of Huntington's chorea. *Trans Am Neurol Assoc* 1974;99:240–243.

138. DiFiglia M, Sapp E, Chase K, et al. Aggregation of huntingtin in neuronal intranuclear inclusions and dystrophic neurites in brain. *Science* 1997;277:1990–1993.

139. Davies S, Cozens B, Turmaine M, et al. Formation of neuronal intranuclear inclusions underlies the neurological dysfunction in mice transgenic for the HD mutation. *Cell* 1997;90: 537–548.

140. Gomez-Tortosa E, MacDonald ME, Friend JC, et al. Quantitative neuropathological changes in presymptomatic Huntington's disease. *Ann Neurol* 2001;49:29–34.

141. Young AB, Greenamyre JT, Hollingsworth Z, et al. NMDA receptor losses in putamen from patients with Huntington's disease. *Science* 1988;981–983.

142. Beal MF, Ferrante RJ, Swartz KJ, et al. Chronic quinolinic acid lesions in rats closely resemble Huntington's disease. *J Neurosci* 1991;11(6):1649–1659.

143. Ferrante RJ, Kowall NW, Cipolloni PB, et al. Excitotoxin lesions in primates as a model for Huntington's disease: histopathologic and neurochemical characterization. *Exp Neurol* 1993;119:46–71.

144. Koroshetz WJ, Jenkins BG, Rosen BR, et al. Energy metabolism defects in Huntington's disease and effects of coenzyme Q10. *Ann Neurol* 1997;41:160–165.

145. Horton TM, Graham BH, Corral-Debrinski M, et al. Marked increase in mitochondrial DNA deletion levels in the cerebral cortex of Huntington's disease patients. *Neurology* 1995;45: 1879–1883.

146. Gu M, Gash MT, Mann VM, et al. Mitochondrial defect in Huntington's disease caudate nucleus. *Ann Neurol* 1996;39: 385–389.

147. Ona VO, Li M, Vonsattel JP, et al. Inhibition of caspase-1 slows disease progression in a mouse model of Huntington's disease. *Nature* 1999;399:263–267.

148. Steffan JS, Kazantsev A, Spasic-Boskovic O, et al. The Huntington's disease protein interacts with p53 and CREB-binding protein and represses transcription. *Proc Natl Acad Sci USA* 2000;97:6763–6768.

149. Nucifora FC, Sasaki M, Peters MF, et al. Interference by huntingtin and atrophin-1 with CBP-mediated transcription leading to cellular toxicity. *Science* 2001;291:2423–2428.

150. McCampbell A, Taylor JP, Taye AA, et al. CREB-binding protein sequestration by expanded polyglutamine. *Hum Mol Genet* 2000;9:2197–2202.

151. Novelli A, Reilly JA, Lysko PG, et al. Glutamate becomes neurotoxic via the *N*-methyl-D-aspartate receptor when intracellular energy levels are reduced. *Brain Res* 1988;451:205–212.

152. Duyao M, Auerbach AB, Ryan A, et al. Inactivation of the mouse Huntington's disease gene homolog Hdh. *Science* 1995; 269:407–410.

153. Wellington CL, Leavitt BR, Hayden MR. Huntington disease: new insights on the role of huntingtin cleavage. *J Transm Suppl* 2000;58:1–17.

154. Scherzinger E, Lurz R, Turmaine M, et al. Huntingtin-encoded polyglutamine expansions form amyloid-like protein aggregates in vitro and in vivo. *Cell* 1997;90:549–558.

155. Cooper JK, Schilling G, Peters MF, et al. Truncated N-terminal fragments of huntingtin with expanded glutamine repeats form nuclear and cytoplasmic aggregates in cell culture. *Hum Mol Genet* 1998;7:783–790.

156. Mangiarini L, Sathasivam K, Seller M, et al. Exon 1 of the *HD* gene with an expanded CAG repeat is sufficient to cause a progressive neurological phenotype in transgenic mice. *Cell* 1996;87:493–506.

157. Li XJ. The early cellular pathology of Huntington's disease. *Mol Neurobiol* 1999;20:111–124.

158. Steffan JS, Bodai L, Pallos J, et al. Histone deacetylase inhibitors arrest polyglutamine-dependent neurodegeneration in *Drosophila*. *Nature* 2001;413:739–743.

159. Shoulson I. Huntington's disease: functional capacities in patients treated with neuroleptic and antidepressant drugs. *Neurology* 1981;31:1333–1335.

160. Marshall FJ. Riluzole dosing in Huntington's disease (RID-HD): results of an 8-week double-blind, placebo-controlled, multi-center study by the Huntington Study Group. *19th International Meeting of the World Federation of Neurology. Research Group on Huntington's Disease* 2001;29–30.

161. Rosas HD, Koroshetz W, Jenkins BG, et al. Riluzole therapy in Huntington's disease (HD). *Mov Disord* 1999;14:326–330.

162. Verhagen L, Morris M, Farmer C, et al. A double-blind, placebo-controlled crossover study of the effect of amantadine on chorea in Huntington's disease. *Neurology* 2001;56: A386.

163. Jankovic J, Beach J. Long-term effects of tetrabenazine in hyperkinetic movement disorders. *Neurology* 1997;48:358–362.

164. Jankovic J. Treatment of hyperkinetic movement disorders with tetrabenazine: a double-blind crossover study. *Ann Neurol* 1982; 11:41–47.

165. Jongen PJ, Renier WO, Gabreels FJ. Seven cases of Huntington's disease in childhood and levodopa induced improvement in the hypokinetic-rigid form. *Clin Neurol Neurosur* 1980;82: 251–261.

166. Fernandez HH, Friedman J, Grace J, et al. Donepezil for Huntington's disease. *Mov Disord* 2000;15:173–176.

167. Murman DL, Giordani B, Mellow AM, et al. Cognitive, behavioral, and motor effects of the NMDA antagonist ketamine in Huntington's disease. *Neurology* 1997;49:153–161.

168. Peyser CE, Folstein M, Chase GA, et al. Trial of *d*-alpha-tocopherol in Huntington's disease. *Am J Psychiatry* 1995;152:1771–1775.

169. Shoulson I, Goldblatt D, Charlton M, et al. Huntington's disease: treatment with muscimol; a GABA-mimetic drug. *Ann Neurol* 1978;4:279–284.

170. Kapur S, Remington G. Serotonin-dopamine interaction and its relevance to schizophrenia. *Am J Psychiatry* 1996;153:466–476.

171. Fava M. Psychopharmacologic treatment of pathologic aggression. *Psychiatr Clin North Am* 1997;20:427–451.

172. Como PG, Rubin AJ, O'Brien CF, et al. A controlled trial of fluoxetine in nondepressed patients with Huntington's disease. *Mov Disord* 1997;12:397–401.

173. Moldawsky RJ. Effect of amoxapine on speech in a patient with Huntington's disease. *Am J Psychiatry* 1984;141:150.

174. Ranen NG, Peyser CE, Folstein SE. ECT as a treatment for depression in Huntington's disease. *J Neuropsychiatry Clin Neurosci* 1994;6:154–159.

175. Chacko RC, Corbin MA, Harper RG. Acquired obsessive-compulsive disorder associated with basal ganglia lesions. *J Neuropsychiatry Clin Neurosci* 2000;12:269–272.

176. Jankovic J. Tardive syndromes and other drug-induced movement disorders. *Clin Neuropharmacol* 1995;18:197–214.

177. Schott K, Ried S, Stevens I, et al. Neuroleptically induced dystonia in Huntington's disease: a case report. *Eur Neurol* 1989;29:39–40.

178. Bonuccelli U, Ceravolo R, Maremmani C, et al. Clozapine in Huntington's chorea. *Neurology* 1994;44:821–823.

179. Rosenblatt A, Anderson K, Goumeniouk D, et al. Clinical management of aggression and frontal syndromes in Huntington's disease. In: Bedard MA, Agid Y, Chouinard S, et al, eds. *Mental and behavioral dysfunction in movement disorders.* Totowa, NJ: Humana Press, 2002 (in press).

180. Grove VE, Quintanilla J, DeVaney GT. Improvement of Huntington's disease with olanzapine and valproate. *N Engl J Med* 2000;343:973–974.

181. Kavoussi RJ, Coccaro EF. Divalproex sodium for impulsive aggressive behavior in patients with personality disorder. *J Clin Psychiatry* 1998;59:676–680.

182. Stewart JT. Huntington's disease and propranolol. *Am J Psychiatry* 1993;150:166–167.

183. Armstrong RJ, Watts C, Svendsen CN, et al. Survival, neuronal differentiation, and fiber outgrowth of propagated human neural precursor grafts in an animal model of Huntington's disease. *Cell Transplant* 2000;9:55–64.

184. Nakao N, Itakura T. Fetal tissue transplants in animal models of Huntington's disease: the effects on damaged neuronal circuitry and behavioral deficits. *Prog Neurobiol* 2000;61:313–338.

185. Borlongan CV, Koutouzis TK, Poulos SG, et al. Bilateral fetal striatal grafts in the 3-nitropropionic acid-induced hypoactive model of Huntington's disease. *Cell Transplant* 1998;7:131–135.

186. Bachoud-Levi AC, Bourdet C, Brugieres P, et al. Safety and tolerability assessment of intrastriatal neural allografts in five patients with Huntington's disease. *Exp Neurol* 2000;161:194–202.

187. Philpott LM, Kopyov OV, Lee AJ, et al. Neuropsychological functioning following fetal striatal transplantation in Huntington's chorea: three case presentations. *Cell Transplant* 1997;6:203–212.

188. Hauser RA, Furtado S, Cimino C, et al. Bilateral human fetal striatal transplantation in Huntington's disease. *Neurology* 2002;58:687–695.

189. Bachoud-Levi AC, Remy P, Nguyen JP, et al. Motor cognitive improvements in patients with Huntington's disease after neural transplantation. *Lancet* 2000;356:1975–1979.

190. CAPIT-HD committee, Quinn N, Brown R, et al. Core assessment program for intracerebral transplantation in Huntington's disease (CAPIT-HD). *Mov Disord Soc* 1996;11:143–150.

191. Shoulson I. DATATOP: a decade of neuroprotective inquiry. Parkinson Study Group. Deprenyl and tocopherol antioxidative therapy of parkinsonism. *Ann Neurol* 1998;44:S160–S166.

192. Kremer B, Clark CM, Almqvist EW, et al. Influence of lamotrigine on progression of early Huntington disease: a randomized clinical trial. *Neurology* 1999;53:1000–1011.

193. Feigin A, Kieburtz K, Como P, et al. Assessment of coenzyme Q10 tolerability in Huntington's disease. *Mov Disord* 1996;11:321–323.

194. Huntington Study Group. Safety and tolerability of the free-radical scavenger OPC-14117 in Huntington's disease. *Neurology* 1998;50:1366–1373.

195. Hersch S, Rosas HD. Neuroprotective therapy for Huntington's disease: new prospects and challenges. *Expert Rev Neurother* 2002;1:111–118.

196. Chen M, Ona VO, Ferrante RJ, et al. Minocycline inhibits caspase-1 and caspase-3 and delays mortality in a transgenic mouse model of Huntington's disease. *Nat Med* 2000;6:797–801.

197. Yrjanheikki J, Tikka T, Keinanen R, et al. A tetracycline derivative, minocycline, reduces inflammation and protects against focal cerebral ischemia with a wide therapeutic window. *Proc Natl Acad Sci USA* 1999;96:13496–13500.

198. Ferrante RJ, Andreassen OA, Jenkins BG, et al. Neuroprotective effects of creatine in a transgenic mouse. *J Neurosci* 2000;20:4389–4397.

199. Matthews RT, Yang L, Jenkins BG, et al. Neuroprotective effects of creatine and cyclocreatine in animal models of Huntington's disease. *J Neurosci* 1998;18:156–163.

200. Butler LM, Agus DB, Scher HI, et al. Suberoylanilide hydroxamic acid, an inhibitor of histone deacetylase, suppresses the growth of prostate cancer cells in vitro and in vivo. *Cancer Res* 2000;60:5165–5170.

201. Warrell RP, He L, Richon V, et al. Therapeutic targeting of transcription in acute promyelocytic leukemia by use of an inhibitor of histone deacetylase. *J Natl Cancer Institute* 1998;90:1621–1625.

15

CHOREA

CHRISTOPHER G. GOETZ
STACY HORN

HISTORY

Chorea is derived from a Greek word meaning "to dance." Chorea describes an involuntary hyperkinetic movement disorder consisting of sudden, irregular, purposeless movements that are distally prominent and which, when the upper extremities are involved, are often described as "piano-playing fingers." Chorea may be generalized, hemi-, segmental, or focal. The term chorea has been variously used in neurologic history, and *chorea major* originally was synonymous with the Dancing Mania, a likely psychiatric disorder. The first descriptions of chorea as a disorder with the currently accepted description likely date to the 16th century by Paracelsus and were termed "chorea naturalis." Paracelsus concentrated on the cognitive effects associated with the movements (1), and the involuntary movements themselves were described in more detail by Sydenham in 1686 (2). In the 19th century, chorea was studied by Jean-Martin Charcot and his pupils, but would not be succinctly categorized until William Osler wrote on the subject in 1894 in his monograph *On Chorea and Choreiform Affectations.* Osler was pivotal to differentiating the varied causes of chorea and clearly separated Sydenham's chorea from Huntington's disease (3).

CHARACTERIZATION OF CHOREA

Chorea is characterized as primary, when idiopathic or genetic in origin, or secondary, when related to infectious, immunologic, or medical causes. Inherited diseases such as Huntington's disease, dentatorubropallidoluysian atrophy (DRPLA), and benign hereditary chorea are primary causes of generalized chorea. Sydenham's chorea is a postinfectious disorder that is abrupt in onset following rheumatic fever. The chorea may be generalized or more focal in anatomic distribution. Anoxic brain injury and head trauma can cause generalized or hemichorea depending on the extent and location of the injury. Other secondary causes include inflammatory diseases (e.g., systemic lupus erythematosus

and Hashimoto's thyroiditis), and a number of medications and toxins can also induce the movement disorder as an acute or long-term effect of exposure. Lastly, chorea may be a manifestation of pregnancy.

PATHOPHYSIOLOGY

Movement disorders arise most often from disruption of the basal ganglia or their afferent or efferent pathways. The basal ganglia are anatomically composed of four primary nuclei: the striatum (caudate and putamen), the globus pallidus, the substantia nigra, and the subthalamic nucleus. The striatum interacts with the motor cortex through the indirect and direct pathways to modulate movement. In the prototypic paradigm, activation of the direct pathway facilitates movement, whereas activation of the indirect pathway inhibits movement. Imbalances in the direct and indirect pathways cause abnormalities of movement. Depending on the pathway that is most affected, the movement disorder may be primarily hypokinetic or hyperkinetic. The direct and indirect pathways are depicted in Figs. 15.1 and 15.2.

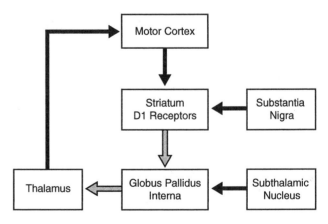

FIG. 15.1. Direct pathway. Each box represents a nucleus of the basal ganglia. *Solid arrows* represent facilitory pathways and *stippled arrows* represent inhibitory pathways.

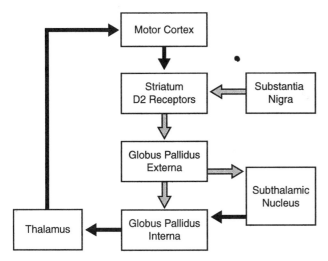

FIG. 15.2. Indirect pathway. Each box represents a nucleus of the basal ganglia. *Solid arrows* represent facilitory pathways and *stippled arrows* represent inhibitory pathways.

All areas of the cortex send excitatory (glutaminergic) projections to the striatum. The striatum also receives input from the substantia nigra pars compacta. Stimulation of the D1 dopamine receptors of the striatum activates the direct pathway and stimulation of the D2 dopamine receptors activates that indirect pathway. The striatum then sends outputs to the other nuclei of the basal ganglia via γ-aminobutyric acid (GABA) medium-spiny neurons (4).

Most physiologic and anatomic evidence suggests that disruption of the indirect pathway either structurally or neurochemically causes chorea. The disruption of the indirect pathway causes a loss of inhibition on the pallidum, allowing excessive movements to occur. Figure 15.3 shows the abnor-

malities in the direct and indirect pathways that allow chorea to occur. Enhanced activity of dopaminergic receptors and excess dopaminergic activity from other mechanisms are proposed mechanisms for the development of chorea at the level of the striatum (5,6). Reasonable strategies to abate indirect pathway–induced chorea would be aimed at decreasing striatal activity by blocking dopamine D2 receptors and depleting dopamine at the presynaptic level.

PRIMARY CHOREA

Huntington's Disease

Huntington's disease is an autosomally dominant inherited neurodegenerative disorder that causes cognitive decline, chorea and other movement disorders, and neuropsychiatric symptoms. George Huntington described the disease in detail in 1872 (7). Huntington's disease is a triplicate repeat disorder of chromosome 4 that causes the production of an abnormal protein called huntingtin (8). There is an inverse correlation between repeat length and age of onset (9). The CAG repeat is unstable and can amplify during gametogenesis. Amplification is more likely with paternal transmission (10). The typical disease progression is over 14 to 17 years (11). Huntington's disease causes a degeneration of the basal ganglia with selective loss of γ-aminobutyric acid (GABA) neurons (12). Whereas chorea is the prototypic movement disorder of Huntington's disease, myoclonus, dystonia, and parkinsonism can be salient features. (See Chapter 14 for additional details.)

Dentatorubropallidoluysian Atrophy

DRPLA is an autosomal dominant neurodegenerative disorder that clinically includes cognitive decline, myoclonus, chorea, dystonia, ataxia, and epilepsy. It was originally described in 1946 (13). The disease is caused by a triplicate repeat expansion on chromosome 12 and, like Huntington's disease, has an inverse correlation between repeat length and age of onset (14,15). Paternal transmission typically shows greater expansion of the repeat size than maternal transmission.

Benign Hereditary Chorea

Benign hereditary chorea is a nonprogressive choreic disorder that begins in early childhood and is not associated with other neurologic deficits. The disease was first reported in the 1960s and has no impact on life expectancy (16,17). This entity has been a subject of controversy because many of the initial families described were later found to have other diseases, such as Huntington's disease. Recent reports have linked this autosomal dominant disorder to chromosome 14q (18).

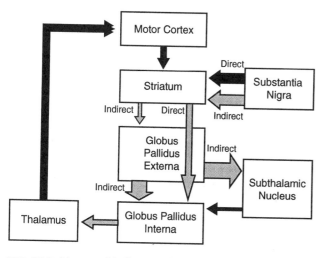

FIG. 15.3. Direct and indirect pathways in chorea. Each box represents a nucleus of the basal ganglia. *Solid arrows* represent facilitory pathways and *stippled arrows* represent inhibitory pathways. The width of the arrow indicates activity of the pathway in the disease state.

Neuroacanthocytosis

Neuroacanthocytosis is a disorder that may be transmitted by autosomal dominant, autosomal recessive, or X-linked inheritance. The disease is marked by the presence of abnormal erythrocytes (acanthocytes) on peripheral smear and neurologic abnormalities including chorea, tics, dystonia, and parkinsonism. The disorder tends to be progressive in nature and most patients die within 15 years of diagnosis. The exact mechanism of disease expression is unknown, but an abnormality in the erythrocyte membranous skeleton results in reduced membrane fluidity and structural abnormalities [19].

SECONDARY CHOREA

Sydenham's Chorea

The acute illness that bears his name was described by Thomas Sydenham in 1686 though he coined the disorder "St. Vitus' Dance." Although earlier clinicians had suggested a relationship between Sydenham's chorea and heart disease, a clear association of this disorder with rheumatic fever did not occur until the 1900s. Today antecedent group A β-hemolytic streptococcal infection is the accepted cause of this disorder, believed to be an autoimmune-mediated inflammatory process that affects the basal ganglia. The occurrence of Sydenham's chorea is now most prevalent in underdeveloped countries.

Sydenham's chorea is an acute onset clinical syndrome that includes chorea, dysarthria, weakness, and behavioral changes. The typical patient is aged 5 to 15 years, and the disorder is more prevalent in females [20]. The chorea may be unilateral or generalized, occurs at rest and with activities, but typically remits with sleep [21]. Behavioral changes include depression, anxiety, personality changes, emotional lability, and obsessive-compulsive traits. In some patients, initial chorea is replaced by extreme weakness and reappears as strength returns. Sydenham's chorea can be severe and interfere with activities of daily living, but is typically a self-limited illness with a good prognosis for full recovery. Patients may require symptomatic treatment with neuroleptics or valproic acid [22–24], but treatment is usually short term because in most patients the disease remits spontaneously within 2 to 3 months [21]. Reoccurrence is possible, and prior affected females have an increased risk of reoccurrence during pregnancy (chorea gravidarum) and during female sex hormonal therapy.

Small numbers of patients with Sydenham's chorea have undergone brain single photon emission computed tomography studies during the acute illness. These patients demonstrated striatal hypermetabolism that normalizes with resolution of their clinical syndrome [25,26]. One case report documents a child with persistent cystic changes in the caudate and putamen following Sydenham's chorea [27].

Immune-mediated Chorea

Autoimmune diseases such as systemic lupus erythematosus (SLE) have been causally linked to chorea. Approximately 4% of patients with SLE experience chorea, and the movement disorder is most likely to occur as part of an acute disease exacerbation. The chorea may be generalized or hemi in distribution and, though often mild, may require treatment with neuroleptic medications [28,29].

Multiple reports have linked the antiphospholipid syndrome and chorea. Generalized or hemichorea develops at an average age of 21 years with a predominance in females [30]. Thirty-five percent of patients in one study had cerebral infarctions on neuroimaging studies [31].

Lastly, rare reports of chorea associated with other autoimmune diseases include such disorders as Behçet's disease, polyarteritis nodosa, and isolated angiitis of the central nervous syndrome [32–35].

Hyperthyroidism

Thyrotoxicosis is a medical illness caused by excessive production of thyroid hormones. If left untreated it can cause serious morbidity and mortality. The disease is marked by a hypermetabolic state and may be associated with neurologic findings such as chorea, cognitive decline, myopathy, and tremor. Determination of the underlying cause of the excessive thyroid hormone production and appropriate thyroid control abate the movement disorder [36].

Infectious Chorea

Multiple infectious agents that affect the central nervous system have been associated with chorea. Acute manifestations of bacterial meningitis, encephalitis, tuberculous meningitis, and aseptic meningitis include movement disorders such as chorea, athetosis, dystonia, or hemiballismus [37,38]. Human immunodeficiency virus (HIV) has also been reported to cause chorea, either as the result of HIV encephalitis or as the result of focal opportunistic infections such as toxoplasmosis [39,40].

Drug-induced Chorea

Drug-induced chorea may be an acute phenomenon or the consequence of long-term therapy. Chorea may the result of medications or illicit drug use. The movement disorder does not always remit with discontinuation of the offending drug. Multiple drugs have been implicated in the acute onset of chorea (Table 15.1). When drug-induced chorea occurs, withdrawal of the offending agent is the treatment of choice. Onset of chorea after prolonged use of a medication is termed tardive dyskinesia and occurs with the use of dopamine blocking agents for greater than three months. Tardive dyskinesia is an involuntary, usually choreic, move-

TABLE 15.1. DRUGS KNOWN TO CAUSE ACUTE CHOREA

Anticonvulsant medications
    Phenytoin
    Carbamazepine
    Felbamate
    Valproate
    Gabapentin
Cocaine and cocaine derivatives
Central nervous system stimulants
Estrogens
Lithium
Levodopa
Dopamine agonists
    Pergolide
    Bromocriptine
    Ropinirole
    Pramipexole

ment disorder that typically affects the mouth and tongue causing random and stereotyped tongue protrusions and facial grimacing. At times these movements can be so severe that they interfere with eating and speech. Less commonly, the head, trunk and extremities may be affected with choreiform movements. Dystonic, akathitic, and tic-like movements can also occur. Epidemiological studies show that tardive dyskinesia is more often seen in elderly females and has an incidence of 24%-56% of patients chronically treated with neuroleptics (41). Table 15.2 lists several dopamine-blocking agents. The pathophysiology of tardive dyskinesia is imperfectly understood. The primary theory postulates that the central nervous system dopamine receptors become hypersensitive due to chronic dopaminergic blockade, so that small amounts of dopamine cause dyskinesias as a behavioral manifestation of enhanced striatal dopaminergic activity (42). The most important treatment for tardive dyskinesia is elimination of the offending medication if possible. If the movement disorder persists after

TABLE 15.2. DOPAMINERGIC BLOCKING AGENTS ASSOCIATED WITH TARDIVE DYSKINESIA

Neuroleptic Medications
    Olanzapine
    Quetiapine
    Risperidone
    Chlorpromazine
    Fluphenazine
    Haloperidol
    Loxapine
    Molindone
    Thioridazine
Gastrointestinal Agents
    Metoclopramide
    Prochlorperazine

discontinuation or, if the patient cannot be taken off of the offending drug due to psychiatric or other concerns, a dopamine-depleting agent, such as reserpine or tetrabenazine, may be useful. Patients who require continual neuroleptic treatment due to psychiatric disease should be maintained on the lowest possible dose and may also benefit from the use of atypical neuroleptic medications such as risperidone, quitiepine, or clozapine. Anticholinergic medications may exacerbate tardive dyskinesia and should be eliminated whenever possible.

Structural Lesions

Structural lesions of the striatum can cause choreiform movements. Chorea has been described as the result of head trauma, carbon monoxide poisoning, hypoxia, stroke, and as a post-pump phenomenon after open-heart surgery with bypass procedures (44–49).

Female Hormone–Mediated Chorea

Female hormone–mediated chorea may be generalized or hemilateral. This phenomenon can be seen during pregnancy or may be iatrogenically caused by hormonal therapy. As mentioned previously, a prior history of Sydenham's chorea or cyanotic heart disease may predispose females to this phenomenon. Patients with collagen vascular disease may also be susceptible to hormonally mediated chorea. The proposed mechanism is through the facilitation of dopamine pharmacology by estrogen either at the receptor site or through second messengers. The treatment of choice for medication-induced chorea is elimination of the offending medication. Most patients with chorea gravidarum remit spontaneously with delivery. If chorea is severe and requires treatment during pregnancy, benzodiazepines are the treatment of choice and neuroleptic medications should be avoided due to risks to fetal development.

DIAGNOSIS AND MANAGEMENT OF CHOREA

Given the difficult diagnosis, the comprehensive evaluation of chorea includes a careful history and physical examination focusing on a family history of choreic or degenerative illness, a medication history of potential causative exposures, and signs of other conditions that could cause secondary chorea. Genetic testing, neuroimaging, and blood work for medical diseases may be helpful to confirm the diagnosis.

For primary choreas, based on the pathophysiologic issues discussed, treatment options could focus on dopaminergic, GABAergic, cholinergic, or glutaminergic systems. Dopaminergic antagonists like neuroleptic medica-

TABLE 15.3. MEDICATIONS IN THE MANAGEMENT OF CHOREA

Neuroleptic medications
  Atypical agents
    Clozapine
    Olanzapine
    Quetiapine
    Risperidone
  Typical agents
    Chlorpromazine
    Fluphenazine
    Haloperidol
    Loxapine
    Molindone
    Thioridazine
Dopamine-depleting agents
  Tetrabenazine
  Reserpine
GABAergic agents
  Amantadine

tions are useful but can induce parkinsonism, tardive dyskinesia, or other complications with long-term use. Dopamine-depleting agents may also be useful but may cause depression, parkinsonism, or hypotension. Table 15.3 contains a list of medications used in the management of chorea.

For secondary choreas, the primary treatment concern should focus on the primary causative disorder; if chorea is due to an exogenous agent, the agent should be withdrawn. Hormonal disorders should be corrected, and inflammatory or infectious processes managed appropriately. The drugs used to treat primary chorea can also be used to treat secondary chorea symptomatically.

FUTURE PERSPECTIVES

An accurate animal model of chorea will facilitate neurologic and pathophysiologic studies for primary choreas. Methods of gene repair and stem cell replacement are potential research areas. With such therapies the concept of curing diseases rather than merely managing symptoms can be potentially approached. Already clinical protocols are evaluating agents aimed to protect patients with degenerative diseases against further cell loss. These strategies may alter the natural course of choreic disorders to diminish morbidity and mortality. The development of dopamine antagonists that are not associated with significant side effects, such as parkinsonism, neutropenia, and tardive dyskinesia, will provide safer agents for choreic patients. To date, drugs that alter GABA, acetylcholine, and glutamate function lack the needed specificity to be regularly used, but future drugs developed to target the indirect pathway have therapeutic potential. The clinical observation that levodopa-induced chorea in idiopathic Parkinson's disease patients can be attenuated by neurosurgical intervention with pallidal or subthalamic nucleus deep brain stimulation suggests that similar strategies could be applied to some patients with medically resistant chorea. The growing fields of neurotransplantation and gene therapy also offer potential applications to primary choreas, although these disorders generally embody diffuse pathologic changes that extend beyond the striatum itself.

REFERENCES

1. Sigerist HF. *Four treatises of Tehophratus von Hoehenheim called Paracelsus.* Baltimore: Johns Hopkins Press, 1941.
2. Schechter DC. St Vitus' dance and rheumatic disease. *NY State J Med* 1975;75:1091–1102.
3. Goetz CG. William Osler: on chorea—on Charcot. *Ann Neurol* 2000;47:404–407.
4. Kandel ER, Schwartz JH, Jessell TM, eds. *Principles of neural science,* 4th ed. New York: McGraw-Hill, 2000:853–864.
5. Marconi R, Lefebvre-Caparros D, Bonnet AM, et al. Levodopa-induced dyskinesias in Parkinson's disease phenomenology and pathophysiology. *Mov Disord* 1994;9(1):2–12.
6. Daras M, Koppel BS, Atos-Radzion E. Cocaine-induced choreoathetoid movements ("crack dancing"). *Neurology* 1994;44: 751–752.
7. Huntington G. On chorea. *Med Surg Reporter Philadelphia* 1972;26:317–321.
8. The Huntington's Disease Collaborative Research Group. A novel containing a trinucleotide repeat that is expanded and unstable on Huntington's disease chromosomes. *Cell* 1993; 72:971.
9. Andrew SE, Goldberg YP, Kremer B, et al. The relationship between trinucleotide (CAG) repeat length and clinical features of Huntington's disease. *Nat Genet* 1993;4(4):398–403.
10. Duyao M, Ambrose C, Myers R, et al. Trinucleotide repeat length instability and age of onset in Huntington's disease. *Nat Genet* 1993;4(4):387–392.
11. Roos RAC. Neuropathology of Huntington's chorea. In: Vinken PJ, Bruyn GW, Klawans HL, eds. *Extrapyramidal disorders.* Amsterdam: Elsevier Science, 1986:315.
12. Albin RL, Reiner A, Anderson KD, et al. Preferential loss of striato-external pallidal neurons in presymptomatic Huntington's disease. *Ann Neurol* 1992;31(4):425–430.
13. Titica J, Van Bogaert L. Heredo-degenerative hemiballismus. *Brain* 1946;69:251–263.
14. Koide R, Ikeuchi T, Onodera O, et al. Unstable expansion of CAG repeat in hereditary dentatorubral-pallidoluysian atrophy (DRPLA). *Nat Genet* 1994;6:9–13.
15. Nagafuchi S, Yanagisawa H, Sato K, et al. Dentatorubral and pallidoluysian atrophy expansion of the unstable CAG trinucleotide on chromosome 12p. *Nat Genet* 1994;6:14–18.
16. Harper PS. Benign hereditary chorea: clinical and genetic aspects. *Clin Genet* 1978;13:85–95.
17. Haerer AF, Currier RD, Jackson JF. Hereditary nonprogressive chorea of early onset. *N Engl J Med* 1967;276:1220–1224.
18. Fernandez M, Raskind W, Matsushita M, et al. Hereditary benign chorea: clinical and genetic features of a distinct disease. *Neurology* 2001;57(1):106–110.
19. Stevenson VL, Hardie RJ. Acanthocytosis and neurological disorders. *J Neurol* 2001;248(2):87–94.
20. Lewis-Johnsson J. Chorea: its nomenclature, etiology, and epi-

demiology in a clinical material from Malmhus County. *Acta Paediatr* 1949;76:1910–1944.

21. Marques-Dias MJ, Mercadante MT, Tucker D, et al. Sydenham's chorea. *Psychiatric Clin North Am* 1997;20(4):809–820.
22. Shannon KM, Fenichel GM. Pimozide treatment of Sydenham's chorea. *Neurology* 1990;40(1):186.
23. Alvarez LA, Novak G. Valproic acid in the treatment of Sydenham chorea. *Pediatric Neurology* 1985;1(5):317–319.
24. Shenker DM, Grossman HJ, Klawans JL. Treatment of Sydenham's chorea with Haloperidol. *Dev Med Child Neurol* 1973;15:19–24.
25. Lee PH, Nam HS, Lee KY, et al. Serial brain SPECT images in a case of Sydenham chorea. *Arch Neurol* 1999;56(2):237–240.
26. Dilenge ME, Shevell MI, Dinh L. Restricted unilateral Sydenham's chorea: reversible contralateral striatal hypermetabolism demonstrated on single photon emission computed tomographic scanning. *J Child Neurol* 1999;14(8):509–513.
27. Emery ES, Vieco PT. Sydenham chorea: magnetic resonance imaging reveals permanent basal ganglia injury. *Neurology* 1997;48(2):531–533.
28. Bruyn GW, Padberg G. Chorea and systemic lupus erythematosus. *Eur Neurol* 1984;23:278–290.
29. Khamashta Ma, Gil A, Anciones B, et al. Chorea in systemic lupus erythematosus: association with antiphospholipid antibodies. *Ann Rheumatol Dis* 1988;47:681–683.
30. Asherson RA, Derksen RHWM, Harris EN, et al. Chorea in systemic lupus erythematosus and "lupus-like" disease: association with antiphospholipid antibodies. *Semin Arthr Rheum* 1987;16:253–259.
31. Cervera R, Asherson RA, Font J, et al. Chorea in the antiphospholipid syndrome: clinical, radiologic, and immunologic characteristics of 50 patients from our clinics and the recent literature. *Medicine* 1997;76(3):203–212.
32. Bussone G, La Mantia L, Boiardi A, et al. Chorea in Behçet's syndrome. *J Neurol* 1982;227:89–92.
33. Ford RG, Siekert RG. Central nervous system manifestations of periarteritis nodosa. *Neurology* 1965;15:114–122.
34. Schotland DL, Wolf SM, White HH, et al. Neurological aspects of Behçet's disease. *Am J Med* 1963;34:544–553.
35. Sigal LH. The neurological presentation of vasculitic and rheumatological syndromes. *Medicine* 1987;66:157–180.
36. Dabon-Almirante CL, Surks MI. Clinical and laboratory diagnosis of thyrotoxicosis. *Endocrinol Metab Clin North Am* 1998;27(1):25–35.
37. Burstein L, Breningstall GN. Movement disorders in bacterial meningitis. *J Pediatr* 1986;109(2):260–264.
38. Alarcon F, Duenas G, Cevallos N, et al. Movement disorders in 30 patients with tuberculous meningitis. *Mov Disord* 2000;15(3):561–569.
39. Pardo J, Marcos A, Bhathal H, et al. Chorea as a form of presentation of human immunodeficiency virus–associated dementia complex. *Neurology* 1998;50(2):568–569.
40. Gallo BV, Shulman LM, Weiner WJ, et al. HIV encephalitis presenting with severe generalized chorea. *Neurology* 1996;46(4):1163–1165.
41. Tepper SJ, Haas JF. Prevalence of tardive dyskinesia. *J Clin Psychiatry* 1979;40(12):508–516.
42. Klawans HL. The pharmacology of tardive dyskinesias. *Am J Psychiatry* 1973;130:82–86.
43. Rangwani SR, Gupta S, Burke WJ, et al. Improvement of debilitating tardive dyskinesia with risperidone. *Ann Clin Psychiatry* 1996;8:27–29.
44. Limperopoulos C, Majnemer A, Shevell MI, et al. Neurodevelopmental status of newborns and infants with congenital heart defects before and after open heart surgery. *J Pediatrics* 2000;137(5):638–645.
45. Robinson RO, Samuels M, Pohl KR. Choreic syndrome after cardiac surgery. *Arch Dis Child* 1988;63:1466–1469.
46. Lee BC, Hwang SH, Chang GY. Hemiballismus-hemichorea in older diabetic women: a clinical syndrome with MRI correlation. *Neurology* 1999;52(3):646–648.
47. Scott BL, Jankovic J. Delayed-onset progressive movement disorders after static brain lesions. *Neurology* 1996;46(1):68–74.
48. Robin JJ. Paroxysmal choreoathetosis following head injury. *Ann Neurol* 1977;2:447–448.
49. Schwartz A, Henneriei M, Weggener OH. Delayed choreoathetosis following acute carbon monoxide poisoning. *Neurology* 1985;35:98–99.

BALLISM

FRANCISCO GRANDAS

Ballism is a term derived from a Greek word meaning "to throw." It refers to a relatively rare hyperkinetic movement disorder characterized by involuntary, irregular, wide-amplitude, flinging, violent, coarse, and poorly patterned movements due to contraction of the proximal limb and associate axial muscles (1,2).

According to its topographic distribution ballism can be classified as (a) monoballism—ballism confined to one extremity; (b) hemiballism—ballism involving one side of the body; (c) paraballism—ballism concerning the lower limbs; (d) bilateral ballism—ballism involving both sides of the body (1).

Bilateral ballism is extremely rare. In fact, there are scarcely 20 cases reported in the literature (2–6).

The incidence of hemiballism is not yet established. The figure of 1 in 500,000 of the general population has been proposed (7), which may explain the small size of the reported series. For instance, Dewey and Jankovic (8) found only 21 cases out of 3,084 patients evaluated in a movement disorders clinic of a large American hospital over a 9-year period, and more recently Vidakovic et al. (9) reported 25 patients with hemiballism seen in Belgrade from 1983 to 1992.

The boundaries between ballism and chorea are blurred. Chorea is characterized by continuous, random, jerking movements involving mainly distal muscles. However, ballistic and choreiform movements may coexist in many patients, and it is not uncommon for ballism to evolve into more distal and lower amplitude chorea (8). Furthermore, both chorea and ballism can be observed in the same animal models of induction of dyskinesias (10). Thus, chorea and ballism are currently viewed as parts of the clinical spectrum of the same basic disease processes (8), and consequently the term hemiballism-hemichorea is frequently used in the literature.

PATHOPHYSIOLOGY

In 1927, Martin (11) reported a patient with hemiballism attributed to a lesion in the contralateral subthalamic nucleus (STN), or corpus Luysi. Since then, many cases of hemiballism have been described in association with focal lesions of the STN or its pathways, as demonstrated by neuroimaging techniques or postmortem pathologic studies (1,12). In addition, contralateral hemiballism-hemichorea can be elicited in monkeys by electrolytic lesions of STN, destroying at least 20% of the nucleus (13), or by small excitotoxic lesions of the STN by injecting ibotenic acid into its dorsolateral region (14). Moreover, Crossman et al. (15) produced hemiballism-hemichorea in the monkey by injecting bicucculine—a γ-aminobutyric acid (GABA) antagonist—into the STN, thus inducing a depolarization block of subthalamic neurons resulting in functional inactivation of the nucleus.

These clinical and experimental observations have reinforced the idea that the STN has a key role in the pathophysiology of ballism.

According to the classical model of basal ganglia function, selective damage of the STN or its connections induces hemiballism due to reduced excitatory drive from the STN to the internal segment of the globus pallidus and substantia nigra pars reticulata, which results in decreased pallidothalamic inhibition, leading to enhanced thalamocortical activation.

However, the concept that a STN lesion inexorably causes ballism has been challenged by the apparent paradox of the functional surgery on the STN for the treatment of Parkinson's disease.

Although high-frequency stimulation of the STN in parkinsonian patients may induce a variety of dyskinesias, including ballistic movements (16), two recent papers have reported a low incidence of hemiballism in patients who underwent unilateral STN lesions for the treatment of Parkinson's disease with severe motor complications (17,18).

Why did not all these patients develop hemiballism? Two possible explanations have been proposed: Guridi and Obeso (19) suggested that the parkinsonian state is characterized by an increased threshold for the induction of dyskinesias after STN lesioning; on the other hand, Lozano (20) pointed out that hemiballism did not occur because the lesions probably extended beyond the limits of the STN, involving the pallidofugal pathways as well. The latter hypothesis is consistent with findings from experimental studies in monkeys, in which lesions involving both the STN and the internal segment of the globus pallidus or the pallidal fugal pathways did not induce ballism (21). In addition, the resolution of hemiballism in humans with pallidotomy (22) also supports this reasoning. Thus, the integrity of the pallidum (internal segment) or its outflow seems necessary for ballism to occur.

Ballism has also been associated with lesions of the basal ganglia outside the STN or its pathways, such as caudate nucleus, putamen, thalamus, or the external segment of the globus pallidus (1,12,23).

Several recent neurophysiologic observations have shed light on the complexity of basal ganglia dysfunction in ballism. Microelectrode recordings in the basal ganglia of patients with hemiballism have shown reduced mean discharge rates in both segments of the globus pallidus. Neurons in the internal segment of the globus pallidus demonstrated irregularly grouped discharges and intermittent pauses, and very few responded to passive manipulations of the limbs (22,24). The irregularity in pallidal activity probably interferes with thalamocortical signal transmission and disrupts the normal spatiotemporal pattern of cortical neuronal activity—perhaps due to alteration of temporal coding or to development of uncontrolled increases in synchronization—leading to errors in cortical output and disordered motor control (24).

More striking is the rare association between ballism and cortical lesions, involving usually the parietal cortex (9,25–27). In one of these cases (27), a parietal cerebral infarction was demonstrated by magnetic resonance imaging (MRI), but a single photon emission computed tomography (SPECT) study using ^{99}Tc-hexamethylpropyleneamineoxime (HMPAO) showed a global reduction of perfusion in the ipsilateral hemisphere, including the basal ganglia. Therefore, basal ganglia ischemia might have had an additional role in causing the ballistic movements.

Of more difficult understanding are the unusual reported patients with hemiballism secondary to ipsilateral lesions of the STN or the striatum (28–30). In some cases, the majority of vascular etiology, the possibility of bilateral lesions could not be completely ruled out by neuroimaging techniques. Nevertheless, bilateral connections between the pedunculopontine nucleus and the STN, bilateral cortical projections, or even commissural connections between both STNs have been postulated as possible causes of the ipsilateral presentation of hemiballism in these patients (28–30).

Bilateral ballism has been related to bilateral lesions of the basal ganglia, as well as to immunologic or metabolic disorders in which a widespread neurologic impairment can be expected (9,31,32).

ETIOLOGY

Most cases of ballism result from structural lesions. Virtually any lesion properly situated in the STN, its connections, or in the other aforementioned structures may induce ballism (Table 16.1). Stroke, which is the most common cause of hemiballism, is responsible for the disorder in 50% to 75% of cases (8,9,12), usually consisting of infarction of lacunar type or, less often, hemorrhage. In general, it has been estimated that hemiballism occurs in 0.5% of strokes (33).

The rarer vascular causes include arteriovenous malformation (34), venous angioma (35), and subarachnoid hem-

TABLE 16.1. ETIOLOGY OF HEMIBALLISM

A) Structural Lesions
  Vascular
  - Infarction[a]
  - Hemorrhage
  - Arteriovenous malformation
  - Transient ischemic attack
  Neoplastic
  - Astrocytoma
  - Meningioma
  - Ependymal cyst
  - Metastasis[a]
  - Paraneoplastic syndrome
  Infectious
  - AIDS
  - Toxoplasmosis
  - Tuberculoma
  - Syphilis
  - Cryptococcal meningitis
  - Influenza A
  - Encephalitis
  Demyelinating lesions in multiple sclerosis[a]
  Immunologic disorders
  - Sydenham's chorea
  - Systemic lupus erythematosus
  - Behçet's disease
  - Antiphospholipid antibody syndrome
  - Fisher's and Guillain-Barré syndromes[a]
  Complication of neurosurgical procedure
  - Stereotactic functional surgery for Parkinson's disease
  - Intraventricular meningioma
  - Ventriculoperitoneal shunting[a]
  Head trauma
  Bilateral basal ganglia calcifications
  Neurodegenerative disorders[a]
B) Metabolic Disorders
  Nonketotic hyperglycemia[a]
  Hypoglycemia
  Hypocalcemia (hypoparathyroidism)
  Drugs:
  - Oral contraceptives[a]
  - Phenytoin
  - Ibuprofen
  - Levodopa

[a]Reported cases of bilateral ballism as well.

orrhage (36). In addition, brief episodes of hemiballism may be a manifestation of transient ischemic attack (37), theoretically in either carotid or vertebrobasilar territories. This region of the STN receives its vascular supply from the carotid artery via the anterior choroidal artery as well as from the basilar artery via the posterior choroidal artery (1), albeit neuroimaging studies have shown that some of these transient episodes are based on permanent infarcts (38).

Besides common vascular risk factors such as hypertension or diabetes mellitus, intravenous heroin overdose (39), marked hypotension during spinal anesthesia (40) and liver transplantation (41) have also been related to stroke-induced hemiballism.

Neoplastic lesions causing ballism include primary tumors such as astrocytoma or meningioma (12,25,30), ependymal cyst (42), and metastases of different tumor types (1,4,43). Recently, Kujawa et al. (44) reported a patient with ballistic-choreic movements as a paraneoplastic syndrome of renal cancer, in whom a biopsy specimen of basal ganglia showed focal encephalitic changes but not malignant neoplasma.

There have been a number of patients with ballism secondary to AIDS and cerebral toxoplasmosis (8,45–47). Other reported infectious causes of ballism are tuberculoma, syphilis (1), cryptococcal meningitis (48), encephalitis (8,9), influenza A infection (49), and minor infections in children with static encephalopathy (50).

Ballism has also been caused by demyelinating lesions in multiple sclerosis (32,51). There are reported cases of ballism associated with immunologic disorders such as Sydenham's chorea (9,52), systemic lupus erithematosus (8,9), Behçet's disease (1), antiphospholipid antibody syndrome (53), and with overlapping Fisher's and Guillain-Barré syndromes (5).

Iatrogenic hemiballism may occur as a complication of stereotactic operations for Parkinson's disease (1,16,19). It has been described associated with intraventricular meningioma surgery (54) and with shunt insertion in a patient with normal-pressure hydrocephalus (55).

Several cases of ballism are related to head trauma, some times following a trivial head injury (1,56,57). However, in one of these patients the autopsy showed a lesion of the posterior portion of the medial segment of the globus pallidus and atrophy of STN (56). Other structural lesions related to ballism are bilateral basal ganglia calcifications and tuberous sclerosis (9).

There are a few reports of ballism associated with neurodegenerative disorders (58–60). In these cases ballism was part of a more widespread clinical picture, reflecting nerve cell loss and gliosis in a variety of structures including the substantia nigra, globus pallidus and STN.

Besides structural lesions, ballism has been reported in the context of metabolic disorders (Table 16.1). Among them, nonketotic hyperglycemia deserves special consideration due to the increasing number of cases describing this association (1,61–64). This syndrome is characterized by the occurrence of hemiballism-hemichorea of sudden onset in elderly, poorly controlled diabetic patients, who are in a nonketotic hyperglycemic state. In these patients a contralateral striatal hyperintensity is seen on T1-weighted MRI, usually associated with hypointensity on T2-weighted images (61). The nature of this MRI abnormality is controversial. Some authors (62) suggested petequial hemorrhages secondary to metabolic changes in the basal ganglia whilst others have found contralateral basal ganglia hypoperfusion using SPECT techniques (63). It has been speculated that selective damage of GABA/enkephalin-containing inhibitory neurons in the striatum may occur under condition of ischemia and nonketotic hyperglycemia, leading to disinhibition of the external segment of the globus pallidus and to inhibition of the STN (61). The necropsy of one of such patients showed multiple foci of recent infarcts associated with reactive astrocytes in the putamen contralateral to the hemiballism (64).

Isolated cases of hemiballism related to hypoglycemia (65) and hypocalcemia secondary to idiopathic hypoparathyroidism (66) have been reported.

Finally, there are patients who have experienced drug-induced ballism. The offending drugs were oral contraceptives, phenytoin, ibuprofen, and levodopa (in parkinsonian patients) (1,2). It has been suggested that patients with pre-existing basal ganglia abnormalities are more susceptible to suffer drug-induced hemiballism (2).

CLINICAL FEATURES AND PROGNOSIS

Ballism is one of the most striking hyperkinesias that can be seen in clinical neurology. The clinical picture of ballism in itself seems to be independent of the many known causes that can induce this abnormal involuntary movements, classically described as uncontrollable jerking, flinging, flailing or kicking (1). Ballistic movements are mainly proximal with large rotatory displacements of extremities, in some cases so violent that can provoke damage of the limbs if they bump against bed rails, furniture or walls, as well as lead to progressive exhaustion in some patients. These throwing movements diminish or disappear during sleep, generally increase with anxiety and are evident at rest. Some patients can voluntarily suppress the movements for brief periods of time, but the majority are functionally impaired for motor activities such as walking or eating. Arm and leg may be equally affected, but usually ballistic movements predominate in one extremity.

Ballism may co-exist with a wide variety of neurological and neuropsychological symptoms reflecting the extent of the lesions of the underlying disease (1). Besides chorea, other abnormal involuntary movements such as dystonia, facial and oromandibular-lingual dyskinesias, parkinsonism, bradykinesia or myoclonus may be seen in patients with ballism (8,9).

The onset of ballism is related to the underlying disease. Thus, ballism of vascular origin usually begins suddenly whereas ballistic movements of subacute onset and progressive course point to inflammatory, metabolic or neoplastic etiologies (8,9). In some patients ballism presents as paroxysmal recurrent attacks, as a type of transient ischemic attack (37) or as a manifestation of systemic lupus erythematosus (8).

The age of onset of ballism also depends on the underlying disease. Stroke-induced ballism commonly occurs in the elderly, whereas ballism related to infectious or inflammatory factors generally develops in younger patients (9).

As mentioned above, neuroimaging techniques—CT and especially MRI—can demonstrate structural lesions in patients with ballism. Even in metabolic disorders it is possible to show basal ganglia abnormalities by MRI or metabolic or perfusion changes in these structures by PET or SPECT techniques. However, in about one third of the cases reported in recent series of patients with ballism, no structural lesions could be demonstrated by neuroimaging techniques (8,9).

In contrast to the older literature in which ballism was associated with a bad prognosis, mainly due to infectious complications or exhaustion (1), modern series have shown that ballism has, in general, a relatively good prognosis (8,9). Nevertheless, the outcome of patients with this motor disorder depends to a great extent on the underlying disease. Thus, many patients with stroke-induced ballism may improve in the course of their illness; such patients may even experience spontaneous remissions, as may those with immunologic diseases, such as central nervous system lupus (8,9), or metabolic disorders, such as nonketotic hyperglycemia, in whom correction of hyperglycemia results in reduction of the abnormal movements (67). In contrast, patients with ballistic movements due to metastatic neoplasms, AIDS, or infectious complications of AIDS have had an ominous outcome (8,9).

THERAPY

Whenever possible, the management of ballism should be directed to the underlying causes. For example, hemiballism related to lupus erythematosus may respond to corticoids (8), subcortical abscesses can improve with antibiotics or surgery (8), and hemiballism secondary to a basal ganglia arteriovenous malformation may disappear after radiosurgery (34).

Although perhaps overemphasized in classical descriptions of ballism, supportive care is important in the clinical management of this disorder. Measures to prevent accidental self-injury by padding furniture and bed rails or by using soft restraints, in addition to other general measures regarding hydration, nutrition, or reduction of medical complications, should be considered in individual patients. These supportive measures are, nevertheless, adjunctive to pharmacologic or surgical treatments directed to the symptomatic relief of ballism.

Pharmacologic Treatment

Due to the rarity of ballism no pharmacologic placebo-controlled studies involving a significant number of patients are available. Information about the efficacy of different drugs comes from reports of small series or single cases. Moreover, spontaneous remission of this movement disorder must be taken into consideration when assessing any clinical improvement putatively related to drugs.

Several drugs have been reported to be successful in the treatment of patients with ballism. Among them, clinical amelioration has been consistently associated with the use of antidopaminergic drugs, mainly haloperidol (1 to 5 mg/day), although other striatal dopamine receptor blockers, such as perphenazine, chlorpromazine, pimozide, risperidone, and the substituted benzamides tiapride and sulpiride, have also been reported to relieve ballism either partially or completely (1,2,8,9,68). In addition, a handful of patients have experienced stable improvement after taking the atypical neuroleptic clozapine, at a dosage of about 50 mg/day, with regular monitoring of white cell counts (69,70). Usually, the response to dopamine receptor–blocking agents can be seen in a few days.

Presynaptic monoamine depleters, such as reserpine and tetrabenazine, have also improved ballistic movements in some patients (1). The latter drug has the advantage of a reduced risk of development of tardive dyskinesia when given chronically, which makes tetrabenazine (50 to 125 mg/day) a suitable drug for long-term management ballism.

The rationale for antidopaminergic drugs is that dopaminergic activity inhibits STN neuronal firing and, therefore, a decrease in dopaminergic activity should result in reduction of the ballistic movements (2).

Another possible pharmacologic approach is based on increasing GABAergic neurotransmission. Since this inhibitory neurotransmitter is involved in the control of basal ganglia ouput—projections from the internal segment of globus pallidus to thalamus are GABAergic—an augmented GABAergic tone might reduce the activity of thalamocortical projections and therefore could reduce ballistic movements. Indeed, some benzodiazepines (diazepam, clonazepam), progabide, sodium valproate, and gabapentine—all drugs with GABAergic properties—have been reported to bring about improvement in patients with ballism (1,2,8,71), although in other cases the clinical response to sodium valproate was inconsistent (72).

Isolated cases of ballism have ameliorated with a miscellany of drugs, including amitriptyline and trihexyphenidyl hydrochloride (8).

Recently, Dressler et al. (73) injected type A botulinum toxin into selected muscles of a patient with hemiballism, obtaining a reduction of involuntary movements after 5 days and full therapeutic effect after 2 weeks, without systemic side effects.

Surgical Treatment

The modern functional stereotactic surgery, implemented by recent advances in neuroimaging and neurophysiologic techniques, has become a real therapeutic option with low morbidity for patients with persistent disabling ballism refractory to medical therapy.

Stereotactic thalamotomy, targeting the ventralis intermedius nucleus, has been reported to improve hemiballism, with mild persistent deficits (contralateral weakness) (74). A combined lesion of the base of the ventrolateral thalamus plus the zona incerta also induced persistent improvement of hemiballism in several cases, with mild morbidity (75). The reason for targeting this area was to include in the lesion the projections from the medial pallidum to the ventrolateral thalamus as well, as the lenticular fasciculus and the ansa lenticularis pass between the zona incerta and the basal thalamus (75).

Besides ablative procedures, chronic high-frequency stimulation of the ventrolateral complex of the thalamus was also successful in controlling contralateral hemiballism in a few patients (76,77).

Finally, Krauss and Mundinger (75) and Suarez et al. (22) have reported, in patients with unremitting and medically intractable hemiballismus, a reduction and even abolition of involuntary movements after pallidotomy, involving the internal segment of the nucleus, without significant side effects.

REFERENCES

1. Buruma OJ, Lakke JP. Ballism. In: Vinken PJ, Bruyn GW, Klawans HL, eds. *Handbook of clinical neurology,* vol 49. Amsterdam: Elsevier, 1986:369–380.
2. Shanon KM. Hemiballismus. *Clin Neuropharmacol* 1990;13: 413–425.
3. Walker FO, Hunt P. Ballism: an association with ventriculo-peritoneal shunting. *Neurology* 1990;40:1004.
4. Laing RW, Howell SJ. Acute bilateral ballism in a patient with intravascular dissemination of gastric carcinoma. *Neuropathol Appl Neurobiol* 1992;18:201–205.
5. Odaka M, Yuki N, Hirata K. Bilateral ballism in a patient with overlapping Fisher's and Guillain-Barré syndromes. *J Neurol Neurosurg Psychiatry* 1999;67:206–208.
6. Knirsh UI, Bachus R, Gosztonyi G, et al. Clinicopathological study of atypical motor neuron disease with vertical gaze and ballism. *Acta Neuropathol* 2000;100:342–346.
7. Meyers R. Ballism. In: Vinken PJ, Bruyn GW, eds. *Handbook of clinical neurology,* vol 6. Amsterdam: Elsevier, 1968:476–490.
8. Dewey RB, Jankovic J. Hemiballism-hemichorea: clinical and pharmacological findings in 21 patients. *Arch Neurol* 1989;46: 862–870.
9. Vidakovic A, Dragasevic N, Kostic S. Hemiballism: report of 25 cases. *J Neurol Neurosurg Psychiatry* 1994;57:945–949.
10. Mitchell IJ, Sambrook MA, Crossman AR. Subcortical changes in the regional uptake of [^{3}H]-2-deoxyglucose in the brain of the monkey during experimental choreiform dyskinesia elicited by injection of a gamma-aminobutyric acid antagonist into the subthalamic nucleus. *Brain* 1985;108:405–422.
11. Martin JP. Hemichorea resulting from a local lesion of the brain (the syndrome of the body of Luys). *Brain* 1927;50: 637–651.
12. Lee MS, Marsden CD. Review: movement disorders following lesions of the thalamus or subthalamic region. *Mov Disord* 1994; 9:493–507.
13. Whittier JR, Mettler FA. Studies on subthalamus of rhesus monkeys: hyperkinesia and other physiological effects of subthalamic lesions, with special reference to the subthalamic nucleus of Luys. *J Comp Neurol* 1949;90:319–372.
14. Hamada Y, DeLong MR. Excitotoxic acid lesions of the primate subthalamic nucleus result in transient dyskinesias of the contralateral limbs. *J Neurophysiol* 1992;68:1850–1858.
15. Crossman AR, Sambrook MA, Jackson A. Experimental hemichorea/hemiballism in the monkey: studies on the intracerebral site of action in a drug-induced dyskinesia. *Brain* 1984;107: 579–596.
16. Limousin P, Pollak P, Hoffmann D, et al. Abnormal involuntary movements induced by subthalamic nucleus stimulation in parkinsonian patients. *Mov Disord* 1996;11:231–235.
17. Alvarez A, Macias R, Guridi J, et al. Dorsal subthalamotomy for Parkinson's disease. *Mov Disord* 2001;16:72–78.
18. Barlas O, Hanagasi H, Imer M, et al. Do unilateral ablative lesions of the subthalamic nucleus in parkinsonian patients lead to hemiballism? *Mov Disord* 2001;16:306–310.
19. Guridi J, Obeso JA. The subthalamic nucleus, hemiballismus and Parkinson's disease: reappraisal of a neurosurgical dogma. *Brain* 2001;124:5–19.
20. Lozano AM. The subthalamic nucleus: myth and opportunities. *Mov Disord* 2001;16:183–184.
21. Carpenter MB, Whittier JR, Mettler FA. Analysis of choreoid hyperkinesia in the rhesus monkey. *J Comp Neurol* 1950;92: 93–322.
22. Suarez JL, Metman LV, Reich SG, et al. Pallidotomy for hemiballismus: efficacy and characteristics of neuronal activity. *Ann Neurol* 1997;42:807–811.
23. Kulisevsky J, Berthier ML, Pujol J. Hemiballismus and secondary mania following a right thalamic infarction. *Neurology* 1993;43: 1422–1424.
24. Vitek JL, Chockkan V, Jian-Yu Z, et al. Neuronal activity in the basal ganglia in patients with generalized dystonia and hemiballismus. *Ann Neurol* 1999;46:22–35.
25. Gilon D, Constantini S, Reches A. Hemiballism as a presentation of a meningioma. *Eur Neurol* 1990;30:277–278.
26. Ferbert A, Rickert HB, Biniek R, et al. Complex hyperkinesia during recovery from left temporoparietal cortical infarction. *Mov Disord* 1990;5:78–82.
27. Mizushima N, Matsumoto YC, Amakawa T, et al. A case of hemichorea-hemiballism associated with parietal lobe infarction. *Eur Neurol* 1997;37:65–66.
28. Borgohain R, Singh AK, Thadani R, et al. Hemiballismus due to an ipsilateral striatal haemorrhage: an unusual localization. *J Neurol Sci* 1995;130:22–24.
29. Crozier S, Lehericy S, Verstichel P, et al. Transient hemiballism/hemichorea due to an ipsilateral subthalamic nucleus infarction. *Neurology* 1996;46:267–268.
30. Krauss JK, Pohle T, Borremans J. Hemichorea and hemiballism associated with contralateral hemiparesis and ipsilateral basal ganglia lesions. *Mov Disord* 1999;3:497–501.
31. Hoogstraten MC, Lakke JP, Zwarts MJ. Bilateral ballism: a rare syndrome. *J Neurol* 1986;233:25–29.
32. Masucci EF, Saini N, Kurtzke JK. Bilateral ballism in multiple sclerosis. *Neurology* 1989;39:1641–1642.
33. Ghika-Schmid F, Ghika J, Regli F, et al. Hyperkinetic movement disorders during and after acute stroke: the Lausanne Stroke Registry. *J Neurol Sci* 1997;146:109–116.
34. Kurita H, Kawamoto S, Sasaki T, et al. Relief of hemiballism

from a basal ganglia arteriovenous malformation after radiosurgery. *Neurology* 1999;52:188–190.

35. Burke L, Berenberg RA, Kim KS. Choreo-ballismus: a nonhemorrhage complication of venous angiomas. *Surg Neurol* 1984; 21:245–248.

36. Muenter MD. Hemiballismus. *Neurology* 1984;34[Suppl 1]:129.

37. Margolin DI, Marsden CD. Episodic dyskinesias and transient cerebral ischemia. *Neurology* 1982;32:1379–1380.

38. Defebvre L, Destee A, Cassim F, et al. Transient hemiballism and striatal infarct. *Stroke* 1990;21:967–968.

39. Vila N, Chamorro A. Ballistic movements due to ischemic infarcts after intravenous heroin overdose: report of two cases. *Clin Neurol Neurosurg* 1997;99:259–262.

40. Itoh H, Shibata K, Nitta E, et al. Hemiballism-hemichorea from marked hypotension during spinal anesthesia. *Acta Anaesthesiol Scand* 1998;42:133–135.

41. Provenzale JM, Glass JP. MRI in hemiballism due to subthalamic nucleus hemorrhage: an unusual complication of liver transplantation. *Neuroradiology* 1996;38[Suppl 1]:75–77.

42. Bejar JM, Kepes J, Koller WC. Hemiballism and tremor due to ependymal cyst. *Mov Disord* 1992;7:370–372.

43. Zianinia T, Resnik E. Hemiballism abd brain metastases from squamous cell carcinoma of the cervix. *Gynecol Oncol* 1999;75:289–292.

44. Kujawa KA, Niemi VR, Tomasi MA, et al. Ballistic-choreic movements as the presenting feature of renal cancer. *Arch Neurol* 2001;58:1133–1135.

45. Nath A, Jankovic J, Pettigrew LC. Movement disorders and AIDS. *Neurology* 1987;37:37–41.

46. Sanchez-Ramos JR, Factor S, Weiner W, et al. Hemichorea-hemiballismus associated with acquired immune deficiency syndrome and cerebral toxoplasmosis. *Mov Disord* 1989;4:266–273.

47. Martínez-Martin P. Hemichorea-hemiballism in AIDS. *Mov Disord* 1990;5:180.

48. Namer IJ, Tan E, Akalin E, et al. A case of hemiballismus during cryptococcal meningitis. *Rev Neurol* 1990;146:153–154.

49. Yoshikawa H, Oda Y. Hemiballismus associated with influenza A infection. *Brain Dev* 1999;21:132–134.

50. Beran-Koehn MA, Zupanc ML, Patterson MC, et al. Violent recurrent ballism associated with infections in two children with static encephalopathy. *Mov Disord* 2000;15:570–574.

51. Riley D, Lang AE. Hemiballism in multiple sclerosis. *Mov Disord* 1988;3:88–94.

52. Konagaya M, Konagaya Y. MRI in hemiballism due to Sydenham's chorea. *J Neurol Neurosurg Psychiatry* 1992;55:238–239.

53. Okun MS, Jummani RR, Carney PR. Antiphospholid-associated recurrent chorea and ballism in a child with cerebral palsy. *Pediatr Neurol* 2000;23:62–63.

54. Krauss JK, Borremans JJ, Pohle T, et al. Movement disorders following nonfunctional neurosurgery. *J Neurosurg* 1999;90:883–890.

55. Walker FO, Hunt VP. Ballism: an association with ventriculoperitoneal shunting. *Neurology* 1990;40:1004.

56. King RB, Fuller C, Collins GH. Delayed onset of hemidystonia and hemiballismus following head injury: a clinicopathological correlation. *J Neurosurg* 2001;94:309–314.

57. Chaynes P, Bousquet P, Fabre N, et al. Transient hemiballismus secondary to minimal head trauma. *Rev Neurol* 2001;157: 323–324.

58. Knirsch UI, Bachus R, Gosztonyi G, et al. Clinicopathological

59. Calopa M, Ferrer I, Villanueva P, et al. Degeneración bilateral y asimétrica del estriado como causa de hemibalismo senil. *Neurologia* 1997;12:92–95.

60. Steiger MJ, Pires M, Scaravilli F, et al. Hemiballism and chorea in a patient with parkinsonism due to a multisystem degeneration. *Mov Disord* 1992;7:71–73.

61. Hashimoto T, Hanyu N, Yahikozawa H, et al. Persistent hemiballism with striatal hyperintensity on T1-weighted MRI in a diabetic patient: a 6-year follow-up study. *J Neurol Sci* 1999; 165:178–181.

62. Oerlemans WG, Moll LC. Non-ketotic hyperglycemia in a young woman presenting as hemiballismus-hemichorea. *Acta Neurol Scan* 1999;100:411–414.

63. Chang MH, Li JY, Lee SR, et al. Non-ketotic hyperglycemic chorea: a SPECT study. *J Neurol Neurosurg Psychiatry* 1996;60: 428–430.

64. Ohara S, Nakagawa S, Tabata K, et al. Hemiballism with hyperglycemia and striatal T1-MRI hyperintensity: an autopsy report. *Mov Disord* 2001;16:521–525.

65. Sweeney BJ, Edgecombe J, Churchill DR, et al. Choreoathetosis/ballismus associated with pentamidine-induced hypoglycemia in a patient with the acquired immunodeficiency syndrome. *Arch Neurol* 1994;51:723–725.

66. Dragasevic N, Petkovic-Medved B, Stevel M, et al. Paroxysmal hemiballism and idiopathic hypoparathyroidism. *J Neurol* 1997; 244:388–401.

67. Lee BC, Hwang SH, Chang GY. Hemiballismus-hemichorea in older diabetic women: a clinical syndrome with MRI correlation. *Neurology* 1999;52:646–648.

68. Evidente VG, Gwin-Hardy K, Caviness JN, et al. Risperidone is effective in severe hemichorea/hemiballismus. *Mov Disord* 1999; 14:377–379.

69. Bashir K, Manyam BV. Clozapine for the control of hemiballismus. *Clin Neuropharmacol* 1994;17:477–480.

70. Stojanovic M, Sternic N, Kostic VS. Clozapine in hemiballismus: report of two cases. *Clin Neuropharmacol* 1997;20:171–174.

71. Kothare SV, Pollack P, Kulberg AG, et al. Gabapentine treatment in a child with delayed-onset hemichorea/hemiballismus. *Pediatr Neurol* 2000;22:68–71.

72. Sethi KD, Patel B. Inconsistent response to divalproex sodium in hemichorea/hemiballism. *Neurology* 1990;40:1630–1631.

73. Dressler D, Wittstock M, Benecke R. Treatment of persistent hemiballism with botulinum toxin type A. *Mov Disord* 2000;15: 1281–1282.

74. Cardoso F, Jankovic J, Grossman RG, et al. Outcome after stereotactic thalamotomy for dystonia and hemiballismus. *Neurosurgery* 1995;36:501–507.

75. Krauss JK, Mundinger F. Functional stereotactic surgery for hemiballism. *J Neurosurg* 1996;85:278–286.

76. Tsubokawa T, Katayama Y, Yamamoto T. Control of persistent hemiballismus by chronic thalamic stimulation. *J Neurosurg* 1995;82:501–505.

77. Siegfried J, Lippitz B. Chronic electrical stimulation of the VL-VP complex and of the pallidum in the treatment of movement disorders: personal experience since 1982. *Stereotact Funct Neurosurg* 1994;62:71–75.

17

NEUROLOGIC ASPECTS OF WILSON'S DISEASE: CLINICAL MANIFESTATIONS AND TREATMENT CONSIDERATIONS

PETER LEWITT
RONALD PFEIFFER

Progressive hepatolenticular degeneration, or Wilson's disease (WD), though only a rare cause of movement disorders, occupies an important place in the history of neurology. Over the past century, it has evolved from a confusing, heterogeneous syndrome to a disease entity whose molecular identity is becoming rapidly ascertained. In a 1912 monograph, S. A. Kinnier Wilson, a young neurologist at the National Hospital in Queen Square, elucidated the key features of this previously unrecognized disease (1). His report defined this disorder from extensive analysis of four cases together with reexamination of six cases previously studied by others. Initially termed "progressive lenticular degeneration" and now synonymous with Wilson's name, WD represents one of medical science's successes in deciphering the biochemical and molecular biological basis for a systemic disease.

WD can take on a puzzling array of clinical findings that can be easy to overlook. In Wilson's day, several syndromes had been described corresponding to the same disorder he defined. These included entities termed "tetanoid chorea" by Gowers (2), "pseudosclerosis" by Westphal (3), and Strümpell (4), and "Wohl Lues hereditaria tarde" by Homen (5). Wilson's 1912 report correctly established the relationship between liver involvement and the central nervous system (CNS) disease, and characterized the pathologic changes unique to this disorder. He also offered insights into the basis for the distinctive types of clinical impairment. In his monograph, Wilson made no mention of the corneal opacification now recognized as nearly always present in WD with CNS involvement, nor did he have an inkling as to the role of copper despite tissue color changes suggestive of the presence of this metal. Nonetheless, the description of "progressive lenticular degeneration" initiated a flood of clinical and laboratory research, which eventually transformed this illness from a disabling and ultimately fatal condition to a disorder with several treatment options and the potential for presymptomatic diagnosis.

Since WD is inherited as an autosomal recessive disorder, carriers of the gene develop the disease only if they are homozygous. The gene appears to be fully penetrant: all individuals homozygous for WD will develop some form of the disease (and their siblings have a 25% risk of doing so). It is extremely unlikely for consecutive generations to be affected, although this has been described (6). Inheritance of the WD gene does not appear to dictate the pattern of predilection for different sites of organ involvement, age of onset, or disease severity. The gene for WD has been estimated to be carried in 1 of every 40,000 births. Based on this estimate, the number of homozygotes in the United States would be approximately 5,000 to 6,000 cases and the carrier frequency may be as great as 1% of the population. Hence, the risk for relatives of an affected patient is 1 in 200 for offspring, 1 in 600 for nieces and nephews, and 1 in 800 for first cousins (7).

In the past decade, linkage analysis studies in affected families have shown that there is a single disease locus for WD, residing on chromosome 13 (8). Most aspects of clinical heterogeneity (i.e., hepatic versus neurologic presentations) probably do not seem to be determined by features of genetic heterogeneity (at least at the level of the gene locus) (7). The discovery of the human gene locus at a single marker interval, 13q14.3 (9), identified a mutation in copper- and membrane-binding ATPase called ATP7B. ATP7B is essential for the normal distribution of copper. A large variety of ATP7B mutation types (including frameshift, splice site, missense, and nonsense) can lead to WD (10). A further advance in studying the pathophysiology of WD has been aided by the discovery of an animal homologue, a genetic form of hepatitis in the Long Evans Cinnamon rat (11,12). With this model, which is susceptible to systemic toxicity from copper excess resembling that found in WD, various therapeutic interventions such as hepatocyte transplantation can be explored (13).

The pathophysiology of WD has a unitary theme in a systemic defect of copper metabolism. Copper derived from the diet is normally excreted into the bile (14). All patients with WD are unable to excrete copper to an adequate extent (15–17). The defect in copper excretion is likely a problem of protein complexing, though the exact mechanism has not been determined. WD is not necessarily due to the defect in the production of ceruloplasmin, a liver-derived copper-binding protein whose serum concentrations are generally (but not always) decreased in WD. While a useful diagnostic marker of the disease, ceruloplasmin is generated by a structural gene residing on chromosome 3. Since the gene for WD is on chromosome 13, other mechanisms need to be invoked if a defect in ceruloplasmin synthesis is also involved in the pathophysiology of WD (18).

WD provided the first example of a progressive neurologic deterioration that could be explained by a neurotoxic mechanism linked to a biological defect (19). The disease appears to be solely the outcome from excessive deposition of a dietary mineral, copper, whose presence in trace amounts is necessary for life. Massive amounts of copper are deposited throughout the body at sites where damage to tissues is observed, as shown by radiolabeled copper studies (20). Though WD is a systemic disorder, correction of copper excretion by means of normalizing liver function can produce full recovery, as first demonstrated by successful outcomes with autologous hepatic transplantation (21). However, removing systemic copper by any means can interrupt progression of WD and often succeeds at reversing neurologic deficits. It is unclear if any additional toxicity is conferred by the increased cerebral uptake of iron also demonstrable in WD (22).

TABLE 17.1. SYSTEMIC MANIFESTATIONS OF WILSON'S DISEASE

Brain (atrophy, necrosis, gliosis, demyelination, central pontine myelinolysis)
Liver (cirrhosis, acute hepatitis)
Ophthalmologic (corneal Kayser-Fleischer rings; star-burst cataract of lens)
Heart (cardiomyopathy)
Kidney (renal lithiasis, hematuria, hypercalcuria, nephrocalcinosis) (218,219)
Anemia (acute hemolytic, thrombocytopenia, Heinz body anemia) (220–222)
Bone and joint disorders (rickets, osteoarthritis, recurrent arthritis, bone fragmentation, chondrocalcinosis, osteoporosis, spinal degeneration, spontaneous fractures, spontaneous rupture of Achilles tendon) (38,52,223–228)
Hypoparathyroidism
Hemosiderosis (229)
Pancreatic exocrine and endocrine impairment (99)
Splenic rupture (230)
Acute rhabdomyolysis (231)

Copper is largely bound to protein throughout the body. Brain and liver, the two organs most susceptible to copper toxicity, exert the greatest avidity for copper. Within the brain, gray matter shows high affinity for copper deposition (23). The damage copper can produce throughout the body can result in a number of clinical syndromes, as listed in Table 17.1. These manifestations of WD can begin monosymptomatically or simultaneously with other clinical features. Although its usual clinical presentations are unmistakable, WD has been observed to start in an extremely limited manner. It has been described with focal, asymmetric features, sometimes without further deficit over several years of follow-up (24,25). Missing the opportunity for diagnosis when its signs and symptoms are mild is one of the greatest challenges posed by this treatable disorder (26,27).

MOTOR FEATURES OF NEUROLOGIC IMPAIRMENT

In addition to a thorough description of hepatolenticular degeneration as a clinical syndrome, Wilson gave a detailed analysis of its pathologic imprint on the brain. He further provided a correlation between the motor disorders and the selectivity of its damage to basal ganglia structures. These impairments include dystonic or choreic involuntary movements, tremor, dysarthria, and rigidity. Although the initial presentation of WD can be only one category of movement disorder, the typical case usually involves combinations of each of these motor features. Rarely, other types of movement disorder (such as essential tremor) can coexist in a family with WD (28).

Almost half of all WD patients with neurologic disease first experience problems in their second or third decade of life (25,26). For neurologic involvement in WD, the age of presentation tends to be older than with purely hepatic disease. However, initial neurologic presentations of WD have been described at less than age 5 years or more than age 50 have been described (29–33). Most commonly, juvenile-onset WD tends to present with hepatic damage, whereas older individuals with WD are more likely to have neurologic symptomatology early in the disorder. In younger individuals WD tends to have a more rapid course than in adults (34). Considerable heterogeneity in clinical features can be found in familial involvement in WD. Another puzzling aspect of WD is the marked variety in neurologic presentations. Even with its propensity for asymmetric or focal deficits, virtually all cases of WD have some degree of bilateral pathologic change in the lenticular nuclei. The broad range of neurologic impairments in WD can also be attributed to the sometimes extensive pathologic change beyond the boundaries of the basal ganglia.

A major challenge for an early diagnosis of WD is the recognition of subtle initial clinical features. Variable signs and symptoms that are intermittent or hard to categorize can result in delayed diagnosis. It is important to recognize that in WD the excess copper load can be quite severe even in patients with only mild neurologic impairments. Also, patients with severe liver damage may be lacking any systemic illness or evidence of CNS involvement. Even certain abrupt systemic manifestations of WD (such as hemolytic anemia or liver failure) can appear with little or no change in neurologic impairment. A sudden or gradual decline in hepatic function caused by WD can by itself generate an extrapyramidal movement disorder and encephalopathy apart from the direct damage that copper deposition can inflict on the brain. Pathologic examination can readily distinguish the two disorders. Unlike changes found in WD, hepatic encephalopathy usually is characterized by neuronal damage with a pseudoulegyric pattern but lacking the necrotic changes in the putamen or frontal gyri as found in WD (35) (see below).

Typically, neurologic WD presents insidiously with tremor, dystonia, rigidity, dysarthria, drooling, dysphagia, unsteady gait, and mental deterioration (36). Less commonly, the neurologic syndrome can present more suddenly in association with an irregular fever, emaciation, and a seemingly toxic state. Among the most common initial signs are dysarthria [described by Wilson (37) as "a trifling indistinctness of speech"], clumsiness of the hands, and mental change ("a childishness seen in facile laughter, or irritability, or caprice"). Another series of neurologic WD (44 cases) found 12 presenting predominantly with basal ganglia–related abnormalities, 6 with cerebellar impairment, and 17 with a combination of these (38). Others have made similar observations with the types of neurologic dysfunction (39). The experience of Walshe and Yealland (26) indicated that parkinsonian signs appeared in almost half the patients. Approximately one quarter of presentations involved a "pseudosclerotic" syndrome, resembling a common pattern of multiple sclerosis involvement by causing cerebellar outflow tremor and speech ataxia. The remainder of patients in the latter study (mostly children) presented with primarily choreic or dystonic features. The disruption of dopaminergic neurotransmission in striatal structures, as demonstrated in neuroimaging studies, is probably responsible for the development of parkinsonian features, dystonia, and dyskinesia in WD (40).

Tremor in one or both hands is probably the most common initial symptom of WD (41,42). Tremor can be unilateral or bilateral, near constant or paroxysmal, or initiated only during specific motor tasks. Most commonly the limbs and the head are affected. The tremor in WD can affect limbs at rest, with postural maintenance, or during movement (or any combination of these). Though the action tremor can resemble that observed with cerebellar dysfunction, other signs (such as dysdiadochokinesis, nystagmus, or the Holmes rebound sign) are generally lacking. One characteristic pattern of tremor in WD involves a coarse, irreg-

ular, to-and-fro movement elicited by action. When the arms are held forward and flexed horizontally, this maneuver can bring out a proximal component of tremor activity with a "wing-beating" quality. The types of tremor found in parkinsonism and or dystonia may also occur in WD. Less commonly, tremor presents in the trunk or in the tongue (37,43). Familial (essential-type) tremor with dominant inheritance has been described as a confounding diagnostic feature in a family also affected with WD (44).

Motor dysfunction in the territory of the bulbar musculature is prominent in WD and in one series (45) was more common than tremor as an initial feature. Drooling, dysarthria, cranial dystonia, and pharyngeal dysmotility (46) all can be observed. Other types of motor impairment can involve the cranial region, especially when dystonic features develop elsewhere in the body (45). Among these are facial grimacing, blepharospasm, and tongue dyskinesia (47). A fixed, "sardonic" smile with retracted lips and opened jaw was illustrated in Wilson's original report (36) and is still a highly typical feature. This facial dystonia can often progress to impair closure of the mouth. Spasmodic movements of dystonia can also occur in cranial or cervical musculature. The varieties of dystonia in WD include generalized, segmental, or multifocal patterns, such as bilateral foot dystonia (48).

Virtually all untreated patients are affected by progressive disturbance of speech. Speech can be disturbed in several ways due to impaired motor control of lip, tongue, and pharyngeal muscles. In Wilson's 1955 description, dysarthria in this disorder "reproduces the slurring but not the staccato element of multiple sclerosis" and can progress to complete anarthria. Lesser degrees of speech impairment include indistinct articulation, loss of consonant production, a "whispering dysphonia" (49), and marked slowing in the cadence of speech (34,50). Walshe and Yealland (26) have commented on a characteristic inspiratory laugh in WD which "once heard, is never forgotten."

In early WD, there can be other types of motor impairment, some of which can be difficult to categorize. Patients tend to become clumsy and slowed at everyday tasks. Handwriting and other limb movements may reflect loss of dexterity, as evidenced by the fingers' diminished ability to tap rapidly (51). Trunk titubation, a change of posture, or a disturbance of gait are commonly observed as subtle features in mild cases. Muscle cramps with distal dysesthesias may be experienced (52). WD can also present with a typical unilateral or bilateral parkinsonian syndrome. Sometimes, clinical features initially observed do not correspond to the basal ganglia involvement, which is nearly always found in the brain. For example, ataxia has been described as the only clinical manifestation in a chronic case of WD (32). Sometimes an early manifestation of WD is an unusual task-specific difficulty, such as inability to maintain a particular head posture or to protrude the tongue (34). Sustained, abnormal postures characteristic of dystonia are especially common and, in addition to the bulbar region, can affect the trunk and limbs. The intensity of rigid dystonic posturing can be so great as to require tendon release for relieving disability.

The basis for clinical heterogeneity in presenting features is not understood (53), although it has long been recognized that some patients develop predominantly dystonic or parkinsonian features, and others are affected more with bulbar dysfunction and tremor. For this reason, WD should be highly suspected with respect to any number of categories of movement disorder. Spasticity usually does not develop although some patients exhibit hyperreflexia and Babinski signs. An early manifestation of WD can be pseudobulbar palsy with involuntary bouts of crying or laughter (54). The latter problems, when advanced, can be highly disabling. Other types of movement disorders, such as tics and myoclonus, are generally not observed. However, in one case of WD that presented as a tremor disorder, there was also episodic truncal myoclonus, priapism, and seminal ejaculation that occurred several times per day (55).

SEIZURES

In Wilson's 1912 monograph, instances of epilepsy are described. Though seizures are not a common occurrence in WD, some reports have documented either focal or major motor seizures at any stage of the disorder (56,57). Seizures have been described in cases lacking other evidence for CNS involvement, and are more common in juvenile WD patients. One large series of cases found the prevalence of seizures in a WD group to be 6.2% (58). The latter prevalence corresponds to an approximately tenfold increase over seizure occurrence in the general population. In some reports, convulsions begin to occur at initiation of decoppering treatment. Seizures sometimes can be confused with other paroxysmal movements, such as tremors or dystonia, which sometimes occur as intermittent events in WD.

BEHAVIORAL AND MENTAL STATUS FEATURES

A spectrum of changes in behavior and mental status can occur in WD. Among these are anxiety, mood alterations, impulsivity, as well as other psychiatric disorders. Wilson's original case reports included the description of "emotionalism," though he regarded such behavioral features to be transient. However, subsequent study of WD has shown how commonly this disorder produces an affliction of the mind. Such impairment can be evident in disturbances of school performance, personality, or behavior. Prominent abnormalities on the Minnesota Multiphasic Personality Inventory (MMPI) and other evaluations of personality traits may be found (59). Other early signs of WD include

a decline in memory function or cognitive abilities (60–62). Some aspects of neuropsychological performance tend not to be impaired, such as rate of information processing (63). Patients with WD have been described to exhibit schizophreniform or paranoid features, sometimes with hallucinations or delusional thinking (64,65). Psychiatric disorders in WD without psychotic manifestations include depression or other mood disorders, lethargy, nightmares, disinhibited behavior (such as inappropriate laughter), or loss of insight (27,62,66).

As many as 20% of patients with WD developed some form of psychiatric disturbance as an initial feature (67,68). Other studies have estimated an even greater incidence of psychiatric disturbance, such as moderate to severe depressive traits (69,70). Prior to a confirmed diagnosis of WD, another series found that 17 of 34 patients had received psychiatric treatment for various disorders, including schizophrenia, depression, and anxiety (71). Depression can be a presenting feature (72). With other types of neurologic involvement, the likelihood of a behavioral disorder is much increased. Among these are behaviors such as impulsiveness, self-injuriousness, suicidal ideation, aggressiveness, sexual preoccupations, and childishness (64). Other behavioral disturbances include irritability and a low threshold for anger. A decline in schoolwork or work performance is almost always evident (70). Antisocial or criminal behavior may occur (73). Case reports of WD appearing with anorexia nervosa (74), hypersomnia (75), or with catatonia (76) have been described. When untreated, patients with WD can experience progressive decline in cognitive abilities as a consequence of neuropathologic changes throughout the brain or as a secondary consequence of liver failure. Dementia from WD is usually irreversible. A striking finding in one study was the lack of correlation between the extent of copper toxicity and the features of neuropsychological impairments in both symptomatic and asymptomatic WD patients (71).

OPHTHALMOLOGIC FEATURES

Opaque or mottled bands of pigmentation in the peripheral cornea are characteristic of WD when it involves the CNS (77,78). Although this feature escaped recognition by Wilson, these corneal rings were discovered prior to description of hepatolenticular degeneration. Independent reports by Kayser (79) and by Fleischer (80) are the basis for the eponym now applied to these distinctive changes in the cornea, caused by deposition of copper. Eventually, clinicians came to recognize the strong connection between the corneal pigmentation and the progressive neurologic and hepatic disorder described by Wilson.

Kayser-Fleischer rings have a brownish or greenish tint, and generally arise in the periphery of the cornea. Though usually they appear uniformly concentric around the cornea, these rings can be especially prominent at the upper pole (and can require lifting of the eyelid for recognition). Rarely, Kayser-Fleischer rings can be unilateral (32,81). Kayser-Fleischer rings can often be identified without magnification or special illumination, especially in individuals with blue irises. However, a definitive analysis for the presence or absence of these rings requires a careful ophthalmologic slit-lamp examination. With this magnified view of the eye, another characteristic finding in WD can be discerned, if present. The "sunflower" cataract is an opacification in the lens (82). Though a less common finding in WD than the Kayser-Fleischer ring (83), sunflower cataracts have the same significance. Using Scheimpflug photography, the clinical course of corneal and lens opacification can be followed (84).

Copper-containing granules compose the Kayser-Fleischer ring, which develops primarily in Descemet's membrane of the cornea. These rings and the sunflower cataract arise simultaneously with the onset of neurologic manifestations of WD (83). The intensity of the rings tends to decrease with institution of decoppering therapy (85) or after liver transplantation (86), occasionally disappearing from view. The majority of cases of CNS WD demonstrate Kayser-Fleischer rings. In exceptional circumstances, they can be absent in otherwise typical cases of WD (26,31,87,144–146). One report described Kayser-Fleischer rings developing only after the start of penicillamine in a subject whose clinical picture was otherwise highly typical of WD (88). Other disorders rarely give rise to corneal deposits very similar in appearance to Kayser-Fleischer rings (89). These conditions include cirrhosis and other forms of biliary obstruction (90).

In WD, the eye may be affected in other ways. As an early feature of the disorder, reading may be impaired (91), possibly due to gaze distractibility or difficulty in fixation (36,92). Among the types of abnormal eye movements are a defect of supranuclear accommodation (93), a disturbance of smooth pursuit, nystagmus, episodic diplopia, and impaired convergence (25,26). Apraxia of eyelid opening (94) and slowed saccadic pursuit (95) have also been described. Presentations of neurologic WD with oculogyric crisis (96) and with progressive visual loss (97) have been described.

NEUROPATHOLOGY OF WILSON'S DISEASE

Much of Wilson's 1912 monograph on hepatolenticular degeneration was devoted to detailed pathologic analysis of the distinctive changes produced in the brain. While the distribution and severity of histologic changes can differ among cases, pathologic involvement is usually most extensive in the basal ganglia, where there can be cystic or cavitary degeneration. The massive necrosis that can be found in the gross pathology of the cut brain (24,35,98) explains why neurologic impairments are often irreversible. As is evi-

dent from neuroimaging studies, the lenticular nuclei are the major targets of atrophic changes. The symmetric shrinkage of the putamen is sometimes the consequence of necrotic changes that tend to be especially prominent laterally. The entire putamen can be shrunken with cavitary necrosis and a cystic or granular appearance. Tissues in the striatum can take on a brown, red, or yellow color, though not the greenish hue sometimes seen in corneas. The pallidum may also exhibit discoloration, but these structures tend not to undergo degeneration. Flattening of the caudate nucleus may occur, though more atrophy in the putamen is usually found. Cystic or cavitary necrosis can occur beyond the lenticular nuclei in claustrum, extreme capsule, thalamus, subthalamic nucleus, and red nucleus (24,99,100). About 10% of cases have atrophic or degenerative changes beyond the lenticular nuclei (98).

Elsewhere in the brain, WD can be associated with dilation of the lateral ventricles and generalized brain atrophy. Rarely, the major brunt of pathologic change is found in cerebral cortical gray and white matter (101–104). Degenerative changes have been described to be most prominent in the superior and middle frontal gyri. Similar degrees of damage can extend as far back as the temporal and parietal cortex. In some cases of WD, damage to myelin has been the predominant pathologic picture. Sometimes the loss of white matter is so extensive as to suggest the presence of demyelinating disease (101,103,104). Another picture of the CNS pathology of WD involves atrophy in the brainstem and cerebellar folia (105). Atrophy can show a predilection for the superior vermis and the dentate nucleus (106). White matter lesions with the appearance of central pontine myelinolysis have been described in otherwise typical cases of WD (35,107–109), including development after liver transplantation (110).

On microscopy, pathologic change in WD tends to be more widespread than might be suspected from inspection of the cut brain. In particular, deeper layers of cerebral cortex and adjacent white matter are often the most affected regions. Prominent changes include capillary endothelial swelling and proliferation of glia (especially those of Alzheimer type II) (62,98). Gliosis is most abundant in putamen and can also be present in globus pallidus and caudate nucleus whether or not cavitary or necrotic changes are present. Most cases of severe WD show extensive evidence of damage to myelinated fibers in association with Alzheimer type II gliosis extending diffusely throughout cerebral white matter. A variety of degenerative changes in glia have been described (98), including spongy changes of white matter.

Though a distinctive pathologic change, Alzheimer type II glia are not specific to WD. When observed in other forms of chronic hepatic disease in association with encephalopathy, they may not be as prominently configured in the lenticular nuclei as in WD. Another pathologic finding in most cases of WD is the Opalski cell, which appears to be derived from glia (111). Opalski cells are large, rounded cells with periodic acid–Schiff–positive staining for cytoplasmic granules and an irregularly shaped nucleus. The most common locations for Opalski cells are the cerebral cortex cells and the boundaries of lenticular nuclei cavity. When they are found in this configuration together with Alzheimer type II glia, the pathologic diagnosis of WD is almost certain. Alzheimer type I cells can also be found in WD. In one study, their presence was highly correlated to the extent of reactive astrogliosis and inversely proportional to the severity of Alzheimer type II changes (112). Opalski cells and Alzheimer I and II glia may be involved in a copper detoxification process, since they express the copper binding protein metallothionein (111).

Other types of neuronal damage may be found throughout the brain, especially for larger neurons. The cerebellar pathology of WD most often consists of prominent damage to white matter surrounding the dentate nuclei and extensive (but nonspecific) loss of Purkinje cells (62). Two reports of cerebral cortex electron microscopy in WD have been published (113,114). In addition to typical degenerative changes in neurons, myelin, glia, and axons, Hirano bodies and protoplasmic astrocytes (probably Alzheimer type II) were also found. In cortical neurons, spheroid bodies were prominent. Similar changes have appeared in the lower brainstem sensory nuclei in WD (115).

The impact of decoppering treatment was analyzed in the brains of eleven WD subjects treated chronically with penicillamine (109). For five of the patients neurologic features of WD had fully resolved, and the other patients achieved marked clinical improvement. Despite continued copper chelation therapy, brain content of copper was greatly increased over control values for eight of the nine brains studied. Furthermore, prominent neuropathologic changes typical of WD were evident in each of the penicillamine-treated patients despite their good neurologic outcomes. These results indicate that chelation therapy with penicillamine does not normalize brain copper content or avert either the gross or microscopic pathology associated with CNS WD. The severity of neuropathologic change and regional cerebral copper content was only weakly correlated.

NEUROPHYSIOLOGIC FINDINGS

Disruption of central conduction pathways can provide a sensitive clue to the impact of WD on the CNS. In general, this disorder does not have pathognomonic findings on any form of neurophysiologic testing, though the results of testing for evoked responses can be useful in the workup of WD (116). Usually, the electroencephalogram has not been informative, though generalized slowing and focal abnormalities may be found (117). Most cases of WD studied by electroencephalographic spectral analysis and topographic mapping have shown slowing or epileptiform activity (118). One study of evoked potentials (EPs) revealed that most WD patients with neurologic involvement had one or more findings of a prolonged EP, as did almost half of those lacking other evidence for CNS involvement (119). Delayed conduction of sensory EPs can show a variety of patterns (117). Whether or not clinical signs are present, patients with WD can have abnormal visual EPs, especially with respect to the P100 waveforms (120–122). Studies of brainstem auditory EPs have shown no abnormality (121) or else prolongation (122). A study comparing all three types of EPs found that those of brainstem auditory and somatosensory pathways were more likely to be delayed than those from the visual pathways (123). In the latter study, prolongation of an EP was determined in all severely affected patients and almost all of those moderately affected by neurologic WD. An abnormal EP was also found in more than half of those judged to be mildly affected and in 4 of 24 lacking any other clinical evidence for CNS involvement. Hence, EP can be highly sensitive to WD in the brain or spinal cord. Brainstem auditory and somatosensory EPs may also show changes in response to therapy for WD (119). Abnormalities of pattern-reversal visual evoked responses and flash electroretinograms can undergo improvement with treatment of WD (124).

Another approach that has been used for studying damage to central conduction pathways has been the study of motor EPs following magnetic stimulation of the motor cortex and the spinal roots (125). Subjects with neurologic WD, whether with demyelination or extrapyramidal features, have shown diminished or absent cortically evoked motor responses (126–128). In one reported case of WD, abnormal electromyographic responses evoked by transcranial magnetic brain stimulation were the only strongly abnormal neurophysiologic finding (129). These magnetically elicited motor responses became normal after a course of decoppering therapy.

DIAGNOSTIC TESTING FOR WILSON'S DISEASE

With the recent identification of the genetic abnormality in WD, a simple diagnostic blood test may become available for even the presymptomatic stage of the illness (130). Until that time, the clinician must rely on a battery of tests that vary with disease stage. Of course, clinical suspicion of this disorder is always an indispensable first step, regardless of the available laboratory tests. The protean nature of WD's clinical presentations will always make its diagnosis a challenge. Because of the pleomorphic clinical character of WD, the diagnosis should be considered in any young or even middle-aged individual presenting with unexplained hepatic, psychiatric, or neurologic dysfunction—especially if the neurologic dysfunction involves basal ganglia or cerebellar function.

Liver Biopsy for Hepatic Copper Content

Liver biopsy is the most sensitive and accurate test for the diagnosis of WD. Hepatic copper content is significantly elevated in virtually all individuals with WD. Even asymptomatic, or presymptomatic, individuals will have marked elevations of hepatic copper. In WD, the major elevation of hepatic copper generally exceeds 250 μg per gram of dry tissue.

Although elevated hepatic copper content is a sensitive diagnostic finding in WD, there may be alternative explanations. Obstructive liver diseases, such as primary biliary cirrhosis, biliary atresia, extrahepatic biliary obstruction, primary sclerosing cholangitis, intrahepatic cholestasis of childhood, Indian childhood cirrhosis, and even chronic active hepatitis, also result in elevated hepatic copper (131–135). Copper content lower than expected—but still elevated beyond the threshold of 100 μg/g—may be found in WD if the biopsy is obtained when copper is being released from the liver into the systemic circulation (62).

As an invasive procedure, liver biopsy is associated with a small but real morbidity. Therefore, it should be reserved for situations in which other noninvasive studies do not provide the answer. Liver biopsy is thus the diagnostic test of choice in the individual presenting solely with hepatic dysfunction, since at this stage the copper load may not have been released from the liver into the general circulation. The clinician should always keep in mind that a single determination of hepatic copper content might be misleading in WD (136).

Serum Ceruloplasmin

Serum ceruloplasmin determination is a simple and useful screening test for WD. Ceruloplasmin concentrations are reduced in the majority of individuals with WD, though not in all. For 5% to 15% of WD cases, serum ceruloplasmin concentrations may be in a low normal or only slightly subnormal range (62,137). It is also helpful to remember that because ceruloplasmin is an acute-phase reactant, it is transiently elevated during pregnancy, during estrogen administration, or during infectious or inflammatory disorders (138). In such circumstances, the diagnosis of WD may be obscured by a normal serum ceruloplasmin concentration (139). Furthermore, ceruloplasmin deficiency is not unique to WD and can be found in a variety of other disorders, including Menkes' disease, protein-losing enteropathy, nephrotic syndrome, sprue, and other situations in which protein and total calorie intake are insufficient (138,140).

Because of these limitations, ceruloplasmin determination should not be relied on as the sole screening study for the diagnosis of WD. However, a serum ceruloplasmin level greater than 30 mg/dL (141) or 40 mg/dL (142) virtually excludes the possibility of WD.

24-Hour Urinary Copper Excretion

Urinary copper excretion serves as another useful screening study for WD. However, urinary copper concentrations may be completely normal in asymptomatic WD cases or in presentations limited to hepatic dysfunction. In the latter circumstance, copper may still be accumulating in the liver and not exiting into the circulation. In individuals with neurologic or psychiatric dysfunction, urinary copper levels consistently tend to exceed 100 μg/day. Obstructive liver disease, such as primary biliary cirrhosis, may also produce elevation of urinary copper (132,143).

Slit-lamp Examination

As discussed above, corneal copper deposition in the form of Kayser-Fleischer rings is an indispensable and sensitive clue to the diagnosis of WD. In fact, the lack of Kayser-Fleischer rings almost always excludes the diagnosis of neurologic or psychiatric WD (62). This rule is only rarely transgressed. Cases in which Kayser-Fleischer rings are absent in the face of typical neurologic symptoms are known (31,88,144,145) but are exceptional (146). Although Kayser-Fleischer rings may sometimes be easily seen by direct observation, a magnified slit-lamp examination by an experienced ophthalmologist is often necessary to visualize the deposited copper. Kayser-Fleischer rings tend not to be present in individuals with purely hepatic manifestations of WD because in this situation, the accumulating copper has not yet escaped the liver.

Serum Free (Unbound) Copper

Serum copper concentrations, which are measurements of both bound and unbound copper, provide only limited diagnostic value for WD because total serum copper concentrations largely reflect the quantity of the copper-transporting protein ceruloplasmin. Serum copper concentrations are reduced in WD in direct correlation to ceruloplasmin reduction (62,141,147). Determination of nonceruloplasmin and, therefore, free (unbound) serum copper can be of value because this measurement represents the potentially toxic fraction of serum copper, which increases once the copper storage capabilities of the liver are exceeded (39,141).

Radioactive Copper Studies

After an oral dose of ^{64}Cu, a normal individual will have an initial rise in the serum radioactive label as it enters the blood and is complexed with albumin and amino acids. The isotope concentration then drops as the ^{64}Cu is cleared from the blood by the liver. A secondary rise peaks at 48 hours from incorporation of ^{64}Cu into newly synthesized ceruloplasmin, which is then released into the bloodstream.

In WD, this secondary rise is not seen, even in individuals with normal or near-normal ceruloplasmin levels.

Thus, while this study is not necessary as a screening tool for WD, it can be useful in confirming the diagnosis of WD in the few individuals for whom serum ceruloplasmin concentrations are inconclusive (148).

Neuroimaging Procedures

Abnormalities on magnetic resonance imaging (MRI) are present in virtually all individuals with WD who display neurologic dysfunction (149,150). Increased signal intensity on T2-weighted images, sometimes with a central core of decreased signal intensity, is the characteristic abnormality. Such findings most consistently involve the basal ganglia (151). Several other MRI abnormalities have been described as characteristic of WD, such as the "face of the panda" sign in the midbrain (152) and the "bright claustrum" sign (153), but these are not consistently present. Abnormal MRI findings can improve or vanish with treatment of WD (154,155). Computed tomography (CT) may also expose abnormalities in WD, but less reliably than MRI. Other aspects of neuroimaging studies, including positron emission tomography (PET) and single photon emission computed tomography (SPECT), are reviewed in Chapter 42.

Cerebrospinal Fluid Copper

Copper concentration in cerebrospinal fluid (CSF) is elevated in WD with neurologic dysfunction, but this test has not been used routinely nor has it been validated for the diagnosis of WD. There are indications that CSF copper offers an accurate reflection of the brain's copper load (156). During treatment for WD, CSF copper content slowly returns to normal (157). Sequential CSF copper content determinations can also provide evidence for noncompliance (158).

Genetic Testing

Testing for the *WD* gene, located on 13q14.3, is becoming widely used to augment clinical diagnosis. However, the diversity of mutations in the *ATP7B* gene in WD is a limit to the utility of genetic testing. The techniques involved include analysis of DNA markers amplified by polymerase chain reaction and single-strand conformational analysis (159). Cases of WD diagnosed by gene markers can lack other diagnostic features, such as Kayser-Fleischer rings (145,146). Successful recognition of WD at a presymptomatic stage is a goal for avoiding tissue damage that can precede even the earliest clinical signs and symptoms of WD.

GUIDELINES TO DIAGNOSTIC TESTING

Generally, in WD subjects with symptoms or signs only of hepatic dysfunction, Kayser-Fleischer rings will be lacking if neurologic or psychiatric features have not developed. Furthermore, urinary copper tends not to be elevated because copper has not started to be disgorged from the liver. Serum ceruloplasmin concentrations also cannot be relied on as a diagnostic measure. Hence, in these circumstances, liver biopsy becomes necessary for pathologic analysis and determination of hepatic copper content.

Once typical forms of neurologic or psychiatric dysfunction have appeared, liver biopsy for diagnostic purposes is generally not necessary. The diagnosis of WD can be developed by the reduced serum ceruloplasmin, the elevated urinary copper excretion, and the appearance of Kayser-Fleischer rings. Only in those unusual instances where ceruloplasmin is normal or marginally reduced might liver biopsy be required. If biopsy is not possible or if the results of biopsy are inconclusive, a radiolabeled copper incorporation study may be useful.

MANAGEMENT OF WILSON'S DISEASE

The management of WD is an arduous task that requires long-term commitment and constant vigilance on the part of both patient and physician. The lifelong compliance required for successful therapy is a major challenge for many patients. At present, all treatment for WD—with the exception of liver transplantation—is strictly empirical and needs to be continued without pause. In the face of situations like pregnancy (160) or rapid progression of neurologic disease, modification of the treatment regimen may be necessary. Four primary approaches to the management of WD are available. For each patient, the ideal treatment modality (or modalities) can vary greatly.

Dietary Therapy

Although copper can be found in small amounts in many comestibles, such foods as chocolate, nuts, shellfish, mushrooms, and liver have an especially high content. Eliminating liver from the diet might seem to be a logical strategy, but strict attempts to eliminate all copper from the diet results in an unpalatable product and offers no definite advantage beyond what can be achieved by simply foregoing high-copper-content foods (161). It is important to note that individuals with WD who have adopted strict lactovegetarian diets have achieved adequate control of copper balance without additional therapy, presumably from reduced dietary copper bioavailability by the fiber and phytates abundant in the lactovegetarian diet (162). However, such a diet is poorly tolerated. Another dietary issue is the presence of copper in drinking water (161,163), use of water softeners [which increase the copper content of the water (141)], and elemental copper present in health food vitamin/mineral supplements.

Inhibition of Intestinal Copper Absorption

In recent years, the treatment for WD has been advanced by several innovative approaches to achieving adequate copper balance by limiting absorption of copper via the gut. Prior attempts to decrease dietary copper absorption through the use of potassium iodide or potassium sulfide met with little success, but newer approaches utilizing zinc or tetrathiomolybdate are very promising (see below).

Zinc

By itself, zinc has no direct effect on copper absorption. However, it acts indirectly on metallothionein, a protein with several physiologic roles. Metallothionein binds zinc for transport and helps to maintain its homeostasis (164). Present in many body tissues (including liver and brain), metallothionein is also found in intestinal mucosal cells (enterocytes). Metallothionein avidly binds copper (165). In the gut this protein exerts its therapeutic effect on copper balance in WD. When persistently increased amounts of zinc enter the intestine, metallothionein formation is induced in the enterocytes and excess zinc is bound by the metallothionein, thus maintaining zinc homeostasis. However, the increased amount of metallothionein in the enterocyte is also capable of binding copper since this metal is absorbed through the enterocytes. The net effect of zinc administration is a negative copper balance. The trapped copper remains in the enterocyte (along with zinc) until the cell is sloughed and excreted in the feces (163,166). Furthermore, both dietary copper and copper secreted into the gastrointestinal tract via saliva and gastric juices are trapped and ultimately eliminated (166). The induction of metallothionein by zinc is a relatively slow process (requiring 1 to 2 weeks to evolve) and results in a relatively small negative copper balance (167).

For the treatment of WD, either zinc sulfate or zinc acetate may be employed. A dosage of 50 mg (elemental zinc) three times daily is generally used. However, a total daily dosage of 75 mg is probably sufficient (168,169). The marketed tablets of zinc sulfate (220 mg) contain 50 mg of elemental zinc. It is important to administer zinc on an empty stomach separated from food intake by at least one hour (170).

Zinc is generally tolerated without any difficulty. However, gastric irritation may occur, especially with zinc sulfate (163,171). Sideroblastic anemia, probably resulting from impaired iron utilization, has also been described from zinc therapy (172). Transient elevations of serum amylase, lipase, and alkaline phosphatase have also been attributed to zinc (169. Reductions of high-density lipoprotein cholesterol in men by approximately 20% and total cholesterol in both men and women by about 10% have been noted as well (167,173).

The virtues of zinc as a therapeutic agent in the treatment of WD have been strongly advocated by Brewer and by Hoogenraad. Despite strong evidence based on clinical experience, the role of zinc administration in the management of WD has not been established to everyone's satisfaction (174). The extremely low incidence of toxicity makes zinc an ideal therapy for the individual with WD who has not yet developed clinical symptoms (163,175). Its place in symptomatic WD is been less certain. The slow onset of action of zinc probably makes it unsuitable as initial therapy for the patient with neurologic symptoms (176), but Brewer has enthusiastically promoted the use of zinc as "maintenance" therapy following initial decoppering with more potent agents (27,167,176). Other investigators, less convinced about the efficacy of zinc, suggest that zinc therapy be limited to individuals who have been unable to tolerate penicillamine or trientine (141,174).

Brewer and colleagues have also addressed the question of utilizing zinc concomitantly with other agents, such as penicillamine, with different mechanisms of action. They reported that even when zinc and penicillamine are given at different times during the day, an interaction occurs: urinary copper excretion increases though fecal copper excretion decreases, thus canceling any benefit derived from combining the two drugs (163).

Tetrathiomolybdate

Ammonium tetrathiomolybdate (TM) actually bridges two categories of mechanism of action in the treatment of WD. Though still experimental, TM has sufficient promise to merit discussion here. TM acts in the gut lumen, where it limits gastrointestinal absorption of copper by forming a tripartite complex with dietary copper and albumin, thus rendering the copper unavailable for absorption (177). This mechanism is especially active if TM is administered with meals. A second mode of action of TM becomes active when TM is administered without food. In this situation, TM is readily absorbed into the bloodstream and there forms the same tripartite complex with albumin and unbound (free) copper, thus trapping and holding the copper in an inactive, nontoxic state (177).

In order to take advantage of this potential dual mechanism of action, TM has been administered in a regimen of six doses daily (three doses with and three doses between meals) (177). Mealtime doses were 20 mg, whereas intermeal doses ranged from 20 to 60 mg. Utilized in this manner, TM produces a prompt and significant reduction in free copper in the plasma (177). In most instances, TM has been tolerated without difficulty. However, reversible bone marrow suppression has been reported (171), which may be the result of impaired erythropoiesis as a consequence of bone marrow copper depletion (George Brewer, personal communication).

TM has not been utilized as a long-term agent in the management of WD, and has been given as an 8-week course, followed by a switch to zinc maintenance therapy (176). It may be especially important to avoid long-term TM administration in children and adolescents, since TM has been shown to damage epiphyses in growing bone in rats (171,178). Clinical experience with TM has suggested that deterioration in neurologic function following initiation of TM therapy is much less common than with penicillamine (179).

Copper Chelation Therapy

The modern era of WD therapy began in 1951 with the introduction of British anti-Lewisite (BAL, dimercaprol) as the first effective copper-chelating agent in the management of WD (180,181). The necessity of parenteral administration and the frequent occurrence of adverse effects were serious limits to use of BAL in the management of WD. BAL has now been replaced by orally administered copper-chelating agents, first penicillamine and then trientine.

Penicillamine

Penicillamine (dimethylcysteine), a metabolic byproduct of penicillin, was introduced into clinical usage shortly after the discovery of excess copper deposition in the pathophysiology of WD (182). Penicillamine avidly chelates copper. The complexed copper is excreted in the urine, initially producing a robust cupriuresis that diminishes with prolonged administration as the excess body load of copper is corrected. Penicillamine is the most potent agent available for the management of WD, although chronic treatment presents many possible adverse outcomes. Because alternatives to penicillamine are available, strong arguments have been made to avoid use of this drug based on the dangers of exacerbation in neurologic impairments and the high frequency of other adverse outcomes (179). Despite this, penicillamine is still widely used as a first-line treatment for initial and long-term management of WD (183).

Acute sensitivity reactions develop in 20% to 30% of individuals placed on penicillamine (184,185). These reactions tend to occur within 2 weeks of initiation of treatment and are characterized by skin rash, fever, or lymphadenopathy with associated laboratory abnormalities (eosinophilia, leukopenia, and thrombocytopenia). Fatal agranulocytosis may occur (186). In the face of an acute sensitivity reaction, penicillamine should be discontinued until the rash clears. Subsequently, it may possible to reintroduce penicillamine, beginning with very low doses and slowly escalating. One formula for reintroducing penicillamine consists of using prednisone 30 mg daily 2 days before the start of penicillamine at a reduced dosage of 125 mg daily. Penicillamine is then increased by 125 mg at 3-day intervals to reach a daily intake of 500 mg. Over the next month, prednisone is gradually tapered and discontinued while penicillamine is progressively increased by 250 mg at 2- to 3-day intervals to reach a target dose of 1,000 mg daily (187). Despite such

measures, 5% to 20% of WD patients will be unable to tolerate penicillamine (27).

A formidable array of potential complications can accompany the long-term use of penicillamine. Various dermatologic problems may develop. Urticaria affects as many as one-third of treated patients (185). Recurrent subcutaneous bleeding following incidental trauma can result in characteristic brownish skin discoloration, termed penicillamine dermatopathy (188). Penicillamine-induced inhibition of collagen and elastin cross-linking may be responsible for the subcutaneous bleeding (189). Impaired wound healing may also complicate chronic penicillamine therapy (190). Reduction of penicillamine dosage to 250 to 500 mg daily during perioperative periods may help to dampen this tendency (62). Other penicillamine-induced problems that have been described include nephrotic syndrome (191), Goodpasture's syndrome (192), a lupus-like syndrome (193,194), a myasthenia gravis–like syndrome (195,196), acute polyarthritis (52), thrombocytopenia (62), retinal hemorrhage (197), dysgeusia (161,198), and IgA deficiency (199). The adverse effects associated with chronic penicillamine administration may first appear after years of therapy.

Penicillamine can trigger neurologic deterioration after the start of therapy. This outcome has led to some disenchantment with using penicillamine as a primary treatment for WD (176,200). Neurologic deterioration may occur in 22% to 52% of persons receiving penicillamine (171). Moreover, when this neurologic deterioration occurs, half of patients will never regain their baseline neurologic status (201). Status dystonicus with a lethal outcome has been reported (202). Emergence of neurologic dysfunction in previously neurologically asymptomatic individuals has also been described (177,203). The mechanism for this neurologic deterioration is not clear but could be due to excessive systemic mobilization of copper that can be taken up in the brain.

There is considerable difference of opinion regarding the appropriate dosage of penicillamine. Although doses of 1,000 to 2,000 mg daily have usually been recommended, more modest doses have been advised, such as a starting dose of 250 mg daily (161,163). Penicillamine should be taken with meals. Supplemental pyridoxine has often been administered with penicillamine, although the need for it has not been established.

Improvement in function following initiation of treatment with penicillamine may not be discernible for 2 to 3 months. Because of this lag in clinical response, it is important to educate patients and their families so that treatment will be maintained and disillusionment in the lack of immediate effect will be avoided. Although virtually all clinical features of WD parameters may improve with penicillamine therapy, some deficits, such as dystonia and a fixed facial grimace, may be more resistant. Improvement may continue for as long as 1 to 2 years with continued therapy. Even abnormalities on neuroimaging that appear to be structural may improve with penicillamine therapy (149,150,204).

Trientine

Triethylene tetramine dihydrochloride (trientine) is an avid copper-chelating agent. It has been utilized in the management of WD since the late 1960s (205–208), though it became available in the United States only recently. Although similar in action to penicillamine, trientine is not quite as potent a chelating agent. This characteristic makes trientine a preferred agent over penicillamine in the opinion of some experts (176). However, most reserve trientine for use in individuals who have been unable to tolerate penicillamine. Trientine is generally administered three times a day, with total daily dose ranging from 750 to 2,000 mg daily. As with penicillamine, trientine should be administered with food.

Adverse effects appear to be less common with trientine than with penicillamine. Among the observed reactions to this drug are colitis, duodenitis (209), sideroblastic anemia (210), and lupus nephritis (207). As with penicillamine, neurologic deterioration may develop following initiation of trientine therapy (209).

Liver Transplantation

Experience with orthotopic liver transplantation in the management of WD has accumulated over the past two decades. As a potentially curative treatment, orthotopic liver transplantation has obvious advantage over symptomatic treatment such as copper chelation. Improvement for hepatic, neurologic, psychiatric, and ophthalmologic aspects of the disorder all may be achieved from orthotopic liver transplantation. Indeed, experience has shown that copper metabolism normalizes following orthotopic liver transplantation and chelation therapy may be discontinued (211,212). Although orthotopic liver transplantation has generally been conducted with WD patients experiencing fulminant hepatic failure (for whom mortality otherwise will be 100%), this procedure has also been performed on individuals with chronic, severe hepatic insufficiency (211). Dramatic clinical improvement can be achieved from successful liver transplantation (213). One-year survival rates of 80% or greater have been documented (211,212,214,215). This success rate has led some investigators to consider orthotopic liver transplantation in individuals with stable hepatic function but deterioration in neurologic function despite trials of appropriate medications (216). Extracorporeal porcine hepatic tissue is also undergoing investigation in WD and other disorders of hepatic failure (217).

REFERENCES

1. Hoogenraad TU. S.A. Kinnier Wilson (1878–1937). *J Neurol* 2001;248:71–72.
2. Gowers WR. Tetanoid chorea. In: *A manual of disease of the nervous system.* Philadelphia: P Blakiston, 1888:1059.
3. Westphal C. Über eine dem Bilde der cerebrospinalen grauen Degeneration ähnliche Erkrankung des centralen Nervensystems ohne anatomischen Befund, nebst einigen Bermerkungen über paradoxe Contraction. *Arch Psychiatr Nervenkrank* 1883; 14:87–134.
4. Strümpell A. Über die Westphal'sche Pseudosklerose und über diffuse Hirnsklerose, inbesondere bei Kindern. *Deutsch Z Nervenheilk* 1898;12:115–149.
5. Homen EA. Eine eigenthümliche bei drei Geschwistern auftretende typische Krankheit unter der Form einer progressiven Dementia, in Verbindung mit ausgedehnten Gefässveränderungen (Wohl Lues hereditaria tarda). *Arch Psychiatr Nervenkrank* 1892;24:191–228.
6. Firnesz G, Szonyi L, Ferenci P, et al. Wilson disease in two consecutive generations: an exceptional family. *Am J Gastroenterology* 2001;96:2269–2271.
7. LeWitt PA, Brewer GJ. Wilson's disease (progressive hepaticolenticular degeneration). In: Calne DB, ed. *Neurodegenerative disorders.* Philadelphia: WB Saunders, 1994:667–683.
8. Houwen RH, Roberts EA, Thomas GR, et al. DNA markers for the diagnosis of Wilson disease. *J Hepatol* 1993;17:269–276.
9. Tanzi RE, Petrukhin K, Chernov I, et al. The Wilson disease gene is a copper transporting ATPase with homology to the Menkes disease gene. *Nat Genet* 1993;5:344–350.
10. Loudianos G, Lovicu M, Solinas P, et al. Delineation of the spectrum of Wilson disease mutations in the Greek population and the identification of six novel mutations. *Genet Test* 2000; 4:399–402.
11. Sasaki N, Hayashizaki Y, Muramatsu M, et al. The gene responsible for LEC hepatitis, located on rat chromosome 16, is the homolog to the human Wilson disease gene. *Biochem Biophys Res Commun* 1994;202:512–518.
12. Yamaguchi Y, Heiny ME, Shimizu N, et al. Expression of the Wilson disease gene is deficient in the Long-Evans Cinnamon rat. *Biochem J* 1994;301[pt 1]:1–4.
13. Malhi H, Irani AN, Rajvanshi P, et al. KAPT channels regulate mitogenically induced proliferation in primary rat hepatocytes and human liver cell lines: implications for liver growth control and potential therapeutic targeting. *J Biol Chem* 2000;275: 26050–26057.
14. Cartwright GE, Wintrobe MM. Copper metabolism in normal subjects. *Am J Clin Nutr* 1964;14:224–232.
15. O'Reilly S, Weber PM, Oswald M, et al. Abnormalities of the physiology of copper in Wilson's disease. III: the excretion of copper. *Arch Neurol* 1971;25:28–32.
16. Frommer DJ. Defective biliary excretion of copper in Wilson's disease. *Gut* 1974;15:125–129.
17. Gibbs K, Walshe JM. Biliary excretion of copper in Wilson's disease. *Lancet* 1980;2:538–539.
18. Iyengar V, Brewer GJ, Dick Rd, et al. Studies of cholecystokinin-stimulated biliary secretions reveal a high molecular weight copper-binding substance in normal subjects that is absent in patients with Wilson's disease. *J Lab Clin Med* 1988; 111:267–274.
19. Cumings JN. The copper and iron content of brain and liver in the normal and in hepatolenticular degeneration. *Brain* 1948;71:410–415.
20. Walshe JM, Potter G. The pattern of whole body distribution of radioactive copper (^{67}Cu, ^{64}Cu) in Wilson's disease and various control groups. *Q J Med* 1977;46:445–462.
21. Groth CG, Dubois RS, Corman J, et al. Hepatic transplantation in Wilson's disease. *Birth Defects* 1973;9:106–108.
22. Bruehlmeier M, Leenders KL, Vontobel P, et al. Increased cerebral iron uptake in Wilson's disease: a 52Fe-citrate PET study. *J Nucl Med* 2000;41:781–787.

23. Warren PJ, Earl CJ, Thompson RHS. The distribution of copper in human brain. *Brain* 1960;83:709–717.
24. Dastur DK, Manghani DK. Wilson's disease: inherited cuprogenic disorder of liver, brain, kidney. In: Goldensohn E, Appel SH, eds. *Scientific foundations of neurology.* Philadelphia: Lea & Febiger, 1977:1033–1051.
25. Sternlieb I, Giblin DR, Scheinberg IH. Wilson's disease. In: Marsden CD, Fahn S, eds. *Movement disorders 2.* New York: Butterworth, 1985:288–302.
26. Walshe JM, Yealland M. Wilson's disease: the problem of delayed diagnosis. *J Neurol Neurosurg Psychiatr* 1992;55: 692–696.
27. Brewer GJ, Yuzbasiyan-Gurkan V. Wilson disease. *Medicine* 1992;71:139–164.
28. Quinn NP, Marsden CD. Coincidence of Wilson's disease with other movement disorders in the same family. *J Neurol Neurosurg Psychiatry* 1986;49:221–222.
29. Fitzgerald M, Gross JB, Goldstein NP, et al. Wilson's disease of late adult onset. *Mayo Clin Proc* 1975;50:438–442.
30. Czlonkowska A, Rodo M. Late onset Wilson's disease. *Arch Neurol* 1981;38:729–730.
31. Ross ME, Jacobson IM, Dienstag JL, et al. Late onset Wilson's disease with neurologic involvement in the absence of Kayser-Fleischer rings. *Ann Neurol* 1985;17:411–413.
32. Madden JW, Ironside JW, Triger DR, et al. An unusual case of Wilson's disease. *Q J Med* 1985;55:63–73.
33. Pilloni L, Lecca S, Coni P, et al. Wilson's disease with late onset. *Dig Liver Dis* 2000;32:180.
34. Purdon Martin J. Wilson's disease. In: PJ Vinken, GW Bruyn, HL Klawans, eds. *Handbook of clinical neurology.* New York: American Elsevier, 1968:267–278.
35. Shiraki H. Comparative neuropathologic study of Wilson's disease and other types of hepatocerebral disease. In: Bergsma D, Scheinberg IH, Sternlieb I, eds. *Wilson's disease.* (Birth defects original article series, vol 4.) New York: The National Foundation–March of Dimes, 1968:64–73.
36. Wilson SAK. Progressive lenticular degeneration: a familial nervous disease associated with cirrhosis of the liver. *Brain* 1912;34:295–509.
37. Wilson SAK. Progressive lenticular degeneration (hepatolenticular degeneration, Wilson's disease). In: Bruce AN, ed. *Neurology,* 2nd ed. Baltimore: Williams & Wilkins, 1955:941–967.
38. Dobyns WB, Goldstein NP, Gordon H. Clinical spectrum of Wilson's disease (hepatolenticular degeneration). *Mayo Clin Proc* 1979;54:35–42.
39. Stremmel W, Meyerrose K-W, Niederau K, et al. Wilson disease: clinical presentation, treatment, and survival. *Ann Intern Med* 1991;115:720–726.
40. Barthel H, Sorger D, Kuhn HJ, et al. Differential alteration of the nigrostriatal dopaminergic system in Wilson's disease investigated with [123I]ss-CIT and high-resolution SPET. *Eur J Nucl Med* 2001;28:1656–1663.
41. Walshe JM. Wilson's disease (hepatolenticular degeneration). In: PJ Vinken, GW Bruyn, HL Klawans, eds. *Handbook of clinical neurology,* vol 27. New York: American Elsevier, 1976: 379–414.
42. Walshe JM. Wilson's disease. In: PJ Vinken, GW Bruyn, HL Klawans, eds. *Handbook of clinical neurology.* New York: American Elsevier, 1986:223–238.
43. Topaloglu H, Gucuyener K, Orkun C, et al. Tremor of tongue and dysarthria as the sole manifestation of Wilson's disease. *Clin Neurol Neurosurg* 1990;92:295–296.
44. Nicholl DJ, Ferenci P, Polli C, et al. Wilson's disease presenting in a family with an apparent dominant history of tremor. *J Neurol Neurosurg Psychiatry* 2001;70:514–516.
45. Starista-Rubinstein S, Young AB, Kluin K, et al. Clinical assessment of 31 patients with Wilson's disease: correlations with structural changes on magnetic resonance imaging. *Arch Neurol* 1987;44:365–370.
46. Gulyas AE, Salazar-Grueso EF. Pharyngeal dysmotility in a patient with Wilson's disease. *Dysphagia* 1988;2:230–234.
47. Liao KK, Wang SJ, Kwan SY, et al. Tongue dyskinesia as an early manifestation of Wilson disease. *Brain Devel* 1991;13: 451–453.
48. Svetel M, Kozic D, Stefanova E, et al. Dystonia in Wilson's disease. *Mov Disord* 2001;16:719–723.
49. Parker N. Hereditary whispering dysphonia. *J Neurol Neurosurg Psychiatry* 1985;48:218–224.
50. Berry WR, Darley FL, Aronson AE, et al. Dysarthria in Wilson's disease. *J Speech Hearing Res* 1974;17:169–183.
51. Davis LJ, Goldstein NP. Psychologic investigation of Wilson's disease. *Mayo Clin Proc* 1974;49:409–499.
52. Golding DN, Walshe JM. Arthropathy of Wilson's disease: study of clinical and radiological features in 32 patients. *Ann Rheum Dis* 1977;36:99–111.
53. Denny-Brown D. Hepato-lenticular degeneration (Wilson's disease). *N Engl J Med* 1964;270:1149–1156.
54. Mingazzini G. Über das Zwangsweinen und lachen. *Klin Wochenschr (Wien)* 1928;41:998–1002.
55. Nair KR, Pillai PG. Trunkal myoclonus with spontaneous priapism and seminal ejaculation in Wilson's disease. *J Neurol Neurosurg Psychiatry* 1990;53:174.
56. Smith CK, Mattson RH. Seizures in Wilson's disease. *Neurology* 1967;17:1121–1123.
57. Chu N-S. Clinical, CT, and evoked potential manifestations in Wilson's disease with cerebral white matter involvement. *Clin Neurol Neurosurg* 1989;91:45–51.
58. Dening TR, Berrios GE, Walshe JM. Wilson's disease and epilepsy. *Brain* 1988;111:1139–1155.
59. Portala K, Westermark K, Ekselius L, et al. Personality traits in treated Wilson's disease determined by means of the Karolinska Scales of Personality (KSP). *Eur Psychiatry* 2001;16:362–371.
60. Knehr CA, Bearn AG. Psychological impairment in Wilson's disease. *J Nerv Ment Dis* 1956;124:251–255.
61. Goldstein NP, Ewert JC, Randall RV, et al. Psychiatric aspects of Wilson's disease (hepatolenticular degeneration): results of psychometric tests during long-term therapy. *Am J Psychiatry* 1968;124:1555–1561.
62. Scheinberg IH, Sternlieb I. *Wilson's disease: major problems in internal medicine,* vol 23. Philadelphia: WB Saunders, 1984.
63. Littman E, Medalia A, Senior G, et al. Rate of information processing in patients with Wilson's disease. *J Neuropsychiatr Clin Neurosci* 1995;7:68–71.
64. Dening TR. Psychiatric aspects of Wilson's disease. *Br J Psychiatry* 1985;147:677–682.
65. Scheinberg IH, Sternlieb I, Richman J. Psychiatric manifestations of Wilson's disease. *Birth Defects Orig Art Ser* 1968;4: 85–86.
66. Hawkes ND, Mutimer D, Thomas GA. Generalised oedema, lethargy, personality disturbance, and recurring nightmares in a young girl. *Postgrad Med J* 2001;77:529,537–539.
67. Medalia A, Scheinberg IH. Psychopathology in patients with Wilson's disease. *Am J Psychiatry* 1989;146:662–664.
68. Jackson GH, Meyer A, Lippmann S. Wilson's disease: psychiatric manifestations may be the clinical presentation. *Postgrad Med* 1994;95:135–138.
69. Portala K, Westermark K, von Knorring L, et al. Psychopathology in treated Wilson's disease determined by means of CPRS expert and self-ratings. *Acta Psychiatr Scand* 2000;101:85–86, 104–109.

70. Akil M, Brewer GJ. Psychiatric and behavioral abnormalities in Wilson's disease. *Adv Neurol* 1995;65:171–178.

71. Rathbun JK. Neuropsychological aspects of Wilson's disease. *Int J Neurosci* 1996;85:221–229.

72. Keller R, Torta R, Lagget M, et al. Psychiatric symptoms as late onset of Wilson's disease: neuroradiological findings, clinical features and treatment. *Ital J Neurol Sci* 1999;20:49–54.

73. Kaul A, McMahon D. Wilson's disease and offending behaviour—a case report. *Med Sci Law* 1993;33:353–358.

74. Gwirtsman HE, Prager J, Henkin R. Case report of anorexia nervosa associated with Wilson's disease. *Int J Eating Disord* 1993;13:241–244.

75. Firneisz G, Szalay F, Halasz P, et al. Hypersomnia in Wilson's disease: an unusual symptom in an unusual case. *Acta Neurol Scand* 2001;101:286–288.

76. Davis EJ, Borde M. Wilson's disease and catatonia. *Brit J Psychiatry* 1993;162:256–259.

77. Heckmann JG, Lang CJ, Neundorfer B, et al. Neuro/Images: Kayser-Fleischer corneal ring. *Neurology* 2000;54:1839.

78. Patel AD, Bozdech M. Wilson disease. *Arch Ophthalmol* 2001;119:1556–1557.

79. Kayser B. Über einen Fall von angeborener grünlicher Verfärbung der Cornea. *Klin Monatsb Augenheilk* 1902;40:22–25.

80. Fleischer B. Über eine der "Pseudosklerose" nahestehende bisher unbekannte Krankheit (gekenn zeichnet durch Tremor, psychische Störungen, braunliche Pigmententierung, bestimmter Gewebe, insobesondere suh der Hornhautperipherie, Lebercirrhose). *Deutsch Z Nervenheilkr* 1912;44:179–201.

81. Innes JR, Strachan IM, Triger DR. Unilateral Kayser-Fleischer ring. *Br J Ophthalmol* 1979;70:469–470.

82. Goyal V, Tripathi M. Sunflower cataract in Wilson's disease. *J Neurol Neurosurg Psychiatry* 2000;69:133.

83. Wiebers DO, Hollenhorst RW, Goldstein NP. The ophthalmologic manifestations of Wilson's disease. *Mayo Clin Proc* 1977; 52:409–416.

84. Obara H, Ikoma N, Sasaki K, et al. Usefulness of Scheimpflug photography to follow up Wilson's disease. *Ophthalmic Res* 1995;27[Suppl 1]:100–103.

85. Sussman W, Sternlieb IH. Disappearance of Kayser-Fleischer rings. *Arch Ophthalmol* 1969;82:738–741.

86. Song HS, Ku WC, Chen CL. Disappearance of Kayser-Fleischer rings following liver transplantation. *Transplant Proc* 1992; 24:1483–1485.

87. Heckmann J, Saffer D. Abnormal copper metabolism: another "non-Wilson's" case. *Neurology* 1988;38:1493–1594.

88. Weilleit J, Kiechl SG. Wilson's disease with neurological impairment but no Kayser-Fleischer rings. *Lancet* 1991;337:1426.

89. Frommer D, Morris J, Sherlock S, et al. Kayser-Fleischer-like rings in patients without Wilson's disease. *Gastroenterology* 1977;72:1331–1335.

90. Fleming CR, Dickson ER, Wahner HW, et al. Pigmented corneal rings in non-Wilsonian liver disease. *Ann Intern Med* 1977;86:285–288.

91. Hyman NM, Phuapradit P. Reading difficulty as a presenting symptom in Wilson's disease. *J Neurol Neurosurg Psychiatry* 1979;42:478–480.

92. Lennox G, Jones R. Gaze distractibility in Wilson's disease. *Ann Neurol* 1989;25:415–417.

93. Klinqele TG, Newman SA, Burde RM. Accommodation defect in Wilson's disease. *Am J Ophthalmol* 1980;90:22–24.

94. Keane JR. Lid-opening apraxia in Wilson's disease. *J Clin Neuro-Ophthalmol* 1988;8:31–33.

95. Kirkham TH, Kamin DF. Slow saccadic eye movements in Wilson's disease. *J Neurol Neurosurg Psychiatry* 1974;37:191–194.

96. Lee MS, Kim YD, Lyoo CH. Oculogyric crisis as an initial manifestation of Wilson's disease. *Neurology* 1999;52:1714–1715.

97. Gow PJ, Peacock SE, Chapman RW. Wilson's disease presenting with rapidly progressive visual loss: another neurologic manifestation of Wilson's disease? *J Gastroenterol Hepatol* 2001;16: 699–701.

98. Schulman S. Wilson's disease. In: Minkler J, ed. *Pathology of the nervous system*. New York: McGraw-Hill, 1968:1139–1151.

99. Owen CA Jr. *Wilson's disease: the etiology, clinical aspects, and treatment of inherited toxicosis*. Park Ridge, NJ: Noyes Publications, 1981:1–215.

100. Duchen LW, Jacobs JM. Nutritional deficiencies and metabolic disorders. In: Adams JH, Corsellis JAN, Duchen LW, eds. *Greenfield's neuropathology*, 4th ed. New York: John Wiley & Sons, 1984:595–599.

101. Schulman S, Barbeau A. Wilson's disease: a case with almost total loss of cerebral white matter. *J Neuropathol Exp Neurol* 1963;22:105–119.

102. Richter RB. Pallidal component in hepatolenticular degeneration. *J Neuropathol Exp Neurol* 1948;7:1–18.

103. Ishino H, Takashi M, Hayashi Y, et al. A case of Wilson's disease with enormous cavity formation of cerebral white matter. *Neurology* 1972;22:905–909.

104. Miyakawa T, Murayama E. An autopsy case of the "demyelinating typ" of Wilson's disease. *Acta Neuropathol* 1976;35: 235–241.

105. Miskolczy D. Wilson'she Krankheit und Kleinhirn. *Arch Psych Nervenkr* 1932;97:27–63.

106. Bielschowsky M, Hallervorden J. Symmetrische Einschmelzungsherde in Stirnhim beim Wilson Pseudosklerose Komplex. *J Psych Neurol* 1931;42:177–189.

107. Popoff N, Budzilovich G, Goodgold A, et al. Hepatocerebral degeneration: its occurrence in the presence and in the absence of abnormal copper metabolism. *Neurology* 1965;15:919–930.

108. Seitelberger F. Zentrale pontin Myelinolyse. *Schweiz Arch Neurol Neurochir Psych* 1973;112:285–297.

109. Horoupian DS, Sternlieb I, Scheinberg IH. Neuropathological findings in penicillamine-treated patients with Wilson's disease. *Clin Neuropathol* 1988;7:62–67.

110. Lui CC, Chen CL, Chang YF, et al. Subclinical central pontine myelinolysis after liver transplantation. *Transplant Proc* 2000;32:2215–2516.

111. Bertrand E, Lewandowska E, Szpak GM, et al. Neuropathological analysis of pathological forms of astroglia in Wilson's disease. *Folia Neuropathol* 2001;39:73–79.

112. Ma KC, Ye ZR, Fang J, et al. Glial fibrillary acidic protein immunohistochemical study of Alzheimer I and II astrogliosis in Wilson's disease. *Acta Neurol Scand* 1988;78:290–296.

113. Foncin JF. *Pathologie ultrastructurale de la glie chez l'homme*. Proceedings of the 6th International Congress of Neuropathology. Paris: Masson et Cie, 1970:377–390.

114. Anzil AP, Herrlinger H, Blinzinger K, et al. Ultrastructure of brain and nerve biopsy tissue in Wilson disease. *Arch Neurol* 1974;31:94–100.

115. Jellinger K. Neuroaxonal dystrophy: its natural history and related disorders. In: Zimmerman HM, ed. *Progress in neuropathology*, vol 2. New York: Grune & Stratton, 1973: 129–180.

116. Chu N-S. Sensory evoked potentials in Wilson's disease. *Brain* 1986;109:491–506.

117. Giagheddu M, Tamburini G, Piga M, et al. Comparison of MRI, EEG, Eps, and ECD-SPECT in Wilson's disease. *Acta Neurol Scand* 2001;103:71–81.

118. Chu N-S, Chu CC, Tu SC, et al. EEG spectral analysis and topographic mapping in Wilson's disease. *J Neurol Sci* 1991;106:1–9.

119. Grimm G, Oder W, Prayer L, et al. Evoked potentials in assessment and follow-up of patients with Wilson's disease. *Lancet* 1990;336:963–964.

120. Aiello I, Sau GF, Cacciotto R, et al. Evoked potentials in patients with non-neurological Wilson's disease. *J Neurol* 1992; 239:65–68.

121. Butinar D, Trontelj JV, Khuraibet AJ, et al. Brainstem auditory evoked potentials in Wilson's disease. *J Neurol Sci* 1990;95: 163–169.

122. Satishchandra P, Swamy HS. Visual and brain stem auditory evoked responses in Wilson's disease. *Acta Neurol Scand* 1989; 79:108–113.

123. Grimm G, Madl C, Katzenschlager R, et al. Detailed evaluation of evoked potentials in Wilson's disease. *EEG Clin Neurophysiol* 1992;82:119–124.

124. Satishchandra P, Ravishankar Naik K. Visual pathway abnormalities Wilson's disease: an electrophysiological study using electroretinography and visual evoked potentials. *J Neurol Sci* 2000;176:13–20.

125. Perretti A, Pellecchia MT, Lanzillo B, et al. Excitatory and inhibitory mechanisms in Wilson's disease: investigation with magnetic motor cortex stimulation. *J Neurol Sci* 2001;192: 35–40.

126. Chu N-S. Motor evoked potentials in Wilson's disease: early and late motor responses. *J Neurol Sci* 1990;99:259–269.

127. Meyer BU, Britton TC, Benecke R. Wilson's disease: normalization of cortically evoked motor responses with treatment. *J Neurol* 1991;238:327–330.

128. Berardelli A, Inghilleri M, Priori A, et al. Involvement of corticospinal tract in Wilson's disease: a study of three cases with transcranial stimulation. *Mov Disord* 1990;5:334–337.

129. Meyer BU, Britton TC, Bischoff C, et al. Abnormal conduction in corticospinal pathways in Wilson's disease: investigation of nine cases with magnetic brain stimulation. *Mov Disord* 1991;6: 320–323.

130. Maier-Dobersberger T, Mannhalter C, Rack S, et al. Diagnosis of Wilson's disease in an asymptomatic sibling by DNA linkage analysis. *Gastroenterology* 1995;109:2015–2018.

131. Smallwood RA, Williams HA, Rosenauer VM. Liver copper levels in liver disease: studies using neutron activation analysis. *Lancet* 1968;2:1310–1313.

132. LaRusso NF, Summerskill WH, McCall JT. Abnormalities of chemical tests for copper metabolism in chronic active liver disease: differentiation from Wilson's disease. *Gastroenterology* 1976;70:653–655.

133. Benson GD. Hepatic copper accumulation in primary biliary cirrhosis. *Yale J Biol Med* 1979;52:83–88.

134. Evans J, Newman S, Sherlock S. Liver copper levels in intrahepatic cholestasis of childhood. *Gastroenterology* 1978;75:875–878.

135. Tanner MS, Portmann B, Mowat AP, et al. Increased hepatic copper concentration in Indian childhood cirrhosis. *Lancet* 1979;1:1203–1205.

136. Song YM, Chen MD. A single determination of liver copper concentration may misdiagnose Wilson's disease. *Clin Biochem* 2000;33:589–590.

137. Yuce A, Kocak N, Ozen H, et al. Wilson's disease patients with normal ceruloplasmin levels. *Turk J Pediatr* 1999;41:99–102.

138. Gibbs K, Walshe JM. A study of the ceruloplasmin concentrations found in 75 patients with Wilson's disease, their kinships and various control groups. *Q J Med* 1979;48:447–463.

139. Sternlieb I, Scheinberg IH. Chronic hepatitis as a first manifestation of Wilson's disease. *Ann Intern Med* 1972;76:59–64.

140. Weiner WJ, Lang AE. *Movement disorders: a comprehensive survey*. Mt. Kisco, NY: Futura, 1989:257–291.

141. Yarze JC, Martin P, Munoz SJ, et al. Wilson's disease: current status. *Am J Med* 1992;92:643–654.

142. Snow B. Laboratory diagnosis and monitoring of Wilson's disease. *Neurological aspects of Wilson's disease*. American Academy of Neurology Course Number 411, 1995:25–30.

143. Frommer DJ. Urinary copper excretion and hepatic copper concentrations in liver disease. *Digestion* 1981;21:169–178.

144. Oder W, Grimm G, Kollegger H, et al. Neurological and neuropsychiatric spectrum of Wilson's disease: a prospective study of 45 cases. *J Neurol* 1991;238:281–287.

145. Vidaud D, Assouline B, Lecoz P, et al. Misdiagnosis revealed by genetic linkage analysis in a family with Wilson disease. *Neurology* 1996;46:1485–1486.

146. Demirkiran M, Jankovic J, Lewis RA, et al. Neurologic presentation of Wilson disease without Kayser-Fleischer rings. *Neurology* 1996;46:1040–1043.

147. Cumings JN. Trace metals in the brain and in Wilson's disease. *J Clin Pathol* 1968;21:1–7.

148. Sternlieb I, Scheinberg IH. The role of radiocopper in the diagnosis of Wilson's disease. *Gastroenterology* 1979;77:138–142.

149. Thuomas KA, Aquilonius SM, Bergstrom K, et al. Magnetic resonance imaging of the brain in Wilson's disease. *Neuroradiology* 1993;35:134–141.

150. Roh JK, Lee TG, Wie BA, et al. Initial and follow-up brain MRI findings and correlation with the clinical course in Wilson's disease. *Neurology* 1994;44:1064–1068.

151. Magalhaes ACA, Caramelli P, Menezes JR, et al. Wilson's disease: MRI with clinical correlation. *Neuroradiology* 1994;36: 97–100.

152. Hitoshi S, Iwata M, Yoshikawa K. Midbrain pathology of Wilson's disease: MRI analysis of three cases. *J Neurol Neurosurg Psychiatry* 1991;54:624–626.

153. Sener RN. The claustrum on MRI: normal anatomy, and the bright claustrum as a new sign in Wilson's disease. *Pediatr Radiol* 1993;23:594–596.

154. Alanen A, Komu M, Penttinen M, et al. Magnetic resonance imaging and proton MR spectroscopy in Wilson's disease. *Br J Radiol* 1999;72:749–756.

155. Stefano Zagami A, Boers PM. Disappearing "face of the giant panda." *Neurology* 2001;56:665.

156. Hartard C, Weisner B, Dieu C, et al. Wilson's disease with cerebral manifestations: monitoring therapy by CSF copper concentration. *J Neurol* 1993;241:101–107.

157. Stuerenburg HJ. CSF copper concentrations, blood–brain barrier function, and ceruloplasmin synthesis during the treatment of Wilson's disease. *J Neural Transm* 2000;107:321–329.

158. Stuerenburg HJ, Eggers C. Early detection of non-compliance in Wilson's disease by consecutive copper determination in cerebrospinal fluid. *J Neurol Neurosurg Psychiatry* 2000;69: 701–702.

159. Butler P, McIntyre N, Mistry PK. Molecular diagnosis of Wilson disease. *Mol Genet Metab* 2001;72:223–230.

160. Furman B, Bashiri A, Wiznitzer A, et al. Wilson's disease in pregnancy: five successful consecutive pregnancies of the same woman. *Eur J Obstet Gynecol Reprod Biol* 2001;96:232–234.

161. Shoulson I, Goldblatt D, Plassche W, et al. Some therapeutic observations in Wilson's disease. *Adv Neurol* 1983;37:239–246.

162. Brewer GJ, Yuzbasiyan-Gurkan V, Dick R, et al. Does a vegetarian diet control Wilson's disease? *J Am Coll Nutr* 1993;12: 527–530.

163. Brewer GJ, Yuzbasiyan-Gurkan V. Wilson's disease. In: Klawans HL, Goetz CG, Tanner CM, eds. *Textbook of clinical neuropharmacology and therapeutics*. New York: Raven Press, 1992: 191–205.

164. Ebadi M. Metallothionein and other zinc-binding proteins in brain. *Meth Enzymol* 1991;205:363–387.

165. Day FA, Panemangalore M, Brady FO. In vivo and ex vivo effects of copper on rat liver metallothionein. *Proc Soc Exp Biol Med* 1981;168:306–310.

166. Brewer GJ, Hill GM, Prasad AS, et al. Oral zinc therapy for Wilson's disease. *Ann Intern Med* 1983;99:314–320.

167. Brewer GJ, Yuzbasiyan-Gurkan V, Lee DY. Molecular genetics and zinc-copper interactions in human Wilson's disease and canine copper toxicosis. In: Prasad AS, ed. *Essential and toxic trace elements in human health and disease: an update.* New York: Wiley-Liss, 1993:129–145.

168. Brewer GJ, Yuzbasiyan-Gurkan V, Johnson V, et al. Treatment of Wilson's disease with zinc. XI: Interaction with other anti-copper agents. *J Am Coll Nutr* 1993;12:26–30.

169. Brewer GJ, Yuzbasiyan-Gurkan V, Johnson V, et al. Treatment of Wilson's disease with zinc. XII: Dose regimen requirements. *Am J Med Sci* 1993;305:199–202.

170. Brewer GJ, Yuzbasiyan-Gurkan V, Dick R. Zinc therapy of Wilson's disease. 8: Dose response studies. *J Trace Elem Exp Med* 1990;3:227–234.

171. Walshe JM, Yealland M. Chelation treatment of neurological Wilson's disease. *Q J Med* 1993;86:197–204.

172. Simon SR, Branda RF, Tindle BH, et al. Copper deficiency and sideroblastic anaemia associated with zinc ingestion. *Am J Hematol* 1988;28:181–183.

173. Hooper PL, Visconti L, Garry PJ, et al. Zinc lowers high-density lipoprotein-cholesterol levels. *JAMA* 1980;244:1960–1961.

174. Lipsky MA, Gollan JL. Treatment of Wilson's disease: in D-penicillamine we trust—what about zinc? *Hepatology* 1987;7:593–595.

175. Brewer GJ, Yuzbasiyan-Gurkan V, Lee DY, et al. Treatment of Wilson's disease with zinc. 6: Initial treatment studies. *J Lab Clin Med* 1989;114:633–638.

176. Brewer GJ. Practical recommendations and new therapies for Wilson's disease. *Drugs* 1995;50:240–249.

177. Brewer GJ, Dick RD, Johnson V, et al. Treatment of Wilson's disease with ammonium tetrathiomolybdate. I: Initial therapy in 17 neurologically affected patients. *Arch Neurol* 1994;51:545–554.

178. Spence JA, Suttle NF, Wenham G, et al. A sequential study of the skeletal abnormalities which develop in rats given a small dietary supplement of ammonium tetrathiomolybdate. *J Comp Pathol* 1980;90:139–153.

179. Brewer GJ. Penicillamine should not be used as initial therapy in Wilson's disease. *Mov Disord* 1999;14:551–554.

180. Denny-Brown D, Porter H. The effect of BAL (2,3 dimercaptopropanol) on hepatolenticular degeneration (Wilson's disease). *N Engl J Med* 1951;245:917–925.

181. Cumings JN. The effects of BAL in hepatolenticular degeneration. *Brain* 1951;74:10–22.

182. Walshe JM. Penicillamine: a new oral therapy for Wilson's disease. *Am J Med* 1956;21:487–495.

183. Walshe JM. Penicillamine: the treatment of first choice for patients with Wilson's disease. *Mov Disord* 1999;14:545–550.

184. Sternlieb I, Scheinberg IH. Penicillamine therapy in hepatolenticular degeneration. *JAMA* 1964;189:748–754.

185. Haggstrom GC, Hirschowitz BI, Flint A. Long-term penicillamine therapy for Wilson's disease. *South Med J* 1980;73:530–531.

186. Corcos JM, Soler-Bechera J, Mayer K, et al. Neutrophilic agranulocytosis during administration of penicillamine. *JAMA* 1964;189:265–268.

187. Chan C-Y, Baker AL. Penicillamine hypersensitivity: successful desensitization of a patient with severe hepatic Wilson's disease. *Am J Gastroenterol* 1994;89:442–443.

188. Sternlieb I, Fisher M, Scheinberg IH. Penicillamine-induced skin lesions. *J Rheumatol* 1981;8[Suppl 7]:149–154.

189. Nimni ME. Mechanism of inhibition of collagen cross-linking by penicillamine. *Proc R Soc Med* 1977;70[Suppl 3]:65–72.

190. Morris JJ, Seifter E, Rettura G, et al. Effect of penicillamine upon wound healing. *J Surg Res* 1969;9:143–149.

191. Hirschman SZ, Isselbacher KJ. The nephrotic syndrome as a complication of penicillamine therapy of hepatolenticular degeneration (Wilson's disease). *Ann Intern Med* 1965;62:1297–1300.

192. Sternlieb I, Bennett B, Scheinberg IH. D-Penicillamine induced Goodpasture's syndrome in Wilson's disease. *Ann Intern Med* 1975;82:673–675.

193. Walshe JM. Penicillamine and the SLE syndrome. *J Rheumatol* 1981;8[Suppl 7]:155–160.

194. Lin HC, Hwang KC, Lee HJ, et al. Penicillamine induced lupus-like syndrome: a case report. *J Microbiol Immunol Infect* 2000;33:202–204.

195. Czlonkowska A. Myasthenia syndrome during penicillamine treatment. *Br Med J* 1975;2:726–727.

196. Narayanan CS, Behari M. Generalized myasthenia gravis following use of D-pencillamine in Wilson's disease. *J Assoc Physicians (India)* 1999;47:648.

197. Bigger JF. Retinal hemorrhages during penicillamine therapy of cystinuria. *Am J Ophthalmol* 1968;66:954–955.

198. Henkin RI, Keiser HR, Jaffe IA, et al. Decreased taste sensitivity after D-penicillamine reversed by copper administration. *Lancet* 1967;2:1268–1271.

199. Proesman W, Jaeken J, Eckels R. D-Penicillamine-induced IgA deficiency in Wilson's disease. *Lancet* 1976;2:804–805.

200. Brewer GJ, Turkay A, Yuzbasiyan-Gurkan V. Development of neurologic symptoms in a patient with asymptomatic Wilson's disease treated with penicillamine. *Arch Neurol* 1994;51:304–305.

201. Brewer GH, Terry CA, Aisen AM, et al. Worsening of neurological syndrome in patients with Wilson's disease with initial penicillamine therapy. *Arch Neurol* 1987;44:490–494.

202. Svetel M, Sternic N, Pejovic S, et al. Penicillamine-induced lethal status dystonicus in a patient with Wilson's disease. *Mov Disord* 2001;16:568–569.

203. Glass JD, Reich SG, DeLong MR. Wilson's disease: development of neurological disease after beginning penicillamine therapy. *Arch Neurol* 1990;47:595–596.

204. Williams FJB, Walshe JM. Wilson's disease: an analysis of the cranial computerized tomographic appearances found in patients and the changes in response to treatment with chelating agents. *Brain* 1981;104:735–752.

205. Walshe JM. The management of penicillamine nephropathy in Wilson's disease: a new chelating agent. *Lancet* 1969;2:1401–1402.

206. Walshe JM. Copper chelation in patients with Wilson's disease: a comparison of penicillamine and triethylene tetramine hydrochloride. *Q J Med* 1973;42:441–452.

207. Walshe JM. Treatment of Wilson's disease with trientine (triethylene tetramine) dihydrochloride. *Lancet* 1982;1:643–647.

208. Walshe JM. Assessment of the treatment of Wilson's disease with triethylene tetramine 2HCL (Trien 2HCl). In: Sarkar B, ed. *Biological aspects of metal related diseases.* New York: Raven Press, 1983:243–261.

209. Dahlman T, Hartvig P, Lofholm M, et al. Long-term treatment of Wilson's disease with triethylene tetramine dihydrochloride (trientine). *Q J Med* 1995;88:609–616.

210. Condamine L, Hermine O, Alvin P, et al. Acquired sideroblastic anaemia during treatment of Wilson's disease with triethylene tetramine dihydrochloride. *Br J Hematol* 1993;83:166–168.

211. Schilsky ML, Scheinberg IH, Sternlieb I. Liver transplantation for Wilson's disease: indications and outcome. *Hepatology* 1994;19:583–587.

212. Rela M, Heaton ND, Vougas V, et al. Orthotopic liver transplantation for hepatic complications of Wilson's disease. *Br J Surg* 1993;80:909–911.

213. Bax RT, Hassler A, Luck W, et al. Cerebral manifestation of

Wilson's disease successfully treated with liver transplantation. *Neurology* 1998;51:863–865.

214. Chen CL, Kuo YC. Metabolic effects of liver transplantation in Wilson's disease. *Transplant Proc* 1993;25:2944–2947.

215. Emre S, Atillasoy EO, Ozdemir S, et al. Orthotopic liver transplantation for Wilson's disease: a single-center experience. *Transplantation* 2001;72:1232–1236.

216. Mason AL, Marsh W, Alpers DH. Intractable neurological Wilson's disease treated with orthotopic liver transplantation. *Dig Dis Sci* 1993;38:1746–1750.

217. Mazariegos GV, Kramer DJ, Lopez RC, et al. Safety observations in phase I clinical evaluation of the Excorp Medical Bioartificial Liver Support System after the first four patients. *ASAIO J* 2001;47:471–475.

218. Laufer J, Passwell J, Lotan D, et al. Screening for Wilson's disease in the investigation of hematuria. *Isr J Med Sci* 1992;28: 367–369.

219. Hoppe B, Newhaust A, Superti-Furga A, et al. Hypercaluria and nephrocalcinosis, a feature of Wilson's disease. *Nephron* 1993; 65:460–462.

220. Deiss A, Lee GR, Cartwright GE. Hemolytic anemia in Wilson's disease. *Ann Intern Med* 1970;73:413–418.

221. Goldman M, Ali M. Wilson's disease presenting as Heinz-body hemolytic anemia. *Can Med Assoc J* 1991;145:971–972.

222. Prella M, Baccala R, Horisberger JD, et al. Haemolytic onset of Wilson disease in a patient with homozygous truncation of ATP7B at Arg1319. *Br J Haematol* 2001;114:230–232.

223. Kabra SK, Bagga A, Malkani I. Wilson's disease presenting with refractory rickets. *Ind Pediatr* 1990;27:395–397.

224. Feller ER, Schumacher HR. Osteoarticular changes in Wilson's disease. *Arthr Rheum* 1972;15:259–266.

225. Hu R. Severe spinal degeneration in Wilson's disease. *Spine* 1994;19:372–375.

226. Menerey KA, Eider W, Brewer GJ, et al. The arthropathy of Wilson's disease: clinical and pathologic features. *J Rheumatol* 1988;15:331–337.

227. Olsen BS, Helin P, Mortensen HB. Recurrent arthritis in a child: a rare manifestation of Wilson's disease. *Ugeskr Laeger* 1996;158:4305–4306.

228. Balint G, Szebenyi B. Hereditary disorders mimicking and/or causing premature osteoarthritis. *Bailliere's Best Pract Res Clin Rheumatol* 2000;14:219–250.

229. Knisely A. Massive haemosiderosis in Wilson's disease. *Histopathology* 2001;39:323.

230. Ahmed A, Feller ER. Rupture of the spleen as the initial manifestation of Wilson's disease. *Am J Gastroenterol* 1996;91: 1454–1455.

231. Propst A, Propst T, Feichtinger H, et al. Copper-induced acute rhabdomyolysis in Wilson's disease. *Gastroenterology* 1995;108: 885–887.

18

NEUROPATHOLOGY OF PARKINSONIAN DISORDERS

DENNIS W. DICKSON

The most common parkinsonian disorders can be assigned to one of two categories based on biochemical and structural abnormalities in either tau protein or synuclein. As a group these disorders have been termed *tauopathies* and *synucleinopathies* (1). Tau protein, which is the major component of neurofibrillary tangles (NFTs) in Alzheimer's disease (AD), was initially considered a neuronal protein, but tau-positive glial lesions are increasingly recognized in parkinsonian disorders (2). The recent discovery of mutations in the *tau* gene, located on chromosome 17, and their relationship to frontotemporal dementia with parkinsonism (FTDP-17) (3) has lead to renewed interest in tau and development of animal models of tau pathology (4) that offer promise for improved diagnosis and management of these disorders. Synuclein was discovered as a non-amyloid component of senile plaques in AD (5). Interest in synuclein was fueled by the discovery that its gene, which is located on chromosome 4, was mutated in rare familial forms of Parkinson's disease (PD) (6). Subsequently, α-synuclein was shown to be present in Lewy bodies (LBs) (7) and glial inclusions in multiple system atrophy (MSA) (8).

Although tau and synuclein are neuronal proteins, they are also expressed in pathologic astrocytes and oligodendroglia. They are heat-stable proteins with potential for protein–protein interactions (reviewed in 9). In addition to their physiologic binding partners (e.g., binding of tau to tubulin), they also have a tendency to self-associate to form pathologic fibrils, and known mutations in each molecule favor fibril formation. The best characterized posttranslational modification of tau and synuclein is phosphorylation. Many protein kinases have been shown to phosphorylate tau, but only a limited set of kinases phosphorylate synuclein (reviewed in 10). Phosphorylation of tau modifies its binding to tubulin, but little is known about the effects of phosphorylation of synuclein. Tau and synuclein in pathologic lesions are ubiquitinated (11). Although ubiquitination may merely be an adaptive cellular response, it may also have a role in the normal life cycle of

these molecules and contribute directly to pathogenesis of the inclusions. Given evidence that parkin, another molecule involved in familial juvenile-onset parkinsonism, is a ubiquitin ligase and involved in proteasome-mediated proteolysis (12), additional studies are required to understand the role of ubiquitin in normal cellular physiology of tau and synuclein and in parkinsonian disorders.

Synuclein and tau inclusions in neurons and glia are the neuropathologic hallmarks of the major parkinsonian disorders. Tau is present in NFTs as well as other neuronal inclusions in the tauopathies. Similarly, synuclein is present not only in LBs and Lewy neurites, but also Lewy-like neuronal inclusions in MSA. Tau-positive glial inclusions include oligodendroglial coiled bodies, tufted astrocytes, and astrocytic plaques (2). Synuclein-positive oligodendroglial cytoplasmic inclusions are the histopathologic hallmark of MSA (13).

SYNUCLEINOPATHIES

Lewy Body Disorders–Parkinson's Disease and Dementia with Lewy Bodies

In this discussion, Parkinson's disease (PD) and dementia with Lewy bodies (DLB) are used as clinical terms, whereas Lewy body disease (LBD) is used as a pathologic term. The clinical features of PD are bradykinesia, rigidity, tremor, postural instability, autonomic dysfunction, and bradyphrenia. The most common pathologic finding in PD is LBD, but occasionally progressive supranuclear palsy (PSP), MSA, or other disorders are clinically mistaken for PD. The clinical features of DLB include dementia, extrapyramidal signs, visual hallucinations, and a fluctuating course (14). The pathologic findings in DLB include LBs and varying degrees of Alzheimer-type pathology. Overlap between these two clinical syndromes is vexing in that dementia can occur late in the course of PD. Whether DLB and dementia in PD are distinct clinicopathologic entities is an area of current study.

Lewy Bodies and Lewy Neurites

LBs are concentric hyaline cytoplasmic inclusions in specific vulnerable populations of neurons (Fig. 18.1). While most LBs are single and spherical, some neurons have multiple or pleomorphic LBs. In some regions of the brain, such as the dorsal motor nucleus of the vagus, similar inclusions within neuronal processes are referred to as intraneuritic LBs. Intraneuritic LBs can be detected in routine histopathologic preparations and should be distinguished from Lewy neurites, which are not visible in routine histopathology. Lewy neurites were first described in the hippocampus (15) but are also found in other regions of the brain, including amygdala, cingulate gyrus, and temporal cortex.

Ultrastructural studies of LBs demonstrate non-membrane-bound, granulofilamentous structures. The central region of the LB is usually amorphous dense material that lacks discernible detail, whereas the periphery has radially arranged 10-nm-diameter filaments (16). At the electron microscopic level, Lewy neurites also have 10-nm filaments, but they lack a dense core and the filaments are more haphazardly arranged (15).

Neurons that are most vulnerable to LBs include the monoaminergic neurons of the substantia nigra, locus ceruleus, and dorsal motor nucleus of the vagus, as well as cholinergic neurons in the basal forebrain. LBs are rarely detected in the basal ganglia or thalamus, but are common in the hypothalamus, especially the posterior and lateral

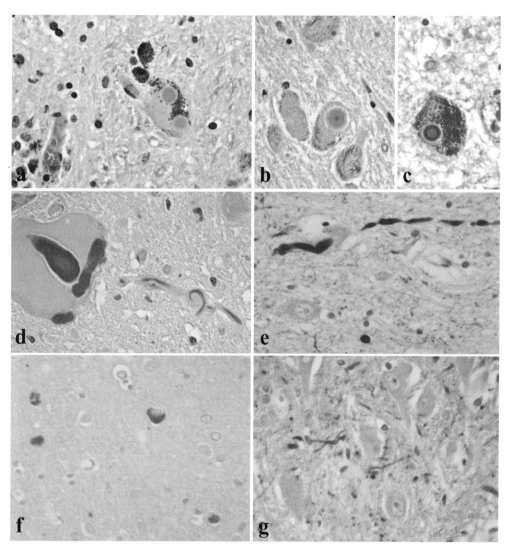

FIG. 18.1. Lewy bodies (LBs) are concentric hyaline inclusions in pigmented neurons of the substantia nigra **(a)** and other brainstem nuclei, such as the dorsal raphe **(b)**. They are immunostained with ubiquitin **(c)**. LBs are also found within neuritic processes such as in the dorsal motor nucleus of the vagus **(d)** and in the basal forebrain **(e)**. Synuclein immunostaining reveals intraneuritic LBs (E) cortical LBs **(f)** and Lewy neurites in the hippocampus **(g)**.

hypothalamus, and the brainstem reticular formation. The oculomotor nuclear complex is also vulnerable. In the pons, the dorsal raphe and subpeduncular nuclei are often affected, but neurons of the pontine base are not. LBs have not been described in the cerebellar cortex. In the spinal cord, the neurons of the intermediolateral cell column are most vulnerable. LBs can be found in the autonomic ganglia, including submucosal ganglia of the lower esophagus.

In contrast to typical or classical LBs, cortical LBs are more difficult to detect with routine histology. They tend to be found in small nonpyramidal neurons in lower cortical layers. Similar lesions in the substantia nigra are referred to as "pale bodies." Ultrastructural studies of cortical LBs demonstrate poorly organized granulofilamentous structures rather than the radial arrangement of filaments in classical LBs. Not all cortical regions are equally vulnerable to cortical LBs. The frontal and temporal multimodal association and limbic cortices are most vulnerable, with the amygdala being the most vulnerable of all. LBs are only rarely detected in primary cortices. Regions with the densest accumulation of cortical LBs are the insular cortex and parahippocampal and cingulate gyri.

Both classical and cortical LBs share the immunocytochemical characteristics. Antibodies to neurofilament were first to be shown to label LBs (17), but most neurofilament antibodies label only a subset of LBs. Ubiquitin is present in most classical and cortical LBs (18), but the most specific method of detecting LBs and Lewy neurites is synuclein immunocytochemistry (19).

Only a few biochemical studies on LBs have been reported due to the paucity of LBs in a given volume of brain tissue and their solubility properties. Lewy bodies are structurally unstable and disrupted upon attempted bio-chemical purification (20). Initial biochemical studies suggested that a major protein constituent of LBs was a 68-kd protein that had cross-reactivity with neurofilament protein (21). More recent studies suggest that the major structural component of LBs is α-synuclein (22), and in vitro studies have demonstrated that α-synuclein aggregates to form filaments similar to those seen in LBs (23).

Pathology of Parkinson's Disease

The brain is usually grossly unremarkable until the brainstem is sectioned; then loss of neuromelanin pigmentation in the substantia nigra and locus ceruleus becomes apparent (Fig. 18.2). The histologic correlate of pigment loss is neuronal loss in the substantia nigra pars compacta. In typical PD, as in most other disorders associated with parkinsonism, the neuronal loss is usually most marked in the ventrolateral tier of neurons, which is known to project to the striatum. Striatal pathology is not apparent with routine histologic methods. Neuronal loss in the substantia nigra is accompanied by astrocytosis and microglial activation. Neuromelanin pigment is often found in the cytoplasm of macrophages, and occasionally neurons can be detected undergoing neuronophagia, or phagocytosis by macrophages. In residual neurons LBs and pale bodies are found. Similar pathology is also played out in the locus ceruleus and the dorsal motor nucleus of the vagus. The basal forebrain is also vulnerable to neuronal loss and LBs. The neocortex usually does not have LBs, but limbic areas, particularly the amygdala, may have some. Depending on the age of the individual, varying degrees of Alzheimer-type pathology may be detected; however, if the person is not demented, such pathology usually falls within the range

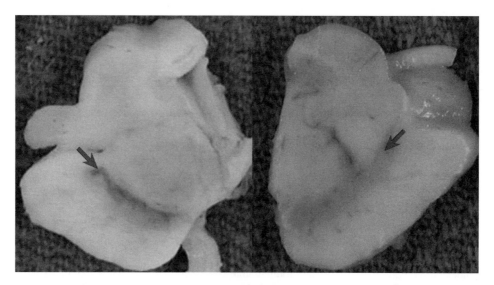

FIG. 18.2. The midbrain of a control *(left)* and PD cases *(right)*. Note black pigment in the substantia nigra in the normal but loss of pigment in PD *(arrows)*.

expected for his or her age. Some individuals many have abundant senile plaques, but few or no NFTs and a low NFT stage (see below).

Diffuse Lewy Body Disease and the Neuropathology of Dementia in Parkinson's Disease

In the London Parkinson brain bank series, pathologic findings considered to account for dementia in PD included subcortical pathology (39%), coexistent AD (29%), and diffuse LBD (26%) (24). The basal forebrain cholinergic system is the subcortical region most often implicated in dementia, and neurons in this region are damaged in both AD and LBD. Neuronal loss in the basal nucleus is consistently found in PD, especially PD with dementia (25). As previously mentioned, the basal nucleus is also vulnerable to LBs. Not surprisingly, cholinergic deficits are found in LBD (26). Cholinergic deficits may contribute to dementia in PD in those patients who do not have concurrent AD or cortical LBs.

Although recent studies have shown that virtually all PD brains have a few cortical LBs (24), they are usually not widespread and not numerous in nondemented PD cases (27–29). When found in PD, cortical LBs are usually detected in the limbic cortices (e.g., cingulate gyrus) and not detected in association cortices of the frontal, temporal, and parietal lobes. In contrast, several studies have shown that cortical LBs can be numerous and widespread in PD with dementia (27–29). Furthermore, the density of cortical LBs has been shown to correlate with severity of dementia in some studies (30). Patients with widespread cortical Lewy bodies are said to have diffuse Lewy body disease (DLBD). Kosaka and co-workers were the first to use the term DLBD, and he subsequently subdivided DLBD into pure and common forms. The latter is associated with coexistent Alzheimer-type pathology (31). Some investigators use the term DLBD for cases in which cortical LBs are found in the absence of any Alzheimer-type pathology, referring to cases with LBs and Alzheimer-type pathology as Lewy body variant of AD (32). Brains with cortical LBs confined to the limbic lobe are classified as "transitional LBD," whereas those with LBs confined to brainstem and diencephalon are said to have "brainstem LBD." Nondemented PD subjects have brainstem or, occasionally, transitional LBD, whereas PD patients with dementia have DLBD or transitional LBD.

The entorhinal cortex is unusually susceptible to degeneration in parkinsonian disorders as well as in aging and AD. In the AD staging scheme of Braak and Braak (33), the entorhinal cortex is among the first areas of the brain to show NFTs. In this staging scheme, six stages are described, with the initial stages being clinically silent. In most cases of DLBD the Braak stage is lower (stage IV or less) than in comparably demented subjects with AD (stage IV or

greater), but usually more than in nondemented controls (stage III or less) (34).

Senile plaques are complicated lesions composed of extracellular deposits of amyloid and localized glial and neuronal changes (35). Given the fact that development of senile plaques is nearly inevitable with aging, it is not surprising that many patients with DLBD, especially those age 60 years or older, have variable numbers of senile plaques. Since clinicopathologic studies have shown that some clinically normal elderly people may have many senile plaques but no NFTs (35), a diagnosis of AD requires the presence of both senile plaques and NFTs (36). Furthermore, there are striking morphologic differences between senile plaques in aging compared with AD. In AD senile plaques differ not only in the nature of the amyloid peptides and reactive glial changes, but also in the presence of neuritic elements (i.e., neuritic plaques). In aging and most cases of DLBD, the most prevalent type of plaques are so-called "diffuse plaques," whereas neuritic plaques are the hallmark of AD. The importance of neuritic plaques and NFTs has been adopted by National Institute of Aging/Reagan Institute criteria in pathologic diagnosis of AD (36). This makes a diagnosis of AD in the setting of LBD more stringent. No longer is it possible to diagnose AD in a someone with dementia and LBs who has plaques but no NFTs; thus, the concept of Lewy body variant of AD must be revisited.

Lewy Bodies in Aging and Alzheimer's Disease

Postmortem studies of asymptomatic elderly humans demonstrate LBs, most often limited to pigmented brainstem nuclei, in up to 10% of the elderly population (37). A certain degree of parkinsonism is practically synonymous with motor aging, and it is possible that the structural correlate of age-related extrapyramidal signs may be incidental brainstem LBs. However, this remains hypothetical. The pathologic substrate of extrapyramidal signs occurring late in the course of otherwise typical AD has been the focus of only a limited number of pathologic studies. While it is commonly assumed that LBs account for extrapyramidal features in AD, NFT in the substantia nigra were the best correlate in one study (38).

Multiple System Atrophy

The term *multiple system atrophy* is used for a nonheritable neurodegenerative disease characterized by parkinsonism, cerebellar ataxia, and idiopathic orthostatic hypotension. The concept of MSA unifies three separate entities: olivopontocerebellar atrophy, Shy-Drager syndrome, and striatonigral degeneration. MSA has an average age of onset between age 30 and 50 years and a disease duration that runs in the decades (39). In contrast to other spinocerebellar degenerations, there is no known genetic risk factor or genetic locus in MSA.

Neuropathology of Multiple System Atrophy

The MSA brain shows varying degrees of atrophy of cerebellum, cerebellar peduncles, pons, and medulla, as well as atrophy and discoloration of the posterolateral putamen and loss of pigment in the ventrolateral substantia nigra (Fig. 18.3). The histopathologic findings include neuronal loss, gliosis, and microvacuolation, involving the putamen, substantia nigra, cerebellum, olivary nucleus, pontine base, and intermediolateral cell column of the spinal cord. White matter inevitably shows demyelination, with the brunt of the changes affecting white matter tracts in affected areas. Recent immunohistochemical studies suggest that white matter pathology may be more widespread than previously suspected (40).

Lantos and co-workers first described oligodendroglial inclusions in MSA and named them glial cytoplasmic inclu-

sions (GCIs) (13). GCIs can be detected with silver stains, such as the Gallyas stain, but are best seen with antibodies to synuclein, where they appear as flame- or sickle-shaped inclusions in oligodendrocytes (Fig. 18.4). In addition to synuclein immunoreactivity, GCIs are consistently immunoreactive for ubiquitin and variably immunoreactive for tubulin, α–B crystallin, and tau (13). At the ultrastructural level, GCIs are non-membrane-bound cytoplasmic inclusions composed of filaments (7 to 10 nm) and granular material that often coats the filaments making precise measurements difficult (41). GCIs are distinctly different from the oligodendroglial inclusions, so-called coiled bodies (42), that are found in the tauopathies (see below). Most tau antibodies readily stain coiled bodies, but GCIs are usually negative. GCIs are specific for MSA and have not been found in other neurodegenerative diseases. In addition to GCIs, synuclein-immunoreactive lesions are also detected

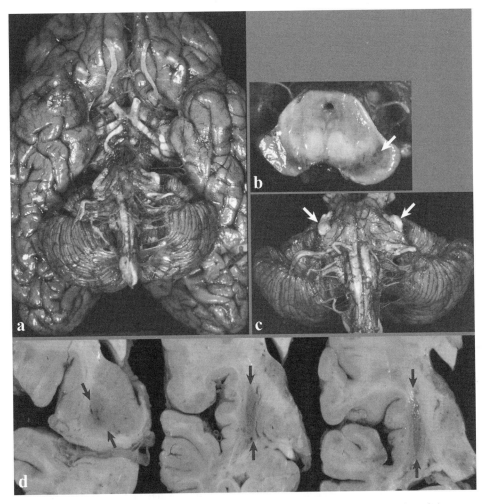

FIG. 18.3. The base of the brain in multiple system atrophy shows marked atrophy of the pons **(a)** with loss of pigment in the lateral part of the substantia nigra **(b,** *arrow*). Note the relative prominence of the trigeminal nerves *(arrows* in **c)** due to pontine atrophy. On coronal sections there is atrophy and discoloration in the lateral putamen *(arrows)* with a gradient of severity that increases the more caudal one goes (left to right).

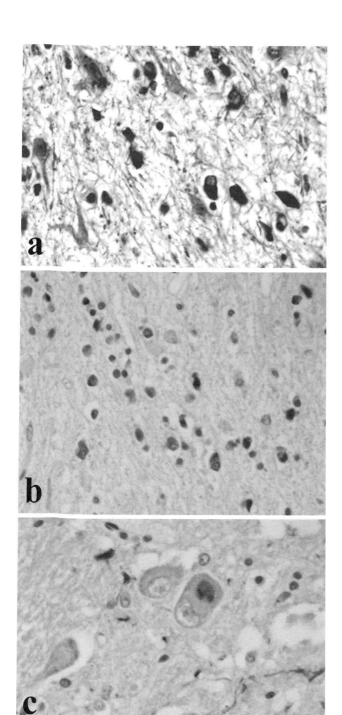

FIG. 18.4. Gallyas silver stain reveals dense, round to crescent-shaped glial cytoplasmic inclusions (GCIs) in multiple system atrophy **(a)** and numerous GCIs in affected areas with synuclein immunostains **(b)**. Synuclein also occasionally reveals Lewy-like neuronal inclusions **(c)** and neuritic processes *(lower right)* in the pontine base.

in some neurons in MSA. Biochemical studies of synuclein in MSA have shown changes in its solubility (43) somewhat similar to solubility changes in tau in the tauopathies.

TAUOPATHIES

Introduction

Tau abnormalities are increasingly felt to play a crucial role in a group of neurodegenerative diseases known as the tauopathies. PSP and CBD are the most common sporadic tauopathies. Other tauopathies include Pick's disease, frontotemporal dementia and parkinsonism linked to chromosome 17 (FTDP-17), postencephalitic parkinsonism (PEP), Guam parkinsonism-dementia complex (Guam PDC), and dementia pugilistica. All tauopathies involve neurodegeneration of specific neuronal populations with filamentous tau protein aggregates in neurons and glia. Many are associated with clinical features of parkinsonism. Some are sporadic (Pick's disease, PSP, CBD, PEP, Guam PDC, dementia pugilistica), whereas others are hereditary (FTDP-17).

PSP and CBD were first reported in the 1960s (44,45), and the term *corticobasal degeneration* was coined in the 1980s (46). Molecular and genetic studies have identified similar changes in PSP and CBD. Furthermore, PSP and CBD share clinical and pathologic features, but notable differences warrant their current separation as clinicopathologic entities. Although individuals with CBD and PSP have bradykinesia, rigidity, and gait abnormalities, neither group has demonstrated a sustained clinical response to levodopa. Rest tremor, one of the cardinal clinical features of PD, is uncommon in PSP and CBD. Motor abnormalities in PSP are usually symmetric, while asymmetry is the hallmark of CBD. Focal cortical signs, such as apraxia and aphasia, are common in CBD but rare in PSP. Dementia is common in CBD and may be one of the most common presentations, but is not prominent in PSP. Supranuclear gaze palsy occurs early in most cases of PSP but is uncommon in CBD.

Pathologically, both PSP and CBD include neuronal and glial lesions composed of tau protein. Although the anatomic distribution of lesions shows overlap, the overall pattern differs (47). Cortical and cerebral white matter is more affected in CBD, whereas diencephalic and brainstem are more affected in PSP. The morphology of the typical neuronal and glial lesions is distinctive in PSP and CBD (48).

On the other hand, biochemical studies of tau protein show indistinguishable alterations in PSP and CBD (49). In both disorders there is evidence of enrichment of abnormal insoluble tau isoforms (4R tau) derived from specific tau mRNA splice forms (splice forms containing exon 10). There is also evidence of similar predisposition with respect to genetic variants in the *tau* gene (50,51).

Neuropathology of Progressive Supranuclear Palsy

Gross examination of the brain often shows frontal and midbrain atrophy. The third ventricle and aqueduct of Sylvius may be dilated. The substantia nigra shows loss of pigment, while the locus ceruleus is better preserved. The subthalamic nucleus is smaller than expected (Fig. 18.5). The superior cerebellar peduncle and the hilus of the cerebellar dentate nucleus may be atrophic and gray due to myelinated fiber loss (Fig. 18.6).

Microscopic findings include neuronal loss and fibrillary gliosis affecting multiple brain regions. The nuclei with the most marked and consistent pathology are the globus pallidus, subthalamic nucleus, and substantia nigra. Other parts of the basal ganglia, diencephalon, and brainstem are affected to a variable degree.

In addition to the changes visible with routine histologic methods, silver stains (e.g., Gallyas stain) or immunostaining for tau reveal NFTs and glial lesions (Fig. 18.7). NFTs in PSP often have a rounded or globose appearance, but flame-shaped NFTs are also detected. Special stains demonstrate a variety of inclusions in both neurons and glia, including pretangles, neuropil threads, and tufts of abnormal fibers. Pretangles are neurons with nonfilamentous granular cytoplasmic tau immunoreactivity that may be precursors to NFTs. Tufts of abnormal fibers, also known as tufted astrocytes, are most common in motor cortex and striatum. They are fibrillary lesions within astrocytes based on double immunolabeling of tau and glial fibrillary acidic protein. Tufted astrocytes account for much of the cortical pathology observed in PSP. Tau immunohistochemistry also reveals tau-positive fibers, so-called neuropil threads, and small round glial cells in the white matter, which are oligodendroglial inclusions based on double immunolabeling with tau and oligodendroglial markers. Thread-like processes in white matter are not as numerous in PSP as in CBD, but in both disorders have been shown with immunoelectron microscopy to be in axons as well as glial processes (52). In gray matter neuropil threads are less common in PSP than in AD and CBD.

The NFTs in PSP may be distinguished from NFTs in AD by the paucity of ubiquitin immunoreactivity. The same is true for CBD. They also have far less fluorescence with thioflavin-S stains. In fact, NFT may be completely missed if thioflavin-S is the only means used to evaluate neuropathology in PSP and CBD. Since NFTs in AD and CBD are composed of tau (53), the observed differences must reflect differences in packing, conformation, or posttranslational modification.

Whereas NFTs in AD are composed mostly of 22-nm-diameter paired helical filaments (PHFs) and a minor com-

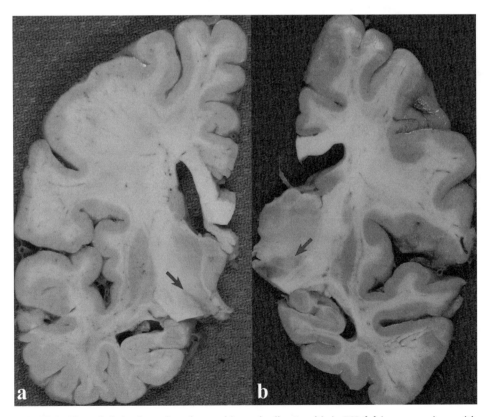

FIG. 18.5. The subthalamic nucleus *(arrows)* is markedly atrophic in PSP **(a)** in comparison with normal **(b).**

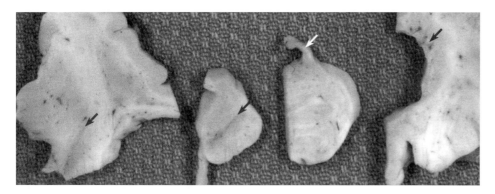

FIG. 18.6. Sections of diencephalon, midbrain, pons, medulla, and cerebellar dentate in progressive supranuclear palsy. Note small subthalamic nucleus *(arrow)*, loss of pigment in the substantia nigra *(arrow)*, atrophy of the superior cerebellar peduncle *(white arrow)* and atrophy and discoloration of the hilus of the dentate nucleus *(arrow)*.

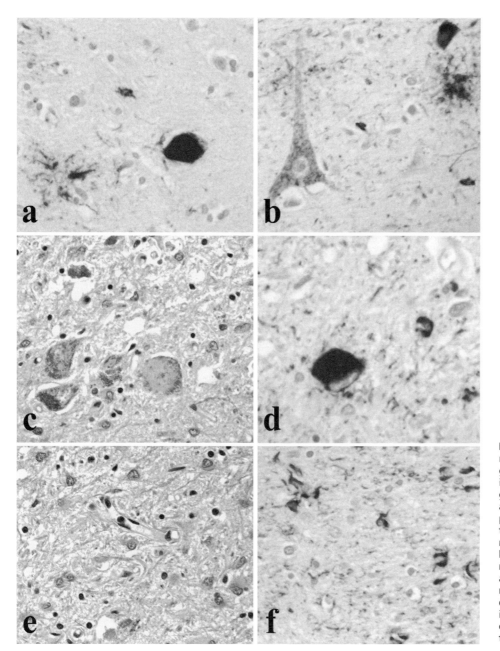

FIG. 18.7. Tau immunostaining reveals a range of lesions in progressive supranuclear palsy, including a globose neurofibrillary tangle (NFT), (**a**, right) and a tufted astrocyte (**a**, left) in the caudate; pretangles (**b**, left), NFTs, and tufted astrocytes (**b**, top right) in motor cortex. The substantia nigra has neuronal loss with extraneuronal neuromelanin pigment (**c**) and NFTs (**d**). The subthalamic nucleus has neuronal loss and dense fibrillary gliosis (**e**). Tau immunostaining shows many coiled bodies in white matter tracts (**f**).

ponent of 15- to 18-nm-diameter straight filaments, NFTs in PSP are composed of 15- to 18-nm straight filaments. The abnormal filaments in glial cells in PSP also contain straight filaments.

The distribution of pathology is highly characteristic of PSP. Pathologic diagnosis is contingent on pathology in specific nuclei and tracts. The globus pallidus and pars reticularis of the substantia nigra may show, in addition to neuronal loss, gliosis, and NFTs, extensive iron pigment deposition and granular neuroaxonal spheroids. The striatum and thalamus, especially ventral anterior and lateral nuclei, may have gliosis. The basal nucleus of Meynert usually has mild cell loss and many pretangles. The brainstem regions that are affected include the superior colliculus, periaqueductal gray matter, oculomotor nuclei, locus ceruleus, pontine nuclei, pontine tegmentum, vestibular nuclei, medullary tegmentum, and inferior olives. The cerebellar dentate nucleus is frequently affected and may show grumose degeneration, a type of neuronal degeneration associated with clusters of degenerating presynaptic terminals around dentate neurons. The dentatorubrothalamic pathway consistently shows fiber loss. The cerebellar cortex is preserved, but there may be mild Purkinje loss with scattered axonal torpedoes. Coiled bodies are common in the cerebellar white matter. The spinal cord is often affected, where neuronal inclusions can be found in anterior horn and intermediolateral cells.

Cortical gray matter is less affected than deep gray matter, but lesions are increasingly recognized in the cortex, especially the peri-rolandic region (54). Neocortical NFTs and tufted astrocytes are concentrated in the motor cortex. Recent studies suggest that cortical pathology may be more widespread in cases of PSP with atypical features, such as

dementia (55). The white matter beneath the motor cortex often has coiled bodies. More widespread cerebral white matter pathology is uncommon in PSP. This contrasts with CBD where white matter lesions are numerous and widespread.

The limbic lobe is preserved in PSP. The neurofibrillary pathology in the hippocampus is variable and not inherent to PSP, but rather more consistent with concurrent age-related pathology. An exception is the frequent involvement of the dentate gyrus granule neurons in PSP (54).

Neuropathology of Corticobasal Degeneration

Gross examination of the brain characteristically reveals subtle asymmetric atrophy of cortical gyri, most marked in pre- and postcentral regions (Fig. 18.8). The atrophy is not as sharply circumscribed or as severe as in Pick's disease. Dorsal frontoparietal atrophy merges with less severe atrophy in ventral frontal and posterior parietal regions, whereas the temporal and occipital cortical regions are usually preserved. The brainstem does not have the consistent atrophy found in PSP, but pigment loss is common in the substantia nigra. In contrast to PSP, the superior cerebellar peduncle and the subthalamic nucleus are also normal on gross examination.

The cerebral white matter in affected areas is often attenuated and may have a gray discoloration. The corpus callosum is sometimes thinned, and the frontal horn of the lateral ventricle is frequently dilated. The anterior limb of the internal capsule may show attenuation as well, but other white matter tracts, such as the optic tract, anterior commissure, and fornix, are preserved.

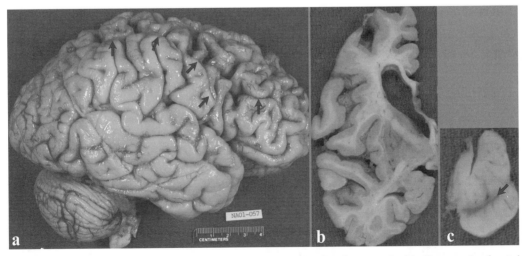

FIG. 18.8. The cortical atrophy in corticobasal degeneration is often most marked in the superior frontal gyrus and superior parietal lobule (**a**, *arrows*). On coronal sections, the frontal horn is dilated, while the temporal horn of the lateral ventricle is normal **(b)**. The lateral part of the substantia nigra *(arrow)* may show pigment loss **(c)**.

Microscopic examination of atrophic regions of the frontoparietal cortex shows moderately severe nerve cell loss with superficial spongiosis, gliosis, and subcortical myelin pallor. Thioflavin-S fluorescence and silver staining fail to reveal senile plaques or NFTs. These findings are not dissimilar to those of nonspecific focal cortical degenerations; however, several histologic features readily distinguish CBD from nonspecific focal cortical degenerations, most notably the presence of many achromatic or ballooned neurons. Ballooned neurons are swollen and vacuolated neurons found in middle and lower cortical layers. They lack apparent Nissl substance, which was the basis for the term *achromasia*. Ballooned neurons in anterior cingulate, amygdala, and claustrum have less diagnostic significance because they can be found in several disorders, most notably argyrophilic grain disease of Braak (56).

Ballooned neurons are strongly immunoreactive for phosphorylated neurofilaments and α–B crystallin (Fig.

18.9). They show variable immunoreactivity for tau and ubiquitin. Ultrastructurally, the cytoplasm of the ballooned neurons contains haphazardly arranged 9- to 16-nm-diameter filaments, interspersed with other cytoplasmic elements.

Neurons in atrophic cortical areas also have pleomorphic tau-immunoreactive lesions. In some neurons, tau is densely packed into a small inclusion body somewhat reminiscent of a Pick body or a small NFT (Fig. 18.9). In other neurons, the filamentous inclusions are more dispersed and disorderly. In contrast to NFTs of AD where lesions are readily detected with a host of diagnostic silver stains and even with thioflavin fluorescent microscopy, the neuronal lesions in CBD are negative with thioflavin-S. Neurofibrillary lesions in brainstem monoaminergic nuclei, such as locus ceruleus and substantia nigra, sometimes resemble globose NFTs but may also be ill-defined amorphous inclusions.

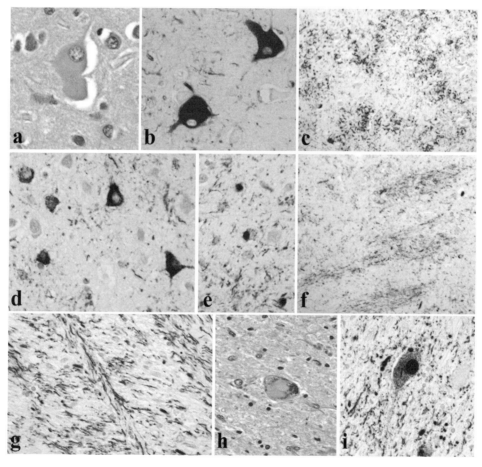

FIG. 18.9. Ballooned neurons have swelling of perikarya and proximal processes **(a)** and immunoreactivity with α-B crystallin **(b)**. Tau immunostaining of the cortex shows annual clusters of cell processes, which are astrocytic plaques **(c)**. Neuronal inclusions are diverse **(d)** and some resemble Pick bodies **(e)**. While matter tracts, such as pencil fibers in the striatum **(f)** and internal capsule near the thalamic fasciculus **(g)**, have many tau-positive thread-like processes. Neurons in the substantia nigra contain eosinophilic corticobasal bodies **(h)** that are tau positive **(i)**.

In addition to fibrillary lesions in perikarya of neurons, the neuropil of CBD invariably contains an assortment of thread-like tau-immunoreactive cell processes (57). A small fraction of thread-like structures are double labeled with neurofilament antibodies, which indicates that many thread-like lesions in CBD are in glial processes. They are usually profuse in affected areas of gray and white matter. The predominance of tau immunoreactivity in cell processes is an important attribute of CBD and a useful feature in differentiating it from other disorders. In other disorders with which CBD can be confused, tau-related pathology is more often located in cell bodies (e.g., NFTs and Pick bodies) and the proximal cell processes of neurons and glia.

The most characteristic tau-immunoreactive astrocytic lesion in CBD is an annular cluster of short stubby processes with fuzzy outlines that may be highly suggestive of a neuritic plaque (57) (Fig. 18.9). These lesions, in contrast to Alzheimer plaques, do not contain amyloid. In further contradistinction, the tau filaments are found in not neuronal but rather glial processes. These lesions are termed *astrocytic plaques*. Astrocytic plaques differ from the tufted astrocytes seen in PSP, and the two lesions do not coexist in the same brain (48). The astrocytic plaque may be the most specific histopathologic lesion of CBD.

In addition to cortical pathology, deep gray matter is consistently affected in CBD. The globus pallidus and putamen show mild neuronal loss with gliosis. The nucleus basalis of Meynert has minimal neuronal loss and pretangles. Thalamic nuclei may also be affected, particularly the ventrolateral nucleus. In the basal ganglia, thread-like processes are often extensive in the pencil fibers of the striatum. There may also be astrocytic plaques in the striatum. Pretangles are common in the striatum and globus pallidus. The internal capsule often has many thread-like processes, especially in the vicinity of the thalamic fasciculus. The subthalamic nucleus usually has a normal neuronal population, but a few neurons may have tau inclusions, and there may be a number of thread-like lesions in the nucleus. Fibrillary gliosis typical of PSP is uncommon in the subthalamic nucleus in CBD.

The substantia nigra usually shows moderate to severe nerve cell loss with extraneuronal neuromelanin and gliosis. Many of the remaining neurons contain NFTs, which have also been termed *corticobasal bodies*. The locus ceruleus and raphe nuclei have similar inclusions. In contrast to PSP where neurons in the pontine base almost always have at least a few NFTs, the pontine base is largely free of NFTs in CBD. On the other hand, tau inclusions in glia and in cell processes are common in the pontine base in CBD. NFTs are also detected in the tegmental gray matter. The cerebellum has mild Purkinje cell loss and axonal torpedoes. There is also mild neuronal loss in the dentate nucleus occurs, but grumose degeneration is much less common than in PSP.

In CBD the filaments have a paired helical appearance at the electron microscopic level, but the diameter is wider and the periodicity longer than the paired helical filaments of AD (58). These structures have been referred to as twisted ribbons. Similar filaments are found in some cases of FTDP-17, particularly those associated with overexpression of specific isoforms of tau containing exon 10 (59). Similar to PSP, tau in CBD is enriched in tau isoforms containing the domain encoded by exon 10 of the *tau* gene (4R tau).

Neuropathology of Other Parkinsonian Disorders with Neurofibrillary Tangles

Several other disorders with parkinsonism are associated with NFTs and can be considered among the tauopathies. These are uncommon disorders that in some cases have nearly disappeared, but they are discussed from a historical perspective.

Postencephalitic Parkinsonism

Parkinsonism following encephalitis lethargica during the influenza pandemic between 1916 and 1926 is known as postencephalitic parkinsonism (PEP) (60). The acute stage of illness was characterized by a somnolent state, for which the disorder is named, that in some cases progressed to coma. Other clinical features included oculomotor palsy, myoclonus, and masked facies. During the recovery phase parkinsonian rigidity developed, with the most characteristic clinical features being oculogyric crises (60). The pathology in the acute stage was characterized by inflammation and hyperemia that was widespread, but marked in basal ganglia and brainstem. Neuronal loss was present in the locus ceruleus, substantia nigra, oculomotor nuclei, and lentiform nucleus. Dystrophic calcification was also described in affected areas (60). Evaluation of brains of subjects long after the disease occurred has revealed NFTs in cortex, basal ganglia, thalamus, hypothalamus, substantia nigra, brainstem tegmentum, and cerebellar dentate nucleus (61,62). The distribution of the pathology overlaps with PSP, and in recent studies it has not been possible to distinguish the two disorders by histopathologic analysis alone (61,62). Biochemical studies of tau that accumulates in PEP has not been reported, but the NFTs resemble those seen in AD so it is reasonable to assume that abnormal tau in PEP is composed of a mixture of 3R and 4R tau. Tau-immunopositive glial lesions have not been reported in PEP.

Guam Parkinsonism-Dementia Complex

An unusually high incidence of PDC has been reported in the native Chamorro population of Guam since the 1950s (63). Some individuals also have amyotrophic lateral sclerosis (ALS), and the natives refer to the complex of PDC with ALS as "lytico-bodig." The incidence of the disorder has declined in recent years for unknown reasons, and the eti-

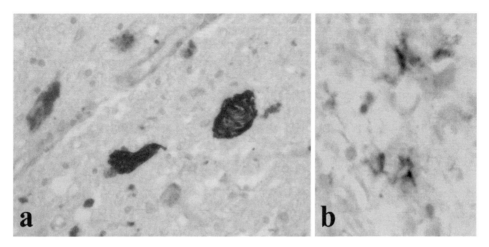

FIG. 18.10. In Guam parkinsonism-dementia complex there is marked neuronal loss in the substantia nigra, and Gallyas silver stain reveals neurofibrillary tangles in the few residual neurons **(a)**. The silver stain also reveals granular hazy astrocytes in parkinsonism-dementia complex **(b)**. (Slides courtesy of Asao Hirano, Montefiore Hospital, The Bronx, New York.)

ology remains unknown despite intensive epidemiologic and genetic research. The disorder has a geographic distribution on Guam, but the basis for this is not known. Some studies suggest that ALS on Guam is no different from ALS in other populations (64). On the other hand, PDC and the pathologic substrate of PDC, namely, widespread cortical and brainstem NFTs, is distinctly different from PD with dementia.

The gross findings in PDC are notable for cortical atrophy affecting frontal and temporal lobes, as well as atrophy of the hippocampus and the tegmentum of the rostral brainstem (65). These areas typically have neuronal loss and gliosis with many NFTs in residual neurons. Extracellular NFTs are also numerous. In the cortex NFTs show a different laminar distribution from that of AD, with more NFTs in superficial cortical layers in Guam PDC and in lower cortical layers in AD (66). The hippocampus has severe pathology with numerous NFTs. Interestingly, NFTs are also found in nondemented Chamorros at a higher frequency than in Western populations (67). The substantia nigra and locus ceruleus have neuronal loss and NFTs (Fig. 18.10). The basal nucleus and large neurons in the striatum are also vulnerable to NFTs. Lewy bodies are not detected, but some neurons in the amygdala may have synuclein-immunoreactive lesions (68). Biochemically and morphologically, NFTs in Guam PDC are indistinguishable from those in AD (69). Immunohistochemically, they are similar, with all antibodies that have been tested to tau and other NFT-associated molecules; at the electron microscopic level, the filaments in the NFTs are 22-nm-diameter paired helical filaments; and biochemically, they contain insoluble tau composed of a mixture of 3R and 4R tau. Recently, an unusual type of tau-immunoreactive astrocyte, so-called granular hazy inclusions, has been noted in Guam PDC

(70). The significance of the glial lesions in Guam PDC awaits conformation because most other disorders with glial lesions have had accumulation of non-AD tau.

Dementia Pugilistica

An akinetic rigid syndrome with dysarthria and dementia is sometimes the long-term outcome of repeated closed-head trauma as is seen in professional boxers. The pathology on gross examination, other than lesions that can be attributed to trauma (e.g., subdural membrane and cortical contusions), is characterized by fenestration or cavum of the septum pellucidum (71). The substantia nigra may also show pigment loss. Microscopically, there are NFTs that are similar to those found in AD. They are found in brainstem monoaminergic nuclei, but also in the cortex and hippocampus. In the cortex they may be clustered around blood vessels (72). At the electron microscopic level, they are composed of paired helical filaments; biochemically, the abnormal insoluble tau extracted from affected brain regions is composed of a mixture of 3R and 4R tau (73).

REFERENCES

1. Hardy J, Gwinn-Hardy K. Genetic classification of primary neurodegenerative disease. *Science* 1998;282:1075–1078.
2. Chin SSM, Goldman JE. Glial inclusions in CNS degenerative diseases. *J Neuropathol Exp Neurol* 1996;55:499–508.
3. Hutton M, Lendon CL, Rizzu P, et al. Association of missense and 5′-splice-site mutations in *tau* with the inherited dementia (FTDP-17). *Nature* 1998;393:702–705.
4. Lewis J, McGowan E, Rockwood J, et al. Neurofibrillary tangles, amyotrophy and progressive motor disturbance in tau mutant (P301L) transgenic mice. *Nat Genet* 2000;25:402–405.
5. Iwai A, Masliah E, Yoshimoto M, et al. The precursor protein of

non-Aβ component of Alzheimer's disease amyloid is a presynaptic protein of the central nervous system. *Neuron* 1995;14:467–475.

6. Polymeropoulos MHC, Leroy E, Ide SE, et al. Mutation in the alpha-synuclein gene identified in families with Parkinson's disease. *Science* 1997;276:2045–2047.

7. Spillantini MG, Schmidt ML, Lee VM, et al. Alpha-synuclein in Lewy bodies. *Nature* 1997;388:839–840.

8. Arima K, Ueda K, Sunohara N, et al. NACP/α-synuclein immunoreactivity in fibrillary components of neuronal and oligodendroglial cytoplasmic inclusions in the pontine nuclei in multiple system atrophy. *Acta Neuropathol* 1998;96:439–444.

9. Dickson DW. Tau and synuclein and their role in neuropathology. *Brain Pathol* 1999;9:657–661.

10. Dickson DW. α-Synuclein and the Lewy body disorders. *Curr Opin Neurol* 2001;14:423–432.

11. Dickson DW, Yen S-H. Ubiquitin, the cytoskeleton and neurodegenerative diseases. In: Mayer RJ, Brown IR, eds. *Heat shock or stress proteins and the nervous system.* London: Academic Press, 1994:235–262.

12. Kitada T, Asakawa S, Hattori N, et al. Mutations in the parkin gene cause autosomal recessive juvenile parkinsonism. *Nature* 1998;392:605–608.

13. Lantos PL. The definition of multiple system atrophy: a review of recent developments. *J Neuropathol Exp Neurol* 1998;57:1099–1111.

14. McKeith IG, Galasko D, Kosaka K, et al. Clinical and pathological diagnosis of dementia with Lewy bodies (DLB): report of the Consortium on Dementia with Lewy Bodies International Workshop. *Neurology* 1996;47:1113–1124.

15. Dickson DW, Ruan D, Crystal H, et al. Hippocampal degeneration differentiates diffuse Lewy body disease (DLBD) from Alzheimer's disease: light and electron microscopic immunocytochemistry of CA2-3 neurites specific to DLBD. *Neurology* 1991;41:1402–1409.

16. Galloway PG, Mulvihill P, Perry G. Filaments of Lewy bodies contain insoluble cytoskeletal elements. *Am J Pathol* 1992;140:809–815.

17. Goldman JE, Yen S-H, Chiu F-C, et al. Lewy bodies of Parkinson's disease contain neurofilament antigens. *Science* 1983;221:1082–1084.

18. Kuzuhara S, Mori H, Izumiyama N, et al. Lewy bodies are ubiquitinated: a light and electron microscopic immunocytochemical study. *Acta Neuropathol* 1988;75:345–353.

19. Irizarry MC, Growdon W, Gomez-Isla T, et al. Nigral and cortical Lewy bodies and dystrophic nigral neurites in Parkinson's disease and cortical Lewy body disease contain α-synuclein immunoreactivity. *J Neuropathol Exp Neurol* 1998;57:334–337.

20. Iwatsubo T, Yamaguchi H, Fujimuro M, et al. Purification and characterization of Lewy bodies from the brains of patients with diffuse Lewy body disease. *Am J Pathol* 1996;148:1517–1529.

21. Pollanen MS, Bergeron C, Weyer L. Detergent-insoluble Lewy body fibrils share epitopes with neurofilament and tau. *J Neurochem* 1992;58:1953–1956.

22. Baba M, Nakajo S, Tu PH, et al. Aggregation of alpha-synuclein in Lewy bodies of sporadic Parkinson's disease and dementia with Lewy bodies. *Am J Pathol* 1998;152:879–884.

23. Conway KA, Harper JD, Lansbury PT. Accelerated in vitro fibril formation by a mutant alpha-synuclein linked to early-onset Parkinson disease. *Nat Med* 1998;4:1318–1320.

24. Hughes AJ, Daniel SE, Blankson S, et al. A clincopathologic study of 100 cases of Parkinson's disease. *Arch Neurol* 1993;50:140–148.

25. Whitehouse PJ, Hedreen JC, White CL III, et al. Basal forebrain neurons in dementia of Parkinson disease. *Ann Neurol* 1983;13:243–248.

26. Dickson DW, Davies P, Mayeux R, et al. Diffuse Lewy body dis-

ease: neuropathological and biochemical studies of six patients. *Acta Neuropathol* 1987;75:8–15.

27. Mattila PM, Roytta M, Torikka H, et al. Cortical Lewy bodies and Alzheimer-type changes in patients with Parkinson's disease. *Acta Neuropathol* 1998;95:576–582.

28. Hurtig HI, Trojanowski JQ, Galvin J, et al. Alpha-synuclein cortical Lewy bodies correlate with dementia in Parkinson's disease. *Neurology* 2000;54:1916–1921.

29. Apaydin H, Ahlskog JE, Parisi JE, et al. Parkinson's disease neuropathology: later-developing dementia and loss of the levodopa response. *Arch Neurol* 2002;59:102–112.

30. Lennox G, Lowe JS, Landon M, et al. Diffuse Lewy body disease: correlative neuropathology using anti-ubiquitin immunocytochemistry. *J Neurol Neurosurg Psychiatry* 1989;52:1236–1247.

31. Kosaka K. Diffuse Lewy body disease in Japan. *J Neurol* 1990;237:197–204.

32. Hansen L, Salmon D, Galasko D, et al. Lewy body variant of Alzheimer's disease: a clinical and pathological entity. *Neurology* 1990;40:1–8.

33. Braak H, Braak E. Neuropathological staging of Alzheimer-related changes. *Acta Neuropathol* 1991;82:239–259.

34. Jellinger KA, Bancher C. Dementia with Lewy bodies: relationships to Parkinson's and Alzheimer's diseases. In: Perry RH, McKeith IG, Perry EK, eds.: *Dementia with Lewy bodies.* Cambridge: Cambridge University Press, 1996:268.

35. Dickson DW. Pathogenesis of senile plaques. *J Neuropathol Exp Neurol* 1997;56:321–354.

36. Hyman BT, Trojanowski JQ. Consensus recommendations for the postmortem diagnosis of Alzheimer disease from the National Institute on Aging and the Reagan Institute Working Group on diagnostic criteria for the neuropathological assessment of Alzheimer disease *J Neuropathol Exp Neurol* 1997;56:1095–1097.

37. Forno LS. Concentric hyaline intraneuronal inclusions of Lewy body type in the brains of elderly persons (50 incidental cases): relationship to parkinsonism. *J Am Geriatr Soc* 1969;17:557–575.

38. Liu Y, Stern Y, Chun MR, et al. Pathological correlates of extrapyramidal signs in Alzheimer's disease. *Ann Neurol* 1997;41:368–374.

39. Wenning GK, Tison F, Ben Shlomo Y, et al. Multiple system atrophy: a review of 203 pathologically proven cases. *Mov Disord* 1997;12:133–147.

40. Matsuo A, Akiguchi I, Lee GC, et al. Myelin degeneration in multiple system atrophy detected by unique antibodies. *Am J Pathol* 1998;153:735–744.

41. Kato S, Nakamura H. Cytoplasmic argyrophilic inclusions in neurons of pontine nuclei in patients with olivopontocerebellar atrophy: immunohistochemical and ultrastructural studies. *Acta Neuropathol* 1990;79:584–594.

42. Braak H, Braak E. Cortical and subcortical argyrophilic grains characterize a disease associated with adult onset dementia. *Neuropathol Appl Neurobiol* 1989;15:13–26.

43. Dickson DW, Liu W-K, Hardy J, et al. Widespread alterations of alpha-synuclein in multiple system atrophy. *Am J Pathol* 1999;155:1241–1251.

44. Steele JC, Richardson JC, Olszewski J. Progressive supranuclear palsy: a heterogenous degeneration involving the brainstem, basal ganglia and cerebellum with vertical gaze and pseudobulbar palsy, nuchal dystonia, and dementia. *Arch Neurol* 1964;10:333–339.

45. Rebeiz JJ, Kolodny EH, Richardson EP Jr. Corticodentatonigral degeneration with neuronal achromasia. *Arch Neurol* 1968;18:20–33.

46. Gibb WRG, Luthert PJ, Marsden CD. Corticobasal degeneration. *Brain* 1989;112:1171–1192.

47. Feany MB, Mattiace LA, Dickson DW. Neuropathologic overlap of progressive supranuclear palsy, Pick's disease and corticobasal degeneration. *J Neuropathol Exp Neurol* 1996;55:53–67.
48. Komori T. Tau-positive glial inclusions in progressive supranuclear palsy, corticobasal degeneration, and Pick's disease. *Brain Pathol* 1999;9:663–679.
49. Buee L, Delacourte A. Comparative biochemistry of tau in progressive supranuclear palsy, corticobasal degeneration, FTDP-17 and Pick's disease. *Brain Pathol* 1999;9:681–693.
50. Baker M, Litvan I, Houlden H, et al. Association of an extended haplotype in the tau gene with progressive supranuclear palsy. *Hum Mol Genet* 1999;8:711–715.
51. Di Maria E, Tabaton M, Vigo T, et al. Corticobasal degeneration shares a common genetic background with progressive supranuclear palsy. *Ann Neurol* 2000;47:374–377.
52. Arima K, Nakamura M, Sunohara N, et al. Ultrastructural characterization of the tau-immunoreactive tubules in the oligodendroglial perikarya and their inner loop processes in progressive supranuclear palsy. *Acta Neuropathol* 1997;93:558–566.
53. Schmidt ML, Huang R, Martin JA, et al. Neurofibrillary tangles in progressive supranuclear palsy contain the same tau epitopes identified in Alzheimer's disease PHF-tau. *J Neuropathol Exp Neurol* 1996;55:534–539.
54. Hof PR, Delacourte A, Bouras C. Distribution of cortical neurofibrillary tangles in progressive supranuclear palsy: a quantitative analysis of six cases. *Acta Neuropathol* 1992;84:45–51.
55. Bigio EH, Brown DF, White CL III. Progressive supranuclear palsy with dementia: cortical pathology. *J Neuropathol Exp Neurol* 1999;58:359–364.
56. Tolnay M, Probst A. Ballooned neurons expressing alpha B-crystallin as a constant feature of the amygdala in argyrophilic grain disease. *Neurosci Lett* 1998;246:165–168.
57. Feany MB, Dickson DW. Widespread cytoskeletal pathology characterizes corticobasal degeneration. *Am J Pathol* 1995;146:1388–1396.
58. Dickson DW, Liu W-K, Ksiezak-Reding H, et al. Neuropathologic and molecular considerations. In: Litvan I, Goetz CG, Lang AE, eds. *Corticobasal degeneration and related disorders.* (Advances in Neurology, vol 82.) New York: Lippincott Williams & Wilkins, 2000:9–27.
59. Spillantini MG, Bird TD, Ghetti B. Frontotemporal dementia and parkinsonism linked to chromosome 17: a new group of tauopathies. *Brain Pathol* 1998;8:387–402
60. Oppenheimer DR. Disease of the basal ganglia, cerebellum, and motor neurons. In: Blackwood W, Corsellis JAN, eds. *Greenfield's neuropathology*, 3rd ed. London: Edward Arnold, 1976:609–622.
61. Geddes JF, Hughes AJ, Lees AJ, et al. Pathological overlap in cases of parkinsonism associated with neurofibrillary tangles: a study of recent cases of postencephalitic parkinsonism and comparison with progressive supranuclear palsy and Guamanian parkinsonism-dementia complex. *Brain* 1993;116:281–302.
62. Litvan I, Hauw JJ, Bartko JJ, et al. Validity and reliability of the preliminary NINDS neuropathologic criteria for progressive supranuclear palsy and related disorders. *J Neuropathol Exp Neurol* 1996;55:97–105.
63. Hof PR, Nimchinsky EA, Buee-Scherrer V, et al. Amyotrophic lateral sclerosis/parkinsonism-dementia complex of Guam: quantitative neuropathology, immunohistochemical analysis of neuronal vulnerability, and comparison with related neurodegenerative disorders. *Acta Neuropathol* 1994;88:397–404.
64. Oyanagi K, Makifuchi T, Ohtoh T, et al. Amyotrophic lateral sclerosis of Guam: the nature of the neuropathological findings. *Acta Neuropathol* 1994;88:405–412.
65. Oyanagi K, Makifuchi T, Ohtoh T, et al. Topographic investigation of brain atrophy in parkinsonism-dementia complex of Guam: a comparison with Alzheimer's disease and progressive supranuclear palsy. *Neurodegeneration* 1994;3:301–304.
66. Hof PR, Perl DP, Loerzel AJ, et al. Neurofibrillary tangle distribution in the cerebral cortex of parkinsonism-dementia cases from Guam: differences with Alzheimer's disease. *Brain Res* 1991;564:306–313.
67. Anderson FH, Richardson EP Jr, Okazaki H, et al. Neurofibrillary degeneration on Guam: frequency in Chamorros and non Chamorros with no known neurological disease. *Brain* 1979;102:65–77.
68. Yamazaki M, Arai Y, Baba M, et al. Alpha-synuclein inclusions in amygdala in the brains of patients with the parkinsonism-dementia complex of Guam. *J Neuropathol Exp Neurol* 2000;59:585–591.
69. Buee-Scherrer V, Buee L, Hof PR, et al. Neurofibrillary degeneration in amyotrophic lateral sclerosis/parkinsonism-dementia complex of Guam. Immunochemical characterization of tau proteins. *Am J Pathol* 1995;146:924–932.
70. Oyanagi K, Makifuchi T, Ohtoh T, et al. Distinct pathological features of the Gallyas- and tau-positive glia in the parkinsonism-dementia complex and amyotrophic lateral sclerosis of Guam. *J Neuropathol Exp Neurol* 1997;56:308–316.
71. Graham DI, Gennarelli TA. Trauma. In: Graham DI, Lantos PL, eds. *Greenfield's Neuropathology,* 6th ed. London: Arnold, 1997:197-263.
72. Geddes JF, Vowles GH, Nicoll JA, et al. Neuronal cytoskeletal changes are an early consequence of repetitive head injury. *Acta Neuropathol* 1999;98:171–178.
73. Schmidt ML, Zhukareva V, Newell KL, et al. Tau isoform profile and phosphorylation state in dementia pugilistica recapitulate Alzheimer's disease. *Acta Neuropathol* 2001;101:518–524.

TREMORS: DIFFERENTIAL DIAGNOSIS, PATHOPHYSIOLOGY, AND THERAPY

GÜNTHER DEUSCHL
JENS VOLKMANN

A practical definition of tremor refers to a rhythmic, mechanical oscillation of at least one functional body region. Although neurologists are mainly confronted with pathologic tremors, one should keep in mind that any movement is accompanied by normal physiologic tremor. This mostly invisible oscillation is assumed to be necessary for fast movements as the onset of voluntary movements coincides usually with the peak of the tremor burst in normal tremor. The limits between normal and pathologic tremors can be difficult to define. A scientific approach would be to define the normal range according to amplitude and frequency with a quantitative measurement. A more pragmatic clinical approach is to define abnormal tremor whenever it is visible to the naked eye or if any frequencies occur that are lower than normal tremor.

PHENOMENOLOGY AND TERMINOLOGY OF TREMOR

Clinical analysis and classification of tremor depends critically on a definition of the activation conditions during which tremor occurs because, for example, the term "resting tremor" will otherwise be used with a very different meaning by clinicians. The following definitions and related criteria are based on the consensus statement of the Movement Disorder Society on tremor (1).

Resting tremor occurs in a body part that is not voluntarily activated and is completely supported against gravity. The amplitude of tremor must increase during mental and sometimes motor activation (counting backward, Stroop test, gait, movements of the contralateral hand), and diminish or even disappear during the onset of voluntary activation (1); moreover, it must reoccur after a certain time period (2).

Mental activation triggers the amplitude of many tremors, but only resting tremor is triggered in the relaxed limbs. Resting tremor often responds to dopaminergic treatment. However, exceptions to this general rule exist, and careful studies of this problem are not available. Resting tremor is a separate tremor entity generated by central mechanisms unique to this symptom.

Action tremor is any tremor occurring upon voluntary contraction of muscle. This includes postural, isometric, and kinetic tremor.

Postural tremor is present while an individual is voluntarily maintaining a position against gravity. A rare variant of postural tremor is *position-specific postural tremor* or *position-sensitive tremor*. *Isometric tremor* occurs as a result of muscle contraction against a rigid stationary object (e.g., a heavy table). This form of force tremor can occur in isolation or together with other tremor symptoms and may be the cause of separate complaints.

Kinetic tremor is tremor that occurs during any voluntary movement. Kinetic tremor may occur in non-goal-directed and goal-directed movements.

Simple kinetic tremor occurs during voluntary movements that are not goal directed and is contrasted with tremor during goal-directed movements ("intention tremor").

Intention tremor is present when the amplitude increases during visually guided movements toward a target and typical fluctuations of the amplitude (velocity) of the tremor occur.

Whenever a tremor increases substantially during the pursuit of a target or goal, it can be assumed that a disturbance of the cerebellum or its afferent or efferent pathways exists (3). Typically, tremor amplitude fluctuates significantly as the target is approached. It may be difficult to distinguish between intention tremor and ataxia in some patients.

Task-specific kinetic tremor may appear or become exacerbated during specific activities. Occupational tremors and primary writing tremor are examples of this kind of tremor.

CLINICAL ASSESSMENT OF TREMOR PATIENTS

The description of a particular tremor should include the following aspects (1): topography of tremor (head, chin, jaw, vocal cords, upper/lower extremity, body, etc.); activation condition of tremor (rest, posture, non-goal-directed movements, goal-directed movements, eventually specific tasks); and frequency of tremor (low: <4 Hz; medium: 4 to 7 Hz; high: >7 Hz). The general neurologic examination has a great impact on the differential diagnosis of tremor. For obvious reasons the presence of akinesia, rigidity (including Froment's sign for the upper and lower extremity and coactivation sign of psychogenic tremor), postural abnormalities, dystonia, spasticity, ataxia, and/or signs of neuropathy should be documented. Specific information from the medical history should include onset of tremor, family history, alcohol sensitivity, associated diseases, medications, and drug use/abuse.

Several rating scales have been proposed. Generally, it is necessary to distinguish between resting and action tremors, which are associated with different complaints. Moreover, specific problems arise from the variability of tremor. For resting tremors the Unified Rating Scale for Parkinson's Disease (UPDRS) (4) with some supplementary questions (5) have been proposed. For postural and intention tremor two partially overlapping scales have been proposed (6,7) including a motor score and a disability scale. A number of excellent instruments for the assessment of essential tremor (ET) are available (8–12).

SYNDROMIC CLASSIFICATION AND MANAGEMENT OF TREMOR

From a clinical standpoint a classification of tremor would be desirable that would allow us to identify the etiology by means of the clinical features of a tremor. But tremors of different causes can have a very similar clinical presentations, making such an approach unsuccessful. On the other hand, some etiologies (e.g., parkinsonian tremor or ET) can have variable clinical expressions, and in these cases the tremor, together with other symptoms, can suggest the diagnosis. Thus, we can separate some distinct tremor syndromes that either are common or can be considered phenomenologic entities from a clinical point of view. The Movement Disorder Society has proposed a classification that in some cases implies a clear-cut etiology but in others describes a syndrome leaving the etiology open. The different syndromes in this classification are defined on the basis of clinical observations without additional laboratory tests. Some tremors might escape classification under this scheme; these are labeled "unclassified tremors." The clinical classification, the frequency range, and the activating conditions are summarized in Fig. 19.1. Some of the etiologic factors in tremor are listed in Table 19.1.

As our knowledge of the pathogenesis and pathophysiology of most tremors is limited, almost all of the tremor drug treatments have been discovered by chance. However, many treatment strategies have been confirmed in careful double-blind studies, at least for the most common tremor.

NORMAL TREMOR

Physiologic tremor is present in every normal subject during posture and action. Its frequency for hand tremor is between 6 and 12 Hz. Normal finger tremor can sometimes be seen with the naked eye. Mechanical and sometimes central oscillations cause this tremor (13–15).

Enhanced physiologic tremor (EPT) is a visible, predominantly postural, high-frequency tremor of short duration (<2 years). Evidence of a neurologic disease related to tremor must be excluded. This definition covers many tremor etiologies, typically those elicited by endogenous or exogenous intoxication producing postural tremor (Table 19.1). These tremors are usually reversible, provided that the cause is identified and corrected for. The term was originally introduced to describe a condition defined by physiologic measurements that applies to various tremor etiologies (13,16). We propose to extend it to the above-mentioned clinical definition because these tremors share the same clinical criteria and a common category for these reversible tremors is needed. Some standard laboratory tests that may be considered for etiologic diagnosis in these patients are summarized in Table 19.2. This type of tremor overlaps with the category of drug-induced and toxic tremors (see below).

Pathophysiology

The mechanism underlying EPT is mainly mechanical tremor aggravated by reflex activation or central oscillations (17). Sometimes central tremor oscillations detectable on an electromyogram are invariant to peripheral loading of the extremity. One mechanism for increasing tremor amplitudes may be activation of these normal central oscillations by drugs, as has been shown for amitriptyline (18).

Treatment

When causal treatment is not available or fails to suppress tremor sufficiently, propranolol or another beta blocker is recommended.

Therapeutic studies are available for a few specific tremors classified as EPTs. Valproate tremors seem to respond to propranolol (19) and acetazolamide (20) but not to amantadine, cyproheptadine, diphenhydramine, and benztropine (19). The general treatment of persons with hyperthyroidism has been addressed in various studies (for review, see 21), but no study has specifically addressed the

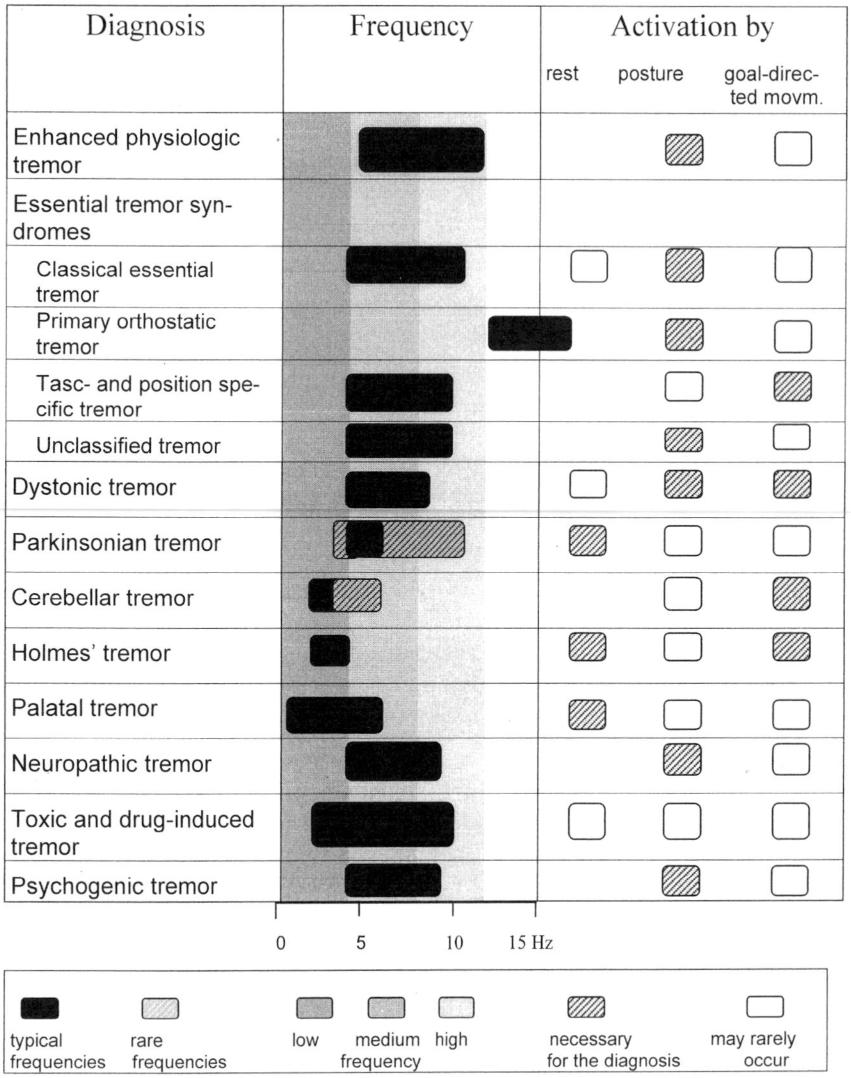

Diagnosis	Frequency	Activation by — rest	posture	goal-directed movm.
Enhanced physiologic tremor			necessary	may rarely occur
Essential tremor syndromes				
Classical essential tremor		may rarely occur	necessary	may rarely occur
Primary orthostatic tremor			necessary	may rarely occur
Tasc- and position specific tremor			may rarely occur	necessary
Unclassified tremor			necessary	may rarely occur
Dystonic tremor		may rarely occur	necessary	necessary
Parkinsonian tremor		necessary	may rarely occur	may rarely occur
Cerebellar tremor			may rarely occur	necessary
Holmes' tremor		necessary	may rarely occur	necessary
Palatal tremor		necessary	may rarely occur	may rarely occur
Neuropathic tremor			necessary	may rarely occur
Toxic and drug-induced tremor		may rarely occur	may rarely occur	may rarely occur
Psychogenic tremor			necessary	may rarely occur

Frequency axis: 0   5   10   15 Hz

Legend: typical frequencies; rare frequencies; low / medium / high frequency; necessary for the diagnosis; may rarely occur

FIG. 19.1. Clinical forms of tremors (1).

clinical management of tremor. The following drugs and dosages have been applied in these patients: propranolol (160 mg daily), atenolol (200 mg daily), metoprolol (200 mg daily), acebutolol (400 mg daily), oxprenolol (160 mg daily), nadolol (80 mg daily), and timolol (20 mg daily). Lithium tremor has also been shown to respond to beta blockers (22). Tremor in drug-induced parkinsonism does not respond to propranolol (23). Some patients with postural tremors in the setting of peripheral neuropathies respond to propranolol.

ESSENTIAL TREMOR SYNDROMES

The definition of ET has evolved into two different meanings in recent years. On the one hand, the term describes a tremor syndrome classically defined by a monosymptomatic tremor that often is hereditary (24–26). This is the most common movement disorder. On the other hand, there are tremors of unknown origin ("idiopathic" or "essential") but with distinct clinical characteristics, which usually can be separated from classical ET on clinical grounds but are also considered ETs. To cover these two groups in a single classification, the Movement Disorder Society (1) in its consensus statement proposed separating these tremors into "classical" ET and the other well-defined but nevertheless idiopathic tremor syndromes. In addition, individuals whose tremor cannot be classified unequivocally receive a diagnosis of "indeterminate postural tremor syndrome."

Classical Essential Tremor

Classical ET is a monosymptomatic, predominantly postural and action tremor that tends to progress slowly over a years. The diagnostic criteria and the differential diagnoses

TABLE 19.1. ETIOLOGIC CLASSIFICATION OF TREMOR

1. Hereditary, degenerative, and idiopathic diseases	
Parkinson's disease	R, P
Pallidonigral degeneration	P
Multiple system atrophy	
Olivopontocerebellar atrophy	R, P, I
Striatonigral degeneration	R, P, I
Wilson's disease	R, P, I
Progressive pallidum atrophy	R
Huntington's disease	R, P, I
Benign hereditary chorea	P, I
Fahr's disease	R, I
Paroxysmal dystonic choreoathetosis	I
Familial intention tremor and lipofuscinosis	I
Ramsay Hunt syndrome	P, I
Ataxia telangiectasia	P
Dystonia musculorum deformans	P
Segawa's dystonia	P
Spasmodic torticollis	P
Meige's disease	P
Essential myoclonus and tremor	P, I
Essential tremor	P, I
Hereditary chin tremor	P, I
Task-specific tremors:	
Writer's tremor	
Voice tremor	
Golfer's tremor ("yips")	
Laughing tremor	
Klinefelter's syndrome	P, I
2. Cerebral diseases of various causes	
Infectious diseases and other inflammations	
Multiple sclerosis	R, P, I
Neurolues	
Neuroborreliosis	
HIV infection	P
FSME	P, I
Small pox, measles	P
Typhus	P
Space-occupying lesions	
Tumors	R, P, I
Cysts	R, P, I
Hematoma	R, P, I
Arteriovenous malformations	R, P, I
Cerebrovascular insults	R, P, I
Trauma	R, P, I
3. Metabolic diseases	
Hyperthyroidism	P
Hyperparathyroidism	R, P
Magnesium deficiency	R, P
Hypocalcemia	R, I
Hyposodiumemia	P
Hypoglycemia	P
Disturbed liver function (chronic hepatocerebral degeneration)	P, I
Hepatic encephalopathy	P, I
Kidney disturbances	P, I
Vitamin B$_{12}$ deficiency	R, P, I
Eosinophilia-myalgia syndrome	P, I
4. Peripheral neuropathies and similar disorders	
Charcot-Marie-Tooth	P, I
Roussy-Levy syndrome	P
Chronic demyelinating neuropathies	P
Guillain-Barré syndrome	P
Gammopathy (IgM, IgG)	P
Malabsorption neuropathy	P
Polyneuropathy of various origins (diabetes, uremia, porphyria)	P
HIV-associated neuropathy	P
Spinal muscle atrophy	P
5. Toxins	
Nicotine	P
Mercury	P, (R, I)
Lead	P, (R, I)
Carbon monoxide	P, (R, I)
Manganese	P, (R, I)
Arsenic	P, (R, I)
Cyanide	P
Naphthalene	P, I
Alcohol	P, I
Phosphor	P, (R, I)
Toluene	P
DDT	P, (R, I)
Lindane	P, I
Kepone	P, I
Dioxins	P
6. Drugs	
Centrally acting substances	
Neuroleptics	R, P
Reserpine	R, P
Tetrabenazine	R, P
Metoclopramide	R, P
Antidepressants (especially tricyclics)	P
Lithium	R, P, I
Cocaine	P
Alcohol	P, I
Sympathomimetics	
Adrenaline	P, I
Bronchodilators (β$_2$ agonists, e.g., Formoterol)	P, I
Theophylline	P
Caffeine	P
Teeine	P
Dopamine	P
Steroids	
Progesterone (methoxyprogesterone)	R, P
Antiestrogens (tamoxifen)	P
Adrenocorticosteroids	P
Miscellaneous	
Valproate	P
Perhexilene	R, P
Antiarrhythmics (amiodarone)	P
Mexiletine, procainamide	P
Calcitonin	P
Thyroid hormones	P
Cytostatics (vincristine, adriablastin, cytosine arabinoside, ifosfamide)	P, I
Immunodepressants (cyclosporin A)	P
7. Others	
Emotions (anxiety, stress)	P
Fatigue	P
Cooling	P
Trauma of the periphery/sympathetic	
Reflex sympathetic dystrophy	P, I
High-pressure neurologic syndrome	P
Withdrawal of drugs	P
Withdrawal of alcohol	P, I
Withdrawal of cocaine	R
Psychogenic tremor	R, P, I

FSME, Frühsommer-Meningoencephalitis; DDT, dichlorodiphenyltrichloroethane.
Modified after Deuschl G, Koester B. Diagnose und Behandlung des Tremors. In: Conrad B, Ceballos-Baumann AO, eds. Bewegunsstörungen in der Neurologie. Stuttgart: Thieme Verlag, 1996:222–253.

TABLE 19.2. LABORATORY CHECK OF SYMPTOMATIC TREMORS

TRH
Na+, K+, Ca2+, Cl–
γ-GT, GOT, GPT, cholinesterase
Creatinine, urea, glucose
Cortisol[a], parathormone[a]
24-hr copper excretion + ceruloplasmin[a]
Toxicologic tests[a]

[a]Tests to be performed only when clinically suggested.
T3, triiodothyronine; T4, thyroxine; TRH, thyroid-releasin hormone; GT, glucaronyl transferase; GPT, glutamate-pyruvate transaminase; GOT, glutamate oxaloacetate transaminase.

are listed in Table 19.3. It is the most common movement disorder. Prevalence rates vary between 0.4% and 5.6% (27,28). In 60% of patients the condition is autosomal dominant. The responsible gene or, more likely, different genes have not yet been identified, although linkage has been found in different families on chromosome 2 (29), 3 (30), and 4 (31). In about 50% to 70% of patients symptoms improve with ingestion of alcohol (32). The condition may begin very early in life but the incidence increases above age 40 years, with the mean age of onset between 35 and 45 years in different studies and an almost complete penetrance at age 60 (24,26). The topographic distribution [meta-analysis of 891 patients from the literature (24–26,32–35)] shows hand tremor in 94%, head tremor in 33%, voice tremor in 16%, jaw tremor in 8%, facial tremor in 3%, leg tremor in 12%, and tremor of the trunk in 3% of the patients. In some topographic regions (e.g., head, voice, and chin) tremor may occur in isolation (36).

The severity of tremor increases gradually over years. All patients are disabled to some extent, and most are socially handicapped due to the tremor. Up to 25% of patients seeking medical attention must change jobs or retire from work (26,32). It is interesting that earlier descriptions have emphasized that ET is not made strikingly worse during goal-directed movements (13,37). In fact, ET is mainly a postural tremor, though rarely resting tremors do occur (16,38–40). But in almost half of patients intention tremor (41) occurs together with other subtle signs of cerebellar dysfunction, such as ataxia and movement overshoot. Often

these patients also have a disturbance of tandem gait that may be clinically visible (42).

Pathophysiology

Classical ET is most likely due to central oscillations (16,17) arising in the Guillain-Mollaret triangle. The inferior olive is believed to function abnormally in this condition.

Treatment (Table 19.4)

Tremor of the Hands

Propranolol and primidone are clearly the drugs of first choice for this indication and both have been carefully studied (for review, see 43). Propranolol was introduced in 1971 (44) for the management of ET. Drugs with predominantly β1 effects have been shown to be less effective than those acting on the β2 receptor, and none has proved superior to propranolol. Only 25% of patients maintain their initial good response for 2 years. Contraindications are cardiac insufficiency or arrhythmia and diabetes. As propranolol acts on the peripheral (reflex) component of tremors it is efficacious for many tremors, such as Parkinson's, cerebellar, and so forth (45,46). Primidone is effective for ET (47) but tachyphylaxia may occur. The major problems are early adverse effects with nausea, dizziness, sedation, and headache. The combination of propranolol and primidone is recommended whenever the use of one drug is insufficient. Gabapentin was also found to be effective in two double blind-studies (48,49), but another double-blind study showed no convincing effect (50). Acetazolamide and methazolamide are not significantly better than placebo (51). Alprazolam is helpful in ET (52). Clonazepam is recommended for patients with predominantly action and intention tremor in ET (53) but not effective in uncomplicated ET (54). Botox 50 U or 100 U has a significant but clinically limited effect especially on motor function (55). Surgery is the accepted treatment for patients resistant to medical treatment who are experiencing severe disability. Two multicenter studies have shown that thalamic deep brain stimulation is effective (56–58), and one study has shown that deep brain stimulation of the nuclear ventralis

TABLE 19.3. GUIDELINES FOR THE DIAGNOSIS OF ESSENTIAL TREMOR (185,186)

Core Criteria	Secondary Criteria	Red Flags
1. Bilateral action tremor of the hands and forearms (but not rest tremor) 2. Absence of other neurologic signs, with the exception of the cog-wheel phenomenon 3. May have isolated head tremor with no abnormal posture	1. Long duration (>3 yr) 2. Family history 3. Beneficial response to ethanol	1. Unilateral tremor, focal tremor, leg tremor, gait disturbance, rigidity, bradykinesia, rest tremor 2. Sudden or rapid onset 3. Current drug treatment that might cause or exacerbate tremor 4. Isolated head tremor with abnormal posture (head tilt or turning)

TABLE 19.4. MANAGEMENT OF ESSENTIAL TREMOR

	Drug	Dosage	Remarks
1st choice	Propranolol	(30–320 mg, 3 doses) (standard or long acting)	Contraindications: cardiac, pulmonary, diabetes, etc. Hand and head tremor
1st choice	Primidone	(62.5–500 mg, single dose in the evening)	Hand and head tremor Preferentially for patients with age >60 years
1st choice	Combination: Propranolol/primidone	Maximal dosage for each	Try always before using 2nd and 3rd choice drugs
2nd choice	Gabapentine	1,800–2,400 mg daily	Conflicting results of three studies: one without, two with benefit!
2nd choice	Clonazepam	0.75–6 mg	For predominant kinetic tremor
3rd choice	Clozapine	Test: 12.5 mg, 30–50 mg daily	Less well-documented effect than for Parkinson's disease
Last choice	Surgery		VIM stimulation

intermedius of the thalamus (VIM) has a better effect than VIM thermocoagulation and fewer side effects (59). Appropriate selection of patients for surgery is a crucial factor for achieving a good therapeutic effect.

Head and Voice

Pharmacologic management of essential head and voice tremor is less efficient than that of hand tremor. Propranolol and primidone, alone or in combination, has been recommended (33,60) for essential head tremor. Clonazepam is often recommended for this indication, but careful studies are not available. One of the promising therapies for head tremor is the local injection of botulinum toxin (61), but further studies are needed. Deep brain stimulation is also effective for head and voice tremor, but usually bilateral VIM stimulation is necessary (57,62–64).

VARIANTS OF ESSENTIAL TREMOR

The following clinical entities can be separated on clinical grounds, although much of the pathophysiologic background of these tremors remains unknown and reclassification may eventually be needed.

Primary Writing Tremor and Other Task- or Position-specific Tremors

Tremor during writing without other manifestations of tremor or other neurologic disease is called primary writing tremor. After the initial observation (65), two forms of writing tremor have been described (66):

1. Tremor appearing during writing only (type A, task-specific tremor).
2. Tremor occurring when the hand position to be used for writing is adopted (type B, position-specific tremor).

There are several other conditions that fit the category of task- or position-specific tremors. Subjects suffering from these tremors are mostly individuals who perform motor activities at the highest level, such as musicians or sportsmen. Such individuals develop tremor in their professional activity (e.g., piano playing) while other skilled movements (eating, handling delicate objects, etc.) remain unaffected. Common examples are tremors in golfers (67,68) or those occurring in pianists (69,70).

Pathophysiology

The pathophysiologic interpretation of these syndromes is controversial. The relation between dystonic tremor and writing tremor is not clearly defined, though some interpret the latter as a form of focal dystonia (71). Other researchers have not found evidence for dystonia and instead consider writing tremor to be an idiopathic condition separate from dystonia, such as a specific overuse syndrome or a focal form of ET (72).

Treatment

Management of task-specific tremors is difficult. Propranolol and local injections of botulinum toxin have been proposed. Often physical therapy, abstinence from the tremor-producing tasks, and subsequent retraining is the best approach to treatment. There is one report about successful treatment of a patient with drug-resistant primary writing tremor by thalamic deep brain stimulation (73).

Isolated Voice Tremor

The clinical diagnosis of isolated voice tremor can be put forward if the tremor is limited to the voice alone. Such isolated voice tremor (74) occurs in two variants. The first resembles spasmodic dysphonia with dysponic and trembling voice and is often considered to be a form of focal dystonia of the vocal cord (75,76). The second presents with a pure voice tremor and is considered to be a form of ET (25,26,32,77). Dystonic voice tremor is more likely if the tremor is not present during emotionally charged speaking or singing. In our experience this feature is not present in voice tremor in the setting of ET. Voice tremor also occurs in cerebellar disease or classical ET together with other tremor manifestations; thus, it does not fit the definition of isolated voice tremor. The pathophysiology of voice tremor is unknown.

Treatment

This is another condition that is difficult to treat. Essential voice tremor can sometimes be improved with propranolol or primidone. Dystonic voice tremor can often be successfully managed with local injections of botulinum toxin in the vocal cord (78,79). This has also been shown for essential voice tremor (80). Thalamic deep brain stimulation does often reduces voice tremor (81), but isolated voice tremor is rarely an indication for surgery.

Isolated Chin Tremor

Isolated chin tremor is a rare, autosomal dominant syndrome characterized by attacks of high-frequency tremor of the mentalis muscles or of the chin typically starting in early childhood (82). A genetic linkage has been found (83). It may be reclassified in the future as a myoclonus or channelopathy rather than a tremor. Low-frequency chin tremors often occur in Parkinson's disease and sometimes occur in ET.

Treatment

Reports on treatment for chin trembling are rare. In most cases, specific treatment is not necessary. One patient has been treated with botulinum toxin (84).

Primary Orthostatic Tremor

Primary orthostatic tremor is a unique tremor syndrome (85,86) observed only in patients older than 40 years. Due to its unusual clinical presentation, many patients are still considered to have a psychiatric condition.

Primary orthostatic tremor is characterized by a subjective feeling of unsteadiness during stance (but only in severe cases during gait). Some patients experience sudden falls. None of the patients have problems when sitting or lying down. The clinical findings are sparse, often limited to a visible or sometimes only palpable fine-amplitude rippling of the leg (quadriceps) muscles. The diagnosis can be confirmed by electromyographic (EMG) recordings (e.g., from the quadriceps femoris muscle) with a typical 13- to 18-Hz pattern. All of the leg, trunk, and even arm muscles show this pattern when standing, which in many cases is absent during tonic innervation when sitting and lying (87–89).

The diagnosis is critically dependent on the EMG demonstration of this pattern because individuals experiencing other tremors during stance (e.g., essential, parkin-

sonian, or cerebellar tremors of the legs) may present with similar complaints.

Pathophysiology

There is strong evidence that primary orthostatic tremor is a central tremor because the high-frequency EMG pattern is highly coherent in all of the trembling muscles. Recent studies have shown that orthostatic tremor may also be present during maneuvers that do not involve stance (90), and that the time relation of the muscle jerks shows a task-specific plasticity (91) since all of the muscles on both sides of the body are involved and are coherent. This is the strongest evidence for a central tremor. The oscillator of this tremor is unknown. Due to the unique coherence of the muscles on both sides and the fact that resetting of the tremor was only possible with electrical stimulation over the posterior fossa but not over the cortex, this tremor is considered to be a brainstem tremor.

Treatment

Orthostatic tremor has been documented to be responsive to clonazepam and primidone. Valproate and propranolol were applied in single cases with variable success. L-dopa has been efficacious in some patients (92). According to small double-blind studies (93,94) and our own experience, gabapentin seems to have the best and most consistent beneficial effect. Meanwhile we use it as the drug of first choice for orthostatic tremor (1,800 to 2,400 mg daily).

Indeterminate Postural Tremor Syndrome

Some patients have a predominantly postural tremor that would qualify as classical ET except that additional neurologic signs of uncertain significance are present. Such signs (e.g., mild extrapyramidal features such as hypomimia, decreased arm swing, or mild bradykinesia) are not sufficient to make the diagnosis of a recognizable neurologic disorder. It may be impossible to definitely classify the patient because the significance of the associated neurologic signs is not yet apparent. By labeling these patients as having an indeterminate tremor syndrome the problems associated with an incorrect diagnosis or conflicting diagnoses are thus avoided and the neurologist remains open minded about the therapeutic options. For example, the differentiation between early parkinsonism and ET can be impossibly difficult in some elderly patients but may become clear with the passage of time.

Dystonic Tremor

Dystonic tremor is an entity that is still under debate, and different definitions have been proposed by clinicians (95–97). Tremor in dystonia has been proposed as a "forme fruste" of ET (98). However, it is not yet clear if they share common genes—the *DYT1* locus has already been excluded (99)—or at least pathophysiologic mechanisms.

But there are clinical features that differentiate these tremors. Dystonic tremor is defined (1) as a postural/kinetic tremor usually not seen during complete rest occurring in an extremity or body part that is affected by dystonia. Usually these are focal tremors with irregular amplitudes and variable frequencies (mostly less than 7 Hz).

Some patients exhibit focal tremors even without overt signs of dystonia. Such patients have been included among those with dystonic tremors (100) because some of them develop dystonia. In many patients with dystonic tremors antagonistic gestures lead to a reduction of the tremor amplitude. This is well known for dystonic head tremor in the setting of spasmodic torticollis (dystonic head tremor) showing tremor reduction when the patient touches the head or lifts an arm (101), whereas essential head tremor does not show this sign (97).

Dystonic tremor and *tremor associated with dystonia* can be different because unspecific postural tremors occur in extremities not involved in dystonia. Hand tremor in patients with otherwise uncomplicated idiopathic spasmodic torticollis is a typical example of this (101). *Dystonia gene–associated tremor* may be another special form of tremor. This is an isolated tremor in patients with a dystonic pedigree.

Pathophysiology

The pathophysiology of tremors in dystonia is unknown. It may be related to the same basal ganglia abnormality as dystonia itself (17).

Treatment

As dystonic extremity tremors are rare and have just recently been established as a clinical entity, detailed drug trials are rare. A positive effect of propranolol was described in studies of dystonic head tremor. The effectivity of botulinum toxin for dystonic head (102) and hand (55) tremor as well as in tremulous spasmodic dysphonia is already well documented. Patients severely affected by generalized dystonia have been successfully treated with deep brain stimulation of the pallidum or ventrolateral thalamus (103). Tremor associated with dystonia and dystonia gene–associated tremor often respond to medication for classical ET.

Tremors in Parkinson's Disease

Most patients with Parkinson's disease present with tremor. Resting tremor with pill-rolling is typical. Besides resting tremor, up to 40% of patients have different forms of postural and action tremor (104–106), which can occur in isolation or together with resting tremor. Thus, tremor in Parkinson's disease (PD) cannot be generally defined by the tremor characteristics itself. Tremor in Parkinson's disease is assumed if the patient has Parkinson's disease according to the brain bank criteria, including bradykinesia, and if the patient has any form of pathologic tremor.

A wide range of clinical presentations of tremors can be found in Parkinson's disease. For reasons of clinical simplicity they have been subdivided strictly according to their clinical symptoms (1).

Type I: Classical Parkinsonian Tremor—Resting Tremor or Resting and Postural/Action Tremor with the Same Frequency

Pure resting tremor occurs in a significant number of patients. The frequency of pure resting tremor is mostly 4 to 6 Hz, but in the early stage of the disease much higher resting tremor frequencies can be found (107,108). In other patients the resting tremor is combined with a kinetic tremor of the same frequency. Its amplitude is increasing with mental stress, contralateral movement, or during gait. Upon initiation of a voluntary movement the tremor is suppressed but it reoccurs after a few seconds with the hands outstretched (1,2). The clinical observations fit with the hypothesis that this postural/kinetic tremor (with similar frequencies for rest and postural/kinetic tremors) is a continuation of the resting tremor under postural and/or action conditions. The frequencies for resting and postural/action tremor can be considered to be equal if they do not differ by more than 1.5 Hz. With some experience this frequency difference can be seen clinically.

Type II: Resting and Postural/Action Tremors of Different Frequencies

A mild form of action tremor is present in almost every parkinsonian patient. This can be seen during slow flexion/extension movements. Sometimes this postural/action tremor can be extremely disabling. This is often considered to be an enhanced physiologic tremor.

Some patients have a predominant postural tremor in addition to resting tremor. The postural/action tremor has a frequency higher than, and nonharmonically related to, that of the resting tremor. This form is rare (less than 15% of patients with Parkinson's disease) and has often been described as a combination of ET and Parkinson's disease (107,108). Some of these patients had their postural tremor long before the onset of other symptoms of Parkinson's disease.

Type III: Pure Postural/Action Tremor

Isolated postural and action tremors are rare but do occur in PD. They have been assigned as ET variants or have been

TABLE 19.5. CLINICAL CRITERIA TO SEPARATE ESSENTIAL AND PARKINSONIAN TREMOR

	Essential Tremor	Parkinson's Disease
Hereditary tremor	+++	–
Head tremor	+++	–
Voice tremor	+++	–
Sensitivity to alcohol	+++	–
Classical resting tremor	+	++
Predominant unilateral tremor	+	+++
Leg tremor	+	+++
Rigidity (not only Fromment's sign)	+	++
Sensitivity to L-dopa	–	+++

found to be indistinguishable from enhanced physiologic tremor. A relationship between this form of tremor and rigidity seems possible (105).

Only the resting tremor component is by itself a positive diagnostic criterion for Parkinson's disease according to the brain bank criteria, but other tremors are often seen in Parkinson's disease. The differential diagnosis between Parkinson's disease and classical ET can be difficult, especially in the early stage of the condition. It has been estimated that 20% of patients with ET are misdiagnosed for Parkinson's disease and vice versa. Some of the differential diagnostic criteria are summarized in Table 19.5.

Type IV: Monosymptomatic Tremor at Rest

Some patients exhibit a resting and postural tremor without overt signs of bradykinesia or rigidity. Thus, the clinical findings are not sufficient to justify a diagnosis of Parkinson's disease, although there is positron emission tomography (PET) evidence that these patients have a dopaminergic deficit (109) and—similar to that in full-blown Parkinson's disease—the distance between substantia nigra and the red nucleus was reduced (110). Treatment of such patients is often difficult. Thus, monosymptomatic tremor at rest is defined (1) by the following criteria:

1. Pure or predominant resting tremor.
2. No signs of bradykinesia, rigidity, or problems with stance stability sufficient to justify a diagnosis of Parkinson's disease.
3. Tremor duration of at least 2 years.

Pathophysiology

Dopamine depletion in the striatum is the hallmark of PD, but the pathophysiology of parkinsonian tremor is still under debate. The most extreme hypotheses argue about peripheral versus central nervous system (CNS) origin, intrinsic cellular oscillator versus network oscillators, and basal ganglia–based pathophysiology versus cerebellothalamic-based pathophysiology. Recent studies support the

view that parkinsonian symptoms are most likely due to abnormal synchronous oscillating neuronal activity in the basal ganglia. Peripheral factors have a minor role in the generation, maintenance, and modulation of PD tremor and other signs. The most likely candidates producing these oscillations are the weakly coupled neural networks of the basal ganglia–thalamocortical loops. However, present evidence supports the view that the basal ganglia loops are influenced by other neuronal structures and systems, and that tuning of these loops by cerebellothalamic mechanisms and by other modulator neurotransmitter systems entrains the abnormal synchronized oscillations. Resting tremor in Parkinson's disease is most likely due to abnormal central oscillators in the basal ganglia (17,111). The pathophysiology of action tremors in Parkinson's disease is unknown.

Treatment

Due to the different forms of tremor in PD the clinical characteristics of the tremor have to be taken into account. Our personal approach to the treatment of patients is included in Tables 19.6 and 19.7.

L-dopa is the most effective treatment for the majority of symptoms in Parkinson's disease. Among the tremors in Parkinson's disease mainly the resting tremor is improved, but other forms may also respond. Generally, the effect on tremor is highly variable in patients with Parkinson's disease and the tremor may even worsen. All of the available double-blind studies of different dopamine agonists failed to demonstrate a superior effect of one or the other agonist on tremor although all of them obviously have a significant effect. For pramipexol an open study has shown a favorable effect on tremor (112). Although management of tremors with anticholinergics is often recommended, only a few double-blind studies have been done. The anticholinergic bornaprine has been found effective in two double-blind studies (113,114). Trihexyphenidyl has been tested alone and compared with amantadine and L-dopa (106). Possible side effects are dry mouth, visual disturbances, constipation, glaucoma, disturbance of micturition, and memory deficits. Especially in elderly subjects, confusional states can occur that are reversible after cessation of the drug. Discontinuation may induce a severe rebound effect.

The favorable effect of clozapine on resting tremor has been confirmed in several studies (115,116), even when other drugs failed (117). No tolerance has been observed over 6 months. The dosage was 18 to 75 mg. Major side effects are sedation and leukopenia (the latter as a serious complication).

Functional neurosurgery is a useful treatment for some patients who cannot be treated otherwise. Thalamic thermocoagulation or deep brain stimulation of the VIM improves tremor but does not improve akinesia. Lesional surgery cannot be applied bilaterally due to speech disturbances (but deep brain stimulation can) and is therefore no

TABLE 19.6. DOSAGES OF VARIOUS SUBSTANCES APPLIED FOR THE MANAGEMENT OF TREMOR[a]

	Initial Dose (mg)	Increase in Steps of	Maximal Dose (mg)
L-dopa			
L-dopa + benserazide	62.5	62.5 mg/d	750
L-dopa + carbidopa	50	50 mg/d	600
Dopamine agonists			
Bromocriptine	5	5 mg/w	20
Lisuride	0.1	0.1 mg/w	1.2
α-Dihydroergocryptine	10	10 mg/w	90
Pergolide	0.15	0.5 mg/w	3.0
Pramipexole	1.5	0.5 mg/w	4.5
Ropinirole	3	3.0 mg/w	15
Cabaserile	2	1 mg/w	6
Anticholinergics			
Bornaprine	3	3 mg/w	12
Biperidene	1	2 mg/w	12
Metixen	7.5	7.5 mg/w	60
Trihexyphenidyl	1	2 mg/w	10
β-blockers			
Propranolol	30	30 mg/w	240
Nadolol	10	30 mg/w	120
Miscellaneous			
Amantadine	100	100 mg/d	300
Primidone	62.5	125 mg/d	500
Clonazepam	0.5	0.5 mg/d	6
Alprazolam	0.75	0.75 mg/d	4
Clozapine	12.5	12.5 mg/d	75

[a]For some substances (e.g., anticholinergics), a slow titration is strictly recommended.

longer the surgical treatment of first choice (59). Pallidotomy as well as stimulation of the pallidum improves tremor as well. Subthalamic nucleus stimulation improves tremor (118) along with akinesia and rigidity, and is therefore the preferred surgery. However, double-blind studies are still needed.

Cerebellar Tremor Syndromes

Cerebellar tremor is often used synonymously with intention tremor, although various clinical forms of tremor have been described in cerebellar disorders (119,120). There is general agreement that the most *common form of cerebellar tremor* is intention tremor.

The following conditions have to be fulfilled for the diagnosis of cerebellar tremor:

1. Pure or dominant intention tremor, often unilateral
2. Tremor frequency below 5 Hz (mostly below 4 Hz)
3. Postural tremor possibly present, but no resting tremor

Another tremor that is most likely due to pathology of the cerebellum or its afferent/efferent pathways is known as *titubation*. It is a slow-frequency oscillation of the whole body and/or head depending on postural innervation. Dur-

TABLE 19.7. SUGGESTIONS FOR THE MANAGEMENT OF TREMORS IN PARKINSON'S DISEASE

Tremor Type	First Step	Second Step	Third Step
Classical parkinsonian tremor or monosymptomatic rest tremor	L-dopa Dopamine agonists Anticholinergics	Amantadine Propranolol Clozapine	STN stimulation
Rest and postural tremor with different frequencies	Propranolol Primidone	Dopamine Dopamine agonists Anticholinergics Clozapine	STN stimulation
Isolated action tremor	Propranolol Anticholinergics	Amantadine	

STN, subthalamic nucleus.

ing movement the amplitude usually increases, and individuals afflicted with this tremor are severely incapacitated (119). The most common causes for intention tremor and titubation are multiple sclerosis, brain trauma with infratentorial damage, and (hereditary) ataxias. Both intention tremor and titubation are symptomatic tremors. The most extensive study of tremor in multiple sclerosis (MS) has confirmed that rest tremor never occurs in MS and that about 50% of MS patients suffer from cerebellar tremor, with 27% exhibiting significant disability and 10% incapacitating tremors (121).

All other forms of tremor (postural tremor, stance tremors, etc.) are only accepted as being of cerebellar origin if other signs of cerebellar dysfunction are also observed. Cerebellar tremor can be considered as a symptomatic tremor. The major differential diagnoses are atypical forms of ET and some symptomatic tremor etiologies, such as Wilson's disease. The pathophysiologic basis of cerebellar tremor is believed to be abnormal feedforward or feedback mechanisms (long-loop reflexes).

Treatment

Cerebellar tremors are difficult to treat and good results are rare. Double-blind studies are rare. Studies with cholinergic substances, such as physostigmine and lecitine (a precursor of choline), have shown improvement in some patients but failure in the majority. Studies with isoniazid failed to show significant results (122). 5-Hydroxytryptophan (5-HTP) has been found to be effective in some patients (123). Another recent proposal has been to administer amantadine. Open studies or single-case observations have shown favorable results with: propranolol, clonazepam, carbamazepine, tetrahydrocannabiol, and trihexyphenidyl. Limited improvements have been observed after loading of the shaking extremity, but patients adapt rapidly to the added weight. Probably the best symptomatic improvement can be obtained with thalamotomy and recently also with stereotactic high-frequency stimulation in selected patients (124–127). However, the functional outcome after stereotaxy varies greatly depending on the presence of other motor symptoms of the disease. In a recent study (128), patients with MS tremor with a frequency greater than 3 Hz and significant tremor-related disabilities were found to respond favorably. Accelerometric recordings have helped in this study to distinguish patients with tremor from those with ataxia.

Holmes Tremor (Rubral Tremor, Midbrain Tremor, Myorhythmia, Benedikt's Syndrome)

These tremors are due to a lesion of the CNS mainly of the midbrain (129,130). In order to avoid definitions that include topographic relations, the Consensus Statement of the Movement Disorder Society has proposed to label this well-defined tremor as Holmes tremor, because G. Holmes was among the first to describe this tremor (131). The following criteria define this tremor (1):

1. The presence of both resting and intention tremor. In many patients postural tremor is also present. The tremor rhythm is often not as regular as for other tremors, giving the impression of jerky movements.
2. Slow frequency, mostly below 4.5 Hz.
3. If the date of the lesion is known (e.g., in case of a cerebrovascular accident), a variable delay between the lesion and the first occurrence of the tremor is typical (mostly 2 weeks to 2 years).

This is among the most disabling forms of tremor because it disturbs rest as well as all kinds of voluntary and involuntary movements. It mainly affects the hands and proximal arm, and is usually unilateral.

Pathophysiology

It is generally accepted that this is a symptomatic tremor due to lesions that seemingly are centered in the brainstem/cerebellum and thalamus. However, lesions of the involved fiber tracts in other regions may cause a similar clinical phenomenology.

The pathophysiologic basis of Holmes tremor is a combined lesion of the cerebellothalamic and nigrostriatal systems. Autopsy data (132), PET data (133), and clinical observations (130,134) suggest that it develops following a combined lesion of these two pathways. Central oscillators cause this tremor. It seems likely that the rhythm of resting tremor is usually blocked during voluntary movements by the cerebellum. If this cerebellar compensation is absent, the rhythm of rest tremor spills into movements (134), thereby producing a low-frequency intention tremor.

Involuntary Movements after Thalamic Stroke

A specific tremor syndrome associated with thalamic lesions that was investigated in the past was recently further analyzed by modern imaging techniques (96,135,136). The label *thalamic tremor* (135) has been used for this novel entity. A more detailed study has shown this tremor to be part of a specific dystonia-athetosis-chorea-action tremor following lateral posterior thalamic stroke (136). The combination of tremor, dystonia, and a severe sensory loss seems to be the important clue for the diagnosis in conjunction with this stroke. The tremor itself is a mixture of action tremor with an intentional component and dystonia in the setting of a well-recovered severe hemiparesis. Proximal segments are often involved. This tremor syndrome also develops with a certain delay after the initial insult.

Treatment of Holmes Tremor and Thalamic Tremor

No generally accepted therapy is available. Nevertheless, the treatment success rate is higher than for patients with cerebellar tremor. Some patients respond to levodopa, anticholinergics, or clonazepam. The effect of functional neurosurgery for this tremor syndrome is poorly documented. Such patients have been operated, but their diagnosis was posttraumatic tremor or post-stroke tremor, and the clinical features are not described in detail. Therefore, additional controlled studies are necessary.

PALATAL TREMOR SYNDROMES

Palatal tremor was originally classified as palatal myoclonus (137). However, because it is rhythmic it has been reclassified as a tremor with two forms (138,139): symptomatic and essential.

Symptomatic palatal tremor (SPT) is characterized by the following features (1):

1. Preceding brainstem/cerebellar lesion with subsequent olivary pseudohypertrophy (which can be demonstrated by magnetic resonance imaging).
2. Rhythmic movements of the soft palate (levator veli palatini) and often other brainstem-innervated or extremity muscles. This is clinically visible as a rhythmic movement of the edge of the palate.

Essential palatal tremor (EPT) is characterized by:

1. Absent CNS lesion and absent olivary pseudohypertrophy.
2. Rhythmic movements of the soft palate (tensor veli palatini), usually with an ear click. The tensor contraction is visible as a movement of the roof of the palate. Extremity or eye muscles are not involved.

The pathophysiologic basis is believed to be autonomous oscillations of the inferior olive in SPT (140) and is unknown for EPT.

Besides these two classical forms, additional rhythmic movement disorders of the palate and neighboring structures may occur that have not yet been classified.

Treatment

The disability of patients with SPT is mostly due to other clinical symptoms of the underlying cerebellar lesion. The rhythmic palatal movement in SPT does not cause discomfort or disability for the patient except when the eyes are involved or when an extremity tremor is present.

Oscillopsia treatment is difficult. Individual patients have been described as having a favorable response to clonazepam. Other oral drugs that have been proposed are trihexyphenidyl and valproate. Botulinum toxin has been used for the management of oscillopsia. The toxin can be injected into the retrobulbar fat tissue or specific muscles can be targeted selectively (141,142). So far no controlled studies are available. In our experience, this treatment is helpful for some patients but is not always acceptable for long-term use.

For the management of extremity tremors, only single case reports have described a favorable response to clonazepam (143) or trihexyphenidyl (144).

The only complaint of patients with EPT is the ear click. A number of medications have been reported as effective: valproate (145), trihexyphenidyl (144), and flunarizine (146). Recently, sumatriptan was found effective in a few patients (147–149), but was ineffective in another (150). The antagonism of serotonin (5-hydroxytryptamine, 5-HT) receptors may thus play a role at least for some patients. As a long term therapy this drug is not suited for various reasons. Presently the most established therapy for the click is injection of botulinum toxin into the tensor veli palatini (151). Low dosages of botulinum toxin (e.g., 4 to 10 units Botox) are injected under EMG guidance either transpalatally or transnasally. The critical point is to ascertain by endoscopic and electromyographic means that the tip of the needle is definitely placed within the tensor muscle. Spread of botulinum toxin in the soft palate can otherwise cause severe side effects. Although we have never seen such complications in our patients, it must be mentioned that the injection of botulinum toxin into the palatal muscles in rabbits has been introduced as an animal model for middle ear infections.

DRUG-INDUCED AND TOXIC TREMOR SYNDROMES

Drug-induced tremors may present with the whole range of clinical features of tremors depending on the drug and probably on the individual predisposition of the patients. The most common form is enhanced physiologic tremor following, for example, sympathomimetics or antidepressants (Table 19.1). Another common form is parkinsonian tremor following neuroleptic or, more generally, antidopaminergic drugs (dopamine receptor blockers, dopamine-depleting drugs such as reserpine, flunarizine, etc.). Intention tremor may occur following lithium intoxication or administration of certain substances. The withdrawal tremor from alcohol or other drugs has been characterized as enhanced physiologic tremor, with tremor frequencies mostly greater than 6 Hz. However, this has to be separated from the intention tremor of chronic alcoholism, which is most likely related to cerebellar damage following alcohol ingestion (152). This often comes with a 3-Hz stance tremor that has been assigned to anterior lobe damage due to chronic alcoholism (153). The etiologies of toxic tremors are summarized in Table 19.1.

A specific variant is *tardive tremor* associated with long-term neuroleptic therapy (154,155). The risk factors for development of this tremor are not well known, but many clinicians believe that patients with ET, older age, and female sex have a higher risk of developing this tremor. Its frequency range is 3 to 5 Hz; it is most prominent during posture but is also present at rest and during goal-directed movements.

Treatment

The treatment for these tremors is usually stopping of medication or toxin ingestion. Treatment attempts for tardive tremor have been with trihexyphenidyl or clozapine.

TREMOR SYNDROMES IN PERIPHERAL NEUROPATHY

Several peripheral neuropathies tend to be more often associated with the development of tremor than others. Dysgammaglobulinemic neuropathies, Guillain-Barré syndrome and chronic inflammatory demyelinating neuropathies (CIDP) are the most common causes, but many other neuropathies have been found to be associated with tremor (156,157) (Table 19.1). The tremors are mostly of the postural and action types. The frequency in hand muscles can be lower than in proximal arm muscles. It should be mentioned that abnormal position sense is not a necessary condition for the diagnosis. The pathophysiology of this tremor is believed to be due to the abnormal interaction of peripheral and central factors (158).

Treatment

No convincing therapies are reported for this type of tremor. Successful management of the neuropathy rarely improves the tremor. In our experience, propranolol and primidone, at doses similar to those for ET, have been helpful for some patients.

PSYCHOGENIC TREMOR

Psychogenic tremors have different clinical presentations. The following criteria suggest a diagnosis of psychogenic tremor (159–161):

1. Sudden onset of the condition and/or remissions.
2. Unusual clinical combinations of resting and postural/intention tremors.
3. Decrease of tremor amplitude during distraction.
4. Variation of tremor frequency during distraction or during voluntary movements of the contralateral hand.

5. "Coactivation sign" of psychogenic tremor.
6. Somatization in the patient's history.

These patients present either with obvious whole-body shaking or with predominant extremity tremor, although there is an overlap between these manifestations in some cases. The diagnosis is easy in the patients exhibiting generalized body shaking. These movements usually cease spontaneously during examination because they are exhausting for the patient. The other group with predominant extremity tremor is more difficult to diagnose and needs careful examination for the criteria listed above. We consider the coactivation sign of psychogenic tremor especially helpful, as such tremors may often last for hours and cannot be a voluntary oscillation. These patients seem to use a physiologic mechanism known as clonus to produce this rhythmic movement just by co-contracting antagonistic muscles. The pathophysiologic basis is therefore possibly a spinal rhythmic oscillation elicited by coactivation (162,163). Thus, we consider coactivation to be a necessary condition to develop these extremity tremors. The prognosis is often poor (164).

Treatment

No studies on the treatment effects in psychogenic tremor are available (159). Psychotherapy is helpful in a minority of patients. During the First World War thousands of patients were treated with hypnosis, and we have no doubt that the treatment was successful at that time (162). Today such treatment is only of limited value. We recommend physiotherapy aimed at decontracting the muscles during voluntary movements. In addition, we administer propranolol at medium or high doses to desensitize the muscle spindles, which are needed to maintain the clonus mechanism in these patients.

DIFFERENTIAL DIAGNOSIS

Rhythmic Myoclonus and Cortical Tremor/Myoclonus

Rhythmic myoclonus is a syndrome that has been proposed by several authors (165) as intermittent brief muscle jerks, irregular or rhythmic, arising in the CNS with a low frequency (usually less than 5 Hz) and topographically limited to segmental levels.

This type of hyperkinesia is not yet well defined, and the present definition is preliminary. Rhythmic myoclonus cannot be clearly distinguished from tremor (especially from myorhythmia/rubral tremor and thalamic tremor). Sometimes the driving muscle contractions are very brisk, so that there are longer pauses between the individual jerks. This has been put forward as a feature for the differential diagnosis (165). The present definition also does not distinguish epilepsia partialis continua from rhythmic myoclonus.

Cortical tremor is considered a specific form of rhythmic myoclonus (166,167). It presents with high-frequency, irregular, tremor-like postural and action myoclonus. Electrophysiologic tracings show the typical features of cortical myoclonus with a related electroencephalographic spike preceding the EMG jerks and often enhanced long-loop reflexes and/or giant somatosensory evoked potentials. This form is mostly hereditary but has also been described in corticobasal degeneration (168,169) and even following focal lesions or celiac disease (170).

Clonus

Clonus is a rhythmic movement mostly around one joint (but sometimes of a whole extremity) elicited through the stretch reflex loop and increasing in strength (or amplitude) as a result of maneuvers affecting the stretch reflex (163). Clonus is only rarely misinterpreted as tremor. On clinical examination passive stretching of the muscles increases the force of clonus but not of tremor. This is the best criterion separating the conditions. In terms of pathophysiology, it is still debated if clonus is also dependent on a central oscillator or based on segmental reflex circuits only.

Asterixis (Negative Myoclonus)

Asterixis is a negative myoclonus with sudden lapses of innervation. When the EMG pauses are long (>200 ms), typical flapping tremor during tonic contraction result. When the pauses are shorter, the clinical phenomenology may resemble a somewhat irregular high-frequency enhanced physiologic tremor.

Asterixis can occur either as a focal or a generalized condition and is usually a symptomatic movement disorder. Unilateral asterixis is often due to focal lesions of the contralateral hemisphere, and bilateral asterixis is commonly due to endocrine dysfunction, intoxication, or certain types of focal lesion (171). The diagnosis should be confirmed with polymyographic recordings from different muscles of one extremity showing synchronous pauses of innervation.

Epilepsia Partialis Continua

Epilepsia partialis continua (EPC) is a focal epilepsy that produces mostly low-frequency rhythmic jerks of an extremity. Thus, it can be misinterpreted as tremor. Resting and, rarely, postural/intention tremors (e.g., Holmes tremor) may resemble EPC. Lack of a history of tremor, a medical history of epilepsy and presence of electroencephalographic spikes, short EMG bursts, and jerk-locked averaging are helpful in identifying this disorder.

PATHOPHYSIOLOGY OF TREMORS

The clinical spectrum of tremors is broad. Nevertheless, the pathophysiologic principles underlying these different entities are limited. A full description of our present knowledge of the origin of tremor is beyond the scope of this chapter (for reviews, see 17 and 111), but the basic principles will be summarized briefly.

Four mechanisms have been proposed to produce tremor:

1. Mechanical oscillations of the extremity.
2. Reflexes eliciting and maintaining oscillations.
3. Abnormally functioning central oscillators.
4. Tremulous central motor command due to alteration of central feedforward or feedback loops.

There is much evidence that one these mechanisms is the main cause of a particular type of tremor. However, several of these mechanisms may occur addictive in a patient (172).

The first mechanism is based on simple mechanical properties of any mass-spring system: A mass (extremity) coupled with a spring of a certain stiffness (joint and muscles) will oscillate after mechanical perturbation. Thus, the hand or arm held against gravity will oscillate with a resonance frequency that can be demonstrated with lightweight accelerometers. The resonance frequency differs for the various joints mainly due to the different mass of the oscillating mechanical parts: fingers, approximately 20 Hz; hand, 7 to 9 Hz; forearm, 3 to 4 Hz; shoulder, 1 to 2.5 Hz (16). Several factors have been identified that mediate the initial perturbations of this passive system. These include cardioballistic oscillations of the extremities, unsteadiness of any postural innervation, and unfused contractions of single motor units that cause a rhythmic modulation of the muscle force. These unfused contractions of the motor units cause a rhythmic activation of the muscle-tendon system that is subsequently synchronized to the resonance frequency. In technical terms, the extremity is behaving like a damped oscillator. The resonance frequency can be determined when the frequency of postural tremor is measured with a sensitive accelerometer. This becomes more evident if loading the extremity reduces the resonance frequency.

The second mechanism is reflex activation of tremor. The basic idea is that the oscillation of a limb will activate muscle receptors that elicit several afferent volleys. These volleys will evoke stretch reflexes activating the muscles through homonymous and heteronymous pathways. If this reflex burst is appropriately timed it can represent the next burst of muscle activity of a tremor rhythm. This subsequently elicits the next afferent volley and thereby produces ongoing tremor. Such a reflex mechanism can be enhanced by two mechanisms: first, by synchronizing or increasing the afferent volley producing a stronger reflex response, and second by increasing the reflex gain. In fact, it is likely that such mechanisms exist in humans. For example, adrenaline and thyroid hormones sensitize the muscle spindles, leading to a more synchronized and stronger afferent volley and thereby increasing tremor amplitude.

The third mechanism producing tremor is through a central oscillator. Specific cell populations within the CNS have the capacity to fire repetitively due to special properties of the membrane potential (173). For example, cell groups in the thalamus can fire in the "relay mode"; that is, they show normal spatial and temporal summation of the membrane potential, including spikes, as long as they get input from other sources. However, under certain circumstances they can fire in an "oscillating mode" being characterized by specific changes of the membrane conductance for calcium. Cells of the inferior olive show continuous spontaneous activity based on this mechanism. Oscillation of single cells within the CNS is not a sufficient condition to produce a visible tremor in the periphery. But if several cells are synchronized, a strong synchronized volley can reach the motoneuronal pool, thus producing muscle tremor. One mechanism synchronizing the activity of a cell group is electrotonic coupling through gap junctions between different cells, as has been demonstrated for the inferior olive. If this coupling is strong, rhythmic activation of one cell will activate other cells. This is probably not the only mechanism synchronizing rhythmic activity in a group of cells. Other possibilities, such as internal loops or abnormal coherence between cells of the basal ganglia (174) mediating synchronized activity may exist. It is likely that central oscillators are the most important factor for the origin of pathologic tremors.

Whether the tremor of a particular patient is due to a central or a reflex mechanism can be assessed by comparing the frequencies of EMG synchronization when the extremity is loaded or unloaded (see Fig. 19.2).

As a fourth mechanism it has been proposed that abnormal functioning of the cerebellum might produce tremor (175,176). This may not necessarily refer to activation of a cerebellar oscillator but more likely relates to altered characteristics of feedforward or feedback loops. Cooling or lesioning experiments have shown that deep cerebellar nuclei have to be affected to produce this type of abnormality. It has been well established in animals (176,177) and humans that one of the striking abnormalities in cerebellar dysfunction is delay of the second and third phases of the triphasic pattern of ballistic movements (177,178) or delay of the reflexes regulating stance control (179). During goal-directed movements this causes the breaking movement to occur late thus producing an overshoot, resulting in a quasi-rhythmic movement compatible with intention tremor. However, this does not exclude the existence of a separate central oscillator related to cerebellar tremor.

ELECTROPHYSIOLOGIC TOOLS FOR DIAGNOSIS AND MONITORING OF TREMORS

Electromyography of Tremors

The diagnosis of tremors can be confirmed by EMG examination. Surface electromyography is sufficient and needle recordings are rarely necessary. Electromyography is the best method to identify the muscles and limb segments involved in tremor (16). The EMG assessment of tremors is the most reliable method to diagnose primary orthostatic tremor and to confirm or exclude asterixis in patients with high-frequency irregular "tremors."

Electromyography can be helpful in the diagnosis of dystonic tremor and in assessing the tremor frequency for various tremors. The value of EMG examinations is limited for the differential diagnosis of essential and parkinsonian tremors.

Quantitative Tremor Analysis

Analysis of the accelerogram and electromyography of hand tremor with spectral analysis can be used to assess the frequency and amplitude of tremor during standardized maneuvers. This helps to quantify both the amplitude and the frequency of tremor for documentation or objective control of treatment. It may also be used for diagnostic purposes. This procedure is well established (16). The mathematical and technical requirements are not trivial and bear some pitfalls (180). It can be assessed if the tremor of a particular patient is due to a central or a reflex mechanism by comparing the frequency of EMG synchronization (15) when the extremity is loaded with 1,000 g or unloaded (Fig. 19.2). Meanwhile a special computer program for this analysis has been developed (181). The results of these tests can be interpreted in the following way:

1. No synchronization of the electromyogram despite rhythmic oscillation of the limb, recorded with accelerometry. The frequency of oscillation decreases when an inertial load is applied to the limb because the resonance frequency of the hand–mass system is lowered. The EMG spectrum is flat because there is no significant contribution from the stretch reflex or central oscillation at the time of tremor recording. This is characteristic of normal mechanical tremor (Fig. 19.2a).
2. Synchronization is found in the electromyogram, and the frequency of the accelerometry and electromyogra-

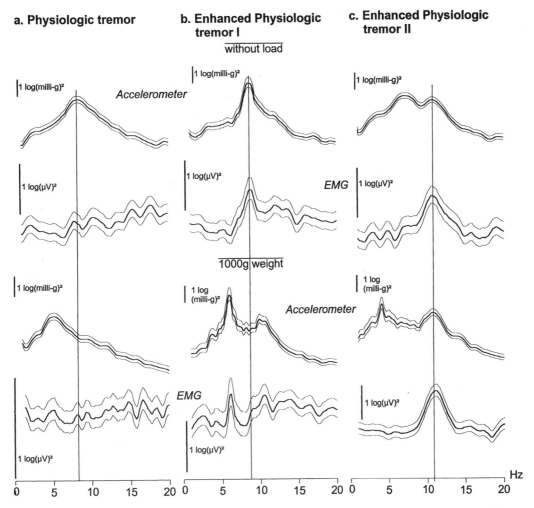

FIG. 19.2. Representative examples of spectral analysis of hand tremor recordings in normal subjects. The first and third tracings in each row show the spectrum of accelerometry, and the second and fourth tracings show the spectrum of the extensor electromyogram. The records without and with a weight of 1,000 g attached to the dorsum of the hand are shown. A majority of normal subjects have no peak in the electromyogram, and the accelerometer–peak (corresponding to the resonance–frequency) has a lower frequency after loading **(a)**. For some patients the frequency of the electromyographic peak decreases with the accelerometer peak **(b)**, indicating that this portion of the tremor is attributable to reflex activation. In this example there is an additional central component at 11 Hz. Finally, a significant portion of normal subjects have a central tremor component **(c)**. This is assumed because electromyographic synchronization appears at a frequency of 11.5 Hz with corresponding peaks in the spectrum of the accelerogram. The weight-dependent resonance component shows a lower frequency after loading.

phy both decrease and are equal. Hence, the oscillating musculoskeletal system dictates the frequency of motor-unit entrainment through somatosensory feedback (reflexes). This is the outcome in some patients with enhanced physiologic tremor (Fig. 19.2b).

3. In the unloaded condition, limb oscillation and electromyography have the same or slightly different frequencies, but in the loaded condition the frequency of the accelerometric peak decreases away from the frequency of the electromyogram. The latter oscillation is

interpreted as a central oscillation. This is the most common outcome in patients with mild ET, but identical results are obtained from some normal people with prominent 8- to 12-Hz tremor (Fig. 19.2c).

4. The mechanical oscillation and EMG entrainment have the same frequency in the loaded and unloaded condition. This is a sign of definite pathologic central oscillations and occurs in almost all central tremors. Higher harmonics may occur but are of no diagnostic value (Fig. 19.3a–c).

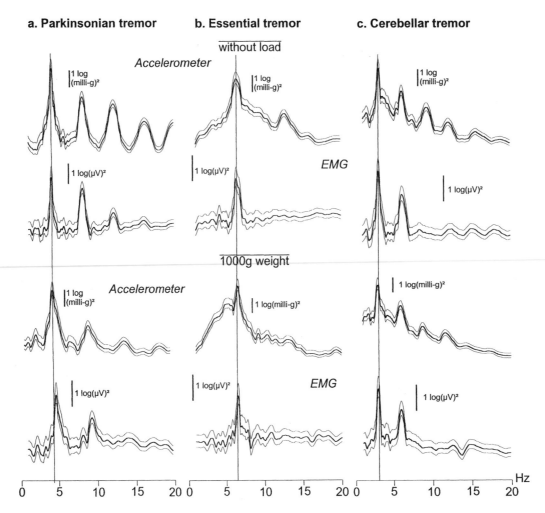

FIG. 19.3. Examples of spectral analysis of hand tremor in patients. Typical parkinsonian tremor **(a)** shows a dominant frequency with several upper harmonics. Loading does not change the frequency. Similar findings can be obtained in patients with essential tremor **(b)**. Cerebellar tremor **(c)** also shows mostly constant frequencies after loading. Load-independent constant frequencies in the electromyographic spectrum are interpreted to reflect a central tremor generator.

Graphic Tablet Analysis

Graphic tablets have been introduced for the analysis of writing tremor and to measure the severity of action and intention tremor (182,183). They can be used for diagnostic purposes and especially for treatment monitoring.

Long-term Recordings of Tremor

Long-term recording of tremor electromyograms has been tested for one or several days. This is of special interest for the study of drug effects (184).

CONCLUSION

Significant advances have been achieved in tremor research during the last decade. Most tremor syndromes have been defined clinically. Still, nowadays many clinical studies are hampered by the fact that inhomogeneous patient populations are included. Advances in the treatment of tremors have also been significant. New medications and especially surgical techniques, including deep brain stimulation, permits treatment of patients who otherwise could not be treated. Although the pathophysiology of tremor remains unclear for many of conditions, we are confident that progress in this field will result in improvements in the rational therapy of tremor in the near future.

REFERENCES

1. Deuschl G, Bain P, Brin M, et al. Consensus statement of the Movement Disorder Society on tremor. *Mov Disord* 1998;13: 2–23.
2. Jankovic J, Schwartz KS, Ondo W. Re-emergent tremor of

Parkinson's disease. *J Neurol Neurosurg Psychiatry* 1999;67:
646–650.

3. Hallett M. Overview of human tremor physiology. *Mov Disord* 1998;13:43–48.

4. Fahn S, Elton RL. Unified Rating Scale for Parkinson's disease. In: Fahn S, Marsden CD, eds. *Recent developments in Parkinson's disease.* London: Macmillan, 1987:153–163, 293–304.

5. Zimmermann R, Deuschl G, Hornig A, et al. Tremors in Parkinson's disease: symptom analysis and rating. *Clin Neuropharmacol* 1994;17:303–314.

6. Fahn S, Tolosa E, Marin C. Clinical rating scale for tremor. In: Jankovic J, Tolosa E, eds. *Parkinson's disease and movement disorders.* Baltimore: Williams & Wilkins, 1993:271–280.

7. Bain PG, Findley LJ, Atchison P, et al. Assessing tremor severity. *J Neurol Neurosurg Psychiatry* 1993;56:868–873.

8. Louis ED, Ford B, Bismuth B. Reliability between two observers using a protocol for diagnosing essential tremor. *Mov Disord* 1998;13:287–293.

9. Louis ED, Ford B, Wendt KJ, et al. A comparison of different bedside tests for essential tremor. *Mov Disord* 1999;14:462–467.

10. Louis ED, Wendt KJ, Albert SM, et al. Validity of a performance-based test of function in essential tremor. *Arch Neurol* 1999;56:841–846.

11. Louis ED, Barnes LF, Wendt KJ, et al. Validity and test–retest reliability of a disability questionnaire for essential tremor. *Mov Disord* 2000;15:516–523.

12. Louis ED, Pullman SL. Comparison of clinical vs. electrophysiological methods of diagnosing of essential tremor. *Mov Disord* 2001;16:668–673.

13. Marsden CD. Origins of normal and pathologic tremor. In: Findley LJ, Capildeo R, eds. *Movement disorders: tremor.* London: Macmillan, 1984:37–84.

14. Deuschl G, Lauck M, Timmer M. Tremor classification and tremor time series. *Chaos* 1995;5:48–51.

15. Raethjen J, Pawlas F, Lindemann M, et al. Determinants of physiologic tremor in a large normal population. *Clin Neurophysiol* 2000;111:1825–1837.

16. Elble RJ, Koller WC. *Tremor.* Baltimore: Johns Hopkins University Press, 1990.

17. Deuschl G, Raethjen J, Lindemann M, et al. The pathophysiology of tremor. *Muscle Nerve* 2001;24:716–735.

18. Raethjen J, Lemke MR, Lindemann M, et al. Amitriptyline enhances the central component of physiological tremor. *J Neurol Neurosurg Psychiatry* 2001;70:78–82.

19. Karas BJ, Wilder BJ, Hammond EJ, et al. Treatment of valproate tremors. *Neurology* 1983;33:1380–1382.

20. Lancman ME, Asconape JJ, Walker F. Acetazolamide appears effective in the management of valproate-induced tremor. *Mov Disord* 1994;9:369.

21. Feely J, Peden N. Use of beta-adrenoceptor blocking drugs in hyperthyroidism. *Drugs* 1984;27:425–446.

22. Gelenberg AJ, Jefferson JW. Lithium tremor. *J Clin Psychiatry* 1995;56:283–287.

23. Metzer WS, Paige SR, Newton JE. Inefficacy of propranolol in attenuation of drug-induced parkinsonian tremor. *Mov Disord* 1993;8:43–46.

24. Larssen T, Sjögren T. Essential tremor: a clinical and genetic population study. *Acta Psychiatr Scand* 1960;36:1–176.

25. Lou JS, Jankovic J. Essential tremor: clinical correlates in 350 patients. *Neurology* 1991;41:234–238.

26. Bain PG, Findley LJ, Thompson PD, et al. A study of hereditary essential tremor. *Brain* 1994;117:805–824.

27. Louis ED, Ottman R, Hauser WA. How common is the most common adult movement disorder? Estimates of the prevalence of essential tremor throughout the world. *Mov Disord* 1998;13:5–10.

28. Louis ED, Ford B, Frucht S, et al. Mild tremor in relatives of patients with essential tremor: what does this tell us about the penetrance of the disease? *Arch Neurol* 2001;58:1584–1589.

29. Higgins JJ, Loveless JM, Jankovic J, et al. Evidence that a gene for essential tremor maps to chromosome 2p in four families. *Mov Disord* 1998;13:972–977.

30. Gulcher JR, Jonsson P, Kong A, et al. Mapping of a familial essential tremor gene, *FET1*, to chromosome 3q13. *Nat Genet* 1997;17:84–87.

31. Farrer M, Gwinn-Hardy K, Muenter M, et al. A chromosome 4p haplotype segregating with Parkinson's disease and postural tremor. *Hum Mol Genet* 1999;8:81–85.

32. Koller WC, Busenbark K, Miner K. The relationship of essential tremor to other movement disorders: report on 678 patients. Essential Tremor Study Group. *Ann Neurol* 1994;35:717–723.

33. Massey EW, Paulson GW. Essential vocal tremor: clinical characteristics and response to therapy. *Southern Med J* 1985;78:316–317.

34. Findley LJ, Gresty MA. Head, facial, and voice tremor. *Adv Neurol* 1988;49:239–253.

35. Louis ED, Ford B, Wendt KJ, et al. Clinical characteristics of essential tremor: data from a community based study. *Mov Disord* 1998;13:803–808.

36. Jankovic J. Essential tremor: clinical characteristics. *Neurology* 2000;54:S21–S25.

37. Findley LJ, Koller WC. Essential tremor: a review. *Neurology* 1987;37:1194–1197.

38. Koller WC. Diagnosis and treatment of tremors. *Neurol Clin* 1984;2:499–514.

39. Lang A, Quinn N, Marsden CD, et al. Essential tremor. *Neurology* 1992;42:1432–1434.

40. Deuschl G, Koester B. Diagnose und Behandlung des Tremors. In: Conrad B, Ceballos-Baumann AO, eds. *Bewegungsstörungen in der Neurologie.* New York: Thieme Verlag, 1996:222–253.

41. Deuschl G, Wenzelburger R, Loffler K, et al. Essential tremor and cerebellar dysfunction clinical and kinematic analysis of intention tremor. *Brain* 2000;123:1568–1580.

42. Stolze H, Petersen G, Raethjen J, et al. The gait disorder of advanced essential tremor. *Brain* 2001;124:2278–2286.

43. Findley LJ. Essential tremor. *Br J Hosp Med* 1986;35:388, 390–392.

44. Winkler GF, Young RR. The control of essential tremor by propranolol. *Transac Am Neurol Assoc* 1971;96:66–68.

45. Koller WC. Long-acting propranolol in essential tremor. *Neurology* 1985;35:108–110.

46. Meert TF. Pharmacological evaluation of alcohol withdrawal-induced inhibition of exploratory behaviour and supersensitivity to harmine-induced tremor. *Alc Alcohol* 1994;29:91–102.

47. Findley LJ, Cleeves L, Calzetti S. Primidone in essential tremor of the hands and head: a double-blind controlled clinical study. *J Neurol Neurosurg Psychiatry* 1985;48:911–915.

48. Gironell A, Kulisevsky J, Barbanoj M, et al. A randomized placebo-controlled comparative trial of gabapentin and propranolol in essential tremor. *Arch Neurol* 1999;56:475–480.

49. Ondo W, Hunter C, Vuong KD, et al. Gabapentin for essential tremor: a multiple-dose, double-blind, placebo-controlled trial [in process citation]. *Mov Disord* 2000;15:678–682.

50. Pahwa R, Lyons K, Hubble JP, et al. Double-blind controlled trial of gabapentin in essential tremor. *Mov Disord* 1998;13:465–467.

51. Busenbark K, Pahwa R, Hubble J, et al. Double-blind controlled study of methazolamide in the treatment of essential tremor [published erratum appears in *Neurology* 1993;43(10):1910]. *Neurology* 1993;43:1045–1047.

52. Huber SJ, Paulson GW. Efficacy of alprazolam for essential tremor. *Neurology* 1988;38:241–243.

53. Biary N, Koller W. Kinetic predominant essential tremor: successful treatment with clonazepam. *Neurology* 1987;37: 471–474.

54. Thompson C, Lang A, Parkes JD, et al. A double-blind trial of clonazepam in benign essential tremor. *Clin Neuropharmacol* 1984;7:83–88.

55. Brin MF, Lyons KE, Doucette J, et al. A randomized, double masked, controlled trial of botulinum toxin type A in essential hand tremor. *Neurology* 2001;56:1523–1528.

56. Koller W, Pahwa R, Busenbark K, et al. High-frequency unilateral thalamic stimulation in the treatment of essential and parkinsonian tremor. *Ann Neurol* 1997;42:292–299.

57. Limousin P, Speelman JD, Gielen F, et al. Multicentre European study of thalamic stimulation in parkinsonian and essential tremor. *J Neurol Neurosurg Psychiatry* 1999;66:289–296.

58. Pahwa R, Lyons KL, Wilkinson SB, et al. Bilateral thalamic stimulation for the treatment of essential tremor. *Neurology* 1999;53:1447–1450.

59. Schuurman PR, Bosch DA, Bossuyt PM, et al. A comparison of continuous thalamic stimulation and thalamotomy for suppression of severe tremor. *N Engl J Med* 2000;342:461–468.

60. Calzetti S, Sasso E, Negrotti A, et al. Effect of propranolol in head tremor: quantitative study following single-dose and sustained drug administration. *Clin Neuropharmacol* 1992;15: 470–476.

61. Pahwa R, Busenbark K, Swanson HE, et al. Botulinum toxin treatment of essential head tremor. *Neurology* 1995;45: 822–824.

62. Pollak P, Benabid AL, Krack P, et al. Deep brain stimulation. In: Jankovic J, Tolosa E, eds. *Parkinson's disease and movement disorders*. Baltimore: Williams & Wilkins, 1998:1085–1102.

63. Koller WC, Lyons KE, Wilkinson SB, et al. Efficacy of unilateral deep brain stimulation of the VIM nucleus of the thalamus for essential head tremor. *Mov Disord* 1999;14:847–850.

64. Ondo W, Almaguer M, Jankovic J, et al. Thalamic deep brain stimulation: comparison between unilateral and bilateral placement. *Arch Neurol* 2001;58:218–222.

65. Rothwell JC, Traub MM, Marsden CD. Primary writing tremor. *J Neurol Neurosurg Psychiatry* 1979;42:1106–1114.

66. Bain PG, Findley LJ, Britton TC, et al. Primary writing tremor. *Brain* 1995;116:203–209.

67. McDaniel KD, Cummings JL, Shain S. The "yips": a focal dystonia of golfers. *Neurology* 1989;39:192–195.

68. Sachdev P. Golfer's cramp: clinical characteristics and evidence against it being an anxiety disorder. *Mov Disord* 1992;7: 326–332.

69. Turjanski N, Pirtosek Z, Quirk J, et al. Botulinum toxin in the treatment of writer's cramp. *Clin Neuropharmacol* 1996;19: 314–320.

70. Ross MH, Charness ME, Sudarsky L, et al. Treatment of occupational cramp with botulinum toxin: diffusion of toxin to adjacent non-injected muscles. *Muscle Nerve* 1997;20:593–598.

71. Elble RJ, Moody C, Higgins C. Primary writing tremor: a form of focal dystonia? *Mov Disord* 1990;5:118–126.

72. Kachi T, Rothwell JC, Cowan JM, et al. Writing tremor: its relationship to benign essential tremor. *J Neurol Neurosurg Psychiatry* 1985;48:545–550.

73. Racette BA, Dowling J, Randle J, et al. Thalamic stimulation for primary writing tremor. *J Neurol* 2001;248:380–382.

74. Hachinski VC, Thomsen IV, Buch NH. The nature of primary vocal tremor. *Can J Neurol Sci* 1975;2:195–197.

75. Aminoff MJ, Dedo HH, Izdebski K. Clinical aspects of spasmodic dysphonia. *J Neurol Neurosurg Psychiatry* 1978;41: 361–365.

76. Barkmeier JM, Case JL, Ludlow CL. Identification of symptoms for spasmodic dysphonia and vocal tremor: a comparison of expert and non-expert judges. *J Commun Disord* 2001;34: 21–37.

77. Koller WC, Glatt S, Biary N, et al. Essential tremor variants: effect of treatment. *Clin Neuropharmacol* 1987;10:342–350.

78. Blitzer A, Brin MF, Stewart C, et al. Abductor laryngeal dystonia: a series treated with botulinum toxin. *Laryngoscope* 1992; 102:163–167.

79. Ludlow CL. Treatment of speech and voice disorders with botulinum toxin. *JAMA* 1990;264:2671–2675.

80. Warrick P, Dromey C, Irish J, et al. The treatment of essential voice tremor with botulinum toxin A: a longitudinal case report [in process citation]. *J Voice* 2000;14:410–421.

81. Taha JM, Janszen MA, Favre J. Thalamic deep brain stimulation for the treatment of head, voice, and bilateral limb tremor. *J Neurosurg* 1999;91:68–72.

82. Danek A. Geniospasm: hereditary chin trembling. *Mov Disord* 1993;8:335–338.

83. Jarman PR, Wood NW, Davis MT, et al. Hereditary geniospasm: linkage to chromosome 9q13-q21 and evidence for genetic heterogeneity. *Am J Hum Genet* 1997;61:928–933.

84. Gordon K, Cadera W, Hinton G. Successful treatment of hereditary trembling chin with botulinum toxin. *J Child Neurol* 1993;8:154–156.

85. Pazzaglia P, Sabattini L, Lugaresi E. Su di un singolare disturbo della stazione eretta (osservatione di tre casi). *Riv Freniatria* 1970;96:450–457.

86. Heilman KM. Orthostatic tremor. *Arch Neurol* 1984;41:880–881.

87. Thompson PD, Rothwell JC, Day BL, et al. The physiology of orthostatic tremor. *Arch Neurol* 1986;43:584–587.

88. Deuschl G, Lücking CH, Quintern J. Orthostatischer Tremor: Klinik, Pathophysiologie und Therapie. *Z EEG-EMG* 1987;18: 13–19.

89. McManis PG, Sharbrough FW. Orthostatic tremor: clinical and electrophysiologic characteristics. *Muscle Nerve* 1993;16: 1254–1260.

90. Boroojerdi B, Ferbert A, Foltys H, et al. Evidence for a non-orthostatic origin of orthostatic tremor. *J Neurol Neurosurg Psychiatry* 1999;66:284–288.

91. McAuley JH, Britton TC, Rothwell JC, et al. The timing of primary orthostatic tremor bursts has a task-specific plasticity. *Brain* 2000;123:254–266.

92. Wills AJ, Brusa L, Wang HC, et al. Levodopa may improve orthostatic tremor: case report and trial of treatment. *J Neurol Neurosurg Psychiatry* 1999;66:681–684.

93. Onofrj M, Thomas A, Paci C, et al. Gabapentin in orthostatic tremor: results of a double-blind crossover with placebo in four patients. *Neurology* 1998;51:880–882.

94. Evidente VG, Adler CH, Caviness JN, et al. Effective treatment of orthostatic tremor with gabapentin. *Mov Disord* 1998;13: 829–831.

95. Jedynak CP, Bonnet AM, Agid Y. Tremor and idiopathic dystonia. *Mov Disord* 1991;6:230–236.

96. Vidailhet M, Jedynak CP, Pollak P, et al. Pathology of symptomatic tremors. *Mov Disord* 1998;13:49–54.

97. Masuhr F, Wissel J, Muller J, et al. Quantification of sensory trick impact on tremor amplitude and frequency in 60 patients with head tremor [in process citation]. *Mov Disord* 2000;15: 960–964.

98. Marsden CD. Dystonia: the spectrum of the disease. *Res Publ Assoc Res Nerv Ment Dis* 1976;55:351–367.

99. Dürr A, Stevanin G, Jedynak CP, et al. Familial essential tremor and idiopathic torsion dystonia are different genetic entities. *Neurology* 1993;43:2212–2214.

100. Rivest J, Marsden CD. Trunk and head tremor as isolated manifestations of dystonia [see comments]. *Mov Disord* 1990;5: 60–65.

101. Deuschl G, Heinen F, Kleedorfer B, et al. Clinical and polymyographic investigation of spasmodic torticollis. *J Neurol* 1992;239:9–15.
102. Jankovic J, Schwartz K. Botulinum toxin treatment of tremors. *Neurology* 1991;41:1185–1188.
103. Coubes P, Roubertie A, Vayssiere N, et al. Treatment of DYT1-generalised dystonia by stimulation of the internal globus pallidus. *Lancet* 2000;355:2220–2221.
104. De Jong H. Action tremor in Parkinson's disease. *J Nerv Ment Dis* 1926;64:1ff.
105. Findley LJ, Gresty MA, Halmagyi GM. Tremor, the cogwheel phenomenon, and clonus in Parkinson's disease. *J Neurol Neurosurg Psychiatry* 1981;44:534–546.
106. Koller WC. Pharmacologic treatment of parkinsonian tremor. *Arch Neurol* 1986;43:126–127.
107. Deuschl G, Lücking CH. Tremor and electrically elicited long-latency reflexes in early stages of Parkinson's disease. In: Riederer P, ed. *Early diagnosis and preventive therapy of Parkinson's disease.* New York: Springer-Verlag, 1989:103–110.
108. Koller WC, Vetere OB, Barter R. Tremors in early Parkinson's disease. *Clin Neuropharmacol* 1989;12:293–297.
109. Brooks DJ, Playford ED, Ibanez V, et al. Isolated tremor and disruption of the nigrostriatal dopaminergic system: an 18F-dopa PET study [see comments]. *Neurology* 1992;42:1554–1560.
110. Chang MH, Chang TW, Lai PH, et al. Resting tremor only: a variant of Parkinson's disease or of essential tremor. *J Neurol Sci* 1995;130:215–219.
111. Deuschl G, Raethjen J, Baron R, et al. The pathophysiology of parkinsonian tremor: a review. *J Neurol* 2000;247[Suppl 5]:V33–V48.
112. Kunig G, Pogarell O, Moller JC, et al. Pramipexole, a nonergot dopamine agonist, is effective against rest tremor in intermediate to advanced Parkinson's disease. *Clin Neuropharmacol* 1999;22:301–305.
113. Cantello R, Riccio A, Gilli M, et al. Bornaprine vs placebo in Parkinson disease: double-blind controlled cross-over trial in 30 patients. *Ital J Neurol Sci* 1986;7:139–143.
114. Piccirilli M., D'Alessandro P, Testa A, et al. Bornaprine in the treatment of parkinsonian tremor. *Rivista di Neurologia* 1985;55:38-45.
115. Pakkenberg H, Pakkenberg B. Clozapine in the treatment of tremor. *Acta Neurol Scand* 1986;73:295–297.
116. Fischer PA, Baas H, Hefner R. Treatment of parkinsonian tremor with clozapine. *J Neural Transm* 1990;2:233–238.
117. Jansen EN. Clozapine in the treatment of tremor in Parkinson's disease. *Acta Neurol Scand* 1994;89:262–265.
118. Krack P, Pollak P, Limousin P, et al. Stimulation of subthalamic nucleus alleviates tremor in Parkinson's disease. *Lancet* 1997;350:1675.
119. Fahn S. Cerebellar tremor: clinical aspects. In: Findley LJ, Capildeo R, eds. *Movement disorders: tremor.* London: Macmillan, 1984:355–364.
120. Hallett M, Massaquoi SG. Physiologic studies of dysmetria in patients with cerebellar deficits. *Can J Neurol Sci* 1993;20 Suppl 3:S83–S92.
121. Alusi SH., Worthington J, Glickman S, et al. A study of tremor in multiple sclerosis. *Brain* 2001;124:720–730.
122. Hallett M, Ravits J, Dubinsky RM, et al. A double-blind trial of isoniazid for essential tremor and other action tremors. *Mov Disord* 1991;6:253–256.
123. Rascol A, Clanet M, Montastruc JL, et al. L-5-H-tryptophan in the cerebellar syndrome treatment. *Biomedicine* 1981;35:112–113.
124. van Manen J. Stereotaxic operations in cases of hereditary and intention tremor. *Acta Neurochirurg* 1974;21:49–55.
125. Jankovic J, Cardoso F, Grossman RG, et al. Outcome after stereotactic thalamotomy for parkinsonian, essential, and other types of tremor. *Neurosurgery* 1995;37:680–686.
126. Geny C, Nguyen JP, Pollin B, et al. Improvement of severe postural cerebellar tremor in multiple sclerosis by chronic thalamic stimulation. *Mov Disord* 1996;11:489–494.
127. Lozano AM. Vim thalamic stimulation for tremor. *Arch Med Res* 2000;31:266–269.
128. Alusi SH, Aziz TZ, Glickman S, et al. Stereotactic lesional surgery for the treatment of tremor in multiple sclerosis: a prospective case-controlled study. *Brain* 2001;124:1576–1589.
129. Ferbert A, Gerwig M. Tremor due to stroke. *Mov Disord* 1993;8:179–182.
130. Krack P, Deuschl G, Kaps M, et al. Delayed onset of "rubral tremor" 23 years after brainstem trauma. *Mov Disord* 1994;9:240–242.
131. Holmes G. On certain tremors in organic cerebral lesions. *Brain* 1904;27:327–375.
132. Masucci EF, Kurtzke JF, Saini N. Myorhythmia: a widespread movement disorder. Clinicopathological correlations. *Brain* 1984, 107:53–79.
133. Remy P, de Recondo A, Defer G, et al. Peduncular "rubral" tremor and dopaminergic denervation: a PET study [see comments]. *Neurology* 1995;45:472–477.
134. Deuschl G, Wilms H, Krack P, et al. Function of the cerebellum in parkinsonian rest tremor and Holmes' tremor. *Ann Neurol* 1999;46:126–128.
135. Miwa H., Hatori K, Kondo T, et al. Thalamic tremor: case reports and implications of the tremor-generating mechanism. *Neurology* 1996;46:75–79.
136. Kim JS. Delayed onset mixed involuntary movements after thalamic stroke: clinical, radiological and pathophysiological findings. *Brain* 2001;124:299–309.
137. Lapresle J. Rhythmic palatal myoclonus and the dentato-olivary pathway. *J Neurol* 1979;220:223–230.
138. Deuschl G, Mischke G, Schenck E, et al. Symptomatic and essential rhythmic palatal myoclonus. *Brain* 1990;113:1645–1672.
139. Deuschl G, Toro C, Valls SJ, et al. Symptomatic and essential palatal tremor. 1. Clinical, physiological and MRI analysis. *Brain* 1994;117:775–788.
140. Lapresle J. Palatal myoclonus. *Adv Neurol* 1986;43:265–273.
141. Repka MX, Savino PJ, Reinecke RD. Treatment of acquired nystagmus with botulinum neurotoxin A. *Arch Ophthalmol* 1994;112:1320–1324.
142. Leigh RJ, Averbuch HL, Tomsak RL, et al. Treatment of abnormal eye movements that impair vision: strategies based on current concepts of physiology and pharmacology. *Ann Neurol* 1994;36:129–141.
143. Bakheit AM, Behan PO. Palatal myoclonus successfully treated with clonazepam [letter] [see comments]. *J Neurol Neurosurg Psychiatry* 1990;53:124.
144. Jabbari B, Scherokman B, Gunderson CH, et al. Treatment of movement disorders with trihexyphenidyl. *Mov Disord* 1989;4:202–212.
145. Borggreve F, Hageman G. A case of idiopathic palatal myoclonus: treatment with sodium valproate. *Eur Neurol* 1991;31:403–404.
146. Cakmur R, Idiman E, Idiman F, et al. Essential palatal tremor successfully treated with flunarizine. *Eur Neurol* 1997;38:133–134.
147. Scott BL, Evans RW, Jankovic J. Treatment of palatal myoclonus with sumatriptan. *Mov Disord* 1996;11:748–751.
148. Jankovic J, Scott BL, Evans RW. Treatment of palatal myoclonus with sumatriptan. *Mov Disord* 1997;12:818.
149. Gambardella A, Quattrone A. Treatment of palatal myoclonus with sumatriptan [letter]. *Mov Disord* 1998;13:195.
150. Pakiam AS, Lang AE. Essential palatal tremor: evidence of het-

erogeneity based on clinical features and response to sumatriptan. *Mov Disord* 1999;14:179–180.

151. Deuschl G, Lohle E, Heinen F, et al. Ear click in palatal tremor: its origin and treatment with botulinum toxin. *Neurology* 1991; 41:1677–1679.

152. Lefebre-D'Amour M., Shahani BT, Young RR. Tremor in alcoholic patients. *Progr Clin Neurophysiol* 1978;5:160–164.

153. Diener HC, Dichgans J. Pathophysiology of cerebellar ataxia. *Mov Disord* 1992;7:95–109.

154. Stacy M, Jankovic J. Tardive tremor. *Mov Disord* 1992;7:53–57.

155. Ebersbach G, Traci F, Wissel J, et al. Tardive jaw tremor. *Mov Disord* 1997;12:460–462.

156. Smith IS. The natural history of chronic demyelinating neuropathy associated with benign IgM paraproteinaemia. A clinical and neurophysiological study. *Brain* 1994;117:949–57.

157. Ghosh A, Young AC. Early tremor seen in IgG-paraproteinaemic neuropathy. *J Neurol* 2001;248:225–226.

158. Bain PG, Britton TC, Jenkins IH, et al. Tremor associated with benign IgM paraproteinaemic neuropathy. *Brain* 1996;119:789–799.

159. Koller W, Lang A, Vetere OB, et al. Psychogenic tremors. *Neurology* 1989;39:1094–1099.

160. Deuschl G, Koster B, Lucking CH, et al. Diagnostic and pathophysiological aspects of psychogenic tremors. *Mov Disord* 1998; 13:294–302.

161. Kim YJ, Pakiam AS, Lang AE. Historical and clinical features of psychogenic tremor: a review of 70 cases. *Can J Neurol Sci* 1999; 26:190–195.

162. Kretschmer E. Die Gesetze der willkürlichen Reflexverstärkung in ihrer Bedeutung für das Hysterie- und Simulationsproblem. *Zsch Neurol Psychiat* 1918;41:354–385.

163. Jung R. Physiologische Untersuchungen über den Parkinsontremor und andere Zitterformen beim Menschen. *Zsch Neurol Psychiat* 1941;173:263–332.

164. Scheidt CE, Köster B, Deuschl G. Diagnose, Symptomatik und Verlauf des psychogenen Tremors. *Nervenarzt* 1996;198–204.

165. Silfverskiöld BP. Rhythmic myoclonias including spinal myoclonus. In: Fahn S, Marsden CD, VanWoert M, eds. *Advances in neurology*. New York: Raven Press, 1986:275–285.

166. Ikeda A, Kakigi R, Funai N, et al. Cortical tremor: a variant of cortical reflex myoclonus. *Neurology* 1990;40:1561–1565.

167. Toro C, Pascual LA, Deuschl G, et al. Cortical tremor. A common manifestation of cortical myoclonus. *Neurology* 1993;43:2346–2353.

168. Chen R, Ashby P, Lang AE. Stimulus-sensitive myoclonus in akinetic-rigid syndromes. *Brain* 1992;115:1875–1888.

169. Thompson PD, Day BL, Rothwell JC, et al. The myoclonus in corticobasal degeneration. Evidence for two forms of cortical reflex myoclonus. *Brain* 1994;44:578–591.

170. Fung VS, Duggins A, Morris JG, et al. Progressive myoclonic ataxia associated with celiac disease presenting as unilateral cortical tremor and dystonia [In Process Citation]. *Mov Disord* 2000;15:732–734.

171. Kim JS. Involuntary movements after anterior cerebral artery territory infarction. *Stroke* 2001;32:258–261.

172. Young RR, Hagbarth KE. Physiological tremor enhanced by manoeuvres affecting the segmental stretch reflex. *J Neurol Neurosurg Psychiatry* 1980;43:248–256.

173. Llinas R. Rebound excitation as the physiological basis for tremor: a biophysical study of the oscillatory properties of mammalian central neurons in vitro. In: Findley LJ, Capildeo R, eds. *Movement disorders: tremor*. London: Macmillan, 1984:339–351.

174. Bergman H, Feingold A, Nini A, et al. Physiological aspects of information processing in the basal ganglia of normal and parkinsonian primates. *Trends Neurosci* 1998;21:32–38.

175. Elble RJ, Randall JE. Motor-unit activity responsible for 8- to 12-Hz component of human physiological finger tremor. *J Neurophysiol* 1976;39:370–383.

176. Flament D, Hore J. Comparison of cerebellar intention tremor under isotonic and isometric conditions. *Brain Res* 1988;439:179–186.

177. Hore J, Wild B, Diener HC. Cerebellar dysmetria at the elbow, wrist, and fingers. *J Neurophysiol* 1991;65:563–571.

178. Hallett M, Shahani BT, Young RR. EMG analysis of patients with cerebellar deficits. *J Neurol Neurosurg Psychiatry* 1975;38:1163–1169.

179. Mauritz KH, Schmitt C, Dichgans J. Delayed and enhanced long latency reflexes as the possible cause of postural tremor in late cerebellar atrophy. *Brain* 1981;104:97–116.

180. Timmer J, Lauk M, Pfleger W, et al. Cross-spectral analysis of physiological tremor and muscle activity. I. Theory and application to unsynchronized electromyogram. *Biol Cybern* 1998; 78:349–357.

181. Lauk M, Timmer T, Lucking CH, et al. A software for recording and analysis of human tremor. *Comput Meth Programs Biomed* 1999;60:65–77.

182. Elbl, RJ, Sinha R, Higgins C. Quantification of tremor with a digitizing tablet. *J Neurosci Meth* 1990;32:193–198.

183. Elble RJ, Brilliant M, Leffle K, et al. Quantification of essential tremor in writing and drawing. *Mov Disord* 1996;11:70–78.

184. Spieker S, Loschmann P, Jentgens C, et al. Tremorlytic activity of budipine: a quantitative study with long-term tremor recordings. *Clin Neuropharmacol* 1995;18:266–272.

185. Bain P, Brin B, Deuschl G, et al. Criteria for the diagnosis of essential tremor. *Neurology* 2000;54:S7.

186. Elble RJ. Diagnostic criteria for essential tremor and differential diagnosis. *Neurology* 2000;54:S2–S6.

MYOCLONUS AND STARTLE SYNDROMES

HIROSHI SHIBASAKI

Myoclonus is defined as sudden, brief, jerky, shock-like, involuntary movements arising from the central nervous system and involving the extremities, face, and trunk. Most myoclonic jerks are caused by abrupt muscle contraction *(positive myoclonus)*, but abrupt movements are also caused by sudden cessation of muscle contraction associated with the silent period of the electromyographic (EMG) discharges *(negative myoclonus)* (1).

Myoclonus can be classified according to various parameters, but it is commonly classified with respect to the underlying physiologic mechanism or causative factor (2). According to its possible origin in the central nervous system, myoclonus is classified in three main categories: cortical, subcortical, and spinal (Table 20.1) (2). Of these three categories, cortical myoclonus is most commonly encountered, and it is most important because patients with this form of myoclonus also tend to suffer from intractable generalized convulsions. This is mainly related to the fact that cortical myoclonus in most cases is based on the pathologic hyperexcitability of the sensory cortex, the motor cortex, or both. Moreover, cortical myoclonus is more often disabling to patients and intractable to treatment than other forms of myoclonus. Cortical myoclonus is seen in a variety of diseases and syndromes (Table 20.2) (2). Progressive

myoclonus epilepsies (PMEs) have various diseases as the underlying cause and are mostly hereditary (3). There are significant differences in the relative frequency of those diseases among different regions of the world. There has been significant advance in the genetic studies of hereditary diseases causing PME (3).

As for the term *Ramsay Hunt syndrome,* which used to be applied to PMEs of undetermined causation, in 1990 the Marseille Consensus Group (4) recommended that it be discarded. The last two categories of PMEs listed in Table 20.2 now replace Ramsay Hunt syndrome; these disorders are referred to as *PMEs of unknown etiology* when seizures are frequent and severe, and as *progressive myoclonic ataxias* when seizures are infrequent and mild. Celiac disease was added as a cause of progressive myoclonic ataxia (5). The neuropathologic findings reported in one autopsied case of celiac disease consisted of atrophy of cerebellar hemispheres but no abnormality in the cerebrum (5). Guerrini et al. (6)

TABLE 20.1. PATHOPHYSIOLOGIC CLASSIFICATION OF MYOCLONUS

Cortical
  Spontaneous cortical myoclonus
  Cortical reflex myoclonus
  Epilepsia partialis continua
Subcortical
  Essential myoclonus
  Periodic myoclonus
  Dystonic myoclonus
  Reticular reflex myoclonus
  Startle syndrome
  Drug-induced myoclonus
Spinal

TABLE 20.2. DISEASES UNDERLYING CORTICAL MYOCLONUS

Progressive myoclonus epilepsy
  Myoclonus epilepsy with ragged-red fibers
  Lipidosis
  Lafora's disease
  Neuronal ceroid lipofuscinosis
  Unverricht-Lundborg disease
  Familial adult myoclonic epilepsy
  Celiac disease
  Angelman's syndrome
  Progressive myoclonus epilepsies of unknown cause
  Progressive myoclonic ataxias
Juvenile myoclonic epilepsy
Postanoxic myoclonus (Lance-Adams syndrome)
Alzheimer's disease
Creutzfeldt-Jakob disease (advanced stage)
Metabolic encephalopathy
Corticobasal ganglionic degeneration
Olivopontocerebellar atrophy
Rett's syndrome

reported Angelman's syndrome as a cause of PME. Furthermore, they demonstrated cortical reflex myoclonus in nine of ten patients with Rett's syndrome (7).

As will be described in detail later in this chapter, the pathophysiology of cortical myoclonus can be studied by using various electrophysiologic techniques (2). In contrast, the diagnosis of subcortical myoclonus largely depends on exclusion of cortical myoclonus. As listed in Table 20.1, the subcortical myoclonus contains various subgroups, and some of them share common features with other kinds of involuntary movements such as tremor and dystonia. Quinn (8) in 1996 reviewed the literature related to essential myoclonus and hypothesized that hereditary essential myoclonus and dominantly inherited myoclonic dystonia, both of which dramatically respond to alcohol, might be the same disease, although the proof must come from genetic studies. Startle syndrome was categorized into subcortical myoclonus because it was demonstrated to be based on the stimulus-sensitive hyperexcitability of lower brainstem centers (9). However, in this chapter it will be dealt with as an independent category, with special emphasis placed on the recent advance in its genetic studies.

Various drugs have been reported to cause myoclonic jerks. These include anticonvulsants such as vigabatrin and valproate, chronically abused alcohol, methyl ethyl ketone, the anesthetic agent propofol, the antipsychotic drug clozapine, the antidiarrheic bismuth subsalicylate, and serotomimetic agents such as trazodone, isocarboxazide, and methylphenidate hydrochloride. Most drug-induced myoclonus is dose dependent. Although detailed electrophysiologic findings have not been reported, most of them seem to be of subcortical origin because the electroencephalogram (EEG) does not show any myoclonus-related spike.

Since the next chapter of this volume is devoted to the pharmacology and management of myoclonus, this aspect of myoclonus will not be discussed here. Similarly, although the genetic study of inherited myoclonus-dystonia has advanced rapidly in recent years, this issue will be discussed in the chapter on dystonia (Chapter 23). Segmental and spinal myoclonus, also discussed in the previous volume, will not be covered here due to lack of progress in the field.

PATHOPHYSIOLOGY OF CORTICAL OR CORTICAL REFLEX MYOCLONUS

Myoclonus of cortical origin is clinically characterized by brief jerks of extremity and facial muscles that are enhanced by posturing and actions (movements) and are commonly sensitive to stimulus. Electrophysiologically it is characterized by (a) an associated EMG discharge of very short duration (usually less than 50 ms), (b) an EEG spike preceding the myoclonus by a short interval (20 ms in case of hand myoclonus) and localized to the area of the contralateral central region corresponding to the involved muscle (around C3 or C4 of the International 10–20 System in the case of hand myoclonus), and (c) pathologic enhancement of early cortical components of the somatosensory evoked responses, often accompanied by enhanced long-latency, long-loop EMG response (C-reflex) (2,10–13).

Most electrophysiologic studies suggest abnormal hyperexcitability of the sensory or motor cortex, or both, underlying the cortical myoclonus. Among various sensory modalities, most patients are predominantly sensitive to the somesthetic stimuli, although some patients show the increased sensitivity to photic stimuli as well (14,15).

Hyperexcitability of the Somatosensory Cortex

Giant somatosensory evoked potentials (SEPs) are attributable to pathologic enhancement of components of SEPs seen in normal subjects but not to the development of abnormal SEP components (12,13,16,17). By analyzing the scalp distribution and the time relationship of the subcomponents of giant SEPs following electric stimulation of the peripheral nerves in patients with cortical reflex myoclonus, Ikeda et al. (17) in 1995 demonstrated that not only the components P30 and N30, which are derived from the tangentially oriented dipole source within area 3b in the posterior bank of the central sulcus, but also the components P25 and N35, which are localized to the central region probably arising from the radially oriented dipole source(s) in the crown of the postcentral gyrus (area 1 or 2), are enhanced to different degrees depending on the individual patient (Fig. 20.1). By using a specially devised instrument for selectively activating the muscle afferents, Mima et al. (18) in 1997 demonstrated that in some patients with cortical reflex myoclonus the proprioception-induced SEPs are also enhanced. In view of the previously reported experimental data suggesting that the impulses arising from muscle afferents arrive at area 3a, 1, and 2 and that those from tactile inputs mainly arrive at area 3b, the above finding is in agreement with the conclusion drawn by Ikeda et al. (17) based on the scalp distribution of giant SEPs following electric stimulation of the peripheral nerve trunk. In contrast with this, nociceptive stimuli presented with CO_2 laser beam did not enhance the pain SEP even in those patients who showed giant SEP in response to electric stimulation of the peripheral nerves (19). However, previous studies using pain SEP were focused on the N2 and P2 components because of the technical difficulty in recording an earlier component, N1, which is most likely generated in the primary somatosensory cortex. As the N2 and P2 components are believed to be generated in the second somatosensory cortex (SII) (20), the above finding suggests that the SII is not hyperreactive in cortical myoclonus.

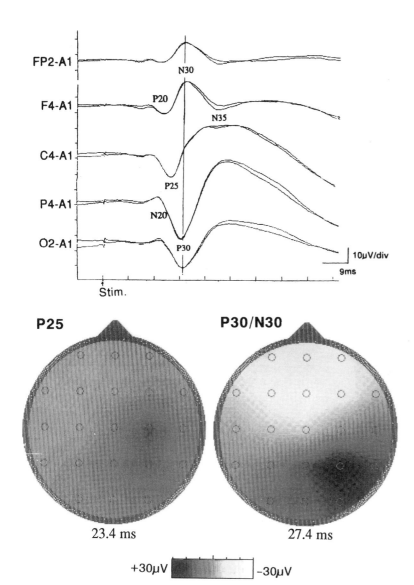

FIG. 20.1. Waveforms of somatosensory evoked potentials (SEPs) to the left median nerve stimulation *(top)* and scalp topography of each component of giant SEPs *(bottom)* in a patient with cortical reflex myoclonus. P25 and N35 are seen as a single positive and negative peak, respectively, at the right peri-rolandic area. N30-P30 is seen as a pair of two fields of opposite polarities across the right central fissure. (From Ikeda A, Shibasaki H, Nagamine T, et al. Peri-rolandic and fronto-parietal components of scalp-recorded giant SEPs in cortical myoclonus. *Electroenceph Clin Neurophysiol* 1995; 96:300–309, with permission.) (See color section.)

Hyperexcitability of the Primary Motor Cortex

The temporal and spatial relation between cortical myoclonus and its EEG correlates can be studied by the use of jerk-locked back averaging technique (21). This technique often discloses the myoclonus-related cortical activity that is not detectable on the conventional EEG-EMG polygraphic record. Certain similarities between the EEG spike preceding the spontaneous cortical myoclonus and the giant SEP following electric stimulation of the peripheral nerve have been pointed out in terms of waveform, time relation to the EMG discharge (spike to spontaneous myoclonus versus giant SEP to C-reflex), and topography on the scalp (10,12,22). This observation led us to postulate that the giant SEP seen in cortical reflex myoclonus might contain the motor or "efferent" component in it

(10,12,22). This concept was substantiated by recent studies of giant SEPs by using magnetoencephalography (MEG). Although the main component of the giant somatosensory evoked magnetic fields was generated in area 3b, a certain component (P25m) was shown to originate from the precentral gyrus, thus supporting the above hypothesis (Fig. 20.2) (23).

As for the MEG correlates of premyoclonus spike, Uesaka et al. (24) in 1996 studied six patients with cortical reflex myoclonus and one with epilepsia partialis continua by MEG. The spike was estimated as a single-current dipole in the postcentral gyrus in five of the six patients with cortical reflex myoclonus, and in the remaining patient two dipoles were detected, one each in the precentral and postcentral gyrus. These facts suggested the possible origin of cortical myoclonus also in the postcentral gyrus. In the patient with epilepsia partialis con-

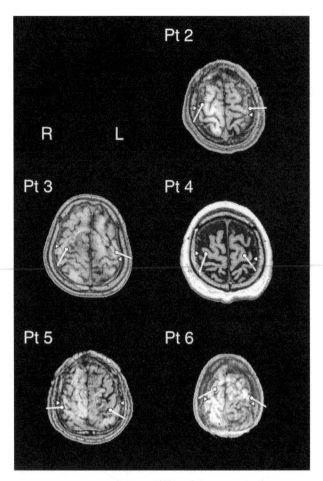

FIG. 20.2. Equivalent current dipole (ECD) sources of the P25m component calculated from the averaged magnetoencephalographic responses to electric stimulation of the median nerves at wrist in five patients with cortical reflex myoclonus. The sources are located in the precentral gyrus in all cases. The ECD sources of the initial cortical component N20m were localized in the postcentral gyrus in all cases (data not shown). White spots and bars indicate the location of the ECD sources and their direction. Triangles show the central sulcus. (From Mima T, Nagamine T, Nishitani N, et al. Cortical myoclonus: sensorimotor hyperexcitability. *Neurology* 1998;50:933–942, with permission.)

tinua, a single dipole was estimated in the precentral gyrus (24). Mima et al. (25) in 1998 studied six patients with cortical myoclonus due to various causes by jerk-locked back averaging of MEG and identified the generator source of the premyoclonus activity in the contralateral precentral gyrus in all the cases, although the direction of the current flow was different among cases (Figs. 20.3 and 20.4). This finding confirmed the important role of the precentral cortex in generating spontaneous myoclonus although the activation pattern may not be consistent among patients. In some patients, jerk-locked back averaging of MEG disclosed myoclonus-related cortical activity that was not detectable on the jerk-locked averaged EEG (Fig. 20.3) (25).

Recently, Silen et al. (26) analyzed the reactivity of the approximately 20-Hz cortical rhythm to electric stimulation of the peripheral nerves as an index for the functional state of the primary motor cortex in patients with Unverricht-Lundborg PME, which is due to mutation of the cystatin B gene in chromosome 21, by using MEG. In the patient group they found a loss of significant rebounds of the cortical rhythm, which occur following a transient decrease of the rhythm in response to the stimulation in normal subjects (Fig. 20.5) (26). The approximately 20-Hz rebounds, believed to reflect increased cortical inhibition, were interpreted as indicating decreased GABAergic inhibition in the motor cortex in this condition (26).

Brown et al. (27) in 1991, by analyzing the time relation among myoclonic jerks of various muscles and that between those myoclonic jerks and the EEG correlates in patients with cortical myoclonus, suggested the spread of myoclonus-related cortical activities through the motor strip within one hemisphere as well as across the two hemispheres through the corpus callosum. In 1996 they extended their study to clarify the excitability of the motor cortex by using transcranial magnetic stimulation in two groups of patients with cortical myoclonus; one group consisted of spreaders (patients with multifocal and bilateral or generalized cortical myoclonus) and the other of nonspreaders (patients with just multifocal cortical myoclonus) (28). They found lower motor thresholds to single magnetic shocks at rest in spreaders than in nonspreaders or healthy subjects. Furthermore, by using paired magnetic stimulation at interstimulus intervals of 1 to 6 ms, they found less ipsilateral inhibition and less transcallosal inhibition in the spreaders than in the nonspreaders or healthy subjects. These findings were interpreted to suggest that abnormalities in ipsilateral and transcallosal inhibition may facilitate the spread of the cortical myoclonic activity responsible for bilateral and generalized jerks (28).

Rhythmicity of Cortical Myoclonus

Cortical myoclonus is usually irregular. However, in some cases it involves the same muscles repetitively, and even rhythmically, thus clinically resembling tremor. Recently, three conditions have attracted attention in this regard: familial adult myoclonic epilepsy (FAME), corticobasal ganglionic degeneration, and Angelman's syndrome. FAME has been reported mainly in Japan under various names, such as benign epilepsy with essential myoclonus, benign familial myoclonic epilepsy, cortical tremor, and familial cortical myoclonic tremor (29). It is characterized by autosomal dominant inheritance, relatively late onset, relatively benign postural-action myoclonus involving small muscles of hands resembling essential tremor, and

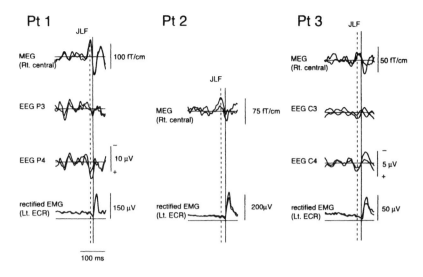

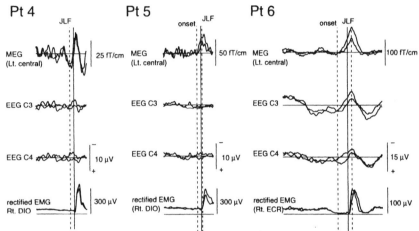

FIG. 20.3. Waveforms of magnetoencephalograms and electroencephalograms that were simultaneously recorded and back-averaged with respect to the onset of hand myoclonus in six patients with cortical myoclonus. In Patient 4 (Pt 4) and Patient 5 (Pt 5), the back-averaged electroencephalograms show no myoclonus-related activity, whereas the corresponding magnetoencephalograms show a cortical activity time-locked to myoclonus. (From Mima T, Nagamine T, Ikeda A, et al. Pathogenesis of cortical myoclonus studied by magnetoencephalography. *Ann Neurol* 1998;43:598–607, with permission.)

only rare generalized convulsions, but it fulfills all the electrophysiologic criteria of cortical reflex myoclonus (29). Recently, the genetic locus of this disease was defined on chromosome 8q24 (30).

The second condition is the myoclonic jerks seen in patients with corticobasal ganglionic degeneration. This is characterized by rigid akinetic syndrome associated with apraxia, myoclonic jerks, and cortical sensory loss, all of which start asymmetrically. Electrophysiologic abnormalities are also quite asymmetric. One of the unique features of electrophysiologic findings in this condition is a slightly shorter latency of the C-reflex or evoked myoclonus by peripheral stimulation as compared with the ordinary form of cortical reflex myoclonus (31). Another feature is reduction of the SEP amplitudes except for the initial cortical component (N20 in the case of median nerve stimulation at wrist) (31,32). The latter finding is compatible with the cortical sensory loss that is clinically demonstrated in the majority of these cases. Furthermore, both the spontaneous and reflex myoclonus tend to repeat themselves at an

approximate rate of once every 70 to 90 ms, or they may occur as trains of jerks. Because this interval is too long for the reverberating circuit between the cortex and the periphery, it is believed to be due to the repetitive excitation of the sensorimotor cortex (29,31,32). Lu et al. (32) in 1998 studied two patients with this disease by transcranial magnetic stimulation of the motor cortex and found shortening of the induced EMG silent period predominantly on the affected side, suggesting impairment of the inhibitory system in the motor cortex.

As for the third condition, Guerrini et al. (6) in 1996 reported 11 patients, aged 3 to 28 years, with Angelman's syndrome, which is due to lack of genetic contribution from maternal chromosome 15q11-13. It manifests severe mental retardation, ataxic gait, tremors, and jerky movements. It is noteworthy that this chromosomal region encompasses three $GABA_A$ receptor subunit genes. All patients exhibited quasi-continuous rhythmic myoclonus mainly involving hands and face, accompanied by rhythmic 5- to 10-Hz EEG activity. Burst-locked

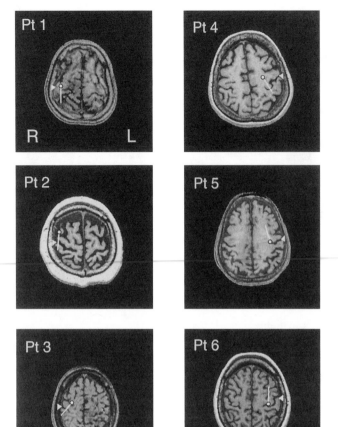

FIG. 20.4. Equivalent current dipole (ECD) sources of cortical activity preceding myoclonus of hand in six patients with cortical myoclonus, calculated from the magnetic fields obtained by jerk-locked back averaging (the same data as shown in Fig. 20.3). The sources are located in the precentral cortex in all cases, although the direction of the current dipole is different (posterior in the first four cases and anterior in the last two cases). Triangles indicate the central sulcus. (Cited from Mima T, Nagamine T, Ikeda A, et al. Pathogenesis of cortical myoclonus studied by magnetoencephalography. *Ann Neurol* 1998;43:598–607, with permission.)

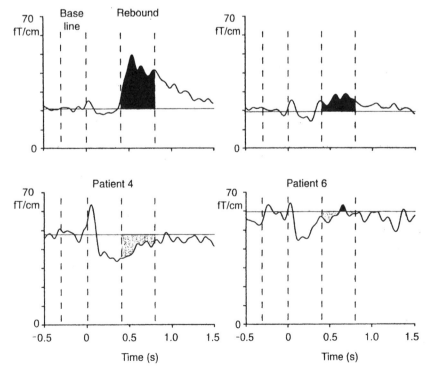

FIG. 20.5. Stimulus-related changes in the approximately 20-Hz mu rhythm level of normal subjects (Controls 1 and 6) and two patients with Unverricht-Lundborg PME. Light gray shadowed areas show the suppression and dark gray shadowed areas the rebounds 400 to 800 ms after stimulus (time 0). (From Silen T, Forss N, Jensen O, et al. Abnormal reactivity of the ~20-Hz motor cortex rhythm in Unverricht-Lundborg type progressive myoclonus epilepsy. *NeuroImage* 2000;12: 707–712, with permission.)

EEG averaging disclosed a premyoclonus transient preceding the burst by 19 ± 5 ms. Although no giant SEP or C-reflex was observed, it was thought to arise in the cortex.

In relation to the rhythmicity of cortical myoclonus, Brown et al. (33) in 1999 studied eight patients with cortical myoclonus by analyzing the coherence between EEG and EMG activities. In addition to significant coherence between the EMG and the contralateral and vertex EEG in the frequency ranges reported in normal subjects (15 to 30 Hz and 30 to 60 Hz), which they found in six patients, they also found significant coherence at higher frequencies (up to 175 Hz) in three of them. They further estimated the conduction time from the cortex to the muscles of the forearm, hand, and foot to be 14, 25, and 35 ms, respectively. Thus, the cortical drive seems to synchronize muscle discharges over a broader range of frequencies in some cases as compared with normal subjects.

NEGATIVE MYOCLONUS

Negative myoclonus, or asterixis, occurs when a muscle contraction is suddenly interrupted. It can be either cortical or subcortical in origin (1). It is often seen in association with metabolic or toxic encephalopathy, but unilateral asterixis is seen most commonly in association with ischemic or hemorrhagic disorders, especially those involving the thalamus. Within the thalamus, ventral lateral or lateral posterior thalamus seems to be responsible for the unilateral pure asterixis (34). Lance and Adams (35) in 1963 clearly documented in their patients with posthypoxic myoclonus the association of positive myoclonus with the EEG spike and that of the EMG silent period (negative myoclonus) with the EEG slow wave, suggesting its cortical origin. In 1994, we reported four cases of negative myoclonus elicited by peripheral stimulation, with or without associated positive myoclonus (36). In those cases, presentation of a single electric shock to the median nerve at wrist while the wrist was maintained in extended position evoked the giant SEP on the EEG and a clear silent period on the EMG, resulting in sudden wrist-drop. It was clearly noted in those cases that the larger the SEP, the longer was the duration of the induced EMG silent period or the more prominent was the induced negative myoclonus. Moreover, the EMG silent period was elicited also in the opposite (nonstimulated) hand only when the giant SEP was recognized also at the hemisphere ipsilateral to the stimulus. This may be explained by postulating, as in the case of positive myoclonus, the interhemispheric spread of the silent period–related cortical activity through the corpus callosum (27). Thus, this stimulus-sensitive negative

myoclonus seems to be mediated by the transcortical reflex mechanism, probably based on the abnormal hyperexcitability of inhibitory components of the motor cortex (36).

As regards the stimulus-sensitive negative myoclonus, Gambardella et al. (37) in 1996 reported a patient with photosensitive epilepsy in whom photoparoxysmal EEG response was sometimes accompanied by loss of postural tone in both arms. This is considered to be an example of photic cortical reflex negative myoclonus.

As for the generating mechanism of cortical negative myoclonus, a possible role of the frontal cortex anterior to the motor cortex has been proposed. Rubolli et al. (38) in 1995 reported a patient with epileptic negative myoclonus. By using the spike averaging technique, they demonstrated one negative peak at the contralateral central region and the following negative peak at the contralateral frontal region. The latter of the two negative peaks preceded the onset of the EMG flattening by 30 ms. That peak was always associated with the epileptic negative myoclonus, but the earlier peak was not necessarily so. Baumgartner et al. (39) in 1996 reported a patient manifesting brief repetitive lapses in postural tone of the right upper extremity while the ictal EEG showed repetitive left frontal spikes much more anterior to the central sulcus as determined by the N20 component of the median nerve SEP. The EEG transient preceded the onset of the EMG silent period by 20 to 40 ms. They further demonstrated a marked regional hyperperfusion in the left middle frontal gyrus by single photon emission computed tomography during the epileptic negative myoclonus. These findings were interpreted to suggest that the epileptic negative myoclonus might be generated by an epileptic activity in the premotor area (39). Lüders et al. (40) found that two cortical areas—one on the mesial frontal cortex and the other on the lateral frontal convexity just in front of the face motor area—interrupt the ongoing muscle contraction or repetitive movements when stimulated with a train of high frequency (50-Hz) electric shocks. However, the relation between these negative motor areas and negative myoclonus has not been clarified.

Negative motor area might be present also in the primary sensorimotor cortex. Noachtar et al. (41) in 1997 reported a patient with focal epileptic negative myoclonus who was studied with subdurally placed electrodes. In that case, repetitive spikes in the postcentral gyrus were consistently followed by an EMG silent period in the contralateral arm with a latency of about 20 to 30 ms. In patients with medically intractable epilepsy who underwent presurgical evaluation with subdural electrodes, Ikeda et al. (42) in 2000 found that some areas of the sensorimotor cortex elicit pure silent period without associated positive motor response when stimulated with a single electric shock.

STARTLE SYNDROME

Startle syndrome is a group of diseases characterized by exaggerated startle responses to sudden unexpected stimuli. Familial startle disease or hyperekplexia is an autosomal dominant disorder characterized by muscular rigidity in the neonatal period and exaggerated startle response to sudden, unexpected acoustic or tactile stimuli. Recently, it has drawn particular attention of many investigators, especially in relation to its genetic pathogenesis (43).

Ryan et al. (44) in 1992 performed systematic linkage analysis in a large family with hyperekplexia and found the polymorphic genetic marker locus mapped to chromosome 5q33-q35. The same authors further identified point mutations in the gene encoding the α_1 subunit of the inhibitory glycine receptor *(GLRA1)* in hyperekplexia patients from four families (45). All mutations occurred in the same base pair of exon 6 and resulted in the substitution of an uncharged amino acid (leucine or glutamine) for arginine in codon 271. A group of neurologists in Leiden made a linkage analysis in 44 Dutch patients with hyperekplexia. They were divided into groups of 28 patients with the major form, associated with stiffness, and 16 patients with the minor form, unassociated with stiffness. The point mutation of the gene encoding GLRA1 was found exclusively in the major form, indicating that the minor form is not a different expression of the same genetic defect but may be merely an excessive form of normal startle response (46). Shiang et al. (47) in 1995 reported families with hyperekplexia showing a different mutation that changed tyrosine at amino acid 279 to cysteine, and also patients with atypical clinical features or absent family history of hyperekplexia who did not have mutation in the gene encoding GLRA1. Rajendra et al. (48) in 1994 showed that the mutation in hyperekplexia profoundly reduces the sensitivity of receptor currents activated by agonist glycine as well as the binding affinity of glycine to the mutant glycine receptors, thus reducing the efficacy of glycinergic inhibitory neurotransmission. In 1999, Saul et al. (49) reported a pedigree showing dominant transmission of hyperekplexia who was found to have another point mutation of *GLRA1* with the substitution of P250, which was located in the intracellular M1-M2 loop. They showed that recombinant $\alpha1P^{250T}$ receptors displayed dramatic alterations in chloride conductance, suggesting an important role of glycine receptor channel gating in the pathogenesis of this syndrome (49).

With regard to the site of action of inhibitory glycine receptors, blockade of the inhibitory glycine receptors in the caudal pontine reticular formation did not affect the acoustic startle response in rats, suggesting that deficiency of glycine receptors in the pontine reticular nucleus might not be involved in the human startle disease (50). Recently,

Pierce et al. (51) found mutations of glycine receptor gene in calves showing stimulus-sensitive myoclonus with autosomal recessive inheritance. Immunohistochemically by using monoclonal antibody to α and β subunits of the glycine receptors, they demonstrated a loss of cell surface immunoreactivity in spinal neurons of the myoclonic animals (51).

Physiologically the startle responses in hyperekplexia have been shown to involve the same structures as the physiologic startle responses seen in normal subjects. The only difference is the excessive response and subnormal habituation resulting in widespread elevated gain of vestigial withdrawal reflexes in the patients (9,52,53). The pattern of the startle EMG responses starting from the sternocleidomastoid muscles and spreading both rostrally and caudally suggests the medulla oblongata as the most likely reflex center (9). At the spinal level, Floeter et al. (54) in 1996 demonstrated diminished reciprocal inhibition between flexor and extensor muscles of the forearm, but normal recurrent inhibition of the soleus H reflex, in patients with hereditary hyperekplexia with mutation in *GLRA1*. Based on these findings, they postulated that disynaptic reciprocal inhibition in humans is mediated through glycinergic interneurons.

SUMMARY

Myoclonus has been extensively studied by using various kinds of electrophysiologic techniques. Among others, the recent application of MEG to the investigation of the generator source of giant SEP and premyoclonus cortical activity in cortical reflex myoclonus elucidated the complex involvement of precentral and postcentral gyrus. As in other fields of clinical neurology, there have been remarkable advances in the genetic and molecular aspects of myoclonus, especially with regard to hyperekplexia or hereditary startle syndrome. Hyperekplexia was found to be mainly caused by the point mutation of the gene encoding GLRA1, although there seems to be different mutations depending on families. Abnormalities of channel gating in GLRA1 have been extensively studied. Although electrophysiologically the startle response seen in hyperekplexia is an exaggerated form of the physiologic startle response present in normal subjects, the precise site of dysfunction remains to be elucidated.

REFERENCES

1. Shibasaki H. Pathophysiology of negative myoclonus and asterixis. *Adv Neurol* 1995;67:199–209.
2. Shibasaki H. AAEE minimonograph #30: Electrophysiological studies of myoclonus. *Muscle Nerve* 2000;23:321–335.
3. Serratosa JM, Gardiner RM, Lehesjoki AE, et al. The molecular

genetic bases of the progressive myoclonus epilepsies. *Adv Neurol* 1999;79:383–398.

4. Marseille Consensus Group. Classification of progressive myoclonus epilepsies and related disorders. *Ann Neurol* 1990;28: 113–116.

5. Bhatia KP, Brown P, Gregory R, et al. Progressive myoclonic ataxia associated with coeliac disease: the myoclonus of cortical origin, but the pathology is in the cerebellum. *Brain* 1995;118:1087–1093.

6. Guerrini R, De Lorey TM, Bonanni P, et al. Cortical myoclonus in Angelman syndrome. *Ann Neurol* 1996;40:39–48.

7. Guerrini R, Bonanni P, Parmeggiani L, et al. Cortical reflex myoclonus in Rett syndrome. *Ann Neurol* 1998;43:472–479.

8. Quinn NP. Essential myoclonus and myoclonic dystonia. *Mov Disord* 1996;11:119–124.

9. Brown P, Rothwell JC, Thompson PD, et al. The hyperekplexias and their relationship to the normal startle reflex. *Brain* 1991;114:1903–1928.

10. Shibasaki H, Yamashita Y, Kuroiwa Y. Electroencephalographic studies of myoclonus: myoclonus-related cortical spikes and high amplitude somatosensory evoked potentials. *Brain* 1978;101: 447–460.

11. Hallett M, Chadwick D, Marsden CD. Cortical reflex myoclonus. *Neurology* 1979;29:1107–1125.

12. Shibasaki H, Yamashita Y, Neshige R, et al. Pathogenesis of giant somatosensory evoked potentials in progressive myoclonic epilepsy. *Brain* 1985;108:225–240.

13. Kakigi R, Shibasaki H. Generator mechanisms of giant somatosensory evoked potentials in cortical reflex myoclonus. *Brain* 1987;110:1359–1373.

14. Shibasaki H, Neshige R. Photic cortical reflex myoclonus. *Ann Neurol* 1987;22:252–257.

15. Kanouchi T, Yokota T, Kamata T, et al. Central pathway of photic reflex myoclonus. *J Neurol Neurosurg Psychiatry* 1997;62:414–417.

16. Shibasaki H, Nakamura M, Nishida S, et al. Wave form decomposition of "giant SEP" and its computer model for scalp topography. *Electroenceph Clin Neurophysiol* 1990;77:286–294.

17. Ikeda A, Shibasaki H, Nagamine T, et al. Peri-rolandic and fronto-parietal components of scalp-recorded giant SEPs in cortical myoclonus. *Electroenceph Clin Neurophysiol* 1995;96: 300–309.

18. Mima T, Terada K, Ikeda A, et al. Afferent mechanism of cortical myoclonus studied by proprioception-related SEPs. *Electroenceph Clin Neurophysiol* 1997;104:51–59.

19. Kakigi R, Shibasaki H, Neshige R, et al. Pain-related somatosensory evoked potentials in cortical reflex myoclonus. *J Neurol Neurosurg Psychiatry* 1990;53:44–48.

20. Kanda M, Nagamine T, Ikeda A, et al. Primary somatosensory cortex is actively involved in pain processing in human. *Brain Res* 2000;853:282–289.

21. Shibasaki H, Kuroiwa Y. Electroencephalographic correlates of myoclonus. *Electroenceph Clin Neurophysiol* 1975;39:455–463.

22. Shibasaki H, Kakigi R, Ikeda A. Scalp topography of giant SEP and premyoclonus spike in cortical reflex myoclonus. *Electroenceph Clin Neurophysiol* 1991;81:31–37.

23. Mima T, Nagamine T, Nishitani, N, et al. Cortical myoclonus: sensorimotor hyperexcitability. *Neurology* 1998;50:933–942.

24. Uesaka Y, Terao Y, Ugawa Y, et al. Magnetoencephalographic analysis of cortical myoclonic jerks. *Electroenceph Clin Neurophysiol* 1996;99:141–148.

25. Mima T, Nagamine T, Ikeda A, et al. Pathogenesis of cortical myoclonus studied by magnetoencephalography. *Ann Neurol* 1998;43:598–607.

26. Silen T, Forss N, Jensen O, et al. Abnormal reactivity of the ~20-Hz motor cortex rhythm in Unverricht-Lundborg type progressive myoclonus epilepsy. *NeuroImage* 2000;12:707–712.

27. Brown P, Day BL, Rothwell JC, et al. Intrahemispheric and inter-

hemispheric spread of cerebral cortical myoclonic activity and its relevance to epilepsy. *Brain* 1991;114:2333–2351.

28. Brown P, Ridding MC, Werhahn KJ, et al. Abnormalities of the balance between inhibition and excitation in the motor cortex of patients with cortical myoclonus. *Brain* 1996;119:309–317.

29. Terada K, Ikeda A, Mima T, et al. Familial cortical myoclonic tremor as a unique form of cortical reflex myoclonus. *Mov Disord* 1997;12:370–377.

30. Plaster NM, Uyama E, Uchino M, et al. Genetic localization of the familial adult myoclonic epilepsy (FAME) gene to chromosome 8q24. *Neurology* 1999;53:1180–1183.

31. Thompson PD, Day BL, Rothwell JC, et al. The myoclonus in corticobasal degeneration: evidence for two forms of cortical reflex myoclonus. *Brain* 1994;117:1197–1207.

32. Lu CS, Ikeda A, Terada K, et al. Electrophysiological studies of early stage corticobasal degeneration. *Mov Disord* 1998;13: 140–146.

33. Brown P, Farmer SF, Halliday DM, et al. Coherent cortical and muscle discharge in cortical myoclonus. *Brain* 1999;122: 461–472.

34. Tatu L, Moulin T, Martin V, et al. Unilateral pure thalamic asterixis: clinical, electromyographic, and topographic patterns. *Neurology* 2000;54:2339–2342.

35. Lance JW, Adams RD. The syndrome of intention or action myoclonus as a sequel to hypoxic encephalopathy. *Brain* 1963; 86:111–136.

36. Shibasaki H, Ikeda A, Nagamine T, et al. Cortical reflex negative myoclonus. *Brain* 1994;117:477–486.

37. Gambardella A, Aguglia U, Oliveri RL, et al. Photic-induced epileptic negative myoclonus: a case report. *Epilepsia* 1996;37: 492–494.

38. Rubboli G, Parmeggiani L, Tassinari CA. Frontal inhibitory spike component associated with epileptic negative myoclonus. *Electroenceph Clin Neurophysiol* 1995;95:201–205.

39. Baumgartner C, Podreka I, Olbrich A, et al. Epileptic negative myoclonus: an EEG-single-photon emission CT study indicating involvement of premotor cortex. *Neurology* 1996;46: 753–758.

40. Lüders HO, Dinner DS, Morris HH, et al. Cortical electrical stimulation in humans: the negative motor areas. *Adv Neurol* 1995;67:115–129.

41. Noachtar S, Holthousen H, Lüders HO. Epileptic negative myoclonus: subdural EEG recordings indicate a postcentral generator. *Neurology* 1997;49:1534–1537.

42. Ikeda A, Ohara S, Matsumoto R, et al. Role of primary sensorimotor cortices in generating inhibitory motor response in humans. *Brain* 2000;123:1710–1721.

43. Rajendra S, Schofield PR. Molecular mechanisms of inherited startle syndromes. *Trends Neurosci* 1995;18:80–82.

44. Ryan SG, Sherman SL, Terry JC, et al. Startle disease, or hyperekplexia: response to clonazepam and assignment of the gene (STHE) to chromosome 5q by linkage analysis. *Ann Neurol* 1992;31:663–668.

45. Shiang R, Ryan SG, Zhu YZ, et al. Mutations in the alpha 1 subunit of the inhibitory glycine receptor cause the dominant neurologic disorder, hyperekplexia. *Nature Genet* 1993;5:351–358.

46. Tijssen MA, Shiang R, van Deutekom J, et al. Molecular genetic reevaluation of the Dutch hyperekplexia family. *Arch Neurol* 1995;52:578–582.

47. Shiang R, Ryan SG, Zhu YZ, et al. Mutational analysis of familial and sporadic hyperekplexia. *Ann Neurol* 1995;38:85–91.

48. Rajendra S, Lynch JW, Pierce KD, et al. Startle disease mutations reduce the agonist sensitivity of the human inhibitory glycine receptor. *J Biol Chem* 1994;269:18739–18742.

49. Saul B, Kuner T, Sobetzko D, et al. Novel GLRA1 missense mutation (P250T) in dominant hyperekplexia defines an intra-

cellular determinants of glycine receptor channel gating. *J Neurosci* 1999;19:869–877.

50. Koch M, Friauf E. Glycine receptors in the caudal pontine reticular formation: are they important for the inhibition of the acoustic startle response? *Brain Res* 1995;671:63–72.

51. Pierce KD, Handford CA, Morris R, et al. A nonsense mutation in the α1 subunit of the inhibitory glycine receptor associated with bovine myoclonus. *Mol Cell Neurosci* 2001;17:354–363.

52. Chokroverty S, Walczak T, Hening W. Human startle reflex: technique and criteria for abnormal response. *Electroenceph Clin Neurophysiol* 1992;85:236–242.

53. Matsumoto J, Fuhr P, Nigro M, et al. Physiological abnormalities in hereditary hyperekplexia. *Ann Neurol* 1992;32:41–50.

54. Floeter MK, Andermann F, Andermann E, et al. Physiological studies of spinal inhibitory pathways in patients with hereditary hyperekplexia. *Neurology* 1996;46:766–772.

NEUROPHARMACOLOGY AND TREATMENT OF MYOCLONUS

SANTIAGO GIMÉNEZ-ROLDÁN

The term *myoclonus* literally means "quick muscle movement." It describes sudden, abrupt, brief, shock-like involuntary movements caused by muscular contractions (positive myoclonus) or sudden, brief lapses of muscle contraction in active postural muscles (negative myoclonus; asterixis) (1,2). The term does not make reference to the nature of the underlying disorder or its mechanism, or even to the anatomic source of the phenomenon. To address the neuropharmacologic basis in the management of myoclonus one must first understand the role of the neurotransmitter systems involved. The second step is to clarify the cause of the disorder because in some disorders myoclonus may resolve following treatment of the underlying cause. Nevertheless, most patients with myoclonus are treated purely on a symptomatic basis. Therefore, it may be useful to establish a few practical guidelines for the treatment of such patients. Finally, the properties and applications of the most common antimyoclonic drugs will be described.

NEUROPHARMACOLOGY OF MYOCLONUS

The two neurotransmitters most clearly implicated in the pathophysiology of myoclonus to date are serotonin (5-hydroxytryptamine; 5-HT) and γ-aminobutyric acid (GABA). There are data supporting major involvement by glycine. However, there is evidence that many other neurotransmitters appear to be involved in experimental models and possibly in humans as well.

Serotonergic System

Implication of the serotonin system in some forms of myoclonus was demonstrated in 1971 by Lhermitte et al., who eclectically investigated the response to 13 different drugs by a single patient who had recovered from intraoperative cardiac arrest (3). The optimal response was observed following intravenous infusion of the serotonin precursor 5-hydroxytryptophan (5-HTP). The therapeutic

effect of 5-HTP on hypoxic action myoclonus, a syndrome for which 88 cases were reported by Fahn in 1986 (2), was subsequently confirmed by many other investigators.

Serotonin Precursors

Serotonin, an inhibitory neurotransmitter, is formed from the amino acid tryptophan. Serotonin does not cross the blood–brain barrier and therefore cannot be administered in the management of central nervous system (CNS) disorders. Though tryptophan, the immediate precursor of serotonin, does cross the blood–brain barrier, the active transport system for tryptophan is not far from saturation. Tryptophan is hydroxylated to 5-HTP by tryptophan 5-hydroxylase, an enzyme specific to serotonergic cells. Conversion to serotonin also occurs by decarboxylation in catecholaminergic cells containing L-aromatic amino acid decarboxylase, an enzyme widely distributed in the brain that is also used by L-3,4-dihydroxyphenylalanine for conversion to dopamine. As a result, L-HTP has become an important treatment for posthypoxic myoclonus and is sometimes useful in other myoclonic disorders as well.

Drugs Promoting Serotonin Activity

Theoretically, 5-HT activity in the brain could also be enhanced by preventing serotonin breakdown by selective monoamine oxidase A (MAO-A) inhibitors or by drugs that inhibit reuptake of 5-HT released at nerve terminals. Sodium valproate and clonazepam, two effective antimyoclonic drugs in humans and in rats (in the latter with regard to auditory-induced muscle jerks following cardiac arrest) (4), probably involve serotonergic activity (5) though the precise mechanisms of action of these drugs are not entirely clear. As presynaptic uptake is the principal means of terminating 5-HT activity, there may be a role for serotonin uptake inhibitors, such as fluoxetine, paroxetine, fluvoxamine, zimeldine, and sertraline, in the management of myoclonus.

Selective 5-HT₂ Receptor Agonists

The therapeutic effect of 5-HTP on posthypoxic action myoclonus in humans appears to occur only after conversion to serotonin (6) and subsequent activation of 5-HT receptors. Several subtypes of serotonin receptors have been proposed on the basis of binding, autoradiographic, and functional studies (7). A number of factors point to 5-HT₂ receptors in the cerebral cortex as a candidate target for the antimyoclonic action of 5-HTP in posthypoxic stimulus-sensitive cortical myoclonus. The number of labeled 5-HT₂ receptors in the cortex of cardiac-arrested rats with myoclonus decreases, a change thought to relate to death of cortical GABAergic neurons on which 5-HT₂ receptors are found (8) (Fig. 21.1).

Myoclonus Associated with Increased Serotonergic Transmission

The various strategies outlined above for increasing serotonergic transmission are postulated on an underlying state of serotonergic deficiency. The alternative possibility is that 5-HT receptors might become supersensitive under certain circumstances. This would explain the paradox of patients whose myoclonus is aggravated by 5-HTP, as was the case in a few patients with posthypoxic

myoclonus (9,10), lipid storage disease (11), and essential myoclonus (11).

An animal model of posthypoxic myoclonus in the rat, as devised by Truong, provides interesting information on the effects of serotonergic receptors. Serotonin receptor populations are discretely and differentially distributed in the brain. Seven 5-HT receptor antagonists with different activity on serotonergic receptors subtypes were assessed in the rat model. Two of the seven drugs (methiotepin, a 5-HT₁ᵦ/₁ᴅ₂ antagonist, and mesulergine, a 5-HT₂ᴀ/₂ᴮ antagonist) were effective in inhibiting myoclonus and therefore are candidates for therapeutic trials in Lance-Adams syndrome. The paradox in Lance-Adams syndrome is that a movement disorder may be aborted by a serotonergic drug, such as 5-HTP, as well as selected serotonergic receptor antagonists. Several hypotheses have been offered that might be confirmed by new techniques, such as 2-deoxyglucose autoradiography, to identify functionally activated areas and experimental lesions with the serotonergic toxin 5,7-dihydroxytryptamine (12).

The role of tetrabenazine in the treatment of persons with myoclonus is also equivocal as this benzoquinolizine compound depletes cerebral monoamines and also blocks dopamine receptors in rat brain. Marked improvement following administration of tetrabenazine has been reported in patients with spinal segmental myoclonus.

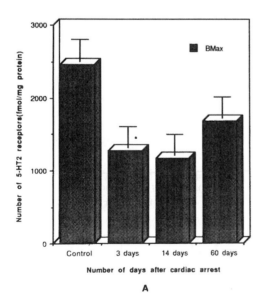

A

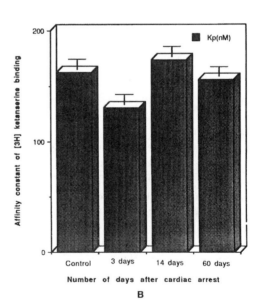

B

FIG. 21.1. 5-HT₂ receptor binding parameters in cortical membranes of rats. **A:** At 3 and 14 days after cardiac arrest, the number of 5-HT₂ receptors as labeled by [³H]ketanserine was decreased to almost one half of those in controls, but the number of 5-HT₂ receptors increased by 60 days after cardiac arrest. **B:** In contrast, no significant changes were found in the affinity constant of 5-HT₂ receptors. Values are mean ± SEM in triplicate determinations from five to eight rats. (Adopted from Jaw SP, et al. Involvement of S-HT₂ receptors in posthypoxic stimulus-sensitive myoclonus in rats. *Pharmacol Biochem Behav* 1994;49:129–131, with permission.)

GABAergic System

Both cortical and subcortical myoclonus appear related to altered GABAergic mechanisms. Thus, epileptic photosensitive myoclonus in the baboon *Papio papio*, which corresponds to epileptic cortical myoclonus, is effectively suppressed by benzodiazepine drugs, such as lorazepam. On the other hand, injection of the GABA antagonist bicuculline (a $GABA_A$ antagonist) in the dorsal and lateral portion of the putamen in primates causes repetitive and predictable jerks in the contralateral limbs. Disinhibition of GABAergic systems may cause disruption of activity in $GABA_A$ receptors at different levels of the neuraxis, resulting in myoclonus (13). Clonazepam and valproic acid, two of the most potent antimyoclonic drugs, are thought to enhance GABAergic transmission.

Observations on patients with different types of myoclonus are somewhat paradoxical, as in hereditary dystonia with alcohol-sensitive myoclonus. Ethanol is thought to exert some of its effects by acting on the GABA receptor–chloride channel complex, yet responsiveness to alcohol does not predict benefit from drugs thought to enhance GABA transmission, nor is it specific for that particular condition (14,15). Linkage studies in alcohol-responsive myoclonic dystonia have so far ruled out any causative role for mutations in 13 subunits of the $GABA_A$ receptor (16). The effect of vigabatrin, a $GABA_T$ inhibitor ($GABA_T$ is the enzyme that intervenes in the breakdown of GABA), may also appear somewhat paradoxical in this context. This drug raises the concentration of GABA in cerebrospinal fluid (CSF) yet may induce myoclonus at toxic levels, an effect that has also been observed in other anticonvulsants (17).

Glycinergic System

Like GABA, glycine is also an inhibitory neurotransmitter in the brainstem and spinal cord of mammals and appears to be involved in spinal spasticity, stiff-person syndrome, and hyperekplexia. Some experimental observations suggest a role for glycine in brainstem and spinal myoclonus. The insecticide dichlorodiphenyltrichloroethane (DDT) elicits stimulus-sensitive myoclonus by displacing glycine from brainstem receptors, also without decreasing the total glycine concentration in the brain (18).

Dorsal horn interneurons are abnormally hyperactive in some forms of spinal myoclonus (19), and hence relatively normal α motor neurons are driven to discharge by abnormal activity in involved spinal circuits (20). Physiologic studies of spinal inhibitory pathways in patients with hereditary hyperekplexia, where a point mutation in the α_1 subunit of the strychnine-sensitive glycine receptor has been identified, suggest that disynaptic reciprocal inhibition in humans is mediated through glycinergic interneurons (21). So far, open-label studies with milacemide, a glycine pro-

drug that increases glycine concentrations in the brain and prevents DDT-induced myoclonus, have been performed on humans but failed to relieve posthypoxic myoclonus and propriospinal myoclonus.

Dopaminergic System

Involvement of dopamine neurotransmission is unlikely to be critical in most types of myoclonus. Nevertheless, parkinsonian patients undergoing levodopa therapy may experience myoclonic jerks during periods of drowsiness (22), though infrequently. Amantadine-induced "voice" myoclonus has also being reported (23). Intravenous lisuride reduced the severity of myoclonic jerking in patients with cortical myoclonus (24). As lisuride has both dopaminergic and serotonergic properties, the specific neuropharmacologic mechanism that was implicated is unclear.

Excitatory Amino Acids

In photically induced myoclonus in the baboon *Papio papio*, a primate model of generalized myoclonus, two competitive *N*-methyl-D-aspartate (NMDA) antagonists, CGP-37849 and CGP-39551, administered *per os* were prolongedly effective (25).

Cholinergic Neurotransmission

Myoclonus induced by intermittent light stimulation In baboons resembles photosensitive epilepsy in humans and is readily suppressed by clonazepam, valproate, and 5-HTP. The neurophysiologic features correspond to epileptic cortical myoclonus. Another type of myoclonus is never accompanied by EEG abnormalities and may be improved by injection of lorazepam, a benzodiazepine with a blocking effect on photosensitivity. Electrophysiologically this type of myoclonus resembles reticular reflex myoclonus. It appears to be dependent on the cholinergic system, as evidenced by the fact that it may be improved by anticholinergics whereas it is aggravated by physostigmine (26).

Essential myoclonus in humans, whether hereditary or sporadic, may respond to anticholinergic medication, though this has not been the experience of other workers (27). Palatal myoclonus has been relieved by high-dose trihexyphenidyl, a condition now assumed to represent a form of focal tremor rather than myoclonus (28). Both sumatriptan (29) and flunarizine (30) have been reported as beneficial.

Adrenergic System

The development of multifocal myoclonus shortly after the introduction of carvedilol, a new nonselective β-adrenergic blocking agent with α_1 blocking activity for the management of congestive heart failure and hypertension (31), and salbutamol, a selective preferential β_2 agonist, in patients with respiratory insufficiency (32) implicates the adrenergic system in the pathophysiology of myoclonus.

CLINICAL APPROACH TO MANAGEMENT OF MYOCLONUS

Myoclonus Is Sometimes Difficult to Recognize

Although recognition of sudden, brief muscle jerks as myoclonus is usually not difficult, careful diagnosis is an essential first step toward proper treatment. Details of differentiation from other movement disorders, particularly tics and dystonic spasms, are outside the scope of this chapter. Pathologic startle syndromes are also considered elsewhere in this book. Though asterixis (negative myoclonus) involves cortical mechanisms, it is not associated with electroencephalographic discharges or epileptic seizures. Asterixis should be distinguished from negative epileptic myoclonus, which is thought to be generated in the middle frontal gyrus, corresponding to Brodmann's area 6, and may respond to clonazepam.

Cortical myoclonus clinically appearing as tremulousness, also termed cortical tremor and polymyoclonus, and made worse by action represents another potential cause of confusion. The movements are characterized by rhythmic electromyographic bursts (<50 ms) at 9 to 18 Hz, synchronous in agonist and antagonist muscles, which are preceded by an electroencephalographic potential on back-averaging studies.

Recognition of the Underlying Cause Is Occasionally an Important Step Toward Treatment

Toxic Agents and Systemic Metabolic Disturbances

Toxic agents and systemic metabolic disturbances are among the most common causes of "curable" myoclonus. The list of poisonous substances and drugs that may cause myoclonus (Table 21.1) is long and ever growing. Creutzfeldt-Jakob disease was wrongly suspected in bismuth subsalicylate poisoning from an over-the-counter remedy for gastrointestinal complaints (33). Recover occur when bismuth preparations are withheld but may be accelerated with the metal chelator dimercaprol (34). Poisoning by methyl ethyl ketone in a printer was another identified curable cause of alcohol-sensitive progressive myoclonic encephalopathy (15).

TABLE 21.1. POTENTIAL CAUSES OF "CURABLE" MYOCLONUS

Etiology	Diagnostic Clues	Treatment
Drug induced[a]	Drug exposure	Dose reduction or discontinuation
	Plasma drug levels of anticonvulsants	Dimercaprol may accelerate in the toxic range
	Renal failure in meperidine toxicity	recovery in bismuth salts encephalopathy
	Drowsiness in levodopa-induced myoclonus	
Toxic myoclonus[b]	History of exposure	Withdrawal from the source of poisoning
Metabolic encephalopathies[c]	Laboratory evidence of organ failure	Correction of the underlying systemic or metabolic abnormality
Biotin-responsive encephalopathy with myoclonus, ataxia, and seizures	Plasma biotin levels	Oral biotin 3–20 mg/d
Opsoclonus-myoclonus syndrome	Serum antineuronal antibodies. An underlying cancer may be found	High-dose steroids or IV cyclophosphamide
Infantile polymyoclonus	Neuroblastoma	ACTH, IV immunoglobulins cyclophosphamide plasma exchange
Hashimoto's encephalopathy	High serum antithyroglobulin antibodies	Steroids
Psychogenic myoclonus	Incongruent or incompatible clinical features. Bereitschafts potential	Comprehensive psychiatric and neurologic approach

[a]Includes levodopa, antidepressants (including fluoxetine), lithium, antibiotics (penicillin, cefepime, imipenen, cefuroxime), opioids, antineoplastics (prednimustine and others), anticonvulsants (including vigabatrin, lamotrigine and gabapentin), anesthetics (e.g., fentanyl), beta-blocking agents (salbutamol, carvedilol), insoluble bismuth salts, methaqualone, antihistamines, diclofenac, saline emetics, benzodiazepine withdrawal and water-soluble contrast medias. Self-limiting myoclonus following parenteral cobalamine may be observed in nutritional cobalamin deficiency and in congenital transcobalamin deficiency.
[b]Includes methylbromide poisoning, DDT, heavy metals, clembuterol, gasoline sniffing, toxic oil syndrome, chloralose, and methyl ethyl ketone.
[c]Includes hepatic failure, renal failure, dialysis syndrome, hyponatremia, hypoglycemia, and nonketotic hyperglycemia.

Opsoclonus-Myoclonus Syndrome

Opsoclonus-myoclonus syndrome (OMS) consists of a combination of involuntary multidirectional saccadic movements of the eyes and multifocal and reflex myoclonus, almost always associated with pancerebellar ataxia. Usually in adults it is either paraneoplastic or an idiopathic condition. The currently known antineuronal antibodies are not consistently found in OMS but when present they favor a paraneoplastic origin (35). In children, OMS is associated with neuroblastoma and ganglioneuroblastoma in about half of the cases, with the remainder being presumably viral in origin (36).

High-dose steroids may bring about a faster recovery than spontaneous remission in adults with idiopathic OMS, but oral cyclophosphamide (150 mg/day) may afford a useful alternative. Idiopathic OMS improved dramatically after intravenous immunoglobulins (35). Immunotherapy appears more effective in children with neuroblastoma than in adult patients with cancer. Removal of the underlying tumor in infants—usually a small, nonmetastasizing, mediastinal neuroblastoma—is beneficial, though temporary worsening following surgery may occur, possibly due to the release of antigens during the operation. Children usually respond rapidly to adrenocorticotropic hormone (ACTH) administered in tapering doses for many weeks, but relapses on discontinuation are common. A somewhat more rapid response has been recorded in cases treated with intravenous immunoglobulins and plasmapheresis with concomitant immunosuppression (37). When the association with neuroblastoma is unclear, corticosteroid treatment should be cautiously considered before the results of enterovirus search in CSF by polymerase chain reaction are available. This is because corticosteroids may potentiate coxsackie virus infection and patients may otherwise recover spontaneously under symptomatic treatment (36).

Hashimoto's Myoclonic Encephalopathy

Hashimoto's myoclonic encephalopathy is another, perhaps underdiagnosed, treatable disorder with an immune basis (38). It is characterized by a subacute syndrome of confusion, apathy, rigidity and akinesia, myoclonus, and sometimes complex partial seizures. Anticonvulsants may cause a paradoxical aggravation of the disorder, whereas administration of steroids brings about rapid neurologic improvement. Crucial to the diagnosis is the finding of high titers of antithyroglobulin antibodies.

Postmalaria Encephalopathy

Following recovery from successfully treated *Plasmidum falciparum* malaria, some patients develop a progressive encephalopathy characterized by word-finding difficulties, generalized stimulus-sensitive myoclonus, and postural tremor. The condition continues to deteriorate until a corticosteroid, such as intravenous methylprednisolone (100 mg/day for 3 days with subsequent tapering for 10 days), is introduced (39).

Myoclonus Associated to Peripheral Mononeuropathy

Rhythmic focal or segmental myoclonus is often of spinal origin. However, peripheral nerve lesions related to scarred defects in subcutaneous tissue or tumors may cause rhythmic or semirhythmic myoclonus. In two cases, excision of the scar or section of the nerve provided marked improvement or resolution (40,41).

Chronic hiccup is caused by diaphragmatic and intercostal muscle contractions and concurrent glottic closure. The cause of hiccup may be peripheral (i.e., gastric distention and mediastinal masses) or central (i.e., damage to vagal nuclei and n. tractus solitarius at the medulla). Opiate-related hiccup has been recently described (42). Management of this bothersome condition may be difficult. Chlorpromazine and baclofen may be useful. Interestingly, eight patients who developed chronic hiccup following brainstem infarction became symptom free within 48 hours following gabapentin administration (400 mg tid) (43).

Psychogenic Myoclonus

This represents the psychogenic movement disorder most commonly seen in some specialized clinics (44) and one of the few of examples of "curable" myoclonus. An integrated team approach seems to be the most effective means for management (45).

Symptomatic Treatment of Myoclonus: Single-drug Therapy Should Be the First Choice, But Polytherapy Is Likely to Be the Best Final Option

Evidence from the literature indicates that at least five drugs (valproate, clonazepam, 5-HTP, primidone, and piracetam) are particularly effective, if not completely exclusive, in the management of cortical reflex and reticular reflex myoclonus. Sodium valproate may be the drug of choice to start with. Clonazepam is probably equally effective, but drowsiness is an inconvenient side effect and instability, already present in many patients with myoclonus, may worsen.

Administration of 5-HTP in posthypoxic myoclonus was fashionable some years ago, when the pharmacologic and biochemical implications of the serotonergic system in this condition were shown. The efficacy of 5-HTP is probably less than that of valproate and clonazepam. Currently, some authors have suggested that association with carbidopa is not indispensable for clinical use of 5-HTP. Piracetam may be a good option for patients already under polytherapy with persistent residual myoclonus as it is virtually devoid of side effects.

Patients may become myoclonus free as a result of a single-drug treatment. However, unlike epilepsies, where the trend is toward the use of anticonvulsant drugs as monotherapy, most patients with action myoclonus reported by Obeso et al. (46) required concurrent administration of three or even four drugs. The rationale for the use of multiple drugs is that they might act synergistically on the various pathophysiologic mechanisms that presumably concur in a single patient.

Electrophysiologic Investigations and Cerebrospinal Fluid Biochemistry May Be Helpful Factors But Are Rarely Crucial to Drug Choice

Reticular and cortical reflex myoclonus are distinct in electrophysiologic terms. However, it is unclear whether they also differ with regard to response to various antimyoclonic drugs. Cortical reflex myoclonus, particularly when muscle jerks are elicited by action, usually responds to single-drug treatment or, more often, to a combination of drugs. Anticholinergics have been suggested, but clonazepam is probably the drug of choice. At present, determination of 5-hydroxyindolacetic acid concentrations in CSF may provide an indicator rather than a conclusive criterion for deciding the use of serotonin enhancers.

Epilepsy Syndromes with Prominent Myoclonus Are Associated with Specific Problems in Terms of Prognosis and Management

When etiology is considered, the term *epileptic myoclonus* is applied to patients in whom seizures predominate and in whom, at least initially, there is no associated progressive encephalopathy. Instead, myoclonic jerks may be the only manifestation of epilepsy or, more commonly, myoclonus may occur in combination to other epileptic seizures. The prognostic, therapeutic, and sometimes etiologic problems associated with this group of epilepsies go beyond the scope of this chapter. Aside from its cause, epilepsia partialis continua is notoriously resistant to available antiepileptic drugs. Patients with reading epilepsy commonly complain of jerking of the jaw, which may respond dramatically to clonazepam. Generalized epilepsies, whether idiopathic or cryptogenic, associating myoclonic jerks compose a relatively poorly defined group of epileptic syndromes in infancy, childhood, and adolescence. Valproic acid is in most cases the first-choice drug (Table 21.2), but the prognosis is strikingly uneven.

Spinal Myoclonus May Respond to Antimyoclonic Agents Effective in Cortical and Reticular Myoclonus

Two different types of spinal myoclonus have been identified. In rhythmic segmental spinal myoclonus, jerks are confined to muscles innervated by a few spinal segments. Propriospinal myoclonus causes more extensive jerks in which many segments are involved, linked by activity in long propriospinal pathways. An early report mentioned some effectiveness of diazepam, but clonazepam appears to be the drug of choice in both forms of spinal myoclonus. If clonazepam fails, it is appropriate to try other drugs such as tetrabenazine, trihexyphenidyl, carbamazepine, or levodopa because these drugs have provided varying degrees of improvement in some cases (47).

Not All Anticonvulsants Are Antimyoclonic

Progressive myoclonus epilepsy of the Unverricht-Lundborg type (Baltic myoclonus) may even be made worse by phenytoin. Carbamazepine is also thought to aggravate some forms of myoclonus. It has been suggested that the

TABLE 21.2. MANAGEMENT AND PROGNOSIS OF MAJOR PRIMARY EPILEPTIC MYOCLONUS SYNDROMES

Epileptic Syndrome	Prognosis	First-choice Drug	Second-choice Drug
Benign myoclonic epilepsy of infancy	Excellent	Valproic acid	—
Severe myoclonic epilepsy in infancy	Poor to very poor		Phenobarbital Valproic acid, clonazepam, piracetam
Lennox-Gastaut syndrome	Poor	Valproic acid Felbamate Lamotrigine	Carbamazepine and clonazepam may aggravate some types of seizures
Myoclonic-astatic epilepsy (Doose's epilepsy)	Good to poor	Valproic acid	Primidone, clonazepam
Epilepsy with myoclonic absences	Good to poor	Valproic acid plus ethosuximide	Phenobarbital
Juvenile myoclonic epilepsy of Janz (Drug dependency)	Good	Valproic acid	Clonazepam, primidone

disease appeared to progress more rapidly, caused intellectual deterioration, and even shortened disease course to death due to a "toxic" effect of phenytoin.

ANTIMYOCLONIC DRUGS

The main drugs used in the management of myoclonus are shown in Table 21.3. Five of these drugs have been most consistent in showing antimyoclonic action.

Sodium Valproate

Due to its good overall tolerance and broad range of effectiveness, sodium valproate is probably the drug of choice to initiate symptomatic treatment in the vast majority of myoclonus cases. This is also the drug of choice in some epileptic syndromes, such as juvenile myoclonic epilepsy. The drug is most effective in the treatment of posthypoxic action myoclonus and Baltic myoclonus. A recent review of the literature reports improvement in 45% of patients administered valproate compared with 51% of patients receiving clonazepam (48).

The usual daily starting dose is 15 mg/kg. Doses as high as 2.5 to 3.0 g/day were required in some patients. Gastrointestinal side effects are among the most frequently encountered adverse effects of valproate, though they can be reduced by administering the medication after meals or by using the enteric-coated formulation. Weight gain, alopecia, and tremor have been observed fairly often. Idiosyncratic reactions, such as pancreatitis, hyperammonemia, and hepatotoxicity, are rare but may prove fatal. It should also be remembered that, due to drug interactions, patients receiving phenobarbitone or primidone may develop somnolence when valproate is introduced. Currently, the most frequently favored explanation of the mechanism of action of valproate is that it enhances GABA function. It is possible that the drug has multiple mechanisms, accounting for its clinical efficacy against a variety of myoclonus and seizure types (49).

Clonazepam

Clonazepam has multiple pharmacologic actions, which may explain why this drug is effective in many forms of myoclonus, though rarely in brainstem myoclonus. There is strong evidence supporting clonazepam's ability to potentiate GABAergic transmission through a direct effect on benzodiazepine receptors at the ionophore–GABA receptor complex. Clonazepam is particularly effective in absence seizures, myoclonic seizures, and status epilepticus. It is markedly useful in some reflex epilepsies, such as startle-induced seizures and jaw myoclonus in reading epilepsy. The remarkable potency of clonazepam as an antimyoclonic agent may be attributable to simultaneous action on both the GABAergic and serotonergic systems, the two neurotransmission systems most directly implicated in the neuropharmacology of myoclonus.

L-5-Hydroxytryptophan

Myoclonus following posthypoxic encephalopathy is the disorder most likely to benefit from treatment with 5-HTP. The intention or action myoclonus is the component of the syndrome that is most responsive to serotonergic-promoting drugs. In humans, plasma levels of hydroxytryptophan can be increased tenfold by pretreatment with a decarboxylase inhibitor; therefore, as in the case of levodopa, administration of 5-HTP with a peripheral decarboxylase inhibitor, such as carbidopa or benserazide, has been recommended.

TABLE 21.3. DRUG TREATMENT FOR MYOCLONUS

Drug	Starting Dose (Daily)	Usual Dose (Daily)	Maximal Dose
Often useful			
Valproic acid	200	600–1,500	2,600
Clonazepam	0.5	6–12	20
Piracetam	800	10–16	24[a]
5-HTP (plus carbidopa)	100	0.5–1.5	3[a]
Primidone	125	325–750	1,500
Sometimes useful			
Trihexyphenidyl	1	6–15	60
Tetrabenazine	25	75–150	200
Clobazam	10	20–30	60
Propranolol	40	120–240	240
Methysergide	1	3–6	6
Fluoxetine	20	20–60	60
Clomipramine	10	30–150	250
Opiates (methadone)	20	20	20

Doses are given in mg/d, except those marked [a] in g/d.

Nevertheless, as already mentioned, some authors do not regard this combination as indispensable. The recommended starting dose for 5-HTP is 100 mg/day, followed by gradual increments up to 400 to 2,000 mg/day, depending on side effects and effectiveness. The total dose may be divided and taken as 4 to 6 doses throughout the day.

The levorotatory form of 5-HTP has few side effects, particularly gastrointestinal disturbances, if the capsules are taken after meals and the dosage is increased gradually. Dyspnea and fainting may occur. Larger doses cause euphoria or may even precipitate a manic state, whereas discontinuance has sometimes resulted in lasting depression. The effect of 5-HTP on seizures varies, but it should be remembered that they may occasionally be aggravated. Increased serum concentrations and phenobarbital toxicity have been observed. Decreasing efficacy after years of continuous use may occur, perhaps due to down-regulation of 5-HT$_2$ serotonin receptors.

Piracetam

Piracetam is a drug with a somewhat paradoxical history and enigmatic mechanisms. It does not bind to any known receptor system and does not specifically affect any enzyme or transporter system. It has been proposed that piracetam increases cell fluidity by binding to phospholipidic molecules in neuronal membranes, which might explain its mode of action (50). This drug modifies facilitatory I-wave interactions at the motor cortex in a way similar to that of GABAergic drugs (51). Still, the efficacy of piracetam in the management of myoclonus is beyond question and levetiracetam, an L isomer with marked antiepileptic action and a broader spectrum than piracetam, shows promise (52).

The beneficial effect of piracetam is not limited to posthypoxic myoclonus; it is also effective in the management of cortical action myoclonus, regardless of cause. Piracetam is mostly beneficial in association with other antimyoclonic drugs as add-on medications, though it has been reported to be useful in monotherapy (53). Moreover, when administered as monotherapy, it may improve electrophysiologic abnormalities but has no useful clinical effect (54) (Fig. 21.2).

The optimal dosage of piracetam in the treatment of myoclonus has not been determined. The range varied widely in the initial studies, but it is now clear that doses as high as 24 g/day may be safely administered. Withdrawal seizures following piracetam discontinuation may occur. In a few instances, patients under polytherapy were reported to have developed thrombocytopenia and leukopenia.

Primidone

Primidone, typically in combination with other antimyoclonic drugs, has been effective in the management of severe action myoclonus. The presence of two active metabolites, phenobarbital and phenylethylmalonamide (PEMA), with demonstrated independent anticonvulsant activity distinguishes primidone from most other conventional antiepileptic drugs. Primidone appears to act on the efferent side of the motor cortex, as it markedly improves action myoclonus, but somatosensory evoked potentials (SEPs) become larger in amplitude. In contrast, clonazepam usually reduces the amplitude of giant SEPs and associated reflex myoclonus.

New Therapies for Myoclonus

Stiff-man syndrome and progressive encephalomyelopathy with rigidity and myoclonus are immune-mediated disorders. Patients refractory to oral antispasticity medications, such as the GABA neuromodulator diazepam or baclofen, a GABA$_B$ agonist, and immunosuppression may improve receiving intrathecal baclofen via pump (55). They often require dosages much higher than those with spasticity. Pump malfunction resulting in inaccurate dosing proved life threatening in two of eight patients.

Focal myoclonus associated with thoracodorsal neuropathy responded for years to botulinum toxin type A infiltra-

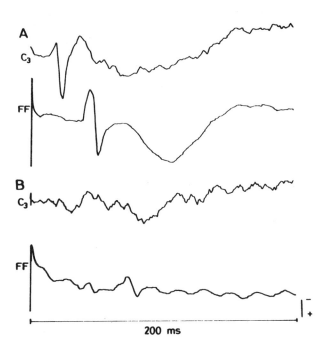

FIG. 21.2. Somatosensory evoked potentials (SSEPs) and electromyographic (EMG) activity after a 10-mA digital nerve electrical stimulus (delivered at the start of the sweep). **A:** Before treatment. **B:** After piracetam (18 g daily PO) for 7 days. At the higher intensity of stimulus there is a large cortical and muscle response before treatment. While the patient was taking piracetam the same strength of stimulus produced much smaller SSEPs and minimal reflex muscle activity. Vertical calibration line represents 10 μV for SSEPs and 200 μV for electromyograms. (From Obeso JA, Artieda J, Quinn N, et al. Piracetam in the treatment of different types of myoclonus. *Clin Neuropharmacol* 1988;11: 529–536.)

tions (41). Eight children and adolescents with myoclonus secondary to a variety of conditions received electromyographically directed botulinum toxin type A infiltrations (56). Myoclonus was generalized in five of these patients, requiring infiltration in as many as 15 muscles. Unaided locomotion was achieved in one patient, but the long-term benefits of this procedure are unknown. Botulinum toxin was also effective for several months in a patient with stimulus-sensitive spinal segmental myoclonus related to a posttraumatic pseudomeningocele and brachial plexus injury sustained 32 years before (57).

CONCLUDING REMARKS

In the last few years we have learned that many neurotransmitter systems are implicated in myoclonus. This explains the polytherapy currently in vogue for the treatment of many patients with severe myoclonus, particularly involving action-induced muscle jerks. The involvement of GABAergic and serotonergic mechanisms in myoclonus is well known. Identification of serotonin receptor subtypes in the cerebral cortex is a promising finding. However, manipulation of glycine transmission and the excitatory amino acids may bring new and effective drugs in the near future. Piracetam has gained a reputation, even when its specific mechanism of action in myoclonus remains somewhat mysterious.

REFERENCES

1. Marsden CD, Hallett M, Fahn S. The nosology and pathophysiology of myoclonus. In: Marsden CD, Fahn S, eds. *Movement disorders.* Boston: Butterworth & Co, 1981:196–248.
2. Fahn S. Posthypoxic action myoclonus: literature review update. In: Fahn S, Marsden CD, Van Woert, M, eds. *Myoclonus.* Advances in neurology, vol 43. New York: Raven Press, 1986: 157–169.
3. Lhermitte F, Peterfalvi M, Marteau R, et al. Analyse pharmacologique d'un cas de myoclonies d'intention et d'action postanoxiques. *Rev Neurol (Paris)* 1971;124:21–31.
4. Truong DD, Matsumoto RR, Schwartz PH, et al. Novel rat cardiac arrest model of posthypoxic myoclonus. *Mov Disord* 1994;9: 201–206.
5. Biggs CS, Pearce BR, Fowler LJ, et al. Regional effects of sodium valproate on extracellular concentrations of 5-hydroxytryptamine, dopamine, and their metabolites in the rat brain: an in vivo microdyalisis study. *J Neurochem* 1992;59:1702–1708.
6. Pranzatelli MR, Galvan I, Tailor PT. Human brainstem serotonin receptors: characterization and implications for subcortical myoclonus. *Clin Neuropharmacol* 1996;19:507–514.
7. Julius D. Molecular biology of serotonin receptors. *Annu Rev Neurosci* 1991;14:335–360.
8. Kawai K, Nitecka L, Ruetzler CA, et al. Global cerebral ischemia associated with cardiac arrest in the rat. I: Dynamics of early neuronal changes. *J Cereb Blood Flow Metab* 1992;12:238–249.
9. Fahn S. Posthypoxic myoclonus: review of the literature and report of two new cases with response to valproate and estrogens. *Adv Neurol, vol 26.* New York: Raven Press, 1979:49–84.
10. Giménez-Roldán S, Mateo D, Muradas V, et al. Clinical, biochemical, and pharmacological observations in patient with postasphyxic myoclonus: association with serotonin hyperactivity. *Clin Neuropharmacol* 1988;11:151–160.
11. Growdon JH, Young RR, Shahani BT. L-5-Hydroxytryptophan in the treatment of several different syndromes in which myoclonus is prominent. *Neurology* 1976;26:1135–1140.
12. Goetz CG, Vu TQ, Carvey PM, et al. Posthypoxic myoclonus in the rat: natural history, stability, and serotonergic influences. *Mov Disord* 2000;15[Suppl 1]:39–46.
13. Matsumoto RR, Truong DD, Nguyen KD, et al. Involvement of GABA-A receptors in myoclonus. *Mov Disord* 2000;15[Suppl 1]: 47–52.
14. Jain S, Tamer SK, Hiran S. Beneficial effect of alcohol in hereditary cerebellar ataxia with myoclonus (progressive myoclonic ataxia): report of two siblings. *Mov Disord* 1996;11:751–752.
15. Ortí-Pareja M, Jiménez-Jiménez FJ, Miquel J, et al. Reversible myoclonus, tremor, and ataxia in a patient exposed to methyl ethyl ketone. *Neurology* 1996;46:272.
16. Gasser T, Bereznai B, Müller B, et al. Linkage studies in alcohol-responsive myoclonic dystonia. *Mov Disord* 1996;11:363–370.
17. Neufeld MY, Vishnevska S. Vigabatrin and multifocal myoclonus in adults with partial seizures. *Clin Neuropharmacol* 1995;18: 280–283.
18. Truong DD, García de Yébenes J, Pezzoli G, et al. Glycine involvement in DDT-induced myoclonus. *Mov Disord* 1988;3: 77–87.
19. Di Lazzaro V, Restuccia D, Nardone R, et al. Changes in spinal cord excitability in a patient with rhythmic segmental myoclonus. *J Neurol Neurosurg Psychiatry* 1996;61:641–644.
20. Simon ES. Involvement of glycine and GABA-A receptors in the pathogenesis of spinal myoclonus: in vitro studies in the isolated neonatal rodent spinal cord. *Neurology* 1995;45:1883–1892.
21. Floeter MK, Andermann F, Andermann E, et al. Physiological studies of spinal inhibitory pathways in patients with hereditary hyperekplexia. *Neurology* 1996;46:766–772.
22. Klawans HL, Goetz C, Weiner WJ. 5-Hydroxytryptophan-induced myoclonus in guinea pigs and the possible role of serotonin in infantile spasms. *Neurology* 1973;23:1234–1240.
23. Pfeiffer RF. Amantadine-induced "vocal" myoclonus. *Mov Disord* 1996;11:104–105.
24. Obeso JA, Rothwell JC, Quinn NP, et al. Cortical reflex myoclonus responds to intravenous lisuride. *Clin Neuropharmacol* 1983; 6:231–240.
25. Chapman AG, Graham JL, Patel S, et al. Anticonvulsant activity of two orally active competitive *N*-methyl-D-aspartate antagonists, CGP 37 849 and CGP 39 551, against sound-induced seizures in DBA/2 mice and photically induced myoclonus in *Papio papio. Epilepsia* 1991;32:578–587.
26. Rektor I, Svejdová M, Silva-Barrat C, et al. The cholinergic system-dependent myoclonus of the baboon *Papio papio* is a reticular reflex myoclonus. *Mov Disord* 1993;8:28–32.
27. Quinn NP. Essential myoclonus and myoclonic dystonia. *Mov Disord* 1996;11:119–124.
28. Deuschl G, Toro C, Valls-Solé J, et al. Symptomatic and essential palatal tremor. I: Clinical, physiological, and MRI analysis. *Brain* 1994;117:775–788.
29. Scott BL, Evans RW, Jankovic J. Treatment of palatal myoclonus with sumatriptan. *Mov Disord* 1996;11:748–751.
30. Cakmur R, Idiman E, Idiman F, et al. Essential palatal tremor successfully treated with flunarizine. *Eur Neurol* 1997;38:133–134.
31. Fernández HH, Friedman JH. Carvedilol-induced myoclonus. *Mov Disord* 1999;14:702.
32. Micheli F, Cersósimo MG, Scorticati MC, et al. Myoclonus secondary to albuterol (salbutamol) instillation. *Neurology* 2000;54: 2022–2023.

33. Gordon MF, Abrams RI, Rubin DB, et al. Bismuth subsalicylate toxicity as a cause of prolonged encephalopathy with myoclonus. *Mov Disord* 1995;10:220–222.

34. Molina JA, Calandre L, Bermejo F. Myoclonic encephalopathy due to bismuth salts: treatment with dimercaprol and analysis of CSF transmitters. *Acta Neurol Scand* 1989;79:200–203.

35. Bataller L, Graus F, Saiz A, et al., for the Spanish Opsoclonus-Myoclonus Study Group. Clinical outcome in adult-onset idiopathic or paraneoplastic opsoclonus-myoclonus. *Brain* 2001;124:437–443.

36. Tabarki B, Palmer P, Lebon P, et al. Spontaneous recovery of opsoclonus-myoclonus syndrome caused by enterovirus infection. *J Neurol Neurosurg Psychiatry* 1998;64:406–407.

37. Yiu VWY, Kovithavongs T, McGonigle LF, et al. Plasmapheresis as an effective treatment for opsoclonus-myoclonus syndrome. *Pediatr Neurol* 2001;24:72–74.

38. Ghika-Schmid F, Ghika J, Regli N, et al. Hashimoto encephalopathy: an underdiagnosed treatable condition? *Mov Disord* 1996;11:555–562.

39. Schnorf H, Diserens K, Schnyder H, et al. Corticosteroid-responsive postmalaria encephalopathy characterized by motor aphasia, myoclonus, and postural tremor. *Arch Neurol* 1998;55:417–420.

40. Glocker FX, Deuchsl G, Volk B, et al. Bilateral myoclonus of the trapezius muscles after distal lesion of an accessory nerve. *Mov Disord* 1996;11:571–575.

41. Carnero-Pardo C, Sánchez Alvarez JC, Gómez Camello A, et al. Myoclonus associated with thoracodorsal neuropathy. *Mov Disord* 1999;13:971–972.

42. Lauterbach EC. Hiccup and apparent myoclonus after hydrocodone: review of the opiate-related hiccup and myoclonus literature. *Clin Neuropharmacol* 1999;22:87–92.

43. Moretti T, Torre P, Antonello RM, et al. Treatment of chronic hiccup: new perspectives. *Eur J Neurol* 1999;6:617–620.

44. Monday K, Jankovic J. Psychogenic myoclonus. *Neurology* 1993;43:349–352.

45. Williams DT, Ford B, Fahn S. Phenomenology and psychopathology related to psychogenic movement disorders. In: Weiner WJ, Lang AE, eds. *Behavioral neurology of movement disorders.* Advances in neurology, vol 65. New York: Raven Press, 1995:231–257.

46. Obeso JA, Artieda J, Quinn N, et al. Piracetam in the treatment of different types of myoclonus. *Clin Neuropharmacol* 1988;11:529–536.

47. Jankovic J, Pardo R. Segmental myoclonus: clinical and pharmacologic study. *Arch Neurol* 1986;43:1025–1031.

48. Frutch S, Fahn S. The clinical spectrum of posthypoxic myoclonus. *Mov Disord* 2000;15[Suppl. 1]:2–7.

49. Bruni J, Williams LJ, Wilder BJ. Treatment of postanoxic intention myoclonus with valproic acid. *Can J Neurol Sci* 1979;6:39–42.

50. Mäller WE, Eckert GP, Eckert A. Piracetam: novelty in a unique mode of action. *Pharmacopsychiatry* 1999;32[Suppl]:2–9.

51. Wischer S, Paulus W, Sommer M, et al. Piracetam affects facilitatory I-wave interaction in the human motor cortex. *Clin Neurophysiol* 2001;112:275–279.

52. Shorvon SD. Piracetam. In: Shorvon S, Dreifuss F, Fish D, et al., eds. *The treatment of epilepsies.* Oxford: Blackwell Science, 1996:466–470.

53. Ikeda A, Shiwasaki H, Tashiro K, et al., and the Myoclonus/Piracetam Study Group. Clinical trial of piracetam in patients with myoclonus: nationwide multi-institution study in Japan. *Mov Disord* 1996;11:691–700.

54. Obeso JA, Artieda J, Rothwell JC, et al. The treatment of severe action myoclonus. *Brain* 1989;112:765–777.

55. Stayer C, Tronnier V, Dressnandt J, et al. Intrathecal baclofen therapy for stiff-man syndrome and progressive encephalomyelopathy with rigidity and myoclonus. *Neurology* 1997;49:1591–1597.

56. Awaad Y, Tayem H, Elgamal A, et al. Treatment of childhood myoclonus with botulinum toxin type A. *J Child Neurol* 1999;14:781.

57. Lagueny A, Tison F, Burbaud P, et al. Stimulus-sensitive spinal segmental myoclonus improved with injections of botulinum toxin type A. *Mov Disord* 1999;14:182–185.

TICS AND TOURETTE'S SYNDROME

JOSEPH J. JANKOVIC

Tourette's syndrome (TS) is a neurologic disorder manifested by motor as well as vocal or phonic tics that in most cases start in childhood and are often accompanied by obsessive-compulsive disorder (OCD), attention deficit-hyperactivity disorder (ADHD), poor impulse control, and other comorbid behavioral problems (1,2). Once considered a rare psychiatric curiosity, TS is now recognized as a relatively common and complex neurobehavioral disorder. Many notable historical figures, including Dr. Samuel Johnson and possibly Wolfgang Amadeus Mozart, are thought to have been afflicted with TS.

The clinical expression of this genetic disorder varies from one individual to another, fluctuations in symptoms are seen within the same individual, and different manifestations occur in various family members (3). This variable expression from one individual to another, even within members of the same family, contributes to diagnostic confusion. Without a specific biologic marker, the diagnosis depends on a careful evaluation of the patient's symptoms and signs by an experienced clinician. However, many patients remain undiagnosed or their symptoms are wrongly attributed to habit, allergies, asthma, dermatitis, hyperactivity, nervousness, and many other conditions (4,5).

PHENOMENOLOGY OF TICS

Tics, the clinical hallmark of TS, are relatively brief and intermittent movements (motor tics) or sounds (vocal or phonic tics). The term *phonic tic* is preferable because not all sounds produced by TS patients involve the vocal cords. Although both types of tics must be present for the diagnosis of TS, this division into motor and phonic tics is arbitrary because phonic tics are actually motor tics involving respiratory, laryngeal, pharyngeal, oral, and nasal musculature. Motor tics typically consist of sudden, often repetitive, movements, gestures, and utterances that mimic fragments of normal behavior (1). To better understand the categorization of tics and how they fit in the general schema of movement disorders, it might be helpful to provide a simple classification of movements. All movements can be categorized into one of four classes: 1. *voluntary*: a. **intentional** (planned, self-initiated, internally generated), b. **externally triggered** (in response to some external stimulus, e.g., turning head toward a loud noise or withdrawing hand from a hot plate); 2. *semivoluntary (unvoluntary)*: a. induced by **inner sensory stimulus** (e.g., need to "stretch" a body part), b. induced by **unwanted feeling or compulsion** (e.g., compulsive touching or smelling); 3. *involuntary*: a. **nonsuppressible** (e.g., reflexes. seizures, myoclonus), b. **suppressible** (tics, tremor, dystonia, chorea, stereotypy); and 4. *automatic* (learned motor behaviors performed without conscious effort, e.g., walking or speaking). Automatic, learned behaviors appear to be encoded in the sensorimotor portion of the striatum (6), which may also have a role in the generation of tics as learned voluntary motor skills may be incorporated into a tic repertoire.

Tics may be *simple* or *complex*. *Simple motor tics* involve only one group of muscles, causing a brief, jerk-like movement. They are usually abrupt in onset and rapid ("clonic tics"), but they may be slower causing a briefly sustained abnormal posture ("dystonic tics") or an isometric contraction ("tonic tics") (7). Examples of simple clonic motor tics include blinking, nose twitching, and head jerking. Simple dystonic tics include blepharospasm, oculogyric movements, bruxism, sustained mouth opening, torticollis, and shoulder rotation; the tensing of abdominal or limb muscles is an example of tonic tic. Dystonic (and tonic) muscle contraction may be responsible for "blocking" tics. These tics are due to prolonged tonic or dystonic tics that interrupt ongoing motor activity, such as speech, or they may be due to a sudden inhibition of motor activity. Others and we have drawn attention to the presence of tics and dystonia in the same family, providing evidence for a possible etiologic relationship between TS and primary dystonia (8).

Motor (particularly dystonic) and phonic tics are preceded by premonitory sensations in more than 80% of patients. This premonitory phenomenon consist of localizable sensations or discomforts, such as a "burning feeling" in the eye before a blink, "tension or crick in the neck" relieved by stretching of the neck or jerking of the head, "feeling of tightness or constriction" relieved by arm or leg extension, "nasal stuffiness" before a sniff, "dry or sore throat" before throat clearing or grunting, and "itching" before a rotatory movement of the scapula. The observed movement or sound sometimes occurs in response to these premonitory phenomena, and this "intentional" or "unvoluntary" component of the movement may be a useful feature differentiating tics from other hyperkinetic movement disorders, such as myoclonus and chorea. Chee and Sachdev (9) suggest that "sensory tics," which we and others refer to as premonitory sensations, "represent the subjectively experienced component of neural dysfunction below the threshold for motor and phonic tic production." Besides the local or regional premonitory sensations, this premonitory phenomenon may be nonlocalizable, less specific, and poorly described feeling, such as an urge, anxiety, anger, and other psychic sensations. Many patients report that they have to repeat a particular movement in order to relieve the uncomfortable urge until "it feels good." The "just right" feeling has been associated with compulsive behavior and as such the "unvoluntary" movement may be regarded as a "compulsive tic."

Complex motor tics consist of coordinated, sequenced movements resembling normal motor acts or gestures that are inappropriately intense and timed. They may be seemingly nonpurposeful, such as head shaking or trunk bending, or they may seem purposeful, such as touching, throwing, hitting, jumping, and kicking. Additional examples of complex motor tics include gesturing "the finger" and grabbing or exposing one's genitalia (copropraxia) or imitating gestures (echopraxia). Burping, vomiting, and retching have been described as part of the clinical picture of TS, but it is not clear whether this phenomenon represents a complex tic or some other behavioral manifestation of TS (10). Complex motor tics may be difficult to differentiate from compulsions, which frequently accompany tics, particularly in TS. A complex, repetitive movement may be considered a compulsion when it is preceded by, or associated with, a feeling of anxiety or panic, as well as an irresistible urge to produce the movement or sound because of fear that if it is not promptly or properly executed "something bad" will happen. However, this distinction is not always possible, particularly when the patient is unable to verbalize such feelings. Some coordinated movements resemble complex motor tics but may actually represent "pseudovoluntary" movements ("parakinesias") designed to camouflage the tics by incorporating them into seemingly purposeful acts, such as adjusting one's hair during a head jerk.

Simple phonic tics typically consist of sniffing, throat clearing, grunting, squeaking, screaming, coughing, blowing, and sucking sounds. *Complex phonic tics* include linguistically meaningful utterances and verbalizations, such as shouting of obscenities or profanities (coprolalia), repetition of someone else's words or phrases (echolalia), and repetition of one's own utterances, particularly the last syllable, word, or phrase in a sentence (palilalia). Some TS patients

also manifest sudden and transient cessation of all motor activity (blocking tics) without alteration of consciousness.

In contrast to other hyperkinetic movement disorders, tics are usually intermittent, and may be repetitive and stereotypic (Table 22.1). Tics may occur as short-term bouts or bursting, or long-term waxing and waning (11). They vary in frequency and intensity, often changing distribution. Typically tics can be volitionally suppressed, although this may require intense mental effort. Suppressibility, while typical of tics, has been well documented in other hyperkinetic movement disorders, but to lesser degree. Using functional magnetic resonance imaging (MRI), Peterson et al. (12) showed decreased neuronal activity during periods of suppression in the ventral globus pallidus, putamen, and thalamus. There was increased activity in the right caudate nucleus, right frontal cortex, and other cortical areas normally involved in the inhibition

TABLE 22.1. DIFFERENTIAL DIAGNOSIS OF TICS

Classification	Differential Diagnosis
A. *Simple motor tics*	
1. Clonic	Myoclonus
	Chorea
	Seizures
2. Dystonic	Dystonia
	Athetosis
3. Tonic	Muscle spasms and cramps
B. *Complex motor tics*	Mannerisms
Stereotypies	
Restless legs	
Seizures	

Phenomenology	
Abrupt	Myoclonus
Chorea	
Hyperreflexia	
Paroxysmal dyskinesia	
Seizures	
Sensory phenomenon	Akathisia stereotypy
(urge → relief)	Restless legs syndrome
	Dystonia
Perceived as voluntary	Akathisia
Suppressibility	All hyperkinesias but less than tics
Decrease with distraction	Akathisia
	Psychogenic movements
Increase with stress	Most hyperkinesias
Increase with relaxation (after period of stress)	Parkinsonian tremor
Multifocal, migrate	Chorea
	Myoclonus
Fluctuate spontaneously	Paroxysmal dyskinesias
	Seizures
Present during sleep	Myoclonus (segmental)
	Periodic movements
	Painful legs/moving toes
	Other hyperkinesias
	Seizures

of unwanted impulses (prefrontal, parietal, temporal, and cingulate cortices). Besides temporary suppressibility, tics are also characterized by suggestibility, exacerbation with stress, excitement, boredom, fatigue, and with an exposure to heat. Tics may also increase during relaxation after a period of stress.

In contrast to other hyperkinetic movement disorders that are usually completely suppressed during sleep, motor and phonic tics may persist during all stages of sleep (13, 14). Many patients, when they are concentrating on mental or physical tasks (such as when playing a video game or during orgasm), note a reduction in their tics. Others have increased frequency and intensity of their tics when distracted, especially when they no longer have the need to suppress the tics. Tics are also typically exacerbated by dopaminergic drugs and by CNS stimulants, including methylphenidate and cocaine (15). Finally, it should be noted that there is a broad spectrum of movements that may be present in patients with TS and these may be confused with tics, such as akathisia, chorea, dystonia, compulsive movements, and fidgeting as part of hyperactivity associated with ADHD (7,16,17).

CLINICAL FEATURES OF TOURETTE'S SYNDROME

Motor Symptoms

TS, the most common cause of tics, is manifested by a broad spectrum of motor and behavioral disturbances. This clinical heterogeneity often causes diagnostic difficulties and presents a major challenge in genetic linkage studies. To aid in the diagnosis of TS, the Tourette's Syndrome Classification Study Group (TSCSG) (18) formulated the following criteria for definite TS: (a) both multiple motor and one or more phonic tics must be present at some time during the illness, although not necessarily concurrently; (b) tics must occur many times a day, nearly every day, or intermittently throughout a period of more than a year; (c) the anatomic location, number, frequency, type, complexity, or severity of tics must change over time; (d) onset must be before age 21; (e) involuntary movements and noises cannot be explained by other medical conditions; and (f) motor and/or phonic tics must be directly witnessed by a reliable examiner at some point during the illness or be recorded by videotape or cinematography. Probable TS type 1 meets all the criteria except the second and/or fourth, and probable TS type 2 meets all the criteria except the first; it includes either single motor tic with phonic tics or multiple motor tics with possible phonic tics. In contrast to the criteria outlined by the *Diagnostic and Statistical Manual of Mental Disorders,* 4th ed. (DSM-IV) (19), the TSCSG criteria do not include a statement about "impairment." There is considerable controversy about the DSM-IV criterion requiring that "marked distress or significant impairment in

social, occupational or other important areas of functioning" be present. Therefore, patients with mild tics that do not produce impairment would not satisfy the diagnostic criteria for TS according to DSM-IV. That particular criterion will be deleted from the DSM-V edition. Kurlan (20) suggested another set of diagnostic criteria for genetic studies and introduced the term "Tourette disorder" for patients who have "functional impairment." However, this does not take into account the marked fluctuation in symptoms and severity; some patients may be relatively asymptomatic at one time and clearly functionally impaired at another time. The Tourette Syndrome Association's International Genetic Collaboration developed the Diagnostic Confidence Index (DCI), which consists of 26 "confidence factors" with weightings given to each of them and a total maximal score of 100. The most highly weighted diagnostic confidence factors include history of coprolalia, complex motor or vocal tics, a waxing and waning course, echo phenomenon, premonitory sensations, an orchestrated sequence, and age at onset. The DCI was found to be a useful instrument in assessing lifetime likelihood of developing TS (21). Several instruments, some based on ratings of videotapes, have been developed to measure and quantitate tics, but they all have some limitations (22,23).

The clinical criteria are designed to assist in accurate diagnosis, in genetic linkage studies, and in differentiating TS from other tic disorders (Table 22.2) (16). There is a body of evidence to support the notion that many, if not all, patients with other forms of idiopathic tic disorders represent one end of the spectrum in a continuum of TS. The most common and mildest of the idiopathic tic disorders is the "transient tic disorder" (TTD) of childhood. This disorder is essentially identical to TS except the symptoms last for less than a year and therefore the diagnosis can be made only in retrospect. "Chronic multiple tic disorder" (CMTD) is also similar to TS, but the patients have only motor or, less commonly, only phonic tics lasting at least a year. "Chronic single tic disorder" (CSTD) is the same as CMTD, but the patients have only single motor or phonic tic. This separation into TTD, CMTD, and CSTD seems artificial because all can occur in the same family and probably represent a variable expression of the same genetic defect.

Although the TSCSG diagnostic criteria require that onset occur before the age of 21, nearly all patients with TS have symptoms before age 12. In 36% to 48% of patients the initial symptom is eye blinking, followed by tics involving the face and head. Blink rate in persons with TS is about double that in normal, age-matched controls (24). During the course of the disorder, nearly all patients exhibit tics involving the face or head; two thirds have tics in the arms; and half have tics involving the trunk or legs. According to one study, the average age at onset of tics is 5.6 years, and the tics usually become most severe at age 10; by 18 years half of the patients are tic free (25). In a study of 58 adults

TABLE 22.2. CAUSES OF TICS

I. Primary
  A. *Sporadic*
    1. Transient motor *or* phonic tics (<1 yr)
    2. Chronic motor *or* phonic tics (>1 yr)
    3. Adult-onset (recurrent) tics
    4. Tourette's syndrome
    5. Primary dystonia
  B. *Inherited*
    1. Tourette's syndrome
    2. Huntington's disease
    3. Primary dystonia
    4. Neuroacanthocytosis
    5. Hallervorden-Spatz
    6. Tuberous sclerosis
    7. Wilson's disease
    8. Duchenne's muscular dystrophy
II. Secondary
  A. Infections: encephalitis, Creutzfeldt-Jakob disease, neurosyphilis, Sydenham's chorea
  B. Drugs: amphetamines, methylphenidate, pemoline, levodopa, cocaine, carbamazepine, phenytoin, phenobarbital, lamotrigine, antipsychotics and other dopamine receptor blocking drugs (tardive tics, tardive tourettism)
  C. Toxins: carbon monoxide
  D. Developmental: static encephalopathy, mental retardation syndromes, chromosomal abnormalities, autistic spectrum disorders (Asperger's syndrome)
  E. Chromosomal disorders: Down's syndrome, Kleinfelter's syndrome, XYY karyotype, fragile X, triple X, 9p mosaicism, partial trisomy 16, 9p monosomy, citrullinemia, Beckwith-Wiedemann syndrome
  F. Other: head trauma, stroke, neurocutaneous syndromes, schizophrenia, neurodegenerative diseases
III. Related Manifestations and Disorders
    1. Stereotypies/habits/mannerisms
    2. Self-injurious behaviors
    3. Motor restlessness
    4. Akathisia
    5. Compulsions
    6. Excessive startle
    7. Jumping Frenchman

diagnosed with TS during childhood, Goetz et al. (26) found that tics persisted in all patients but were moderate or severe in only 24%, although 60% had moderate or severe tics during the course of the disorder. Tic severity during childhood had no predictive value for the future course, but patients with mild tics during the preadult period had mild tics during adulthood. Although the vast majority of tics in adults represent recurrences of childhood-onset tics, rare patients may have their first tic occurrence during adulthood (27). In these adults with new-onset tics, it is important to search for secondary causes, such as infection, trauma, cocaine use, and neuroleptic exposure (16,27). Poor motor control, which can lead to poor penmanship and, at times, almost illegible handwriting, may contribute to the academic difficulties faced by many patients with TS. Tics, though rarely disabling, can be quite troublesome for TS patients because they cause embarrassment, interfere with social interactions, and at times can be quite painful or uncomfortable. Rarely, they can cause secondary neurologic deficits, such as compressive cervical myelopathy in patients with violent head and neck tics (28).

Vocalizations have been reported as the initial symptom in about one third of all patients, with throat clearing being the most common initial phonic tic (29). Phonic tics can be troublesome for patients and those around them, particularly when they consist of loud, shrieking sounds. In addition to involuntary noises, some patients have speech dysfluencies that resemble developmental stuttering, and up to half of all patients with developmental stuttering have been thought to have undiagnosed TS (30). Coprolalia, perhaps the most recognizable and certainly one of the most distressing symptom of TS, is actually present in only half of patients. When describing the distress caused by his severe coprolalia, one of our patients remarked that immediately after shouting an obscenity he reaches out with his hand in an attempt to "catch the word and bring it back before others can hear it." This symptom appears to be markedly influenced by cultural background. Although in one retrospective analysis of 112 children with TS only 8% exhibited coprolalia (Goldenberg et al., 1994), the true prevalence of coprolalia in TS children and adults is only about 50% in the U.S. population, even when mental coprolalia (without actual utterance) is included. Coprolalia has been reported to occur in only 26% of Danish and 4% of Japanese patients (29). Copropraxia has been found in about 20% of patients, echolalia in 30%, echopraxia in 25%, and palilalia in 15%.

Except for the presence of tics, the neurologic examination in patients with TS is usually normal. In one case-control study, TS patients were found to have a shorter duration of saccades, but the saccades were performed with a greater mean velocity than normal controls and were associated with fewer correct antisaccade responses, suggesting a mild oculomotor disturbance in TS (31). Although the ability to inhibit reflexive saccades is normal, TS patients make more timing errors, indicating an inability to appropriately inhibit or delay planned motor programs (32).

Behavioral Symptoms

In addition to motor and phonic tics, patients with TS often exhibit a variety of behavioral symptoms, particularly ADHD and OCD (Fig. 22.1). The diagnosis of ADHD and OCD is based on clinical history; there are no laboratory or other tests that reliably diagnose these neurobehavioral disorders (33,34) (Table 22.3). These comorbid behavioral conditions often interfere with learning and with academic and work performance. In contrast to tics, ADHD and obsessional symptom severity are significantly associated with impaired social and emotional adjustment

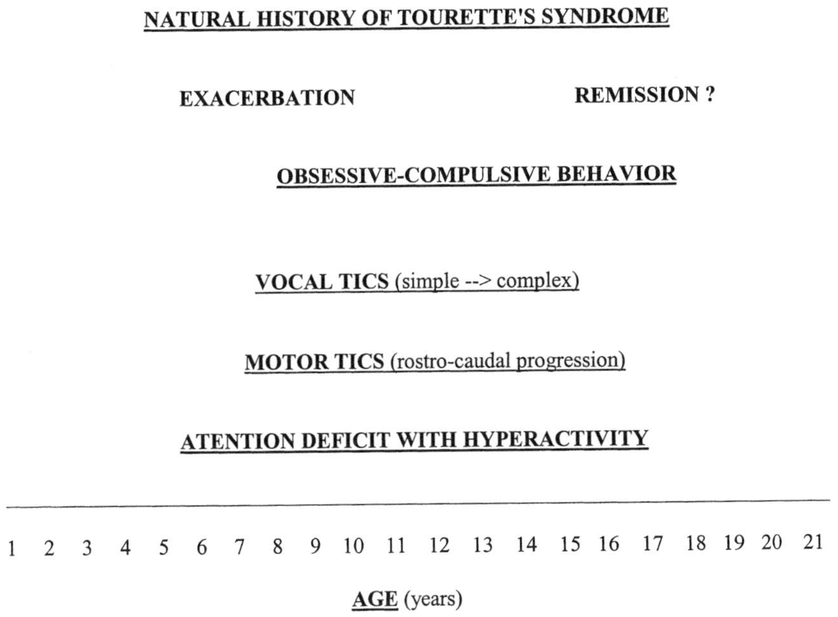

NATURAL HISTORY OF TOURETTE'S SYNDROME

EXACERBATION   REMISSION ?

OBSESSIVE-COMPULSIVE BEHAVIOR

VOCAL TICS (simple --> complex)

MOTOR TICS (rostro-caudal progression)

ATENTION DEFICIT WITH HYPERACTIVITY

1   2   3   4   5   6   7   8   9   10 11 12 13 14 15 16 17 18 19 20 21

AGE (years)

FIG. 22.1. Progression of symptoms during the course of Tourette's syndrome.

(35). The clinician should be skilled not only in the recognition and management of ADHD, but also in documenting the ADHD-related deficits (36). Such documentation is essential for parents and educators to provide the optimal educational setting for the affected individual.

Since nearly all studies on the frequency of associated features have been based on a population of TS patients referred to physicians (usually specialists), there is a selection bias; therefore, accurate figures on the prevalence of these behavioral disorders in TS patients are not available. It has been estimated that 3% to 6% of the school-aged population suffers from ADHD (34), and probably a majority of patients with TS have had symptoms of ADHD, OCD, or both sometime during the course of their illness (37). The symptoms of ADHD may be the initial manifestations of TS and may precede the onset of motor and phonic tics by about 3 years. Despite growing publicity about ADHD, there is little evidence of widespread overdiagnosis or overtreatment of this disorder (34).

There are three types of ADHD: predominantly inattentive, predominantly hyperactive-impulsive, and combined (Table 22.3) (38). Although attention deficit is certainly

TABLE 22.3. ATTENTION DEFICIT–HYPERACTIVITY DISORDER/HYPERKINETIC DISORDER (ICD-10 AND DSM-IV)

Inattention (IN)	Hyperactivity (H)	Impulsivity (IMP)
Fails to attend to details	Fidgets with hands or feet	Talks excessively
Difficulty sustaining attention	Leaves seat in classroom	Blurts out answers
Does not seem to listen	Runs about or climbs	Difficulty waiting turn
Fails to finish	Difficulty playing quietly	Interrupts or intrudes on others
Difficulty organizing tasks	Motor excess ("on the go")	
Avoids sustained effort	Talks excessively	
Loses things		
Distracted by external stimuli		
Forgetful		

ADHD Diagnostic Subtypes (DSM-IV)
Combined: six or more from the IN domain and six or more from the H/IMP domain
Inattentive: six or more from the IN domain and fewer than six from the H/IMP domain
Hyperactive/impulsive: six or more from H/IMP domain and fewer than six from the IN domain

HKD (ICD-10)
Six or more from the IN domain, three or more from the H domain, one or more from the IMP domain

ADHD, attention deficit–hyperactivity disorder; HKD, hyperkinetic disorder; ICD-10, *International Classification of Diseases*, 10th ed.; DSM-IV, *Diagnostic and Statistical Manual of Mental Disorders*, 4th ed.

one of the most common and disabling symptoms of TS, in many patients the inability to pay attention is due not only to a coexistent ADHD but also to uncontrollable intrusions of thoughts. Some patients are unable to pay attention because of a compulsive fixation of gaze. For example, while sitting in a classroom or a theater or during a conversation their gaze becomes fixed on a particular object and, despite concentrated effort, they are unable to break the fixation. As a result, they miss the teacher's lesson or a particular action in a play. Another reason for impaired attention in some TS patients is mental concentration exerted in an effort to suppress tics. Yet another cause for inattention is the sedative effect of anti-TS medications. It is, therefore, important to determine which mechanism or mechanisms are most likely responsible for the patient's attention deficit. Although genetics clearly has a key role in the mechanism of ADD and ADHD, the gene(s) or other causes have not been fully elucidated. In a genome scan of 106 families including 128 affected sibling pairs with estimated heritability of 60% to 80%, multipoint MLS values above 1 suggested the possibility of a gene locus on chromosomes 4, 9, 10, 11, 12, 16, and 17 (39). One study showed that children and adolescents with ADHD, as compared to those without ADHD, are more likely to have major injuries and asthma, and their 9-year medical costs are double (40).

Although OCD frequently occurs alone without other features of TS (41), it is now well accepted that OCD is a part of the spectrum of neurobehavioral manifestations in TS (41,42). OCD, with an estimated lifetime prevalence of 2% to 3% (43) and an incidence of 0.55 per 1,000 person-years (44), is one of the most common causes of disability. The instrument used most frequently to measure the severity of OCD is the Yale-Brown Obsessive Compulsive Scale (45). A distinction should be made between obsessive-compulsive symptoms or traits, obsessive-compulsive personality disorder, and OCD. Obsessions are characterized by intense, intrusive thoughts, such as concerns about bodily wastes and secretions; unfounded fears; need for exactness, symmetry, evenness, and/or neatness; excessive religious concerns; perverse sexual thoughts; and intrusions of words, phrases, or music. Compulsions consist of subjective urge to perform meaningless and irrational rituals, such as checking, counting, cleaning, washing, touching, smelling, hoarding, and rearranging. Leckman et al. (46) have drawn attention to the frequent occurrence of the "just right" perception in patients with OCD and TS. While obsessional slowness accounts for some of the school problems experienced by TS patients, cognitive slowing ("bradyphrenia") is also a contributing factor (47). In contrast to primary OCD in which the symptoms relate chiefly to hygiene and cleanliness, the obsessive symptoms associated with TS usually involve concerns with symmetry, violent aggressive thoughts, forced touching, fear of harming self or others, and need for saying or doing things "just right" (48). A principal-components factor analysis of 13 categories used

to group types of obsessions and compulsions in the Yale-Brown Obsessive Compulsive Scale symptom checklist identified the obsessions and checking and the symmetry and ordering factors as particularly common in patients with tic disorders (49). In addition to an idiopathic sporadic or familial disorder and TS, OCD has been reported to occur as a result of a variety of lesions in the frontal-limbic-subcortical circuits (50,51). Although both ADHD and OCD are regarded as integral findings of the syndrome, only OCD has been shown to be genetically linked to TS (52). A pathogenic link between TS and OCD is also suggested by the finding in one study that 59% of 54 patients with OCD had a lifetime history of tics and 14% fulfilled the criteria for TS during the 2- to 7-year follow-up (53).

One of the most troublesome symptoms of TS is poor impulse control manifested sometimes by inability to control anger as a result of which many patients may exhibit frequent, and sometimes violent, temper outbursts and rages. Indeed, many behavioral symptoms of TS, including some complex tics, coprolalia, copropraxia, and many behavioral problems, can be explained by loss of normal inhibitory mechanisms (disinhibition) manifested by poor impulse control. Rarely, TS patients exhibit inappropriate sexual aggressiveness, as well as antisocial, oppositional, and even violent, unlawful, or criminal behavior. Indeed, TS serves as a model medical disorder that may predispose one to engage in uncontrollable and offensive behaviors that are misunderstood by the law-abiding community and legal justice system. The social and legal aspects of TS have yet to be investigated, but there is growing concern regarding media misrepresentation that attributes violent criminal behavior in certain individuals to TS. Although TS should not be used as an "excuse" to justify unlawful or criminal behaviors, studies are needed to determine whether TS-related symptoms and neurobehavioral comorbidities predispose individuals with TS to engage in such behaviors. Often the avolitional nature of behaviors in response to involuntary internal thought and emotional patterns is supported by the subsequent remorse and lack of secondary gain. This suggests that the preponderance of unlawful acts committed by TS patients are not premeditated but may result from a variety of TS-related mechanisms, such as poor impulse control, OCD associated with addictive behavior (e.g., drugs, alcohol, gambling), ADD and distractibility (e.g., motor vehicle accidents). In one study, TS accounted for 2% of all cases referred for forensic psychiatric investigation in Stockholm, Sweden between 1990 and 1995; 15% of offenders had ADHD, 15% had PDD, and 3% had Asperger's syndrome (54).

Focal frontal lobe dysfunction, demonstrated in TS by various functional and imaging studies, has been associated with impulsive subtype of aggressive behavior (55). It has been postulated that impulse disorders stem from exaggerated reward-, pleasure-, or arousal-seeking brain centers, resulting in failure of inhibition. Animal studies of rats with lesions of the nucleus accumbens core, the brain region noted for reward and reinforcement, showed that the lesioned rats preferred small immediate rewards to larger delayed rewards (56). In addition to the ventromedial prefrontal cortices, lesions in the amygdala have also been known to cause alteration in decision making processes and a disregard for consequences (57).

One of the most distressing symptoms of TS is a self-injurious behavior, reported in up to 53% of all patients (29,58). A common form of self-injurious behavior is damage of skin by compulsive biting, scratching, cutting, engraving, hitting (particularly in the eye and throat), often accompanied by an irresistible urge (obsession) (4). Thus, self-injurious behavior appears to be related to OCD, which has treatment implications.

The *TS* gene(s) may, in addition to tics, ADHD, and OCD, be expressed in a variety of behavioral manifestations, including learning and conduct disorders, schizoid and affective disorders, antisocial behaviors, oppositional defiant disorder, anxiety, depression, conduct disorder, severe temper outbursts, rage attacks, impulse control problems, inappropriate sexual behavior, and other psychiatric problems (59). Personality disorder and depression has been reported in 64% of patients with TS (60). Besides comorbid behavioral conditions, TS has been reported to be frequently associated with migraine headaches, which may be related to the coexistent OCD (61). Tourette International Consortium Database, which at the time of publication in 2000 included information on 3,500 patients with TS collected from 64 centers from around the world, showed that only 12% of patients with TS had no other disorders; ADHD was seen in 60%, symptoms of OCD in 59%, anger control problems in 37%, sleep disorder in 25%, learning disability in 23%, mood disorder in 20%, anxiety disorder in 18%, and self-injurious behavior in 14% (62).

PATHOGENESIS

Neurophysiology

Although the pathogenic mechanisms of TS are unknown, the weight of evidence supports organic rather than psychogenic origin (63,64). Despite the observation that some tics may be, at least in part, voluntary, physiologic studies suggest that tics are not mediated through normal motor pathways utilized for willed movements. About 20% of patients with TS have exaggerated startle responses, which may fail to habituate with repetition (65). Using back-averaging techniques, Karp et al. (66) documented premotor negativity in two of five patients with simple motor tics. Although the investigators could not correlate the presence of Bereitschaftspotential with the premonitory sensation, the physiology of the premovement phenomenon requires further studies.

Functional MRI studies in patients with TS have shown decreased neuronal activity during periods of suppression in the ventral globus pallidus, putamen, and thalamus and increased activity in the right caudate nucleus, right frontal cortex, and other cortical areas normally involved in the inhibition of unwanted impulses (prefrontal, parietal, temporal, and cingulate cortices) (67). In another study utilizing functional MRI, Serrien et al. (68) showed marked reduction or absence of activity in secondary motor areas while the patients attempted to maintain a stable grip-load force control (68). The authors interpreted the findings as ongoing activation of the secondary motor areas reflecting patients' involuntary urges to move. In a study of children with ADHD, functional MRI showed increased frontal activation and reduced striatal activation on various tasks, and an enhancement of striatal function after treatment with methylphenidate (69). Transcranial magnetic stimulation (TMS) studies have demonstrated shortened cortical silent period and defective intracortical inhibition (determined in a conditioning test paired-stimulus paradigm) in patients with TS (70) and OCD (71), thus providing possible explanation for intrusive phenomena. Subsequent studies utilizing the same technique have demonstrated that patients with tic-related OCD have more abnormal motor cortex excitability than OCD patients without tics (72). TMS studies have also demonstrated that TS children have a shorter cortical silent period but their intracortical inhibition is not different from that of controls, although intracortical inhibition is reduced in children with ADHD (73). There is evidence of additive inhibitory deficits, as demonstrated by reduced intracortical inhibition and shortened cortical silent period in children with TS and comorbid ADHD.

Sleep studies have provided additional evidence that some tics are truly involuntary (13,14). Polysomnographic studies in TS patients recorded motor and phonic tics in various stages of sleep and have found that some patients with TS have alterations of arousal; decreased percentage of stage 3/4 (slow-wave) sleep; decreased percentage of rapid eye movement (REM) sleep; paroxysmal events in stage 4 sleep with sudden intense arousal, disorientation, and agitation; restless legs syndrome; periodic leg movement of sleep; and other sleep-related disorders, including sleep apnea, enuresis, sleep walking and sleep talking, nightmares, myoclonus, bruxism, and other disturbances (74–76).

Neuroimaging

Although standard anatomic neuroimaging studies in TS are unremarkable, using special volumetric, metabolic, blood flow, ligand, and functional imaging techniques, several interesting findings have been reported that have strong implications for the pathophysiology of TS (67). Careful volumetric MRI studies have suggested that the normal asymmetry of the basal ganglia is lost in TS. Frederickson et al. (77) found evidence of smaller gray matter volumes in left frontal lobes of patients with TS, further supporting the findings of loss of normal left–right asymmetry. Quantitative MRI studies have found subtle but possibly important reduction in the volume of caudate nuclei in patients with TS. In ten pairs of monozygotic twins, the right caudate was smaller in the more severely affected individuals, providing evidence for the role of "environmental events" in the pathogenesis of TS (78). In contrast, corpus callosum has been found to be larger in children with TS than in normal controls (79). Subsequent study showed that this finding was gender related and was present only in boys with TS (80).

Positron emission tomography (PET) scanning has shown variable rates of glucose utilization in basal ganglia as compared with controls. In one study, ^{18}F-fluorodeoxyglucose (FDG) PET has shown evidence of increased metabolic activity in the lateral premotor and supplementary motor association cortices and in the midbrain (pattern 1), and decreased metabolic activity in the caudate and thalamic areas (limbic basal ganglia–thalamocortical projection system) (pattern 2) (81). Pattern 1 is reportedly associated with tics, and pattern 2 correlates with the overall severity of TS. In contrast to dystonia, characterized by lentiform nucleus–thalamic metabolic dissociation, attributed to overactivity of the direct striatopallidal inhibitory pathway, the pattern of TS is characterized by concomitant metabolic reduction in striatal and thalamic function. The authors suggested that this pattern could be explained by a reduction in the indirect pathway resulting in reduction in subthalamic nucleus activity. Using event-related $[^{15}O]H_2O$ PET combined with time-synchronized audio- and videotaping in six patients with TS, Stern et al. (82) found increased activity in the sensorimotor, language, executive, paralimbic, and frontal-subcortical areas that were temporarily related to the motor and phonic tics and the irresistible urge that precedes these behaviors. Rauch et al. (83) showed bilateral medial temporal (hippocampal/parahippocampal) activation on PET in patients with OCD, as compared with normal controls, and absence of activation of inferior striatum, seen in normal controls. Various neuroimaging studies have also demonstrated moderate reduction in the size of the corpus callosum, basal ganglia (particularly caudate and globus pallidus), and frontal lobes (84), and striatal hypoperfusion (69) in patients with ADHD.

Neurochemistry

Neurochemical studies of TS have been hampered by the unavailability of postmortem brain tissue. Biochemical abnormalities in the few postmortem brains that have been studied include low serotonin, low glutamate in the internal globus pallidus, and low cyclic adenosine monophos-

phate (cAMP) in the cortex (85). An alteration in the central neurotransmitters in TS has been also suggested chiefly because of relatively consistent responses to modulation of the dopaminergic system. Dopamine antagonists and depletors generally have an ameliorating effect on tics, whereas drugs that enhance central dopaminergic activity exacerbate tics. Low cerebrospinal fluid homovanillic acid, coupled with a favorable response to dopamine receptor–blocking drugs, has been interpreted as evidence in support of the notion that tics and TS are due to supersensitive dopamine receptors; however, postmortem binding studies of dopamine receptors have failed to provide support for this hypothesis (85).

Functional neuroimaging studies have been used to aid in the understanding of neurotransmitter and receptor alterations in TS. Using $[^{123}I]\beta$-carboxymethoxy-3-β-(4-iodophenyl)tropane (CIT) single photon emission computed tomography (SPECT), Malison et al. (86) demonstrated a mean of 37% increase in binding of this dopamine transporter ligand in the striatum in five adult patients with TS, as compared with age-matched controls. In contrast, Heinz et al. (87) found no difference in $[^{123}I]\beta$-CIT binding in the midbrain, thalamus or basal ganglia between 10 TS patients and normal control subjects. There was, however, a significant negative correlation between the severity of phonic tics and β-CIT binding in the midbrain and thalamus. In another study involving 12 adult TS patients, β-CIT scans showed evidence of increased dopamine transporter binding (88). Combining SPECT and MRI, Wolf et al. (89) found 17% greater binding of IBZM, a D2 receptor ligand, in the caudate (but not putamen) nucleus in five of the more affected monozygotic twins discordant for TS. It is important to note that two of the five subjects were taking neuroleptics for up to 6 weeks prior to the SPECT studies. Nevertheless, these findings, if confirmed by other studies of neuroleptic-naive patients, support the notion that the presynaptic dopamine function is enhanced in TS. This may, in turn, lead to a reduced inhibitory pallidal output to the mediodorsal thalamus. However, the observation that in patients with Parkinson's disease the severity of childhood-onset tics was not influenced by the development of parkinsonism or by its treatment with levodopa argues against the role of dopamine in the pathogenesis of TS symptoms (90). This is supported by the results of PET ligand studies showing normal D2 receptor density (91). Furthermore, Meyer et al. (92) used PET imaging of (+)-α-$[^{11}C]$dihydrotetrabenazine to determine the density of vesicular monoamine transporter type 2 (VMAT2), a cytoplasm-to-vesicle transporter linearly related to monoaminergic nerve terminal density unaffected by medications, in 8 TS patients and 22 controls. This study showed no significant difference in terminal density between patients and controls, thus failing to provide support for the concept of increased striatal innervation. However, these studies do not exclude the possibility of abnormal regulation of dopamine release and uptake.

In a small sample of TS patients, PET studies have demonstrated a 25% increase in accumulations of fluorodopa in the left caudate ($p = 0.03$) and a 53% increase in right midbrain ($p = 0.08$) (93). These findings indicate possible dopaminergic dysfunction in the cells of origin and in the dopaminergic terminals, suggesting increased activity of dopa decarboxylase.

Despite some limitations and inconsistencies, the imaging, ligand, and biochemical studies provide support for the hypothesis that the corticostriatothalamocortical circuit has an important role in the pathogenesis of TS and related disorders (1,67). The dorsolateral prefrontal circuit, which links Brodmann's areas 9 and 10 to the dorsolateral head of the caudate, appears to be involved with "executive functions" (manipulation of previously learned knowledge, abstract reasoning, organization, verbal fluency, and problem solving; it is closely related to intelligence, education, and social exposure) and "motor planning." An abnormality in this circuit has been implicated in ADHD. The lateral orbitofrontal circuit originates in the inferior lateral prefrontal cortex (area 10) and projects to the ventral medial caudate. An abnormality to this circuit is associated with personality changes, mania, disinhibition, and irritability. Lastly, the anterior cingulate circuit arises in the cingulate gyrus (area 24) and projects to the ventral striatum, which also receives input from the amygdala, hippocampus, medial orbitofrontal cortex, entorhinal and perirhinal cortices. A variety of behavioral problems, including OCD, may be linked to an abnormality in this circuit.

Reduced metabolism or blood flow to the basal ganglia, particularly in the ventral striatum, most often in the left hemisphere, has been demonstrated in a majority of studies involving TS subjects. These limbic areas are thought to be involved in impulse control, reward contingencies, and executive functions, and these behavioral functions appear to be abnormal in most patients with TS. Future imaging and ligand studies should include children, a population that has been largely excluded because of ethical considerations. The studies should also rigorously characterize comorbid disorders and take into consideration potential confounding variables, such as the secondary effects of chronic illness, medications, and so forth.

IMMUNOLOGY

The potential role of immunologic mechanisms and specifically antineuronal antibodies is currently being explored in a variety of neurologic disorders, including TS (94,95). Several studies have suggested that exacerbations of TS symptoms correlated with an antecedent group A β-hemolytic *Streptococcus* (GABHS) infection (demonstrated by elevated antistreptococcal titers) and the presence of serum antineuronal antibodies. Epitopes of streptococcal M proteins have

been found to cross-react with human brain, particularly the basal ganglia, and may be pathogenetically important in various neurologic disorders, such as Sydenham's chorea, TS-like syndrome, dystonia, and parkinsonism (96). Development of dyskinesias (paw and floor licking, head and paw shaking) and phonic utterances has been reported in rodents after the microinfusion of dilute IgG from TS subjects into their striatum, and intrastriatal microinfusion of TS sera or gamma immunoglobulins (IgG) in rats produced stereotypies and episodic utterances, analogous to involuntary movements seen in TS (95). In ten patients with poststreptococcal acute disseminated encephalomyelitis (PSA-DEM) following exposure to GABHS, Dale et al. (96) showed antibasal ganglia antibodies in all with three—60, 67, and 80 kd—dominant bands. Furthermore, MRI showed hyperintense basal ganglia in 80% of the patients. The B lymphocyte antigen D8/17 is considered to be a marker for rheumatic fever but is also frequently overexpressed in patients with tics, OCD, and autism (97). In one study, children and adults with TS had significantly higher serum levels of antineuronal antibodies against putamen, but not caudate or globus pallidus, in comparison with controls (98). However, the potential relevance of this finding has been questioned because there is no relationship between the presence of antineuronal antibodies and age at onset, severity of tics, or presence of comorbid disorders. Trifiletti and Packard (99) have confirmed the presence of a specific brain protein with a molecular weight of 83 kd that is recognized by antibodies in the serum of 80% to 90% of patients with TS or OCD (99). They concluded that there might be a subset of patients with TS and OCD, perhaps up to 10% of all cases, in whom a streptococcal infection triggers the onset of symptoms. In a large case-control study of 150 patients with tics and 150 controls, Cardona and Orefici (100) found a correlation between the occurrence of tics and prior exposure to streptococcal antigens and also found that the severity of tic disorder correlates with the magnitude of the serologic response to streptococcal antigens measured by ASO titers (38% of children with tics compared with 2% of control subjects had ASO titers ≥500 IU ($p < 0.001$). In another study involving 25 adult patients with TS and 25 healthy controls, increased antibody titers against streptococcal M12 and M19 proteins were found in the TS group as compared with healthy controls (101).

Variably referred to as pediatric autoimmune neuropsychiatric disorders associated with strep infections (PANDAS) or pediatric infection-triggered autoimmune neuropsychiatric disorders (PITANDS), this area is one of the most controversial topics in the pediatric neurologic and psychiatric literature (99,102). Nevertheless, the concept of "postinfectious" OCD is gradually seeping into the literature, even though definite proof is still lacking (103). Untreated GABHS infection is often complicated by rheumatic fever, within 10 to 14 weeks, and by Sydenham's chorea, within several months. Several studies have provided evidence for an overlap between TS and Sydenham's chorea with tics and OCD being manifested in both disorders. It is, therefore, not clear whether TS and OCD are independent sequelae of GABHS or whether the observed symptoms of TS and OCD are manifestations of Sydenham's chorea. Although this intriguing hypothesis requires further study, plasmapheresis (PEX), intravenous IgG, and immunosuppressant therapies are currently being investigated in the management of TS. In a study of 30 children in whom OCD or tics were presumably triggered or exacerbated by GABHS, there were striking improvements in various measures of OCD after intravenous immunoglobulin (IVIG) and in tics after plasma exchange (104). Twenty-nine children with PANDAS were randomized in a partially double-blind fashion (no sham PEX) to an IVIG, IVIG placebo (saline), PEX group. One month after treatment, the severity of obsessive-compulsive symptoms were improved by 58% and 45% in the PEX and IVIG groups, respectively, compared with only 3% in the IVIG control. In contrast, tic scores were only improved after PEX treatment; reductions of 49% (PEX), 19% (IVIG), and 12% (IVIG placebo) were noted. Improvements in both tics and obsessive-compulsive symptoms were sustained for 1 year. However, there was no control PEX group, and the control comparisons were limited to the 1-month visit. Furthermore, there was no relationship between rate of antibody removal and therapeutic response. Until the results of this study are confirmed these treatment modalities are not justified in patients with TS. Furthermore, because of uncertainties about the possible cause-and-effect relationship between GABHS and tics and OCD, an antibiotic treatment for acute exacerbations of these symptoms is currently considered unwarranted (102).

GENETICS

Finding a genetic marker, and ultimately the responsible gene, has been the highest priority in TS research during the past decade. Unfortunately, despite a concentrated effort by many investigators, the *TS* gene has thus far eluded this intensive search. A systematic genome scan using 76 affected sib-pair families with a total of 110 sib-pairs showed two regions, 4q and 8p, with a lod score of 2.38 and 2.09, respectively; four additional regions, on chromosomes 1, 10, 13, and 19, had a lod score greater than 1.0 (105). McMahon et al. (106) examined 175 members of a large, four-generation, TS family as well as 16 spouses who married into this family. Interestingly, they found evidence of TS in 36% of the family members and in 31% of the married-in spouses (some form of tic was found in 67% and 44%, respectively). Multivariate analysis showed that tics were more severe in the offspring of both parents with tics. This study raises the possibility of assortative mating (like marry like) in TS in contrast to random, nonassortative

mating presumed in the general population. Thus bilineal transmission may lead to frequent homozygosity and high density of TS in some families. Using rigorous diagnostic criteria, we found that 25% of our TS patients had both parents with some features of TS: tics, 8%; OCB, 4%; and ADD, 12% (107). We compared our TS patients with a control population of 1,142 students, observed in second-, fifth-, and eighth-grade classrooms. In contrast to 5% frequency of ADD in one parent of controls, the occurrence of tics in at least one parent of TS cases was 31%, ADD 45%, and OCB 41%. Among all parents of TS cases, tics were present in 24%, OCB in 25%, and ADD in 34%, whereas only 3% of parents of controls exhibited ADD. Bilineal transmission violates the standard principle of one-trait-one-locus and may explain why a gene marker has not yet been identified in TS despite intense collaborative research effort. Our results are similar to those of Lichter et al. (108) who found bilineal transmission in 6% of patients; tics or OCB represented bilineally in 22%. In a large family study and segregation analysis, Walkup et al. (109) provided evidence for a mixed model of inheritance rather than a simple autosomal model of inheritance. This complex model of inheritance suggests that the majority of TS patients have two copies of the gene, one from each parent. This is consistent with the observation that many TS patients have both parents affected.

Twin studies, showing 89% concordance for TS and 100% concordance for either TS or CMTD, provide strong support for the genetic etiology of TS (85). How much influence environmental factors have on the phenotypic expression of this disorder is not known. Leckman et al. (110) in a search for nongenetic factors in the pathogenesis of TS found that maternal life stress, nausea, and vomiting during the first trimester of pregnancy were some of the perinatal factors that influenced the expression of the *TS* gene. In a study of 16 pairs of monozygotic twins, 94% of whom were concordant for tics, low birth weight was a strong predictor of tic severity, supporting a relationship between birth weight and phenotypic expression of *TS* (111).

EPIDEMIOLOGY

Discovery of a disease-specific marker will be helpful not only in improving our understanding of this complex neurobehavioral disorder but also in clarifying the epidemiology of TS (112). The prevalence rates have varied markedly and have been estimated to be as high as 4.2% when all types of tic disorders are included (113). There are many reasons for this wide variation, the most important of which are different ascertainment methods, different study populations, and different clinical criteria. Since about one third of patients with tics do not recognize their presence, it is difficult to derive more accurate prevalence figures for TS without a well-designed door-to-door survey. Our own observational study involved 1,142 children in second, fifth, and eighth grades of general school population, among whom 8 (0.7%) had some evidence of TS (107). In another school-based study involving 167 randomly selected 13- and 14-year-olds in U.K. high schools, the prevalence of TS based on DSMIII-R was estimated at 3%, but 18% screened positive for tics (114). Kurlan et al. (115) found that 27% of 341 special-education students had tics, compared with 19.7% of 1,255 students in regular classroom programs; the incidence of TS was 7% and 3.8%, respectively.

HYPOTHESIS

A unifying hypothesis for the pathogenesis suggests that TS represents a developmental disorder resulting in dopaminergic hyperinnervation of the ventral striatum and the associated limbic system. Although highly speculative, it is possible that the genetic defect in TS somehow interferes with normal apoptosis during development, resulting in the increased innervation of the ventral striatum and other limbic areas (116). This implies that the genetic defect somehow interferes with the programmed cell suicide needed to control cell proliferation in normal development and growth. The link between the basal ganglia and the limbic system may explain the frequent association of tics and complex behavioral problems, and a dysfunction in the CSTC circuitry seems to provide the best explanation for the most fundamental behavioral disturbance in TS, namely, loss of impulse control and a state of apparent "disinhibition." There are currently no animal models of TS, except for some families of horses with "equine self-mutilation syndrome" with features resembling human TS (117). However, future genetic studies should provide insights into the pathogenesis of this complex neurobehavioral disorder and lead to animal models on which this and other hypotheses can be tested.

TREATMENT

The first step in the management of patients with TS is proper education of the patients, relatives, teachers, and other individuals who frequently interact with the patient regarding the nature of the disorder. School principals, teachers, and students can be helpful in implementing the therapeutic strategies. In addition, the parents and the physician should work as partners in advocating the best possible school environment for the child. This may include extra break periods and a refuge area to "allow" release of tics, waiving time limitations on tests or adjusting timing of tests to the morning, and other measures designed to relieve stress. National and local support groups, particularly the

Tourette Syndrome Association, can provide additional information and can serve as a valuable resource for the patient and his or her family (Appendix). Counseling and behavioral modification may be sufficient for those with mild symptoms. However, medications may be considered when symptoms begin to interfere with peer relationships, social interactions, academic or job performance, or activities of daily living. Because of the broad range of neurologic and behavioral manifestations and the varying severity of TS, treatment must be individualized and tailored specifically to the needs of the patient (Tables 22.4 and 22.5) (118,119,120).

Before discussing pharmacologic therapy of TS symptoms it is appropriate to make a few remarks about behavioral therapy (121). Different forms of behavioral modification have been recommended since the disorder was first described, but until recently, very few studies of behavioral

TABLE 22.4. PHARMACOLOGY OF TOURETTE'S SYNDROME

Drugs	Initial Dosage (mg/d)	Clinical Effect
Dopamine receptor blockers		*Tics*
1. Fluphenazine	1	+++
2. Pimozide	2	+++
3. Haloperidol	0.5	+++
4. Risperidone	0.5	++
5. Ziprasidone	20	++
6. Thiothixene	1	++
7. Trifluoperazine	1	++
8. Molindone	5	++
Dopamine depleters		*Tics*
1. Tetrabenazine	25	++
CNS stimulants		*ADHD*
1. Methylphenidate	5	+++
2. Concerta	18	+++
3. Metadate CD	20	+++
4. Metadate ER	20	+++
5. Ritalin SR	20	+++
6. Adderall	10	+++
7. Pemoline	18.75	++
8. Dextroamphetamine	5	++
9. Dexedrine spansules	20	++
		Impulse control
Noradrenergic drugs		*ADHD*
1. Clonidine	0.1	++
2. Guanfacine	1.0	++
Serotonergic drugs		*OCD*
1. Fluoxetine	20	+++
2. Clomipramine	25	+++
3. Sertraline	50	+++
4. Paroxetine	20	+++
5. Fluvoxamine	50	+++
6. Venlafaxine	25	+++

+, minimal improvement; ++, moderate improvement; +++, marked improvement.
ADHD, attention deficit–hyperactivity disorder; OCD, obsessive-compulsive disorder.

TABLE 22.5. TREATMENT STRATEGIES IN TOURETTE'S SYNDROME

TICS	OCD	ADD/ADHD
Fluphenazine	Imipramine	Clonidine
Pimozide	Clomipramine	Imipramine
Haloperidol	Fluoxetine	Nortriptyline
Thiothixene	Sertraline	Desipramine
Trifluoperazine	Nefazodone	Deprenyl
Molindone	Fluvoxamine	Bupropion
Sulpiride	Paroxetine	Guanfacine
Tiapride	Venlafaxine	Carbamazepine
Flunarizine	Citalopram	Methylphenidate
Dextroamphetamine	Lithium	Adderal
Olanzapine	Buspirone	Pemoline
Risperidone	Clonazepam	Modafinil
Quetiapine	Trazodone	Atomoxetine
Clozapine	Clonazepam	Mecamylamine
Tetrabenazine		Neurosurgery
Pergolide		
Nicotine		
Naltrexone		
Flutamide		
Cannabinoid		
Botulinum toxin		

OCD, obsessive-compulsive disorder; ADD, attention deficit disorder; ADHD, attention deficit–hyperactivity disorder.

treatments had been subjected to rigorous scientific scrutiny. Most of the reported studies suffer from poor or unreliable assessments, small sample size, short follow-up, lack of controls, no validation of compliance, and other methodologic flaws. Given these limitations, the following behavioral techniques have been reported to provide at least some benefit: (a) massed (negative) practice (voluntary and effortful repetition of the tic leads to a buildup of a state termed "reactive inhibition" at which point the subject is forced to rest and not perform the tic due to an accumulation of "negative habit"; (b) operant techniques/contingency management (tic-free intervals are positively reinforced, and tic behaviors are punished); (c) anxiety management techniques (relaxation training); (d) exposure-based treatment (desensitization to address tic triggering phenomena, such as premonitory sensory urges); (e) awareness training (direct visual feedback, self-monitoring, and awareness enhancement techniques, such as saying the letter "T" after each tic); and (f) habit reversal training, consisting of reenactment of tic movements while looking in a mirror, training to detect and increase awareness of one's tics, identification of high-risk situations, training to isometrically contract the tic-opposing muscles, and recognition of and resistance to tic urges (121). It is not clear whether patients without preominory urges would benefit from this form of therapy. There is also some concern whether the mental effort required to fully comply with habit reversal training could actually interfere with the patient's attention and learning. Given the demands on

time and effort by the patient, the therapist, and parents, it is not surprising that even if effective, the benefits of habit reversal training are usually only temporary. However, the above-described therapies may be useful ancillary techniques in patients whose response to other therapies, including pharmacotherapy, is not entirely satisfactory.

Management of Tics

The goal of treatment should not be to completely eliminate all tics but to achieve a tolerable suppression. Because of the variability of tics in terms of severity, frequency, and distribution, the assessment of efficacy of a therapeutic intervention on tics is often quite problematic. A number of tic rating scales have been utilized, but none of them are ideal. Although at-home videotapes can be used to capture tics that are not appreciated by patients or when patients are examined in the clinic, video-based tic rating scales have many shortcomings (22).

Despite these limitations, controlled and open trials have found that of the pharmacologic agents used for tic suppression, the dopamine receptor–blocking drugs (neuroleptics) are clearly most effective (59,120) (Tables 22.4 and 22.5). Haloperidol (Haldol) and pimozide (Orap) are the only neuroleptics actually approved by the U.S. Food and Drug Administration for the management of TS. In one randomized, double-blind, controlled study pimozide was found to be superior to haloperidol with respect to efficacy and side effects (122). We prefer fluphenazine (Prolixin) as the first-line anti-tic pharmacotherapy because it appears to have a lower incidence of sedation and other side effects. If fluphenazine fails to adequately control tics, we substitute risperidone (Risperdal) or pimozide. We usually start with fluphenazine, risperidone, and pimozide at 1 mg at bedtime and increase by 1 mg every 5 to 7 days. If these drugs fail to adequately control tics, then we try haloperidol, thioridazine (Mellaril), trifluoperazine (Stelazine), molindone (Moban), or thiothixene (Navane). Risperidone, a neuroleptic with both dopamine and serotonin blocking properties, has been shown to be effective in reducing tic frequency and intensity in most (123) but not all studies (124). It is not clear whether the atypical neuroleptics, such as clozapine (Clozaril), olanzapine (Zyprexa), or quetiapine (Seroquel), will be effective in the management of tics and other manifestations of TS. Quetiapine, a dibenzothiazepine that blocks not only D1 and D2 receptors but also $5\text{-}HT_{1A}$ and $5\text{-}HT_2$ receptors, has been reported to provide beneficial effects in some patients with TS, but the clinical improvement may not be sustained. Ziprasidone (Geodon), the most recently studied atypical neuroleptic, a potent blocker of both D2 and D3 as well as $5\text{-}HT_{2A}$, $5\text{-}HT_{2C}$, $5\text{-}HT_{1A}$, $5\text{-}HT_{1D}$, and α_1 receptors, was found to decrease tic severity by 35% as compared with 7% change in the placebo group (125). Similar to pimozide, ziprasidone may prolong the QT interval but has an advantage over other atypical neuroleptics in that it is less likely to cause weight gain. The clinical significance of prolonged QT interval is controversial, but it may be associated with "torsades de pointes," which can potentially degenerate into ventricular fibrillation and sudden death. Besides pimozide and ziprasidone, other drugs that can prolong QT interval include haloperidol, risperidone, thioridazine, and desipramine. Tetrabenazine, a monoamine-depleting and dopamine receptor–blocking drug, is a powerful anti-tic drug, but regrettably, it is not readily available in the United States (126). This drug has been found very effective in the management of TS and has an advantage over conventional neuroleptics in that it does not cause tardive dyskinesias. Drugs used in the management of tics include sulpiride, tiapride, metoclopramide, piquindone, and others (120).

The side effects associated with neuroleptics, such as sedation, depression, weight gain, and school phobia, seem to be somewhat less common with fluphenazine than with haloperidol and the other neuroleptics (123). The most feared side effects of chronic neuroleptic therapy include tardive dyskinesia and hepatotoxicity. In addition, pimozide may prolong the QT interval, and therefore patients treated with the drug must undergo an electrocardiographic examination before starting therapy. We repeat the electrocardiographic examination about 3 months later and annually thereafter. It is important to note that certain antibiotics, such as clarithromycin, can raise the blood levels of pimozide and indirectly contribute to the drug's cardiotoxicity. Tardive dyskinesia, usually manifested by stereotypic involuntary movements, is only rarely persistent in children. However, tardive dystonia, a variant of tardive dyskinesias most frequently encountered in young adults, may persist and occasionally progresses to a generalized and disabling dystonic disorder. Other movement disorders associated with neuroleptics include bradykinesia, akathisia, and acute dystonic reactions (127). Therefore, careful monitoring of patients is absolutely essential and, whenever possible, the dosage should be reduced or even discontinued during periods of remission or during vacations.

Several nonneuroleptic treatments have been reported to be effective in the treatment of tics. In one study, 24 patients with TS (ages 7 to 17), who were medication free for 4 weeks prior to treatment, were randomized to receive either placebo or pergolide (150 to 300 µg daily) for 6 weeks, followed by a 2-week washout, and then crossed over to the other treatment arm (128). Although the authors conclude that "pergolide appears to be a safe and efficacious treatment for TS in children," this result may seem paradoxical in view of the well known beneficial effects of dopamine receptor blockers. However, it is possible that the observed effects of dopamine agonists could be mediated by their action on dopamine D2 autoreceptors, thus reducing endogenous dopamine turnover.

Clonazepam is another drug that is sometimes useful in patients with TS, particularly in the management of clonic

tics. Since some of the premonitory sensations resemble obsessions and the tics may be viewed as "compulsive" movements, anti-OCD medications may also be helpful. Management of the premonitory sensations may lead to improvement of these tics. Since sex steroids affect the expression of *TS* gene and modulate multiple neurotransmitter systems, antiandrogens have been tried in the treatment of patients with TS. Flutamide, an acetanilide nonsteroidal androgen antagonist, has been found in one double-blind, placebo-controlled study to modestly and transiently reduce motor, but not phonic, tics with a mild improvement in associated symptoms of OCD (129). Because of potentially serious side effects, such as diarrhea and fulminant hepatic necrosis, this drug should be reserved for those patients in whom tics remain a disabling problem despite optimal anti-tic therapy. Ondansetron, a selective 5-HT$_3$ antagonist at 8 to 16 mg/day for 3 weeks, has been associated with a decrease in severity of tics (130). Baclofen, GABA$_B$ autoreceptor agonist, has been found to markedly decrease the severity of motor and phonic tics in 95% of 264 patients with TS (131); however, a double-blind, placebo-controlled, crossover trial of nine patients with TS showed that the beneficial response to baclofen was due to improvement in overall impairment score rather than a reduction of tic activity (132). Donepezil, a noncompetitive inhibitor of acetylcholinesterase, has been reported anecdotally to suppress tics (133).

Ever since the discovery that cannabinoids markedly potentiate neuroleptic-induced hypokinesis in rats and that their effects on the extrapyramidal motor system may be mediated through a nicotinic cholinergic receptors, there has been growing interest in nicotine as a treatment for various movement disorders, including TS (134,135). Mecamylamine (Inversine), an antihypertensive agent with central antinicotinic properties, was initially shown to improve tics as well as behavioral problems in 11 of 13 patients with TS at doses up to 5 mg/day (134). However, a subsequent double-blind, placebo-controlled study failed to demonstrate a significant benefit on the symptoms associated with TS (136). Finally, there have been several anecdotal reports of marijuana helping various symptoms of TS. This is consistent with the finding that cannabinoid receptors are densely located in the output nuclei of the basal ganglia and that activation of these receptors increases GABAergic transmission and inhibition of glutamate release (137). Some patients clearly benefit when taking the cannabinoid analog dronabinol (Marinol) at a dosage of 2.5 to 10 mg twice a day.

Motor tics may be successfully managed with botulinum toxin (BTX) injections in the affected muscles. Such focal chemodenervation ameliorates not only the involuntary movements but also the premonitory sensory component. We initially treated ten TS patients with BTX injections into the involved muscles, and all experienced moderate to marked improvement in the intensity and frequency of their tics (138). Subsequent experience with a large number of patients has confirmed the beneficial effects of BTX injections in the management of motor and phonic tics, including severe coprolalia (139,140). Furthermore, those patients in whom premonitory sensations preceded the onset of tics noted lessening of these sensory symptoms. The benefits last on the average 3 to 4 months, and there are usually no serious complications. In a study of 35 patients treated for troublesome or disabling tics in 115 sessions, the mean peak effect response was 2.8 (range 0 to 4) (140). The mean duration of benefit was 14.4 weeks (up to 45). Latency to onset of benefit was 3.8 days (up to 10). Mean duration of tics prior to initial injections was 15.3 years (range 1 to 62) and mean duration of follow-up was 21.2 months (range 1.5 to 84). Twenty-one of 25 (84%) patients with notable premonitory sensory symptoms derived marked relief of these symptoms from BTX (mean benefit: 70.6%). Patients reported an overall global response of 62.7%. We concluded that BTX is effective and well tolerated in the management of tics. An additional and consistent finding was the relief of disturbing premonitory sensations. In a placebo-controlled study of 18 patients with simple motor tics, Marras et al. (141) found a 39% reduction in the number of tics per minute within 2 weeks after injection with BTX, as compared with a 6% increase in the placebo group. In addition, there was a significant reduction in "urge scores" with BTX compared with an increase in the placebo group. However, this preliminary study lacked the power to show significant differences in other measured variables, such as severity score, tic suppression, pain, and patient global impression. Furthermore, the full effect of BTX may not have been appreciated at only 2 weeks; a single treatment protocol does not reflect the clinical practice of evaluating patients after several adjustments in dose and site of injection; and the patients complaints were relatively mild since they "did not rate themselves as significantly compromised by their treated tics" at baseline (142). A larger sample and longer follow-up will be needed to further evaluate the efficacy of BTX in the management of tics and to demonstrate that this treatment offers clinically meaningful benefit.

Surgical treatment of TS is controversial, and the overall experience of stereotactic surgery in the management of tics has been somewhat disappointing. Experience with 17 patients, median age 23 years (range 11 to 40), treated between 1970 and 1998 was reviewed by Babel et al. (143). Unilateral zona incerta and VL/LM lesioning was used, and occasionally second surgery on the contralateral side was performed. The authors concluded that the procuder(s) "sufficiently" reduced both motor and phonic tics. Transient complications were reported in 68% of patients, and only one patient suffered permanent complications. Although stereotactic surgery has not been found generally useful in the management of tics (see discussion of surgical treatment of OCD), a preliminary report of a 42-year-old

man with severe motor and phonic tics controlled by high-frequency deep brain stimulation of thalamus is quite encouraging (144). Although this initial observation must be confirmed by a controlled trial before it can be recommended even to severely affected patients, it suggests that stimulation of the nucleus oralis internus may inhibit the overactivity of the nucleus and its associated frontal cortex, thus reducing motor and phonic tics.

Management of Behavioral Symptoms

Attention Deficit-hyperactivity Disorder

Behavioral modification, school and classroom adjustments, and other approaches described above may be useful in selected patients for the management of behavioral problems associated with TS. However, pharmacologic therapy is required when the symptoms of ADHD impair interpersonal relationships and interfere with academic or occupational performance (145). The NIMH Collaborative Multimodal Treatment Study of Children with ADHD found medication superior to behavioral treatment (146).

Central nervous system (CNS) stimulants, such as methylphenidate (Ritalin), controlled-release methylphenidate (Concerta), controlled-delivery methylphenidate (Metadate CD), dexmethylphenidate (Focalin), *d*-amphetamine (Dexedrine), a mixture of amphetamine salts with a 75:25 ratio of *d*- and *l*-amphetamine (Adderall), and pemoline (Cylert), are clearly the most effective agents in the management of ADHD. The initial dose for methylphenidate is 5 mg in the morning, and the dose can be gradually advanced up to 20 to 60 mg/day (0.3 to 0.7 mg/kg per dose). Methylphenidate has been found useful not only in the management of attention deficit but also as a short-term therapy for conduct disorders (147). *d*-Amphetamine doses are usually one half of those of methylphenidate. Pemoline should be given as a single morning dose that is approximately six times the daily dose of methylphenidate. These drugs usually have a rapid onset of action but also have a relatively short half-life. The long-acting preparations, such as Ritalin SR (20 mg), are less reliable and less effective than two doses of standard preparation. Dexedrine Spansule has the advantage of greater range of available doses (5, 10, 15 mg). Some studies (148,149) suggest that *l*-amphetamine is better tolerated, produces less anorexia and sedation, and may be longer lasting than methylphenidate and can be administered as a one-time (morning) dose. Only future studies will determine the utility of the new formulation of methylphenidate using a novel controlled-release delivery system designed for once-daily oral dosing (Concerta: 18 to 36 mg methylphenidate; Metadate CD: 20 mg methylphenidate). Metadace CD is formulated to release 6 mg of methylphenidate from immediate-release (IR) and 14 mg from extended-release (ER) beads. Tolerance, while rare, is more likely to occur with the long-acting formulations, but this has not been demonstrated in patients with ADHD. In addition to the possible development of tolerance, potential side effects of these stimulant drugs include nervousness, irritability, insomnia, anorexia, abdominal pain, and headaches. In one study, *d*-amphetamine was found to cause more insomnia and negative emotional symptoms than methylphenidate (150). Pemoline can rarely produce chemical hepatitis and even fulminant liver failure. Liver enzymes should be assessed before administration, but because the onset of hepatitis is unpredictable, routine laboratory studies are not useful. The parents should be instructed to notify the physician if nausea, vomiting, lethargy, malaise, or jaundice appears. Although growth retardation has been suggested by some studies, this effect, if present at all, is minimal and probably clinically insignificant.

CNS stimulants may exacerbate or precipitate tics in up to 25% of patients. However, if the symptoms of ADHD are troublesome and interfere with a patient's functioning, it is reasonable to use these CNS stimulants and titrate the dosage to the lowest effective level (Tables 22.4 and 22.5). More recent studies suggest that while CNS stimulants may exacerbate tics when are introduced into the anti-TS treatment regimen, with continued use these drugs can be well tolerated without tic exacerbation (151–154). The dopamine receptor–blocking drugs can be combined with the CNS stimulants if the latter produce unacceptable exacerbation of tics. If one stimulant is ineffective or poorly tolerated, another stimulant should be tried.

While initially thought to work by raising brain levels of dopamine, more recent studies have suggested that methylphenidate's beneficial effects on ADHD are mediated via the serotonin system (155). A strain of mice with inactivated gene for dopamine transporter (DAT) has been described to exhibit behavioral symptoms similar to those in children with ADHD. Their hyperactivity was markedly ameliorated by methylphenidate, and this improvement correlated with an increase in brain serotonin. Other investigators have provided evidence that ADHD is a "noradrenergic disorder" (156). Although it has been suggested that long-term use of CNS stimulants may lead to substance abuse, some studies have demonstrated that untreated ADHD is a significant risk factor for substance abuse and that management of ADHD with CNS stimulants significantly reduces the risk for substance use disorder (157).

The α_2 agonists and tricyclic antidepressants are also useful in the management of ADHD, particularly if CNS stimulants are not well tolerated or are contraindicated. Clonidine (Catapres), a presynaptic α_2-adrenergic agonist used as an antihypertensive because it decreases plasma norepinephrine, improves symptoms of ADHD and impulse control. Although a multicenter controlled clinical trial showed that clonidine is an effective anti-tic drug (154), our experience has suggested that the perceived benefit may be due not to a specific anti-tic efficacy but rather to a nonspecific anxiolytic effect or its beneficial effect on comorbid disorders (see below). The usual starting dose is 0.1 mg at bedtime, and the dosage is gradually increased up to 0.5 mg/day in three divided doses. The drug is also available as a transdermal patch (Catapres TTS-1, TTS-2, TTS-3, corresponding to 0.1, 0.2, and 0.3 mg) that should be changed once a week, using a different skin location. Side effects include sedation, light-headedness, headache, dry mouth, and insomnia. Because of its sedative effects, some clinicians use clonidine as a nighttime soporific agent. Although the patch can cause local irritation, it seems to cause fewer side effects than oral clonidine.

Another drug increasingly used in the management of ADHD and impulse control problems is guanfacine (Tenex), available as 1-mg or 2-mg tablets. The initial dose is 0.5 mg at bedtime with gradual increases, as needed, to final doses up to 4 to 6 mg/day. Pharmacologically similar to clonidine, guanfacine may be effective in patients in whom clonidine failed to control the behavioral symptoms. Guanfacine may have some advantages over clonidine in that it has a longer half-life, appears to be less sedating, and produces less hypotension. It also seems to be more selective for the α_2-noradrenergic receptor and binds more selectively to the postsynaptic α_{2A}-adrenergic receptors located in the prefrontal cortex. Although both clonidine and guanfacine appear to be effective in the management of attention deficit with and without hyperactivity, they appear to be particularly useful in the management of oppositional, argumentative, impulsive, and aggressive behavior. The most frequently encountered side effects include sedation, dry mouth, itchy eyes, dizziness, headaches, fatigability, and postural hypotension. We have also found deprenyl or selegiline (Eldepryl), a monoamine oxidase B inhibitor, to be effective in controlling the symptoms of ADHD without exacerbating tics (158). It is not clear how deprenyl improves symptoms of ADHD, but the drug is known to metabolize into amphetamines. Other drugs frequently used in relatively mild cases of ADHD include imipramine (Tofranil), nortriptyline (Pamelor), and desipramine (Norpramin). Because of potential cardiotoxicity, electrocardiographic or cardiologic evaluation may be needed before initiation of desipramine therapy, and follow-up electrocardiography should be performed every 3 to 6 months. It is not yet known whether nonstimulant drugs, such as modafinil or atomoxetine (inhibitor of presynaptic norepinephrine transporter) (159), will be useful in the management of ADHD associated with TS.

Obsessive-compulsive Disorder

The role of cognitive-behavioral psychotherapy in the management of OCD has not been well defined, but this approach is gaining more acceptance particularly when used in combination with pharmacotherapy (41,160). Although imipramine and desipramine have been reported to be useful in the management of OCD, the most effective drugs are the selective serotonin uptake inhibitors (SSRIs) (161). These include fluoxetine (Prozac), fluvoxamine (Luvox), clomipramine (Anafranil), paroxetine (Paxil), sertraline (Zoloft), venlafaxine (Effexor), and citalopram (Celexa). The initial dosage of clomipramine is 25 mg at bedtime, and the dosage can be gradually increased up to 250 mg/day, using 25-, 50-, or 75-mg capsules after meals or at bedtime. Fluoxetine, paroxetine, and citalopram should be started at 20 mg after breakfast, and the dosage can be increased up to 80 mg/day. In contrast to clomipramine and fluvoxamine, the other SSRIs should be started as a morning (after breakfast) dose. Although comparative trials have been lacking, meta-analyses have provided some useful information. In one such analysis, venlafaxine was found to be particularly effective in the management of depression and inducing remission as compared with the other SSRIs, possibly because of its dual effect by inhibiting both serotonin and noradrenaline (162). In addition to its antidepressant and anti-OCD effects, fluvoxamine has been found to be an effective treatment for children and adolescents with social phobia and anxiety, a relatively common comorbidity in patients with TS (163). Sudden explosive attacks of rage, which occur in a considerable proportion of patients with TS, have been found to respond to SSRIs, such as paroxetine (163). Certain drugs, such as lithium and buspirone, have been reported to augment the SSRIs, but there is little information about the potential synergistic effects of different SSRIs. When a combination of drugs, or polypharmacy, is used, it is prudent to discuss with the patients potential adverse reactions, including the serotonin syndrome (confusion, hypomania, agitation, myoclonus, hyperreflexia, sweating, tremor, diarrhea, and fever), withdrawal phenomenon, and possible extrapyramidal side effects.

In patients with extremely severe and disabling OCD in whom optimal pharmacologic therapy has failed, psychosurgery, limbic leucotomy or cingulotomy, or anterior capsulotomy may be considered as a last resort (164). Although some pilot studies suggest that stereotactic infrathalamic lesions or deep brain stimulation can improve OCD (144), long-term results are lacking.

REFERENCES

1. Leckman J, Cohen D, Goetz C, et al. Tourette syndrome: pieces of the puzzle. In: Cohen DJ, Jankovic J, Goetz CG, eds. *Tourette syndrome*. Advances in neurology, vol 85. Philadelphia: Lippincott Williams & Wilkins, 2001:369–390.
2. Jankovic J. Tourette's syndrome. *N Engl J Med* 2001;345: 1184–1192.
3. Kurlan R. Hypothesis II: Tourette's syndrome is part of a clinical spectrum that includes normal brain development. *Arch Neurol* 1994;51:1145–1150.
4. Jankovic J, Sekula SL, Milas D. Dermatological manifestations of Tourette's syndrome and obsessive-compulsive disorder. *Arch Dermatol* 1998;134:113–114.
5. Hogan MB, Wilson NW. Tourette's syndrome mimicking asthma. *J Asthma* 1999;36:253–256.
6. Jog MS, Kubota Y, Connolly CI, et al. Building neural representations of habits. *Science* 1999;286:1745–1749.
7. Jankovic J. Phenomenology and classification of tics. *Neurol Clin North Am* 1997;15:267–275.
8. Németh AH, Mills KR, Elston JS, et al. Do the same genes predispose to Gilles de la Tourette syndrome and dystonia? Report of a new family and review of the literature. *Mov Disord* 1999;14:826–831.
9. Chee K-Y, Sachdev P. A controlled study of sensory tics in Gilles de la Tourette syndrome and obsessive-compulsive disorder using a structured interview. *J Neurol Neurosurg Psychiatry* 1997; 62:188–192.
10. Rickards H, Robertson MM. Vomiting and retching in Gilles de la Tourette syndrome: a report of ten cases and a review of the literature. *Mov Disord* 1997;12:531–535.
11. Peterson BS, Leckman JF. The temporal dynamics of tics in Gilles de la Tourette syndrome. *Biol Psychiatry* 1998;44: 1337–1348.
12. Peterson BS, Skudlarski P, Anderson AW, et al. A functional magnetic resonance imaging study of tic suppression in Tourette syndrome. *Arch Gen Psychiatry* 1998;54:326–333.
13. Rothenberger A, Kostanecka T, Kinkelbur J, et al. Sleep and Tourette syndrome. In: Cohen D, Jankovic J, Goetz C, eds. *Tourette syndrome*. Advances in neurology, vol 85. Philadelphia: Lippincott Williams & Wilkins, 2001:245–260.
14. Hanna PA, Jankovic J. Sleep and tic disorders. In: Chokroverty S, Hening Walters A, eds. *Sleep and movement disorders*. Woburn, MA: Butterworth-Heinemann, 2002 (in press).
15. Cardoso FEC, Jankovic J. Cocaine related movement disorders. *Mov Disord* 1993;8:175–178.
16. Jankovic J. Differential diagnosis and etiology of tics. In: Cohen DJ, Jankovic J, Goetz CG, eds. *Tourette syndrome*. Advances in neurology, vol 85. Philadelphia: Lippincott Williams & Wilkins, 2001:15–29.
17. Kompoliti K, Goetz CG. Hyperkinetic movement disorders misdiagnosed as tics in Gillles de la Tourette syndrome. *Mov Disord* 1998;13:477–480.
18. The Tourette Syndrome Classification Study Group. Definitions and classification of tic disorders. *Arch Neurol* 1993;50: 1013–1016.
19. *Diagnostic and statistical manual of mental disorders,* 4th ed. Washington, DC: American Psychiatric Association, 1994: 100–105.
20. Kurlan R. Diagnostic criteria for genetic studies of Tourette syndrome. *Arch Neurol* 1997;54:517–518.
21. Robertson MM, Banerjee S, Kurlan R, et al. The Tourette Syndrome Diagnostic Confidence Index. Development and clinical associations. *Neurology* 1999;53:2108–2112.
22. Goetz CG, Leurgans S, Chumara TA. Home alone: methods to maximize tic expression for objective videotape assessments in Gilles de la Tourette syndrome. *Mov Disord* 2001;16:693–697.
23. Goetz CG, Kampoliti K. Rating scales and quantitative assessment of tics. In: Cohen DJ, Jankovic J, Goetz CG, eds. *Tourette syndrome*. Advances in neurology, vol 85. Philadelphia: Lippincott Williams & Wilkins, 2001:31–42.
24. Tulen JHM, Azzolini M, De Vries JA, et al. Quantitative study of spontaneous eye blinks and eye tics in Gilles de la Tourette's syndrome. *J Neurol Neurosurg Psychiatry* 1999;67:800–802.
25. Leckman JF, Zhang H, Vitale A, et al. Course of tic severity in Tourette syndrome: the first two decades. *Pediatrics* 1998;102: 14–19.
26. Goetz CG, Tanner CM, Stebbins GT, et al. Adult tics in Gilles

de la Tourette's syndrome: description and risk factors. *Neurology* 1992;42:784–788.

27. Chouinard S, Ford B. Adult onset tic disorders. *J Neurol Neurosurg Psychiatry* 2000;68:738–743.

28. Krauss JK, Jankovic J. Severe motor tics causing cervical myelopathy in Tourette's syndrome. *Mov Disord* 1996;11:563–566.

29. Robertson MM. The Gilles de la Tourette syndrome: the current status. *Br J Psychiatry* 1989;154:147–169.

30. Abwender DA, Trinidad K, Jones KR, et al. Features resembling Tourette's syndrome in developmental stutterers. *Brain and Language* 1998;62:455–464.

31. Farber RH, Swerdlow NR, Clementz BA. Saccadic performance characteristics and the behavioural neurology of Tourette's syndrome. *J Neurol Neuorsurg Psychiatry* 1999;66:305–312.

32. LeVasseur AL, Flanagan JR, Riopelle RJ, et al. Control of volitional and reflexive in Tourette's syndrome. *Brain* 2001;124:2045–2058.

33. Swanson JM, Sergeant JA, Taylor E, et al. Attention-deficit hyperactivity disorder and hyperactivity disorder. *Lancet* 1998;351:429–433.

34. Goldman LS, Genel M, Bezman RJ, et al. Diagnosis and treatment of attention-deficit/hyperactivity disorder in children and adolescents. *JAMA* 1998;279:1100–1107.

35. Carter AS, O'Donnell DA, Schultz RT, et al. Social and emotional adjustment in children affected with Gilles de la Tourette's syndrome associations with ADHD and family functioning. *J Child Psychol Psychiatry* 2000;41:215–223.

36. Richard MM, Finkel MF, Cohen MD. Preparing reports documenting attention deficit/hyperactivity disorder for students in post-secondary education: what neurologists need to know. *Neurologist* 1998;4:277–283.

37. Coffey BJ, Park KS. Behavioral and emotional aspects of Tourette syndrome. *Neurol Clin North Am* 1997;15:277–290.

38. Dulcan M, and the AACAP Works Group on Quality Issues. Practice parameters for the assessment and treatment of children, adolescents, and adults with attention-deficit/hyperactivity disorder. *J Am Acad Child Adolesc Psychiatry* 1997;36:10 (Suppl):85S–121S.

39. Smalley SL, Fisher SE, Francks C, et al. Genome-wide scan in attention deficit hyperactivity disorders (AHD). *Am J Hum Genet* 2001;69:535(abst).

40. Leibson CL, Katusic SK, Barbaresi WJ, et al. Use and costs of medical care for children and adolescents with and without attention-deficit/hyperactivity disorder. *JAMA* 2001;285:60–66.

41. Micallef J, Blin O. Neurobiology and clinical pharmacology of obsessive-compulsive disorder. *Clin Neuropharmacol* 2001;24:191–207.

42. Stein D. The neurobiology of obsessive-compulsive disorder. *Neuroscientist* 1996;2:300–305.

43. Snider LA, Swedo SE. Pediatric obsessive-compulsive disorder. *JAMA* 2000;284:3104–3106.

44. Nestadt G, Bienvenu OJ, Cai G, et al. Incidence of obsessive-compulsive disorder in adults. *J Nerv Ment Dis* 1998;186:401–406.

45. Scahill L, Riddle MA, McSwiggin-Hardin M, et al. Children's Yale-Brown Obsessive Compulsive Scale: reliability and validity. *J Am Acad Child Adolesc Psychiatry* 1997;36:844–852.

46. Leckman JF, Walker DE, Goodman WK, et al. "Just right" perceptions associated with compulsive behavior in Tourette's syndrome. *Am J Psychiatry* 1994;151:675–680.

47. Singer HS, Schuerholz LJ, Denckla MB. Learning difficulties in children with Tourette's syndrome. *J Child Neurol* 1995;10:558–561.

48. Eapen V, Robertson MM, Alsobrook JP, et al. Obsessive-compulsive symptoms in Gilles de la Tourette syndrome and obsessive compulsive disorder: differences by diagnosis and family history. *Am J Med Genet* 1997;74:432–438.

49. Leckman JF, Grice DE, Boardman J, et al. Symptoms of obsessive-compulsive disorder. *Am J Psychiatry* 1997;154:911–917b.

50. Berthier ML, Kulisevsky J, Gironell A, et al. Obsessive-compulsive disorder associated with brain lesions: clinical phenomenology, cognitive function, and anatomic correlates. *Neurology* 1996;47:353–361.

51. Kwak CH, Jankovic J. Tourettism and hemidystonia secondary to stroke. *Mov Disord* 2002 (in press).

52. Alsobrook JP, Pauls DL. The genetics of Tourette syndrome. *Neurol Clin N Am* 1997;15:381–394.

53. Leonard H. Tourette syndrome and obsessive compulsive disorder. In: Chase T, Friedhoff A, Cohen DJ, eds. *Tourette's syndrome.* Advances in neurology. New York: Raven Press, 1992:83–94.

54. Siponmaa L, Kristiansson M, Jonson C, et al. Juvenile and young adult mentally disordered offenders: the role of child neuropsychiatric disorders. *J Am Acad Psychiatry Law* 2001;29:420–426.

55. Brower M, Price B. Neuropsychiatry of frontal lobe dysfunction in violent and criminal behavior: a critical review. *J Neurol Neurosurg Psychiatry* 2001;71:720–726.

56. Cardinal R, Pennicott D, Sugathapala C, et al. Impulsive choice induced in rats by lesions of the nucleus accumbens core. *Science* 2001;292:2499–2501.

57. Bechara A, Tranel D, Damasio H. Characterization of the decision-making deficit of patients with ventromedial prefrontal cortex lesions. *Brain* 2000;123:2189–2202.

58. Robertson M, Doran M, Trimble M, et al. The treatment of Gilles de la Tourette syndrome by limbic leucotomy. *J Neurol Neurosurg Psychiatry* 1990;53:691–694.

59. Robertson MM. Tourette syndrome, associated conditions, and the complexities of treatment. *Brain* 2000;123:425–462.

60. Robertson MM, Banerjee S, Fox Hiley PJ, et al. Personality disorder and psychopathology in Tourette's syndrome: a controlled study. *Br J Psychiatry* 1997;171:283–286.

61. Kwak C, Jankovic J. Migraine headache in Tourette syndrome. *Ann Neurol* 2001;50(Suppl 1):S21–S22.

62. Freeman RD, Fast DK, Burd L, et al. Tourette Syndrome International Database Consortium. An international perspective on Tourette syndrome—selected findings from 3,500 individuals in 22 countries. *Dev Med Child Neurol* 2000;42:436–447.

63. Leckman JF, Peterson BS, Anderson GM, et al. Pathogenesis of Tourette's syndrome. *J Child Psychol Psychiatry* 1997;38:119–142a.

64. Palumbo D, Maughan A, Kurlan R. Hypothesis III: Tourette syndrome is only one of several causes of a developmental basal ganglia syndrome. *Arch Neurol* 1997;54:475–483.

65. Stell R, Thickbroom GW, Mastaglia FL. The audiogenic startle response in Tourette's syndrome. *Mov Disord* 1995;10:723–730.

66. Karp BI, Porter S, Toro C, et al. Simple motor tics may be preceded by a premotor potential. *J Neurol Neurosurg Psychiatry* 1996;61:103–106.

67. Peterson BS. Neuroimaging studies of Tourette syndrome: a decade of progress. In: Cohen DJ, Jankovic J, Goetz CG, eds. *Tourette syndrome.* Advances in neurology, vol 85. Philadelphia: Lippincott Williams & Wilkins, 2001:179–196.

68. Serrien DJ, Nirkko AC, Loher TJ, et al. Movement control of manipulative tasks in patients with Gilles de la Tourette syndrome. *Brain* 2002;125:290–300.

69. Vaidya C, Austin G, Kirkorian G, et al. Selective effects of methylphenidate in attention deficit hyperactivity disorder: a functional magnetic resonance study. *Proc Natl Acad Sci USA* 1998;95:14494–14499.

70. Ziemann U, Paulus W, Rothenbgerger A. Decreased motor inhibition in Tourette's disorder: evidence from transcranial magnetic stimulation. *Am J Psychiatry* 1997;154:1277–1284

71. Greenberg BD, Ziemann U, Harmon A, et al. Decreased neuronal inhibition in cerebral cortex in obsessive-compulsive disorder on transcranial magnetic stimulation. *Lancet* 1998;352: 881–882.

72. Greenberg BD, Ziemann U, Cora-Locatelli G, et al. Altered cortical excitability in obsessive-compulsive disorder. *Neurology* 2000;54:142–147.

73. Moll GH, Heinrich H, Troo GE, et al. Children with comorbid attention-deficit-hyperactivity disorder and tic disorder: evidence for additive inhibitory deficits with the motor systems. *Ann Neurol* 2001;49:393–396.

74. Voderholzer U, Müller N, Haag C, et al. Periodic limb movements during sleep are a frequent finding in patients with Gilles de la Tourette's syndrome. *J Neurol* 1997;244:521–520.

75. Picchietti DL, Underwood DJ, Farris WA, et al. Further studies on periodic limb movement disorder and restless legs syndrome in children with attention-deficit hyperactivity disorder. *Mov Disord* 1999;14:1000–1007.

76. Chokroverty S, Jankovic J. Restless legs syndrome: a disease in search of identity. *Neurology* 1999;52:907–910.

77. Frederickson KA, Cutting LE, Kates WR, et al. Disproportionate increases of white matter in right frontal lobe in Tourette syndrome. *Neurology* 2002;58:85–89.

78. Hyde TM, Stacey ME, Copoola R, et al. Cerebral morphometric abnormalities in Tourette's syndrome: a quantitative MRI study of monozygotic twins. *Neurology* 1995;45:1176–1182.

79. Baumgardner TL, Singer HS, Denckla MB, et al. Corpus callosum morphology in children with Tourette syndrome and attention. *Neurology* 1996;47:477–482.

80. Mostofsky SH, Wendlandt J, Cutting L, et al. Corpus callosum measurement in girls with Tourette syndrome. *Neurology* 1999; 53:1345–1347.

81. Eidelberg D, Moeller JR, Antonini A, et al. The metabolic anatomy of Tourette's syndrome. *Neurology* 1997;48:927–934.

82. Stern E, Silbersweig DA, Chee K-Y, et al. A functional neuroanatomy of tics in Tourette syndrome. *Arch Gen Psychiatry* 2000;57:741–748.

83. Rauch SL, Savage CR, Alpert NM, et al. Probing striatal function in obsessive-compulsive disorder: a PET study of implicit sequence learning. *J Neuropsychiatry Clin Neurosci* 1997;9: 568–573.

84. Filipek P, Semrud-Clikeman M, Steinggard RJ, et al. Volumetric MRI analysis comparing subjects having attention deficit-hyperactivity disorder with normal controls. *Neurology* 1997; 48:589–601.

85. Singer HS. Current issues in Tourette syndrome. *Mov Disord* 2000;15:1051–1063.

86. Malison RT, McDougl CJ, van Dyck CH, et al. (^{123}I)β-CIT SPECT imaging of striatal dopamine transporter binding in Tourette's disorder. *Am J Psychiatry* 1995;152:1359–1361.

87. Heinz A, Knable MB, Wolf SS, et al. Tourette's syndrome. (I-123)β-CIT SPECT correlates of vocal tic severity. *Neurology* 1998;51:1069–1074.

88. Müller-Vahl KR, Berding G, Brücke T, et al. Dopamine transporter binding in Gilles de la Tourette syndrome. *J Neurol* 2000;247:514–520.

89. Wolf S, Jones DW, Knable MB, et al. Tourette syndrome: prediction of phenotypic variation in monozygotic twins by caudate nucleus D2 receptor binding. *Science* 1996;273: 1225–1227.

90. Kumar R, Lang AE. Coexistence of tics and parkinsonism: evidence for non-dopaminergic mechanisms in tic pathogenesis. *Neurology* 1997;49:1699–1701.

91. Turjanski N, Sawle GV, Playford ED, et al. PET studies of the presynaptic and postsynaptic dopaminergic system in Tourette's syndrome. *J Neurol Neurosurg Psychiatry* 1994;57:688–692.

92. Meyer P, Bohnen NI, Minshima S, et al. Striatal presynaptic monoaminergic vesicles are not increased in Tourette's syndrome. *Neurology* 1999;53;371–374.

93. Ernst M, Zametkin AJ, Jons PH, et al. High presynaptic dopaminergic activity in children with Tourette's disorder. *J Am Acad Child Adolesc Psychiatry* 1999;38:86–94.

94. Hallett JJ, Kiesling LS. Neuroimmunology of tics and other childhood hyperkinesias. *Neurol Clin North Am* 1997;15: 333–344.

95. Hallett JJ, Harling-Berg CJ, Knopf PM, et al. Anti-striatal antibodies in Tourette syndrome cause neuronal dysfunction. *J Neuroimmunol* 2000;111:195–202.

96. Dale R, Church AJ, Cardoso F, et al. Poststreptococcal acute disseminated encephalomyelitis with basal ganglia involvement and auto-reactive antibasal ganglia antibodies. *Ann Neurol* 2001;50:588–595.

97. Hoekstra PJ, Bijzet J, Limburg PC, et al. Elevated D8/17 expression on B lymphocytes, a marker of rheumatic fever, measured with flow cytometry in tic disorder patients. *Am J Psychiatry* 2001;158:605–610.

98. Singer HS, Giuliano JD, Hansen BH, et al. Antibodies against human putamen in children with Tourette syndrome. *Neurology* 1998;50:1618–1624.

99. Trifiletti RR, Packard AM. Immune mechanisms in pediatric neuropsychiatric disorders: Tourette's syndrome, OCD, and PANDAS. *Child Adolesc Psychiatr Clin North Am* 1999;8: 767–775.

100. Cardona F, Orefici G. Group A streptococcal infections and tic disorders in an Italian pediatric population. *J Pediatr* 2001;138: 71–75.

101. Müller N, Kroll B, Schwartz MJ, et al. Increased titers of antibodies against streptococcal M12 and M19 proteins in patients with Tourette's syndrome. *Psychiatry Res* 2001;101:187–193.

102. Kurlan R. Tourette's syndrome and APANDAS@. Will the relation bear out? *Neurology* 1998;50:1530–1534.

103. Leonard H, Swedo SE, Garvey M, et al. Postinfectious and other forms of obsessive-compulsive disorder. *Child Adolesc Psychiatr Clin North Am* 1999;8:497–511.

104. Perlmutter SJ, Leitman SF, Garvey MA, et al. Therapeutic plasma exchange and intravenous immunoglobulin for obsessive-compulsive disorder and tic disorders in childhood. *Lancet* 1999;354:1153–1158.

105. The Tourette Syndrome Association International Consortium on Genetics. A complete genome screen in sib-pairs affected by Gilles de la Tourette syndrome. *Am J Hum Genet* 1999;65: 1428–1436.

106. McMahon WM, van der Wetering BJ, Filoux F, et al. Bilineal transmission and phenotypic variations of Tourette's disorder in a large pedigree. *J Am Acad Child Adolesc Psychiatry* 1996;35: 672–680.

107. Hanna PA, Janjua FN, Contant CF, et al. Bilineal transmission in Tourette syndrome. *Neurology* 1999;53:813–818.

108. Lichter DG, Dmochowski J, Jackson LA, et al. Influence of family history on clinical expression of Tourette's syndrome. *Neurology* 1999;52:308–316.

109. Walkup JT, LaBuda MC, Singer HS, et al. Family study and segregation analysis of Tourette syndrome: evidence for a mixed model of inheritance. *Am J Hum Genet* 1996;59:684–693.

110. Leckman JF, Dolnansky ES, Hardin MT, et al. Perinatal factors in the expression of Tourette's syndrome: an exploratory study. *J Am Acad Child Adolesc Psychiatry* 1990;29:220–226.

111. Hyde TM, Aaronson BA, Randolph C, et al. Relationship of birth weight to the phenotypic expression of Gilles de la

Tourette's syndrome in monozygotic twins. *Neurology* 1992;42: 652–658.

112. Scahill L, Tanner C, Dure L. The epidemiology of tics and Tourette syndrome in children and adolescents. In: Cohen DJ, Jankovic J, Goetz CG, eds. *Tourette syndrome.* Advances in neurology, vol 85. Philadelphia: Lippincott Williams & Wilkins, 2001:261–272.

113. Costello EJ, Angold A, Burns BJ, et al. The Great Smokey Mountains Study of Youth: goals, design, methods, and the prevalence of DSM-III-R disorders. *Arch Gen Psychiatry* 1996; 53:1129–1136.

114. Mason A, Banerjee S, Zeitlin H, et al. The prevalence of Tourette syndrome in a mainstream school population. *Dev Med Child Neurol* 1998;40:292–296.

115. Kurlan R, McDermott MP, Deeley C, et al. Prevalence of tics in schoolchildren and association with placement in special education. *Neurology* 2001;57:1383–1388.

116. Itoh K, Suzuki K, Bise K, et al. Apoptosis in the basal ganglia of the developing human nervous system. *Acta Neuropathol* 2001;101:92–100.

117. Dodman NH, Normile JA, Shuster L, et al. Equine self-mutilation syndrome (57 cases). *JAVM* 1994;204:1219–1223.

118. Jankovic J. Gilles de la Tourette syndrome. In: Rakel RE, ed. *Conn's current therapy.* Philadelphia: WB Saunders, 1999: 915–919.

119. Lang AE. Update on the treatment of tics. In: Cohen DJ, Jankovic J, Goetz CG, eds. *Tourette syndrome.* Advances in neurology, vol 85. Philadelphia: Lippincott Williams & Wilkins, 2001:355–362.

120. Jimenez-Jimenez FJ, Garcia-Ruiz PJ. Pharmacological options for the treatment of Tourette's disorder. *Drugs* 2001;61: 2207–2220.

121. Piacentini J, Chang S. Behavioral treatment for Tourette syndrome and tic disorders. In: Cohen DJ, Jankovic J, Goetz CG, eds. *Tourette syndrome.* Advances in neurology, vol 85. Philadelphia: Lippincott Williams & Wilkins, 2001:319–332.

122. Sallee FR, Nesbit L, Jackson C, et al. Relative efficacy of haloperidol and pimozide in children and adolescents. *Am J Psychiatry* 1997;154:1057–1062.

123. Bruun RD, Budman CL. Risperidone as a treatment for Tourette's syndrome. *J Clin Psychiatry* 1996;57:29–31.

124. Robertson MM, Scull DA, Eapen V, et al. Risperidone in the treatment of Tourette syndrome: a retrospective case note study. *J Psychopharmacol* 1996;10:317–320.

125. Sallee FR, Kurlan R, Goetz CG, et al. Ziprasidone treatment of children and adolescents with Tourette's syndrome: a pilot study. *J Am Acad Child Adolesc Psychiatry* 2000;39:292–299.

126. Jankovic J, Beach J. Long-term effects of tetrabenazine in hyperkinetic movement disorders. *Neurology* 1997;48:358–362.

127. Jankovic J. Tardive syndromes and other drug-induced movement disorders. *Clin Neuropharmacol* 1995;18:197–214.

128. Gilbert DL, Sethuraman G, Sine L, et al. Tourette's syndrome improvement with pergolide in a randomized, double-blind crossover trial. *Neurology* 2000;54:1310–1315.

129. Peterson BS, Zhang H, Anderson GM, et al. A double-blind, placebo-controlled, crossover trial of an antiandrogen in the treatment of Tourette's syndrome. *J Clin Psychopharmacol* 1998;18:324–331.

130. Toren P, Laor N, Cohen DJ, et al. Ondansetron treatment in patients with Tourette's syndrome. *Int Clin Psychopharmacol* 1999;14:373–376.

131. Awaad Y. Tics in Tourette syndrome: new treatment options. *J Child Neurol* 1999;14:316–319.

132. Singer HS, Wendlandt J, Krieger M, et al. Baclofen treatment in Tourette syndrome: a double-blind, placebo-controlled, crossover trial. *Neurology* 2001;56:599–604.

133. Hoopes SP. Donezepil for Tourette's disorder and ADHD. *J Clin Psychopharmacol* 1999;19:381–382.

134. Sanberg PR, Shytle RD, Silver AA. Treatment of Tourette's syndrome with mecamylamine. *Lancet* 1998;352:705–706.

135. Hughes JR, Goldstein MG, Hurt RD, et al. Recent advances in the pharmacotherapy of smoking. *JAMA* 1999;281:72–76.

136. Silver AA, Shytle RD, Sheehan D, et al. A multi-center, double-blind placebo controlled safety and efficacy study of mecamylamine (Inversine) monotherapy for Tourette syndrome. *J Am Acad Child Adolesc Psychiatry* 2001;40:1103–1110.

137. Müller-Vahl KR, Kolbe H, Schneider U, et al. Cannabis in movement disorders. *Forsch Komplementarmed* 1999;6(Suppl 3):23–27.

138. Jankovic J. Botulinum toxin in the treatment of dystonic tics. *Mov Disord* 1994;9:347–349.

139. Scott BL, Jankovic J, Donovan DT. Botulinum toxin into vocal cord in the treatment of malignant coprolalia associated with Tourette's syndrome. *Mov Disord* 1996;11:431–433.

140. Kwak CH, Hanna PA, Jankovic J. Botulinum toxin in the treatment of tics. *Arch Neurol* 2000;57:1190–1193.

141. Marras C, Andrews D, Sime EA, et al. Botulinum toxin for simple motor tics: a randomized, double-blind, controlled clinical trial. *Neurology* 2001;56:605–610.

142. Kurlan R. New treatments for tics? *Neurology* 2001;56: 580–581.

143. Babel TB, Warnke PC, Ostertag CB. Immediate and long term outcome after infrathalamic and thalamic lesioning for intractable Tourette's syndrome. *J Neurol Neurosurg Psychiatry* 2001;70:666–671.

144. Vandewalle V, Van Der Linden C, Groenegen HJ, et al. Stereotactic treatment of Gilles de la Tourette syndrome by high frequency stimulation of thalamus. *Lancet* 1999;353:724.

145. Riddle MA, Carlson J. Clinical psychopharmacology for Tourette syndrome and associated disorders. In: Cohen DJ, Jankovic J, Goetz CG, eds. *Tourette syndrome.* Advances in neurology, vol 85. Philadelphia: Lippincott Williams & Wilkins, 2001:343–354.

146. The MTA Cooperative Group. A 14-month randomized clinical trial of treatment strategies for attention-deficit/hyperactivity disorder: the MTA Cooperative Group—Multimodal Treatment Study of Children with ADHD. *Arch Gen Psychiatry* 1999;56:1073–1086.

147. Klein RG, Abikoff H, Klass E, et al. Clinical efficacy of methylphenidate in conduct disorder with and without attention deficit hyperactivity disorder. *Arch Gen Psychiatry* 1997; 54:1073–1080.

148. Manos MJ, Short EJ, Findling RL. Differential effectiveness of methylphenidate and Adderall[R] in school-age youths with attention-deficit/hyperactivity disorder. *J Am Acad Child Adolesc Psychiatry* 1999;38:813–819.

149. Pliszka SR, Browne RG, Olvera RL, et al. A double-blind, placebo-controlled study of Adderall and methylphenidate in the treatment of attention-deficit/hyperactivity disorder. *J Am Acad Child Adolesc Psychiatry* 2000;39:619–626.

150. Efron D, Jarman F, Barker M, et al. Side effects of methylphenidate and dextroamphetamine in children with attention deficit hyperactivity disorder: a double-blind, crossover trial. *Pediatrics* 1997;100:662–666.

151. Gadow KD, Sverd J, Sprafkin J, et al. Long-term methylphenidate therapy in children with comorbid attention-deficit hyperactivity and chronic multiple tic disorder. *Arch Gen Psychiatry* 1999;56:330–336.

152. Law SF, Schachtar RT. Do typical clinical doses of methylphenidate cause tics in children treated for attention-deficit hyperactivity disorder? *J Amer Acad Child Adolesc Psychiatry* 1999;38:944–951.

153. Kurlan R. Methylphenidate to treat ADHD is not contraindicated in children with tics. *Mov Disord* 2002;17:5–6.

154. The Tourette's Syndrome Study Group. Treatment of ADHD in children with tics: a randomized controlled trial. *Neurology* 2002 (in press).

155. Gainetdinov RR, Wetsel WC, Jones SR, et al. Role of serotonin in the paradoxical calming effect of psychostimulants in hyperactivity. *Science* 1999;283:397–401.

156. Biederman J, Spencer T. Attention-deficit/hyperactivity disorder (ADHD) as a noradrenergic disorder. *Biol Psychiatry* 1999;46:1234–1242.

157. Biederman J, Wilens T, Mick E, et al. Pharmacotherapy of attention-deficit/hyperactivity disorder reduces risk of substance abuse disorder. *Pediatrics* 1999;104:e20b.

158. Feigin A, Kurlan R, McDermott MP, et al. A controlled trial of deprenyl in children with Tourette's syndrome and attention deficit hyperactivity disorder. *Neurology* 1996;46:965–968.

159. Michelson D, Faries D, Wernicke J, et al. Atomoxetine in the treatment of children and adolescents with attention-deficit/hyperactivity disorder: a randomized, placebo-controlled, dose-response study. *Pediatrics* 2001;108:1–9.

160. March JS, Franklin M, Nelson A, et al. Cognitive-behavioral psychotherapy for pediatric obsessive-compulsive disorder. *J Child Psychology* 2001;30:8–18.

161. Grados MA, Riddle MA. Pharmacologic treatment of childhood obsessive-compulsive disorder: from theory to practice. *J Child Psychology* 2001;30:67–79.

162. Thase ME, Entsua AR, Rudolph RL. Remission rates during treatment with venlafaxine or selective serotonin reuptake inhibitors. *Br J Psychiatry* 2001;178:234–241.

163. The Research Unit on Pediatric Psychopharmacology Anxiety Study Group. Fluvoxamine for the treatment of anxiety disorders in children and adolescents. *N Engl J Med* 2001;344:1279–1285.

163. Bruun RD, Budman CL. Paroxetine treatment of episodic rages associated with Tourette's disorder. *J Clin Psychiatry* 1998;59:581–584.

164. Rauch SL, Baer L, Cosgrove GR, et al. Neurosurgical treatment of Tourette's syndrome: a critical review. *Compr Psychiatry* 1995;36:141–156.

APPENDIX

Tourette Syndrome Association (TSA)
42-40 Bell Boulevard
Bayside, NY 11361
Tel: 718-224-2999
http://neuro-www2.mgh.harvard.edu/tsa/tsamain.nclk

Related Web Sites

http://www.ed.gov
http://www.nih.gov
http://www.wemove.org
Obsessive Compulsive Foundation
http://www.ocfoundation.org
Children and Adults with Attention Deficit Disorder
http://www.chadd.org

Additional Web Sites

http://www.cw.bc.ca
http://www.medscape.com

DYSTONIC DISORDERS

JOSEPH J. JANKOVIC
STANLEY FAHN

HISTORICAL PERSPECTIVE

The primary objective of this chapter is to provide an updated review on the diagnosis, classification, etiology, and pathophysiology of dystonia. Therapeutic approaches will be covered separately (see Chapter 24). One of the earliest descriptions of dystonia was provided by Gowers in 1888, who coined the term *tetanoid chorea* to describe the movement disorder in two siblings later found to have Wilson's disease (1) (Table 23.1). The term *dystonia musculorum deformans*, coined by Oppenheim in 1911, was criticized because fluctuating muscle tone was not necessarily characteristic of the disorder, the term "musculorum" incorrectly implied that the involuntary movement was due to a muscle disorder, and not all patients became deformed. Until recently, the term *torsion dystonia* has been used in the literature, but since "torsion" is part of the definition of dystonia, the term torsion dystonia seems redundant and hence the simple term dystonia is preferred.

PHENOMENOLOGY OF DYSTONIA AND DIFFERENTIAL DIAGNOSIS

Dystonia is currently defined as a neurologic syndrome characterized by involuntary, sustained, patterned, and often repetitive muscle contractions of opposing muscles, causing twisting movements or abnormal postures. Traditional descriptions of dystonia emphasize that the muscle contractions are sustained and rapid dystonic movements are often not recognized. These rapid movements resemble myoclonus, and the term *myoclonic dystonia* is sometimes applied when the movements are fast and repetitive. Myoclonic dystonia, a rapid dystonic movement, should be differentiated from the syndrome of *myoclonus-dystonia*, an autosomal dominant, alcohol-responsive disorder manifested by coexisting dystonia and myoclonus, where the myoclonus occurs in body parts not necessarily affected by dystonia (2,3).

A characteristic feature of dystonia that helps to distinguish it from the other hyperkinetic movement disorders is the fact that dystonic movements, whether slow or rapid, are repetitive and patterned. The term "patterned" refers to the repeated involvement of the same group of muscles. Thus, a patient with cervical dystonia manifested by torticollis to the left tends to always have the same abnormal pattern and direction of movement (i.e., turning of the head to the left) during the course of the disease. Although additional muscles may subsequently be involved, the pattern usually remains the same. This is in contrast to chorea, which consists of brief movements that occur continuously and flow randomly from one body part to another. Tics are brief and intermittent movements (motor tics) or sounds (vocal tics) (4). In contrast to dystonia, tics can be more easily suppressed, are usually abrupt rather than continual, and are often preceded by a subjective, compulsive urge or sensation (premonitory sensation) that is temporarily relieved after the tic has been executed. The phenomenology of tics ranges from brief, lightning-like jerks ("clonic tics") to more sustained contractions ("tonic" or "dystonic tics"). Although these latter tics resemble dystonic movements, they can be differentiated easily from dystonic movements, particularly when clonic tics or other features of Tourette's syndrome are present.

The diagnosis of dystonia is often complicated by the coexistence of tremor. Two basic types of tremor can occur in patients with dystonia: postural (essential-like) and dystonic. Postural tremor in the hands, phenomenologically identical to essential tremor (ET), is present in a quarter of patients with cervical dystonia (5). Whether the hand tremor seen in 10% to 85% of patients with cervical dystonia represents an enhanced physiologic tremor, ET, dystonic tremor, or some other form of postural tremor is unknown. Although patients referred to a movement disorders clinic have disorders more severe and atypical than the general population of patients with ET-like tremor, the true prevalence of dystonia in patients with ET tremor is clearly higher than in the general population. Furthermore, a number of large families have been described in which some members have only ET while others have only dystonia and still others have the combination of dystonia and ET (6). Münchau et al. (7) studied 11 patients with classic ET and compared them to 19 patients with cervical dystonia and arm tremor. They found that the latency of second agonist burst during ballistic wrist flexion movements occurred later in ET patients than in those with

TABLE 23.1. MILESTONES IN THE HISTORY OF DYSTONIA

Year	Author	Description
1887	Wood	Facial and oromandibular dystonia
1888	Gowers	"Tetanoid chorea"—2 siblings, later found to have Wilson's disease
1901	Destarac	"Torticollis spasmodique"—a 17-year-old girl with torticollis, tortipelvis, writer's cramp, foot cramps, improved by sensory tricks, exacerbated by motor activity
1903	Leszynsky	Hysterical spasms and gait
1908	Hunt	"Myoclonia of the trunk," "tic spasms," hystericia
1908	Schwalbe	Hereditary "tonic, crampus" syndrome, maladie des tics—rapid movements; recognized the familial nature of dystonia in Jewish siblings (Lewin family); used scopolamine
1911	Ziehen	"Torsion neurosis"—did not believe it to be hysterical; observed that "convulsive movements increased during voluntary movement" and during emotional excitement
1911	Oppenheim	"Dystonia musculorum deformans" and "dysbasia lordotica progressive," "monkey" or "dromedary" gait, "mobile spasms," sustained posturing, spasms, fluctuating muscle tone, rapid movement resembling tremor, chorea and athetosis
1911	Flatau and Sterling	"Progressive torsion spasm"—noted hereditary, repetitive pattern, "jerky"; Jewish patients of high intelligence; objected to the term "deformans" because not all patients become disfigured and objected to the term "musculorum" because it implied a muscle condition
1912	Fraenkel	Rapid, twisting, sustained movement, tortipelvis
1912	Wilson	"Hepatolenticular degeneration"—"clonic" or "tic-like" spasms, "choreiform and athetoid" movements
1916	Hunt	Slow, twisting or clonic, rhythmic movements
1919	Mendel	"Torsion dystonia"—review of literature; 33 patients; "a morbid disease entity"
1920	Taylor	"Dystonia lenticularis," postural ("myostatic") and kinetic forms of dystonia
1926	Davidenkow	"Myoclonic dystonia"—rapid "tic-like" movements
1929	Wimmer	"Not a disease but only a syndrome"—seen in Wilson's disease, postencephalitic, perinatal brain damage
1944	Herz	Idiopathic dystonia as a disease entity—15 personal cases and 105 from the literature; "slow, long-sustained, turning movements"; alternating "myorhythmia" or "very rapid, tic-like twitchings"
1958	Cooper	Thalamotomy
1959	Zeman	Autosomal dominant
1960	Zeman et al.	Formes frustes of dystonia
1962	Denny-Brown	"Fixed or relatively fixed attitude"
1967	Zeman and Dyken	No specific neuropathology in dystonia brains
1976	Marsden	Blepharospasm is a form of focal dystonia
1983	Fahn	High-dose anticholinergic therapy
1983	Jankovic and Patel	Blepharospasm–oromandibular dystonia secondary to rostral brainstem–diencephalic lesion
1985	Scott et al.	Botulinum toxin for blepharospasm
1989	Ozelius et al.	Gene for autosomal dominant dystonia linked to chromosome 9q32–34 (*DYT1*)
1989		Botulinum toxin type A approved by the U.S. Food and Drug Administration
1994	Ichinose et al.	Mutations in the GTP-cyclohydrolase 1 gene on chromosome 14q22.1–22.2 in autosomal dominant dopa-responsive dystonia
1995		Mutation in the *TH* gene on chromosome 11p15.5 causes autosomal recessive form of dopa-responsive dystonia
1996		Third International Dystonia Symposium
1997	Ozelius et al.	Dystonia gene (*DYT1*) encodes an ATP-binding protein
1999	Nygaard et al.	A gene for myoclonus-dystonia mapped to chromosome 7q21–q23
1999		Botulinum toxin type A and botulinum toxin type B approved for the management of cervical dystonia by the U.S. Food and Drug Administration
2001	Zimrich et al.	Myoclonic dystonia localized to 7q21 gene coding for ε-sarcoglycan

arm tremor–associated cervical dystonia. Furthermore, the latter group had a greater variability in reciprocal inhibition than the ET group. Patients with normal presynaptic inhibition had onset of their arm tremor simultaneously with their cervical dystonia (mean age 40 years), whereas patients with reduced or absent presynaptic inhibition had onset at an earlier age (mean 14 years) and the interval between the onset of the tremor and of cervical dystonia was longer (mean 21 years). These findings suggest that the mechanisms of arm tremor in patients with ET and cervical dystonia are different. In some patients, head and trunk tremor (usually of slow, 2- to 5-Hz frequency) may precede the onset of dystonia and may be the initial manifestation of focal dystonia (dystonic tremor) (8). Certain task-specific (e.g., writing) tremors may actually represent forms of focal dystonia (9). Rarely, cerebellar and parkinsonian tremors can be associated with dystonia, and dystonia may be the presenting finding of Parkinson's disease or other parkinsonian disorders such as progressive supranuclear palsy and corticobasal degeneration (10,11).

Dystonia is either a symptom of an underlying disorder or a specific disease entity (Table 23.2). When no etiologic factor can be identified, the dystonia is referred to as *pri-*

TABLE 23.2. ETIOLOGIC CLASSIFICATION OF DYSTONIA

I. *Primary dystonia*
   A. Sporadic
   B. Inherited (all autosomal dominant)
      Classic (Oppenheim's) dystonia (common in Ashkenazi Jews, DYT1—9q34)
      Childhood- and adult-onset cranial-cervical-limb dystonia (DYT6—8p21–22)
      Adult-onset cervical and other focal dystonia (DYT7—18p)
II. *Secondary dystonia (dystonia-plus syndromes)*
   A. Sporadic
      Parkinson's disease
      Progressive supranuclear palsy
      Multiple system atrophy
      Corticobasal degeneration
   B. Inherited
      1. Autosomal dominant
         Dopa-responsive dystonia (DRD) (DYT5—GTP cyclohydrolase I 14q22.1)
         Dystonia-myoclonus (11q23)
         Alternating hemiplegia of childhood
         Dystonia-ataxia (SCA types 3 and 6)
      2. Autosomal recessive
         Dopa-responsive dystonia (11p11.5)
         Tyrosine hydroxylase deficiency (chromosome –21)
         Biopterin deficiency diseases
         Aromatic amino acid decarboxylase deficiency
            (dopamine agonist–responsive dystonia)
III. *Heredogenerative diseases* (typically not pure dystonia)
   A. X-linked recessive
      Lubag (X-linked dystonia-parkinsonism, DYT3—Xq12–Xq21)
      Pelizaeus-Merzbacher disease
      Lesch-Nyhan syndrome
      Dystonia-deafness (Xq22)
      Deafness, dystonia, retardation, blindness
   B. Autosomal dominant
      Rapid-onset dystonia-parkinsonism
      Juvenile parkinsonism-dystonia
      Huntington's disease (*IT15*–4p16.3)
      Spinocerebellar degenerations (SCA1–SCA8)
      Dentatorubropallidoluysian atrophy
      Hereditary spastic paraplegia with dystonia
      Thalamo-olivary degeneration with Wernicke's
         encephalopathy
   C. Autosomal recessive
      Wilson's disease (Cu-ATPase–I3q14.3)
      Neurodegeneration with brain iron accumulation type 1 or
         pantothenate kinase–associated neurodegeneration
         (formerly Hallervorden-Spatz disease–20p12.3–p13)
      Hypoprebetalipoproteinemia, acanthocytosis, retinitis
         pigmentosa, and pallidal degeneration (HARP syndrome)
      Ataxia telangiectasia
      Associated with metabolic disorders
      1. Amino acid disorders
         Glutaric acidemia
         Methylmalonic acidemia
         Homocystinuria
         Hartnup disease
         Tyrosinosis
      2. Lipid disorders
         Metachromatic leukodystrophy
         Ceroid lipofuscinosis
         Niemann-Pick type C (dystonic lipidosis, "sea blue" histiocytosis)
         Gangliosidoses G_{M1}, G_{M2} variants
         Hexosaminidase A and B deficiency
      3. Other metabolic disorders
         Biopterin deficiency diseases
         Triose phosphate isomerase deficiency
         Aromatic amino acid decarboxylase deficiency
            (dopamine agonist–responsive dystonia)

   Biotin-responsive basal ganglia disease
   D. Mitochondrial
      Leigh's disease
      Leber's disease
   E. Unknown inheritance
      Neuroacanthocytosis
      Rett's syndrome
      Intraneuronal inclusion disease
      Infantile bilateral striatal necrosis
      Familial basal ganglia calcifications
      Hereditary spastic paraplegia with dystonia
      Deletion of 18q
   Due to a known specific cause
      Perinatal cerebral injury and kernicterus: athetoid cerebral
         palsy, delayed-onset dystonia
      Infection: viral encephalitis, encephalitis lethargica, Reye's
         syndrome; subacute sclerosing panencephalitis;
         Creutzfeldt-Jakob disease; HIV infection
      Other: tuberculosis, syphilis, acute infectious torticollis
      Drugs: levodopa and dopamine agonists, dopamine
         receptor—blocking drugs, fenfluramine, anticonvulsants,
         flecainide, ergots, some calcium channel blockers
      Toxins: MN, CO, CS_2, cyanide, methanol, disulfiram,
         3-nitropropionic acid, wasp sting toxin
      Metabolic: hypoparathyroidism
      Paraneoplastic brainstem encephalitis
      Vitamin E deficiency
      Primary antiphospholipid syndrome
      Cerebrovascular or ischemic injury, Sjögren's syndrome
      Multiple sclerosis
      Central pontine myelinolysis
      Brainstem lesions
      Spinal cord lesions
      Syringomyelia
      Brain tumor
      Arteriovenous malformation
      Head trauma and brain surgery (thalamotomy)
      Lumbar stenosis
      Peripheral trauma (with causalgia)
      Electrical injury
IV. *Other hyperkinetic syndromes associated with dystonia*
   A. *Tic disorders with dystonic tics*
   B. *Paroxysmal dyskinesias*
      1. Paroxysmal kinesigenic dyskinesia (16p11.2–q12.1)
      2. Paroxysmal nonkinesigenic dyskinesia (2q33–35)
      3. Paroxysmal exertional dyskinesia (16p12–q12)
      4. Paroxysmal hypnogenic dyskinesia (20q13.2–13.3)
V. *Psychogenic*
VI. *Pseudodystonia*
      Atlantoaxial subluxation
      Syringomyelia
      Arnold-Chiari malformation
      Trochlear nerve palsy
      Vestibular torticollis
      Posterior fossa mass
      Soft-tissue neck mass
      Congenital postural torticollis
      Congenital Klippel-Feil syndrome
      Isaacs' syndrome
      Sandifer's syndrome
      Satoyoshi's syndrome
      Stiff-man syndrome
      Dupuytren's contractures
      Trigger digits
      Ventral hernia

SCA, spinocerebellar ataxia; DRD, dopa-responsive dystonia.

mary dystonia. Primary dystonia can be either sporadic or inherited, and is not associated with any cognitive, pyramidal, cerebellar, or sensory abnormalities. When there is an associated neurologic abnormality, such as parkinsonism, dementia, corticospinal tract signs, and other disturbances besides dystonia, the term *dystonia-plus* may be appropriate (Table 23.2).

CLASSIFICATION OF DYSTONIA

Dystonia can be classified according to (a) severity, (b) clinical characteristics, (c) distribution, (d) age at onset, and (e) etiology (12) (Fig. 23.1).

Classification by Severity

Dystonic movements can occur at rest but are usually exacerbated by voluntary motor activity ("action dystonia"). One form of action dystonia is the task-specific focal dystonia present only during specific activity. This type of dystonia is exemplified best by writer's cramp (graphospasm) (13). Other specific activities known to induce dystonic movements or postures include holding a cup or utensils in certain positions, cutting food, typing, and other skilled actions required in certain occupations or sports, including playing musical instruments, such as piano, violin, and embouchure (14), auctioneering (15), and other specific activities (16). The severity of dystonia varies from a task- or position-specific dystonia to "status dystonicus" and "dystonic storm," causing a breakdown of the contracting muscles and a life-threatening myoglobinuria (17).

The intensity of dystonic movements can be influenced by various conditions. For example, voluntary motor activity, such as walking, running, writing, talking, and performing specific motor tasks, can intensify dystonia. Furthermore, dystonia often increases with stress and fatigue. On the other hand, dystonic movements can be sometimes relieved by rest, self-hypnosis, and various sensory tricks ("geste antagonistique") or counterpressure, such as touching the chin or the occiput to help overcome torticollis (18). Patients with generalized dystonia, particularly involving the trunk and legs, note marked improvement when they walk backward. Rarely, dystonia improves during activity. With this so-called paradoxical dystonia, the patient actively moves the affected body part in an attempt to relive the dystonia. This voluntary movement can be mistaken for restlessness or akathisia, particularly when the dystonia affects the trunk. The type of dystonia that is most typically relieved by voluntary movement, such as speaking,

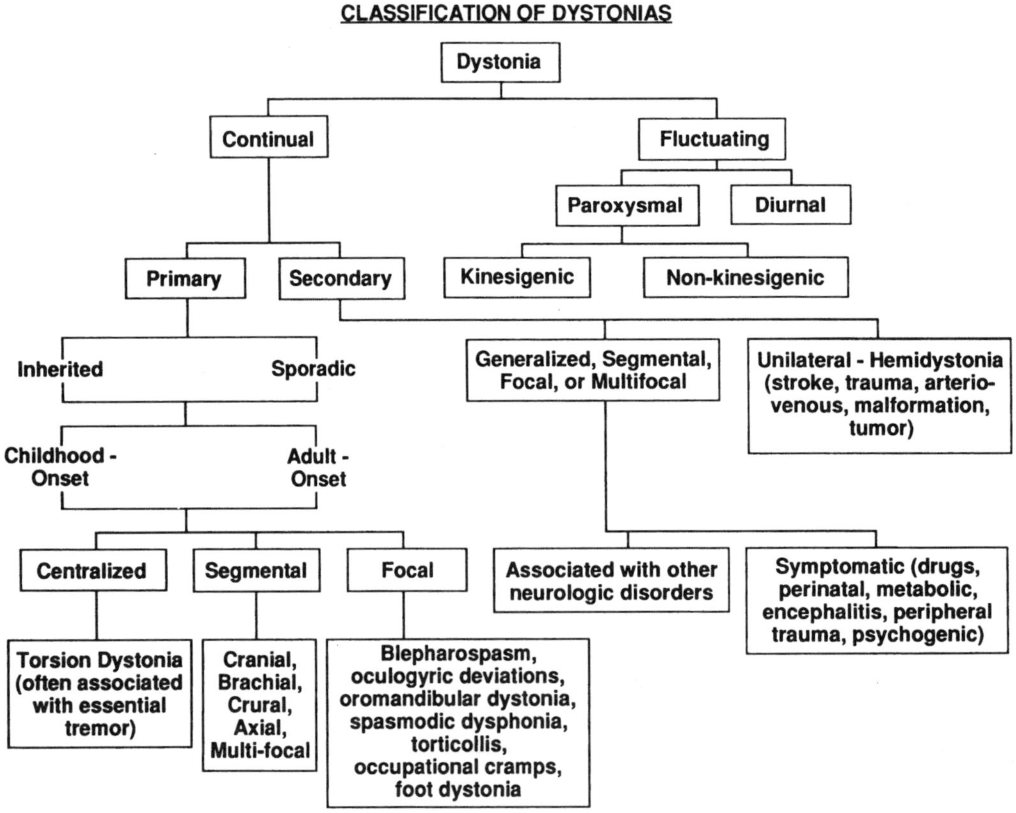

CLASSIFICATION OF DYSTONIAS

FIG. 23.1. Algorithm for the classification of dystonias.

is blepharospasm. Dystonic movements usually cease during sleep but may be recorded during lighter stages of sleep; however, dystonic postures may persist during all stages of sleep.

Classification by Clinical Characteristics

While dystonic movements are usually continual, the timing and intensity of the movements can be influenced by various factors, including emotion, fatigue, relaxation, and motor activity. In some patients dystonia fluctuates so much that it may be almost absent in the morning and become pronounced and disabling in the afternoons and evenings. This diurnal dystonia may be associated with parkinsonian features and characteristically improves dramatically with L-dopa therapy; hence the term *dopa-responsive dystonia* (DRD) (19). The genetics and classification of DRD will be discussed later.

Another type of fluctuating dystonia is paroxysmal dystonia, characterized by sudden onset or an exacerbation of dystonic movements lasting seconds to hours (20; also see Chapter 29) (Table 23.3). We favor a classification for this group of disorders that is based chiefly on precipitating events, which categorizes the attacks as either nonkinesigenic or kinesigenic paroxysmal dyskinesias. In contrast to paroxysmal nonkinesigenic dystonia (PND), which occurs unpredictably without any particular precipitant, paroxysmal kinesigenic dystonia (PKD) is induced by a sudden movement. In addition, paroxysmal exertional dystonia (PED) follows prolonged physical exertion, and paroxysmal hypnogenic dystonia (PHD) occurs only during sleep. These paroxysmal episodes usually last only a few seconds to minutes and may be exacerbated by stress, extreme temperatures, menses, and other factors. Some paroxysmal dystonias are also associated with seizures and ataxia. The relationship between paroxysmal dystonia and epilepsy is further supported by the observation that dystonic movements can occur during certain seizures ("ictal dystonia")

(21) and that PKD responds well to anticonvulsant drugs (20).

Besides the idiopathic fluctuating dystonias there are many other causes of paroxysmal or fluctuating dystonias, including seizures, multiple sclerosis, thyrotoxicosis, migraines, transient ischemic attacks, aminoacidurias, and other metabolic disorders (Table 23.2). Inherited errors of metabolism, such as aromatic amino acid decarboxylase deficiency, should be considered in patients with fluctuating (diurnal) dystonia, particularly if it starts in infancy and if accompanied by axial hypotonia, athetosis, ocular convergence spasm, oculogyric crises, and limb rigidity (22). Patients with aromatic amino acid decarboxylase deficiency fail to respond to levodopa but may obtain substantial benefit from dopamine agonists. The disorder is inherited in an autosomal recessive pattern and the gene maps to 7p12.1-p12.3. Levodopa therapy, acute dystonic reactions to neuroleptics, and gastroesophageal reflux are other examples of intermittent fluctuating dystonia. Another example of intermittent paroxysmal dystonia is "oculogyric crisis," characterized by a sudden, transient, conjugate eye deviation, often seen as part of the postencephalitic parkinsonism syndrome, Tourette's syndrome, drug-induced dystonia, or tardive dyskinesia (23). There are many other causes of paroxysmal dystonias, and these should be pursued particularly in patients with atypical features (24).

Classification by Distribution

Dystonia may be classified according to distribution into one of five categories:

1. Focal dystonia affects a single body part and is exemplified by cervical dystonia (torticollis); occupational cramp (e.g., writer's cramp); foot dystonia; oculogyric deviations; blepharospasm; oromandibular, lingual, pharyngeal, and laryngeal dystonia (spasmodic dysphonia); and some forms of bruxism and trismus.

TABLE 23.3. PAROXYSMAL DYSKINESIAS

	PKD	PND	PED
Male/female ratio	4:1	3:2	1:2 (?)
Age at onset (yr)	5–15 (1–35)	<5 (0–25)	2–20
Inheritance	AD, sporadic	AD, sporadic	AD
Duration of attacks	<5 min	Minutes-hours	5–30 min
Frequency of attacks	100/d–1/mo	3/d–2/yr	1/d–1/mo
Associated features	Dystonia, chorea, epilepsy	Chorea, dystonia, ataxia	Dystonia, chorea
Asymmetry	++	+	
Ability to suppress attacks	+++	+++	
Inducing or precipitating factors	Sudden movement; startle; hyperventilation; fatigue; stress	Alcohol; caffeine; exercise; excitement	Prolonged exercise, stress, caffeine, fatigue
Medical therapy	Phenytoin; carbamazepine; barbiturates; acetazolamide	Clonazepam;oxazepam	

AD, autosomal dominant; PKD, paroxysmal kinesigenic dyskinesia (dystonia); PND, paroxysmal nonkinesigenic dyskinesia (dystonia); PED, paroxysmal exertional dyskinesia (dystonia).

2. Segmental dystonia affects one or more contiguous body parts. Examples of segmental dystonia include craniocervical dystonia, characterized by the combination of blepharospasm, facial-oromandibular, lingual, pharyngeal, laryngeal, and cervical dystonia. Other categories of segmental dystonia include brachial (one or both arms with or without the involvement of axial or cranial muscles), crural (one leg plus trunk or both legs), and axial (neck and trunk with or without cranial muscles).

3. Multifocal dystonia involves two or more noncontiguous body parts (such as a combination of oromandibular dystonia and dystonia of a leg).

4. Generalized dystonia consists of segmental crural dystonia and dystonia in at least one additional body part (Figs. 23.2 and 23.3).

5. Hemidystonia (unilateral dystonia) involves only half of the body and is usually associated with a structural lesion in the contralateral basal ganglia, particularly the putamen (Figs. 23.4 and 23.5).

Based on a combined series of about 8,000 patients with dystonia evaluated at the Movement Disorders Clinic at Baylor College of Medicine (Houston) and Columbia-Presbyterian Medical Center (New York) about two thirds of patients have focal dystonia, one fourth have segmental, and one fourth have either generalized hemidystonia or multifocal dystonia. Cervical dystonia represents about half of all patients, cranial dystonia (blepharospasm and oromandibular dystonia) one fourth, and laryngeal or limb dystonia one fourth. However, this distribution may not be typical for the

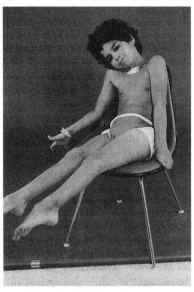
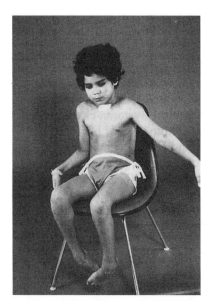
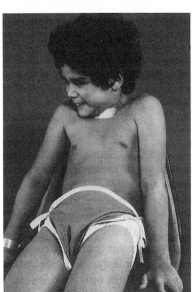
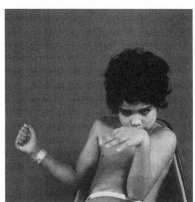

FIG. 23.2. An 8-year-old boy with severe inherited generalized dystonia causing myoglobinuria. Tracheostomy was performed because he required prolonged paralysis with curare to prevent further rhabdomyolysis. (Jankovic and Penn, 1982.)

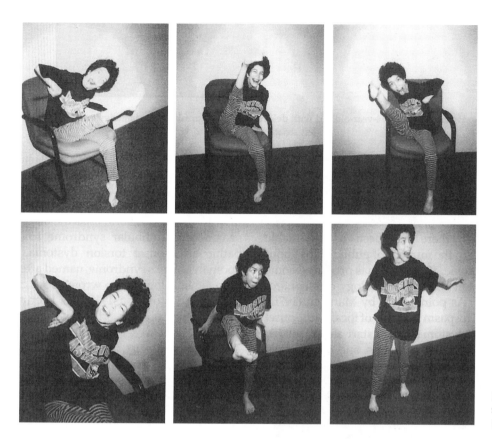

FIG. 23.3. A 33-year-old woman with severe, generalized primary dystonia, progressive since age 4.

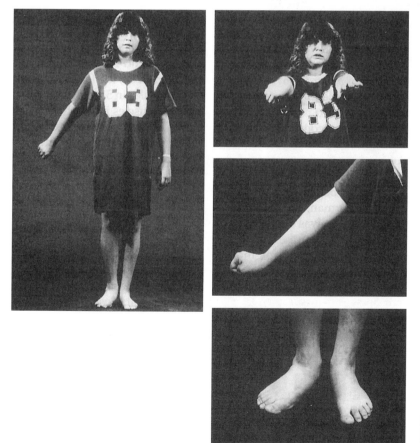

FIG. 23.4. A 14-year-old girl with delayed-onset progressive right hemidystonia due to left striatal injury at age 2.

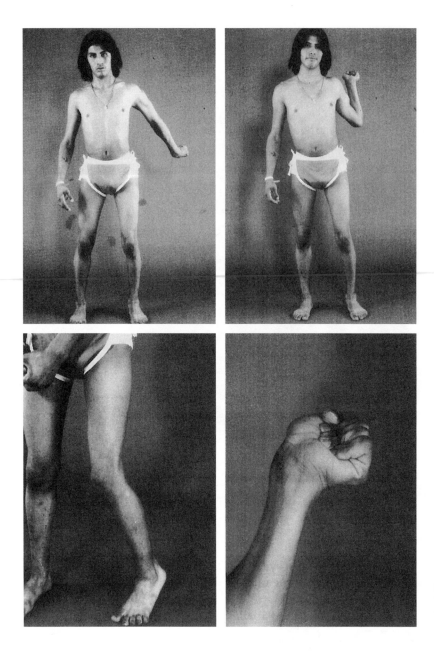

FIG. 23.5. Dystonic abduction and extension of the left arm and flexion of the left hand associated with left hemidystonia due to right putamenal postencephalitic lesion.

general population of dystonic individuals because, by virtue of referral to a specialty clinic, this population is biased toward more severe and atypical cases. It is likely, for example, that dystonic writer's cramp is much more common in the general population than is indicated by these figures. Several rating scales, including the Toronto Western Spasmodic Torticollis Scale (TWSTRS) (25,26), Barry-Albright Dystonia (BAD) Scale (27), Unified Dystonia Rating Scale (UDRS), and Blepharospasm Disability Scale (28), are currently used to assess the severity of dystonia.

Cranial Dystonia

Since craniocervical structures are most frequently affected by dystonia, the characteristic clinical features of craniocer-

vical dystonia will be emphasized. Blepharospasm, an involuntary bilateral eye closure produced by spasmodic contractions of the entire (pretarsal, preseptal, and periorbital) orbicularis oculi muscles, is often accompanied by dystonic movements of the eyebrows and of the paranasal, facial, masticatory, labial, lingual, oral, pharyngeal, laryngeal, and cervical muscles (Fig. 23.6). Blepharospasm usually affects women (3:1 in comparison to men) older than 50 years (29). Blepharospasm is often exacerbated by exposure to bright light, wind, and air pollution, as well as by movement and stress. Although some patients with blepharospasm may seem somewhat anxious and talkative, there is no evidence that blepharospasm is associated with any overt psychopathology (30). When it occurs only in response to certain stimuli, such as sudden visual threat or

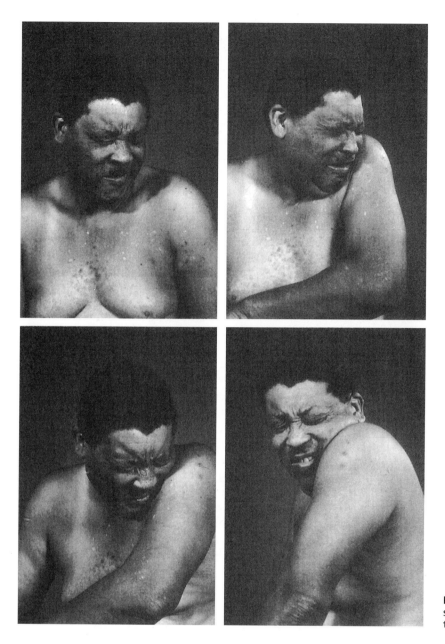

FIG. 23.6. Patient with craniocervical dystonia showing blepharospasm, oromandibular dystonia, torticollis, and left shoulder shrug.

auditory or tactile stimuli, the term *reflex blepharospasm* is used. Reflex blepharospasm is also seen in premature infants and patients with various parkinsonian syndromes, nondominant temporoparietal lobe lesions (Fisher's sign), and a variety of ocular disorders, including blepharitis, conjunctivitis, iritis, and dry-eye syndrome. Eventually patients have difficulty reading, watching television, driving, and performing other daily activities that depend on normal vision. Various "tricks," such as pulling on an upper eyelid, pinching the neck, talking, humming, or singing, can transiently relieve the involuntary eye closure in some patients. Because of the fluctuating symptoms, exacerbation by emotional stimuli, and frequent association with logorrhea, anxiety, and depression, there is a tendency to label blepharospasm as a psychogenic problem.

A form of focal adult-onset torsion dystonia, blepharospasm can start as an isolated movement of the eyelids. If blepharospasm occurs alone, without the involvement of other craniocervical structures, then the term "essential blepharospasm" might be appropriate. However, in the vast majority of blepharospasm patients, the other facial, pharyngeal, or cervical muscles are also involved, and therefore the term "craniocervical dystonia" best describes the condition. The eponym Meige's syndrome, named after the French neurologist who wrote about craniocervical dystonia in 1910, has been used in the literature to describe this movement disorder. However, Horatio Wood, a Philadelphia neurologist, described facial and oromandibular dystonias in 1887, 23 years before Meige. Therefore, the generic term craniocervical dystonia is more appropriate for this disorder.

In addition to dystonia, other conditions can lead to closure of the eyelids, such as ptosis due to weakness or paralysis of the levator palpebrae muscle or the smooth muscle of Müller. Some patients are unable to open their eyes because they cannot "activate" the levator palpebrae muscles. This is analogous to the motor blocks or the freezing phenomenon experienced by some, and the terms "apraxia of eyelid opening" and "eyelid freezing" have been used to describe this disorder. Apraxia of eyelid opening may occur in isolation without any other motor deficits, or it may be combined with blepharospasm or associated with parkinsonian disorders. The inability to open one's eyes has been attributed to absence of contraction or even inhibition of the levator palpebrae (despite compensatory frontalis contraction), but others have argued that this sign was caused by isolated contraction of the pretarsal orbicularis oculi. In some cases electromyographic recording from the levator palpebrae and orbicularis oculi muscles is required to differentiate this persistent pretarsal orbicularis oculi contraction from the levator inhibition.

Oromandibular dystonia may cause jaw closure with trismus and bruxism, or involuntary jaw opening or deviation, interfering with speaking and chewing and often causing severe pain or discomfort due to secondary temporomandibular joint syndrome (31–33) (Fig. 23.7). Many patients have noted that various maneuvers (sensory tricks) and dental prosthetic devices relieve their jaw spasms, particularly jaw closure dystonia (34). Oromandibular dystonia may follow jaw injury or surgery and may be complicated by secondary dental wear and temporomandibular joint syndrome (35). Besides primary or peripherally induced dystonia, oromandibular dystonia may be associated with or secondary to a variety of neurodegenerative disorders, such as neuroacanthocytosis (36), Huntington's

disease (36), and brainstem lesions (37). Oromandibular dystonia should be differentiated from hemifacial or hemimasticatory spasm, tetany, tetanus, trismus, and mechanical disorder of the jaw or the temporomandibular joint (32,38).

Blepharospasm is usually idiopathic, but many cases are associated with lesions in the rostral brainstem or the basal ganglia (39). A variety of lesions in this area, including stroke, multiple sclerosis, encephalitis, thalamotomy, hydrocephalus, as well as autoimmune and other disorders, can produce craniocervical dystonia. An abnormal excitatory drive from the basal ganglia to the facial and other motor brainstem nuclei has been proposed as a mechanism of the blepharospasm seen after lesions in the midbrain-diencephalic area (40). Some support for this hypothesis is provided by neurophysiologic studies demonstrating increased amplitude and duration of the R1 and R2 blink response and increased duration of the corneal reflex in blepharospasm patients. In addition, acoustic reflex abnormalities have been found in 87% of patients with craniocervical dystonia (41).

As in other forms of dystonia, genetic factors might also be important in craniocervical dystonia. Besides idiopathic or familial forms, some patients with craniocervical dystonia have secondary dystonias (42). These include drug-induced dystonia, such as that seen after withdrawal from dopamine-blocking agents (tardive dystonia) (43,44) or caused by levodopa and other drugs known to produce abnormal involuntary movements. Furthermore, an injury to or surgery on the eye, jaw, teeth, and other facial structures can trigger blepharospasm or oromandibular dystonia (35). A corneal lesion has been found to enhance the gain of blink reflex and as such has been proposed as an animal model for dystonic blepharospasm (45). Postmortem stud-

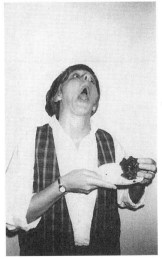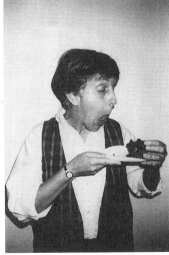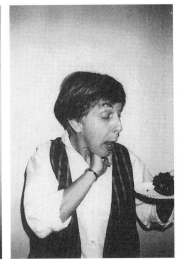

FIG. 23.7. Patient with oromandibular jaw-opening dystonia that interferes with her ability to eat.

ies of brains of patients with craniocervical dystonia usually show no specific pathology. Some postmortem studies of brains of patients with primary adult-onset dystonia have demonstrated a significant increase in copper levels and a reduction of copper-transporting Menkes protein in the lentiform nuclei (as well as reduced Menkes mRNA copies and lower copper levels in leukocytes) compared with controls (46).

Cervical Dystonia

Cervical dystonia is the most common form of focal dystonia encountered in a movement disorders clinic (47). In addition to turning (torticollis), flexing (anterocollis), or extending (retrocollis) of the neck, the head might be shifted forward or off the midline to either side, or tilted toward one shoulder (Fig. 23.8). Frequently, the shoulder is elevated and displaced anteriorly on the side toward which the chin is pointing. In 300 patients with cervical dystonia studied at Baylor College of Medicine (Houston), 61% of whom were women, the mean age was 49.7 years and the mean duration of dystonia 7.8 years (48). Torticollis was present in 82%, laterocollis in 42%, retrocollis in 29%, and anterocollis in 25%. Majority (66%) of the patients had a combination of these abnormal postures; in addition, scoliosis was present in 39%. In addition to cervical involvement, 16% of patients had oral dystonia, 12% mandibular dystonia, 10% hand/arm dystonia, and 10% blepharospasm.

While in some patients the head deviation produced by cervical dystonia is constant, the majority display "spasmodic" contractions of the neck muscles causing rhythmic, jerky movements of the head in the direction of the most active muscles. These muscles can be identified readily by palpation, which reveals not only the active contractions but also hypertrophy (Fig. 23.9). However, if not performed properly, such an examination can be misleading and may fail to differentiate between the agonist and compensating antagonist muscles, both of which typically contract simultaneously in dystonia. In order to identify the most involved muscles, we find it helpful to instruct the patient to close his or her eyes and to allow the head to "draw" or deviate into the most comfortable position without any active volitional resistance. Electromyographic (EMG) recordings of the cervical muscles can be helpful in such an evaluation (49). Blocking the active contraction of the agonist by local injection of an anesthetic or by botulinum toxin (BTX) causes a reduction in the activity in the antagonist muscle. On the other hand, paralyzing the antagonist muscles should not alter the contraction of the agonist.

Patients with cervical dystonia have been found to have an increased risk of secondary degenerative changes of the upper cervical spine, particularly on the side ipsilateral to the head tilt (50). This cervical arthritis can contribute to the pain, limitation of head movement, and poor response to BTX and surgical therapy. Evidence of secondary cervical radiculopathy was noted in 32% of the patients at Baylor (48). One patient developed left arm paralysis due to a thoracic outlet syndrome produced by a hypertrophied left sternocleidomastoid muscle (Fig. 23.9). The arm weakness improved after a myotomy of the muscle. Torticollis accompanied by pain seems to have a less favorable prognosis and response to therapy than painless torticollis. Some investigators have also postulated central mechanisms for the pain associated with cervical dystonia (51). In addition to pain,

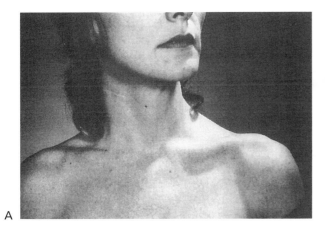
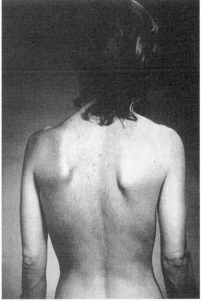

FIG. 23.8. A: Patient with torticollis that persists even after right sternocleidomastoid myectomy. **B:** Same patient with torticollis showing the segmental involvement of the upper trunk and left scapula.

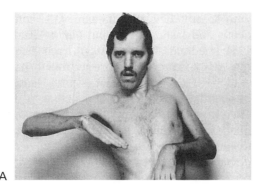
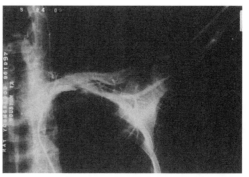

A

B

FIG. 23.9. A: A 23-year-old schizophrenic man with tardive torticollis and a hypertrophy of the left sternocleidomastoid muscle causing marked left arm weakness and atrophy due to thoracic outlet syndrome. **B:** An arteriogram showing occlusion of the left subclavian artery, compressed by enlarged left neck muscles.

some patients with cervical dystonia also have dysphagia due to delayed swallow initiation (52).

Cervical dystonia is often exacerbated during periods of stress or fatigue and is usually relieved by relaxation and various sensory maneuvers. Although some series have reported that up to 23% of patients with spasmodic torticollis achieve spontaneous and lasting remission, a remission rate of 10% is probably more accurate. Remission, if it occurs, is most frequently noted during the first 3 years after the onset of symptoms and is more likely in patients with spasmodic or "jerky" dystonia than in patients with constant neck deviation. However, in the vast majority of patients cervical dystonia is a lifelong disorder, and in about 20% of patients it progresses to segmental or generalized dystonia. Similar to other forms of dystonia, the abnormal muscle contractions that produce head deviation can be temporarily controlled by a variety of sensory tricks, such as touching the chin, face, or back of the head. In a study of 50 patients with Cervical dystonia known to have at least one sensory trick, 54% of them had two to five tricks and 82% had a reduction of head deviation at least 30% (53). While this observation suggests that cervical dystonia can be influenced by altering the proprioceptive input, the exact mechanism of the "counterpressure," "sensory trick," or "geste antagoniste" phenomenon is not known (18). In one study of patients with cervical dystonia, using H$_2$^{15}O positron emission tomography (PET), Naumann et al. (54) found that keeping the head in primary position by application of a sensory trick decreased motor cortical activation (including the anterior part of the supplementary motor cortex) contralateral to the side to which the head tends to turn. In addition, the sensory trick is associated with increased activation of the parietal cortex ipsilateral to the direction of dystonic head rotation.

The pathophysiologic mechanisms underlying cervical dystonia have not been elucidated. While some studies have suggested primary disturbance in the vestibular system, other studies concluded that the "vestibular hyperactivity" noted in some patients with cervical dystonia was "secondary" (55). Some investigators found that patients with torticollis seemed to relate "straight ahead" to the orientation of their trunks rather than their heads, thus implying faulty processing of the afferent signals from the vestibular apparatus and from proprioceptors in the neck (56). It is possible that when torticollis patients utilize a sensory trick they provide needed additional proprioceptive input to restore their head position. The repetitive head movement seen particularly in phasic cervical dystonia may result in disruption of normal vestibular input and a perception if impaired dynamic equilibrium (57). An involvement of the midbrain in the pathogenesis of cervical dystonia has been suggested by reports of torticollis secondary to midbrain lesions and posterior fossa and spinal cord tumors (58).

Similar to other forms of idiopathic dystonia, genetic mechanisms seem to have an important role in the pathogenesis of cervical dystonia. A family history of some movement disorder was present in 44% (dystonia in 20% and tremor in 32%) of the patients studied at Baylor (48) and a family history of dystonia was present in 12% of the Columbia-Presbyterian patients (59). Tardive dystonia was the cause in 6%, and 11% had onset of their dystonia after a neck trauma. Central and peripheral trauma has been implicated not only in the etiology of some cases of cervical dystonia, but also in other forms of focal dystonia (60,61). In contrast to the mobile dystonic posture, seen typically in patients with primary dystonia, the posttraumatic, peripherally induced dystonia is often characterized by a fixed posture, absence of sensory tricks and activation maneuvers, focal muscle hypertrophy, and severe causalgia, sometimes referred to as "complex regional pain syndrome" (CRPS) (60).

Laryngeal Dystonia (Spasmodic Dysphonia)

The career of a teacher, a trial attorney, or a professional singer can be prematurely terminated with the development of spasmodic dysphonia. Despite growing evidence in support of neurologic origin, the symptoms are still too often attributed to psychogenic causes. Dystonia of the larynx may cause excessive and uncontrolled closing of the vocal folds (adductor spasmodic dysphonia), producing effortful and strained voice interrupted by frequent breaks in phonation (voiceless pauses). The abductor form of spasmodic dysphonia is much less common, consisting of prolonged vocal fold openings producing breathy and whispering voice and phonatory pauses extending into vowels. Adductor spasmodic dysphonia is caused by hyperadductions of the thyroarytenoid vocalis complex, and the abductor form of spasmodic dysphonia is due to contractions of the posterior cricoarytenoid muscle. Whereas nearly all cases of adductor spasmodic dysphonia are thought to represent a form of focal dystonia, many cases of abductor dysphonia are thought to be of psychogenic origin. Spasmodic dysphonia often begins as a task-specific focal (laryngeal) dystonia affecting either the speaking voice or the singing voice, but the symptoms usually progress to involve both speaking and singing voice. Many patients with spasmodic dysphonia also have voice tremor, and in some cases isolated voice tremor precedes the onset of spasmodic dysphonia by several years. Patients with spasmodic dysphonia may also complain of difficulties breathing, and respiratory muscles may be affected in dystonia even without laryngeal involvement (62).

Respiratory involvement in dystonia may be manifested by deep inspiratory gasps, loud breathing, respiratory arrests, and respiratory dysregulation.

Limb Dystonia

Idiopathic limb dystonia usually starts as an action dystonia, whereas secondary dystonia may begin as dystonia at rest. The task-specific, focal dystonia seen in many occupational cramps is the most common example of idiopathic arm dystonia. This type of focal dystonia often occurs in association with writing, typing, and feeding; during certain sports-related activities; and during the playing of musical instruments (13,14). Like cervical dystonia, the distal, focal, task-specific dystonias are often associated with either dystonic or essential-type tremor. Such dystonic tremor occurs only during a specific action, and the tremor may not be evident when arms are outstretched in front of the body or when placed in any other position.

The legs are involved quite often in children as the initial site of primary generalized dystonia; however, they are affected only rarely in adult dystonic patients. When dystonia affects the foot of an adult one should consider the possibility of Parkinson's disease or a parkinsonian syndrome as the cause (10). The striatal foot deformity, with unilateral equinovarus dystonic posture of the foot and extension of the big toe (sometimes confused with Babinski's sign), may

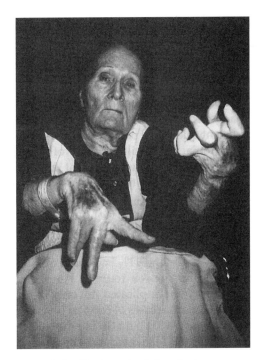

FIG. 23.10. "Striatal" dystonic deformity in a woman with Parkinson's disease.

be seen in as many as half of patients with Parkinson's disease. Besides the striatal foot, some Parkinson's patients have a striatal hand deformity, often confused with rheumatoid arthritis (Fig. 23.10). We have also observed patients in whom foot or leg dystonia was the initial manifestation of the stiff-man syndrome, associated with positive antibodies against glutamic acid dehydrogenase (63).

Trunk Dystonia

Trunk dystonia can result in scoliosis, lordosis, kyphosis, tortipelvis, and opisthotonic posturing (Fig. 23.11). At onset, the truncal movements may be seen during walking or running, but in the advanced stages of disease the trunk deformities become fixed and present even when the patient is sitting or lying. As a result of trunk dystonia many patients have a very bizarre gait, phenomenologically linked to gaits of various animals; hence the terms "dromedary-like," "monkey-like," and "duck-like" gait. Various sensory tricks, such as placing hands in pockets, behind the neck or back, or on the hip, might enable the patient to walk relatively normally. Also, running or walking backward or dancing might improve the truncal dystonia and dystonic gait. A study of 18 patients with adult-onset, severe, predominantly axial primary dystonia showed that, similar to the other adult-onset dystonias, this form of dystonia tends to remain focal (64).

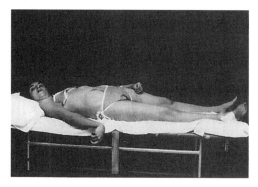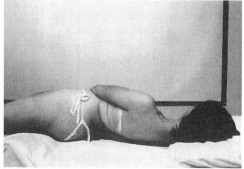

FIG. 23.11. Young woman with severe generalized, predominantly trunk, tardive dystonia.

Hemidystonia

In contrast to other types of dystonias, which are usually idiopathic, about 75% of patients with hemidystonia have computed tomography (CT) or magnetic resonance imaging (MRI) evidence of contralateral basal ganglia lesion, a history of hemiparesis, or both. Infarction or hemorrhage involving the basal ganglia, particularly the putamen, preceded onset of hemidystonia in one third of patients; other causes included perinatal trauma, head trauma, infarction, thalamotomy, encephalitis, AIDS, neurodegenerative disorders, arteriovenous malformation, and porencephalic cyst (Fig. 23.5) (65–68). In 190 cases of hemidystonia reviewed by Chuang et al. (68), stroke, trauma, and perinatal injury were responsible for most cases. While a relatively long delay of several years is somewhat typical for dystonia related to perinatal injury (69,70), the latency between the acute lesion and subsequent onset of dystonia is often less than 6 months in adult patients. It has been postulated that contralateral dystonia results from striatal lesions, particularly in the putamen or the striatopallidothalamic pathway (70). Because the corticospinal tract is spared for the most part, the abnormal input into the premotor cortex is expressed as dystonic movements. Rarely, hemidystonia may be associated with hemiparkinsonism and hemiatrophy (10,68,71).

Classification by Age at Onset

Whereas childhood-onset dystonias often become generalized, adult-onset dystonias tend to remain focal or segmental. In the majority of patients with childhood-onset dystonia, the disorder progresses into generalized dystonia, whereas patients with adult-onset movements only rarely manifest generalized dystonia.

ETIOLOGY

When dystonia occurs as an isolated neurologic disorder without any evidence of cognitive abnormalities, seizures, weakness, sensory or cerebellar deficit, and without other movement disorders, it is classified as primary dystonia (previously referred to as idiopathic torsion dystonia). Primary dystonia can be either sporadic or inherited. The genetic forms of dystonia will be discussed later.

Secondary dystonias, caused by a specific structural or metabolic etiologic factor, are usually associated with additional neurologic findings; therefore, the secondary dystonias are often classified as "dystonia-plus" syndromes (10,42). Whereas primary dystonia usually begins gradually as an action dystonia, secondary dystonias often begin suddenly and occur at rest from the onset (Table 23.4). Secondary dystonia may occur after a specific event such as head trauma, encephalitis, stroke, brain surgery, or exposure to certain drugs or toxins, and in association with a variety of systemic and neurodegenerative disorders (42,72). Virtually any metabolic or structural lesion of the brain, particularly if it involves the putamen, other basal ganglia, rostral brainstem, and upper cervical lesions have been associated with dystonia (Table 23.1). In a multivariate analysis of 202 patients with adult-onset primary dystonia, the Italian Movement Disorders Study Group identified the following

TABLE 23.4. SECONDARY (SYMPTOMATIC) DYSTONIA

1. Etiologic history: perinatal problems, encephalitis, head/neck trauma, peripheral injury, toxin/drug exposure
2. Sudden onset and rapid progression
3. Onset in infancy
4. Cranial onset in childhood
5. Onset in legs in adulthood
6. Abnormal neurologic findings: dementia, apraxia, seizures, ocular/visual disturbance, ataxia, weakness, amyotrophy, spasticity, areflexia, sensory deficit, parkinsonism, dysautonomia, systemic and skeletal abnormalities
7. Hemidystonia
8. Fixed posture
9. Early speech involvement
10. Evidence for psychogenic etiology
11. Abnormal brain imaging
12. Abnormal laboratory studies

for the development of dystonia: head or facial trauma with loss of consciousness, family history of dystonia, family history of tremor, and local body injury and dystonia of the same body part (73). Although genetic predisposition has been suggested to play a role in some cases of secondary dystonia, the presence of the DYT1 haplotype does not seem to contribute to secondary dystonia (74).

Of the secondary dystonias, Wilson's disease is particularly important to recognize because early treatment can result in a complete or nearly complete abolishment of neurologic and liver problems associated with this autosomal recessive disease (75; also see Chapter 17). In one study, dystonia was found in 10 of 27 (37%) patients with Wilson's disease and was the presenting sign in 4 (15%) (75). All children and young adults with dystonia should have their serum ceruloplasmin tested and should have a slit-lamp examination. If the results are abnormal or questionable, then 24-hour urine copper excretion and a liver biopsy for morphology and copper content should be carried out.

One of the most important causes of secondary dystonia is drug-induced dystonia. The dopamine receptor–blocking drugs or neuroleptics (e.g., the major tranquilizers, metoclopramide) can cause not only an acute transient dystonic reaction but a persistent dystonic disorder (tardive dystonia) (43,76). Brain injury is another important cause of dystonia (61). In some cases, there may be a latency of several months or years from the time of the brain injury to the onset of dystonia (69,70). Among the metabolic causes of dystonia, homocysteinuria has been attracting more attention, particularly because homocysteinuria has been associated with dystonia and patients with primary dystonia have been found to have abnormally high levels of plasma homocysteine in comparison with age- and sex-matched controls (77).

Besides central etiologic factors, which presumably account for the vast majority of dystonias, peripherally induced dystonia caused by an injury to a nerve or a nerve root, often associated with reflex sympathetic dystrophy, is being increasingly recognized as an important cause of focal and segmental dystonia (60,78), although this is still a topic of debate (79).

About 40% of all patients with dystonia have been previously misdiagnosed as having a psychogenic illness, but less than 5% have a psychogenic cause (80). The differentiation between psychogenic and neurologic dystonia represents one of the most formidable challenges facing the clinical neurologist. Because primary dystonia is not associated with any laboratory abnormalities, diagnosis of psychogenic dystonia must be based on positive criteria; it is not sufficient to merely exclude other causes. Certain clues usually provide evidence of a psychogenic etiology (Table 23.5). These include false weakness, false sensory symptoms, multiple somatizations, self-inflicted injuries, bizarre movements or pseudoseizures, obvious psychiatric illness, and other features that are incongruous with typical dystonia

TABLE 23.5. PSYCHOGENIC DYSTONIA

1. Incongruous (nonpatterned) movements and postures
2. Markedly fluctuating or intermittent dystonia
3. Inconsistent weakness
4. Inconsistent sensory deficit
5. Multiple somatizations (pain)
6. Self-inflicted injuries
7. Psychiatric disturbance
8. Response to placebo and suggestions
9. Marked distractibility
10. Other abnormal movements, including bizarre gait

(81; also see Chapter 36). Relief of dystonia with psychotherapy, powerful suggestion, placebo, or physiotherapy virtually excludes a neurologic cause because complete and permanent remissions are rare in "organic" forms of dystonia. Improvement under hypnosis or with amobarbital is not particularly helpful because both can ameliorate even neurologic dystonia. On the other hand, acute exacerbation and relief of the dystonia by a powerful suggestion coupled with intravenous or oral placebo provides important support for the diagnosis of psychogenic dystonia (82). Some patients with psychogenic dystonia undergo a variety of invasive and surgical procedures, and may develop Munchausen's syndrome. Using PET functional imaging, Halligan et al. (83) found that hypnotic paralysis and conversion hysteria activated the contralateral anterior cingulate and orbitofrontal cortex, which, they suggested, represented neural activity responsible for inhibiting the subject's voluntary attempt to move the limb. This may provide clues as to the psychophysiologic mechanisms of conversion or psychogenic disorders, including psychogenic dystonia.

GENETICS

Despite the variable presentation and phenotypic heterogeneity of dystonia, many families with genetic forms of dystonia have been genetically characterized, and a genetic classification of dystonia is rapidly evolving (Table 23.6). Most cases of childhood-onset dystonia are inherited, usually in an autosomal dominant pattern. The most important advance in the understanding of autosomal dystonia has been identification of a DNA marker (TOR1A, DYT1) in the q32-34 region of chromosome 9 in a large non-Jewish kindred (84). Subsequently, a 3-bp (GAG) deletion was identified in the fifth exon of the *TOR1A* gene in the 9q34 locus coding for a novel 332-amino-acid, ATP-binding protein, termed torsinA, resulting in a loss of a pair of glutamic acid residues (85). This important discovery not only enabled DNA testing for the abnormal *TOR1A (DYT1)* gene but launched a fruitful research into the cellular mechanisms of this form of dystonia. In addition to the 3-bp GAG deletion, an 18-bp deletion that would remove 6-

TABLE 23.6. GENETIC CLASSIFICATION OF DYSTONIAS

Type of Dystonia	Chromosome Gene Mutation	Pattern of Inheritance	Onset Age	Distribution Additional Features	Comment
DYT1	9q34, GAG deletion TorsinA 18—bp deletion in one case of dystonia, myoclonus, tics, and parkinsonism	AD	<40	limbs	Primary, penetrance: 30% AJ, 70% NJ
DYT2	NM	AR			Spanish Gypsies
DYT3	Xq13	X-linked	<55	parkinsonism (including larynx, stridor), limb	Filipinos (Lubag), cranial mosaic striatal gliosis
DYT4	NM	AD		whispering dysphonia	Australian family
DYT5	14q22.1 GTP cyclohydrolase (many mutations)	AD	<16	gait disorder, parkinsonism diurnal fluctuation	Dopa-responsive (DRD), F>M
DYT6	8p21–q22	AD	A,C	cranial (dysarthria/dysphonia), cervical limb	Primary, Mennonite. 30% penetrance
DYT7	18p	AD	A	cervical, cranial, spasmodic dysphonia, hand tremor	Primary, German families
DYT8	2q33–q25	AD	C	choreoathetosis paroxysmal	
DYT9	1p	AD	C	ataxia, spasticity	paroxysmal, Episodic
DYT10	NM	AD	C	choreoathetosis paroxysmal, kinesigenic	
DYT11	11q23 (D2 receptor)	AD	C	myoclonus	alcohol-responsive
DYT12	19q13	AD	A,C	parkinsonism	rapid-onset
DYT13	1p36.13–36.32	AD	C,A	Cranial-cervical, upper limb	Primary, Italian
Other Genetic Dystonias					
Myoclonus-dystonia	7q21–q31	AD	A,C	myoclonus	alcohol-responsive
Wilson's disease	13,ATP7B	AR	A,C	tremor, other movement disorders	liver disease, copper deposition
Hallervorden-Spatz disease	20p12.3–p13 PANK2 pantothenate kinase	AR	A,C	dementia, seizures	iron deposition
Amino acid decarboxylase deficiency	7p12.1–p12.3	AR	C	dystonia, hypotonia oculogyric deviations	

A, Adult onset; AJ, Ashkenazi Jewish; AD, autosomal dominant; AR, autosomal recessive; CO, childhood onset; NJ, non-Jewish; NM, not mapped.

amino-acid residues close to the carboxy terminus of torsinA was discovered in one patient with dystonia, myoclonus, and tics (86).

TOR1A, which encodes torsinA is a member of a large gene family including *TOR1B*, *TOR2A*, and *TOR2B*. TorsinA is expressed widely in the brain, particularly in the hippocampus, substantia nigra compacta, and cerebellum (87,88). Although the function of torsinA is still not fully understood and its role in the pathogenesis of primary dystonia remains unknown, the protein is a 332-amino-acid member of the AAA+ (ATPases *a*ssociated with a variety of cellular *a*ctivities) superfamily of chaperone proteins with ATPase activity predominantly expressed in dopaminergic neurons (89). AAA+ ATPases share Mg^{2+}-ATP binding domain, an AAA-specific region of homology, and a typical six-membered oligomeric ring structure (90). This doughnut-like ring is situated in the lumen of the endoplasmic reticulum, with each monomer tethered to the endoplasmic

reticulum membrane via the N terminus. The loss of glutamic acid residue in the C terminus apparently prevents closure of the ring or prevents interaction with some partner protein. The wild-type torsinA protein is found throughout the cytoplasm and neurites with a high degree of colocalization with the endoplasmic reticulum. In contrast, the mutant protein forms multiple, large inclusions composed of endoplasmic reticulum–derived membrane whorls in cultured cells (91,92), but not in the brains of patients with DYT1 dystonia (93). However, no alterations in torsinA immunohistochemistry, such as cytoplasmic aggregations or colocalization of torsinA with endoplasmic reticulum, have been found in brains of patients with DYT1 dystonia (93). TorsinA has been found in Lewy bodies, which are cytoplasmic inclusions typically found in patients with Parkinson's disease (94). It is also of interest that the protein has 25% to 30% homology to the 100/Clp proteases family of heat-shock proteins (HSPs), which are normally responsible for protecting the cells from variety of stresses (e.g., heat, trauma, toxins). It is, therefore, interesting to speculate whether central or peripheral trauma somehow alters the brain's HSP and eventually leads to the expression of dystonia in an individual who otherwise would be asymptomatic (nonpenetrant) (60,95). TorsinA also shares features with ATPases that are involved in vesicle fusion, mitochondrial function, and protein translocation. Thus, current evidence suggests that the mutant torsinA interferes with the integrity of the endoplasmic reticulum, membrane trafficking, downstream regulation of vesicular release, and metabolic-energy processes of the cells (90,91). Some preliminary results in PC12 cell lines suggest that torsinA may have a neuroprotective role in making the cells more resistant to the effects of the proteasome inhibitor MG132 (Shashidharan, personal communication, 2002). TOR1A "knock-in" and "knock-down" mice have demonstrated some subtle behavioral changes manifested by increased reactivity in the open field and deficient response habituation, but no dystonia; the knock-out mice do not survive (Dauer, personal communication, 2002).

The single GAG deletion mutation in the *TOR1A (DYT1)* gene is apparently responsible for the vast majority of typical early-onset dystonia, and it accounts for approximately 90% of such cases in the Ashkenazi Jewish population (96). The mutation was probably introduced in the Ashkenazi Jewish population about 350 year ago in Lithuania or Byelorussia (97). This population has a five- to tenfold increase in incidence of early-onset dystonia compared with a control population, and the estimated frequency of the disease in this population is 1:3,000 to 1:9,000. The *DYT1* GAG mutation may be detected even in patients with primary dystonia without family history (98). About one third of those carrying the *DYT1* gene express it clinically (30% to 40% penetrance). However, using [18F]fluorodeoxyglucose PET, Eidelberg et al. (95) found an abnormal metabolic pattern in asymptomatic carriers of the *DYT1* gene that was similar to that of symptomatic individuals, indicating that the penetrance of the *DYT1* gene is considerably greater than previously assumed.

Typically DYT1 dystonia presents as a childhood-onset dystonia usually starting in the foot or hand and gradually progressing to generalized dystonia. However, there are many exceptions to this typical presentation; the phenotype may range from simple focal dystonia, such as writer's cramp, to cervical dystonia, to severe, life-threatening dystonia ("dystonic storm") (17,99). An analysis of clinical features and genetic status of 267 patients with primary dystonia indicated that the clinical feature most highly correlated with *DYT1* GAG deletion carrier status in patients with onset of dystonia before age 26 (100). Using this age at onset limit, the specificity of the DYT1 test is 63% in Ashkenazi Jews and 43% in non-Jews. In addition to testing for *DYT1* mutation in patients with primary dystonia whose age of onset is earlier than 26 years, Bressman et al.

(100) recommend the use of this test in patients with onset after age 26 if there are affected relatives who exhibit dystonia at an early age.

In addition to the DYT1 dystonia, several other genetic forms of primary torsion dystonia have been identified and designated as DYT6, DYT7, and DYT13. A gene locus in the 8p21-q22 region has been identified in a large German-American Mennonite family with craniocervical and limb dystonia (101). This dystonia, designated as DYT6, 8p21-q22, is clinically similar to DYT1 although the involvement is more generalized and it includes the head and neck. A DYT7 designation was assigned to the locus on chromosome 18p in a German family with adult-onset, autosomal dominant inheritance predominantly manifested by cervical dystonia and spasmodic dysphonia (102). However, subsequent studies by the same group caused some doubts about this association (103). Three patients monosomic for large parts of chromosome 18p displayed a syndrome of mental retardation, mildly dysmorphic appearance, short stature, and dystonia. Two patients showed blepharospasm, oromandibular dystonia, and cervical dystonia, whereas the third exhibited cervical dystonia, axial dystonia, arm rigidity, and dystonic posturing of the right upper extremity. Genetic analysis revealed that the common deleted area spanned a 49.6-centimorgan distance, and included the DYT7 locus. The authors note that "dystonia in these patients may be caused by haploinsufficiency of the *DYT7* gene, a new dystonia gene on 18p, or may result from developmental brain anomalies" (104). Another genetic primary torsion dystonia, designated DYT13 and mapped to chromosome 1p36.13-36.22 in an Italian family, is manifested as craniocervical or upper limb dystonia (105). In addition to these gene abnormalities, several studies have demonstrated various polymorphisms, including the dopamine receptor D5 gene (106).

In one family with myoclonic dystonia (also referred to as myoclonus-dystonia), the gene locus was mapped to 7q21-q31 (107). The average age at onset was 6 to 8 years with action-induced myoclonus or dystonia. The myoclonus was usually not startle sensitive, but in all patients it was alcohol responsive. Symptoms tend to stabilize in adulthood although some have developed associated psychiatric symptoms such as depression, anxiety, and obsessive-compulsive disorder. Another family with alcohol-responsive myoclonus-dystonia syndrome has been recently reported to have a Val154→Ile missense mutation in the D2 dopamine receptor (DRD2) gene on chromosome 11q23 and has been designated DYT11, but this mutation was not found in five other families with myoclonus-dystonia syndrome (2). In contrast, positive lod scores were found in all three families with myoclonus-dystonia and one with essential myoclonus, indicating that chromosome 7q21-q31 is a major locus for myoclonus-dystonia syndrome (108). Using a positional cloning approach, Zimprich et al. (109) identified five different heterozygous loss-of-function mutations in the 7q21 gene for ε-sarcoglycan (SGCE), expressed in all brain regions examined. SGCE is one of five members of the sarcoglycan family encoding transmembrane components of trophin-glycoprotein complex, which links that cytoskeleton to the extracellular matrix. It is possible that the loss of SGCE alters the normal neuronal architecture, leading to changes in "wiring" of the normal neuronal circuitry. The 7q and 11q23 loci have been excluded in a large Canadian family with autosomal dominant dystonia-myoclonus, but a linkage to a novel 5-Mb region on chromosome 18p11 has been identified (110).

DRD, designated as DYT5 and inherited in an autosomal dominant pattern, typically presents during early childhood (onset 1 to 12 years) with foot dystonia during walking or running; later, patients may show signs of parkinsonism. The gene for the most common form of DRD was mapped to a locus on chromosome 14 by Nygaard et al. (111) in 1993, and the following year Ichinose et al. (112) discovered four independent mutations in the GTP-cyclohydrolase 1 (GCH1) gene (113). GCH1 is the enzyme that catalyzes the first step in the synthesis of tetrahydrobiopterin (BH_4), the natural cofactor for tyrosine hydroxylase (TH), tryptophan hydroxylase, and phenylalanine hydroxylase (113). This gene defect results in impaired synthesis of dopamine by nigral neurons without degeneration (hypomelanization without neuronal cell loss) (114). GCH1 mutation seems to have a higher penetrance in women than men, thus accounting for the female preponderance in this disorder (115). In about 40% of families, members affected with DRD do not appear to have the GCH1 mutation (116), or the mutation may lie outside the coding region (117). Furukawa et al. (118) found a large heterozygous deletion in the *GCH1* gene which cannot be detected by the usual genomic DNA sequence analysis and might account for some "mutation-negative" patients with dominantly inherited DRD. Well over 100 independent mutations in the *GCH1* gene producing different phenotypes have been described (113,119–121). It has been postulated that the decreased GCH1 activity in the autosomal dominant form of DRD may be due to a dominant negative effect of the mutant GCH1, thus inhibiting the expression of the wild-type protein and reducing the normal enzyme activity, which may also account for the phenotypic heterogeneity of DRD (19). As a result of this dominant-negative mechanism, a single mutation may decrease GCH1 activity to less than 50% of normal (122). Another possibility is that the decreased levels of GCH1 mRNA and protein cause inactivation of one allele of the *GCH1* gene (113).

Because of the large number of GCH1 mutations, a simple DNA test as a diagnostic tool is not going to be readily available and, therefore, alternate diagnostic methods are being sought. Endogenous neopterin levels are low in unstimulated lymphoblasts, but this may not be a reliable test for all cases of DRD since GCH1 mutation may not necessarily affect GCH1 enzyme activity (123). Cerebrospinal fluid (CSF) biopterin and neopterin levels are reduced by 20% to 30% in patients with DRD due to GCH1 deficiency. A phenylalanine loading protocol has been proposed to determine if there is a defect in BH_4, which is an essential cofactor not only for TH, but also for phenylalanine hydroxylase (124). Patients with DRD have a significantly higher phenylalanine-to-tyrosine ratio, whereas biopterin levels are decreased at baseline and after a load of 100 mg/kg of oral phenylalanine. It is not yet clear how sensitive and specific this test is as a diagnostic tool for this form of dystonia. Furthermore, it is important to recognize that not all patients with DRD have a defect in the *GCH1* gene (125).

PET studies have a limited usefulness in confirming the diagnosis of DRD, but they may be helpful in differentiating DRD from juvenile Parkinson's disease in that the latter shows evidence of reduced fluorodopa uptake, whereas fluorodopa uptake is usually normal in patients with DRD. [^{123}I]β-CIT single photon emission computed tomography (SPECT) is also normal, indicating normal striatal dopamine transporter (DAT) (126). Interestingly, striatal D2 receptor binding is increased in symptomatic and asymptomatic carriers of the DRD gene mutation, possibly as a homeostatic response to the dopaminergic deficit.

Although diurnal variation, characterized by worsening of symptoms as the day progresses and relief after sleep, is a typical feature of DRD, such marked fluctuation is present only in half of patients with DRD. Because DRD patients often present with developmental motor delay, stiff gait, and marked postural instability, they are often initially misdiagnosed as having cerebral palsy or parkinsonism. Patients with DRD usually continue to respond well to relatively low doses of carbidopa/levodopa (usual dose is 1 to 3 tablets of 25/100 per day) without developing motor fluctuations, although some patients report a wearing-off effect, with recurrence of dystonia and parkinsonism 6 to 8 hours after the last levodopa dose (127). In one study of 20 patients with DRD, 20% of the patients exhibited mild levodopa-induced dyskinesia (128). In contrast to Parkinson's disease, the short-duration response to levodopa dosing seems to develop more slowly and persists for a longer time (129). Most patients with DRD also improve with anticholinergic drugs (130).

GCH1 mutation is occasionally present in patients who do not exhibit the typical symptoms of DRD. The clinical phenotype and spectrum of manifestations of GCH1 mutation have now been extended to include focal dystonia, intermittent dystonia, and dystonia with onset during the first week of life (125,131). However, the clinical spectrum of the DRD phenotype may include parkinsonism with levodopa-induced dyskinesia, spastic paraplegia, scoliosis (132), and absence of dystonia (120). The diagnosis is further complicated by the identification of mutations in the *parkin* gene on chromosome 6 in some patients with otherwise typical DRD (120). In addition to the motor signs, some patients with DRD exhibit a variety of psychiatric symptoms, such as depression and anxiety, and some families also exhibit deafness (133).

Although the presentation and course of DRD is highly variable, at least three types of GCH1 deficiency have been proposed: (a) heterozygote manifested chiefly by limb dystonia responding to levodopa; (b) compound heterozygote manifested by limb dystonia with developmental motor delay responding to the combination of levodopa and BH$_4$; and (c) homozygote manifested by mental retardation, developmental motor delay, limb dystonia and truncal hypotonia, elevated plasma phenylalanine, low plasma and CSF biopterin, responding to the combination of levodopa, BH$_4$, and 5-hydroxytryptophan (134) (Table 23.7). Studies have shown that BH$_4$ and neopterin are markedly decreased in the brains of patients with DRD (135).

About 40% of all patients with otherwise typical DRD with diurnal variation do not have a mutation in the coding region of the *GCH1* gene, and some of these patients may have an autosomal recessive form of DRD due to mutations in the *TH* gene on chromosome 11p15.5 (113,119,136). While in the autosomal dominant DRD the TH enzyme activity is decreased to 2% to 20% of normal, in the autosomal recessive form the activity is reduced to 30% to 40% of normal and the heterozygotes are normal. A point mutation in this gene, inherited in an autosomal recessive pattern, has resulted in 85% to 98% reduction in the activity of TH and parkinsonism/dystonia phenotype (113). Some members of the family with autosomal recessive DRD have severe dysarthria, rigidity, and progressive contractures, only partially relieved by levodopa. The autosomal recessive TH-deficient form of DRD may start in infancy or early childhood and responds completely to low doses of levodopa. In addition to dystonia, patients with autosomal recessive TH deficiency suffer from mental retardation, developmental delay, limb rigidity, truncal hypotonia, parkinsonism, and overt hyperphenylalaninemia. Furukawa et al. (137) described a 10-year-old boy, a compound heterozygote for a novel mutation in the *TH*-gene, who had levodopa responsive spastic paraplegia and whose father had exercise-induced stiffness.

Other dystonias resulting from inborn errors of metabolism affecting the dopamine biosynthetic pathway include dihydropteridine reductase deficiency and aromatic amino acid decarboxylase deficiency. A disorder with subacute encephalopathy, dysarthria, dysphagia, possible ophthalmoparesis, dystonia, parkinsonism, and quadriparesis responsive to biotin has been described (138). About half of patients with DRD have no family history, and some of these sporadic cases may represent incomplete penetrance of GCH1 mutation or independent de novo mutation (134). The penetrance of GCH1 mutation is much higher in females (87% to 100%) than in males (38% to 55%) and in young individuals.

Besides DRD, dystonia may be associated with parkinsonism in the syndrome "rapid-onset dystonia-parkinsonism" (RDP) (139,140). This autosomal dominant disorder is characterized by rapid development of focal, segmental, or unilateral dystonia, often over a period of hours or days, involving primarily the cranial structures and upper limbs. It is often associated with bulbar symptoms (particularly dysarthria and dysphagia), bradykinesia, postural instability, other parkinsonian features, and depression. The progression is relatively slow and patients respond poorly to dopaminergic therapy. PET studies suggest that there is no degeneration of dopamine nerve terminals and no loss of dopamine reuptake sites. Some members of the RDP family may involve only mild writer's cramp or subtle parkin-

TABLE 23.7. DIFFERENTIAL DIAGNOSIS OF CHILDHOOD DYSTONIA

	Primary Dystonia	DRD	Juvenile PD
Onset	>6	<12	<20
Gender	M = F	F > M	M > F
Foot dystonia	40–60%	100%	>50%
Arm dystonia	45–65%	5–75%	<10%
Axial dystonia	15–65%	5–50%	<5%
Bradykinesia	0	+++	++++
Rest tremor	0	+	+++
Diurnal	0	++	0
L-dopa response	0	++++	+++
Dyskinesias	0	+	+++
Pet F-dopa	NL	NL	
Beta CIT SPECT	NL	NL	
CSF biopterin	NL		
Phenylalanine test	NL	ABNL	NL
Progression	+++	0	++++

DRD, dopa-responsive dystonia; PET, positron emission tomography; SPECT, single photon emission computed tomography; PD, Parkinson's disease.

sonism. Neuroimaging studies are usually normal and CSF homovanillic acid levels have been reported as low. A gene marker on chromosome 19q13 was recently identified in three families with RDP (140,141).

X-linked recessive dystonia, called Lubag's disease and classified as DYT3, has been reported only in natives of Panay Island in the Philippines. The gene causing this form of inherited dystonia has been mapped to the pericentromeric region of the X chromosome, Xq12-Xq21 (142). Some brains of patients of patients with this dystonia-parkinsonism syndrome have been found to have a mosaic pattern of striatal gliosis (143).

Leber's disease is another X-linked recessive disorder has been seen in association with dystonia (144,145); a mitochondrial abnormality has been considered to be the underlying pathogenic mechanism in this disorder. Putaminal necrosis with "striatal slits" on MRI has been reported in some members of a large kindred with Leber's hereditary optic atrophy and "spastic dystonia" (146). Features of Leber's disease, including progressive dystonia and striatal necrosis, have been also observed in Leigh's disease, another mitochondrial striatopallidal disease with yet undetermined genetic defect (147). Another X-linked dystonia, linked to Xq22 locus, is associated with early-onset deafness, cognitive impairment, and corticospinal tract involvement (148,149). Similar to Lubag's, this X-linked dystonia-deafness syndrome is associated with a mosaic pattern of neuronal loss and gliosis in the striatum. Another form of dystonia associated with deafness, as well as blindness and mental retardation, is Mohr-Tranebjaerg syndrome (DFN1/MTS) and has been found to be due to a mutation in the gene on X chromosome that codes for the deafness-dystonia peptide (DDP1). DDP1 is a mitochondrial intermembrane space protein similar to Tim8p, one of five proteins that function as chaperones guiding hydrophobic proteins across the aqueous inner mitochondrial membrane (150,151).

In addition to finding gene markers on chromosomes 8 and 9 for idiopathic dystonia, gene markers or mutations have been identified in a number of secondary dystonias. The Wilson's disease gene has been localized to the long arm of chromosome 13; it encodes copper-transporting P-type ATPase and has been termed *ATP7B* (152). Numerous mutations have been already identified and most patients carry at least two mutations (153). The Wilson's disease gene has a frequency of about 0.005 and a carrier frequency of about 0.01 (see Chapter 17). Linkage analyses initially localized Hallervorden-Spatz disease to the gene on 20p12.3-p13; subsequently, 7-bp deletion and various missense mutations were identified in the coding sequence of gene *PANK2* with homology to pantothenate kinase (154). Because of the recent discovery of Hallervorden's terrible past and his shameless involvement in active euthanasia, the disorder has been renamed neurodegeneration with brain iron accumulation type 1 (NBIA 1) or pantothenate kinase–associated neurodegeneration (PKAN). Finally, many of the spinocerebellar atrophies, particularly type 3 and type 6, have been associated with dystonia (155).

EPIDEMIOLOGY

In a large series of patients with primary dystonia studied in Europe, female predominance was found in all anatomic categories, except for writer's cramp (156). Based on an epidemiologic study in the population living in Rochester, Minnesota, the incidence of dystonia has been estimated to be 2 per million persons per year for generalized dystonia and 24 per million per year for focal dystonia (157). The prevalence of dystonia has been estimated to be 3.4 per 100,000 for generalized and 30 per 100,000 for focal. The prevalence of generalized dystonia among Jews of Eastern European ancestry (Ashkenazi) living in Israel was double that of the U.S. population (6.8/100,000) (158). In the northern England the prevalence of generalized dystonia has been estimated to be 1.42 per 100,000 and 12.9 per 100,000 for focal dystonia (159).

PATHOPHYSIOLOGY OF DYSTONIA

The pathophysiology of dystonia is not well understood, but progress has been made as a result of novel neurophysiologic and imaging techniques (160–162). Excessive co-contraction of antagonist muscles is one of the physiologic hallmarks of dystonia. The co-contraction in dystonia is apparently produced by abnormal synchronization of presynaptic inputs to antagonist motor neuron pools (163). Besides co-contraction, there is an "overflow" of contractions to adjacent or remote muscles, which is particularly noticeable during a volitional movement of the affected limb. The third characteristic of dystonia is the paradoxical contraction of passively shortened muscles (the Westphal's phenomenon). However, this phenomenon is not specific for dystonia and is also seen in spasticity and in parkinsonian disorders. Using the H-reflex technique, reciprocal inhibition, normally a triphasic event lasting up to 1 second, was reduced in several studies of patients with dystonia (162). Although the exact mechanism of this abnormality is not understood, a disturbed presynaptic inhibition of 1A afferents from the flexor muscles has been proposed as a possible explanation. The neurophysiologic findings, including increased duration of both the long latency stretch reflex and the first burst of agonist EMG activity in ballistic movements, suggest that lack of inhibition or excess excitation in both reflex and voluntary movement is the underlying mechanism of dystonia. Abnormalities in early and late long-latency reflex responses have been found in focal dystonia and these can be influenced by BTX injections, suggesting involvement of peripheral mechanisms

(164). Several investigators have demonstrated increased amplitude and duration of the R1 and R2 blink responses not only in patients with blepharospasm but also in those with cervical and other dystonias. These findings have been interpreted as being indicative of enhanced excitatory drive to the rostral brainstem or reduced spinal and brainstem inhibition.

Abnormal processing of muscle spindle input has been suggested as an important element in the pathophysiology of dystonia. Dystonia may be precipitated or exacerbated by vibration that activates sensory fibers, particularly Ia spindle afferents (165). This can be blocked by lidocaine, which blocks the gamma motor neurons. In some studies, however, vibration improves cervical dystonia. Vibration induces presynaptic inhibition and the tonic vibration reflex (TVR), a polysynaptic spinal cord reflex. The observation that dystonic patients have abnormal perception of motion, but not position, in response to a 50-Hz vibratory stimulus was interpreted as evidence for abnormal muscle spindle afferent processing in dystonia (166).

Several studies have suggested that cortical excitability is increased in dystonia (160,167,168). Using transcranial magnetic stimulation (TMS) and recording from the flexor carpi radialis muscles bilaterally, Ikoma et al. (167) found that the area of the motor evoked potentials (MEPs) to the M wave was increased in patients with dystonia, providing evidence of increased cortical motor excitability in dystonia. Using similar techniques, but recording from orbicularis oculi and perioral muscles, Currà et al. (168) found shortened silent period in patients with blepharospasm and other types of cranial dystonia reflecting hyperexcitability of cortical inhibitory neurons in cranial dystonia. This can be modified by BTX injections into dystonic muscles (169). Patients with writer's cramp have been shown to have a deficiency in the negative slope that follows the Bereitschaftspotential, suggesting failure to achieve normal motor cortex activation in dystonia. The deficient activation of the premotor cortex in patients with writer's cramp has been thought to be due to a dysfunction of the premotor cortical network coupled with a loss of inhibition during generation of motor commands (170). Using the Bereitschaftspotential, Yazawa et al. (171) found that patients with focal hand dystonia had abnormal cortical preparatory process for voluntary muscle relaxation or motor inhibition. Studying scalp electroencephalographic (EEG) oscillations in response to self-paced simple index finger abduction movements, Toro et al. (172) found that patients with writer's cramp had less reduction in 20- to 30-Hz EEG (beta rhythm) power compared with controls. Since this EEG activity in the sensorimotor region is related to ongoing muscle activity, the observed abnormality in movement-related EEG desynchronization provides additional evidence for motor cortical involvement in focal dystonia.

More and more studies seem to indicate that the excessive activation of antagonists, overflow into synergists, and prolongation of muscle activation are due to a deficiency of inhibition (173). This has been demonstrated at the level of the motor cortex, brainstem, and spinal cord. TMS studies, using the paired-pulse technique, found evidence of defective intracortical inhibition in patients with dystonia. In addition to a disorder of movement execution, there is growing evidence that dystonia is a sensory disorder as well as a disorder of movement preparation (173). The evidence for the latter includes (a) loss of EEG negativity of the movement-related cortical potential; (b) movement-related EEG desynchronization; (c) deficient contingent negative variation (CNV), which is the EEG period between a warning signal (S1) and a go signal (S2) (172); and (d) inappropriate modulation of the N30 between S1 and S2 in that instead of the normal reduction (gating) of N30 during the premovement period there is no such gating in patients with dystonia (although normal gating does occur during movement) (174).

The role of cortical reorganization in response to altered or repetitive peripheral input in the pathophysiology of dystonia is gaining increased recognition among neurophysiologists, neuroanatomists, and neurobiologists (60,175). Byl et al. (176) provided evidence for involvement of the somatosensory cortex in dystonia. They trained monkeys to perform repetitive hand-grip opening and closing and found, by electrophysiologic mapping of primary somatosensory cortical area 3b, marked dedifferentiation and enlargement of the normal cortical representation of the hand, breakdown of the normal sharply segregated areas of representation, and a change in the cortical topography. Since this cortical area has connections not only with other cortical areas but also with putamen, the alterations described in the above paradigm may have implications for development of peripherally induced movement disorders, such as dystonia, associated with repetitive strain injuries ("overusage syndromes"). Although evidence that anatomic reorganization within the somatosensory cortex leads to a change in function is still lacking (177), it is possible that deafferentation as a result of peripheral injury may not only cause topographic reorganization but may also lead to abnormal function manifested by dystonia. Indeed, Lenz and Byl (178) found that the receptive fields in the ventral caudal (sensory) thalamus were three times larger in patients with dystonia than in those with ET. The notion that abnormal central nervous system plasticity is involved in the development of dystonia is also supported by the alteration in the somatosensory homunculus in patients with focal hand dystonia as demonstrated by topographic mapping using the N20 peak of somatosensory evoked potentials (179). As a result of these and other studies, there is a growing support for the concept of cortical reorganization as a pathogenetic mechanism for some forms of dystonia. According to this notion, environmental experience, such as repetitive motion (e.g., continuous practicing by musicians), prolonged restriction of focal movement, or limb amputation, changes the brain's representation of the periphery. Studies by Merzenich and colleagues (180), as well as by others, have led some investigators to conclude that "fusion of representational zones is at the core of dystonia" (181).

The involvement of basal ganglia and their cortical projections in dystonia is also supported by the finding of reduced glucose metabolism, as demonstrated by PET scans, in the basal ganglia, in the frontal projection field of the mediodorsal thalamic nucleus, and in the frontal cortex of patients with primary dystonia. Blood flow PET and activation studies suggest that the chief alteration in primary dystonia is overactivity of the planning (rostral) portion of the supplemental motor area (SMA), prefrontal area, and caudate nucleus, whereas the motor executive (caudal) portion of the SMA and the motor cortex are underactive. These findings have been interpreted as evidence of thalamofrontal disinhibition and abnormal central sensorimotor processing in dystonia (162). It is of interest that an ablative lesion or high-frequency stimulation of the globus pallidus can produce as well as improve dystonia, suggesting that it is the pattern of discharge in the basal ganglia rather than the location or frequency of discharge that is pathophysiologically relevant to dystonia. Using [^{18}F]fluorodeoxyglucose PET scan, Eidelberg et al. (182) found lentiform-thalamic metabolic dissociation, supporting the notion that dystonic movements may arise from excessive activity of the direct putamenopallidal inhibitory pathway. In a subsequent study, Eidelberg et al. (95) demonstrated two patterns of metabolic abnormality in patients with dystonia: (a) increased activity in the lentiform nuclei, cerebellum, and SMA, found in dystonic patients without evident dystonia during sleep (movement free, or MF), and (b) increased metabolic activity in the midbrain, cerebellum, and thalamus, found only in patients who exhibited dystonia at rest while awake (movement related, or MR). Various neurophysiologic and imaging studies provide additional support for the observation that in dystonia there is reduced pallidal inhibition of the thalamus that may explain the overactivity of medial and prefrontal cortical areas and underactivity of the primary motor cortex (160). In comparison with normal or parkinsonian primates the globus pallidus interna (GPi) discharges in patients with dystonia seem to be lower in frequency and more irregular, with more bursting and pauses, and the receptive fields to passive and active movements seem to be widened (183). Although the physiologic studies, based on lower mean discharge rates in globus pallidus externa (GPe) and GPi suggest an overactivity of both direct (striatum-GPi) and indirect (striatum-GPe-GPi) pathway (184), dopamine receptor ligand studies suggest increased activity in the direct and decreased activity in the indirect pathway. In either case, pallidotomy (184,185) and GPi deep brain stimulation (186) appear to be an effective procedure for patients with dystonia, perhaps because they disrupt the abnormal GPi pattern and thus reduce cortical overactivation, characteristic of dystonia.

PATHOANATOMY AND BIOCHEMISTRY

Although in most patients with dystonia no specific abnormality can be identified by neuroimaging or autopsy studies, there is convincing evidence supporting central origin (basal ganglia, brainstem, or both) for this movement disorder. Lesions, particularly in the putamen and GPi, have been associated with dystonia (66). In one anatomic-clinical study using three-dimensional MRI, "dystonic spasms" were associated with a lesion in the striatopallidal complex, whereas "myoclonic dystonia" was associated with lesions in the thalamus, particularly ventral intermediate and ventral caudal nuclei (187). In another study, using three-dimensional T1-weighted MRI, striatopallidal dystonia was attributed to lesions within the sensorimotor part of the striatopallidal complex and thalamic dystonia was associated with lesions in the centromedian or the ventral intermediate nuclei (70). Imaging studies do not usually show any specific abnormalities, but a 10% enlargement of the putamen was found in patients with focal dystonia (188). Although this finding probably reflects a response to the dystonia, it could also indicate early gliosis in the lentiform nucleus.

Despite high DYT1 mRNA expression in the substantia nigra pars compacta of normal brains, the DYT1 mutation is not associated with significant change in the nigrostriatal DA system, which may explain the lack of response to levodopa (118). Only a mild reduction in striatal [^{18}F]dopa uptake was demonstrated in some patients with familial primary dystonia and in DRD. Perlmutter et al. (189) found about 30% reduction in D2 receptor density as estimated by PET scans of patients with hand dystonia using [^{18}F]spiperone. In patients with secondary dystonia due to midbrain damage, Vidailhet et al. (40) demonstrated evidence of dopaminergic dysfunction using [^{18}F]dopa and three-dimensional MRI. Using two-dimensional J-resolved magnetic resonance spectroscopy to study brain γ-aminobutyric acid (GABA) levels in seven patients with focal dystonia, Levy and Hallett (190) showed a significant decreased in GABA levels in the contralateral sensorimotor cortex and lentiform nucleus.

Biochemical analysis of brains of two patients with generalized childhood-onset dystonia showed a 30% to 80% reduction in norepinephrine concentration in the posterior and lateral hypothalamus and the fourfold increase in the red nucleus (191). Similar biochemical changes were noted in the brain of a 68-year-old woman with a 7-year history of blepharospasm, oromandibular dystonia, spasmodic dysphonia, and anterocollis (192). Neuronal loss in the lateral tegmentum and the compensatory increase in norepinephrine levels (via the locus ceruleus) in the projection areas were hypothesized as an explanation for these changes in norepinephrine. The other neurotransmitters were less affected. Additional postmortem examinations must be performed before it can be concluded that these changes in norepinephrine are pathophysiologically related to dystonia. Although the morphology is normal, copper and manganese content are increased in the lentiform nucleus of brains of three patients with primary adult-onset dystonia (193).

PATHOLOGY

Although autopsy studies of brains of patients with primary dystonia have found no specific pathology, some brains of patients with atypical dystonia have shown a mosaic pattern of striatal gliosis. Similar changes were reported in a 34-year-old Filipino man with X-linked dystonia-parkinsonism (Lubag's disease) (143). Studies of patients with secondary dystonia have identified lesions involving the basal ganglia, particularly putamen, and the rostral brainstem (42).

ANIMAL MODELS OF DYSTONIA

Various animal models of dystonia have implicated a dysfunction in the basal ganglia, thalamus, cerebellum, and brainstem (194). The red nucleus, other rostral brainstem structures, and cerebellum have been implicated in the pathogenesis not only of human dystonia but also of mouse and rat mutant dystonia. Pharmacologically induced dystonia has been studied in monkeys rendered parkinsonian by unilateral infusion of 1-methyl-4-phenyl-1,2,3,6-tetrahydropyridine (MPTP) into the right common carotid artery (195). Using this model, these investigators demonstrated a marked increase in 2-deoxyglucose uptake in the basal ganglia, including the subthalamic nucleus, but decreased uptake in the subcortical structures that receive output from the basal ganglia, such as anterior/ventral lateral thalamic complex and lateral habenula. The authors concluded that dystonia was characterized by increased activity in the basal ganglia outflow pathways. Other studies in MPTP-treated monkeys have provided evidence that D2 receptor stimulation is not only important for antiparkinsonian activity, but it may also result in dystonia; activation of the D1 receptors appears to be important in the genesis of chorea (196). Delayed-onset progressive dystonia has been reported following subacute 3-nitroproprionic acid treatment in monkeys (197).

PSEUDODYSTONIA

Besides dystonia due to central nervous system dysfunction and peripherally induced dystonia, there are many other causes of abnormal postures that resemble dystonia. These syndromes should be differentiated from true dystonia and are classified here as pseudodystonias (Table 23.2). Examples include disorders associated with muscle stiffness and continuous muscle contractions (see Chapter 33), such as stiff-man syndrome (198), Isaacs' syndrome, Satoyoshi's syndrome, and others. Another example of pseudodystonia is flexor tendon entrapment of the digits, also referred to as trigger finger and trigger thumb (177). Characterized by sudden, painful or painless, snapping or locking of the thumb or fingers, this disorder is usually due to thickening of the digits A1 (proximal) annular pulley or other tendon abnormalities at the different finger joints.

REFERENCES

1. Goetz CG, Chmura TA, Lanska DJ. History of dystonia: Part 4 of the MDS-sponsored history of movement disorders exhibit, Barcelona, June 2000. *Mov Disord* 2001;16:339–345.
2. Klein C, Gurvich N, Sena-Esteves M, et al. Evaluation of the role of the D2 dopamine receptor in myoclonus dystonia. *Ann Neurol* 2000;47:369–373.
3. Grimes DA, Bulman D, George-Hyslop PS, et al. Inherited myoclonus-dystonia: evidence supporting genetic heterogeneity. *Mov Disord* 2001;16:106–110.
4. Jankovic J. Tourette's syndrome. *N Engl J Med* 2001;345:1184–1192.
5. Jankovic J. Essential tremor: heterogeneous disorder. *Mov Disord* 2002 (in press).
6. Jankovic J, Beach J, Pandolfo M, et al. Familial essential tremor in four kindreds: prospects for genetic mapping. *Arch Neurol* 1997;54:289–294.
7. Münchau A, Schrag A, Chuang C, et al. Arm tremor in cervical dystonia differs from essential tremor and can be classified by onset age and spread of symptoms. *Brain* 2001;124:1765–1776.
8. Jedynak CP, Bonnet AM, Agid Y. Tremor and idiopathic dystonia. *Mov Disord* 1991;6:230–236.
9. Soland VL, Bhatia KP, Volonte MA, et al. Focal task-specific tremors. *Mov Disord* 1996;11:665–670.
10. Jankovic J, Tintner R. Dystonia and parkinsonism. *Parkinsonism Relat Disord* 2001;8:109–121.
11. Vanek Z, Jankovic J. Dystonia in corticobasal degeneration. *Mov Disord* 2001;16:252–257.
12. Fahn S, Bressman S, Marsden CD. Classification of dystonia. *Adv Neurol* 1998;78:1–10.
13. Jedynak PC, Tranchant C, Zegers de Beyl. Prospective clinical study of writer's cramp. *Mov Disord* 2001;16:494–499.
14. Frucht SJ, Fahn S, Greene PE, et al. The natural history of embouchure dystonia. *Mov Disord* 2001;16:899–906.
15. Scolding NJ, Smith SM, Sturman S, et al. Auctioneer's jaw: a case of occupational oromandibular hemidystonia. *Mov Disord* 1995;10:508–509.
16. Rosenbaum F, Jankovic J. Task-specific focal dystonia and tremor. *Neurology* 1988;38:522–527.
17. Opal P, Tintner R, Jankovic J, et al. Intrafamilial phenotypic variability of the *DYT1* dystonia: from asymptomatic *TOR1A* gene carrier status to dystonic storm. *Mov Disord* 2002 (in press).
18. Jahanshahi M. Factors that ameliorate or aggrevate spasmodic torticollis. *J Neurol Neurosurg Psychiatry* 2000;68:227–229.

19. Segawa M. Hereditary progressive dystonia with marked diurnal fluctuation. *Brain Dev* 2000;22[Suppl]:S65–S80.

20. Jankovic J, Demirkiran M. Classification of paroxysmal dyskinesias and ataxias. In: Frucht S, Fahn S, eds. *Myoclonus and paroxysmal dyskinesias. Advances in Neurology.* Philadelphia: Lippincott Williams & Wilkins, 2002 (in press).

21. Dupont S, Semah F, Boon P, et al. Association of ipsilateral motor automatisms and contralateral dystonic posturing. *Arch Neurol* 1999;56:927–932.

22. Swoboda KJ, Hyland K, Goldstein DS, et al. Clinical and therapeutic observations in aromatic L-amino acid decarboxylase deficiency. *Neurology* 1999;53:1205–1211.

23. FitzGerald P, Jankovic J. Tardive oculogyric crises. *Neurology* 1989;39:1434–1437.

24. Blakeley J, Jankovic J. Secondary paroxysmal dyskinesias. *Mov Disord* 2002 (in press).

25. Comella CL, Stebbins GT, Goetz CG, et al. Teaching tape for the motor section of the Toronto Western Spasmodic Torticollis Scale. *Mov Disord* 1997;12:570–575.

26. Consky ES, Lang AE. Clinical assessments of patients with cervical dystonia. In: Jankovic J, Hallett M, eds. *Therapy with botulinum toxin.* New York: Marcel Dekker, 1994:211–237.

27. Barry, JM VanSwearingen, AL Albright. Reliability and responsiveness of the Barry-Albright Dystonia Scale. *Dev Med Child Neurol* 1999;41404–41411.

28. Lindeboom R, de Haan R, Aramideh M, et al. The blepharospasm disability scale: an instrument for the assessment of functional health in blepharospasm. *Mov Disord* 1995;10: 444–449.

29. Jankovic J. Blepharospasm. In: Gilman S, ed. *Medlink.com.* La Jolla, CA: Arbor Publishing, 2002.

30. Scheidt CE, Schuller B, Rayki O, et al. Relative absence of psychopathology in benign essential blepharospasm and hemifacial spasm. *Neurology* 1996;47:43–45.

31. Wooten-Watts M, Tan E-K, Jankovic J. Bruxism and cranial-cervical dystonia: is there a relationship? *Cranio* 1999;17:1–6.

32. Tan EK, Jankovic J. Bilateral hemifacial spasm: a report of 5 cases and a literature review. *Mov Disord* 1999;14:345–349.

33. Jankovic J. Oromandibular dystonia. In: Gilman S, ed. *Medlink.com.* La Jolla, CA: Arbor Publishing, 1999, 2000, 2001, 2002c.

34. Frucht S, Fahn S, Ford B, et al. A geste antagoniste device to treat jaw-closing dystonia. *Mov Disord* 1999;14:883–886.

35. Sankhla C, Lai E, Jankovic J. Peripherally induced oromandibular dystonia. *J Neurol Neurosurg Psychiatry* 1998;65: 722–728.

36. Tan E-K, Jankovic J, Ondo W. Bruxism in Huntington's disease. *Mov Disord* 2000;15:171–173.

37. Dietrichs E, Heier MA, Nakstad PH. Jaw-opening dystonia presumably caused by a pontine lesion. *Mov Disord* 2000;15: 1026–1028.

38. Wang A, Jankovic J. Hemifacial spasm: clinical correlates and treatments. *Muscle Nerve* 1998;21:1740–1747.

39. Hallett M, Daroff RB. Blepharospasm: report of a workshop. *Neurology* 1996;46:1213–1218.

40. Vidailhet M, Dupel C, Lehericy S, et al. Dopaminergic dysfunction in midbrain dystonia: anatomoclinical study using three-dimensional magnetic resonance imaging and fluorodopa F18 positron emission tomography. *Arch Neurol* 1999;56: 982–989.

41. Lew H, Jordan C, Jerger J, et al. Acoustic reflex abnormalities in cranial-cervical dystonia. *Neurology* 1992;42:594–597.

42. Hartmann A, Pogarell O, Oertel WH. Secondary dystonia. *J Neurol* 1998;245:511–518.

43. Adityanjee, Yeken AA, Jampala VC, et al. The current status of tardive dystonia. *Biol Psychiatry* 1999;45:715–730.

44. Van Harten NP, Kahn RS. Tardive dystonia. *Schizophrenia Bull* 1999;25:741–748.

45. Schicatano EJ, Basso MA, Evinger C. Animal model explains the origins of the cranial dystonia benign essential blepharospasm. *J Neurophysiol* 1997;77:2842–2846.

46. Kruse N, Berg D, Francis MJ, et al. Reduction of Menkes mRNA and copper leukocytes of patients with primary adult-onset dystonia. *Ann Neurol* 2001;49:405–408.

47. Dauer WT, Burke RE, Greene P, et al. Current concepts on the clinical features, aetiology, and management of idiopathic cervical dystonia. *Brain* 1998;121:547–560.

48. Jankovic J, Leder S, Warner D, et al. Cervical dystonia: clinical findings and associated movement disorders. *Neurology* 1991; 41:1088–1091.

49. Deuschl G, Heinen F, Kleedorfer B, et al. Clinical and polymyographic investigation of spasmodic torticollis. *J Neurol* 1992;239:9–15.

50. Chawda SJ, Münchau A, Johnson D, et al. Pattern of premature degenerative changes of the cervical spine in patients with spasmodic torticollis and the impact on the outcome of selective peripheral denervation. *J Neurol Neurosurg Psychiatry* 2000;68: 465–471.

51. Kutvonen O, Dastidar P, Nurmikko T. Pain in spasmodic torticollis. *Pain* 1997;69:279–286.

52. Münchau A, Good CD, McGowan S, et al. Prospective study of swallowing function in patients with cervical dystonia undergoing selective peripheral denervation. *J Neurol Neurosurg Psychiatry* 2001;71:67–72.

53. Muller J, Wissel T, Masuhr F, et al. Clinical characteristics of the geste antagoniste in cervical dystonia. *J Neurol* 2001;248: 478–482.

54. Naumann M, Magyar-Lehmann S, Reiners K, et al. Sensory tricks in cervical dystonia: perceptual dysbalance of parietal cortex modulates frontal motor programming. *Ann Neurol* 2000; 47:322–328.

55. Münchau A, Bronstein AM. Role of the vestibular system in the pathophysiology of spasmodic torticollis. *J Neurol Neurosurg Psychiatry* 2001;71:285–288.

56. Anastasopoulos D, Bhatia K, Bronstein AM, et al. What is straight ahead to a patient with torticollis? *Brain* 1998;121: 91–101.

57. Müller J, Ebersbach G, Wissel J, et al. Disturbance of dynamic balance in phasic cervical dystonia. *J Neurol Neurosurg Psychiatry* 1999;67:807–810.

58. Krauss JK, Toops EG, Jankovic J, et al. Symptomatic and functional outcome of surgical treatment of cervical dystonia. *J Neurol Neurosurg Psychiatry* 1997;63:642–648b.

59. Chan J, Brin MF, Fahn S. Idiopathic cervical dystonia: clinical characteristics. *Mov Disord* 1991;6:119–126.

60. Jankovic J. Can peripheral trauma induce dystonia and other movement disorders? Yes! *Mov Disord* 2001;16:7–12.

61. Krauss JK, Jankovic J. Head injury and posttraumatic movement disorders. *Neurosurgery* 2002 (in press).

62. Lagueny A, Burband P, Le Masson G, et al. Involvement of respiratory muscles in adult-onset dystonia: a clinical and electrophysiologic study. *Mov Disord* 1995;10:708–713.

63. Blum P, Jankovic J. Stiff-person syndrome: an autoimmune disease. *Mov Disord* 1991;6:12–20.

64. Bhatia KP, Quinn NP, Marsden CD. Clinical features and natural history of axial predominant adult onset primary dystonia. *J Neurol Neurosurg Psychiatry* 1997;63:788–791.

65. Krauss JK, Kiriyanthan GD, Borremans JJ. Cerebral arteriovenous malformations and movement disorders. *Clin Neurol Neurosurg* 1999;101:92–99.

66. Münchau A, Mathen D, Cox T, et al. Unilateral lesions of the globus pallidus: report of four patients presenting with focal or

segmental dystonia. *J Neurol Neurosurg Psychiatry* 2000;69: 494–498.

67. Lehéricy S, Grand S, Pollak P, et al. Clinical characteristics and topography of lesions in movement disorders due to thalamic lesions. *Neurology* 2001;57:1055–1066.

68. Chuang C, Fahn S, Fruch SJ. The natural history and treatment of acquire hemidystonia: report of 33 cases and review of literature. *J Neurol Surg Psychiatry* 2002;72:59–67.

69. Scott B, Jankovic J. Delayed-onset progressive movement disorders. *Neurology* 1996;46:68–74.

70. Kim JS. Delayed onset mixed involuntary movements after thalamic stroke: clinical, radiological, and pathophysiological findings. *Brain* 2001;124:299–309.

71. Greene PE, Bressman SB, Ford B, et al. Parkinsonism, dystonia, and hemiatrophy. *Mov Disord* 2000;15:537–541.

72. Janavs J, Aminoff MJ. Dystonia and chorea in acquired systemic disorders. *J Neurol Neurosurg Psychiatry* 1998;65: 436–445.

73. Defazio G, Berardelli A, Abbruzzese G, et al. Possible risk factors for primary adult onset dystonia: a case-control investigation by the Italian Movement Disorders Study Group. *J Neurol Neurosurg Psychiatry* 1998;64:25–32.

74. Bressman SB, de Leon D, Raymond D, et al. Secondary dystonia and the *DYT1* gene. *Neurology* 1997;48:1571–1577.

75. Svetel M, Kozic D, Stefanoval E, et al. Dystonia in Wilson's disease. *Mov Disord* 2001;16:719–723.

76. Jankovic J. Tardive syndromes and other drug-induced movement disorders. *Clin Neuropharmacol* 1995;18:197–214.

77. Müller T, Woitalla D, Hunsdiek A, et al. Elevated plasma levels of homocysteine in dystonia. *Acta Neurol Scand* 2000;101:388–390.

78. Topp KS, Byl NN. Movement dysfunction following repetitive hand opening and closing: anatomical analysis in owl monkeys. *Mov Disord* 1999;14:295–306.

79. Weiner WJ. Can peripheral trauma induce dystonia? No! *Mov Disord* 2001;16:13–22.

80. Owens DG. Dystonia—a potential psychiatric pitfall. *Br J Psychiatry* 1990;156:620–634.

81. Brown P, Thompson PD. Electrophysiologic aids to the diagnosis of psychogenic jerks, spasms, and tremor. *Mov Disord* 2001;16:595–599.

82. Monday K, Jankovic J. Psychogenic myoclonus. *Neurology* 1993;43:349–352.

83. Halligan PW, Athwal BS, Oakley DA, et al. Imaging hypnotic paralysis: implications for conversion hysteria. *Lancet* 2000; 355:986–987.

84. Kramer PL, Ozelius L, de Leon D, et al. Dystonia gene in Ashkenazi Jewish population located on chromosome 9q32-34. *Ann Neurol* 1990;27:114–120.

85. Ozelius LJ, Hewett JW, Page CE, et al. The early onset torsion dystonia gene *[DYT1]* encodes an ATP-binding protein. *Nat Genet* 1997;17:40–48.

86. Leung JC, Klein C, Friedman J, et al. Novel mutation and polymorphisms in the *TOR1A (DYT1)* gene in atypical, early onset dystonia and polymorphisms in dystonia and early onset parkinsonism. *Neurogenetics* 2001;3:133–143.

87. Konakova M, Huynh DP, Yong W, et al. Cellular distribution of torsinA and torsinB in normal human brain. *Arch Neurol* 2001; 58:921–927.

88. Walker RH, Brin MF, Sandu D, et al. Distribution and immunohistochemical characterization of torsinA immunoreactivity in rat brain. *Brain Res* 2001;900:348–354.

89. Ozelius LJ, Page CE, Klein C, et al. The *TOR1A (DYT1)* gene family and its role in early onset torsion dystonia. *Genomics* 1999;62:377–384.

90. Breakfield XO, Kamm C, Hanson PI. TorsinA: movement at many levels. *Neuron* 2001;31:9–12.

91. Hewett J, Gonzalez-Agosti C, Slater D, et al. Mutant torsinA, responsible for early-onset torsion dystonia, forms membrane inclusions in cultured neural cells. *Hum Mol Genet* 2000;9: 1404–1414.

92. Kustedjo K, Bracey MH, Cravatt BF. TorsinA and its torsin dystonia–associated mutant forms are lumenal glycoproteins that exhibit distinct subcellular localizations. *J Biol Chem* 2000;275: 27933–27939.

93. Walker RH, Brin MF, Sandu D, et al. TorsinA immunoreactivity in brains of patients with DYT1 and non-DYT1 dystonia. *Neurology* 2002;58:120–124.

94. Sharma N, Hewett J, Ozelius LJ, et al. A close association of torsinA and alpha-synuclein in Lewy bodies: a fluorescence resonance energy transfer study. *Am J Pathol* 2001;159:339–344.

95. Eidelberg D, Moeller JR, Antonini A, et al. Functional brain networks in DYT1 dystonia. *Ann Neurol* 1998;44:303–312.

96. Valente EM, Warner TT, Jarman PR, et al. The role of DYT1 in primary torsion dystonia in Europe. *Brain* 1998;121: 2335–2339.

97. Risch N, DeLeon D, Ozelius L, et al. Genetic analysis of idiopathic torsion dystonia in Ashkenazi Jews and their recent descent from small founder population. *Nat Genet* 1995;9: 152–159.

98. Brassat D, Camuzat A, Vidailhet M, et al. Frequency of the *DYT1* mutation in primary torsion dystonia without family history. *Arch Neurol* 2000;57:333–335.

99. Kamm C, Naumann M, Mueller J, et al. The *DYT1* GAG deletion is infrequent in sporadic and familial writer's cramp. *Mov Disord* 2000;15:1238–1241.

100. Bressman SB, Sabatti C, Raymond D, et al. The DYT1 phenotype and guidelines for diagnostic testing. *Neurology* 2000;54: 1746–1752.

101. Almasy L, Bressman SB, Raymond D, et al. Idiopathic torsion dystonia linked to chromosome 8 in two Mennonite families. *Ann Neurol* 1997;42:670–673.

102. Leube B, Hendgen T, Kessler KR, et al. Sporadic focal dystonia in northwest Germany: molecular basis on chromosome 18p. *Ann Neurol* 1997;42:111-114.

103. Leube B, Auburger G. Questionable role of adult-onset focal dystonia among sporadic dystonia patients. *Ann Neurol* 1998; 44:984–986.

104. Klein C, Page CE, LeWitt P, et al. Genetic analysis of three patients with an 18p- syndrome and dystonia. *Neurology* 1999; 52:649–651a.

105. Valente EM, Bentivoglio AR, Cassetta E, et al. *DYT13*, a novel primary torsion dystonia locus, maps to chromosome 1p36.13-36.32 in an Italian family with cranial-cervical or upper limb onset. *Ann Neurol* 2001;49:362–366.

106. Placzek MR, Misbahuddin A, Chadhuri KR, et al. Cervical dystonia is associated with a polymorphism in the dopamine (D5) receptor gene. *J Neurol Neurosurg Psychistry* 2001;71:262–264.

107. Nygaard TG, Raymond D, Chen C, et al. Localization of a gene for myoclonus-dystonia to chromosome 7q21-q23. *Ann Neurol* 1999;46:794–798.

108. Vidailhet M, Tassin J, Durif F, et al. A major locus for several phenotypes of myoclonus-dystonia on chromosome 7q. *Neurology* 2001;56:1213–1216.

109. Zimprich A, Grabowski M, Asmus F, et al. Mutations in the gene encoding varepsilon-sarcoglycan cause myoclonus-dystonia syndrome. *Nat Genet* 2001;29:66–69.

110. Grimes DA, Han F, Lang AE, et al. A novel locus for inherited myoclonus-dystonia on 18p11. *Hum Mol Genet* 2002 (in press).

111. Nygaard TG, Wilhelmsen KC, Risch NJ, et al. Linkage mapping of dopa-responsive dystonia (DRD) to chromosome 14q. *Nat Genet* 1993;5:386–391.

112. Ichinose H, Ohye T, Takahi E, et al. Hereditary progressive dys-

tonia with marked diurnal fluctuation caused by mutations in the GTP cyclohydrolase I gene. *Nat Genet* 1994;8:236–242.

113. Ichinose H, Suzuki T, Inagaki H, et al. Molecular genetics of dopa-responsive dystonia. *Biol Chem* 1999;380:1355–1364.

114. Rajput AH, Gibb WRG, Zhong XH, et al. DOPA-responsive dystonia: pathological and biochemical observations in a case. *Ann Neurol* 1994;35:396–402.

115. Furukawa Y, Lang AE, Trugman JM, et al. Gender-related penetrance and de novo GTP-cyclohydrolase I gene mutations in dopa-responsive dystonia. *Neurology* 1998;50:1015–1020b.

116. Nygaard TG, Wooten GF. Dopa-responsive dystonia: some pieces of the puzzle are still missing. *Neurology* 1998;50:853–855.

117. Tamaru Y, Hirano M, Ito H, et al. Clinical similarities of hereditary progressive/dopa responsive dystonia caused by different types of mutations in the GTP cyclohydrolase I gene. *J Neurol Neurosurg Psychiatry* 1998;64:469–473.

118. Furukawa Y, Guttman M, Sparagana SP, et al. Dopa-responsive dystonia due to a large deletion in the GTP cyclohydrolase I gene. *Ann Neurol* 2000;47:517–520.

119. Furukawa Y, Kish SJ. Dopa-responsive dystonia: recent advances and remaining issues to be addressed. *Mov Disord* 1999;14:709–715.

120. Tassin J, Dürr A, Bonnet A-M, et al. Levodopa-responsive dystonia: GTP cyclohydrolase I or parkin mutations? *Brain* 2000; 123:1112–1121.

121. Steinberger D, Korinthenber R, Topka H, et al. Dopa-responsive dystonia: mutation analysis of GCH1 and analysis of therapeutic doses of L-dopa. *Neurology* 2000;55:1735–1737.

122. Hwu W-L, Chiou Y-W, Lai S-Y, et al. Dopa-responsive dystonia is induced by a dominant-negative mechanism. *Ann Neurol* 2000;48:609–613.

123. Bezin L, Nygaard TG, Neville JD, et al. Reduced lymphoblast neopterin detects GTP cyclohydrolase dysfunction in dopa-responsive dystonia. *Neurology* 1998;50:1021–1027.

124. Hyland K, Fryburg JS, Wilson WG, et al. Oral phenylalanine loading in dopa-responsive dystonia: a possible diagnostic test. *Neurology* 1997;48:1290–1297.

125. Bandman O, Valente EM, Holmans P, et al. Dopa-responsive dystonia: a clinical and molecular genetic study. *Ann Neurol* 1998;44:649–656.

126. Jeon BS, Jeong J-M, Park S-S, et al. Dopamine transporter density measured by [123I]β-CIT single-photon emission tomography is normal in dopa-responsive dystonia. *Ann Neurol* 1998; 43:792–800.

127. Dewey RB, Muenter MD, Kishore A, et al. Long-term follow-up of levodopa responsiveness in generalized dystonia. *Arch Neurol* 1998;55:1320–1323.

128. Hwang WJ, Calne DB, Tsui JK, et al. The long-term response to levodopa in dopa-responsive dystonia. *Parkinsonism Relat Disord* 2001;8:1–5.

129. Nutt JG, Nygaard TG. Response to levodopa treatment in dopa-responsive dystonia. *Arch Neurol* 2001;58:905–910.

130. Jarman PR, Bandmann O, Marsden CD, et al. GTP cyclohydrolase I mutations in patients with dystonia responsive to anticholinergic drugs. *J Neurol Neurosurg Psychiatry* 1997;63: 304–308.

131. Steinberger D, Topla H, Fischer D, et al. GCH1 mutation in a patient with adult-onset oromandibular dystonia. *Neurology* 1999;52:877–879.

132. Furukawa Y, Kish SJ, Lang AE. Scoliosis in a dopa-responsive dystonia family with a mutation of the GTP cyclohydrolase I gene. *Neurology* 2000;54:2187.

133. Hahn H, Trant MR, Brownstein MJ, et al. Neurologic and psychiatric manifestations in a family with a mutation in exon 2 of the guanosine triphosphate-cyclohydrolase gene. *Arch Neurol* 2001;58:749–755.

134. Furukawa Y, Kish SJ, Bebin EM, et al. Dystonia with motor delay in compound heterozygotes for GTP-cyclohydrolase I gene mutations. *Ann Neurol* 1998;44:10–16a.

135. Furukawa Y, Nygaard TG, Gutlich M, et al. Striatal biopterin and tyrosine hydroxylase protein production in dopa-responsive dystonia. *Neurology* 1999;53:1032–1041.

136. de Rijk-van Andel JF, Gabreëls FJM, Geurtz B, et al. L-dopa-responsive infantile hypokinetic rigid parkinsonism due to tyrosine hydroxylase deficiency. *Neurology* 2000;55: 1926–1928.

137. Furukawa Y, Graf WD, Wong H, et al. Dopa-responsive dystonia simulating spastic paraplegia due to tyrosine hydroxylase (TH) gene mutations. *Neurology* 2001;56:260–263.

138. Ozand PT, Gascon GG, Essa MA, et al. Biotin-responsive basal ganglia disease: a novel entity. *Brain* 1998;121:1267–1279.

139. Brashear A, DeLeon D, Bressman SB, et al. Rapid-onset dystonia-parkinsonism in a second family. *Neurology* 1997;48.1086.

140. Pittock SJ, Joyce C, O'Keane V, et al. Rapid-onset dystonia-parkinsonism: a clinical and genetic analysis of a new kindred. *Neurology* 2000;55:991–995.

141. Kramer PL, Mineta M, Klein C, et al. Rapid-onset dystonia-parkinsonism: linkage to chromosome 19q13. *Ann Neurol* 1999;46:176–182.

142. Wilhelmsen KC, Weeks DE, Nygaard TG, et al. Genetic mapping of "Lubag" (X-linked dystonia-parkinsonism) in a Filipino kindred to the pericentromeric region of the X chromosome. *Ann Neurol* 1991;2:124–131.

143. Waters CH, Faust PL, Powers J, et al. Neuropathology of Lubag (X-linked dystonia parkinsonism). *Mov Disord* 1993;8: 387–390.

144. Marsden CD, Lang AE, Quinn NP, et al. Familial dystonia and visual failure with striatal CT lucencies. *J Neurol Neurosurg Psychiatry* 1986;49:500–509.

145. Novotny EJ, Gurparkash S, Wallace DC, et al. Leber's disease and dystonia: a mitochondrial disease. *Neurology* 1986;36: 1053–1060.

146. Bruyn GW, Vielvoye GJ, Went LN. Hereditary spastic dystonia: a new mitochondrial encephalopathy? *J Neurol Sci* 1991;103: 195–202.

147. Caparros-Lefebvre D, Destee A, Petit H. Late onset familial dystonia: could mitochondrial deficits induce a diffuse lesioning process of the whole basal ganglia system? *J Neurol Neurosurg Psychiatry* 1997;63:196–203.

148. Hayes MW, Ouvrier RA, Evans W, et al. X-linked dystonia-deafness syndrome. *Mov Disord* 1998;13:303–308.

149. Ujike H, Tanabe Y, Takehisa Y, et al. A family with X-linked dystonia-deafness syndrome with a novel mutation of the *DDP* gene. *Arch Neurol* 2001;58:1004–1007.

150. Koehler CM, Leuenberger D, Merchant S, et al. Human deafness dystonia syndrome is a mitochondrial disease. *Proc Natl Acad Sci USA* 1999;96(5):2141–2146.

151. Swerdlow RH, Wooten GF. A novel deafness/dystonia peptide gene mutation that causes dystonia in female carriers of Mohr-Tranebjaerg syndrome. *Ann Neurol* 2001;50:537–540.

152. Bull P, Thomas GR, Forbes J, et al. The Wilson disease gene is a putative copper transporting P-type ATPase similar to the Menkes disease gene. *Nat Genet* 1993;5:327–337.

153. Xu P, Liang X, Jankovic J, et al. Identification of a high frequency of mutation at exon 8 of *ATP7B* gene in Chinese population with Wilson's disease by fluorescent PCR. *Arch Neurol* 2001;58:1879–1882.

154. Zhou B, Westaway SK, Levinson B, et al. A novel pantothenate kinase gene *(PANK2)* is defective in Hallervorden-Spatz syndrome. *Nat Genet* 2001;28:345–349.

155. Sethi KD, Jankovic J. Dystonia in spinocerebellar ataxia type 6. *Mov Disord* 2002;17:150–153.

156. Epidemiologic Study of Dystonia in Europe (ESDE) Collaborative Group. Sex-related influences on the frequency and age of onset of primary dystonia. *Neurology* 1999;53:1871–1873.

157. Nutt JG, Muenter MD, Melton J, et al. Epidemiology of dystonia in Rochester, Minnesota. In: Fahn S, Marsden CD, Calne DB, eds. *Dystonia.* Advances in neurology, vol. 50. New York: Raven Press, 1988:361–365.

158. Zilber N, Korczyn AD, Kahana E, et al. Inheritance of idiopathic torsion dystonia among Jews. *J Med Genet* 1984;21: 13–20.

159. Duffey P, Butler AG, Hawthorne MR, et al. The epidemiology of primary dystonia in the North of England. In: Fahn S, Marsden CD, DeLong DR, eds. *Dystonia 3.* Advances in neurology, vol 78. Philadelphia: Lippincott–Raven Publishers, 1998: 121–125.

160. Berardelli A, Rothwell JC, Hallett M, et al. The pathophysiology of primary dystonia. *Brain* 1998;121:1195.

161. Crossman AR, Brotchie JM. Pathophysiology of dystonia. In: Fahn S, Marsden CD, DeLong DR, eds. *Dystonia 3.* Advances in neurology, vol 78. Philadelphia: Lippincott–Raven Publishers, 1998:19–25.

162. Hallett M. Physiology of dystonia. *Adv Neurol* 1998;78:11–18.

163. Farmer SF, Sheean GL, Mayston MJ, et al. Abnormal motor unit synchronization of antagonist muscles underlies pathological co-contraction in upper limb dystonia. *Brain* 1998;121:801–814.

164. Naumann M, Reiners K. Long-latency reflexes of hand muscles in idiopathic focal dystonia and their modification by botulinum toxin. *Brain* 1997;120:409–416.

165. Kaji R, Rothwell JC, Katayama M, et al. Tonic vibration reflex and muscle afferent block in writer's cramp. *Ann Neurol* 1995; 38:155–162.

166. Grünewald RA, Yoneda Y, Shipman JM, et al. Idiopathic focal dystonia: a disorder of muscle spindle afferent processing? *Brain* 1997;120:2179–2185.

167. Ikoma K, Sami A, Mercuri B, et al. Abnormal cortical motor excitability in dystonia. *Neurology* 1996;46:1371–1376.

168. Currà A, Romaniello A, Berardelli A, et al. Shortened cortical silent period in facial muscles of patients with cranial dystonia. *Neurology* 2000;54:130–135.

169. Gilio F, Curra A, Lorenzano C, et al. Effects of botulinum toxin type A on intracortical inhibition in patients with dystonia. *Ann Neurol* 2000;48:20–26.

170. Ibánez V, Sadato N, Karp B, et al. Deficient activation of the motor cortical network in patients with writer's cramp. *Neurology* 1999;53:96–105.

171. Yazawa S, Ikeda A, Kaji R, et al. Abnormal cortical processing of voluntary muscle relaxation in patients with focal hand dystonia studied by movement-related potentials. *Brain* 1999;122: 1357–1366.

172. Toro C, Deuschl G, Hallett M. Movement-related electroencephalographic desynchronization in patients with hand cramps: evidence for motor cortical involvement in focal dystonia. *Ann Neurol* 2000;47:456–461.

173. Hallett M. Disorder of movement preparation in dystonia. *Brain* 2000;123:1765–1766.

174. Murase N, Kaji R, Shimazu H, et al. Abnormal premovement gating of somatosensory input in writer's cramp. *Brain* 2000; 123:1813–1829.

175. Meunier S, Garnero L, Ducorps A, et al. Human brain mapping in dystonia reveals both endophenotypic traits and adaptive reorganization. *Ann Neurol* 2001;50:521–527.

176. Byl NN, Merzenich MM, Jenkins WM. A primate genesis model of focal dystonia and repetitive strain injury. I: Learning-induced dedifferentiation of the representation of the hand in the primary somatosensory cortex in adult monkeys. *Neurology* 1996;47:508–520.

177. Moore CEG, Schady W. Investigation of the functional correlates of reorganization within the human somatosensory cortex. *Brain* 2000;123:1883–1895.

178. Lenz FA, Byl NN. Reorganization in the cutaneous core of the human thalamic principal somatic sensory nucleus (ventral caudal) in patients with dystonia. *J Neurophysiol* 1999;82:3204–3212.

179. Bara-Jimenez W, Catalan MJ, Hallett M, et al. Abnormal somatosensory homunculus in dystonia of the hand. *Ann Neurol* 1998;44:828–831.

180. Sanger TD, Merzenich MM. Computational model of the role of sensory disorganization in focal task-specific dystonia. *J Neurophysiol* 2000;84:2458–2464.

181. Elbert T, Heim S. A light and a dark side. *Nature* 2001;411:139.

182. Eidelberg D, Moeller JR, Ishikawa T, et al. The metabolic topography of idiopathic torsion dystonia. *Brain* 1995;118: 1473–1484.

183. Hashimoto T, Tada T, Nakazato F, et al. Abnormal activity in the globus pallidus in off-period dystonia. *Ann Neurol* 2001;49: 242–245.

184. Vitek JL, Chockkan V, Zhang J-Y, et al. Neuronal activity in the basal ganglia in patients with generalized dystonia and hemiballism. *Ann Neurol* 1999;46:22–35.

185. Ondo WG, Desaloms M, Jankovic J, et al. Surgical pallidotomy for the treatment of generalized dystonia. *Mov Disord* 1998;13: 693–698.

186. Krauss JK, Loher TJ, Pohle T, et al. Pallidal deep brain stimulation in patients with cervical dystonia and sever cervical dyskinesias with cervical myelopathy. *J Neurol Neurosurg Psychiatry* 2002;72:249–256.

187. Lehéricy S, Vidailhet M, Dormont D, et al. Striatopallidal and thalamic dystonia: a magnetic resonance imaging anatomoclinical study. *Arch Neurol* 1996;53:241–250.

188. Black KJ, Öngür D, Perlmutter JS. Putamen volume in idiopathic focal dystonia. *Neurology* 1998;51:819–824.

189. Perlmutter JS, Stambuk MK, Markham J, et al. Decreased [^{18}F]spiperone binding in putamen in idiopathic focal dystonia. *Neuroscience* 1997;17:843–850.

190. Levy LM, Hallett M. Impaired brain GABA in focal dystonia. *Ann Neurol* 2002;51:93–101.

191. Hornykiewicz O, Kish SJ, Becker LE, et al. Brain neurotransmitters in dystonia musculorum deformans. *N Engl J Med* 1986;315:347–353.

192. Jankovic J, Svendsen CN, Bird ED. Brain neurotransmitters in dystonia. *N Engl J Med* 1987;316:278–279.

193. Becker G, Berg D, Rausch W-D, et al. Increased tissue copper and manganese content in the lentiform nucleus in primary adult-onset dystonia. *Ann Neurol* 1999;46:260–263.

194. Richter A, Löscher W. Pathophysiology of idiopathic dystonia: findings from genetic animal models. *Progr Neurobiol* 1998; 54:633–677.

195. Mitchell IJ, Luquin R, Boyce S, et al. Neural mechanisms of dystonia: evidence from a 2-deoxyglucose uptake study in a primate model of dopamine agonist-induced dystonia. *Mov Disord* 1990;5:49–54.

196. Boyce S, Rupniak NMJ, Steventon MJ, et al. Differential effects of D1 and D2 agonists in MPTP-treated primates: functional implications for Parkinson's disease. *Neurology* 1990;40:927–933.

197. Palfi S, Leventhal L, Goetz CG, et al. Delayed onset of progressive dystonia following subacute 3-nitroprionic acid treatment in *Cebus apella* monkeys. *Mov Disord* 2000;15:524–530.

198. Murinson BB. Stiff-man syndrome: GABA, GAD, and mechanisms of disease. *Neuroscientist* 2000;6:147–150.

24

TREATMENT OF DYSTONIA

STACY HORN
CYNTHIA L. COMELLA

Dystonia is a central nervous system (CNS) disorder that causes excessive, sustained muscular contractions of both agonist and antagonist muscles. The sustained contractions cause repetitive twisting movements that may be fast or slow (1). Dystonia is often aggravated by activity and may be painful due to the sustained muscular contractions. Treatment for dystonia is required when functional or social impairment occurs. The treatment strategies for dystonia include pharmacologic and nonpharmacologic means and are directed to the type of dystonia present. The pathophysiology of dystonia is incompletely understood and has made therapy less than optimal.

TREATMENT

Treatment strategies are varied and include oral medication, chemodenervation, surgical approaches, limb immobilization and orthosis, and physical therapy. The most effective treatment for secondary dystonia is to focus on the underlying etiologic factor, but standard treatment regimens may be effective when necessary. Medical therapy for dystonia may be effective for generalized, hemi-, segmental, focal, or tardive dystonias. Management of dystonia can be very difficult. Patients do not consistently respond to one type of therapy, and multiple strategies may be necessary before an effective therapy can be found (2). The most common medical therapies for dystonia with their typical dosages are listed in Table 24.1. Each of these therapies will be detailed

in the following paragraphs. A treatment options algorithm is provided in Fig. 24.1.

ORAL MEDICATIONS

Anticholinergic medications have been found to be the most effective oral medication for the treatment of dystonia (3). The first beneficial reports of anticholinergic medications in dystonia occurred in the 1970s (4). Since that time, anticholinergic medications have often been used. Anticholinergic medications are often the first choice of medical therapy used in adults and the second medication trial in most children and adolescents after levodopa. Anticholinergic medications were initially used in an open-label fashion and then double-blind trials were instituted to prove their effectiveness. The initial open-label studies used low dosages of medication. Until high dosages of anticholinergic medications were studied, medical responses were less than optimal. After instituting high-dose anticholinergic therapy, it was found that children are able to tolerate higher dosages of medication than adults and thus had a better clinical response (5). Anticholinergic medications were then shown to be effective in a double-blind prospective crossover trial. In this study, 31 patients with dystonia, primary or secondary, were studied using trihexyphenidyl in dosages up to 30 mg/day. Twenty-two patients had clinical improvement in their dystonia using the Fahn-Marsden scale (6). Anticholinergic medications can be difficult for

TABLE 24.1. FREQUENTLY USED ORAL MEDICATIONS IN THE MANAGEMENT OF DYSTONIA

Medication	Typical Starting Dosage (mg/d)	Typical Therapeutic Dosage (mg/d)
Trihexyphenidyl	1–2	Up to 120
Benztropine	0.5–1	Up to 8
Baclofen	5–10	Up to 120
Clonazepam	0.5–1	Up to 5
Levodopa	100	Up to 800
Tetrabenazine	25	Up to 75

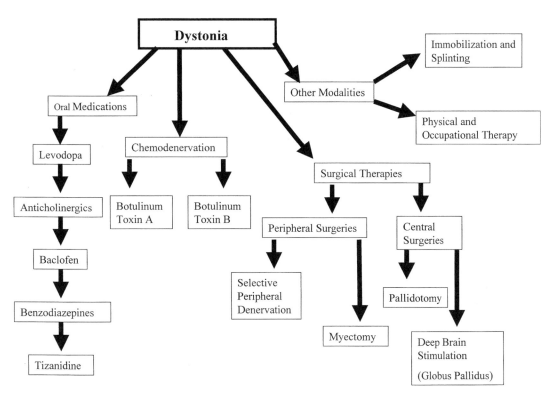

FIG. 24.1. Algorithm of treatment options.

patients to tolerate; therefore, it should be started at a low dose and optimized slowly to clinical effect or intolerable side effects. Children in general can tolerate higher dosages of anticholinergic medications and may need these higher dosages before clinical effect is seen. Fahn has noted that the majority of patients need a minimum of 40 mg/day of trihexyphenidyl for clinical response (7). Children may require dosages of trihexyphenidyl up to 120 mg/day. Open-label trials of anticholinergic medications in adults and children confirmed this clinical suspicion (2,7). Anticholinergic medications are effective in approximately 50% of children and 40% of adults to obtain moderate to marked clinical improvement (7). An open-label trial of anticholinergic medications in 358 patients found a statistically significant difference in treatment effect among patients in terms of the initiation of therapy. It was found that patients treated within 5 years of the onset of their illness were more likely to have a clinical response to anticholinergic medications than patients treated after 5 years of illness (8). Patients with mild dystonia were also found to have a better response to anticholinergic medications than patients with severe disease, such as those who are wheelchair bound (9). No differences in response could be found in terms of gender. Studies have shown that there is no statistically significant difference in therapeutic response to anticholinergic medications between patients with primary or secondary dystonia. Therapeutic response to anticholinergic therapy is thought to wane over time. Greene found a

good therapeutic response for a median of 15 months in all patients, and a median therapeutic response of 38 months for patients with an onset less than 20 years of age (8). Side effects of anticholinergic medications can include memory loss, dry mouth, confusion, hallucinations, exacerbation of acute angle glaucoma, and sedation.

The second medication that will be discussed is the muscle relaxant baclofen. This medication may be useful for generalized, hemi-, segmental, focal, or tardive dystonia. An agonist of GABA, baclofen is thought to work through binding of the L isomer to the $GABA_B$ presynaptic receptor, inhibiting calcium influx and reducing the release of the excitatory transmitters glutamate and aspartate (10). In a retrospective chart review of 358 patients treated for dystonia, 108 patients were treated with baclofen and 20% had a good therapeutic response. The daily dose of baclofen ranged from 25 mg to 120 mg, with an average daily dose of 82 mg. There was no statistically significant difference in therapeutic response between familial and nonfamilial cases of dystonia. Interestingly, patients with blepharospasm had the best response to baclofen when distribution was taken into account. However, this was not statistically significant. Duration of illness prior to institution of therapy did not affect outcome of treatment with baclofen; neither did gender or ethnic background. Patients with an onset of dystonia in adulthood displayed a better response to baclofen than patients with an onset of dystonia in childhood (8). In general, baclofen is less effective than anticholinergic medications for managing dystonia (3). In retrospective studies, 13% of patients with generalized dystonia were found to have a good therapeutic response to baclofen (11). Again, baclofen should be started at low doses and optimized to therapeutic response or untoward side effects. Slow titration schedules may help to prevent side effects. The combination of baclofen and anticholinergics may be very effective for controlling the symptoms of dystonia (12). The side effect profile of baclofen includes sedation, weakness, and memory loss.

Benzodiazepines may be useful for generalized, hemi-, segmental, focal, or tardive dystonia. These medications are thought to work through the enhancement of GABA in the CNS. There are many choices of medications in this class, but the most commonly used is clonazepam due to its long half-life. Benzodiazepines may effectively treat primary, segmental, hemi-, and focal dystonias, but were found to be less effective than anticholinergics or muscle relaxants. Benzodiazepines may be most effective for management of secondary dystonias (8). The typical effective dosage for clonazepam is 2.5 mg to 12 mg per day. No statistical differences were found in treatment responses between ethnic groups or genders. Age of onset of dystonia did not affect treatment outcomes (11). The major side effects of benzodiazepines include sedation and memory loss. These medications may be addictive if taken long term and should always be discontinued slowly to prevent withdrawal. Sudden withdrawal of benzodiazepines can potentially cause seizures.

Levodopa can be a useful agent in dystonia. It is often used as a first-line therapy in cases of childhood- and adolescent-onset dystonia because a small percentage of these patients will have dopa-responsive dystonia. Dopa-responsive dystonia is a childhood- or adolescent-onset dystonia associated with parkinsonism and diurnal fluctuations. These patients have a deficiency of tyrosine hydroxylase and have a dramatic and sustained response to levodopa therapy, with an average dosage of 500 mg to 1,000 mg per day. Full benefit from levodopa has been reported to occur within days of initiation of levodopa. Minor abnormalities of gait may persist after levodopa administration, but most patients achieve a full recovery (13).

Dopamine agonists have also been used in the management of dystonia. Dopamine agonists have been studied in a double-blind crossover trial in eight patients with cervical dystonia. The results of this study did not show statistically significant improvement in the treatment group as compared with placebo. Three patients had improvement while taking a dopamine agonist, but only two patients had sustained improvement for more than a year. No consistent patient demographics could identify responders to this therapy. The major side effects of the dopamine agonists include nausea, orthostasis, confusion, delusions, hallucinations, drowsiness, and memory impairment (14).

Tizanidine has not been extensively studied in dystonia but may be helpful in some patients. Tizanidine is a centrally acting potent noradrenergic α_2-receptor agonist. This chemical causes direct impairment of excitatory amino acid release from spinal interneurons and a concomitant inhibition of the facilitatory ceruleospinal pathway (15). Ten patients with cranial dystonia were studied in an open-label single-blind study using dosages of 28 to 36 mg/day. Five patients did not complete the trial due to untoward side effects. Of the five patients who completed the trial, two patients had unsustained benefit and three patients had no benefit. Tizanidine was found to be ineffective for managing cranial dystonia in this small trial. Side effects were common in this study and included sedation, orthostasis, dry mouth, weakness, nausea, and skin rash. A large-scale double-blind trial will be needed to help ascertain the effectiveness of tizanidine in dystonia (16).

Another medication that may be helpful in the treatment of dystonia is tetrabenazine. Tetrabenazine is a monoamine-depleting and dopamine receptor–blocking medication (17). This medication has not been approved by the U.S. Food and Drug Administration but is available in Canada and Europe. Tetrabenazine has been used in patients with focal, segmental, generalized, and tardive dystonia. Tetrabenazine has been shown to be effective in double-blind crossover studies. Jankovic studied 12 patients with dystonia. Each patient was treated for 3 or more weeks with a maximal dosage of 200 mg/day. Nine patients in this small study had clinical improvement in their dystonia (18). Long-term effects of tetrabenazine on dystonia were then studied. In this study, a total of 201 patients with idiopathic and tardive dystonia were followed for an average of 29 and 35 months, respectively. Of 108 patients with idiopathic dystonia, 62.9% of patients had an initial mild clinical improvement and 45.4% had a mild lasting clinical improvement. Eighty-nine percent of patients with tardive dystonia experienced a mild initial response, and 73% experienced mild response during long-term treatment. The typical therapeutic dosage was 25 to 75 mg/day. The major side effects seen with tetrabenazine include depression, sedation, parkinsonism, orthostatic hypotension, insomnia, and akathisia (19).

Clozapine has been studied in open-label fashion in small numbers of patients with focal, generalized, and tardive dystonia. Clozapine is an atypical centrally acting dopaminergic blocking medication associated with minimal occurrence of drug-induced parkinsonism or dystonia. Clozapine has affinity for multiple receptors, including H1, muscarinic, 5-HT$_2$, 5-HT$_3$, α_1-adrenergic, α_2-adrenergic, D1, D2, and D5. The probable mechanism of efficacy is clozapine's blockage of D1 receptors. The blockage of D1 receptors may reduce the relative overactivity of the direct pathway that occurs in dystonia (20). Since clozapine is an atypical neuroleptic, it has a lower incidence of drug-induced parkinsonism and tardive phenomenon. One study included five patients and found a 30% improvement in their clinical symptoms using the Fahn-Marsden scale.

Patients began to experience clinical improvement after 3 weeks of therapy (21). Patients experienced clinical benefit after taking between 75 and 400 mg/day (21). A second open-label trial consisting of ten patients failed to show clinically statistical benefit in patients with dystonia. In this open-label trial, patients were given 100 mg/day of clozapine (22). The discrepancy between the two studies may be due to dosage differences. A large, double-blind, placebo-controlled trial will be needed to determine the usefulness of this medication in dystonia. The untoward side effects of this medication include life-threatening neutropenia requiring weekly complete blood counts, orthostatic hypotension, and seizures.

CHEMICAL DENERVATION

The paralytic effects of botulinum toxin have been useful in controlling the clinical symptoms of dystonia. Botulinum toxin is the product of an anaerobic bacteria, *Clostridium botulinum*, that is purified and injected into affected muscles. There are seven serotypes of botulinum toxin, A–G. Only two strains are commercially available for clinical use: types A and B. The first clinical use of botulinum toxin was for strabismus in 1980. Botulinum toxin therapy can be useful for treating focal and segmental dystonia. It can also be useful in generalized dystonia in terms of treating focal areas that may be resistant to medications or painful. Botulinum toxin therapy does not alter the underlying CNS dysfunction but does weaken overactive muscles that cause disability and pain. The mechanism of action of botulinum toxin is blockage of the presynaptic release of acetylcholine at the neuromuscular junction. The toxin binds to the presynaptic cholinergic terminals and is then internalized. Once internalized, the toxin inhibits the exocytosis of acetylcholine (23).

Botulinum toxin therapy consisted of botulinum toxin type A, Botox, until 2000 when botulinum toxin type B, Myobloc, was approved for clinical use. Most of our clinical experience to date has been with botulinum toxin A therapy. Clinical effect is typically seen one week after injections and has a duration of approximately 3 to 4 months (24). Botulinum toxin is a foreign protein and may serve as an antigen. In some patients, this may lead to the development of neutralizing antibodies and resistance to the effects of the toxin.

Botulinum toxin type A was initially studied in a randomized, double-blind, placebo-controlled trial for cervical dystonia in 1990. This study was performed in 55 patients and 61% of treated patients showed clinical improvement over the placebo group (25). In 1996, botulinum toxin type A was compared with trihexyphenidyl in a double-blind trial for cervical dystonia. A total of 64 patients were studied in this protocol. This study showed statistically significant improvement of botulinum toxin–treated patients over

trihexyphenidyl–treated patients (26). This therapy is generally well tolerated without any significant systemic effects. The major side effects of botulinum toxin therapy include pain and bruising at the injection site, weakness, dysphagia, and a flu-like syndrome following injection. The high cost of toxin and availability of skilled practitioners to perform this procedure are drawbacks.

Botulinum toxin type B is a serotype that has been used in the management of cervical dystonia. The first study of botulinum toxin type B included 109 patients with botulinum type A responsiveness in a randomized, double-blind, placebo-controlled trial. This trial showed statistically significant clinical improvement in patients treated with botulinum toxin type B over placebo (27). Botulinum toxin type B therapy was also studied in cervical dystonia patients with type A resistance. This study included 77 patients and again showed statistically significant improvement in clinical dystonia over placebo. The clinical effect of botulinum toxin type B was 12 to 16 weeks. The main side effects of botulinum toxin type B include dry mouth, weakness, dysphagia, and pain at the injection site (28).

Both types of botulinum toxin have been proven effective for controlling cervical dystonia. It is not clear if one strain offers any advantage over the other. A large randomized trial comparing botulinum toxin type A and B is being completed to help answer these questions. In the future, other strains of botulinum toxin may be studied to help control the symptoms of dystonia.

SURGICAL THERAPY

Surgical therapies for dystonia are available when medical therapies are inadequate. Surgical therapies include peripheral procedures and CNS procedures. Each of these procedures will be discussed in further detail in the following sections and are listed in Table 24.2.

Patients with cervical dystonia who have developed botulinum toxin resistance or whose symptoms cannot be controlled with medication may benefit from peripheral surgical procedures. Peripheral surgical procedures include rhizotomy, ramisectomy, and myotomy. Rhizotomies and ramisectomies address cervical dystonia by selectively denervating and weakening the overactive musculature. Myotomies attempt to control symptoms of dystonia by partial sectioning of selected muscles. These therapies were employed more frequently prior to the clinical use of botulinum toxin therapy. One retrospective chart review of 58 patients who had undergone rhizotomy for cervical dystonia showed that 85% of patients had a marked improvement in their clinical condition (29,30). A long-term follow-up study of 46 patients with staged, selected peripheral surgical procedures, including rhizotomy, ramisectomy, and myotomy were studied. These patients were followed for an average of 6.5 years postoperatively and assessed using the

TABLE 24.2. SURGICAL THERAPIES IN DYSTONIA

Peripheral surgical procedures
Rhizotomy
Ramisectomy
Myotomy
Intrathecal baclofen
CNS ablative procedures
Pallidotomy
Thalamotomy
Deep brain stimulation procedures
Globus pallidus interna stimulation
Ventrolateral thalamic stimulation

Toronto Western Spasmodic Torticollis Rating Scale (TWSTRS). Forty-eight percent of patients achieved an excellent long-term outcome and 42% of patients had a moderate to mild long-term response to peripheral surgical therapies for cervical dystonia (31). The risks of these procedures include paralysis of arm elevation, neck weakness, and dysphagia.

A peripheral procedure that has been employed in the management of generalized dystonia is intrathecal baclofen. In this procedure, a reservoir with a pump is implanted in the subcutaneous tissue and a specified amount of baclofen is pumped into the intrathecal space via a catheter. Intrathecal baclofen has been effective in the treatment of patients with spasticity for more than a decade, but its effects on primary dystonia are discouraging. Despite case reports of a beneficial response, a retrospective study of 25 patients with severe segmental or generalized dystonia failed to show statistically significant clinical improvement using blinded evaluators of videotapes prior to and after installation of an intrathecal baclofen pump (32,33). A second retrospective trial with blinded evaluators of 14 patients with primary and secondary dystonia again failed to show statistically significant clinical improvement with an intrathecal baclofen pump (34). Two patients with reportedly primary dystonia were clinically improved after implantation of the intrathecal baclofen pump (35,36). The drawbacks and risks of this procedure include overdosage, respiratory depression, pump malfunction, availability, programming errors, infection, cost, and catheter breakage.

Lastly, CNS surgeries may be helpful in controlling the symptoms of dystonia. These therapies are typically reserved for patients who fail medical therapy. CNS surgical procedures for dystonia were found incidentally in the late 1950s. Following ablative treatment for Parkinson's disease, Cooper noted an improvement in the patient's dystonia symptoms. Due to the limited choices for treatment and the varied response, Cooper began to offer ablative procedures to patients with dystonia. This work paved the way for more research into CNS surgical treatments of dystonia.

The first procedures that will be discussed are ablative: thalamotomy and pallidotomy. These procedures are typically useful in patients with generalized dystonia or hemi-

dystonia. Ablative procedures are performed by identifying a desired nucleus in the brain and then creating a small lesion in that area. In these procedures, brain tissue is destroyed.

Thalamotomy was the initial preferred CNS procedure. Targeted nuclei within the thalamus have included the ventral intermedius, the posterior ventromedial, and the posterior ventrolateral. Initial reports by Cooper reported a moderate to marked lasting clinical improvement in 69.7% of patients; however, subsequent reports have failed to reproduce these findings (37). Fifty-five patients undergoing thalamotomy were studied by Andrew. In this retrospective study, 16 patients had generalized dystonia and only 4 patients had a beneficial clinical response to thalamotomy (38). A prospective study by Tasker included 56 patients undergoing thalamotomy. Tasker found that 34% of patients had an improvement of 50% in their clinical symptoms. Tasker noted that patients had an improvement in distal limb mobility but no change in midline symptoms (39). In the studies by Tasker and Andrew, complications included dysarthria, hemiparesis, pseudobulbar palsy, ataxia, paresthesias, and personality changes. These complications were seen more frequently following bilateral procedures.

The second ablative procedure that has been instituted is lesioning of the globus pallidus interna. Again, anecdotal reports of improvement of dystonic symptoms in patients with Parkinson's disease following pallidotomy prompted clinical trials in dystonia. Ondo studied eight patients with generalized dystonia prior to and after pallidotomy in an unblinded fashion. Six patients were noted to have a marked clinical improvement, whereas the other two patients improved, but less dramatically. Interestingly, patients had improvement immediately following surgery but continued to improve over the next 1 to 3 months. Ondo found a decrease in the Unified Dystonia Rating Scale (UDRS) of 62.5%. Adverse events included transient weakness (40).

A small study of 32 patients compared the results of thalamotomy and pallidotomy in patients with dystonia. Although comparison was difficult due to differences in the groups, this study found a statistically significant improvement in pallidotomy patients over thalamotomy patients with primary dystonia (41).

The last procedure to be discussed is deep brain stimulator implantation. This is a relatively new technology that employs identification of the desired nucleus with subsequent implantation of a stimulating wire into that nucleus. The stimulating wire is then burrowed under the skin and connected to a pacemaker placed subcutaneously in the upper chest. The pacemaker can then be adjusted to control the symptoms of dystonia. Experience with this procedure for dystonia has not been extensive. Case reports have found a favorable clinical response (42). A recent retrospective study of 19 patients with medically intractable dystonia reports a favorable response to chronic deep brain stimulation. Patients with primary and secondary dystonia were studied in this group with a minimum of 6 months follow-up. This group of patients was further divided into those receiving thalamic and those receiving pallidal stimulation. Twelve patients were treated with chronic stimulation of the ventrolateral thalamic nucleus. Of these patients, global functional outcome was improved in eight patients, although no significant improvement in dystonia rating scores or disability scores was seen. The second group of patients was treated with chronic stimulation of the globus pallidus interna. This group showed a significant improvement in their dystonia rating scores and disability scores, suggesting that pallidal stimulation may be more effective than thalamic stimulation (43). These study results must be confirmed through examination of a larger homogeneous patient population and blinded evaluation of patients.

Each surgical procedure has its pros and cons. The pros of ablative procedures include less intensive follow-up schedules. The drawbacks of ablative procedures include destruction of brain tissue and a high incidence of side effects with bilateral procedures, including dysarthria, dysphagia, and pseudobulbar palsy. The pros of deep brain stimulation include preservation of brain tissue and the ability to perform bilateral procedures. The drawbacks of these procedures include availability, cost, equipment malfunction, battery changes, and the need for frequent adjustments of the stimulator. Both procedures carry a risk of intracranial hemorrhage and hemiparesis.

IMMOBILIZATION AND ORTHOTIC THERAPIES

A recent article described the effectiveness of prolonged limb immobilization in the management of focal upper extremity dystonia. Eight patients with medically resistant idiopathic focal dystonia were studied in an open-label fashion with focal splinting of the affected limb for 4 to 5 weeks. Each patient underwent six assessments for severity of dystonia and objective motor performance using the Arm Dystonia Disability Scale and Tubiana and Chamagne Score, and subjective improvement using the Self-Rating Score. Each patient was studied at baseline, during the immobilization and following the immobilization. The longest follow-up was 12 months. This study found that at 24 weeks three patients had a moderate objective improvement and four patients had marked objective improvement (44). The proposed mechanism for efficacy involves the pathophysiologic changes that occur in focal upper extremity dystonia. These changes include enlargement and smearing of the cortical areas representing the affected muscles (45–48). Immobilization may possibly promote inactivity-dependent plastic changes in the overrepresented cortical areas and thus help to restore normal cortical representation (49). These initial results are promising, but additional large-scale studies will be needed to confirm these results. The major side effect experienced with limb immobilization is muscular weakness following removal of the splint that gradually improves with activity (44).

A second recent series of case reports describes the usefulness of orthotic devices in the treatment of idiopathic writer's cramp. In each of five patients, a thermoplastic hand orthosis designed to substitute the use of distal musculature for more proximal musculature was constructed for each patient. Adaptation to the devise was reportedly easily achieved and improved the handwriting in each of the five patients. Patients reportedly had immediate reoccurrence of their symptoms when writing without the orthosis (50). Again, a large-scale clinical trial is needed to confirm the efficacy of hand orthosis for writer's cramp.

ADJUNCT THERAPIES

Another treatment option that should be discussed is the use of support groups. Support groups offer a forum for patients and caregivers to share their experiences about disease symptoms and treatments. These groups can be very important sources of emotional support and education.

Lastly, physical and occupational therapy can be helpful adjuncts to treatment plans. Physical therapy can help with gait, transfers, strengthening, and stretching to prevent contractures. Physical therapy can help patients to understand their limitations and to set goals. Physical therapy also teaches patients how to live safely with their disabilities. Occupational therapy can be very helpful in providing devices to assist patients with dystonia. These devices allow patients to regain some of their independence and to perform tasks that would have otherwise been impossible.

FUTURE PERSPECTIVES

The advent of new imaging techniques that allow us to study the function of the brain, as well as animal models, has greatly aided in our understanding of dystonia. Genetic identification of different forms of dystonia has also enhanced our understanding of specific disease processes. As more of these genetic forms with their abnormal gene products are elucidated, our understanding of the pathophysiology of this disease will increase. A greater understanding of the underlying pathophysiology of dystonia may facilitate the creation of new medications. New surgical techniques have allowed us to treat generalized dystonia without destroying valuable brain structures or causing significant side effects. Lastly, on the horizon are treatment strategies such as gene therapy and stem cell research. These therapies are just now being applied to animal models but may become important factors for the treatment of dystonia in the future.

REFERENCES

1. Marsden CD, Harrison MJD. Idiopathic torsion dystonia. *Brain* 1994;97:793–810.
2. Marsden CD, Marion MH, Quinn N. The treatment of severe dystonia in children and adults. *J Neurol Neurosurg Psychiatry* 1984;47:1166–1173.
3. Bressman SB. Dystonia update. *Clin Neuropharmacol* 2000;23(5):239–251.
4. Fahn S. Treatment of dystonia with high dosage anticholinergic medicine. *Neurology* 1979;29:609.
5. Fahn S. High dosage anticholinergic therapy in dystonia. *Neurology* 1983;33:1255–1261.
6. Burke RE, Fahn S, Marsden CD. Torsion dystonia: a double-blind prospective trial of high-dosage trihexyphenidyl. *Neurology* 1986;36:160–164.
7. Fahn S. Generalized dystonia: concept and treatment. *Clin Neuropharmacol* 1986;9[Suppl 2]:S37–S48.
8. Greene P, Shale H, Fahn S. Experience with high dosages of anticholinergic and other drugs in the treatment of torsion dystonia. *Adv Neurol* 1988;50:547–556.
9. Burke RE, Fahn S. Double-blind evaluation of trihexyphenidyl in dystonia. *Adv Neurol* 1983;14:189–192.
10. Davidoff RA. Antispasticity drugs: mechanisms of action. *Ann Neurol* 1985;17:107–116.
11. Greene P, Shale H, Fahn S. Analysis of open-label trials in torsion dystonia using high dosages of anticholinergics and other drugs. *Mov Disord* 1988;3(1):46–50.
12. Greene PE, Fahn S. Baclofen in the treatment of idiopathic dystonia in children. *Mov Disord* 1992;7(1):48–52.
13. Nygaard TG, Marsden CD, Duvoisin RC. Dopa-responsive dystonia. *Adv Neurol* 1988;50:377–384.
14. Teravainen H, Calne S, Burton K, et al. Efficacy of dopamine agonists in dystonia. *Adv Neurol* 1988;50:571–578.
15. Coward DM. Tizanidine: neuropharmacology and mechanism of action. *Neurology* 1994;44[11 Suppl 9]:S6–S10.
16. Lang AE, Riley DE. Tizanidine in cranial dystonia. *Clin Neuropharmacol* 1992;15(2):142–147.
17. Pletscher A, Brossi A, Gey KF. Benzoquinoline derivatives: a new class of monoamine-decreasing drugs with psychotropic action. *Int Rev Neurobiol* 1962;4:275–306.
18. Jankovic J. Treatment of hyperkinetic movement disorders with tetrabenazine: a double-blind crossover study. *Ann Neurol* 1982;11:41–47.
19. Jankovic J, Beach J. Long-term effects of tetrabenazine in hyperkinetic movement disorders. *Neurology* 1997;48(2):358–362.
20. Trugman JM, Leadbetter R, Zalis ME, et al. Treatment of severe axial tardive dystonia with clozapine: case report and hypothesis. *Mov Disord* 1994;9:441–446.
21. Karp BI, Goldstein SR, Chen R, et al. An open trial of clozapine for dystonia. *Mov Disord* 1999;14:652–657.
22. Burbaud P, Guehl D, Lagueny A, et al. A pilot trial of clozapine in the treatment of cervical dystonia. *J Neurol* 1998;245:329–331.
23. Jankovic J, Brin MF. Therapeutic uses of botulinum toxin. *N Engl J Med* 1991;324(17):1186–1194.
24. Jankovic J, Brin MF. Botulinum toxin: historical perspective and potential new indications. *Muscle Nerve* 1997;20[Suppl 6]:S129–S145.
25. Greene P, Kang U, Fahn S, et al. Double-blind, placebo-controlled trial of botulinum toxin injections for the treatment of spasmotic torticollis. *Neurology* 1990;40:1213–1218.
26. Brans JWM, Lindeboom R, Snoek JW, et al. Botulinum toxin versus trihexyphenidyl in cervical dystonia: a prospective, randomized, double-blind controlled trial. *Neurology* 1996;46(4):1066–1072.
27. Brashear A, Lew MF, Dykstra DD, et al. Safety and efficacy of NeuroBloc (botulinum toxin type B) in type A-responsive cervical dystonia. *Neurology* 1999;53(7):1439–1446.
28. Brin MF, Lew MF, Adler CH, et al. Safety and efficacy of NeuroBloc (botulinum toxin type B) in type A-resistant cervical dystonia. *Neurology* 1999;53(7):1431–1438.
29. Friedman AH, Nashold SB, Sharp R, et al. Treatment of spasmotic torticollis with intradural selective rhizotomies. *J Neurosurg* 1993;78(1):46–53.
30. Krauss JK, Koller R, Burgunder JM. Partial myotomy/myectomy of the trapezius muscle with an asleep–awake–asleep anesthetic technique for treatment of cervical dystonia. *J Neurosurg* 1999;91:889–891.
31. Krauss JK, Toups EG, Jankovic J, et al. Symptomatic and functional outcome of surgical treatment of cervical dystonia. *J Neurol Neurosurg Psychiatry* 1997;63:642–648.
32. Ford B, Greene P, Louis ED, et al. Use of intrathecal baclofen in the treatment of patients with dystonia. *Arch Neurol* 1996;53:1241–1246.
33. Albright AL, Barry MJ, Fasick P, et al. Continuous intrathecal baclofen infusion for symptomatic generalized dystonia. *Neurosurgery* 1996;38(5):934–939.
34. Walker RH, Danisi FO, Swope DM, et al. Intrathecal baclofen for dystonia: benefits and complications during six years of experience. *Mov Disord* 2000;15(6):1242–1247.
35. Jaffe MS, Nienstedt LJ. Intrathecal baclofen for generalized dystonia: a case report. *Arch Phys Med Rehab* 2001;82(6):853–855.
36. Paret G, Tirosh R, Ben Zeev B, et al. Intrathecal baclofen for severe torsion dystonia in a child. *Acta Paediatrica* 1996;85(5):635–637.
37. Cooper IS. Twenty-year follow-up on the neurosurgical treatment of dystonia musculorum deformans. *Adv Neurol* 1976;14:423–452.
38. Andrew J, Fowler C, Harrison MJG. Stereotaxic thalamotomy in 55 cases of dystonia. *Brain* 1983;106:981–1000.
39. Tasker RR, Doorly T, Yamashiro K. Thalamotomy in generalized dystonia. *Adv Neurol* 1988;50:615–631.
40. Ondo WG, Desaloms M, Jankovic J, et al. Pallidotomy for generalized dystonia. *Mov Disord* 1998;13(4):693–698.
41. Yosher D, Hamilton WJ, Ondo W, et al. Comparison of thalamotomy and pallidotomy for the treatment of dystonia. *Neurosurgery* 2001;48(4):818–824.
42. Kumar R, Dagher A, Hutchison WD, et al. Globus pallidus deep brain stimulation for generalized dystonia: clinical and PET investigation. *Neurology* 1999;53(4):871–874.
43. Vercueil L, Pollak P, Fraix V, et al. Deep brain stimulation in the treatment of severe dystonia. *J Neurol* 2001;248(8):695–700.
44. Priori A, Presenti A, Cappellari A, et al. Limb immobilization for the treatment of focal occupational dystonia. *Neurology* 2001;57(3):405–409.
45. Byrnes ML, Thickbroom GW, Wilson SA, et al. The corticomotor representation of upper limb muscles in writer's cramp and changes following botulinum toxin injection. *Brain* 1998;121:977–988.
46. Elbert T, Candia V, Alternmuller E, et al. Alteration of digital representations in somatosensory cortex in focal hand dystonia. *Neuroreport* 1998;9:3571–3575.
47. Pujol J, Roset-Llobet J, Rosines-Cubels D, et al. Brain cortical activation during guitar-induced hand dystonia studied by functional MRI. *Neuroimage* 2000;12:257–267.
48. Odergren T, Stone-Elander S, Ingvar M. Cerebral and cerebellar activation in correlation to the action-induced dystonia in writer's cramp. *Mov Disord* 1998;3:497–508.
49. Liepert J, Tegenthoff M, Malin JP. Changes of cortical motor area size during immobilization. *Electroenceph Clin Neurophysiol* 1995;97:382–386.
50. Tas N, Karatas GK, Sepici V. Hand orthosis as a writing aid in writer's cramp. *Mov Disord* 2001;16(6):1185–1189.

25

DRUG-INDUCED DYSKINESIAS

OSCAR S. GERSHANIK

Since this chapter was updated in 1998, a quick search of the literature produced more than 700 new references on the subject of drug-induced dyskinesias covering both clinical and basic research, giving an indication on how vast and important this field has become. As new drugs are being introduced in the market their capacity to induce dyskinesia is being tested in everyday clinical practice. This wealth of new information has unfortunately yielded very little in terms of a better understanding of the pathophysiology of these disorders, nor has it brought us closer to better treatments for problems such as tardive dyskinesia (TD), which stands out as the most emblematic of drug-induced movement disorders. Having made these introductory remarks on recent developments, the broader concepts remain unchanged and still provide a basic framework to understand the issues facing the clinician.

Unfortunately, drugs are still frequently responsible for movement disorders, and different mechanisms are involved in their production, depending on the type of drug. Among them, neuroleptics or any pharmacologic agents capable of either blocking or stimulating dopamine receptors are the ones most commonly associated with this type of disorder (1). Both categories of drugs exert their effects through their action on dopamine receptors within the circuitry of the basal ganglia. Recent developments in basal ganglia physiology and pharmacology have provided new and more compelling evidence of the underlying mechanisms of this type of drug-induced dyskinesias. Other drugs, like central nervous system (CNS) stimulants, certain anticonvulsants, tricyclic antidepressants, estrogens, and so forth, are also capable of inducing movement disorders, through different pathogenetic mechanisms and with a different clinical expression (2).

This chapter will focus on the issue of movement disorders induced by dopamine-blocking agents, most of which have neuroleptic properties and are used in psychiatry as antipsychotics. We will also review those dyskinesias observed with the use of CNS stimulants and other miscellaneous drugs. Levodopa-induced dyskinesias appearing in the course of antiparkinsonian therapy, drug-induced parkinsonism, and neuroleptic malignant syndrome will not be included in this review.

The subject of drug-induced dyskinesias can be approached from two different perspectives. On one hand, drugs can be analyzed individually in their ability to produce a movement disorder, while on the other, the phenomenology can be the starting point of our analysis. We will attempt to combine both approaches in order to provide a comprehensive view of the clinical problem.

Table 25.1 provides an overview of the drugs known to be involved in the production of movement disorders, classified according to the type of motor phenomenon.

DYSKINESIAS INDUCED BY DOPAMINE RECEPTOR BLOCKERS

The administration of drugs having antagonistic effects on striatal dopamine receptors is frequently associated with the development of different types of movement disorders. These disorders are most often seen in psychiatric patients undergoing neuroleptic treatment. In the case of psychotic patients receiving these drugs, dyskinesias are an inherent risk of the treatment, although this risk has been reduced to some extent with the use of the newer generation of atypical antipsychotics. There are, however, numerous other drugs used in internal medicine that share with neuroleptics the ability to block dopamine receptors and are therefore capable of inducing similar movement disorders. Such is the case with benzamides (e.g., metoclopramide, sulpiride, clebopride, veralipride, etc.) used in the treatment of nausea, vomiting, gastrointestinal upset, and menopausal hot flushes. Calcium channel blockers (e.g., flunarizine, cinnarizine, nifedipine, verapamil, diltiazem, etc.) in varying degrees are also responsible for the development of movement disorders similar to those seen with neuroleptics. These drugs have a wide range of applications in clinical practice, from management of vertigo and migraine, to treatment of cardiovascular disorders, to their use as putative cognitive enhancers (1). Antihistamines can also cause dyskinesias that are clinically similar to classic TDs. More recently a new class of antidepressants, the selective serotonin reuptake inhibitors (SSRIs), have been reported as

TABLE 25.1. DRUG-INDUCED DYSKINESIAS

Syndrome	Drugs Responsible	Syndrome	Drugs Responsible
Postural tremor and myoclonus	Sympathomimetics Levodopa Amphetamine Bronchodilators Tricyclic antidepressants Serotonin reuptake inhibitors Lithium carbonate Caffeine Steroids Hypoglycemic agents Amiodarone	*Parkinsonism*	Neuroleptics Benzamides Reserpine Tetrabenazine Methyldopa Calcium channel blockers Isoniazide Serotonin reuptake inhibitors Meperidine
Acute dystonic reactions	Neuroleptics Benzamides (e.g., metoclopramide) Calcium channel blockers (e.g., flunarizine) Tetrabenazine Methamphetamine Cocaine	*Chorea, tardive syndromes*	Neuroleptics Benzamides Calcium channel blockers Levodopa and DA agonists Oral contraceptives Phenytoin and other anticonvulsants
Akathisia	Neuroleptics Benzamides Reserpine Tetrabenazine Levodopa and DA agonists Calcium channel blockers	*Neuroleptic malignant syndrome*	Neuroleptics Withdrawal of antiparkinsonian drugs

being responsible for cases of TD among a wide spectrum of other movement disorders caused by these drugs (3). In some patients the dyskinesias have persisted long after discontinuation of the medication. The risk of developing movement disorders with these drugs could be related to the structural and pharmacologic similarities existing between the antihistamines and the phenothiazines.

The clinical presentation and time of onset of movement disorders resulting from the use of dopamine-blocking or dopamine-depleting agents are quite variable. They include *parkinsonism* as well as motor restlessness *(akathisia)* and the whole range of hyperkinesias *(chorea, stereotypies, myoclonus, dystonia, tics)*. A classification of the different movement

TABLE 25.2. MOVEMENT DISORDERS INDUCED BY DRUGS INTERFERING WITH DOPAMINERGIC TRANSMISSION

Acute dystonic reactions
Acute akathisia
Parkinsonism
Neuroleptic-induced malignant syndrome
Tardive syndromes (tardive dyskinesia)
- *Buccolinguomasticatory syndrome*
- *Stereotypies*
- *Tardive dystonia*
- *Tardive tourettism*
- *Tardive tremor*
- *Tardive myoclonus*
- *Tardive akathisia*

disorders induced by this family of drugs is shown in Table 25.2.

Depending on its appearance in the course of treatment they can be classified as acute, subacute and late or tardive. Acute dystonic reactions often develop soon after the offending drug is introduced, whereas parkinsonism and akathisia have a subacute form of presentation. If exposure to dopamine-blocking agents is prolonged enough (months or years), patients can experience a wide range of movement disorders that are usually grouped together as a syndrome, the so-called tardive syndrome (tardive dyskinesia, tardive myoclonus, tardive tics, tardive dystonia, tardive akathisia). Tardive syndromes often run a persistent course despite cessation of therapy with the offending drug. In some instances they may become permanent and irreversible (2).

ACUTE DYSTONIC REACTIONS

Dystonic postures and movements are usually seen soon after the initiation of neuroleptic therapy. They range from brief jerks to prolonged muscle spasms often involving the craniocervical region (eyes, mouth, throat, neck). Oculogyric crises indistinguishable from those reported in postencephalitic parkinsonism can also occur in the context of acute dystonic reactions. These crises are often associated with psychiatric manifestations, such as exacerbation of pre-existing thought disorders or sudden onset of intrusive thoughts. Involvement of the trunk and limbs, although less common, may be part of the clinical spectrum of acute dystonic reactions, particularly in children, similar to what is seen in idiopathic dystonia. Acute dystonic reactions are often dramatic in their presentation and at times of enough severity to warrant lifesaving measures. This is usually the case when the laryngeal muscles are involved and the patient develops respiratory difficulties (2).

Around 90% of dystonic reactions take place within the first 5 days of neuroleptic therapy. The incidence rate of this disorder ranges from 2.3% to 63% (4). The onset of dystonic symptoms usually occurs 2 to 24 hours after administration of the first dose of the offending drug. Symptom duration is variable, with signs persisting for hours or days, while intensity may oscillate during its course. Clinical manifestations may vary depending on the age of the affected subject. Children may develop generalized dystonic spasms involving the trunk and extremities. Adults, on the other hand, usually present with face, neck, and upper extremity involvement. Dystonic spasms and postures are of abrupt onset, are frequently painful, and may fluctuate in their distribution, affecting different body parts at different times. Common forms of presentation include blepharospasm, oculogyric crises, trismus, jaw deviation, tongue protrusion, torticollis, retrocollis, and abnormal trunk posturing such as lordosis, scoliosis, and even opisthotonus.

Several risk factors have been proposed, including male sex, age younger than 30, type of underlying psychiatric disorder, high neuroleptic dosage and potency of the drug involved, and familial predisposition. Men are more frequently affected than women (2:1) (4). The same is true for children and young adults as they tend to be more prone to develop acute dystonic reactions than elderly subjects. In Kondo's series of schizophrenic patients, young males (≤ 30 years) had an extremely high incidence of this side effect (91.7%), showing a positive correlation with prolactin response after 1 week of treatment and dystonia rating scores. Elderly patients are not entirely free of the risk of having acute dystonic reactions as recently reported (5). A higher incidence of dystonic reactions in patients given neuroleptics for the management of mania than in nonparanoid schizophrenia has been reported. However, these results have been challenged (6) based on a prospective study of neuroleptic-induced dystonia in mania and schizophrenia. Fifty patients with mania and 33 with schizophrenia, all male, age 17 to 45, with no exposure to neuroleptics in the previous month and absence of past or family history of extrapyramidal disorders were included in this prospective study. Twenty-four percent of the patients with mania and 15% of those with schizophrenia developed acute dystonia. Stepwise multiple regression analysis showed that peak neuroleptic dose and age, not primary illness, strongly correlated with dystonic reactions. This study concluded that the apparent difference in incidence could be explained in terms of the higher peak dose of neuroleptics used in the

treatment of acute mania. A certain propensity for the development of acute dystonic reactions has been described in a number of families, suggesting the existence of a genetic predisposition in this disorder. Similarly, relatives of patients with idiopathic dystonia have been suggested to be more prone to suffer from neuroleptic-induced acute dystonia than the general population.

Acute dystonic reactions are undoubtedly more common in individuals receiving high-potency neuroleptics; however, these symptoms are also seen with drugs like metoclopramide, a benzamide class antiemetic. Opposite to what is observed with classic neuroleptics, metoclopramide-induced acute dystonia is more common in young females. Familial predisposition, in some cases with dominance inheritance, has also been reported with this drug. Another antiemetic, domperidone, though known to have very little penetration through the blood–brain barrier has been reported as responsible for acute dystonic reactions in a few cases. Sulpiride, another benzamide class drug, has been recently added to the list of dopamine-blocking agents capable of causing acute dystonic reactions. Acute dystonic reactions have also been reported with miscellaneous drugs such as ranitidine, cimetidine, nefazadone, tiagabine, and mixed cough suppressants.

The pathophysiology of acute dystonic reactions has been linked to a sudden imbalance between striatal dopamine and cholinergic systems causing a relative preponderance of acetylcholine. Hypofunction of dopaminergic transmission would be the underlying mechanism according to this hypothesis. Quite the opposite, a rapid development of increased dopamine turnover secondary to preferential blockade of presynaptic dopamine receptors, with increased dopamine release acting on supersensitive postsynaptic dopamine receptors, has also been proposed (2). However, there is recent experimental evidence that dopamine-depleting agents like α-methylparatyrosine (AMPT) in animal models of acute dystonia fail to prevent and moreover can induce this movement disorder, negating the theory that presynaptic mechanisms have a role in its pathogenesis. This has been supported by a pharmacologic study (7) carried out in normal men (volunteers) who received AMPT in doses of 750 mg PO QID to a maximum of 8.25 g. Five of the 24 subjects (21%) developed acute dystonic reactions between 3½ and 12 hours after the last medication dose. This is the first clinical evidence that catecholamine depletion in the absence of dopamine receptor blockade can induce acute dystonic reactions in normal humans. The possible role of other neurotransmitter systems in the pathogenesis of acute dystonic reactions has also been explored. Blockade of dopaminergic neurotransmission induces striking modifications in the γ-aminobutyric acid (GABA)–mediated putaminopallidal output pathways, with concomitant increase in enkephalin expression. The possible involvement of opioid receptors in the pathogenesis of acute dystonic reactions has been recently proposed.

Matsumoto and Pouw (8) reported significant correlation between binding affinities for both σ1 and σ2 receptors and the tendency of different neuroleptics to produce acute dystonic reactions in humans. The relevance of these findings and their relationship to neuroleptic-induced acute dystonic reactions needs further clarification.

Acute dystonia will resolve spontaneously upon drug withdrawal. This is always the case as there are no documented cases of acute dystonic reactions persisting after the causative agent was removed. The treatment of choice for this disorder is the use of parenteral anticholinergics (biperiden, benztropine) or antihistamines (diphenhydramine). Muscle relaxants, such as diazepam, are also effective in some cases.

AKATHISIA

Akathisia is a very common, very early, and dose-related side effect of neuroleptics (9). It is not exclusive of neuroleptics and other dopamine receptor–blocking drugs, as it has also been described in unmedicated and postencephalitic parkinsonism; even newer atypical neuroleptics, such as risperidone, are no different from haloperidol in their ability to induce akathisia (10). Moreover, nonneuroleptic medications (e.g., SSRI antidepressants) have been reported as a frequent cause of drug-induced akathisia in predisposed individuals (3). Even nonpsychotropic medications can be the cause of akathisia as recently reported with patients receiving interferon-α (11).

Patients experience an aversion to keeping still, associated with a subjective sensation of restlessness and accompanied by complex or stereotyped movements. Affected individuals often complain of a feeling of inner tension in their limbs and body, causing them to shift from one position to another in an attempt to relieve it. The subjective feeling of inner restlessness has been classically referred to the lower extremities, but in some cases it can be localized to other body parts, as in a recently reported case in which the respiratory as well as the suboccipital muscles were those preferentially affected (12,13). Frequently, the treating physician misdiagnoses akathisia for anxiety, hyperactivity, agitation, or even delusional thoughts, related to the underlying primary illness (13). Akathisia also may occur after long-term exposure to neuroleptics, with signs and symptoms persisting chronically. This condition has been described as "tardive akathisia" (see next section, "Tardive Syndromes") to differentiate it from acute neuroleptic-induced akathisia. It is also possible for akathisia to develop late in the course of neuroleptic treatment, coincidental with an increase in dosage or when treatment is changed and a more potent drug is given. A diagnosis of akathisia can only be considered when both subjective and objective features are present. The reported prevalence of this disorder ranges from 9% to 75% of patients receiving neuroleptics. In a comprehensive survey

(14), akathisia was found in 36% of patients undergoing neuroleptic treatment, independent of the presence of other drug-induced movement disorders. According to this study, the incidence of akathisia was disproportionally higher in patients receiving high-potency neuroleptics. In 50% of cases symptoms develop within the first month of treatment with the offending drug, whereas in almost 90% of cases akathisia is present after 2 or 3 months of neuroleptic exposure. The secondary complications of akathisia are numerous. Among them noncompliance and suicidal ideation or behavior are significant (15). Akathisia has also been reported to predict more severe symptoms and poorer treatment response to typical neuroleptics among patients with schizophrenia, to the extent of being associated with symptom exacerbation and a higher risk of developing TD (16,17). It is therefore necessary to treat akathisia as promptly as possible to avoid complications and to allow for a better prognosis of the underlying psychopathology (16). Although incidence studies on akathisia have been predominantly undertaken in patients with schizophrenia and schizoaffective disorders, there is evidence that in patients suffering from bipolar affective disorder the incidence may run as high as 65% (18).

The pathophysiology of akathisia is not completely understood but most likely arises from complex interactions at the cortical-subcortical-spinal level. Blockade of mesocortical dopaminergic receptors as well as noradrenergic and opioid mechanisms have been alternatively proposed as the underlying pathophysiology of this disorder. A relative serotonin (5-hydroxytryptamine, 5-HT)/dopamine imbalance could also be implicated as some of the newer atypical antipsychotics with a moderate to high affinity for the 5-HT_3 receptor subtype have a low propensity to cause akathisia. Genetic risk factors may also play a predisposing role as in patients with homozygosity for the Ser9Gly variant of the dopamine D3 receptor gene *(DRD3)* the incidence of akathisia almost twice that of the nonhomozygous patient population (17). Cases of akathisia secondary to structural brain damage have been reported. In these cases, the lesions were located at the level of the basal ganglia outflow system. It is therefore possible that drug-induced modifications in the function of the pallidal output pathways may underlie the clinical syndrome of neuroleptic-induced akathisia. Iron status as well as ferritin levels have been recently examined in relation to the development of acute akathisia due to their influence on dopamine D2 receptor sensitivity. However, the precise role of this interaction needs to be elucidated, as more recent studies underplay their participation in the pathophysiology of akathisia (19).

Any therapeutic strategy for akathisia should include dose reduction, changing to a lower potency neuroleptic, or drug withdrawal, as these are the most effective treatments for this condition. If these treatments are not possible, numerous medications are available that are variably effective. In some cases, anticholinergics, diphenhydramine, or amantadine also used in the management of a concomitant drug-induced parkinsonism (DIP) are useful (13). Other drugs, like propranolol, clonidine, benzodiazepines, and, more recently, opioid agonists like propoxyphene have been found to be effective in a number of patients. Mianserin, a 5-HT$_2$ antagonist, may be a promising new option, according to a recent report (20); however, attempts with other 5-HT antagonists, such as granisetron, have been less successful (21). Less commonly used drugs, such as buspirone, piracetam, amitriptyline, and dopamine depleters, can be tried in more refractory cases. Ziprasidone, belonging to the new generation of atypical neuroleptics and currently under clinical evaluation, appears to be particularly useful in the management of psychotic agitation and virtually without the risk of akathisia (22).

TARDIVE SYNDROMES

The term *tardive syndromes* applies to persistent, sometimes irreversible, abnormal involuntary movements appearing over the course of prolonged neuroleptic treatment (23,24). They usually present in the form of hyperkinesias involving the orofacial, limb, and truncal regions. Although more frequently associated with the chronic use of antipsychotic drugs, other drugs known to impair dopaminergic transmission in the nigrostriatal system can be responsible for this disorder. Every year, newer compounds are added to the already impressive list of drugs capable of causing tardive syndromes (Table 25.1). Flecainide (a benzamide antiarrhythmic), clenbuterol (a sympathomimetic drug with no known antidopaminergic effects), and the SSRIs, as previously mentioned, are just a few examples of drugs recently associated with the development of tardive syndromes (3). Tardive syndromes have seldom been reported with the use of drugs that interfere with dopaminergic transmission through a presynaptic mechanism, such as reserpine or tetrabenazine. Certain atypical antipsychotics with a peculiar receptor blocking profile (involving serotonergic receptors), such as risperidone and olanzapine, were developed with the idea of preventing the development of TD.

Tardive syndromes can faithfully reproduce almost the entire spectrum of known abnormal involuntary movements of the hyperkinetic type (chorea, dystonia, tics, myoclonus, tremor, etc.). Tardive dyskinesia is the generic denomination most frequently used to identify all clinical forms of this disorder. A more restricted use of the term applies to abnormal movements in the orolinguomandibular, truncal, and limb regions that appear choreatic in nature. This form of presentation, also known as *buccolinguomasticatory syndrome*, was the first type of TD described in the medical literature soon after the introduction of neuroleptics. It is indeed the most common of the tardive syndromes seen in clinical practice, affecting usually the more elderly subjects. The syndrome consists of repetitive stereo-

typed movements of tongue twisting and protrusion, lip smacking and puckering, and chewing movements. The upper facial muscles are less frequently affected by the involuntary movements; however, it is possible to see increased blinking, blepharospasm, arching of the eyebrows, ocular torsion, and deviation. Additional involvement of the trunk and extremities is common although variable in its presentation and severity. Body rocking and swaying motions of the trunk together with pelvic thrusts (copulatory dyskinesia) are sometimes part of the syndrome. Gait can be abnormal, with a broad base, leg jerking, and repetitive irregular flexion and extension of the knees. While standing in place, affected individuals tend to shift their weight from one leg to the other or exhibit pacing or marching in place. The diaphragm and accessory respiratory muscles are often involved, causing a fast and irregular breathing pattern (respiratory dyskinesia). The presence of deep inspirations, tachypnea, and arrhythmic breathing in these patients is often the cause of inadequate referral to a cardiologist or a lung specialist for consultation. In cases in which the dyskinetic movements affect the laryngeal muscles this could be the cause of upper airway obstructive syndrome. In addition, many patients exhibit repetitive grunting and moaning, which is believed to represent the phonic equivalent of the motor manifestations of TD. More complex, seemingly purposeful movement patterns, such as hair, hand, and face rubbing, as well as picking and pulling at clothes, can also be observed in patients with TD. The nature of movements in TD is somewhat different from that in typical chorea in that they tend to be more patterned, repetitive, and stereotypic. Although patients frequently show an apparent restlessness that is indistinguishable from acute or subacute akathisia (tardive akathisia), the subjective component is rarely present and, surprisingly, a large number of patients are unaware of the presence of abnormal involuntary movements. There is a persistent controversy regarding terminology of this disorder, on account of the peculiar nature of the movements observed in this type of TD. The terms *rhythmic chorea, tardive stereotypies,* and *tardive akathisia* have been used indistinctly to describe these movements. Arguments for and against the use of either term abound (2). The presence of an associated parkinsonian syndrome in these patients is quite common and should immediately suggest a drug-induced disorder whenever such a combination is detected. The differential diagnosis of buccolinguomasticatory syndrome should include a variety of other movement disorders, including some that are also related to neuroleptic treatment (e.g., acute or subacute akathisia). A list of alternative diagnoses is provided in Table 25.3.

Dystonic phenomena account for 2% of tardive syndromes found in psychiatric inpatients; however, if milder forms of these disorders are included, the prevalence increases up to 21%. Tardive dystonia has been recognized as a clinical variant of TD. The repertoire of dystonic symp-

TABLE 25.3. DIFFERENTIAL DIAGNOSIS OF THE BUCCOLINGUOMASTICATORY SYNDROME

Spontaneous buccolingual dyskinesias of the elderly
Edentulous dyskinesias
Stereotyped movements in schizophrenia
Drug-induced chorea (including levodopa-induced dyskinesias)
Other choreic syndromes:
  Hereditary choreas (Huntington's disease, neuroacanthocytosis)
  Metabolic and endocrine choreas (hyperparathyroidism, hyperthyroidism, acquired hepatocerebral degeneration)
  Vasculitis (lupus erythematosus, periarteritis nodosa)
  Stroke (basal ganglia lacunae)

toms seen after long-term neuroleptic treatment is indistinguishable from the abnormal movements and postures seen in idiopathic dystonia (25). This movement disorder is characterized by the presence of chronic dystonia in a patient with a history of exposure to antipsychotics or dopamine receptor–blocking drugs preceding or concurrent with the onset of the dystonic. A diagnosis of tardive dystonia is made after exclusion of known causes of secondary dystonia by appropriate clinical and laboratory evaluation, and when no family history of a dystonic movement disorder is present.

The affected population is usually younger than that presenting with the more common form of TD (buccolinguomasticatory syndrome). In the study carried out by Kiriakakis et al. (25), the mean age at onset was 38.3 years. The development of tardive dystonia is dependent on the age of the subject exposed to the causative agent. Therefore, no particular drug can be held responsible for this disorder, which can occur with various drugs having in common dopamine receptor blocking properties. The nature of the underlying disease is not a predisposing factor, as tardive dystonia is seen in psychiatric and nonpsychiatric illnesses as well. Dystonic symptoms may have a focal, segmental, or generalized distribution, as seen in idiopathic dystonia. The generalized forms of dystonia are not common in tardive syndromes. Patients with generalized tardive dystonia are usually much younger at onset than those with segmental or focal dystonia. The most common body regions involved in tardive dystonia are the neck (e.g., torticollis, retrocollis), present in 87% of cases according to Kiriakakis (25); the cranial musculature (e.g., blepharospasm, oromandibular and pharyngeal dystonia); and the trunk (opisthotonus). Oculogyric crises are seen both in acute dystonic reactions and in tardive dystonia. These crises are often recurrent and associated with exacerbation of psychiatric symptomatology (obsessional thoughts and hallucinations). The legs are less often involved. Focal cranial tardive dystonia, developing in elderly patients, can be often identical to primary Meige's syndrome (primary cranial dystonia). The differential diag-

nosis of tardive dystonia should include other disorders presenting with dystonic phenomena, such as idiopathic torsion dystonia, Wilson's disease, and other symptomatic dystonias. Tardive dystonia can be distinguished from idiopathic torsion dystonia on the basis of the clinical examination if the patient has other signs of TD. The combination of different tardive syndromes in the same patient is not unusual (tardive dystonia can coexist with the more common buccolinguomasticatory syndrome and with neuroleptic-induced parkinsonism). However, a positive history of exposure to a dopamine-blocking drug is necessary to make a valid diagnosis of tardive dystonia. In certain clinical situations it may become difficult to diagnose tardive dystonia even though other clinical features suggest this diagnosis. Patients with chronic dystonia and a history of antipsychotic drug treatment often are uncertain about whether the onset of neuroleptic treatment preceded the onset of the movement disorder or the other way around. In some cases, the onset of dystonic symptoms did not take place for weeks or months after the dopamine blocking agents had been discontinued. In other cases, symptoms continued to progress months after neuroleptic therapy had been discontinued. These are but a few examples of the difficulties one may encounter in everyday practice when dealing with tardive syndromes. The course of tardive dystonia is variable and depends, as for TD in general, on the chances of discontinuation of neuroleptic medication. According to Kiriakakis et al. (25), this is a very persistent disorder with a remission rate of only 14% in their series.

Motor and vocal tics following long-term neuroleptic treatment can be occasionally seen as part of the tardive syndrome. This type of clinical presentation has been described and referred to as *tardive tourettism* or *tardive Tourette's syndrome* (26). All three patients included in the original report experienced a sudden onset of abnormal movements and vocalizations in adult life, following chronic neuroleptic therapy. The symptoms were in all respects similar to those seen in primary Tourette's syndrome. Neither the patients nor their relatives had ever experienced tics, vocalizations, or abnormal movements prior to being exposed to neuroleptics. The presence of vocal or phonic tics was indeed essential as the combination of the latter with motor tics is necessary for making a diagnosis of tourettism. One of the patients had simple vocalizations (e.g., barking and clicking noises), whereas in the other two, more complex verbal tics were present, including coprolalia, echolalia, and palilalia. As with TD in general, in two of the affected individuals neuroleptic withdrawal preceded the onset of the disorder. Bharucha and Sethi (27) have published a comprehensive review of the literature on the subject.

In a small number of cases, myoclonus can be the predominant feature of TD (28). The original publication reported the presence of prominent postural myoclonus in the upper extremities in 32 of 133 psychiatric patients who had been under neuroleptic treatment for at least 3 months.

There was a slight male-to-female preponderance in these cases. In addition to myoclonus the patients exhibited other drug-induced movement disorders, such as tremor (27 cases), parkinsonism (7 cases), and orofacial dyskinesias (7 cases). In 6 of the 32 cases electromyographic recordings were performed, and typical positive myoclonic discharges of 30 to 40 msec duration were detected. A positive response to clonazepam was reported in these patients.

In 1992, Stacy and Jankovic added a new entity, tardive tremor, to the clinical spectrum of TD (29). Their cases fulfilled the clinical, diagnostic, and therapeutic response criteria used in defining tardive syndromes. In their five patients, tremor developed during the course of chronic neuroleptic treatment; it was aggravated by and persisted after neuroleptic withdrawal, in a fashion similar to that of other tardive syndromes. Tremor was oscillatory and postural, with a frequency range of 3 to 5 Hz, and involved all four extremities. The head was affected in one case. Other parkinsonian features were not present. Tetrabenazine was effective in reducing tremor in these cases, unlike any other type of tremor. The positive response to tetrabenazine was used by the authors as an additional supportive criteria to ascertain the tardive nature of this disorder.

Painful sensations localized in the oral and genital regions, alone or in association with dyskinesias, have recently been reported as another clinical manifestation of TD (30). These authors reported on 11 patients who developed chronic painful oral or genital sensations in the context of different tardive syndromes. In each case, the pain syndrome became so distressful as to overshadow all other concurrent psychiatric and motor manifestations. Pharmacologic agents used in the management of tardive syndromes proved effective in reducing the painful sensations.

A peculiar type of tremor also related to chronic neuroleptic treatment is the so-called rabbit syndrome. This uncommon neuroleptic-induced movement disorder usually presents as 4- to 6-Hz rhythmic discharges involving the jaw, perinasal, and perioral musculature and mimics the chewing movements of a rabbit. This syndrome is believed to be a form of neuroleptic-induced parkinsonism and, unlike buccolinguomasticatory syndrome, can improve with anticholinergics.

Tardive syndromes, irrespective of the clinical type, are considered in patients presenting with abnormal involuntary movements after at least 3 months of total cumulative neuroleptic exposure (23), although they are more frequently observed after longer periods of exposure (1 to 2 years). They can develop during the course of treatment, after dose reduction (unmasked TD), or even after the causative drug has been withdrawn (covert or withdrawal TD). Cessation of neuroleptic treatment or reduction of dosage is followed by the onset of TD in about 40% of previously asymptomatic patients. Choreic-type dyskinesias can be seen in children after abrupt discontinuation of neuroleptics. They are referred to as "withdrawal dyskinesias"

(withdrawal emergent syndrome). They are usually short-lived, spontaneously remitting, involuntary movements. This syndrome is not believed to be part of the spectrum of TD and should be differentiated from covert or withdrawal TD.

The degree of severity of TD can be quite variable, although, surprisingly, even severely affected patients are often unaware of their disorder. In two recent studies the percentage of patients unaware of the presence of TD ranged from 46.5% to 67.4% (31,32). There was some correlation between this lack of awareness and the presence of cognitive impairment in these patients. Moreover, according to Chong (32), the greater the severity of TD the lesser the chances of being aware of its presence.

Prevalence of TD is also variable, according to different authors, ranging from 17% to 30%. The annual incidence in younger adults is 4% to 5%, whereas in patients over 45 it is greater than 30%. In chronically institutionalized elderly schizophrenic patients, the prevalence has been found to be as high as 60% (33). In a comprehensive survey of a large population of psychiatric inpatients (647), Koshino et al. (34) analyzed the prevalence, clinical phenomenology, and risk factors for TD. In this study, overall prevalence of TD was found to be 22.3%, with older patients being more frequently affected. Interestingly, the dose of neuroleptics in these patients turned out to be lower than that of non-TD cases. Patients with TD had on average a longer duration of disease. There was no correlation between the presence of TD and gender or the nature of the primary psychiatric illness. This study also compared the prevalence of TD with the average prescribed dose of neuroleptics in different countries. The finding of a much lower prevalence (9.3%) of TD (35) in a study conducted on a large population of psychiatric inpatients in Hong Kong raised the possibility of ethnic differences in the prevalence of this disorder. In considering the prevalence of TD one should also be aware of the possibility of occurrence of spontaneous involuntary movements both in psychiatric (stereotypies and orofacial dyskinesias) and in elderly patients (edentulism). In a recent meta-analysis of 14 studies conducted in drug-naive schizophrenic patients, available data suggest a spontaneous dyskinesia rate of approximately 4% in first-episode patients, 12% for those with several years of illness but younger than 30 years, 25% for those between 30 and 50 years, and 40% for those 60 years or older (36). This factor could, in some cases, account for the variability in prevalence figures among different studies.

The natural history of TD can be quite variable, depending on a number of factors. Among these are the maintenance of neuroleptic therapy after the development of abnormal involuntary movements, upward or downward changes in the dose of neuroleptics, change to a lower potency drug, and withdrawal of neuroleptics. In some cases, the involuntary movements may worsen progressively after onset; however, in the majority of patients the intensity of the movements tends to remain constant over time. Spontaneous remission can take place after cessation of therapy. Remission rates have been estimated at 30% to 60%, depending on the length of the observation period. It may take up to 5 years for complete remission to occur. The combination of shorter neuroleptic exposure and age younger than 60 after onset of TD is correlated with a greater likelihood of remission. Dyskinesias, however, may reappear when treatment is reinstituted. In a significant number of patients, dyskinesias may become irreversible despite cessation of neuroleptic treatment. The issue of irreversibility in tardive dyskinesia is controversial due to variability in the follow-up periods considered in the numerous reports dealing with this subject. Among the early reports, a study published in 1964 (37) found that all symptoms of dyskinesias abated more or less completely within 3 years after treatment with neuroleptics was discontinued. During a shorter observation period (7 to 10 months), Degwitz (38), in a series of 237 patients, found that symptoms disappeared after drug cessation in 19%, were reduced in another 19%, were increased in 12%, and remained unchanged in 50%. Crane (39), reporting on 37 patients, found that after 6 to 26 months without drugs, the reduction rate of TDs was much less, with only 10% of patients showing improvement or remission. In older patients, the risk of development and persistence of neuroleptic-induced TD is known to be high. In a more recent study (40), 69 middle-aged and elderly outpatients newly diagnosed with TD were followed in a longitudinal, prospective fashion after neuroleptics had been withdrawn. The authors observed a highly fluctuating early course of TD. Although the cumulative proportion of patients whose TD partially remitted was quite high (56% at 3 months, 80% at 6 months), the cumulative proportion of patients whose TD relapsed (post remission) was also high (33% at 3 months, 54% at 6 months). The fact that TD, in some cases, becomes permanent and irreversible raises the possibility that neuroleptics could not only produce functional changes but may indeed have toxic effects leading to neuropathologic changes on certain neuronal systems (41).

In some cases symptoms may improve or even disappear without drug dosage modification, according to early reports. Heinrich and colleagues (42) followed a group of patients with classical TDs and noticed that after 15 months 40% were asymptomatic. However, this possibility seems remote in the light of more recent follow-up studies. According to these reports, patients maintained on neuroleptics in spite of the presence of abnormal involuntary movements fare differently. A more recent survey from Japan studied the long-term outcome of TD in patients under treatment with neuroleptics assessed at 5 and 11–12 years after the initial evaluation (43). This extended follow-up of 28 patients with TD was performed to elucidate their outcome with continuing medication. All patients showed persistence of TD during the study period; movements were

unchanged in 39.3%, improved in 17.9%, and worsened in 21.4%. Outcome was not correlated with gender, age, duration of primary illness, dose or change in dosage of the neuroleptic. Initial severity of TD showed some relationship to outcome. Another study analyzed both the long-term risk and outcome of TD if neuroleptic medications are continued (44). These authors studied prospectively a cohort of 362 chronic psychiatric outpatients who were free of TD at baseline. On the basis of 5 years of follow-up, the estimated risk of persistent TD was found to be 32% after 5 years of neuroleptic exposure, 57% after 15 years, and 68% after 25 years of exposure. On the same issue, Cavallaro et al. (45) published a study on 125 institutionalized schizophrenic patients receiving continuous neuroleptic treatment who were followed for 3 years. The prevalence of TD rose from 39.2% at the first examination to 52.8% at the last follow-up examination; however, 28.6% of TD-affected patients recovered and 30% improved. These last results have to be cautiously interpreted as TD symptoms may have improved if neuroleptic dosage was increased during the observation period (masked TD).

Older age, female sex, length of drug exposure, duration of illness, cumulative drug exposure, history of affective disorder, cognitive impairment, negative symptoms, diabetes mellitus, early extrapyramidal side effects (parkinsonism), history of electroconvulsive therapy (in some cases), preventive use of antiparkinsonian medications, and clinical indicators of structural brain involvement have been alternatively proposed as risk factors for TD. More recently, and in line with present day concepts on disease pathogenesis, genetic factors have been proposed as predisposing individuals to TD (46).

Yassa et al. (47) performed a study of TD in elderly subjects in the geriatric psychiatry unit of a Canadian hospital. They evaluated the prevalence and risk factors for TD in patients who had never received neuroleptic medication before their first hospitalization. They included 162 patients of whom 99 had received neuroleptics; of these 99 patients, 35 (35.4%) had developed TD. TD was significantly more prevalent in patients with major depression than in those with primary degenerative dementia or psychosis. Similarly, Koshino et al. (34) found a significant age difference between patients with or without TD. These authors found a steady increase in prevalence from 3.7% in the fourth decade to 49.5% in the seventh. Surprisingly, above the seventh decade a decline was observed. There were no differences in prevalence according to sex, contrary to previous reports. According to this study, duration of primary illness but not the type of psychiatric disorder was found to correlate with the presence of TD. In an attempt to explain the decline in prevalence of TD after age 60, Sweet et al. (48) speculated on a possible age-related loss of dopamine receptors as the underlying cause. More recently, Woerner et al. (49) in an assessment of the cumulative incidence rates of TD in patients older than 55 according to length of exposure to neuroleptics found them to be 25%, 34%, and 53% after 1, 2, and 3 years of treatment, respectively. The authors underscore the fact that TD rates for patients beginning treatment with conventional antipsychotics in their fifth decade or later are three to five times higher than what is usual in younger patients.

It is commonly held that women are at greater risk of developing TD. However, in a recent large prospective study involving 706 chronic psychotic patients who were not older than 65 years (UK700 Group), female sex was associated with a lower risk of TD (50).

High neuroleptic dose and concomitant use of neuroleptic and antiparkinsonian drugs (anticholinergics) were both found to be significantly associated with increased risk of TD in a large study involving 1,745 patients (51). These findings have to be seriously considered because the preventive use of antiparkinsonian drugs in neuroleptic-treated patients is common in many countries. An additional significant finding related to treatment modalities and risk of TD is that more than two neuroleptic interruptions in the course of antipsychotic medication have been found to correlate with a threefold increase in the risk of developing TD, contradicting previous indications of intermittent administration of neuroleptics as a valid strategy for the prevention of TD (52).

Diabetes mellitus has been identified as a possible risk factor for TD. In a study involving 160 elderly individuals who were beginning neuroleptic treatment, the cumulative incidence rate for diabetics and nondiabetics was analyzed. Diabetics were found to have more than twice the risk of developing TD than nondiabetics (53).

The contribution of cognitive impairment, negative symptoms, and signs of "organicity" to the risk of developing TD remains controversial. In a study comparing 20 male patients meeting the DSM-III-R criteria for chronic schizophrenia and Shooler and Kane's criteria for TD with 20 age-matched male chronic schizophrenic patients without TD, Davis et al. (54) found a significant association between TD, cognitive impairment, some negative symptoms, and formal thought disorder. Moreover, the severity of TD correlated with the degree of cognitive impairment. The findings of a larger multicenter study performed in Scotland (55) argue against such association. A strong correlation was found between negative symptoms and frontal lobe deficits; however, the statistical correction for the presence of TD as an intervening variable reduced the level of significance of this association. More recently, in a longitudinal study carried out in the Netherlands using a large patient sample (*n* = 708), it was concluded that the development of TD is linked to an illness-related pathologic process, characterized by worsening negative symptoms (56).

The issue of "brain organicity" as an increased risk factor for the development of TD was addressed by Gold et al. (57) in a controlled study on neuropsychological, computed tomographic, and psychiatric symptoms findings in

patients with and without TD. Previous studies had reported that signs of organic brain involvement were more common in TD than in non-TD patients. The authors studied 27 schizophrenic patients with TD and the same number of age-, gender-, and education-matched schizophrenic controls. Patients received neuropsychological testings, psychiatric symptom ratings, and cerebral computed tomography (CT) scans. Patients with TD differed from controls on only 1 of 23 cognitive variables. Moreover, they had significantly smaller ventricular/brain ratios on CT measurements. These results argue against previous theories on organicity and TD. In agreement with the previous study, Sachdev (58) found that although the total dose of neuroleptics significantly correlated with an increased risk of TD in mentally retarded institutionalized patients, other factors, such as gender, brain damage, or level of mental retardation, did not.

However, organicity seems to have a role, at least under certain circumstances, as reported by Hriso et al. (59) who found AIDS patients on neuroleptic therapy to be 2.4 times more likely than controls to develop extrapyramidal symptoms.

Several genes have been proposed as susceptibility factors for the development of TD; their pharmacogenetic impact in the present-day use of antipsychotics was recently reviewed by Ozdemir et al. (60). Many neuroleptics are metabolized by the cytochrome P450 enzyme debrisoquine hydroxylase, and certain polymorphisms of the *CYP2D6* gene encoding this enzyme correlate with the presence of TD in psychiatric patients receiving neuroleptics, according to different studies (60). Similarly, allelic polymorphisms of the dopamine D3 receptor gene *(DRD3)*, specifically the Ser9Gly variant, correlate with increased incidence of TD in patients under neuroleptic treatment (62). Lastly, several studies, recently published, have linked the occurrence of alellic polymorphisms of the serotonin type 2A receptor with a greater risk of TD in patients treated with antipsychotic medication (63). However, these findings could not be replicated in a comparable study conducted in Canada (64).

The pathophysiology of TD remains an enigma, although hypothetical mechanisms for its development abound (46; for a review, see 65). It has been originally attributed to the development of postsynaptic dopamine receptor supersensitivity and increase in the presynaptic turnover of dopamine induced by neuroleptics secondary to chronic dopaminergic blockade. Withdrawal of these drugs or dose reduction would allow these hypersensitive receptors to respond in an exaggerated fashion to normal levels of dopaminergic stimulation. Similar to classic TD, tardive tourettism would be related to the development of hypersensitive dopamine receptors in other dopamine-rich areas, such as the mesolimbic/mesocortical system.

An increased knowledge of basal ganglia functioning has provided alternative explanations, causing the supersensitive receptor hypothesis to come under heavy criticism. Mitchell et al. (66) have proposed TD to be the result of hypoactivity of the subthalamic output pathway to the medial pallidal segment resulting in loss of GABA-mediated inhibition of the thalamocortical outflow. These authors have made significant contributions to the understanding of the pathophysiology of movement disorders. They have functionally mapped the different pathways involved in basal ganglia control of movement and posture. In their study on pathophysiology of TD they have used a primate model of this disorder to investigate changes in 2-deoxyglucose (2-DG) uptake in different brain areas, correlating them with the presence of TD. Neuroleptic-treated dyskinetic animals showed reduced uptake of 2-DG in the medial segment of the globus pallidus and in the ventral anterior and ventral lateral nuclei of the thalamus. In support of this theory, Auchus and Pickel (67) reported sustained modifications in metenkephalin levels, associated with striatopallidal GABA pathways, in animals chronically exposed to neuroleptics. This study analyzed the role of endogenous opioid peptides in the pathophysiology of neuroleptic-induced movement disorders. Met5-enkephalin-like immunoreactivity (MELI) in terminal fields within the globus pallidus and in perikarya of caudate-putamen nuclei of rats chronically treated with haloperidol or clozapine was differentially altered. Significant increases in MELI were found only in haloperidol-treated rats. These differences could explain in part the lack of extrapyramidal side effects seen with clozapine. Using somewhat more refined techniques, Andreassen et al. (68) found that modifications in the number of striatal neurons expressing preproenkephalin messenger RNA (a precursor of metenkephalin) correlated with the development of oral dyskinesias in rats exposed to neuroleptics (an animal model of TD). An increase in this marker was observed only in rats that did not develop pronounced oral dyskinesias during treatment, suggesting that the mechanism by which neuroleptics induce dyskinesias involves a functional disturbance or even damage to a subpopulation on enkephalin expressing striatal neurons. Surprisingly, modifications in enkephalinergic transmission are not accompanied by compensatory changes in postsynaptic neurons measured through μ-opioid binding (69). In a previous study, Delfs et al. (70) had found evidences of decreased GABAergic transmission in the projection neurons of the external globus pallidus in an animal model of TD. The output pathways of the globus pallidus would be differentially affected by typical neuroleptics in contrast to clozapine. Typical neuroleptics would preferentially block D2 dopamine receptors located on GABAergic neurons projecting to the lateral globus pallidus. The repetitive stimulation of the D1 dopamine receptor by endogenous dopamine in the presence of D2 receptor blockade would result in sensitization of the D1-mediated striatal output. This imbalance would be a predisposing factor for the development of TD. These findings have been replicated, at

least in part, in recent studies exploring the effects of traditional (as opposed to new or atypical) antipsychotics on neurotransmission markers in basal ganglia–thalamocortical neural pathways (71). Haloperidol, in contrast to olanzapine and sertindole, showed a broad and potent action in the basal ganglia, inducing GABA$_A$ receptor up-regulation and dopamine D1 down-regulation, as well as changes in the expression of glutamic acid decarboxylase messenger RNA in the substantia nigra pars reticulata as well as the mediodorsal and reticular thalamic nucleii. This shift in the balance of dopamine D1 and D2 receptor–mediated activity was recently explored with modern genetic pharmacology techniques; results showed that blockade of the expression of D1 receptors through oligodeoxynucleotide antisense administration reduced the expression of vacuous chewing movements (VCMs; an animal model of TD) in rats (72).

Excitotoxic mechanisms have also been proposed as having a role in the pathophysiology of TD (73; for a review of experimental evidence in this regard, see 74 and 75). Excess glutamatergic activity could either be the result of lack of dopaminergic inhibition on the corticostriatal terminals or be secondary to increased activity of the subthalamic nucleus. Both mechanisms could eventually lead to structural lesions at the pallidal level. The net result would be a reduction in GABAergic function. It has been shown that glutamate levels are increased in the brain of animals chronically treated with typical neuroleptics. In addition, markers of glutamatergic neurotransmission and oxidative stress have been found to be elevated in the cerebrospinal fluid of schizophrenic patients with TD (73). Moreover, blockade of either glutamate receptors, calcium channels, and nitric oxide significantly reduced VCM in rats exposed to neuroleptics, lending further support to the excitotoxic hypothesis of TD (75). The participation of GABAergic mechanisms in TD is further supported by the finding that progabide and tiagabine (GABA-mimetic drugs) preventively inhibit the development of haloperidol-induced oral dyskinesias in rats. Melatonin, acting on benzodiazepine receptors, has been recently shown to dose dependently reduce the severity of VCM in rats, and this phenomenon has been attributed to an enhancement of GABAergic activity (76). The possibility that up-regulation of adenosine receptors contributes to supersensitive responses mediated by D2 dopamine receptors has been explored in animal models of TD. The role of neurotensin in the development of TD has been examined in animal models of this disorder. Neurotensin has been found to be increased within the ventrolateral striatum of animals chronically exposed to neuroleptics, raising the possibility of using neurotensin antagonists in the treatment of TD. Supersensitivity of D2 dopamine receptors is associated with reduced cyclic adenosine 3′,5′-monophosphate (cAMP). Restoration of cAMP levels through the use of rolipram, a phosphodiesterase inhibitor, significantly reduced dyskinesias in an animal model of TD (77), supporting the hypothesis that this drug may have a therapeutic effect on TD. Cyclic guanosine monophosphate (cGMP) is also suppressed by neuroleptic treatment in rats, together with nitric oxide (both signaling mechanisms appear to be involved in striatal neural plasticity), and these findings correlate with the development of VCM (78). In addition, impairment of cellular energy metabolism through mitochondrial dysfunction caused by neuroleptics has been proposed as a contributory factor to the development of TD. However, according to a recent study (79), mitochondrial ultrastructure and density did not correlate with the occurrence of VCM in rats. There are, nevertheless, a significant number of experimental evidences supporting the existence of structural changes at the striatal level induced by neuroleptic treatment and associated with the development of VCM, such as reduced number of striatal neurons expressing preprosomatostatin mRNA (74); reduced dendritic surface area and changes in the pattern of synaptic organization of dynorphin-positive terminals (80); reduction in striatal symmetric synapses by haloperidol in comparison to olanzapine (81); and modifications in the nerve terminal area and the density of nerve terminal glutamate immunoreactivity (82). Moreover, direct neurotoxic effects of haloperidol have been demonstrated in mouse neuronal cultures and PC-12 cells (83).

Despite the fact that numerous therapeutic strategies have been proposed for the management of TD, none has proved to be significantly effective (for extensive reviews on treatment, see 84 and 85). The best advice in this regard is early recognition and prevention. In psychiatric patients, there should be careful consideration of the real need to initiate neuroleptic treatment, and alternative therapeutic options should be evaluated. Neuroleptics should only be used when there is a clear indication for their prescription, at minimally effective doses and for as short a time as possible. In patients already receiving antipsychotic drugs, a reevaluation for the need for continuing neuroleptic treatment should be done periodically. The first option in patients who have already developed symptoms of TD should be reduction or withdrawal of the neuroleptic, if possible, even though it might exacerbate the involuntary movements initially. Spontaneous remission may occur after drug withdrawal, and this possibility should be considered before specific drug treatments are indicated. If the underlying psychiatric illness warrants the need for maintaining the patient under neuroleptic treatment, an attempt should be made to replace it with drugs that potentially induce less TD, such as thioridazine, risperidone, olanzapine, quetiapine, ziprasidone, or, if possible, clozapine (86–88).

Drugs used in the management of TD include dopamine-depleting agents (reserpine and tetrabenazine) (89), benzodiazepines such as clonazepam in milder forms, GABA mimetics (sodium valproate, baclofen), dopamine agonists in low doses (to stimulate autoreceptors), and a heterogeneous list of other compounds (85).

Both reserpine and tetrabenazine have been shown to be effective in reducing TD, at times dramatically. Both drugs should be initially given at low doses (reserpine: 0.25 mg/day; tetrabenazine: 25 mg/day) and gradually titrated until adequate benefit or undesirable side effect occurs. Effective doses of reserpine are usually around 3 to 5 mg/day; of tetrabenazine 100 to 200 mg/day. Common adverse effects with these drugs are hypotension, mental depression, and parkinsonism. In some cases, tetrabenazine can also induce acute dystonic reactions, as mentioned above.

Clonazepam has been reported to be effective in improving some cases of TD, especially its milder forms, through an indirect effect at the GABA receptor. Other drugs with presumed GABAergic properties have also been tried in the treatment of this syndrome. Baclofen, a putative GABA agonist, has been used, alone or in association with antidopaminergic drugs, with limited success. Sodium valproate, γ-vinyl-GABA, and, more recently, vigabatrin have also shown mild clinical efficacy in small groups of patients. Apomorphine, bromocriptine, and other direct dopamine agonists have been found to be useful in alleviating TDs in some clinical trials. Their beneficial effect on TD has been attributed to direct stimulation of presynaptic dopamine autoreceptors, inhibiting firing and release of dopamine at the nerve terminal.

A variety of other drugs have been proposed as alternative treatment for TD, although most of the reports dealing with them are only anecdotal or limited to the effects observed in a small number of patients. AMPT, an inhibitor of tyrosine hydroxylase that induces depletion of dopamine at the terminal level, has been reported to improve TD either alone or in combination with reserpine. Its use has been limited to experimental studies. A variety of cholinergic agents have also been used in the past, based on the early theories of cholinergic hypofunction in TD. There have been reports of occasional improvement with the use of acetylcholine precursors, such as choline, lecithin, and deanol; cholinesterase inhibitors, such as physostigmine and tacrine; the acetylcholine agonist aerocholine; and with the administration of meclophenoxate, a presumed activator of the cholinergic system. A number of anecdotal reports of uncontrolled studies have shown minimal benefit with the use of propranolol, clonidine, tryptophan, cyproheptadine, opiates, manganese, and carbamazepine. The reported beneficial effect of lithium has not been replicated in other studies. Calcium channel blockers, such as nifedipine or diltiazem, have produced some prolonged benefit in a limited number of patients. The effect of G_{M1} ganglioside, a substance known to promote neuronal plasticity, was compared to placebo on TD patients. A randomized trial including affected young adults and elderly subjects (90) was carried out in two large psychiatric centers. The results of this study showed no significant differences between G_{M1} ganglioside and placebo. Antioxidants such as vitamin E have also been proposed, assuming that oxidative stress linked to iron deposition in the striatum, together with increased lipid peroxidation, is partially responsible for TD (91). In preliminary uncontrolled studies results have been conflicting (92). However, in more recent clinical trials carried out for longer periods and under controlled conditions (93), vitamin E proved effective in improving dyskinesias in TD patients. This effect persisted over time even after placebo substitution. Vitamin B₆ was recently found to be effective in reducing the symptoms of TD in a double-blind, placebo-controlled, crossover study involving a small number of patients (94). In an open-label study involving 20 schizophrenic patients, the 5-HT₃ receptor antagonist ondansetron was also shown to improve TD (95). Melatonin has also been proposed as an alternative treatment modality, although in a recent study supraphysiologic doses of the drug did not prove effective (96).

Tardive dystonia often requires a different therapeutic approach than the more common form of TD. In this case the use of anticholinergics and even dopamine-blocking agents is sometimes required because reserpine and tetrabenazine often fail to bring about symptomatic improvement. Sometimes a combined approach is necessary using anticholinergics and dopamine-depleting drugs together. In almost 50% of cases of tardive dystonia this strategy is effective. Clonazepam has also been reported to be more beneficial for patients with predominantly dystonic symptoms than for those with buccolinguomandibulary syndrome. The atypical neuroleptic clozapine has been reported useful in the treatment of TD in general; however, it appears to be particularly effective in cases with dystonic features. Botulinum toxin injections, a standard form of treatment in idiopathic dystonia, has been used to treat tardive dystonia patients, especially those with focal manifestations. Under extreme circumstances stereotactic pallidotomy has been indicated in severe cases of tardive dystonia. For more information on the clinical aspects and treatment of tardive dystonia, see the review by van Harten and Kahn (97).

DYSKINESIAS INDUCED BY OTHER DRUGS

Phenytoin, among the rest of the antiepileptic drugs, is the most frequently associated with the development of movement disorders. This drug has been reported to induce orofacial chorea, ballismus, dystonia, tremor, asterixis, and myoclonus (98,99). In a review of the literature by Harrison et al. (98), 77 cases had been reported by 1993. Involuntary movements have occurred in some patients with high plasma phenytoin levels, while in 23% of cases phenytoin levels were within the therapeutic range; however, movement disorders occur most often in patients on polytherapy or following an increase in dosage. It should be noted that, according to Harrison (1993), 68% of the patients who developed movement disorders were taking other antiepileptic drugs in combina-

tion with phenytoin. The dyskinesias observed with this drug tend to disappear with dose reduction or withdrawal of the medication. The most common hyperkinesia observed in these patients is choreoathetosis, present in 91% of patients. More than one type of movement disorder may be present in the same patient. It has been suggested that a preexisting lesion in the basal ganglia might be an important predisposing factor for the development of phenytoin-induced dyskinesias. However, in only 12% of patients reported in the literature was a focal structural lesion of the brain identified. There are occasional reports of dyskinesias induced by other antiepileptic drugs, such as ethosuximide (100) and carbamazepine (101). Carbamazepine has also been found responsible for the development of motor and vocal tics in children and dystonic movements in brain-damaged children (102). A recent publication reported on the occurrence of asterixis in a patient receiving gabapentin for postherpetic neuralgia (103).

Tricyclic antidepressants, such as amytriptyline and imipramine, are known to induce dyskinesias both secondary to an acute intoxication and after long-term administration. The most common movement disorders associated with acute exposure to tricyclic antidepressants are choreoathetosis, tremor, and myoclonus; choreatic movements have also been observed in patients under long-term treatment for affective disorders. Involuntary movements usually disappear with drug withdrawal. It has been suggested that both the anticholinergic and serotonin reuptake inhibiting properties of the tricyclic antidepressants could be related to the development of abnormal movements (2).

The more novel class of antidepressants, the SSRIs have also been associated with the development of movement disorders (3). Fluoxetine has been reported to produce myoclonus or more complex movement disorders combining myoclonus, chorea, dystonia, and stereotypies. Gerber and Lynd (3) recently published a compilation of all available data on SSRI-induced movement disorders. They reviewed a total of 127 published reports involving 30 cases of akathisia, 19 of dystonia, 12 of dyskinesia, 6 of TD, 25 of parkinsonism, and 15 cases of mixed disorders. Ten isolated cases of bruxism were also identified, and an additional 10 reports could not be classified. In addition, manufacturers of these drugs provided 49 reports of akathisia, 44 of dystonia, 208 of dyskinesia, 76 of TD, 516 of parkinsonism, and 60 of bruxism. Treatment strategies included discontinuation of the SSRI; dosage reduction; or addition of a benzodiazepine, beta blocker, or anticholinergic. Buspirone, a drug acting as a full agonist at the 5-HT₁ₐ receptor, has been proposed as the preferred treatment for SSRI-induced bruxism (104). Myoclonus can be part of a more serious adverse effect observed with SSRIs, the serotonin syndrome. This is a potentially fatal disorder linked to excessive serotonergic activity. It is characterized by changes in mental status, hypertension, restlessness, myoclonus, hyperreflexia, diaphoresis, shivering, and tremor.

CNS stimulants, such as amphetamines, cocaine, pemoline, and methylphenidate, are also known to induce dyskinetic movements (105). Acute administration of amphetamine rarely produces abnormal involuntary movements, except in cases with preexisting striatal pathology or dysfunction. Chronic exposure to amphetamines and other stimulants may induce orofacial dyskinesias and choreic movements of the trunk and extremities. In some cases the dyskinesias have persisted for years after withdrawal of the drug(s). CNS stimulants used in the treatment of attention deficit-hyperactivity disorder have been implicated in many instances in the development of tics or other dyskinesias, and the close association of treatment and exacerbation of symptoms in some Tourette's syndrome patients seems clear. In most instances, the movement disorders seen with these drugs are transient. The risk of developing chronic tics with the use of CNS stimulants in patients with attention deficit-hyperactivity disorder has not been firmly established. The underlying pathophysiology of amphetamine- and other stimulant-induced dyskinesias is probably related to the induction of a state of postsynaptic dopamine receptor hypersensitivity. Other drugs with stimulant properties, such as β-adrenergic agonists used in the management of respiratory disorders, are also known to produce involuntary movements. Tremor is the most common movement disorder seen with such drugs as terbutaline, bambuterol, albuterol, and salbutamol. Buspirone, a nonbenzodiazepine anxiolytic drug with serotonergic and dopaminergic properties, has been associated with isolated reports of akathisia, orofacial dyskinesias, transient myoclonus, and transient and persistent dystonia. Benzodiazepines, such as diazepam, clorazepate, and lorazepam, rarely have been found to exacerbate or even induce dyskinesias. Acute dystonic reactions have been reported with the use of intravenous midazolam.

Oral contraceptives are occasionally responsible for the development of choreatic movements. The movement disorder usually appears 9 to 60 days after the onset of treatment. The existence of predisposing factors has been discussed as some patients developing chorea with the use of oral contraceptives had a history of rheumatic fever, encephalitis, or chorea gravidarum. It is almost the rule that the involuntary movements disappear a few days after drug withdrawal. Contraceptive-induced dyskinesias are probably related to the antidopaminergic action of estrogen.

Other drugs that occasionally have been reported to induce dyskinesias are cimetidine (associated with terbutaline and theophylline), methyldopa, diazoxide, digoxin, lithium, amoxapine, methadone, tumor necrosis factor, fentanyl, amantadine, and levofloxacin (2,106).

REFERENCES

1. Gershanik O. Drug-induced movement disorders. *Curr Opin Neurol Neurosurg* 1993;6(3):369–376.
2. Gershanik O. Drug-induced dyskinesias. In: Jankovic J, Tolosa E, eds. *Parkinson's disease and movement disorders,* 3rd ed. Baltimore: Williams & Wilkins, 1998.
3. Gerber PE, Lynd LD. Selective serotonin-reuptake inhibitor-induced movement disorders. *Ann Pharmacother* 1998;32(6):692–698.
4. Kondo T, Otani K, Tokinaga N, et al. Characteristics and risk factors of acute dystonia in schizophrenic patients treated with nemonapride, a selective dopamine antagonist. *J Clin Psychopharmacol* 1999;19(1):45–50.
5. Magnuson TM, Roccaforte WH, Wengel SP, et al. Medication-induced dystonias in nine patients with dementia. *J Neuropsychiatry Clin Neurosci* 2000;2(2):219–225.
6. Khanna R, Das A, Damodaran SS. Prospective study of neuroleptic-induced dystonia in mania and schizophrenia. *Am J Psychiatry* 1992;149:4:511–513.
7. McCann UD, Penetar DM, Belenky G. Acute dystonic reaction in normal humans caused by catecholamine depletion. *Clin Neuropharmacol* 1990;13:6:565–568.
8. Matsumoto RR, Pouw B. Correlation between neuroleptic binding to sigma(1) and sigma(2) receptors and acute dystonic reactions. *Eur J Pharmacol* 2000;401(2):155–160.
9. Berardi D, Giannelli A, Barnes TR. Clinical correlates of akathisia in acute psychiatric inpatients. *Int Clin Psychopharmacol* 2000;15(4):215–219.
10. Rosebush PI, Mazurek MF. Neurologic side effects in neuroleptic-naive patients treated with haloperidol or risperidone. *Neurology* 1999;52(4):782–785.
11. Sunami M, Nishikawa T, Yorogi A, et al. Intravenous administration of levodopa ameliorated a refractory akathisia case induced by interferon-alpha. *Clin Neuropharmacol* 2000;23(1):59–61.
12. Hirose S. Restlessness of respiration as a manifestation of akathisia: five case reports of respiratory akathisia. *J Clin Psychiatry* 2000;61(10):737–741.
13. Hirose S. Restlessness in suboccipital muscles as a manifestation of akathisia. *Psychiatry Clin Neurosci* 2001;55(1):81–82.
14. Kahn EM, Munetz MR, Davies MA, et al. Akathisia: clinical phenomenology and relationship to tardive dyskinesia. *Compr Psychiatry* 1993;33:4:233–236.
15. Duncan EJ, Adler LA, Stephanides M, et al. Akathisia and exacerbation of psychopathology: a preliminary report. *Clin Neuropharmacol* 2000;23(3):169–173.
16. Nair CJ, Josiassen RC, Abraham G, et al. Does akathisia influence psychopathology in psychotic patients treated with clozapine? *Biol Psychiatry* 1999;45(10):1376–1383.
17. Eichhammer P, Albus M, Borrmann-Hassenbach M, et al. Association of dopamine D3-receptor gene variants with neuroleptic induced akathisia in schizophrenic patients: a generalization of Steen's study on DRD3 and tardive dyskinesia. *Am J Med Genet* 2000;96(2):187–191.
18. Brune M. The incidence of akathisia in bipolar affective disorder treated with neuroleptics—a preliminary report. *J Affect Disord* 1999;53(2):175–177.
19. Hofmann M, Seifritz E, Botschev C, et al. Serum iron and ferritin in acute neuroleptic akathisia. *Psychiatry Res* 2000;93(3):201–207.
20. Poyurovsky M, Shardorodsky M, Fuchs C, et al. Treatment of neuroleptic-induced akathisia with the 5-HT2 antagonist mianserin: double-blind, placebo-controlled study. *Br J Psychiatry* 1999a;174:238–242.
21. Poyurovsky M, Weizman A. Lack of efficacy of the 5-HT3 receptor antagonist granisetron in the treatment of acute neuroleptic-induced akathisia. *Int Clin Psychopharmacol* 1999b;14(6):357–360.
22. Daniel DG, Potkin SG, Reeves KR, et al. Intramuscular (IM)

ziprasidone 20 mg is effective in reducing acute agitation associated with psychosis: a double-blind, randomized trial. *Psychopharmacology (Berl)* 2001;155(2):128–134.

23. Faurbye A, Rasch PJ, Peterson PB, et al. Neurological symptoms in pharmacotherapy of psychoses. *Acta Psychiatr Scand* 1964;40:10–14.

24. Schooler NR, Kane JM. Research diagnoses for tardive dyskinesia. *Arch Gen Psychiatry* 1982;39:486–487.

25. Kiriakakis V, Bhatia KP, Quinn NP, et al. The natural history of tardive dystonia: a long-term follow-up study of 107 cases. *Brain* 1998;121(Pt 11):2053–2066.

26. Klawans HL, Nausieda PA, Goetz CC, et al. Tourette-like symptoms following chronic neuroleptic therapy. *Adv Neurol* 1982;35:415–418.

27. Bharucha KJ, Sethi KD. Tardive tourettism after exposure to neuroleptic therapy. *Mov Disord* 1995;10(6):791–793.

28. Tominaga H, Fukuzako H, Izumi K, et al. Tardive myoclonus. *Lancet* 1987;1:322.

29. Stacy M, Jankovic J. Tardive tremor. *Mov Disord* 1992;7:1:53–57.

30. Ford B, Greene P, Fahn S. Oral and genital tardive pain syndromes. *Neurology* 1994;4(11):2115–2119.

31. Arango C, Adami H, Sherr JD, et al. Relationship of awareness of dyskinesia in schizophrenia to insight into mental illness. *Am J Psychiatry* 1999;156(7):1097–1099.

32. Chong SA, Remington G, Mahendran R, et al. Awareness of tardive dyskinesia in Asian patients with schizophrenia. *J Clin Psychopharmacol* 2001;21(2):235–237.

33. Byne W, White L, Parella M, et al. Tardive dyskinesia in a chronically institutionalized population of elderly schizophrenic patients: prevalence and association with cognitive impairment. *Int J Geriatr Psychiatry* 1998;13(7):473–479.

34. Koshino Y, Madokoro S, Ito T, et al. A survey of tardive dyskinesia in psychiatric inpatients in Japan. *Clin Neuropharmacol* 1992;15:1:34–43.

35. Chiu H, Shum P, Lau J, et al. Prevalence of tardive dyskinesia, tardive dystonia, and respiratory dyskinesia among Chinese psychiatric patients in Hong Kong. *Am J Psychiatry* 1992;149:8:1081–1085.

36. Fenton WS. Prevalence of spontaneous dyskinesia in schizophrenia. *J Clin Psychiatry* 2000;61[Suppl 4]:10–14.

37. Haddenbrock S. Prolonged hyperkinetic syndrome following long-term treatment with high doses of neuroleptic agents. In: Kranz H, Heinrich K, eds. *Begleitwirkungen und Misserfolge der Psychiatrischen Pharmakotherapie.* Stuttgart: Thieme-Verlag, 1964:54–63.

38. Degwitz R. Extrapyramidal motor disorders following long-term treatment with neuroleptic drugs. In: Crane GE, Gardner R, eds. *Psychotropic drugs and dysfunction of the basal ganglia.* Public Health Service Publication No. 1938. Washington, DC: U.S. Government Printing Office, 1969:22–25.

39. Crane GE, Naranjo ER. Motor disorders induced by neuroleptics. *Arch Gen Psychiatry* 1971;24:179–184.

40. Lacro JP, Gilbert PL, Paulsen JS, et al. Early course of new-onset tardive dyskinesia in older patients. *Psychopharmacol Bull* 1994;30(2):187–191.

41. Harrison PJ. The neuropathological effects of antipsychotic drugs. *Schizophr Res* 1999;30:40(2):87–99.

42. Heinrich K, Wegener I, Bender HJ. Spuate extrapiramidale Hyperkinesen bei neuroleptischer Langzeittherapie. *Pharmakopsychiatr Neuropsychopharmakol* 1968;1:169–195.

43. Koshino Y, Wada Y, Isaki K, et al. A long-term outcome study of tardive dyskinesia in patients on antipsychotic medication. *Clin Neuropharmacol* 1991;14:6:537–546.

44. Glazer WM, Morgenstern H, Doucette JT. Predicting the long-term risk of tardive dyskinesia in outpatients maintained on neuroleptic medications. *J Clin Psychiatry* 1993;54:4.

45. Cavallaro R, Regazzetti MG, Mundo E, et al. Tardive dyskinesia outcomes: clinical and pharmacological correlates of remission and persistence. *Neuropsychopharmacology* 1993;8:3.

46. Sachdev PS. The current status of tardive dyskinesia. *Aust N Z J Psychiatry* 2000;34(3):355–369.

47. Yassa R, Nastase C, Dupont D, et al. Tardive dyskinesia in elderly psychiatric patients: a 5 year study. *Am J Psychiatry* 1992;149:9:1206–1211.

48. Sweet RA, Mulsant BH, Rifai AH, et al. Relation of age to prevalence of tardive dyskinesia. *Am J Psychiatry* 1992;149:1:141.

49. Woerner MG, Alvir JM, Saltz BL, et al. Prospective study of tardive dyskinesia in the elderly: rates and risk factors. *Am J Psychiatry* 1998;155(11):1521–1528.

50. van Os J, Walsh E, van Horn E, et al. Tardive dyskinesia in psychosis: are women really more at risk? UK700 Group. *Acta Psychiatr Scand* 1999;99(4):288–293.

51. Muscettola G, Pampallona S, Barbato G, et al. Persistent tardive dyskinesia: demographic and pharmacological risk factors. *Acta Psychiatr Scand* 1993;87:1.

52. van Harten PN, Hoek HW, Matroos GE, et al. Intermittent neuroleptic treatment and risk for tardive dyskinesia: Curacao Extrapyramidal Syndromes Study III. *Am J Psychiatry* 1998;155(4):565–567.

53. Woerner MG, Saltz BL, Kane JM, et al. Diabetes and development of tardive dyskinesia. *Am J Psychiatry* 1993;150:6.

54. Davis EJB, Borde M, Sharma LN. Tardive dyskinesia and type II schizophrenia. *Br J Psychiatry* 1992;160:253–256.

55. Brown KW, White T. The association among negative symptoms, movement disorders, and frontal lobe psychological deficits in schizophrenic patients. *Biol Psychiatry* 1991;30:12:1182–1190.

56. van Os J, Walsh E, van Horn E, et al. Changes in negative symptoms and the risk of tardive dyskinesia: a longitudinal study. UK700 Group. *Acta Psychiatr Scand* 2000;101(4):300–306.

57. Gold JM, Egan MF, Kirch DG, et al. Tardive dyskinesia: neuropsychological, computerized tomographic and psychiatric symptom findings. *Biol Psychiatry* 1991;30:6:587–599.

58. Sachdev P. Drug-induced movement disorders in institutionalised adults with mental retardation: clinical characteristics and risk factors. *Aust N Z J Psychiatry* 1992;26:2:242–248.

59. Hriso E, Kuhn T, Masdeu JC, et al. Extrapyramidal symptoms due to dopamine-blocking agents in patients with AIDS encephalopathy. *Am J Psychiatry* 1991;148:11:1558–1161.

60. Ozdemir V, Basile VS, Masellis M, et al. Pharmacogenetic assessment of antipsychotic-induced movement disorders: contribution of the dopamine D3 receptor and cytochrome P450 1A2 genes. *J Biochem Biophys Meth* 2001;47(1–2):151–157.

61. Basile VS, Ozdemir V, Masellis M, et al. A functional polymorphism of the cytochrome P450 1A2 (*CYP1A2*) gene: association with tardive dyskinesia in schizophrenia. *Mol Psychiatry* 2000;5(4):410–417.

62. Liao DL, Yeh YC, Chen HM, et al. Association between the Ser9Gly polymorphism of the dopamine D3 receptor gene and tardive dyskinesia in Chinese schizophrenic patients. *Neuropsychobiology* 2001;44(2):95–98.

63. Segman RH, Heresco-Levy U, Finkel B, et al. Association between the serotonin 2A receptor gene and tardive dyskinesia in chronic schizophrenia. *Mol Psychiatry* 2001;6(2):225–229.

64. Basile VS, Ozdemir V, Masellis M, et al. Lack of association between serotonin-2A receptor gene (*HTR2A*) polymorphisms and tardive dyskinesia in schizophrenia. *Mol Psychiatry* 2001;6(2):230–234.

65. Casey DE. Tardive dyskinesia: pathophysiology and animal models. *J Clin Psychiatry* 2000;61[Suppl 4]:5–9.

66. Mitchell IJ, Crossman AR, Liminga U, et al. Regional changes in 2-deoxyglucose uptake associated with neuroleptic-induced

tardive dyskinesia in the Cebus monkey. *Mov Disord* 1992;7:1: 32–37.

67. Auchus AP, Pickel VM. Quantitative light microscopic demonstration of increased pallidal and striatal met5-enkephalin-like immunoreactivity in rats following chronic treatment with haloperidol but not with clozapine: implications for the pathogenesis of neuroleptic-induced movement disorders. *Exp Neurol* 1992;117:1:17–27.

68. Andreassen OA, Finsen B, Ostergaard K, et al. The relationship between oral dyskinesias produced by long-term haloperidol treatment, the density of striatal preproenkephalin messenger RNA and enkephalin peptide, and the number of striatal neurons expressing preproenkephalin messenger RNA in rats. *Neuroscience* 1999;88(1):27–35.

69. Bower CM, Hyde TM, Zaka M, et al. Decreased mu-opioid receptor binding in the globus pallidus of rats treated with chronic haloperidol. *Psychopharmacology (Berl)* 2000;150(3): 260–263.

70. Delfs JM, Ellison GD, Mercugliano M, et al. Expression of glutamic acid decarboxylase mRNA in striatum and pallidum in an animal model of tardive dyskinesia. *Exp Neurol* 1995;133(2): 175–188.

71. Sakai K, Gao XM, Hashimoto T, et al. Traditional and new antipsychotic drugs differentially alter neurotransmission markers in basal ganglia–thalamocortical neural pathways. *Synapse* 2001;39(2):152–160.

72. Van Kampen JM, Stoessl AJ. Dopamine D(1A) receptor function in a rodent model of tardive dyskinesia. *Neuroscience* 2000; 101(3):629–635.

73. Tsai G, Goff DC, Chang RW, et al. Markers of glutamatergic neurotransmission and oxidative stress associated with tardive dyskinesia. *Am J Psychiatry* 1998;155(9):1207–1213.

74. Andreassen OA, Jorgensen HA. Neurotoxicity associated with neuroleptic-induced oral dyskinesias in rats: implications for tardive dyskinesia? *Prog Neurobiol* 2000;61(5):525–541.

75. Naidu PS, Kulkarni SK. Excitatory mechanisms in neuroleptic-induced vacuous chewing movements (VCMs): possible involvement of calcium and nitric oxide. *Behav Pharmacol* 2001;12(3):209–216.

76. Raghavendra V, Naidu PS, Kulkarni SK. Reversal of reserpine-induced vacuous chewing movements in rats by melatonin: involvement of peripheral benzodiazepine receptors. *Brain Res* 2001;904(1):149–152.

77. Sasaki H, Hashimoto K, Maeda Y, et al. Rolipram, a selective c-AMP phosphodiesterase inhibitor, suppresses oro-facial dyskinetic movements in rats. *Life Sci* 1995;56(25):443–447.

78. Bester AM, Harvey BH. Early suppression of striatal cyclic GMP may predetermine the induction and severity of chronic haloperidol-induced vacuous chewing movements. *Metab Brain Dis* 2000;15(4):275–285.

79. Eyles DW, Pond SM, Van der Schyf CJ, et al. Mitochondrial ultrastructure and density in a primate model of persistent tardive dyskinesia. *Life Sci* 2000;66(14):1345–1350.

80. Meredith GE, De Souza IE, Hyde TM, et al. Persistent alterations in dendrites, spines, and dynorphinergic synapses in the nucleus accumbens shell of rats with neuroleptic-induced dyskinesias. *J Neurosci* 2000;20(20):7798–7806.

81. Roberts RC. Effect of chronic olanzapine treatment on striatal synaptic organization. *Synapse* 2001;39(1):8–15.

82. Andreassen OA, Meshul CK, Moore C, et al. Oral dyskinesias and morphological changes in rat striatum during long-term haloperidol administration. *Psychopharmacology (Berl)* 2001; 157(1):11–19.

83. Galili R, Mosberg, Gil-Ad I, et al. Haloperidol-induced neurotoxicity—possible implications for tardive dyskinesia. *J Neural Transm* 2000;107(4):479–490.

84. Soares KV, McGrath JJ. The treatment of tardive dyskinesia—a systematic review and meta-analysis. *Schizophr Res* 1999;39(1): 1–16.

85. Cochrane Database Systematic Reviews.

86. Beasley CM, Dellva MA, Tamura RN, et al. Randomised double-blind comparison of the incidence of tardive dyskinesia in patients with schizophrenia during long-term treatment with olanzapine or haloperidol. *Br J Psychiatry* 1999;174:23–30.

87. Glazer WM. Expected incidence of tardive dyskinesia associated with atypical antipsychotics. *J Clin Psychiatry* 2000;61[Suppl]4: 21–26.

88. Jeste DV, Lacro JP, Bailey A, et al. Lower incidence of tardive dyskinesia with risperidone compared with haloperidol in older patients. *J Am Geriatr Soc* 1999;47(6):716–719.

89. Ondo WG, Hanna PA, Jankovic J. Tetrabenazine treatment for tardive dyskinesia: assessment by randomized videotape protocol. *Am J Psychiatry* 1999;156(8):1279–1281.

90. Sommer BR, Cohen BM, Satlin A, et al. Changes in tardive dyskinesia symptoms in elderly patients treated with ganglioside GM1 or placebo. *J Geriatr Psychiatry Neurol* 1994;7(4): 234–237.

91. Brown K, Reid A, White T, et al. Vitamin E, lipids, and lipid peroxidation products in tardive dyskinesia. *Biol Psychiatry* 1998;43(12):863–867.

92. Barak Y, Swartz M, Shamir E, et al. Vitamin E (alpha-tocopherol) in the treatment of tardive dyskinesia: a statistical meta-analysis. *Ann Clin Psychiatry* 1998;10(3):101–105.

93. Adler LA, Edson R, Lavori P, et al. Long-term treatment effects of vitamin E for tardive dyskinesia. *Biol Psychiatry* 1998;43(12): 868–872.

94. Lerner V, Miodownik C, Kaptsan A, et al. Vitamin B(6) in the treatment of tardive dyskinesia: a double-blind, placebo-controlled, crossover study. *Am J Psychiatry* 2001;158(9):1511–1514.

95. Sirota P, Mosheva T, Shabtay H, et al. Use of the selective serotonin 3 receptor antagonist ondansetron in the treatment of neuroleptic-induced tardive dyskinesia. *Am J Psychiatry* 2000;157(2):287–289.

96. Shamir E, Barak Y, Plopsky I, et al. Is melatonin treatment effective for tardive dyskinesia? *J Clin Psychiatry* 2000;61(8):556–558.

97. van Harten PN, Kahn RS. Tardive dystonia. *Schizophr Bull* 1999;25(4):741–748.

98. Harrison MB, Lyons GR, Landow ER. Phenytoin and dyskinesias: a report of two cases and review of the literature. *Mov Disord* 1993;8(1):19–27.

99. Chi WM, Chua KS, Kong KH. Phenytoin-induced asterixis—uncommon or underdiagnosed? *Brain Inj* 2000;14(9):847–850.

100. Kirschberg GJ. Dyskinesia—an unusual reaction to ethosuximide. *Arch Neurol* 1975;32:137–138.

101. Go T. [Carbamazepine-induced involuntary movements in a girl with localization-related epilepsy.] *No To Hattatsu* 1999;31 (4):366–369.

102. Neglia JP, Glaze DG, Zion TE. Tics and vocalizations in children treated with carbamazepine. *Pediatrics* 1984;73: 841–844.

103. Jacob PC, Chand RP, Omeima el-S. Asterixis induced by gabapentin. *Clin Neuropharmacol* 2000;23(1):53.

104. Bostwick JM, Jaffee MS. Buspirone as an antidote to SSRI-induced bruxism in 4 cases. *J Clin Psychiatry* 1999;60(12): 857–860.

105. Weiner WJ, Rabinstein A, Levin B, et al. Cocaine-induced persistent dyskinesias. *Neurology* 2001;56(7):964–965.

106. Yasuda H, Yoshida A, Masuda Y, et al. [Levofloxacin-induced neurological adverse effects such as convulsion, involuntary movement (tremor, myoclonus and chorea like), visual hallucination in two elderly patients.] *Nippon Ronen Igakkai Zasshi* 1999;36(3):213–217.

SLEEP-RELATED MOVEMENT DISORDERS AND RESTLESS LEGS SYNDROME

CLAUDIA TRENKWALDER

Sleep-related movement disorders are sleep disturbances occurring during the night, but they may also manifest as movement disorders during wakefulness at daytime. Some sleep-related movement disorders are associated with neurodegenerative diseases, such as REM sleep behavior disorder (RBD) with Parkinson's disease (PD), and multiple system atrophy (MSA).

In this chapter, disturbances of REM (rapid eye movement) sleep (1), both idiopathic and secondary RBD associated with neurodegenerative disease (2), are described and followed by "nocturnal dystonia" assigned as nocturnal frontal lobe epilepsy (NFLE) (3,4). The subsequent part of the chapter describes one of the most common movement disorders, restless legs syndrome and periodic limb movements (PLMs) in sleep, two conditions that are closely related.

Hypnic jerks, jactatio capitis, somnambulism, and pavor nocturnus are characteristic sleep-associated motor or behavioral abnormalities but do not manifest as a motor disorder during daytime. Therefore, discussion of these disturbances may be restricted to textbooks of sleep disorders medicine.

REM SLEEP BEHAVIOR DISORDER

Schenck and Mahowald (1) described RBD as a syndrome of excessive motor activity while dreaming, with a loss of the normal voluntary muscle atonia during REM sleep. RBD is classified as a parasomnia (5). Parasomnias, defined as intermittently occurring nocturnal events in association with wake–sleep transition disturbances, occur as REM as well as non-REM (NREM) sleep disorders (Table 26.1).

RBD was first observed in patients with alcohol withdrawal. RBD occurring in otherwise healthy patients is called *idiopathic*, and that associated with an already apparent neurodegenerative disorder is *secondary* (2,6–8).

Definition and Clinical Features: Idiopathic and Secondary Forms of RBD

Symptoms of RBD are frequently reported by patients' bed partners, who observe sometimes-violent behavior during sleep that is typically discordant with the patient's normal behavior during the day (9). During REM sleep, patients move vehemently in association with dream mentation that is often recalled on awakening. These dreams are mostly characterized by nightmares with fights, self-defense, or useless attempts to flee. Violent movements may lead to self-injury or to attacking the bed partner (1). Other movements are stereotypically repeated arm and hand waving associated with polysomnographically recorded increased muscle tone of the chin and limbs (Fig. 26.1). Various abrupt behaviors, including explosive, complex movements associated with yelling and shouting, may occur episodically. Mild forms of RBD

TABLE 26.1. A CLASSIFICATION OF THE PARASOMNIAS

Wake–sleep transition disorders
    Sleep starts (hypnic jerks)
    Rhythmic movement disorder (jactatio capitis nocturna)
Non-REM sleep disorders
    Confusional arousals (nocturnal sleep drunkenness)
    Sleepwalking (somnambulism)
    Sleep terrors (pavor nocturnus, incubus)
    Nocturnal paroxysmal dystonia
REM sleep disorders
    Nightmares (terrifying dreams, anxiety dreams)
    REM sleep behavior disorder
    Sleep paralysis, isolated form
    Painful erections
Light sleep disorders (stage 1, 2, REM)
    Sleep talking
    Bruxism (teeth grinding)
Diffuse sleep disorders (no stage preference)
    Enuresis nocturnus (bed-wetting)

Duration: 30 sec

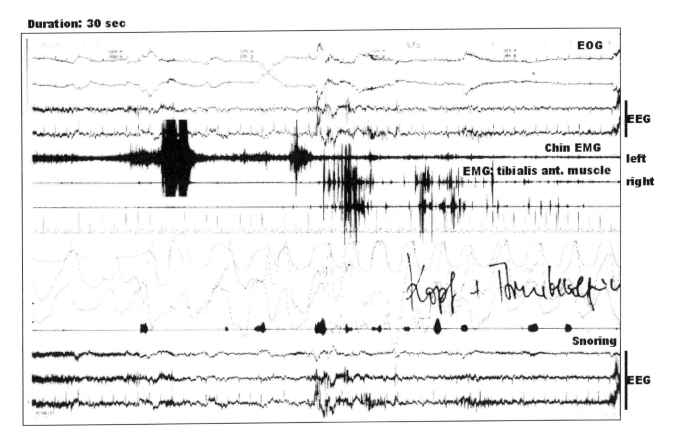

EOG = electrooculogram

FIG. 26.1. Patient with Parkinson's disease and REM sleep behavior disorder, who exhibited severe sleep talking and moving of head and arms during a REM episode as observed here. Electro-oculogram shows typical REM sleep with an increased tone of chin. Electromyogram of tibialis muscles exhibits muscle twitches and single leg movements.

may precede the full-blown syndrome for years and consist of vocalizations during sleep, nonspectacular movements, and vivid dreams (1). Those mild forms are a common finding in patients with parkinsonian syndromes, when investigated polysomnographically (10).

The minimal diagnostic criteria for RBD have been defined by the International Classification of Sleep Disorders as "movements of the limbs or body associated with dream mentation," and at least one of the following criteria: potentially harmful sleep behavior; dreams that appear to be acted out; sleep behavior that disrupts sleep continuity (5).

Idiopathic RBD is a rare disorder that occurs in patients with no other neurologic disorders or any history of psychopharmacologic treatment. However, the first published observation of the syndrome was documented in chronic alcoholics (11). *Secondary RBD* is associated with alcohol consumption, psychopharmacologic treatment, or neurodegenerative disease, especially synucleopathy (2). Recently, however, it has been assumed that idiopathic RBD may reflect the initial manifestation of a neurodegenerative disease and that idiopathic and secondary forms of RBD are closely related. Prospective studies of patients with idiopathic RBD may someday reveal whether a neurodegenerative disease follows after onset of RBD. Initial studies tend to confirm this hypothesis (2,6).

Epidemiology

Approximately 60% of the cases described are idiopathic and not associated with metabolic alterations or psychopharmacologic treatment (9). The syndrome is generally more common in males. Idiopathic RBD is rare, and population-based studies of the prevalence of idiopathic RBD have not been reported.

As recent publications assume that RBD may represent a preclinical state of a neurodegenerative disorder (2,7,12, 13), the increased prevalence of RBD in the elderly may be due to the increased prevalence of neurodegeneration in the elderly. The male preponderance has not been explained sufficiently. The percentage of RBD in PD patients according to polysomnographic criteria is approximately 40% (10), whereas it is up to 80% in patients with MSA (7).

Diagnosis and Differential Diagnosis

The assumption that someone is suffering from RBD derives from the bed partner's complaints and the patient's history. Mild forms are not reported if patients are not questioned specifically. This is especially true for secondary RBD in patients with PD and other neurodegenerative disorders, who fully disclose their sleep problems only when appropriate sleep questionnaires are applied (14). The differential diagnosis may depend on the comorbidity and previously known neurologic disorder of the patient. If, for example, the patient is known to have a parkinsonian syndrome, the differential diagnosis should consider specific parkinsonian motor symptoms during sleep, such as nocturnal akinesia, dystonia, tremor, onset of nightmares versus nocturnal dopaminergic psychosis, or even drug-induced confusional states (10,15). If the history is typical and fulfills the diagnostic criteria of RBD without daytime symptoms of delusions or psychosis, a clinical diagnosis may be sufficient, as RBD is a common nocturnal complaint in parkinsonian syndromes.

The differential diagnosis of idiopathic RBD includes posttraumatic stress syndrome, classic nightmares, sleep talking, sleep terrors, and any kind of epileptic activity with seizures during sleep (9). In these patients the clinical history eventually may be completed by the bed partners, but the definitive diagnosis should not be verified without a polysomnographic study.

Polysomnographic Findings in RBD

Polysomnographic studies show increased phasic and tonic electromyographic activity during REM sleep in RBD patients; this occurred in 97% of a consecutive clinically defined RBD population. Severe abnormal motor behavior and PLMs are frequently associated phenomena in those patients (13).

Although nocturnal episodes tend to decrease with time in parkinsonian patients, maybe due to the progressive neurodegeneration (13), increased muscle tone during sleep persists and is the most consistent polysomnographic finding in RBD. However, the occurrence of PLMs is a common finding in PD patients as well as in MSA patients (7,10) and may be independent of RBD.

All patients with assumed idiopathic RBD by history should be diagnosed with a polysomnographic study. As idiopathic RBD occurs rarely, more common nocturnal movement disorders, such as seizures, must be excluded before a specific treatment for RBD is initiated.

In secondary RBD, associated with neurodegeneration, Eisensehr and colleagues found that a clinical interview does not suffice to diagnose RBD, as only 50% of polysomnographic RBDs could be detected by history and an interview in PD patients (6). However, it is important to differentiate clinically relevant forms of RBD that require treatment from subclinical forms. These mild forms are accompanied by a loss of skeletal muscle atonia during REM sleep and have been observed in more than 50% of patients with PD and MSA (10). Clinically relevant sleep complaints in PD, consisting of frequent sleep disruptions and awakenings, vocalizations, and nocturnal motor symptoms, may not sufficiently be differentiated by history and should be diagnosed by polysomnographic studies more frequently. The use of appropriate sleep questionnaires developed for parkinsonian syndromes (14) may increase the frequency of diagnosing and distinguishing RBD in the future.

Pathophysiology and Etiology

There is increasing evidence that secondary and presumably idiopathic RBDs are closely related to neurodegenerative disorders. RBDs may precede motor symptoms of PD or MSA by years (2,6–8,13). Lewy bodies occurred in a series of ten patients diagnosed with RBD; nine of these were identified with Lewy body disease, one with MSA at autopsy (2). Therefore, the authors suspect RBD as a possible manifestation of an evolving synucleopathy. Neuroimaging studies of dopamine receptors showed a significant reduction of striatal [123]J-IPT binding in five patients with idiopathic RBD as a sign of reduced dopamine release (12), a finding that was confirmed in a larger group of RBD patients compared with PD patients and controls (6).

The neurodegeneration of brainstem nuclei that suppresses muscle tone during REM is thought to cause RBD. The ventromedial medullary zone may promote REM atonia and may be targeted by GABAergic projections of the basal ganglia to midbrain neurons (16). Different patterns of neurodegeneration, dependent on the extent and localization of neuronal cell loss in the dorsolateral pons, may be responsible for atonia in REM sleep and provoke some degree of RBD. In magnetic resonance imaging (MRI) studies, no specific regions could be detected in relation to RBD. Nonspecific periventricular white matter lesions (20 of 52) and cerebral atrophy (24 of 52) were the most prominent findings in 52 patients (13).

Treatment

Clonazepam is the most effective treatment for RBD. A dose of 0.5 to 2 mg at bedtime markedly reduces all symptoms in 90% of cases (1,17), although REM atonia persists (18). A small dose of clonazepam almost immediately suppresses the motor behavior and violent attacks. In a population of RBD patients only 13% did not respond sufficiently to clonazepam (13). A few patients, who also suffered from obstructive sleep apnea syndrome and therefore could not take benzodiazepines, experienced remission without treatment. Two others responded to clozapine (13). Changing the environment of the patient's bed and removing potentially dangerous items may also be advisable for RBD patients and their families.

Reports on treatment of patients with RBD are based mostly on individuals with idiopathic RBD. Clonazepam is efficient in both forms of RBD, according to case reports and clinical experience, although no controlled treatment studies in RBD are available. Therapy with benzodiazepines is mostly described in case series of secondary or idiopathic RBD (1,8,13) without controlled designs or long-term treatment observation.

NOCTURNAL PAROXYSMAL DYSTONIA; NOCTURNAL FRONTAL LOBE EPILEPSY

Definition and Clinical Features

These motor attacks during NREM sleep are characterized by complex behavior with dystonic-dyskinetic movements and may last for several seconds up to an hour, sometimes associated with nocturnal wanderings or stereotyped agitated somnambulism (19,20). Tinuper and co-workers studied three patients with frequent attacks of nocturnal paroxysmal dystonia (NPD) during NREM sleep and detected epileptic discharges occurring periodically every 20 to 40 seconds. They postulated that these episodes might represent frontal lobe seizures (4).

Most cases of NPD could be identified as seizures and assigned as nocturnal frontal lobe epilepsy (NFLE). Three clinical subtypes of NFLE have been distinguished according to the duration and motor phenomena (3). NFLE shows a male preponderance. The onset of symptoms is early (mostly in infancy or in adolescence), and a strong familial association has been found. In some of those families the etiology of the disease was a hereditary channelopathy (21).

Diagnosis

The patient's history of nocturnal motor episodes is often associated with daytime tiredness and poor quality of sleep. Patients with assumed NPD or NFLE have to be recorded by videopolysomnography, as interictal wake and sleep electroencephalograms (EEGs) are mostly normal (19). Abnormal stereotyped, dystonic-like movements during the attack are mandatory for diagnosis. Polysomnographic recordings show that attacks occur exclusively in NREM sleep stage 2, rarely in stage 3 or 4 with desynchronization of EEG. They may be associated with strong vegetative alterations (9). Ictal discharges of frontal origin prove the epileptic etiology of the movement disorder.

Treatment

Carbamazepine controls or at least significantly reduces seizures in about 70% of NFLE patients (3). Other medications are not known to be helpful. As in some patients a channelopathy is the underlying disease, novel therapeutic strategies known to influence potassium channels (21) have to be considered.

RESTLESS LEGS SYNDROME AND PERIODIC LIMB MOVEMENT DISORDER

Restless legs syndrome was first described in 1672 by Sir Thomas Willis, an English physician. Later, in his book *The London Practice of Physick*, he documented patients with RLS symptoms: "Wherefore to some, when being a Bed, they betake themselves to sleep, presently in the Arms and Leggs, Leapings and Contractions of their Tendons, and so great a Restlessness and Tossing of their Members ensue, that the diseased are no more able to sleep than if they were in a place of the greatest torture" (22). During the centuries either the disorder was forgotten or the name was changed several times until Karl A. Ekbom, a Swedish neurologist and surgeon, described the entire spectrum of the disorder and named it "restless legs syndrome" (23). Ekbom had already cited many aspects of the syndrome, including the sleep disturbances, the possible hereditary factor, and the increased prevalence of the syndrome in pregnancy.

Definition and Clinical Features

RLS, as the term is used now, was defined in its present form for the first time by the International Restless Legs Syndrome Study Group (IRLSSG) (24). For the clinical diagnosis of the syndrome, a minimum of *four essential* criteria are obligatory, and characteristics that may frequently occur in RLS patients are mentioned as "additional criteria" (Table 26.2). First, RLS is characterized by a wide range of

TABLE 26.2. DIAGNOSTIC CRITERIA FOR RESTLESS LEGS SYNDROME (24)

Obligatory criteria
  Desire to move the limbs usually associated with paresthesias or dysesthisias *and*
  Motor restlessness *and*
  Symptoms are worse or exclusively present at rest (i.e., lying, sitting), with at least partial and temporary relief by activity *and*
  Symptoms are worse during evening or night
Additional features
  Sleep disturbances and their consequences
  Involuntary movements (periodic limb movements in sleep, involuntary limb movements while awake and at rest)
  Chronic condition (any age, but more severe after middle age)
  Family history
  No neurologic abnormalities in primary RLS
  In secondary RLS, peripheral neuropathy, radiculopathy, and other neurologic disorders may be present

RLS, restless legs syndrome.

sensory symptoms including unpleasant sensations mostly deep in the limbs, occurring unilaterally or bilaterally and spreading from the ankle or knee to sometimes the entire lower or upper limb. With progressive disease an involvement of the arms has been described in up to 48% of patients (25). In some patients pain dominates the picture and may lead to RLS being misdiagnosed as a chronic pain problem. An increasing number of patients complain about the manifestation of the syndrome after a specific peripheral nerve problem, such as radiculopathy, and show a clear preponderance of symptoms in one extremity. Motor restlessness, the second of the four essential criteria, pertains to the patients' general motor activity and a desire to stay active during the day, in order to avoid periods of rest, because RLS symptoms are likely to occur at rest. This brings us to the third criterion: All symptoms, sensory as well as motor, occur mostly when the patient is lying or resting and are stopped by movement, especially walking (24).

The movements in RLS can be divided into two classes: those performed voluntarily to relieve the RLS symptoms, and those performed involuntarily. The involuntary movements are myoclonic jerks mostly in the lower legs, which occur at rest in association with sensory symptoms of RLS. Movements of up to 7 to 10 seconds' duration with repetitive contractions are similar to dyskinesias and may occur periodically or aperiodically mostly in the tibialis muscles or the quadriceps or biceps femoris (26). Most characteristic for RLS are the PLMs during wakefulness, which are described according to the definition of PLMs during sleep and show the typical flexion of the knee and ankle with extension of the big toe in most cases (27,28). Voluntary movements include actions such as pacing, shaking, or rubbing the limbs (24), but these acts usually relieve symptoms only temporarily and generally cannot replace pharmacologic treatment. The clinical diagnosis is based on the symptomatology, the course of the disease, and findings from sleep studies, if available. The fourth criterion—circadian variation of the syndrome—has been derived from the observation that patients complain about RLS mostly in the evening and at night. Some studies have demonstrated that the circadian rhythm itself plays an important role in the manifestation of RLS symptoms and might occur independently from the condition of sleep in RLS (29).

Epidemiology

Recent population-based surveys showed that the prevalence of RLS in adults might range from 5% to 10% or even higher (30–32). In the MEMO study (31), a population-based survey of the elderly population in Germany, there was a higher prevalence of RLS in women (13%) over the age of 65 compared with elderly men (7%). A similar population-based study from the United States (32) found an age-dependent prevalence of RLS between 3% and 13% in the white Caucasian population but no gender-specific

differences. No data are currently available for prevalences in other ethnic groups, such as Asian or black populations.

The prevalence of PLMs among patients with RLS varies widely. The first reports from Lugaresi et al. (33) reveal a prevalence of PLMs of almost 90% in RLS patients. Estimations in the general population vary between 6% in young adults and almost 60% in the elderly (34). These data refer to the occurrence of pure PLMs and do not control for PLM-associated arousals, which may play an important role in RLS.

Diagnoses and Differential Diagnosis

Restless legs syndrome is a clinical diagnosis based on the patient's history and the four essential criteria listed in Table 26.2 (24). Additional technical investigations may support the diagnosis but are not clinically necessary. The differential diagnosis of RLS includes both conditions associated with motor restlessness and disagreeable sensations in the legs. Other differential diagnoses include specific sleep disorders associated with motor symptoms. The most important differential diagnoses are polyneuropathy, radiculopathy (35), the syndrome of painful legs and moving toes (36), and myelopathies or inflammatory disorders of the spinal cord. To differentiate polyneuropathy from RLS it is helpful to concentrate on the criterion of "relief of symptoms by activity." Some patients suffer from both RLS and neuropathy (37), but the number of RLS symptoms among the patient's complaints can be best estimated by the amelioration of symptoms after walking. The syndrome of painful legs and moving toes (36) arises mostly in patients with previous trauma or surgery of the lumbosacral plexus and can be differentiated from RLS by a continuously present pain in the legs that is not substantially improved by activity. Another differential diagnosis of nocturnal motor disorders may include nocturnal panic attacks or myoclonic syndromes of other etiology, such as benign muscle cramps or sleep starts. Patients with other specific sleep disorders, such as sleep apnea syndrome, narcolepsy, or pure periodic limb movement disorder (PLMD), often chiefly complain about daytime fatigue. They have to be distinguished from RLS patients if they report sleep disturbance and polysomnographically show an increased number of PLMs (38).

Periodic Limb Movements and Polysomnography

PLMs in sleep with arousals (Figs. 26.2 and 26.3) occur in about 80% of patients with RLS (38). PLMs in sleep are common but not specific for the diagnosis of RLS. The diagnosis of PLMs is based on the definition of the American Sleep Disorders Association (39) according to which PLMs in sleep are measured by surface electromyography from the tibialis muscle and show muscle activation in a sequence of at least four muscle contractions, each lasting

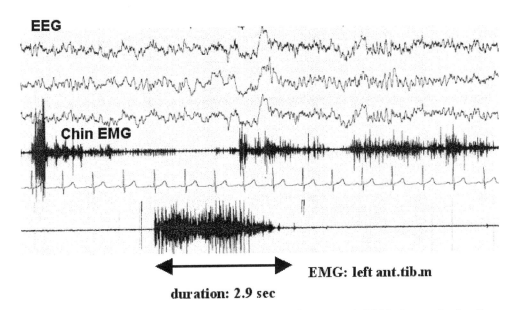

FIG. 26.2. Patient with restless legs syndrome during sleep stage 2. Within 2 seconds after the end of the muscle activity of the left limb the electroencephalogram shows a K-Komplex, a possible sign of an arousal reaction.

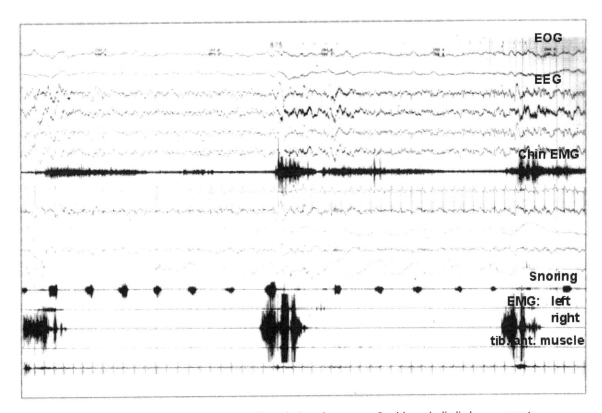

FIG. 26.3. Restless legs syndrome patient during sleep stage 2 with periodic limb movements (PLMs) sequence and associated PLM arousals starting with the beginning of electromyographic activity.

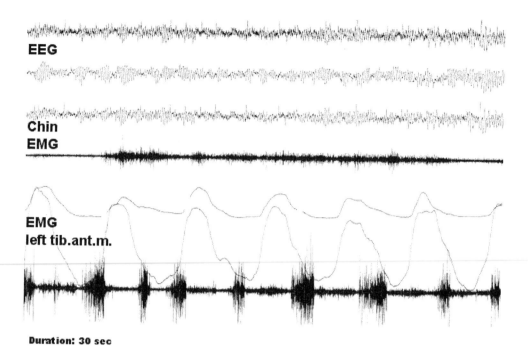

EEG

Chin
EMG

EMG
left tib.ant.m.

Duration: 30 sec

FIG. 26.4. Periodic limb movement (PLM) sequence during wakefulness with normal wake electroencephalogram, recorded during a suggested immobilization test of a patient with restless legs syndrome. Recording with short intermovement intervals of PLMs of the left leg.

0.5 to 5 seconds and recurring at intervals of 5 to 90 seconds. These movements seem similar to the triple-flexion reflex of the hip, knee, and ankles and to Babinski's sign (40). They also occur during relaxed wakefulness, either in rest periods or before falling asleep, and are described as dyskinesias while awake (27). The occurrence of PLMs during wakefulness seems to be a reliable and characteristic phenomenon in RLS patients that can be quantified in the suggested immobilization test (SIT) (41). In this test, patients are asked to lie still and not to move, while the tibialis electromyogram is recorded during wakefulness. Depending on the severity of the syndrome, patients start to complain about sensory symptoms and an urge to move the limbs after 15 to 30 minutes. PLM occur mostly in the same interval (Fig. 26.4) and will be recorded during a period of 1 hour. The SIT is a tool for diagnosing and quantifying RLS and to control treatment (38).

Actigraphy may be another method to measure patients' motor restlessness occurring in RLS. Actigraphic studies can be performed during the night (42), similar to polysomnographic studies of PLM in sleep, or can measure daytime restlessness.

Pathophysiology

Initially, RLS was classified as a peripheral nerve disorder, but in the last two decades scientists mainly have agreed that RLS may have its origin in the central nervous system. Alterations in the complex interactions between peripheral and central structures of the nervous system may play a role and complicate the clinical picture. An increasing number of well-documented patients with symptoms of RLS and associated peripheral nerve diseases such as neuropathies or radiculopathies, as well as patients with obvious central lesions, may illustrate the role of both a central and peripheral contribution to the disease (43,44). Whether there is a primary anatomic locus of the disorder or a general molecular mechanism remains unknown.

The occurrence of PLMs in sleep and the characterization of these movements may give further clues to the pathophysiology: polygraphically recorded PLMs during the day did not elicit cortical activity preceding these movements, thus excluding a primary cortical origin as the source of RLS-associated involuntary movements (28). PLMs in sleep probably result from supersegmental disinhibition phenomena. Recruitment patterns of muscular activity during PLMs when the patient is awake have been found similar to those of slow spinal propagation (26), whereas another investigation measuring 100 consecutive PLMs in sleep in RLS patients could not show stable recruitment patterns (45). Using transcranial magnetic stimulation in a special double-stimulation technique, impaired intracortical inhibition was found in RLS patients in both a foot muscle and a hand muscle, with the latter not involved in the clinical symptoms (46). A recent study of Bara-Jimenez et al. (47) investigated the flexor reflex response in RLS patients while PLMs in sleep occurred, which pointed to an increased disinhibition level. Activated brain areas detected by functional magnetic resonance tomography (fMRT) favor brainstem generators and the involvement of the red nuclei as well as the cerebellum during the occurrence of PLMs (48). The role of the basal ganglia, especially with respect to the efficacy of dopaminergic medication in RLS, remains controversial. Studies using positron emission tomography (PET) and single photon emission computed tomography (SPECT) to investigate the dopaminergic system in RLS patients reported no (49,50) or only subtle alterations of the presynaptic and postsynaptic dopamine receptors (51,52); this is clearly different from the marked changes observed in patients with PD. Comparing RLS patients with aged-matched controls, no difference was found between the postsynaptic striatal binding with iodobenzamide (IBZM-SPECT) and the dopamine transporter binding (IPT-SPECT or β-CIT SPECT) when treated and never-treated RLS patients were compared (50). In a small study, two family members with RLS were investigated while in a state of pain. The regional cerebral blood flow (rCBF-SPECT) was measured with the tracer hexamethylpropyleneamineoxime before and after treatment with L-dopa. There was an increase of blood flow in the thalamus and decrease in the caudate nucleus in both patients occurring only during the states of pain. With respect to the painful sensations that occur in RLS patients, the measured changes may correlate more with the condition of pain than with a primary dopaminergic deficit in RLS (53).

There is increasing evidence that peripheral nerve disorders may be associated with RLS or may increase RLS symptoms. Observations of RLS symptoms in patients with diabetes, cryoglobulinemia, amyloidosis (37,43,54), and other neuropathies confirm this hypothesis. Studies of patients with Charcot-Marie-Tooth disease types 1 and 2 showed RLS in 37% of those with type 2 disease (55). Morphometric analysis of a sural nerve biopsy revealed alterations in myelinated fiber density in patients with RLS, compared with healthy controls, although RLS patients did not reveal a clinically manifest polyneuropathy. The authors suggest that an affection of small unmyelinated fibers may have a role in the development of RLS symptoms (56).

The positive response to L-dopa as well as to opioid treatment points to the involvement of both neurotransmitter systems in the pathophysiology of RLS. This hypothesis is confirmed by the observation that dopamine D2 receptor–blocking agents, such as typical neuroleptics, exacerbate RLS or may induce symptoms (37,58). Although naloxone, a μ-opioid receptor antagonist, mildly provoked RLS symptoms in untreated patients (59), it was a powerful activator of specific RLS symptoms in opioid-pretreated patients (60). One may assume that a provocation of RLS symptoms

by opioid antagonists in never-treated RLS patients is not possible and that the opioidergic tone in RLS may be rather low. Neuroimaging and electrophysiologic studies as well as observations in patients with spinal or peripheral pathologies are in line with the hypothesis that RLS is a disease of dopaminergic dysfunction: even patients with spinal pathologies and RLS could be effectively treated with dopaminergic drugs (34). Furthermore, the RLS symptoms of patients with spinocerebellar ataxia (SCA3) and additional RLS responded sufficiently to L-dopa.

Endocrine investigations in RLS patients revealed an overall normal level and circadian distribution of cortisol, prolactin, and growth hormone (61), although detailed endocrine investigations are still lacking. The worsening of RLS symptoms in the evening and at night is an independent diagnostic criterion of the syndrome and is related more to the time of the day than to sleep itself. The maximum of sensory symptoms as well as PLMs occur between midnight and 2 a.m. in RLS patients with an almost symptom-free interval between morning and noon (24).

Since we know that iron deficiency leads to severe RLS symptoms (62), Allen and colleagues studied the possible contribution of iron deficiency to the pathophysiology of RLS (63). Studies of cerebrospinal fluid measurements in RLS patients showed a deficit of ferritin (63), and MRI studies revealed probable alterations of iron storage in several brain regions in RLS patients (64). The molecular relation of iron deficiency and RLS remains to be determined. Iron supplementation leads to a significant alleviation of symptoms only in iron-deficient RLS patients (65).

Genetic Forms

Ekbom described the familial component of RLS in 1945 (23), although there is a large variation in the numbers of probable cases of familial RLS. In many studies the methodologic problems of defining RLS, and in addition defining a positive family history of RLS, have not been addressed sufficiently. In the study of Montplaisir and co-workers (38), the diagnosis of familial RLS was confirmed not by direct interview but by history; 63% of 127 consecutive RLS patients had affected first-degree relatives. In an additional study involving a direct standardized interview of 300 RLS patients concerning their family history, Winkelmann and co-workers (66) found a definitively positive family history present in 42% of the idiopathic RLS population, with an additional 12% scored as "possibly positive." In a recent segregation analysis of 908 subjects that included RLS patients and their family members, it could be demonstrated by standardized interviews of all subjects that the mean age of onset of RLS varies in clearly differentiated subgroups: in the affected subjects with an age of onset younger than 31 years an autosomal dominant transmission of a single gene was the most likely mode of inheritance; in affected subjects with an older age of onset there was no consistent mode of inheritance and sporadic forms of RLS were more likely (67). This observation is common to many neurologic disorders with "complex inheritance," such as Alzheimer's dementia or PD.

Recently, several large families with RLS have been described in more detail (68). In some of these families there is some evidence for anticipation (earlier age of onset in later generations) (68,69), but an ascertainment bias cannot be excluded. Anticipation may trigger the occurrence of "unstable" mutations similar to those in Huntington's chorea with expanded trinucleotide repeat sequences. A large variability of clinical symptoms has been described in all families with RLS (69,70). In a first study of ten pairs of monozygotic twins with RLS, there was a variable expressivity of RLS symptoms together with a high concordance rate (71). A recent association study investigating the mutations of dopamine receptor genes in RLS patients could not detect specific differences between 92 RLS patients and 182 controls (72). A first and very recent report showed a genetic susceptibility to RLS on chromosome 12q in a large French-Canadian family, which may account for a specific population effect in this family, as supposed by the authors (73).

Secondary Forms

The clinical symptomatology of the secondary RLS closely resembles the phenomena of the idiopathic forms. This could be demonstrated in comparing patients with idiopathic and uremic RLS (74–76). Patients with uremic RLS exhibit a higher PLM-in-sleep index than idiopathic RLS patients when polysomnographic recordings have been compared (75). Uremic RLS is the most common secondary form of RLS, with approximately 20% of dialysis patients suffering from RLS symptoms (74,76). RLS seems to be associated with the increase of uremia and not the start of dialysis (74). No additional parameter could be associated with RLS and uremia. Although an association of RLS with anemia has been postulated in one study in which erythropoietin improved RLS symptoms in dialysis patients (77), this hypothesis has not been confirmed.

Iron deficiency is another common cause of the manifestation or worsening of RLS and may be associated with low levels of ferritin (64). In addition, RLS often occurs in conjunction with rheumatoid arthritis, disturbances of the thyroid metabolism, and pregnancy (78). Some females suffer from RLS for the first time during pregnancy; these patients are often characterized by a positive family history of RLS (66).

Treatment

Treatment is indicated in cases of subjectively reduced quality of life and depends on the extent of the resulting sleep disorder. Before pharmacologic treatment is started, non-pharmacologic measures should be attempted, including sleep hygiene and avoidance of stimulants or aggravating drugs (e.g., caffeine, alcohol, antihistamines, neuroleptics, antidepressants). In the physiologic condition of pregnancy, symptoms may resolve following delivery. In cases of iron deficiency, iron supplementation should be given first. Very low iron and ferritin levels (<20 µg/L) should be managed with intravenous iron. A therapy for the underlying disease should always be attempted before symptomatic treatment is initiated.

Therapy for idiopathic RLS consists of dopaminergic drugs as medication of first choice (79). A single dose of 50 to 100 mg of L-dopa plus a dopa decarboxylase inhibitor (DDCI), such as carbidopa or benserazide, is effective when administered an hour before bedtime (79,80). Single or divided doses of up to 200 to 300 mg of L-dopa per night as short-acting or sustained-release preparations (81) can be titrated individually. Patients with problems of sleep maintenance may benefit from a combination of 100 to 200 mg standard and 100 to 200 mg sustained-release L-dopa preparations (81). Patients with RLS treated with L-dopa have been followed systematically for 2 years, and single cases now for up to 10 years. Thus far, long-term treatment with L-dopa has not resulted in serious side effects, especially not dyskinesias as seen in PD. L-dopa is well tolerated in most patients, and the so-called augmentation phenomenon may be regarded as the most relevant clinical side effect of treatment. The main symptoms consist of an alteration of the clinical symptomatology of RLS after initiation of treatment. These changes may lead to RLS symptoms starting earlier in the day, RLS involving other body parts, and/or increasing severity of symptoms (82).

Those patients with augmentation under levodopa treatment may enjoy substantial improvement when switching to a dopamine agonist (83). Recent studies have shown that various dopamine agonists that have been tested in RLS are an effective treatment for moderate and severe cases. Dopamine agonists should be used in long-term treatment, and a slow titration period is recommended for all agents, especially for the ergot derivatives such as pergolide, bromocriptine, and cabergoline, because of nausea. Bromocriptine, up to 7.5 mg, can be taken 1 to 3 hours before bedtime (84) beginning with 2.5 mg. Pergolide (0.15 to 0.75 mg, start with 0.05 mg) has been used successfully in double-blind studies (85,86). For better tolerability, the combination treatment with domperidone (not available in the United States) is recommended at the beginning. The first controlled, multicenter, long-term study using centrally evaluated polysomnograms showed the benefit of 0.25 to 0.75 mg pergolide for the improvement of subjective sleep quality, severity of RLS, and reduction of PLMs. Long-term results from more than 12 months of treatment show a continuous efficacy of pergolide on RLS symptoms (87). Augmentation seems to be only a minor problem in the treatment with other dopamine agonists (88), but long-term data regarding dopaminergic therapy are only partially available (89). Other dopamine agonists proved efficacious in the management of RLS in open studies. Cabergoline in a single dose of 0.5 to 2 mg reduced both the symptoms and the frequency of PLMs, resulting in improved sleep (90) and improved subjective symptoms. Lisuride (91) and dihydroergocriptine (92) have been shown to be efficient in open trials.

The nonergot dopamine agonists pramipexole and ropinirole alleviated PLMs as well as RLS symptoms both during the day and during sleep. Controlled studies with pramipexole (93) and ropinirole (94) could also prove the efficacy of these nonergot agonists in RLS; side effects such as nausea seem to occur less frequently than with ergot derivatives, but comparative studies have not been done. Recent publications on sleep attacks in PD occurring during treatment with pramipexole suggest that such attacks may also occur in RLS but have not been reported (95).

If dopaminergic agents are not effective or if contraindications do not allow dopaminergic treatment, opioids should be given as medication of second choice. Recent publications confirm not only the efficacy (96,97) but also the long-term beneficial effects (98) of opioids in RLS. In a controlled study of oxycodone for idiopathic RLS, there was improvement of sleep efficiency and motor restlessness using a drug regimen of 5 mg oxycodone 2 hours before bedtime, at bedtime, and in the middle of the night. PLMs in sleep and the overall quality of sleep also improved (96). Sustained-released preparations of opioids seem to improve the therapeutic effect, especially in patients who suffer from daytime symptoms. Opioids are also helpful in acute exacerbations of RLS (e.g., by neuroleptic agents or during immobilization or after surgery). They can be delivered epidurally for rapid relief of symptoms. Patients with a history of addiction to alcohol or drugs should not be treated with opioids.

Because of possible substance dependence, clonazepam (0.5 mg at bedtime) should be prescribed with caution. As with other benzodiazepines, tolerance may develop. Clonazepam reduced RLS symptoms and improved sleep (99).

In recent years, benzodiazepine receptor ligands (e.g., zolpidem) have been prescribed more frequently than benzodiazepines for patients whose main problem is falling asleep. These may be combined with any dopaminergic drug.

Anticonvulsants, such as carbamazepine (100) or gabapentin (101), are second-choice therapy and generally are considered not to be consistently efficacious as first-line agents. To obtain efficacy, it is usually necessary to increase the dosage to as high as that used for epilepsy. Anticonvulsants should be considered when pharmacotherapy is indicated and patients cannot tolerate first-line agents.

Results of a questionnaire study among sleep experts as well as a task force group of the American Sleep Disorders Association indicate agreement that dopaminergic agents followed by opioids and benzodiazepines are the treatment of choice for RLS. In some difficult cases, combination therapies have been considered necessary as well, with agents generally selected from the three favored classes (79).

In the past, many therapies were based on anecdotal observations, few of which have been tested in controlled trials. Many of these therapies can no longer be recommended. They include avoidance of nicotine; avoidance or consumption of caffeine; red wine at bedtime; vitamins; or zinc, dextran, chloroquine. Note that amitriptyline, a drug commonly used for control of neuropathic paresthesia, can exacerbate RLS symptoms; however, there are also observations that it may help in painful forms of RLS (A.S. Walters, personal observation). An initial increase of PLMs in sleep has been observed after treatment with imipramine and trimipramine. Other antidepressants (trazodone, paroxetine) may improve RLS symptoms in certain cases, but can also exacerbate RLS symptoms in some patients (102,103). Controversial effects on the symptoms of RLS were documented under treatment with sertraline, paroxetine, and fluoxetine (104).

PLMs in sleep syndrome in isolation, once known as "nocturnal myoclonus" and renamed periodic limb movement disorder (PLMD, 39), does not necessarily require treatment and does not primarily have any pathologic impact. If daytime fatigue dominates the picture, PLMs in sleep should be suspected and ruled out (105). In positive cases, dopaminergic agents are the first-choice treatment, and L-dopa has been shown to reduce PLMs in sleep (79). Indeed, a medical regimen similar to that for RLS seems justified because PLMs in sleep syndrome is a very common phenomenon in familial and sporadic RLS patients (38). Other agents, such as dopamine agonists, opioids, and anticonvulsants, have been observed to reduce the number of PLMs in pure PLMD. In summary, one may try dopaminergic agents first, followed by clonazepam, anticonvulsants, and opioids.

REFERENCES

1. Schenck C, Mahowald M. A polysomnographic, neurologic, psychiatric and clinical outcome report on 70 consecutive cases with REM sleep behavior disorder (RBD): sustained clonazepam efficacy in 89.5% of 57 treated patients. *Clev Clin J Med*1990;57[Suppl]:10–24.
2. Boeve BF, Silber MH, Ferman TJ, et al. Association of REM sleep behavior disorder and neurodegenerative disease may reflect an underlying synucleinopathy. *Mov Disord* 2001;16: 622–630.
3. Provini F, Plazzi G, Tinuper P, et al. Nocturnal frontal lobe epilepsy: a clinical and polygraphic overview of 100 consecutive cases. *Brain* 1999;122:1017–1031.
4. Tinuper P, Cerullo A, Cirignotta F, et al. Nocturnal paroxysmal dystonia with short-lasting attacks: three cases with evidence for an epileptic frontal lobe origin seizures. *Epilepsia* 1990;31: 549–556.

5. American Sleep Disorders Association. *International classification of sleep disorders, revised: diagnostic and coding manual.* Rochester, MN, 1997.

6. Eisensehr I, Lindeiner H, Jäger M, et al. REM sleep behavior disorder in sleep-disordered patients with versus without Parkinson's disease: is there a need for polysomnography? *J Neurol Sci* 2001;186:7–11.

7. Plazzi G, Corsini R, Provini F, et al. REM sleep behavior disorder in multiple system atrophy. *Neurology* 1997;48:1094–1097.

8. Schenck CH, Mahowald MW. REM sleep parasomnias (Review). *Neurol Clin* 1996;14:697–720.

9. Broughton RJ. Parasomnias. In: Chokroverty S, ed. *Sleep disorders medicine: basic science, technical considerations, and clinical aspects.* Woburn, MA: Butterworth-Heinemann, 1995: 381–400.

10. Wetter TC, Collado-Seidel V, Pollmächer T, et al. Sleep and periodic leg movement patterns in drug-free patients with Parkinson's disease and multiple system atrophy. *Sleep* 2000; 23:361–367.

11. Tachibana M, Tanaka K, Hishikawa Y, et al. A sleep study of acute psychotic states due to alcohol and meprobamate addiction. *Adv Sleep Res* 1975;2:177–205.

12. Eisensehr I, Linke R, Noachtar S, et al. Reduced striatal dopamine transporters in idiopathic rapid eye movement sleep behavior disorder: comparison with Parkinson's disease and controls. *Brain* 2000;123:1155–1160.

13. Olson EJ, Boeve BF, Silber MH. Rapid eye movement sleep behavior disorder: demographic, clinical, and laboratory findings in 93 cases. *Brain* 2000;123:331–339.

14. Chaudhuri KR, Pal S, Bridgman K, et al. Achieving 24-hour control of Parkinson's disease symptoms: use of objective measures to improve nocturnal disability. *Eur Neurol* 2001; 46S1:3–10.

15. Comella CL, Nardine TM, Diederich NJ, et al. Sleep-related violence, injury, and REM sleep behavior disorder in Parkinson's disease. *Neurology* 1998;51:526–529.

16. Rye DB. Contributions of the pedunculopontine region to normal and altered REM sleep. *Sleep* 1997;20:757–788.

17. Schenck C, Hurwitz T, Mahowald M. REM sleep behavior disorder: an update on a series of 96 patients and a review of the world literature. *J Sleep Res* 1993;2:224–231.

18. Lapierre O, Montplaisir J. Polysomnographic features of REM sleep behavior disorder: development of a scoring method. *Neurology* 1992;42:1371–1374.

19. Provini F, Plazzi G, Lugaresi E. From nocturnal paroxysmal dystonia to nocturnal frontal lobe epilepsy. *Clin Neurophysiol* 2000; 2:S2–S8.

20. Montagna P. Nocturnal paroxysmal dystonia and nocturnal wandering. *Neurology* 1992;42:61–67.

21. Lerche H, Jurkat-Rott K, Lehmann-Horn F. Ion channels and epilepsy. *Am J Med Gen* 2001;106:146–159.

22. Willis T. *The London practise of physick.* London: Bassett and Crooke, 1685.

23. Ekbom KA. Restless legs syndrome. *Acta Medica Scand* 1945; 158:4–122.

24. Walters AS, and the International Restless Legs Syndrome Study Group. Toward a better definition of the restless legs syndrome. *Mov Disord* 1995;10:634–642.

25. Michaud M, Chabli A, Lavigne G, et al. Arm restlessness in patients with restless legs syndrome. *Mov Disord* 2000;15: 289–293.

26. Trenkwalder C, Bucher SF, Oertel WH. Electrophysiological pattern of involuntary limb movements in the restless legs syndrome. *Muscle Nerve* 1996;19:155–162.

27. Hening WA, Walters AS, Kavey N, et al. Dyskinesias while awake and periodic movements in sleep in restless legs syndrome: treatment with opioids. *Neurology* 1986;36: 1363–1366.

28. Trenkwalder C, Bucher S, Oertel WH, et al. Bereitschaftspotential in idiopathic and symptomatic restless legs syndrome. *Electroenceph Clin Neurophysiol* 1993;89:95–103.

29. Trenkwalder C, Hening WA, Walters AS, et al. Circadian rhythm of periodic limb movements and sensory symptoms of restless legs syndrome. *Mov Disord* 1999;14:102–110.

30. Lavigne GJ, Montplaisir JY. Restless legs syndrome and sleep bruxism: prevalence and association among Canadians. *Sleep* 1994;17:739–743.

31. Rothdach A, Trenkwalder C, Haberstock J, et al. Prevalence and risk factors of RLS in an elderly population: the MEMO study. *Neurology* 2000;54:1064–1068.

32. Philips B, Young T, Finn L, et al. Epidemiology of restless legs symptoms in adults. *Arch Intern Med* 2000;160: 2137–2141.

33. Lugaresi E, Coccagna C, Tassinari CA, et al. Reliefi poligrafici sui fenomeni motori nella sindrome delle gambe senza riposo. *Riv Neurol* 1965;35:550–561.

34. Ancoli-Israel S, Kripke DM, Klauber MR, et al. Periodic limb movements in sleep in community dwelling elderly. *Sleep* 1991;14:496–500.

35. Walters AS, Wagner M, Hening WA. Periodic limb movements as the initial manifestation of restless legs syndrome triggered by lumbosacral radiculopathy. *Sleep* 1996;19:825–826.

36. Dressler D, Thompson PD, Gledhill RF, et al. The syndrome of painful legs and moving toes. *Mov Disord* 1994;9:13–21.

37. Rutkove SB, Matheson JK, Logigian EL. Restless legs syndrome in patients with polyneuropathy. *Muscle Nerve* 1996;19: 670–672.

38. Montplaisir J, Boucher S, Poirier G, et al. Clinical, polysomnographic, and genetic characteristics of restless legs syndrome: a study of 133 patients diagnosed with new standard criteria. *Mov Disord* 1997;12:61–65.

39. Atlas Task Force of the American Sleep Disorders Association, Guilleminault C, chairman. Recording and scoring leg movements. *Sleep* 1993;16:748–759.

40. Smith RC. Relationship of periodic movements in sleep (nocturnal myoclonus) and the Babinski sign. *Sleep* 1985;8: 239–243.

41. Montplaisir J, Boucher S, Nicolas A, et al. Immobilization tests and periodic leg movements in sleep for the diagnosis of restless leg syndrome. *Mov Disord* 1998;13:324–329.

42. Kazenwadel J, Pollmächer T, Trenkwalder C, et al. New actigraphic assessment method for periodic leg movements (PLM). *Sleep* 1995;18:689–697.

43. Gemignani F, Marbini A, DiGiovanni G, et al. Cryoglobulinaemic neuropathy manifesting with restless legs syndrome. *J Neurol Sci* 1997;152:218–223.

44. Walters AS, Hickey K, Maltzman J, et al. A questionnaire study of 138 patients with restless legs syndrome: the night-walkers-survey. *Neurology* 1996;46:92–95.

45. Provini F, Vetrugno R, Meletti S, et al. Motor patterns of periodic limb movements during sleep. *Neurology* 2001;57 (2):300–304.

46. Tergau F, Wischer S, Paulus W. Motor system excitability in patients with restless legs syndrome. *Neurology* 1999;52: 1060–1063.

47. Bara-Jimenez W, Aksu M, Graham B, et al. Periodic limb movements in sleep: state dependent excitability of the spinal flexor reflex. *Neurology* 2000;54:1609–1616.

48. Bucher SF, Seelos KC, Oertel WH, et al. Cerebral generators involved in the pathogenesis of the restless legs syndrome. *Ann Neurol* 1997;41:639–645.

49. Trenkwalder C, Walters AS, Hening W, et al. Positron emission

tomographic studies in restless legs syndrome. *Mov Disord* 1999;14(1):141–145.

50. Eisensehr I, Wetter TC, Linke R, et al. Normal IPT and IBZM SPECT in drug-naive and levodopa-treated idiopathic restless legs syndrome. *Neurology* 2001;57:1307–1309.

51. Staedt J, Stoppe G, Kogler A, et al. Dopamine D2 receptor alteration in patients with periodic movements in sleep (nocturnal myoclonus). *J Neural Transm* 1993;93:71–74.

52. Turjanski N, Lees AJ, Brooks DJ. Striatal dopaminergic function in restless legs syndrome: ^{18}F-dopa and ^{11}C-raclopride PET studies. *Neurology* 1999;52:932–937.

53. Mountz JM, Bradley LA, Modell JG, et al. Fibromyalgia in women: abnormalities of regional blood flow in the thalamus and the caudate nucleus are associated with low pain threshold levels. *Arthr Rheum* 1995;138:926–938.

54. Salvi F, Montagna P, Plasmati R, et al. Restless legs syndrome and nocturnal myoclonus: initial clinical manifestation of familial amyloid polyneuropathy. *J Neurol Neurosurg Psychiatry* 1990;53:522–525.

55. Gemignani F, Marbini A, Di Giovanni G, et al. Charcot-Marie-Tooth disease type 2 with restless legs syndrome. *Neurology* 1999;52:1064–1066.

56. Iannaccone S, Zucconi M, Marchettini P, et al. Evidence of peripheral axonal neuropathy in primary restless legs syndrome. *Mov Disord* 1995;10:2–9.

57. Walters AS, Hening W. Review of the clinical presentation and neuropharmacology of the restless legs syndrome. *Clin Neuropharmacol* 1987;10:225–237.

58. Kraus T, Schuld A, Pollmächer T. Periodic leg movements in sleep and restless legs syndrome probably caused by olanzapine. *J Clin Psychopharmacol* 1999;19:478–479 [letter].

59. Winkelmann J, Schadrack J, Wetter TC, et al. Opioid and dopamine antagonist drug challenges in untreated restless legs syndrome patients. *Sleep Med* 2001;2:57–61.

60. Walters AS, Hening W. Clinical presentation and neuropharmacology of restless legs syndrome. *Clin Neuropharmacol* 1987;10:225–237.

61. Wetter TC, et al. Endocrine rhythms in patients with restless legs syndrome. *J Neurology* 2002;249(2):146–151.

62. Sun ER, Chen CA, Ho G, et al. Iron and the restless legs syndrome. *Sleep* 1998;21:371–377.

63. Earley CJ, Connor JR, Beard JL, et al. Abnormalities in CSF concentrations of ferritin and transferring in restless legs syndrome. *Neurology* 2000;54:1698–1700.

64. Allen RP, Barker PB, Wehrl F, et al. MRI measurement of brain iron in patients with restless legs syndrome. *Neurology* 2001;66:263–265.

65. Davis BJ, Rajput A, Rajput ML, et al. A randomized, double-blind placebo-controlled trial of iron in restless legs syndrome. *Eur Neurol* 2000;43:70–75.

66. Winkelmann J, Wetter TC, Collado-Seidel V, et al. Frequency and characteristics of the hereditary restless legs syndrome in a population of 300 patients. *Sleep* 2000;23:597–602.

67. Winkelmann J, Müller-Myhsok B, Wittchen HU, et al. Comlex segregation analysis of restless legs syndrome provides evidence for an autosomal dominant mode of inheritance in early age at onset families. *Ann Neurol* 2002.

68. Lazzarini A, Walters AS, Hockey K, et al. Studies of penetrance and anticipation in five autosomal-dominant restless legs syndrome pedigrees. *Mov Disord* 1999;14:111–116.

69. Trenkwalder C, Seidel VC, Gasser T, et al. Clinical symptoms and possible anticipation in a large kindred of familial restless legs syndrome. *Mov Disord* 1996;11:389–394.

70. Walters AS, Pichietti D, Hening W, et al. Variable expressivity in familial restless legs syndrome. *Arch Neurol* 1990;47:1219–1220.

71. Ondo WG, Vuong KD, Wang Q. Restless legs syndrome in monozygotic twins: clinical correlates. *Neurology* 2000;55:1404–1406.

72. Desautels A, Turecki G, Montplaisir J, et al. Dopaminergic neurotransmission and restless legs syndrome: a genetic association analysis. *Neurology* 2001;57:1304–1306.

73. Desautels A, Turecki G, Montplaisir J, et al. Identification of a major susceptibility locus for restless legs syndrome on chromosome 12q. *Am J Hum Genet* 2001;69:1266–1270.

74. Collado-Seidel V, Kohnen R, Samtleben W, et al. Clinical and biochemical findings in uremic patients with and without restless legs syndrome. *Am J Kid Dis* 1998;31:324–328.

75. Wetter TC, Stiasny K, Kohnen R, et al. Polysomnographic sleep measures in patients with uremic and idiopathic restless legs syndrome. *Mov Disord* 1998;13:820–824.

76. Winkelman JW, Chertow GM, Lazarus JM. Restless legs syndrome in end-stage renal disease. *Am J Kidney Dis* 1996;28:372–378.

77. Roger SD, Harris DC, Stewart JH. Possible relation between restless legs and anaemia in renal dialysis patients [letter]. *Lancet* 1991;337:1551.

78. Goodman JDS, Brodie C, Ayida GA. Restless leg syndrome in pregnancy. *Br Med J* 1988;297:1101–1102.

79. Chesson AL, Wise M, Davila D, et al. Practice parameters for the treatment of restless legs syndrome and periodic limb movement disorder. An American Academy of Sleep Medicine Report. Standards of Practice Committee of the Academy of Sleep Medicine. *Sleep* 1999;22:961–968.

80. Trenkwalder C, Stiasny K, Pollmaecher T, et al. L-Dopa therapy of uremic and idiopathic restless legs syndrome: a double-blind, crossover trial. *Sleep* 1995;18:681–688.

81. Collado-Seidel V, Kazenwadel J, Wetter TC, et al. A controlled study of additional sr-L-dopa in L-dopa-responsive restless legs syndrome with late-night symptoms. *Neurology* 1999;52:285–290.

82. Allen RP, Earley CJ. Augmentation of the restless legs syndrome with carbidopa/levodopa. *Sleep* 1996;19:205–213.

83. Winkelmann J, Wetter T, Stiasny K, et al. Treatment of restless legs syndrome with pergolide: an open clinical trial. *Mov Disord* 1998;13:566–569.

84. Walters AS, Hening W, Kavey N, et al. A double-blind randomized crossover trial of bromocriptine and placebo in restless legs syndrome. *Ann Neurol* 1988;24:455–458.

85. Earley CJ, Yaffee JB, Allen RP. Randomized, double-blind, placebo-controlled trial of pergolide in restless legs syndrome. *Neurology* 1998;51:1599–1602.

86. Wetter TC, Stiasny K, Winkelmann J, et al. A randomized controlled study of pergolide in patients with restless legs syndrome. *Neurology* 1999;52:944–950.

87. Stiasny K, Wetter TC, Winkelmann J, et al. Long-term effects in the treatment of restless legs syndrome. *Neurology* 2001;56:1399–1402.

88. Ferini-Strambi L, Oldani A, Castronovo V, et al. RLS augmentation and pramipexole long-term treatment. *Neurology* 2001;56:A20(abstr).

89. Becker PM, Jamieson AO, Brown WD. Dopaminergic agents in restless legs syndrome and periodic limb movements of sleep: response and complications of extended treatment in 49 cases. *Sleep* 1993;16:713–716.

90. Stiasny K, Roebbecke J, Schüler P, et al. The treatment of idiopathic restless legs syndrome (RLS) with the D2-agonist cabergoline—an open clinical trial. *Sleep* 2000;23:349–354.

91. Benes H, Deissler A, Clarenbach P, et al. Lisurid in the management of restless legs syndrome—an extended polysomnographic study. *Mov Disord* 2000;15[Suppl 3]:134.

92. Tergau F, Wischer S, Wolf C, et al. Treatment of restless legs syndrome with dopamine agonist alpha-dihydroergocryptine. *Mov Disord* 2001;16:731–735.

93. Montplaisir J, Nicolas A, Denesle R, et al. Restless legs syndrome improved by pramipexole: a double-blind randomized trial. *Neurology* 1999;52:938–943.

94. Saletu B, Gruber G, Saletu M, et al. Sleep laboratory studies in restless legs syndrome patients as compared with normals and acute effects of ropinirole. 1. Findings on objective and subjective sleep and awakening quality. *Neuropsychobiology* 2000;41:181–189.

95. Frucht S, Rogers JD, Greene PD, et al. Falling asleep at the wheel: motor vehicle mishaps in persons taking pramipexole and ropinirole. *Neurology* 1999;52:1908–1910.

96. Walters AS, Wagner ML, Hening WA, et al. Successful treatment of the idiopathic restless legs syndrome in a randomized double-blind trial of oxycodone versus placebo. *Sleep* 1993;16:327–332.

97. Lauerma H, Markkula J. Treatment of restless legs syndrome with tramadol: an open study. *J Clin Psychiatry* 1999;60:241–244.

98. Walters AS, Winkelmann J, Trenkwalder C, et al. Long-term follow-up on restless legs syndrome patients reated with opioids. *Mov Disord* 2001;16(6):1105–1109.

99. Montagna P, Sassoli de Bianchi L, Zucconi M, et al. Clonazepam and vibration in restless legs syndrome. *Acta Neurol Scand* 1984;69:428–430.

100. Telstad W, Sorensen O, Larsen S, et al. Treatment of the restless legs syndrome with carbamazepine: a double-blind study. *Br Med J* 1984;288:444–446.

101. Happe S, Klösch G, Saletu B, et al. Treatment of idiopathic restless legs syndrome (RLS) with gabapentin. *Neurology* 2001;57:1717–1719.

102. Bakshi R. Fluoxetine and restless legs syndrome. *J Neurol Sci* 1996;142:151–152.

103. Sanz-Fuentenebro FJ, Huidobro A, Tejadas-Rivas A. Restless legs syndrome and paroxetine. *Acta Psychiatrica Scand* 1996;94:482–484.

104. Dimmitt SB, Riley GJ. Selective serotonin receptor uptake inhibitors can reduce restless legs syndrome. *Arch Intern Med* 2000;160:712.

105. Hornyak M, Kotterba S, Trenkwalder C. Indications for performing polysomnography in the diagnosis and treatment of restless legs syndrome. *Somnologie* 2001;5:159–162.

27

ATAXIA AND OTHER CEREBELLAR SYNDROMES

STEVE G. MASSAQUOI
MARK HALLETT

ATAXIA: DEFINITION AND ELEMENTAL KINETIC FEATURES

The term *ataxia*, literally meaning "without order," historically refers to disorganized, poorly coordinated, or clumsy movement. Since the time of Holmes (1) it has been applied more specifically to clumsiness due to lesions of the cerebellum and its immediate connecting pathways, of proprioceptive sensory pathways, or sometimes of the vestibular system. Thus, it may occur in the absence of any abnormality of isometric strength, segmental reflexes, muscular tone, ability to isolate movement of individual body parts, gross motor sequencing, or spatial planning. The clumsiness is also not due to spontaneous involuntary movements. Ataxia may be associated with any voluntary movement and with many reflex movements. It commonly affects upright balance, gait, manual coordination, and speech, yielding stagger, clumsy manipulation, and slurring dysarthria that make the person appear drunk. Indeed, the motor coordination–impairing effects of ethanol are attributed to its specific interference with cerebellar function. Hence, the motor performance of individuals intoxicated with alcohol, aside perhaps from certain errors in judgment, can be considered characteristic of cerebellar ataxia (2). Ataxia may also affect eye movements, swallowing, and breathing rhythms.

Because of the compromise of walking, precision manual coordination, verbal communication, and clarity of vision that results from ataxia, it may be associated with significant loss of independence and occupational function, as well as with social isolation. Depression is a common complication, and injuries sustained in falls and choking episodes are sources of significant physical morbidity.

There is sufficient overlap in morphology, clinical setting, and associated pathologic lesions between cerebellar and so-called sensory ataxia (proprioceptive ataxia) to warrant use of a common general term. The presence of a significant proprioceptive basis for ataxia can be determined most specifically by noting a dramatic worsening of clumsiness with eye closure. Ataxia is confidently attributed specifically to the cerebellum on the basis of bedside testing only when there is ataxia with minimal or no other motor or proprioceptive deficits.

Garcin (3) specifies a third type of ataxia that is related to vestibular dysfunction. *Labyrinthine ataxia* also has some clear clinical similarities to cerebellar ataxia and technically can be considered a type of proprioceptive ataxia. Vestibular ataxia is fairly easily distinguished from cerebellar ataxia when it presents alone. Patients with vestibular ataxia have major gait and balance difficulties but no incoordination of limbs or speech. The difficulty is primarily the impaired sense of head movement and orientation with respect to gravity, as opposed to a general disruption of body movement organization. Because of the usually clearly distinguishing features of labyrinthine ataxia, or labyrinthine disequilibrium, we do not discuss it further in this chapter. See Leigh and Zee for discussion of the evaluation of vestibular disorders (4).

Abnormalities in Tonic Force Control: Hypotonia and Asthenia

Although ataxia is the principal sign and symptom of cerebellar disease, certain abnormalities of steady force production are sometimes associated with cerebellar dysfunction. These are usefully kept in mind during clinical evaluation. Normal individuals have very low, barely perceptible muscle tone when fully relaxed. However, Holmes (1) noted that acutely injured soldiers with penetrating wounds to the cerebellum had further reduced resistance to passive movement and had slackened postures ("attitudes"). Cerebellar hypotonia tended to be characteristic especially of the upper extremities (1) and to normalize gradually over weeks to months depending on the severity of the injury. Gilman et al. (5) showed that in primates this change parallels the recovery of muscle spindle sensitivity that was acutely depressed by loss of cerebellar fusimotor facilitation (6).

Large-scale surgical cerebellar ablation in monkeys is generally reported to produce actual weakness, especially of the extensor muscles (5). In humans, Holmes (1,7) clearly distinguished *asthenia,* the weakness that followed acute massive damage to the cerebellar hemispheres, from *paresis,* which is associated with corticospinal tract lesions. Holmes noted that asthenia did not affect specific muscle groups more than others and was not necessarily associated with changes in tendon reflex sensitivity. Asthenia was noted particularly when strength was tested during movement. Although ataxic patients clearly have difficulty generating force rapidly (discussed below), their strength as indicated by peak isometric force is usually normal (1,8). Thus, although complaints of "weakness" are not rare in cerebellar patients, careful questioning usually reveals the problem to be primarily one of easy fatigability, sluggishness (reduced crispness of motion), and/or a lack of coordination or stability. Holmes also drew attention to the inability of some patients to maintain steady force levels [*astasia* after Luciani; see also Mai et al. (8)]. Indeed, patients sometimes report sudden losses of strength, such as a leg giving out or the tendency of the hand to drop an item suddenly. Holmes (7) attributed these episodes to hypotonia, but their nature remains unclear. As with hypotonia, asthenic weakness is most often seen in the context of acute cerebellar injury, especially, Holmes (7) thought, when deep nuclei were involved. This was presumably related to the abrupt withdrawal of cerebellar facilitation from certain spinal, brainstem, and perhaps cerebral centers (5), which may be referred to as *diaschisis* (9). Recovery usually takes place within weeks to months (1), but its mechanism is not known.

Even in the presence of normal muscular tone and strength, easy fatigability, a second aspect of asthenia (1), is a prominent complaint of many patients with cerebellar ataxia. The fatigue may affect an individual body part but may also be sensed more globally, and most patients report that all aspects of ataxia worsen when they are fatigued. Fatigue in cerebellar patients appears to be central, not muscular, in origin. Electrophysiologic studies of fatigue in nondepressed patients with cerebellar ataxia have shown decreased postexercise facilitation of motor potentials evoked from transcranial magnetic stimulation. This is a central activation defect similar to that seen in patients with depression and chronic fatigue syndrome. As in the latter disorders, patients with cerebellar lesions sometimes complain of decreased concentration and mild difficulties with thinking. In this regard, the fatigue is also qualitatively similar to that seen in multiple sclerosis, dystonia (especially dopa-responsive dystonia), and Parkinson's disease. The general fatigue in cerebellar disease and other movement disorders may be related to the increased mental concentration needed to compensate for degraded automatic motor control. However, considering the possible role of the cerebellum in mental processes (discussed later in the chapter), fatigue in cerebellar disease may also result directly from certain deficits in cerebellum-mediated cognitive support.

Deficits in Force Rate and Movement Amplitude Scaling: Slowed Reactions, Dysmetria, Impaired Check, and Past Pointing

Classical descriptions of cerebellar ataxia have been provided by Babinski, Luciani, Holmes (1,7,10,11) and, more recently, by Garcin (3), Gilman et al. (5), Ito (12), Diener and Dichgans (13) and Lechtenberg (14), who have analyzed the disorder in terms of various clinical signs, including dysmetria, dyssynergia (asynergia, decomposition of movement), dysdiadochokinesia, dysrhythmia, and kinetic (intention) and postural tremors. Largely from his experience with acutely injured soldiers, Holmes ascribed to hypotonia a central role in the genesis of cerebellar signs, including ataxia (11). However, the relations among cerebellar dysfunction, muscle spindle function, and tone abnormalities are complex (5). Although spindle afferents are often depressed in peripheral sensory ataxia and with acute cerebellar injury, they may also be normal in the presence of ataxia. Moreover, various forms of increased tone may be seen in chronically ataxic patients due to anterior lobe lesions, spinal lesions in spinocerebellar degenerations, or basal ganglionic or brainstem lesions in olivopontocerebellar atrophy. To be sure, if tone becomes exaggerated as marked spasticity or rigidity, any ataxia that was noted earlier in the course of the patient's illness may become less apparent.

Characteristically ataxic individuals have particular difficulty in properly generating, guiding, and terminating high-speed movements. Movements accelerate somewhat slowly and are relatively late in onset if executed in reaction to a cue (1). Movements may either transiently arrest prior to reaching their targets (1) or gradually accelerate to excessive speed and overshoot their targets to an abnormal degree. These two types of errors are examples of dysmetria or, more specifically, of hypometria and hypermetria, respectively. At least two distinct motor control abnormalities appear to attribute to dysmetria: force rate inadequacy and step amplitude misscaling. The former causes brief acceleration-sensitive inaccuracies, and the latter, targeting errors that are slightly more sustained.

At a fundamental level, the patient with cerebellar ataxia has difficulty changing voluntary force levels abruptly (1,8). Both acceleration and deceleration are abnormal, as has been noted for many years. In point-to-point movements, for example, this voluntary force rate deficit is generally corroborated by slowness in the buildup and prolongation of the agonist electromyogram (EMG) that is followed by delayed onset of antagonist EMG. The antagonist burst is also typically enlarged, and decelerations are greater than normal. However, the peak magnitude of *jerk,* the rate of change of acceleration and deceleration (related to the rate of change of EMG and force), is reduced. The associated movement characteristically exhibits sluggish onset and transient overshoot, suggesting that hypermetria is the more fundamental form of dysmetria, at least when movements are not directed against gravity. Hypometria has been attributed to compensation for overshoot (discussed later in this chapter), to asthenia in the acute setting (1), to tremor, and to failure of timely relaxation of the antagonist during movement initiation (13,15). Conceivably it also may be due to a fundamental amplitude misscaling (discussed later).

If a patient flexes the elbow strongly against the grasp of the examiner and the examiner suddenly releases, it is difficult for the patient to avoid striking himself or herself with the hand. This sign is called *impaired check* (1). Holmes referred to this as lack of the (normal) rebound phenomenon. Today the term *rebound* is most often used for another pathologic cerebellar sign (see section "Involuntary Movements Associated with Cerebellar Disease"). Impaired check can also be attributed to slowness in the offset of the agonist and delay in the triggering of an antagonist.

In addition to transient overshoot, some patients may show movements that come to rest briefly or nearly come to rest at locations away from the target, most often beyond it. This is known as *past pointing* (5). The sign can be elicited by use of the Barany past-pointing test (5), in which the patient is asked to extend an arm forward, holding it parallel to the floor, and to note its position carefully. Next the patient closes the eyes, points the arm straight up toward the ceiling, and brings the arm rapidly down to a level as close to its original horizontal position as possible. The ataxic patient, without demonstrable proprioceptive deficits, may return at least briefly to a steady position beyond (lower than) the original, as if there is an error in the calculation of the distance moved or to have been moved. Among ataxic patients, past pointing is less consistently observed than is dynamic overshoot, and it is not known whether past pointing is as closely linked to movement acceleration as is dynamic overshoot.

Leigh and Zee (4) point out that in cerebellar disease, saccadic eye movements exhibit both hypometria and, more commonly, hypermetria. As with limb dysmetria, there are two components of point-to-point movement inaccuracy. An abnormality in the eye-driving pulse signal size leads to a transient undershoot or, more often, an overshoot. Thereafter, the eye glides to a steady position via a post-saccadic drift of variable distance and direction. The steady position achieved may be before or beyond the target. This depends on the scaling of the step (eye position holding) signal that follows the pulse. Pulse magnitude abnormalities are attributable to lesions of the dorsal vermis and/or underlying fastigial nucleus. Pulse-step size mismatches are attributed to lesions of the flocculus (and perhaps paraflocculus) (Table 27.1).

Degraded Control of Simple Multijoint Movements: Dyssynergia

In ataxic simple multijoint movements, such as intended straight point-to-point hand movements, there is a breakdown in the normal coordination of joint rotations. This can be viewed as the failure in producing movements properly within the context of other simultaneous movements. Termed *dyssynergia* (1) (or *asynergia*), this is considered a type of movement decomposition (5). Dyssynergia typically causes abnormal curvature of multijoint movements (1). Moreover, the curvature appears to be systematic rather than random (16–18). It is plausible that ataxia is especially apparent in multijoint movements because the control problem is inherently more demanding and/or because the cerebellum has a preferential role in such movements (19). Specific analysis of simple horizontal planar two-joint arm movements supports the impression that the deficits in acceleration and braking observed at single joints [see above and (1,15)] may account at least in part for the observed dyssynergia. It appears that the force rate deficit is accentuated at the joint having the greatest torque rate requirement (16), causing an imbalance in the joint accelerations and in turn to curvature of movement. This suspected mechanism is consistent with the marked worsening of dyssynergia with increases in intended acceleration or deceleration. Bastian et al. (17) and Topka et al. (20) specifically relate multijoint trajectory errors in cerebellar ataxia to deficits in interaction torque compensation. A proposed theoretic model of cerebellar function relates the force production deficit in both single- and multijoint limb movements to a common failure of long-loop feedback control mechanisms (21).

When patients with cerebellar dysfunction are asked to look back and forth between two visual targets, abnormal curvature of the saccades is often noticed in addition to dysmetria. This is presumably due to improper coordination or a transient imbalance between the accelerations produced by the different yoke muscles and thus can be viewed as a form of dyssynergia (the different rotational axes of the muscle pairs can be viewed as separate "joints"). Similarly, cerebellar patients often complain of visual blurring or frank diplopia transiently during visual tracking and immediately following visual refixations. The underlying momentary ocular disconjugation may be visible to the examiner. Apparently this relates to significantly different rates of acceleration and deceleration between the two eyes that exaggerates the normal intrasaccadic divergence (4).

Several investigators have suggested other mechanisms for asynergia that may be additionally or alternatively operative. Conceivably, multijoint movements may sometimes be decomposed voluntarily into multistep single-joint movement components (1) to minimize interaction torques between the joints and thereby simplify control. Dyssynergy might be due to the general difficulties cerebellar patients have with timing tasks (22–24) (see below) yielding problems with coordinating the actions of the dif-

TABLE 27.1. LOCALIZATION OF BEDSIDE SIGNS OF CEREBELLAR PARENCHYMAL LESIONS

Signs and Symptoms	Region Probably Most Involved	Defined or Theorized Abnormality
Ataxia and cognitive and behavioral abnormalities		
Staggering gait, balance difficulties	Anterior vermis, but also seen lateral hemispheric and vestibulocerebellar lesions	Impaired tuning of postural reflexes
Affect and behavior changes	Posterior vermis	Poor scaling of emotional responses
Saccadic dysmetria	Dorsal vermis	Incorrect scaling of saccadic pulse magnitude
Macrosaccadic oscillations	Dorsal vermis, especially fastigial nuclei	Serially dysmetric responses to initial extreme saccadic hypermetria
Saccadic ocular pursuit	Dorsal vermis, especially flocculus and paraflocculus	Inadequate use of retinal slip velocity information for prediction and correction
Cerebellar dysarthria	Especially posterior left hemisphere (contralateral to language nondominant hemisphere) and vermis	Failed muscle synergies and poor context-dependent (language-dependent) triggering of movement (oral dysdiadochokinesia)
Limb ataxia	Lateral hemispheres, especially anterior (including dentate and interposed nuclei) possibly more medial than manual ataxia (i.e., intermediate zone)	Failed muscle synergies and poor context-dependent triggering of movement (dysdiadochokinesia)
Manual ataxia	Lateral hemispheres (including parts of dentate nucleus)	Failed muscle synergies and poor context-dependent triggering of movement (dysdiadochokinesia)
Reduced motion prediction, appreciation of weight, internal "clock" function	Lateral hemispheres and dentate nucleus	Failed generation of predictive and timing signals
Higher cognitive functions	Lateral hemispheres, posterior, and dentate nucleus	Impaired context-dependent triggering of thought and action
Tremor		
Titubation (body, head tremor)	Any zone, perhaps more so for anterior vermis and associated deep nuclei (principally interposed and fastigius)	Same as postural tremor in limbs
Limb action tremor	Dentate and/or interposed nuclei, or cerebellar outflow to ventral thalamus	Poor damping of oscillations in posture and movement related to imbalance between predictive cerebellar and nonpredictive extracerebellar circuits modified by mechanical factors
Symptomatic palatal tremor	Dentate nucleus (and dentatorubro-olivary pathway: two sides of Guillain-Mollaret triangle)	Hyperactivity of inferior olive
Other		
Macro square-wave jerks	Cerebellar outflow	Mechanism unknown
Myoclonus	Dentate nucleus, dentatorubro-olivary pathway, possibly in conjunction with other extracerebellar lesions	Cortical or brainstem hyperexcitivity due to release from Purkinje cell inhibition? Unclear
Gaze-evoked nystagmus	Flocculus and paraflocculus	"Leaky" position control integrator due to failed cerebellar tuning
Autonomic abnormalities	Vermis, fastigial nucleus	Impaired tuning of autonomic reflexes

ferent muscles within the synergy, as suggested by Thach et al. (25).

Abnormalities in Movement Concatenation and Timing: Dysrhythmia, Dysdiadochokinesia, and Impaired Time Interval Assessment

Ataxia also includes the disruption of the normally smooth concatenation and coordination of multistep movement subcomponents. This can be viewed as a failure in producing each movement properly within the context of preceding movements. For repetitive, alternating-direction, single-joint movements, this manifests itself as *dysrhythmia*. For alternating-direction multijoint movements, the problem appears as a failure of coordination of the different single-joint movement components. This yields *dysdiadochokinesia* (or *adiadochokinesia*), a second type of movement decomposition. Clinical testing for dysrhythmia and dysdiadochokinesia typically employs rapidly alternating, oppositely directed movements that increase the visible effects of errors in the timing of movement onsets and offsets. However, when looked for, timing difficulties may be also noted in a variety of other tasks that involve sequential movements.

Bedside testing for dysrhythmia can be done by having the patient tap out a rhythm with a single-joint movement. Tests for dysdiadochokinesia include alternately slapping the palmar and dorsal surfaces of the hand on the thigh, or making rapid pincer movements of the index fingertip to the opposing mid-thumb crease. Accurate slapping or tapping requires precise synchronization of rotations of more than one joint (the elbow and radioulnar joints in the first case, the interphalangeal and metacarpophalangeal joints in the latter). In these two tasks ataxic patients display both an irregular underlying rhythm and inaccurately placed contacts owing to failed multijoint coordination. Dysdiadochokinesia can therefore be seen as a combination of dysrhythmia and dyssynergia.

The timing aberrations that are associated with poor movement concatenation may be due to failure of a cerebellum-dependent clocking mechanism. Theoretically this clock assists in the timely launching and termination of movements with respect to preceding movements (24). The same system may generally help to launch movements in a timely fashion with respect to other events, both external and internal.

INVOLUNTARY MOVEMENTS ASSOCIATED WITH CEREBELLAR DISEASE

The cerebellar signs thus far described are related to trajectory, position, and force control deficits in voluntary movement and posture. However, cerebellar disease also gives rise to involuntary movements that disrupt postural fixation and trajectory smoothness and accuracy. Involuntary movements include tremors, increased body sway, exaggerated postural reactions, myoclonus, and a variety of involuntary eye movements.

Cerebellar Tremors: General Characteristics

Two types of cerebellar tremor are commonly identified: kinetic and postural. These are action tremors. Cerebellar rest tremor, if it exists, is rare (see below). All cerebellar tremors manifest alternating electromyographic bursting in agonist and antagonist muscles.

In cerebellar action tremor, tremor frequency may differ between limbs, and the oscillations are often not synchronous in nonadjacent body parts. The tremors are often exacerbated near the point of attempted fixation if greater effort is made to maintain position precisely, and, as with most tremors, they are worsened by fatigue. Unlike essential tremor, they also worsen with alcohol but not with propranolol. Cerebellar action tremors are often eliminated or improved by eye closure. Although cerebellar action tremors are characteristically modified by visual input, external disturbances, and body mechanical state, their persistence after proprioceptive deafferentation also indicates some inherent instability of

central neural circuits. Several experimental results and models of cerebellar function include the interaction between central and peripheral (delayed) feedback loops that could be consistent with these observations.

Whether true cerebellar rest tremor exists is a matter of controversy. It is clear that some sensitive postural tremors are provoked by minimal voluntary muscular action and thus appear to be present at rest. Symptomatic palatal tremor (SPT) and related body tremors (see 26 and Chapter 19 in this volume) truly occur at rest and are associated with ataxia. However, they are apparently generated by unstable neurons in hypertrophied inferior olivary nuclei rather than by the cerebellum per se. Unlike cerebellar action tremors, these tremors persist during sleep, are relatively synchronized throughout the body, and are comparatively insensitive to peripheral influences.

Kinetic and Postural Tremor

The most commonly seen cerebellar tremor occurs in the extremities as a point-to-point movement is made. Tremor is generally less apparent before the midpoint of the movement and characteristically worsens as the target is approached. Tremor with this type of end-point exacerbation has been called "intention tremor," but the use of this term has been criticized because it refers to a cognitive state that cannot be reliably assessed. The term *kinetic tremor* is preferred for all tremors associated with voluntary movements. However, we still customarily comment on whether a kinetic tremor has end-point exacerbation because this feature is typical of cerebellar system tremor. Kinetic cerebellar tremors range in frequency from 2 to 5 Hz in the proximal extremities and from 5 to 10 Hz in the distal extremities. According to Gilman et al. (5), kinetic tremor appears to be more common at proximal joints.

After the target is reached, cerebellar kinetic tremor may disappear quickly or may persist indefinitely. In the latter situation it blends with cerebellar postural tremor, which by definition occurs upon assumption of a particular posture. Most often this is seen in the extremities when they are held elevated against gravity. It is commonly elicited by having the patient extend the hands gently forward, arms parallel to the floor, with palms down. Somewhat irregular tremors based at any of the upper extremity joints may ensue. Essential tremor may also be observed in this position. However, it has been noted that development or exacerbation of tremor in the hands when they are moved to a position near the nose with the elbows flexed and shoulders abducted (bent arms appearing as wings) is more specific for cerebellar postural tremor. In general, the amplitude of cerebellar postural tremor varies more with position than does essential tremor. The often violent side-to-side tremor of the heel when it is suspended above the contralateral knee while the patient is sitting is another characteristic cerebellar postural tremor.

So-called rubral tremor is an oscillation associated with ataxia, often of the limbs, that appears to occur at rest but is essentially a very sensitive postural tremor. Its name derives from historical reports of lesions at the red nucleus. However, the most common clinical condition in which this 2- to 5-Hz, often violent tremor is seen is probably multiple sclerosis. In at least one such case, the lesion was clearly shown to involve the superior cerebellar peduncle or other portions of cerebellar outflow pathways, not in the red nucleus.

An irregular postural tremor of the head (1) or more regular oscillation of the body as a whole, termed *titubation*, may be seen in association with cerebellar disease. The term titubation has been employed by some clinicians to refer to any head tremor or even to staggering and reeling gait. They recommend that qualifying statements always be used with titubation to clarify its meaning. We advocate that use of the term be restricted to cerebellar postural tremor of the head or trunk if it is to be employed at all. Body titubation is discussed later in relation to postural sway.

Lesions of the dentate, interpositus, and cerebellar outflow via the brachium conjunctivum appear to be most frequently associated with action tremors. Lesions at these sites are also usually associated with ataxia. More specifically, however, injury to the portion of the cerebellar outflow that crosses and ascends, destined for the thalamus, produces predominantly tremor, both kinetic and postural, rather than ataxia. Conversely, damage to the portion of the cerebellar outflow destined for the magnocellular red nucleus and/or the pontine reticular tegmental nucleus primarily gives rise to ataxia. Lesions of the dentate nucleus are reported by some to be most potent in causing tremor. However, impairment of the interpositus in isolation clearly causes tremor as well (19), and some lesions of the dentate are associated with little tremor. In general, lesions of both of these nuclei exacerbate tremor synergistically, and severe action tremor results from lesions of the dentate–interpositus border (19).

Increased Postural Sway and Body Titubation

Ataxic patients also exhibit increased irregular sway and sometimes a more regular body tremor. The characteristics of these involuntary movements vary according to the site of the cerebellar system lesion.

Diener and colleagues have performed extensive studies of postural balance in patients with cerebellar system disease (13,27,28). Ataxic patients, especially those who do not have lesions restricted to the hemispheres, have a tendency to have abnormally larger amplitude body sway when the eyes are closed than when they are open. They are described as having a large "Romberg quotient" (27). Patients with anterior lobe atrophy due to chronic alcohol intake and malnutrition and patients with Friedreich's ataxia have particularly high Romberg quotients. The eyes-closed instabil-

ity is generally greater in Friedreich's patients, who typically have significant proprioceptive loss and may fall without vision. By contrast, although anterior lobe lesion patients tend to oscillate markedly when their eyes are closed, they tend not to fall. With anterior lobe damage there tends to be much more sagittal plane motion, whereas with Friedreich's ataxia there is excessive lateral sway (27).

Patients with vestibulocerebellar lesions display increased omnidirectional low-frequency (about 1 Hz) sway and may fall with eyes either open or closed, and therefore they have a normal Romberg quotient. Patients with hemispheric lesions may exhibit slightly more sway than normal subjects, but balance instability is not prominent. Those with diffuse cerebellar damage exhibit a mixture of characteristics. They may be differentiated from normal subjects on the basis of posturography.

In addition to low-frequency sway, a characteristic 2- to 3-Hz body tremor, termed titubation (also see above), is seen in patients with anterior lobe dysfunction, most prominently when the eyes are closed (27). There is anteroposterior oscillation at the head, hip, and ankle, with the head and hip moving oppositely, so that the center of gravity moves little and balance is maintained despite marked body movement. This postural tremor has been associated with increased duration and amplitude of long-latency stretch responses (13). This is likely related to postural rebound (see below) and appears to be consistent with the observation in patients with alcohol-related cerebellar cortical degeneration of a nonspastic "tightness and tenseness" in the trunk and legs when they stand (29).

Exaggerated Postural Reactions: Rebound

When the patient with cerebellar dysfunction affecting the upper extremities is asked to maintain a steady outstretched arm position and the examiner applies a gentle downward tap, there typically follows a rapid, excessive upward displacement termed *rebound*. The term now has a meaning slightly different from the original; see Holmes (1) and discussion about impaired check, earlier in the chapter. In any case, the same phenomenon is seen as excessive postural responses to platform perturbations observed by Horak and Diener (30) in patients with injury to the anterior lobe. Due to the excessive rate and magnitude of the response, the patient initially yields less than normal to the disturbance but overshoots in the opposite direction. As with rebound seen in the upper extremity, the excessive initial component of the platform postural response does not attenuate (rescale) with repetition. Rebound may occur transiently in normal individuals. However, it vanishes quickly with subsequent disturbances as the normal subject adapts to the disturbance magnitude.

The mechanism of rebound is unknown. It may be partially due to sluggish braking, as occurs with impaired check. However, excessive force in the primary response is at least contributory. Thus, rebound appears to be a form of long-loop hyperresponsiveness that contrasts with the segmental hyperactivity that yields spasticity.

Myoclonus

Myoclonus is described in detail in Chapters 20 and 21 and in Hallett et al. (31). It is a simple, rapid, involuntary jerking that may occur in virtually any body part. Myoclonus is seen in association with ataxia in a number of neurologic conditions. In these cases, it tends to be segmental or multifocal in distribution and is often induced by action and/or sensory stimulation (e.g., the percussion of tendons). Similar to so-called intention tremor, action myoclonus may be exacerbated by increased efforts to maintain a trajectory or posture precisely. Forms that are commonly seen include a fine facial action myoclonus elicited by forced smiling or tight eye closure, a small-amplitude irregular action tremulousness of the fingers, and more violent and disabling multifocal jerking throughout the body that is provoked by movement and posture. When myoclonic jerking is fairly continuous and smaller in amplitude, it may be very difficult at the bedside to differentiate it from cerebellar tremor. However, electrophysiologic testing discloses discrete electromyographic bursts that last less than 50 ms and that are synchronous between agonist and antagonist muscles. Cerebellar tremor shows bursts that are reciprocal and last much longer (at least 100 ms).

Myoclonus related to the cerebellum has the features of either (cerebral) cortical or subcortical (reticular) myoclonus. In nearly all of these cases there appears to be coincidental lesions in the cerebellum and elsewhere in the central nervous system (CNS). In very many cases, a lesion has been found somewhere in the Guillain-Mollaret triangle or no lesion has been found. The serotonergic and GABAergic systems have been implicated in the genesis of forms of action myoclonus; indeed, myoclonus associated with ataxia is often ameliorated by serotonin or γ-aminobutyric acid (GABA) agonists. However, myoclonus has also been associated with excessive serotonergic activity. Thus, the mechanism of cerebellum-related action myoclonus remains to be elucidated.

Involuntary Eye Movements

More than 30 eye signs have been associated with cerebellar disease (1,4,32). In addition to the disorders of saccadic and pursuit eye movements that are apparently analogous to the limb and trunk movement derangements described earlier, many involuntary eye movements appear related to the unique interaction between the cerebellum and specialized oculomotor control circuitry. We note here that gaze-evoked nystagmus and macrosquare-wave jerks are two signs particularly easily noted at the bedside that may indicate cerebellar disease. For more detailed and comprehen-

sive discussions of cerebellar eye signs, see Leigh and Zee (4).

Several models of eye movement control attribute to the cerebellum regulation of the stability of the ocular neural integrator necessary to hold the eyes in eccentric positions. As such, cerebellar failure may be associated with a "leaky" integrator (4) giving rise to gaze-evoked nystagmus, a common eye finding in cerebellar disease. This type of nystagmus has a centripetally directed slow phase with declining velocity and a centrifugally directed fast phase. This sign is characteristic of injury to the flocculus and paraflocculus. However, gaze-evoked nystagmus is not specific for cerebellar disease because it may be produced by lesions of extracerebellar portions of the integrator.

Another important sign associated with cerebellar disease is macrosquare-wave jerks. These rapid, step-like, 5- to 15-degree excursions of the eye followed by return to base position are seen on steady fixation and are often exacerbated by attempted smooth-pursuit tracking. They may occur infrequently, on the order of two to three per minute, or almost continuously. The mechanism of these jerks is not known, but they have been attributed to lesions that disrupt cerebellar outflow (4). To our knowledge, these signs are not seen in proprioceptive (sensory) ataxia, and they are therefore often useful diagnostic findings.

ABNORMALITIES IN MOTOR LEARNING, PERCEPTION, AND MENTAL PROCESSES

Impaired Motor Learning

The rapid adaptability of cerebellar circuit activity (12) is consistent with an important role in many types of motor learning. Indeed, the cerebellar system has been shown to be involved with classical conditioning, adaptation of vestibulo-ocular reflex (VOR) gain, adaptation to rescaled vision, adaptation of limb responses to novel loads, and adaptation of limb trajectories to high speeds. Patients with cerebellar disease were significantly impaired in learning to trace a pattern manually while looking in a mirror, and patients showed a deficit in implicit motor learning by failing to improve performance of manual sequences normally when repeating movement patterns were secretly imbedded. In each case patients were less able to improve movements in terms of automaticity, timing, scaling, or stability and reliability.

There are currently several general views of the cerebellar role in motor learning. A prominent theory advanced by Thompson (33) based on classical conditioning in animals and in humans with cerebellar system lesions suggests that the cerebellum, specifically including the dorsolateral interpositus nucleus, is the exclusive storage site for the memory traces of certain acquired stimulus–response associations. Another widely held view (24,34–36 and others), developed on the basis of cerebral and cerebellar neuronal recordings and blood flow studies (37), suggests that during voluntary motor learning the cerebellum begins to assume a major portion of control. It thereby automates and refines certain actions that were originally directed at least crudely by other CNS circuits. More recent reviews (38) that appear to be supported by positron emission tomography (PET) and functional magnetic resonance imaging (fMRI) studies showing a gradual shift of increased regional blood flow away from the cerebellum to the cerebrum propose that the cerebellum is instrumental primarily in the early phases of motor skill acquisition. Thereafter, cerebral sites become trained and substantially assume control from the cerebellum.

Despite seemingly major differences, these conceptions are not necessarily inconsistent when viewed from the perspective of Ito's cerebellar microcomplexes (12,39). Ito suggests that cerebellar microcomplexes function as adaptable modules that operate in series or in parallel with simple reflex arcs or with voluntary command channels (which may themselves be forward paths within longer feedback loops). Presumably, on the basis of training, the relative strength of the cerebellar path may be adjusted to be small or large with respect to the extracerebellar path. This strength setting is stored until a contrary training event occurs, or perhaps there is a slow decay over time unless reinforced. In command channels particularly, cerebellar side paths may contain fewer synapses and therefore may represent the most direct connections from command-generating or reflex centers to their spinomuscular targets. In these situations the cerebellum would therefore constitute the primary associative connection between input and output, even if other connections existed outside of the cerebellum.

Generally, it appears that good motor performance depends on the integrity and ongoing cooperation of many motor system components. It therefore seems most likely that during motor learning plastic changes occur at both intra- and extracerebellar sites in relative concert. Presumably, these may operate at different rates, and to different extents, depending on the nature of the task.

Disturbances of Temporal Discrimination and Perception: Impaired Time Interval and Motion Assessment, Prediction, and Mass Estimation

Not only are patients with cerebellar dysfunction typically impaired in their production of well-timed movements as described earlier in the section on timing and movement concatenation deficits, but their ability to discriminate especially short time intervals in nonmotor tasks is often compromised. Ivry et al. (40,41) found in particular that patients with lateral hemisphere lesions had difficulties in accurately assessing the difference in time intervals between two pairs of tones, whereas those with medial cerebellar

lesions did not. This observation supports the hypothesized involvement of the lateral hemispheres in an internal clocking mechanism (22,23,40).

Probably closely related to patients' problems with assessment of time intervals is their difficulty with using sensory information to assess and predict motion characteristics. This applies to body parts, as shown by Grill (42), and to external objects (23,24).

The cerebellum appears to be important for prediction both for internal signal transmission delay compensation and visuomotor tracking, although the manner in which it performs or improves prediction in each case is not known. Velocity or velocity-like signal processing has been seen to occur at the interpositus nucleus (43), and various models of cerebellar function incorporate predictive or quasi-predictive operation (44–47).

Motion prediction deficits can often be identified at the bedside by asking the patient to track, with his or her finger, the examiner's finger as it moves slowly back and forth in a smooth motion. A motion that would normally be easy to follow should be used at a speed that would not engender overshoot in a simple point-to-point movement. Patients with cerebellar dysfunction generate movements that frequently lag the examiner and/or overshoot at the direction reversals, presumably because they fail to assess properly the examiner's rate of acceleration and deceleration or the rhythm of the examiner's overall movement. Very slow manual tracking in patients also shows breakdown into a sequence of small movements in staircase pattern that has been attributed to loss of velocity feedback control (48,49).

Patients often report that although they have no change in visual acuity while looking at stationary targets, they find it very difficult to track or focus on rapidly moving objects. They may find it difficult, for example, to read signs from a moving car. Inability to adjust eye pursuit velocity in response to rapid or changing stimulus velocity underlies the saccadic intrusions commonly seen during smooth pursuit in cerebellar disease (4). Here, catch-up saccades are inserted to correct for repeated slippage of the image on the retina, again producing a staircase-like tracking pattern, apparently because of inadequate velocity feedback control. The responsible lesions are typically in the dorsal vermis or especially the flocculus (Table 27.1).

Holmes (1) and Angel (50) have noted in hemiataxic patients a tendency to overestimate the weight of objects in the affected hand. However, Holmes found no difference between the sides in the ability to discriminate accurately between two different weights placed successively in the same hand. Furthermore, Keele and Ivry (23) did not find an abnormality in the perception of static force in cerebellar patients. The explanations favored by Holmes and Angel (50) point out that individuals tend to assess mass, as opposed to force per se, by moving an object back and forth or up and down with their hands, presumably while attempting to relate the applied effort to the rate of acceleration or oscillation frequency (50). Patients have difficulties with the kinesthetic assessment of motion characteristics (42,51) and also may have some element of asthenia that alters (increases) the relation between effort and force and hence between effort and acceleration. Therefore, it is not surprising that patients' assessments of mass may be disturbed secondarily.

Sensory Information Acquisition and Analysis, and Motor Control

The critical role of sensory information in successful motor control has long been recognized. Based on the perceptual deficits that have been noted in cerebellar patients (see above) and the afferent neuroanatomic connections of the cerebellum, it is evident that structure must have an important role in processing sensory information to influence motor performance. However, the nature of this influence has been debated. Although it would appear that improved stability and accuracy of body motion are principal functions, Bower (52) has put forward the controversial suggestion that the cerebellum is primarily concerned with fine control of the acquisition of sensory information rather than control of movement per se. In particular, it may be chiefly designed to coordinate the positioning and movement of tactile sensory surfaces to optimize the information received. This view is motivated in large part by the discovery of prominent paw and perioral as opposed to limb tactile receptive fields in cerebellar hemispheric neurons in animals (52), and by observations in humans that parts of the cerebellum may be particularly active in fMRI studies during sensory discrimination tasks even when a body part is motionless (53).

However, the question of whether the cerebellum is viewed primarily as a sensory information acquisition controller or motor controller is substantially moot from the point of view of feedback control system design, which often incorporates sophisticated afferent signal processing. The job of a feedback-based movement controller is to assess or predict actual body state (position and velocity) at least approximately, and to use this information to control motion in a manner so that state information received comes to match that which was desired. In principle, processed feedback signals derived from a feedback controller can be used for estimation or prediction of body state (54) with or without subsequent movement command. For example, assessment of the slide rate along the skin of a point of surface contact may be useful for control of active tactile exploration, as well as for monitoring the progress of an object slipping from a stationary hand, or the slippage of a gripping hand from a support. Because the detection of slip may be used to monitor as well as to trigger and control subsequent behavior, the distinction between motor control and sensory data acquisition control is not fundamental.

Alterations in Cognitive Function

The general teaching from the time of Holmes until fairly recently has been that, aside possibly from the assessment of mass (discussed earlier), the cerebellum is not involved with cognition. Certainly, complaints of major cognitive dysfunction are not typical in association with cerebellar lesions. Neuropsychological testing does not disclose any consistent abnormalities in visual perception or recognition, selective attention, or recognition memory. The clinical picture of patients with cerebellar ataxia, like that of sensory ataxia, is dominated by the movement executional abnormalities described earlier. However, the fairly common minor complaints of some patients with cerebellar dysfunction that their thinking is not quite as sharp should today be given greater analytic attention. Considerable experimental evidence has now accumulated that the effects of especially lateral cerebellar hemispheric dysfunction include a range of cognitive impairments. Problems with planning, comprehending, and executing a sequence of cognitive activities, as well as certain aspects of word production, attention shifting, and free recall of information recently presented, have been observed. A more detailed review of this work is beyond the scope of this chapter. However, Schmahmann (55) has assembled and reviewed an extensive compilation of the historical and current thinking about the cerebellum and cognition to which the reader is referred.

AUTONOMIC DYSFUNCTION

Many studies have directly implicated especially the medial cerebellum in autonomic function. Among the clearest demonstrations have been those involving control of blood pressure and pulse rate. Cerebellar connections with respiratory and vasomotor function have also been described. Haines et al. have reviewed the anatomic basis for cerebellar involvement in anatomic functions (56).

CLINICAL LOCALIZATION OF ATAXIC SYNDROMES DUE TO FOCAL LESIONS

Intracerebellar Lesions

Many lesions of the cerebellar parenchyma can be associated with ataxia at least transiently. However, stable deficits usually result only from lesions that are large with respect to the lobe in which they occur. This is presumably because of the considerable redundancy, distribution, and plasticity of cerebellar circuits. Detailed cerebellar anatomy and ultrastructure are reviewed in several excellent texts and articles (12,19,57,58). However, for the preceding reasons, it is usually not possible to predict lesion site within the cerebellum with great spatial precision from the bedside examination. Nevertheless, a few clinicoanatomic correlations can be discerned. In general, the phylogenetically older, more medial parts of the cerebellum influence visceral, basic emotional, and simple midline motor functions. The hemispheres are involved in phylogenetically more advanced functions that are usually lateralized. Very basic motor functions, such as postural stabilization and elemental movement control, are mediated by the anterior lobe and its connections. More complex motor and nonmotor functions are mediated by the posterior lobe and its connections. Because natural movements frequently require several levels of control, motor performance can be degraded by cerebellar lesions in a number of different regions. This is one reason for the limited localization value of many cerebellar signs.

On the basis of bedside testing, then, the examiner tends to be able to only distinguish strongly midline from strongly lateral, and strongly anterior from strongly posterior syndromes. Anterior vermal lesions are marked by ataxia of gait and sometimes titubation with little or no limb ataxia, whereas anterior hemispheric lesions produce dysdiadochokinesia (ipsilateral to lesions) with minimal gait disturbance. Behavioral and emotional changes, if due to cerebellar lesions, indicate posterior vermal damage, whereas disrupted nonmotor cognitive functions implicate the posterior hemispheres. In chronic conditions especially, formal neuropsychological testing may be needed to identify the latter. Dysarthria can be caused by vermal or left posterior hemispheric lesions, and Gilman et al. (5) consider the hemispheric site more important. Many oculomotor disturbances are seen in association with cerebellar disease (1,4,32). Leigh and Zee (4) have summarized three eye sign syndromes that when present permit slightly more precise cerebellar localization. Table 27.1 provides a general guide to bedside localization.

In interpreting cerebellar signs, it is useful to keep in mind a few other points. First, although signs that involve only the limbs unilaterally are most often due to lesions of the ipsilateral cerebellar hemispheres (5), this is not uniformly the case. A series of 106 patients having unilateral or predominantly unilateral hemispheric injury (mostly postsurgical cases) was studied by Lechtenberg and Gilman (5). In 22 of 26 (85%) cases with predominantly right limb dysmetria there was right hemisphere damage, and in 37 of 42 (88%) cases with left limb dysmetria there was left hemispheric damage. For dysdiadochokinesia, ipsilateral hemispheric lesions were seen in 11 of 12 (91%) cases with right-predominant signs and 25 of 32 (78%) cases with left-predominant signs. The mechanism of the occasional contralateral hemispheric effects on limb movement is not known. When vermal lesions affected the limbs, the deficits were usually seen bilaterally, and when there was asymmetry of deficit, the left limbs tended to be more severely affected. Overall, tremor was found less often than dysmetria or dysdiadochokinesia, but it occurred with similar rates in vermal and unilateral hemispheric disease.

A second consideration is that certain pathologic processes have a particular predisposition for affecting midline motor function. Gait and balance disability are particularly characteristic of anterior vermal lesions as seen in vitamin (especially thiamine) deficiency, which is often secondary to chronic alcohol intoxication and with tumors, especially in children. Third, because cerebellar tremor is seldom due to lesions of the cerebellar cortex alone, its presence suggests a deep cerebellar nuclear or cerebellar outflow lesion.

Supraspinal Extracerebellar Lesions

Ataxia that has all or most of the features of the ataxia associated with intracerebellar lesions has been described with lesions at several other sites. In each case it can be argued that the lesion interrupts an important flow of information to or from the cerebellum. Clearly, as mentioned earlier, major motor or sensory (especially proprioceptive) abnormalities severely confound the analysis of ataxia. Therefore, we restrict discussion to situations in which weakness, alterations in tone or reflexes, and sensory changes are minor.

Hemiataxia is frequently seen in association with mild pyramidal signs as part of the ataxic hemiparesis syndrome (AHS). Reviewed by Attig (59), it was originally described by Fisher and Cole (60). These first cases were due to lacunar infarcts in the upper basis pontis and corona radiata that presumably damaged corticopontine and corticospinal pathways and caused contralateral limb ataxia, mild to moderate hemiparesis, a Babinski sign, and often dysarthria. Fisher (60) and many authors (59) consider the clumsy-hand dysarthria lacunar syndrome to be a minor variant of AHS. Small hemorrhages, tumors, chronic subdural hematomata, and demyelinating disease may produce the same syndrome. Ataxia, unilateral or bilateral (59), almost always with some minor associated corticospinal deficits, has also been described as a result of focal lesions of the cerebral cortex, internal capsule, lentiform nucleus, thalamus, pons, and cerebellum, as well as subthalamus and cerebral peduncle. Among these locations the posterior limb of the internal capsule and the upper basis pontis appear to be the most commonly involved.

Many sites in the brainstem have been associated with ataxia. Each of these sites has a fairly direct relation to the cerebellar inflow or outflow pathways. Most naturally occurring lesions producing ataxia in the brainstem are associated with other brainstem signs (although isolated gait ataxia may be seen) that admit to the usual localization algorithms. However, a particularly important but uncommon lesion site is the rubro-olivary path, which is close to or within the central tegmental tract. Because of secondary dysfunction of the inferior olives, sometimes associated with olivary hypertrophy and symptomatic palatal tremor, a profound contralateral cerebellar syndrome may result (26).

Sensory, Spinal, and Peripheral Ataxia

In practice, spinal and peripheral nervous system lesions that cause ataxia are often also associated with conscious sensory, especially proprioceptive, deficits. However, it is clear that even severe conscious proprioceptive deficits may be associated with little if any ataxia, as is discussed by Garcin (3). This occurs primarily at thalamic and parietal levels, presumably where proprioceptive paths may be damaged independently of cerebellar inflow or outflow pathways. In the spinal cord it is even more difficult to isolate cerebellar inflow from proprioceptive pathways. Presumably because of interruption of input to the anterior lobe of the cerebellum that is conveyed by fibers from the gracile and main cuneate nuclei, lesions of the dorsal columns are associated with ataxia and proprioceptive deficits even when spinocerebellar tracts are not damaged. Naturally occurring lesions only rarely affect the spinocerebellar tracts in isolation. Pure cerebellar ataxia, without proprioceptive abnormality, has been reported to be due to spinocerebellar tract compromise from penetrating trauma or an angioma (61,62). We are unaware of any experimental studies in which these tracts were selectively lesioned.

Lesions of the peripheral nervous system can also produce severe ataxia. Causes include paraneoplastic and autoimmune disorders, pyridoxine toxicity, acute inflammatory polyradiculitis (acute Guillain-Barré syndrome) and its residua (63–65), and idiopathic conditions. In most cases, there is considerable loss of conscious proprioception as well. Thus, these conditions typically present as sensory ataxia.

The ataxia associated acutely with the Fisher variant of Guillain-Barré syndrome (63,66) is very interesting in this regard. Given the established lesions of nerve roots in Guillain-Barré syndrome, the ataxia is generally thought to have a peripheral mechanism. Yet this syndrome often has no associated conscious proprioceptive deficit and the ataxia generally lacks other characteristics of sensory ataxia. Ropper and Shahani (64) suggest, on the basis of possibly unique reflex silent period alterations, that this may be because there is a dissociation between muscle spindle and cutaneous information transmitted to the CNS. Why this yields ataxia, though, is not clear. They consider also an alternative possibility that Fisher's syndrome involves interruption of only afferents within the dorsal root that are specifically destined for the cerebellum, but they do not favor this mechanism. Complicating the picture further, Iwahashi et al. (67) reported an anticerebellar antibody in Fisher's syndrome, suggesting that the ataxia may not have a peripheral basis after all.

SUMMARY OF ATAXIC DISORDERS

A very large number of pathologic processes may affect the cerebellum and its connections. All result in ataxia, tremor, myoclonus, nystagmus, or other cerebellar eye signs in some combination. We organize these with respect to a practical approach in general medical practice. Although most patients presenting with ataxia will have a sporadic disorder, there has been increasing attention paid to the genetic ataxias because of the recent research advances.

Sporadic Cerebellar Ataxia

Degenerative Cerebellar Ataxia

Multiple system atrophy (MSA) is likely the most common degenerative cerebellar ataxia, certainly in adults. In addition to ataxia, patients have parkinsonism and autonomic dysfunction (including impotence). The disorder can also be called olivopontocerebellar atrophy when the emphasis is on ataxia, striatonigral degeneration when the emphasis is on bradykinesia and rigidity, and Shy-Drager syndrome when the emphasis is on autonomic dysfunction. Early falls are a prominent feature. Variable clinical features include pyramidal signs, tremor, dysarthria, dystonia, and mild dementia. There is typically a poor response to levodopa, but clearly at times there is some response, and this can be confusing. Responses are never dramatic and are usually transient. The pathologic hallmark of the disorder, in addition to neuronal cell loss, is the glial cytoplasmic inclusion (GCI). The findings may include cerebellar and pontine atrophy on MRI, decreased *N*-acetylacetate signal in the cerebellum on magnetic resonance spectroscopy (MRS), and decreased cerebellar metabolism on PET imaging.

Another group of sporadic cerebellar degenerations are the progressive myoclonic epilepsies. In these patients myoclonus and ataxia are difficult to separate clinically.

Stroke

There are a variety of strokes that produce ataxia. These can be due to lesions of the cerebellum or to cerebellar pathways. Ataxic hemiparesis is characterized by both weakness, reflex alterations, and incoordination as described above. Lesions can be in the thalamus and posterior limb of the internal capsule, upper basis pontis and cerebral peduncle, parietal lobe, and (debated) anterior internal capsule and frontal lobe. Hemisensory loss together with hemiataxia is typically due to a thalamic lesion. Isolated gait ataxia can be seen with a lesion of the pontomedullary junction. Ataxia (hemiataxia and/or gait ataxia) with variable cranial nerve involvement can be seen with involvement of several arteries. The superior cerebellar artery affects the upper pontine tegmentum, the anterior inferior cerebellar artery leads to damage of the lateral pontomedullary junction, and the posterior inferior cerebellar artery gives rise to the well-known lateral medullary syndrome.

Mass Lesions

The most common cerebellar mass lesions are hemorrhage near the dentate in the setting of hypertension; edematous swelling of a large cerebellar infarction; tumors—in children, medulloblastoma, astrocytoma, and ependymoma—and in adults, metastatic tumors and hemangioblastoma; abscesses, tuberculomas and other granulomas, and toxoplasmomas. Importantly, large acutely developing cerebellar mass lesions may present with little other than headache, vomiting, and/or gait instability.

In cerebellar hemorrhage, several large series show headache, nausea, vomiting, gait ataxia, and vertigo to be common, though clinical findings are variable.

Abscesses, which are notorious for paucity and variability of signs, may present with headache alone (5) and usually result from infections in or immediately adjacent to the cerebellum. As such, preexisting otitis media is a common cause, and cultures of cerebellar abscesses frequently yield *Streptococcus*, *Staphylococcus*, or *Proteus* (5).

Unsteady gait with cerebellar character is often seen with hydrocephalus. When it develops quickly, secondary to a high-grade ventricular obstruction, hydrocephalus is associated with other signs of increased intracranial pressure, including headache, mental slowing, drowsiness, and vomiting. If, however, hydrocephalus develops more slowly, it may be associated with more normal intracranial pressures (so-called normal pressure hydrocephalus), and ataxia may develop with fewer additional signs, classically perhaps only dementia and incontinence. It has been suggested that compromise of corticopontocerebellar fibers that travel adjacent to the lateral ventricles is the mechanism of ataxia in this setting.

Metabolic/Toxic Factors

Hypoxia damages the cerebellum, particularly the Purkinje cells. Both ataxia and myoclonus may result. Hyperthermia is another cause for Purkinje cell loss. The childhood hyperammonemias may cause intermittent ataxia. Celiac disease or sprue is a gluten-sensitive enteropathy that may be associated with ataxia and possibly myoclonus as well. The gastrointestinal disorder but not necessarily the cerebellar degeneration can be reversed with a gluten-free diet. Interestingly, up to 30% of patients with sporadic ataxia have antigliadin antibodies but no sign of celiac disease (68–70). Antigliadin antibodies are also seen in a similar percentage of patients with genetic ataxias (68). The significance of this is not clear. In some of these patients, there are abnormalities of the white matter and prominent headache; at least these patients have some symptomatic response to a gluten-free diet (71). Vitamin deficiencies, including those of thiamine, vitamin B_{12}, vitamin E, and possibly zinc, can cause cerebellar dysfunction. Wilson's disease is a recessively inherited disorder of copper handling. Ataxia is typically associated with marked tremor and dystonia. Dietary copper restriction and systemic chelation therapy may reverse some symptoms and signs. Hypothyroidism, hypoparathyroidism, and hypoglycemia (insulinoma) have been associated with ataxia.

Toxic injury to the cerebellum can be caused by ethanol. Acute intake of excessive ethanol appears to cause a true ataxia due to reversible interference with cerebellar function, as measured by physiologic studies. Chronic alcoholism, especially when combined with malnutrition, may be associated with irreversible damage of the cerebellar anterior vermis. This leads to particular difficulties with gait and a characteristic prominent anterior-posterior sway when standing. The extent to which the permanent cerebellar lesion is due to alcohol itself or to vitamin deficiencies remains unclear. Other substances/drugs potentially toxic to the cerebellum include thallium, bismuth subsalicylate, methymercury, methylbromide, toluene, phenytoin, carbamazepine, barbiturates, lithium, cyclosporine, methotrexate, and 5-FU. Ataxia can be a component of the serotonin syndrome that can result from therapy with selective serotonin reuptake inhibitors.

Paraneoplastic Cerebellar Degeneration

It is important to keep paraneoplastic cerebellar degeneration (72) in mind because of the potential for instituting life-saving management when it is recognized early. The clinical syndrome is usually that of acute or subacute progression of generalized ataxia resulting in permanent dysfunction. The mechanism appears to be a rapid immunologic destruction of cerebellar tissue elements. In many cases, antibodies are detectable in the serum. There are three types of anti-Purkinje cell antibodies. Anti-Yo (PCA-1) is seen with tumors of breast, ovary, and adnexa. Atypical anticytoplasmic antibody (anti-Tr or PCA-Tr) is seen with Hodgkin's disease and tumors of the lung and colon. Recently, PCA-2 has been identified mostly with lung tumors; 3 of 10 patients had ataxia (73). There are three antineuronal antibodies. Anti-Hu (ANNA-1) can be seen in possible conjunction with encephalomyelitis (74). It is associated with small cell lung tumor and tumors of breast, prostate, and neuroblastoma. Atypical Anti-Hu is seen with tumors of lung, colon, adenocarcinoma, and lymphoma. Anti-Ri (ANNA-2) is found with tumors of breast and ovary. Anti-CV2 (CRMP) antibody is associated with a syndrome of ataxia and optic neuritis (75). It has been seen with small cell lung carcinoma. The CV2 antigen is expressed by oligodendrocytes. Interestingly, this is one syndrome in which improvement has been seen with removal of the tumor. Antibodies directed to a serum protein, Ma1, have been seen in patients with testicular and other tumors (76,77). Ma1 is a phosphoprotein that is highly limited to brain and testis. The antibodies are anti-Ma and anti-Ta (Ta is Ma2). These patients may also have limbic encephalitis. Ma1 is a phosphoprotein that is highly limited to brain and testis. Antibodies directed to amphiphysin have rarely been associated with a cerebellar syndrome (78). This is a marker for small cell lung carcinoma. Antibodies against a glutamate receptor can be seen with cancer, and this causes a pure cerebellar syndrome (79).

In general, the antibodies are markers of cancer and are not specific for cerebellar syndromes. Some cases of paraneoplastic ataxia have no defined associated antibody. Currently, commercial tests for antibodies to Hu, Ma, Ta, Yo, Ri, and CV2 are available.

Infectious and Nonparaneoplastic Autoimmune Causes

Infectious causes include rubella and *Haemophilus influenzae*. Acute postinfectious cerebellitis is generally a childhood condition, most common after varicella. Gerstmann-Sträussler syndrome is an ataxic form of Creutzfeldt-Jakob disease.

Ataxia has been seen in association with anti-GAD antibodies (80). There can be a pure ataxia syndrome and one with an associated peripheral neuropathy. Anti-GAD antibodies are better known for the association with stiff-man syndrome, but the relationship is not clear. In one case with antibodies in the cerebrospinal fluid, the antibody blocked GABAergic transmission in the rat cerebellum. As with stiff-man syndrome, patients can exhibit other forms of autoimmunity.

Cerebellar ataxia is common in multiple sclerosis.

Other Sporadic Cerebellar Ataxic Disorders

Other disorders associated with cerebellar ataxia include Chiari malformations and superficial CNS hemosiderosis.

Genetic Cerebellar Ataxia

One of the most active areas in movement disorder and genetic research is that of the hereditary ataxias. Many of the genes can now be identified using commercial tests. This is helpful, but it is important to remember that genetic testing can have significant consequences, both emotionally and socially for both patient and family. Hence, testing should be done with care and with clear informed consent. Genetic ataxia is the subject of Chapter 37 of this volume, and a very detailed compendium of the genetic ataxic disorders can be found at http://www.neuro.wustl.edu/neuromuscular/ataxia/aindex.html.

RECOVERY FROM CEREBELLAR INJURY AND APPROACHES TO THERAPY

Chronic signs and symptoms of cerebellar injury differ from those of the acute phase. Moreover, signs may disappear entirely, especially when cerebellar damage is sustained early in life or is limited in extent. In general, lasting disability from lesions limited to regions of the cerebellar cortex, especially of the lateral hemispheres, is potentially less profound than that from lesions affecting the deep nuclei.

This may be due to plasticity at other sites within and outside of the cerebellum, combined with the fact that cognitive repercussions of cerebellar injury may not be especially debilitating for many activities of daily living.

Physical Therapy

Weakness, deconditioning, and spasticity are often seen in conjunction with ataxia and contribute substantially to its morbidity. All other factors being equal, stronger, more athletic individuals tend to tolerate moderate ataxia better. However, specific exercises directed to ataxia usually have not been found helpful. The use of added mass to treat certain tremors has been effective in some situations. Hewer et al. (81) found better results in patients who had a tremor frequency greater than 7 Hz. In general, the more severe the tremor in terms of amplitude, the more weight was needed to obtain improvement. Additional mass also improved ataxia of arm movement and of gait up to a point. However, beyond this, increased weight was associated with poorer performance. The optimal weight value varied by individual and was not clearly related to the severity of ataxia. Within the limits of fatigue tolerance, which unfortunately may pose a significant restriction, weight therapy remains a reasonable treatment option for some patients. It is also possible to use devices with incorporated viscous damping (82).

Pharmacotherapy

Several agents have been reported to show some ataxia-reducing effects. Botez et al. found low levels of the dopamine metabolite homovanillic acid in the cerebrospinal fluid of patients with Friedreich's ataxia and olivopontocerebellar atrophy, and in a double-blind trial amantadine produced significant improvements in both movement time and reaction time in patients (83). Unfortunately, this was not associated with functional improvement. Research conducted largely in Japan has emphasized the potential utility of thyrotropin-releasing hormone and many analogs in cerebellar ataxia, but these results are generally not dramatic and have not been widely reproduced.

The dense and widespread distribution of serotonergic terminals throughout the cerebellum and spinocerebellar tracts suggests that serotonin plays a major role in regulating cerebellar function. While some studies have shown benefit in ataxic patients from oral administration of L-5-hydroxytryptophan (L-5-HTP) (84), there have also been a number of negative results (85). Moreover, L-5-HTP therapy has had a fairly high rate of unpleasant gastrointestinal side effects, chiefly nausea and diarrhea, even when administered with a peripheral decarboxylase blocker. In addition, L-5-HTP has been associated with a syndrome resembling eosinophilia-myalgia, although the possible role of contaminants in the preparation was not fully determined. Some attention has shifted to trials of alternative serotonin agonists. Buspirone is a selective serotonin 1A receptor agonist that has been found by Lou et al. (86) in an open-label study, and by Trouillas et al. (87) in both an open and a randomized double-blind study, to produce some small benefit.

There have been reports of a small but persistent improvement in ataxia, and possibly arrest of symptom progression in patients treated with physostigmine, either orally or via a transdermal patch (88). However, double-blind studies have failed to demonstrate significant benefit (89). Anecdotally (90–92), the antioxidant *N*-acetylcysteine has improved ataxia along with a number of other problems encountered in degenerative ataxic conditions. Controlled trials have not been reported.

Management of cerebellar degenerative conditions with various metal-chelating agents has been advocated. While iron chelation therapy has been reported to produce clinical improvement in the rare condition superficial hemosiderosis of the CNS (93), chelation has not been established to have any benefit in idiopathic cerebellar degenerations. Work in yeast suggests that in Friedreich's ataxia an inappropriate accumulation of iron in mitochondria causes excessive oxidative production of free radicals that in turn damages neural, cardiac, and other tissues. This has prompted the consideration of iron chelation therapy and of treatment with antioxidants and free-radical scavengers. Despite the clear link with disordered iron metabolism, the value of iron chelation therapy remains unclear, especially given reports of adverse effects (94). On the other hand, studies using coenzyme Q10 (95) and idebenone (94,96) have yielded mixed but somewhat encouraging results. Although thus far neural injury has not been reversed, cardiac lesions have been improved.

Surgical Techniques

Ablation or high-frequency electrical stimulation of the ventral intermediate nucleus of the thalamus can be effective in reducing cerebellar tremor (97). However, these procedures do not significantly lessen ataxia. Experimental fetal tissue grafts have significantly improved walking and ambulatory posture in genetically ataxic mice (98,99). Apparently, engrafted primordial tissue matures and establishes appropriate connections (100). For ethical, political, as well as scientific reasons, the future of human fetal tissue graft techniques is uncertain.

Gene Therapy

The recent rapid advances in the understanding of the genetic bases of inherited ataxia raise hopes for genetic therapies for these disorders. However, at the moment there are no such therapies for any of the hereditary degenerative ataxias.

ACKNOWLEDGMENTS

The authors thank Joseph Higgins and Jeremy Schmahmann for their thoughtful assistance in the preparation of this chapter.

REFERENCES

1. Holmes G. The symptoms of acute cerebellar injuries due to gunshot injuries. *Brain* 1917;40:461–535.
2. Diener HC, et al. Mechanisms of postural ataxia after intake of alcohol. *Z Rechtsmed* 1983;90:159–165.
3. Garcin R. The ataxias. In: Vinken PJ, Bruyn GW, Klawans HL, eds. *Handbook of neurology.* New York: John Wiley & Sons, 1969:309–355.
4. Leigh JR, Zee DS. *The neurology of eye movements,* 2nd ed. In: Plum F, et al., eds. Contemporary neurology series. Philadelphia: FA Davis, 1991:402.
5. Gilman S, Bloedel JR, Lechtenberg R. Disorders of the cerebellum. In: Plum F, McDowell FH, Baringer R, eds. *Contemporary neurology series,* vol 21. Philadelphia: FA Davis, 1981:415.
6. Gilman S, MacDonald WI. Cerebellar facilitation of muscle spindle activity. *J Neurophysiol* 1967;30(6):1494–1512.
7. Holmes G. Clinical symptoms of cerebellar disease and their interpretation. The Croonian Lectures. II. *Brain* 1922;1: 1177–1182.
8. Mai N, et al. Control of isometric finger force in patients with cerebellar disease. *Brain* 1988;111:973–998.
9. Gerloff C, Altenmuller E, Dichgans J. Disintegration and reorganization of cortical motor processing in two patients with cerebellar stroke. *Electroencephalogr Clin Neurophysiol* 1996;98 (1):59–68.
10. Holmes G. Clinical symptoms of cerebellar disease and their interpretation. The Croonian Lectures. I. *Lancet* 1922;1:1231–1237.
11. Holmes G. The cerebellum of man. *Brain* 1939;62:1–30.
12. Ito M. *The cerebellum and neural control.* New York: Raven Press, 1984:461–464.
13. Diener HC, Dichgans J. Pathophysiology of cerebellar ataxia. *Mov Disord* 1992;7(2):95–109.
14. Lechtenberg R. Ataxia and other cerebellar syndromes. In: Jankovic J, ed. *Parkinson's disease and movement disorders.* Baltimore: Williams & Wilkins, 1993c.
15. Hallett M, et al. Physiological analysis of simple rapid movements in patients with cerebellar deficits. *J Neurol Neurosurg Psychiatry* 1991;53:124–133.
16. Massaquoi SG, Hallett M. Kinematics of initiating a two-joint arm movement in patients with cerebellar ataxia. *Can J Neurol Sci* 1996;23:3–14.
17. Bastian AJ, Martin TA, Keating JG. Cerebellar ataxia: abnormal control of interaction torques across multiple joints. *J Neurophysiol* 1996;76(1):492–509.
18. Topka H, Konczak J, Dichgans J. Coordination of multi-joint arm movements in cerebellar ataxia: analysis of hand and angular kinematics. *Exp Brain Res* 1998;119(4):483–492.
19. Thach WT, et al. Cerebellar output: multiple maps and modes of control in movement coordination. In: Llinas R, Sotelo C, eds. *Ramon Y Cahal Centenary,* 1992b.
20. Topka H, et al. Multijoint arm movements in cerebellar ataxia: abnormal control of movement dynamics. *Exp Brain Res* 1998; 119(4):493–503.
21. Massaquoi SG. Modelling the function of the cerebellum in scheduled linear servo control of simple horizontal planar arm movements. In: *Electrical Engineering and Computer Science.*

PhD thesis, Dept. of Electrical Engineering and Computer Science. Cambridge: Massachusetts Institute of Technology, 1999: 240.

22. Ivry RB, Keele SB. Timing functions of the cerebellum. *J Cogn Neurosci* 1989;1:136–152.
23. Keele S, Ivry R. Does the cerebellum provide a common computation for diverse tasks? *Ann NY Acad Sci* 1990;608: 179–211.
24. Diener HC, et al. Cerebellar dysfunction of movement and perception. *Can J Neurol Sci* 1993;20[Suppl 3]:S62–S69.
25. Thach WT, Goodkin HP, Keating JG. The cerebellum and the adaptive coordination of movement. *Annu Rev Neurosci* 1992; 15:403–442.
26. Deuschl G, et al. Symptomatic and essential palatal tremor I. Clinical, physiological, and MRI analysis. *Brain* 1994;117: 775–788.
27. Diener HC, et al. Characteristic alterations of long loop "reflexes" in patients with Friedreich's ataxia and late atrophy of the anterior cerebellar lobe. *J Neurol Neurosurg Psychiatr* 1984;47:679–685.
28. Diener HC, et al. Associated postural adjustments with body movement in normal subjects and patients with parkinsonism and cerebellar disease. *Rev Neurol (Paris)* 1990;146:555–563.
29. Victor M, Adams RD. A restricted form of cerebellar cortical degeneration in alcoholics. *Arch Neurol* 1959;1:579–688.
30. Horak FB, Diener HC. Cerebellar control of postural scaling and central set in stance. *J Neurophysiol* 1994;72(2):479–493.
31. Hallett M, Marsden CD, Fahn S. Myoclonus. In: Vinken PJ, Bruyn GW, Klawans HL, eds. *Handbook of clinical neurology.* Amsterdam: Elsevier, 1987:609–625.
32. Daroff RB. Eye signs in humans with cerebellar dysfunction. In: Lennerstrand G, Zee DS, Keller EL, eds. *Functional basis of ocular motility disorders.* Oxford: Pergamon, 1982:463–465.
33. Thompson RF. Neural mechanisms of classical conditioning in mammals. *Philos Trans R Soc Lond* 1990;329:161–170.
34. Brindley GS. The use made by the cerebellum of the information that it receives from sense organs. *Int Brain Res Org Bull* 1969;3:80.
35. Sanes JN, Dimitrov B, Hallett M. Motor learning in patients with cerebellar dysfunction. *Brain* 1990;113:103–120.
36. Thach WT. On the specific role of the cerebellum in motor learning and cognition: clues from PET activation and lesion studies in man. In: Harnad S, ed. *BBS special issue: Controversies in neurosciences IV: Motor learning and synaptic plasticity.* Cambridge University Press, 1996:411–431.
37. Doyon J. Functional anatomy of visuomotor skill learning in human subjects evaluated with positron emission tomography. In: Schmahmann JD, ed. *The cerebellum and cognition.* San Diego: Academic Press, 1997:273–294.
38. Bloedel JR, Bracha V. Duality of cerebellar motor and cognitive functions. In: Schmahmann JD, ed. *The cerebellum and cognition.* San Diego: Academic Press, 1997:613–634.
39. Ito M. Cerebellar microcomplexes. In: Schmahmann JD, ed. *The cerebellum and cognition.* Academic Press, 1997:475–487.
40. Ivry R. Cerebellar timing systems. In: Schmahmann JD, ed. *The cerebellum and cognition.* San Diego: Academic Press, 1997: 555–573.
41. Ivry RB, Keele SW, Diener HC. Dissociation of the lateral and medial cerebellum in movement timing and movement execution. *Exp Brain Res* 1988;73:167–180.
42. Grill SG, et al. Disturbances of kinaesthesia in patients with cerebellar disorders. *Brain* 1994;117:1433–1447.
43. Burton JE, Onoda N. Interpositus neuron discharge in relation to a voluntary movement. *Brain Res* 1977;121:167–172.
44. Kawato M, Gomi H. A computational model of four regions of the cerebellum based on feedback-error learning. *Biol Cybern* 1992;68:95–103.

45. Miall RC, Weir DJ, Stein JF. Visuo-motor tracking during reversible inactivation of the cerebellum. *Exp Brain Res* 1987; 65:455–464.
46. Massaquoi SG, Slotine J-JE. The intermediate cerebellum may function as a wave-variable processor. *Neurosci Lett* 1996;215: 60–64.
47. Kettner RE, et al. Prediction of complex two-dimensional trajectories by a cerebellar model of smooth pursuit eye movement. *J Neurophysiol* 1997;77:2115–2130.
48. Beppu H, Suda M, Tanaka R. Analysis of cerebellar motor disorders by visually-guided elbow tracking movements. *Brain* 1984;107:787–809.
49. Beppu H, Nagaoka M, Tanaka R. Analysis of cerebellar motor disorders by visually-guided elbow tracking movements: 2. Contribution of visual cues on slow ramp pursuit. *Brain* 1987; 110:1–18.
50. Angel RW. Barognosis in a patient with hemiataxia. *Ann Neurol* 1980;7(1):73–77.
51. Grill SE, Hallett M, McShane LM. Timing of onset of afferent responses and use of kinesthetic information for control of movement in normal and cerebellar-impaired subjects. *Exp Brain Res* 1997;113:33–47.
52. Bower JM. Control of sensory data acquisition. In: Schmahmann JD, ed. *The cerebellum and cognition.* San Diego: Academic Press, 1997:489–513.
53. Gao J-H, et al. Cerebellum implicated in sensory acquisition and discrimination rather than motor control. *Science* 1996; 272:545–547.
54. Paulin MG. The role of the cerebellum in motor control and perception. *Brain Behav Evolution* 1993;41:39–50.
55. Schmahmann JD, Pandya DN. The cerebrocerebellar system. In: Schmahmann JD, ed. *The cerebellum and cognition.* San Diego: Academic Press, 1997:31–60.
56. Haines DE, et al. Cerebellar-hypothalamic axis: basic circuits and clinical observations. In: Schmahmann JD, ed. *The cerebellum and cognition.* San Diego: Academic Press, 1997.
57. Brodal A. *Neurological anatomy in relation to clinical medicine.* New York: Oxford University Press, 1981.
58. Lechtenberg R. *Handbook of cerebellar diseases.* In: Koller WC, ed. Neurological disease and therapy. New York: Marcel Decker, 1993:73.
59. Attig E. Parieto-cerebellar loop impairment in ataxic hemiparesis: proposed pathophysiology based on an analysis of cerebral blood flow. *Can J Neurol Sci* 1994;21:15–23.
60. Fisher CM. Ataxic hemiparesis: a pathologic study. *Arch Neurol* 1978;35:126–128.
61. Marcolongo F. Varices et anigome de la moelle avec syndrome d'ataxie cerebelleuse. *Rev Neurol* 1932;1:565.
62. Noica M. Syndrome de Brown-Sequard ne presentant que des troubles cerebelleux au lieu de paralysie. *Rev Neurol* 1932;1: 469–472.
63. Fisher CM. An unusual variant of acute idiopathic polyneuritis (syndrome of ophthalmoplegia, ataxia and areflexia). *N Engl J Med* 1956;255:57–65.
64. Ropper AH, Shahani BT. Proposed mechanism of ataxia in Fisher's syndrome. *Arch Neurol* 1983;40:537–538.
65. Sobue G, et al. Sensory ataxia: a residual disability of Guillain-Barré syndrome. *Arch Neurol* 1983;40:86–89.
66. O'Leary CP, Willison HJ. Autoimmune ataxic neuropathies (sensory ganglionopathies). *Curr Opin Neurol* 1997;10: 366–370.
67. Iwahashi T, et al. The detection of anti-cerebellar antibody western blot analysis in serum from a patient with Miller Fisher syndrome. *Arerugi* 1995;44(9):1176–1180.
68. Bushara KO, et al. Gluten sensitivity in sporadic and hereditary cerebellar ataxia. *Ann Neurol* 2001;49:540–543.

69. Burk K, et al. Sporadic cerebellar ataxia associated with gluten sensitivity. *Brain* 2001;124:1013–1019.
70. Pellecchia MT, et al. Idiopathic cerebellar ataxia associated with celiac disease: lack of distinctive neurological features [see comments]. *J Neurol Neurosurg Psychiatry* 1999;66:32–35.
71. Hadjivassiliou M, et al. Headache and CNS white matter abnormalities associated with gluten sensitivity. *Neurology* 2001 (56):385–358.
72. Bolla L, Palmer RM. Paraneoplastic cerebellar degeneration: case report and literature review. *Arch Intern Med* 1997;157:1258–1262.
73. Vernino S, Lennon VA. New Purkinje cell antibody (PCA-2): marker of lung cancer-related neurological autoimmunity. *Ann Neurol* 2000;47:297–305.
74. Lucchinetti CF, Kimmel DW, Lennon VA. Paraneoplastic and oncologic profiles of patients seropositive for type 1 antineuronal nuclear autoantibodies. *Neurology* 1998;50:652–657.
75. de la Sayette V, et al. Paraneoplastic cerebellar syndrome and optic neuritis with anti-CV2 antibodies: clinical response to excision of the primary tumor. *Arch Neurol* 1998(55):405–408.
76. Dalmau J, et al. Ma1, a novel neuron- and testis-specific protein, is recognized by the serum of patients with paraneoplastic neurological disorders. *Brain* 1999;122:27–39.
77. Gultekin SH, et al. Paraneoplastic limbic encephalitis: neurological symptoms, immunological findings and tumour association in 50 patients. *Brain* 2000;123:1481–1494.
78. Saiz A, et al. Anti-amphiphysin I antibodies in patients with paraneoplastic neurological disorders associated with small cell lung carcinoma. *J Neurol Neurosurg Psychiatry* 1999;66:214–217.
79. Sillevis Smitt P, et al. Paraneoplastic cerebellar ataxia due to autoantibodies against a glutamate receptor. *N Engl J Med* 2000;342:21–27.
80. Honnorat J, et al. Cerebellar ataxia with anti-glutamic acid decarboxylase antibodies: study of 14 patients. *Arch Neurol* 2001;58:225–230.
81. Hewer RL, Cooper R, Morgan MH. An investigation into the value of treating intention tremor by weighting the affected limb. *Brain* 1972;95:579–590.
82. Aisen ML, et al. The effect of mechanical damping loads on disabling action tremor. *Neurology* 1993;43:1346–1350.
83. Botez MI, et al. Amantadine hydrochloride in heredeodegenerative ataxias: a double blind study. *J Neurol Neurosurg Psychiatry* 1996;61(3):259–264.
84. Trouillas P, et al. Levorotatory form of 5-hydroxytryptophan in Friedreich's ataxia. *Arch Neurol* 1995;52:456–460.
85. Wessel K, et al. Double-blind crossover study with levorotatory form of hydroxytryptophan in patients with degenerative cerebellar diseases. *Arch Neurol* 1995;52(5):451–455.
86. Lou JS, et al. Use of buspirone for treatment of cerebellar ataxia: an open-label study. *Arch Neurol* 1995;52(10):982–988.
87. Trouillas P, et al. Buspirone, a 5-hydroxytryptamine1A agonist, is active in cerebellar ataxia: results of a double-blind drug placebo study in patients with cerebellar cortical atrophy. *Arch Neurol* 1997(54):749–752.
88. Aschoff JC, Kailer NA, Walter K. Physostigmine in treatment of cerebellar ataxia. *Nervenarzt* 1996;67(4):311–318.
89. Wessel K, et al. Double-blind crossover study with physostigmine in patients with degenerative cerebellar diseases. *Arch Neurol* 1997;54:397–400.
90. Helveston W, et al. Abnormalities of antioxidant metabolism in a case of Friedreich's disease. *Clin Neuropharmacol* 1996;19:271–275.
91. Helveston W, et al. Abnormalities of glutathione peroxidase and glutathione reductase in four patients with Friedreich's disease [letter]. *Mov Disord* 1996;11:106–107.
92. Hurd R, et al. Treatment of four siblings with progressive myoclonus epilepsy of the Unverricht-Lundborg type with N-acetylcysteine. *Neurology* 1996;47:1284–1288.
93. River YH, Gomori JM, Reches A. Superficial hemosiderosis of the central nervous system [see comments in *Mov Disord* 1995;10(5):685]. *Mov Disord* 1994;9(5):559–562.
94. Rustin P, et al. Effect of idebenone on cardiomyopathy in Friedreich's ataxia: a preliminary study. *Lancet* 1999;354(9177):477–479.
95. Lodi R, et al. Antioxidant treatment improves in vivo cardiac and skeletal muscle bioenergetics in patients with Friedreich's ataxia. *Ann Neurol* 2001;49(5):590–596.
96. Schols L, et al. Idebenone in patients with Friedreich ataxia. *Neurosci Lett* 2001;306(3):169–172.
97. Nguyen JP, Degos JD. Thalamic stimulation and proximal tremor: a specific target in the nucleus ventrointermedius thalami. *Arch Neurol* 1993;50(5):498–500.
98. Triarhou LC, Zhang W, Lee WH. Amelioration of the behavioral phenotype in genetically ataxic mice through bilateral intracerebellar grafting of fetal Purkinje cells. *Cell Transplant* 1996;5(2):269–277.
99. Zhang W, Lee WH, Triarhou LC. Grafted cerebellar cells in a mouse model of hereditary ataxia. *Nat Med* 1996;2(1):65–71.
100. Sotelo C, Alvarado-Mallart RM. The reconstruction of cerebellar circuits. *Trends Neurosci* 1991;14(8):350–355.

28

DISORDERS OF GAIT

EVŽEN RŮŽIČKA
JOSEPH J. JANKOVIC

Locomotion is one of the essential vital functions in most animals, and its significance can hardly be underestimated in humans. Bipedal gait, together with speech and language, distinguishes man from his ancestors. However, the newly adopted erect posture necessitated the development of a complex system designed to maintain balance and motor coordination even while the upper extremities were busy performing complex specialized operations.

Gait is defined as a complex motor skill that, when properly executed, requires the integration of mechanisms of locomotion with those of balance, motor control, and musculoskeletal function (1). Pathologic involvement of any particular component of gait, in particular, posture and balance, as well as initiation and maintenance of the rhythmic pattern of advancement of lower extremities, will lead to abnormal locomotion.

Gait disorders are caused by many neurologic and non-neurologic diseases and often reflect a broad category of dysfunctions of the central and peripheral nervous system, musculoskeletal system, or both. In 1950, Švehla reported 2,714 cases of gait disorder seen in more than 20% of all the patients he had examined (2). With regard to the state of the art of the day and time, he confined himself to phenomenologic classification in most of the cases, in particular: peripheral (musculoskeletal) causes, in 18% of the patients; proprioceptive or vestibular involvement, in 15%; cerebral (vascular or tumorous) hemiparesis, in 13%; cerebral or spinal paraplegia, in 12%; parkinsonian gait, in 9%; cerebellar gait, in 8%. In the rest of the cases the disorder could not be unambiguously classified or was thought to be of psychogenic etiology. Nearly half a century later, a study, taking advantage of all modern diagnostic techniques to describe 120 cases of gait disorders in elderly patients referred to neurologic scrutiny, found the following pattern: 18% were due to sensory impairment, 17% to myelopathy, 15% to vascular encephalopathy, 12% to parkinsonism, 7% to hydrocephalus, 7% to cerebellar disorders, and the rest to an assortment of other pathologies (3).

Falls, causally closely connected with gait or balance, are among the salient causes of morbidity and mortality, particularly in the elderly. According to Tinetti (4), 30% of elderly persons suffer at least one fall annually, with the figure being 40% among those older than 80 years and a good 50% among nursing homes residents. Falls also represent an important cause of secondary morbidity and mortality as a result of fractures, other serious injuries, and immobilization.

This chapter aims to provide a review of gait disorders that would be applicable to the medical practice of a clinical neurologist. Only a brief account of the motor physiology of gait will be given as this topic is covered in a number of specialized reviews (5–7). An overview of diagnostic approaches is followed by descriptions of the clinical characteristics of gait disorders and, in particular, their diverse expressions relative to different etiologies organized according to clinical-anatomic classification.

ANATOMIC AND PHYSIOLOGIC FOUNDATIONS OF GAIT: MECHANISMS OF LOCOMOTION AND BALANCE

Locomotion is effected by a continuous stream of integrated signals orchestrating the alternate advancing, loading, and unloading of lower extremities. Rather than a consciously executed motor activity, this learned motor pattern is produced by complex coordinated spinal mechanisms, triggered and modified from brainstem structures and supraspinal motor centers (8). Rhythmic walking movements evolve and persist even in decerebrated or "spinalized" cats and dogs. They arise from rhythmic activity in the network of spinal interneurons constituting the locomotor generator (an equivalent of the generator of the rhythmic movements of the wings in birds or flippers in fishes). Unlike mammalian quadrupeds, whose gait mainly depends on the motor pattern spinal generators (5), automatic gait in primates can be induced by electrical stimulation of the mesencephalic tegmentum (mesencephalic locomotor center), the laterodorsal portion of the ponto-mesencephalic junction including pedunculopontine nucleus (PPN), and the posterior subthalamus (9). The PPN, a cluster of cholinergic neurons in the caudal mesencephalic tegmentum, receives direct bilateral descending projection from the subthalamic nucleus, dorsal and ventral striatum, globus pallidum (GP), and substantia nigra pars reticulata (SNr). The descending projections from the GP and SNr use the inhibitor neurotransmitter γ-aminobutyric acid (GABA) as a mediator, whereas the PPN sends excitatory acetylcholinergic and glutamatergic ascending projections to the striatal nuclei. Though the PPN function has yet to be fully elucidated, it appears to mediate basal ganglia action on the brainstem and spinal cord motor mechanisms, including gait, posture, and balance (10). PPN then seems to represent the principal component of the mesencephalic locomotor center. PPN stimulation in the cat induces stepping and other rhythmic processes, whereas PPN inhibition results in restricted locomotor activity. Elements of spinal stepping have been described in humans with paraplegia (11). It appears that, besides the spinal cord, the dorsal mesencephalon, a counterpart of the brainstem locomotor area in experimental animals, is also active in the course of bipedal locomotion (12). The posterior parietal cortex also plays an important role in locomotion by providing the perception of the body posture, thus helping to maintain normal gait and balance (13).

The two essential prerequisites of erect bipedal gait are (a) *equilibrium*, the ability to keep the body upright and to maintain balance, and (b) *locomotion*, the capacity for rhythmic stepping (14).

Erect posture is ensured by righting and antigravitational reflexes that keep the knees, hips, and back in extension continually adaptable to the head and neck position. This accounts, for example, for the ability to stand up from lying or sitting into the erect position. Postural reflexes depend on vestibular, somatosensory (proprioceptive and tactile), and visual inputs. Afferent stimuli are integrated at spinal, brainstem, and basal ganglia levels. The conventional model of decerebration rigidity on brainstem transsection between the nucleus ruber and vestibular nuclei, marked by extreme extension, is an example of increased antigravitational reflexes. *Equilibrium* is the ability to maintain balance under dynamic conditions in the plane of the direction of locomotion and in the plane at right angles to it. In walking, the mechanisms of equilibrium continually make up for the center of gravity shifts in connection with the forward direction of locomotion and with alternating leg movements. *Anticipatory postural reflexes* ensure adequate adjustment prior to intended voluntary movement. *Reactive postural responses* adapt the body attitude and posture to shifts of the center of gravity and sudden changes of external conditions. Appropriate reflex balancing function requires good *proprioceptive* (source of stretch reflexes) and *visual* as well as *vestibular* (source of vestibulocerebellar reflexes) integration. At least two of the three afferent pathways must remain intact or else the sense of balance fails, as seen in Romberg's sign in which a subject loses balance upon closing the eyes as a result of proprioceptive or vestibular damage.

Stepping is a basic, automatic motor function that appears to be programmed in the brainstem and spinal cord in early stages of development as it is present even before birth. However, the gait mechanisms of adult individuals are under the control of higher regulating centers (situated in the posterior subthalamus, caudal mesencephalon, and pons), which control spinal activity by means of reticulospinal, vestibulospinal, and tectospinal projections in the anterior funiculi of the spinal cord (9). Stepping is initiated by the sole of the foot contact with the supporting surface and by shifting the center of gravity, first sideways over one lower extremity so that the other can be lifted, and then forward in the direction of the advancing extremity. The same mechanisms are engaged in voluntary initiation of walking when the *propulsion force* stimulates the leg to step forward and makes it provide the body with necessary support on touching the ground ahead.

NORMAL POSTURE AND GAIT

Posture and Gait Evolution

Normal gait is man's most spontaneous motor stereotype seen as an objective criterion of adequate postnatal motor development, later to become a characteristic feature of the adult individual's motor personality and behavioral image and, ultimately, a telltale sign of aging.

The phylogenetic evolution by way of quadrupedal to bipedal locomotion is reflected in the ontogenesis of every human individual (7). In the early stages, some of the characteristics of quadrupedal locomotion are preserved, suggesting the presence of a central pattern generator capable of producing automatic movements. The later stages of development of independent coordinated walking are marked by the gradual maturation of supraspinal control mechanisms.

Locomotor-like movements are discernible in utero beginning at postconception week 10. What are known as locomotor automatisms are inborn, rhythmic, gait-like movements elicitable immediately after birth if the newborn is held under the shoulders with his or her feet allowed to touch a support surface (gait automatism). Electromyography will then show *coactivation* of antagonist muscles of the lower extremities (15). The extinction of this pattern as from postnatal week 10 obviously reflects functional changes in the arrangement of the network of spinal circuits. The subsequent period is marked by a quadrupedal posture–locomotion pattern changing into the bipedal pattern as from the age of 7 to 10 months when the child begins to stand up, either without or with minor support. The gait pattern is then characterized by the digitigrade position of the feet. In the load-bearing phase, the leg—positioned vertically—serves the body as a support but fails to provide for advancement. Forward motion requires rotation in the hip of the unloaded extremity. This early spontaneous bipedal locomotion is marked by coactivation of the leg muscle antagonists in the support phase of the walking cycle (explained hereinafter), by low-voltage tonic electromyographic (EMG) activity of the extensors, and by high biphasic potentials reflecting the monosynaptic stretch reflex on the tiptoe touch-down. Sudden stimuli simulating obstacles and floor surface irregularities evoke simple short-latency mono- and oligosynaptic reflexes followed by persisting polysynaptic responses of extensors with the coactivation of antagonists (16).

In the third year of life, the previous "coactivation" pattern is gradually replaced by a pattern of *reciprocal muscle activation* permitting free unassisted walking adaptable to surface ruggedness. The foot touches the ground heel-first in a plantigrade manner. During the load-bearing phase, the body rolls over the support leg and receives forward thrust. This is where the supraspinal mechanisms of locomotion control are already fully activated. The biphasic short-latency stretch reflexes are now suppressed; tonic EMG activity of the leg extensors gathers momentum while polysynaptic responses to sudden stimuli are getting shorter (17). Roughly from age 4 years the gait pattern begins to look like that of adults, though the subsequent period is marked by perfection of coordination of head, neck, and trunk movements; by increasing coordination of leg joint movements; and by growing demands on equilibrium.

Early gait development disorders, typically in association with the diplegic form of cerebral palsy, are noted for the persistence of immature patterns of locomotion, mainly by antagonist coactivation in the standing position, by lowered tonic activity of leg extensors, and by increased excitability of the stretch reflex. This stiff, toe-walking gait (a sign of locomotion development arrested in an immature stage) is quite unlike spastic paraparesis developed in adulthood where the previously developed pattern of reciprocal activation is well preserved (18).

Normal Gait

Characteristic features of a mature gait pattern include upright attitude of the trunk and neck; lower extremities resting on feet set slightly apart; hips, knees, and ankles flexing in coordinated forward locomotion with the pelvis tilting slightly at the corresponding moments, thus allowing the unloaded leg to pass forward without touching the floor; upper extremities swinging freely along the sides in slight semiflexion and performing adequate synkinetic movements relative to the strides of the contralateral legs while the chest, too, makes minor forward excursions toward the swinging arm side. The person's narrow-based walking proceeds straight ahead with the connecting line of the heel touch-down points on the floor running in a straight line while the strides of roughly equal length rhythmically follow one another.

Gait patterns are characteristic of each individual and provide useful information about their personality and cur-

rent psychic state. The walking body posture, the length and regularity of the strides, the touch-down impact, synkinetic movements of upper extremities, and other consciously as well as inadvertently performed and by an observer's equally so perceived features of gait usually permit discrimination between male and female gait, between extroverts and introverts, and between persons feeling joyful and those who are depressed. In addition, there are obvious cultural and ethnic differences in gait patterns, such as between those of Asian, European, Latin, or African origin, or between those living in urban as opposed to rural communities, which may influence the walking cycle parameters and gait characteristics (19,20). Running and jogging may be viewed as variants of accelerated walking wherein the double-support phase disappears and locomotion is effected by a series of jumps with a greater amplitude and with intermittent contact with the ground. The running characteristics may also be genetically or ethnically determined and influenced by the need for optimal energy efficiency. For example, Arab runners traditionally run in an ambling way, that is, with the homolateral extremities moving isochronically, thus easily attaining speed of 10 kilometers per hour over long periods (2).

Changes in Old Age

Changes in the pattern of walking inevitably accompany aging without necessarily reflecting a pathologic involvement of the nervous system (21). According to Tinetti (22), 40% to 50% of nursing home inmates have difficulty walking and suffer from frequent falls. In the course of senescence the elastic harmony of movements characteristic of young individuals wanes, walking becomes progressively slower, and the sense of balance deteriorates. There may be different degrees of bent posture, rigidity of the trunk and extremities, stride shortening, and widening of the leg support base. As people age they turn by moving their head, neck, and trunk "en bloc." This cautious gait and balance pattern is not unlike that of a younger healthy person walking on a slippery surface, in response to feeling unsafe in space and to the threat of falling. Such manifestations may be related to age-related deterioration of sight, proprioception, or vestibular function, and may reflect a weakening of erector muscles, as well as degenerative changes in extremity joints and in the vertebral column. Gaits associated with normal senescence may be difficult to differentiate from gait patterns discussed later, such as "cautious gait," gait of "frontal apraxia," and other abnormal gaits.

GAIT AND BALANCE EXAMINATION

Posture, balance, and gait assessment are not always fully valued as important elements of the basic neurologic examination unless problems with walking and balance are the main reason for the patient's seeking neurologic advice. Nevertheless, a characteristic disorder of gait can prompt diagnosis in the moment the patient enters the consulting room, as is often the case in patients with Parkinson's disease, progressive supranuclear palsy, hereditary motor neuropathy, muscular dystrophy, or psychogenic disorders. Although admittedly highly sophisticated methods of quantitative analysis of gait can be a welcome addition to the clinical facilities for research purposes, simple observation remains the essential approach, the "gold standard" of gait investigation, from which an experienced observer can extract crucial information for differential diagnosis of the particularly gait and balance problem. Using appropriate scales, gait and balance parameters can be clinically quantified (23) (see section "Gait and Balance Scale" and Appendix 1).

Clinical Assessment

Symptoms of balance and gait disorders often tend to be nonspecific. As a rule, the patient complains of sloweddown walking, uncertainty in space, perception of instability when standing or walking, or frequent falls. Finding more about the circumstances of gait or balance problems is essential, especially regarding freezing and falls as these may

TABLE 28.1. CLINICAL EXAMINATION OF POSTURE, BALANCE, AND GAIT

1) Neurologic examination, including assessment of the configuration of lower extremities, their attitude, range of active and passive movement, muscle tone, and strength
2) Getting up from lying to sitting, from sitting to standing positions—looking for possible muscular weakness, disorder of motor coordination
3) Spontaneous stance
   Posture of trunk and extremities
   Base width (distance between the two feet)
4) Maneuvers while standing (*Caution: ensure protection against falling*)
   Stance with feet close together, eyes open
   Romberg test (the same as above, with eyes closed)
   Postural response to external stimuli in the anteroposterior direction—pull test (shoulder-tug test) or push test
   One-limb stance, tandem stance (feet placed toe-to-heel)
5) Spontaneous gait (to be examined in the corridor or some other space offering at least 10 m of freeway)
   Base width, stride length, cadence, fluidity of movements, deviations from given direction
   Start and stop, turning in place and while walking, spontaneously and in response to command
   Walking through constricted passage (doorway), clearing and avoiding obstacles
6) Maneuvers while walking
   Tandem gait (feet placed toe-to-heel)
   Walking with eyes closed (Romberg test while walking)
   Walking backward
   Walking on heels and on tiptoes

TABLE 28.2. BASIC FEATURES CONSTITUTING SYNDROMES OF POSTURE AND GAIT DISORDERS

Muscle weakness
Base width
Stride length
Cadence
Directional deviations
Fluidity of movements
Gait initiation and maintenance
Adaptability

Data from Nutt JG. Classification of part and balance disorders. In: Růžička E, Hallett M, Jankovic J, eds. *Gait disorders.* Philadelphia: Lippincott Williams & Wilkins, 2001:135–141.

not be observed during examination. The comprehensive gait and balance evaluation comprises maneuvers designed to assess the overall execution of the required movement, muscular strength, postural reflexes, and signs of lateral instability (Table 28.1). The phenomenologic classification of gait disorders, partly adopted from recent reviews, is based on integration of observed clinical characteristics (Table 28.2) with known anatomic and etiologic mechanisms (24).

Muscular weakness can usually be detected during neurologic examination of the lower limbs and tends to be brought out on execution of functional changes of position: sitting down, arising from a chair, standing, and, in particular, walking. *Base width* is studied in spontaneous standing and in walking when we take note of the base width changes and any possible *deviations* from the straight pathway suggesting disturbed lateral stability. *Maneuvers while standing* (e.g., feet close together, Romberg's test) will help to reveal minor disturbances of lateral stability. Anteroposterior stability disturbance can be diagnosed with the push and pull (shoulder tug) tests. The gait parameters, such as *stride length, cadence* (number of strides per minute), *gait speed and regularity,* and *fluidity* of walking movements can be all ascertained by observing the subject's "normal" or usual gait. After command the patient to start walking, change direction, stop, we explore gait *initiation, maintenance,* and *adaptation* to changes in environmental conditions (support surface changes, narrow passages, etc.) or to intentional gait changes. *Maneuvers while walking* (tandem gait, walking with closed eyes, walking on heels and tiptoes, walking backward) will expose lateral instability, disorders of proprioception, distal muscle weakness, and psychogenic or dystonic gait. These elements are included in the *gait and balance scale* (GABS) (see below).

Gait Cycle

Quantitative analysis of walking focuses on the time and space segment between two successive points where the heel of the same foot reaches the support surface (Fig. 28.1). This *walking cycle* consists of two regularly alternating

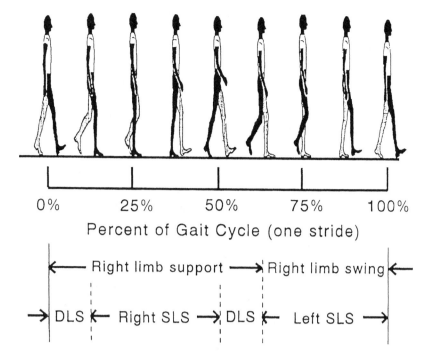

Percent of Gait Cycle (one stride)

$\longleftarrow$ Right limb support $\longrightarrow$ Right limb swing $\longleftarrow$

$\rightarrow$ DLS $\longleftarrow$ Right SLS $\rightarrow$ DLS $\longleftarrow$ Left SLS $\longrightarrow$

FIG. 28.1. Gait cycle. The gait cycle extends from the time of heel–floor contact to the time of next heel–floor contact with the same (right) foot. DLS, double-limb support; SLS, single-limb support. (Reprinted with permission from Elble R. Changes in gait with normal aging. In: Masdeu JC, Sudarsky L, Wolfson L, eds. *Gait disorders of aging: falls and therapeutic strategies.* Philadelphia: Lippincott–Raven, 1997:96.)

phases for either of the two lower extremities. In the example illustrated in Fig. 28.1, the right-foot heel impact opens the *support or stance phase* of the cycle, during which the foot touches the ground and extensor muscle activity predominates (25). As the right great toe leaves the ground, the *swing phase* begins with predominant flexor activity. In terms of time, the support phase covers 60% to 65% of the walking cycle, including 20% to 25% of the *double-support phase.* The rest—35% to 40%—is taken by the swing phase of the cycle. Acceleration results in the shortening of both the support and the swing phases, with the double-support phase being shortened relatively more. The proportion of the particular phases undergoes change in senescence, with the stride length becoming shorter and the relative share of double support growing.

A *stride* comprises the activity of one lower extremity in the course of one walking cycle (between two strikes made by the heel of the same foot). The basic pattern of walking is defined by the stride length and stride duration where the former reflects the dynamic component, the latter the rhythmic component of walking. Cadence indicates the number of strides per minute. The function of equilibrium becomes manifest in the *double-support duration* and in the *step width.* Changes in the above parameters are due to the person's immediate locomotion needs or to adaptation to environmental factors. Any marked variation in the parameters measured in the course of locomotion indicates some kind of gait pattern and equilibrium disorder. Stride-to-stride variability is at its highest in young children, reduced in adolescence, but increasing again in pathologic states such as in Parkinson's and Huntington's diseases.

Kinetic Analysis of Gait

Kinetic quantitative analysis of gait may involve simple tools such as stopwatch and tape measure in order to quantify some of the gait parameters. This may be useful in assessing the effects of a therapeutic intervention or to prospectively follow patients (26). In the *stand-walk-sit test* we ask the patient to stand up on command from sitting on a chair, to walk as quickly as possible to a mark (usually 5 m), to turn around there, and to return and sit down on the chair (27). If, in addition to that, the number of steps is measured simultaneously in the so-called *steps-seconds test* we can also calculate the average stride length and duration (Fig. 28.1). Precision of time and distance measurement is an obvious prerequisite for the reliability of results. Free walking and the above simple tests can be combined with another *simultaneous task* (speaking, counting, etc.). The competitive task exertion can bring out the existing gait disorder and help to identify it (or differentiate it from psychogenic gait disorder). The gait parameters can likewise be influenced by acoustic or visual sensory stimuli with perturbing effects mainly on pathologic gait, though in some cases sensory stimuli may, in contrast, improve gait (e.g., rhythmic visual or acoustic cues in the freezing gait).

Techniques of Gait and Balance Analysis

Although clinical observation and simple kinetic analysis will, as a rule, suffice to identify the gait pattern, it may be necessary for testing the therapeutic effects or for research reasons alone to measure the walking cycle phases (Fig.

28.1) in order to quantify with more precision the posture and gait pattern parameters. This purpose is served by a number of sophisticated technical procedures found of use in laboratories for motion and gait analysis (28).

The most easily available gait analysis technical facility is a *footswitch* attached to each shoe sole. In combination with stationary or mobile registering equipment, footswitches identify the exact moment at which the foot makes contact with the floor, thus revealing the duration of each stride phase and any possible parameter variation between strides. Two or more footswitches attached to each foot will produce further features of gait, such as the time relation between the heel and tiptoe touch-down, and the like. One disadvantage of the switch-based analysis is that it does not allow for identification of the spatial parameters of walking.

Other methods require more specialized motion analysis facilities that are not always readily available (28). *Conductive pathway* provides gait parameters of time but also space (stride length, base width) and their variations. The *treadmill* serves rehabilitation but, when coupled with a suitable recording method, may be also used in gait analysis. Various *cinematic methods* are based on *pictorial motion records* taken from several angles with the motion trajectory visualized by means of marks attached to various body segments. Computer-aided processing of the records then permits a three-dimensional reconstruction of the motion in a system of coordinates using a biomechanical model. The pictorial record can be combined with other simultaneous testing methods, such as *telemetric EMG*. Diagnostic methods for balance testing make use of tilting or foam-covered platforms (29,30). Measurements of internal and external forces transmitted between the lower extremities and the floor while the person examined is standing or walking involve the use of *force plates* working on the piezoelectric principle (28).

Gait and Balance Scale

Various quantitative, computer-based, physiologic gait analyses and platform studies of balance have been used to investigate gait and balance disorders, but their utility in the assessment of these disorders has been limited by relative inaccessibility of these tools in the clinic. There is currently no validated clinical rating scale of gait and balance problems. The proposed list of timed and untimed assessments, referred to as the Gait and Balance Scale (GABS, Appendix 1), is being developed and validated. Other gait rating scales, such as the modified Gait Abnormality Rating Scale (GARS), have been used to quantitate gait and predict the risk of falling (31). The purpose of GABS is to provide a user-friendly instrument that objectively assess gait and balance and can be easily applied in the clinic, analogous to the Unified Parkinson's Disease Rating Scale (UPDRS) (32).

PHENOMENOLOGIC CLASSIFICATION OF GAIT DISORDERS

In the absence of a diagnostic marker, disorders of gait are difficult to classify. Method based on phenomenology, coupled with knowledge about structural and etiologic abnormalities, seems to be the most logical approach to the classification of gait disorders (24) (Tables 28.3 and 28.4). However, specific categorization of the gait disorder may be difficult because of the combination of patterns and mutually overlapping clinical features. Moreover, there is a certain tradition in the use of descriptive labeling designed to characterize each of the gait disorder patterns (33). Thus, for instance, the "stiff gait" pattern may indicate spasticity in pyramidal lesions, dystonia, or rigidity arising from basal ganglia, but also restricted leg movement due to joint and musculoskeletal problems.

For purposes of phenomenologic classification we opted for a division based on the description of the basic features and clinical signs brought out during posture and gait examination (Table 28.2). The most typical, clinically observed disorders of gait may, of course, be made up of several basic elements intertwined in the resulting pattern (Table 28.3). The clinical-anatomic classification then proceeds from the site of the damage usually responsible for the complex gait disorder pattern resulting from a combination of several basic phenomenologic features (more in section "Anatomic-Clinical Classification of Gait Disorders" and Table 28.4).

Gait Disorders Due to Muscular Weakness

Owing to muscular weakness (in primary muscle diseases and in peripheral nerve involvement), motion in the segment and direction concerned is affected by reduced strength. Weakness severe enough to result in abnormalities of gait is usually noticeable during the basic neurologic examination. Depending on whether the proximal or distal muscles of the leg are affected, gait patterns are classified as discussed in the following sections.

Proximal Weakness (Waddling Gait, Duck Gait)

Weakness affects pelvic girdle muscles and proximal muscles of the leg normally responsible for support hip abduction and for keeping the pelvis in horizontal position while walking. Owing to gluteal muscle weakness, the hip tends to tip toward the swing leg. To compensate for this abnormal situation, lumbar hyperlordosis develops with the trunk flexing toward the support leg. The hip and trunk swing from side to side to compensate for the difficulties in lifting the leg. The alternate collapsing

TABLE 28.3. BASIC GAIT DISORDER PATTERNS

Physical Sign	Description	Associated Signs
Hemiparetic gait	Extension and circumduction of one leg	Weakness on the affected side; hyperreflexia; extensor plantar response; flexed arm
Paraparetic gait	Stiffness, extension, adduction, and scissoring of both legs	Bilateral leg weakness, hyperreflexia, spasticity, and extensor plantar responses
Sensory gait	Unsteadiness of walking when visual input is withdrawn	Positive Romberg sign; decreased position sense
Steppage gait	Weakness of foot dorsiflexors; foot-drop; excessive flexion of hips and knees when walking; short strides; unilateral or bilateral	Atrophy of distal leg muscles; decreased ankle reflex; possible sensory loss
Cautious gait[a]	Wide based, careful, slow	Associated often with anxiety, fear of open spaces and fear of falling
Freezing gait[a]	Difficulty initiating a step; freezing; feet almost stuck to floor; turn hesitation; shuffling gait	Hypokinesia; muscular rigidity; grasp reflexes; possible resting tremor, dementia, or urinary incontinence
Propulsive or retropulsive gait[a]	Body's center of gravity appears to be either in front or behind the patient, who is struggling to keep his or her feet up to center of gravity; festination	Hypokinesia; muscular rigidity; postural instability
Ataxic gait	Wide based gait; incoordination; staggering; decomposition of movements	Dysmetria; dysdiadochokinesia; tremor; postural instability
Astasia	Primary balance disorder	Postural instability
Waddling gait	Wide based gait; swaying; toe-walk; lumbar lordosis; symmetric	Proximal muscle weakness of lower extremities
Dystonic gait[a]	Sustained abnormal posture of the foot or leg; distorted gait; hyperflexion of hips	Action-related gait disturbance; atypical presentations
Choreic gait[a]	Irregular, dance-like gait; slow and wide based; spontaneous knee flexion and leg raising	Athetotic and choreic movements of the upper extremities
Antalgic gait	Limping; avoidance of bearing full weight on the affected leg; limitation of range of movement	Pain in lower extremity aggravated by leg, hip, thigh movement and weight bearing
Vertiginous gait	Unsteady gait; falling to one side; postural imbalance	Vertigo; nausea; nystagmus
Psychogenic (hysterical) gait	Bizarre and nonphysiologic gait; different varieties; rare fall or injury	Give-way weakness; Hoover's sign; other signs of conversion

[a]These gaits may be seen in patients with Parkinson's disease.
Reprinted with permission from Jankovic J, Nutt JG, Sudarsky LR. Classification, diagnosis, and etiology of gait disorders. In: Růžička E, Hallett M, Jankovic J, eds. *Gait disorders.* Philadelphia: Lippincott Williams & Wilkins, 2001:119–133.

of the hip gives the impression of waddling, hence the term "duck gait." Due to muscle weakness, arising from a chair is often feasible only with the support of upper extremities. The difficulties are even more conspicuous in getting up from lying or sitting on the ground with the patient forced to lean against the floor, surrounding objects, or his or her own lower extremities ("myopathic climb" or "Gower's sign") (34). Walking upstairs and downstairs will also reveal proximal or distal weakness, respectively.

Distal Weakness (Cock Gait, Steppage, Foot Drop, Flail Foot, Slapping Gait)

The most common pattern of gait disorder due to weakness of the *anterolateral (peroneal)* muscle group of the leg takes the form of footdrop as the patient lifts the foot to clear the ground. While walking, in order to keep the tip of the foot clear of the floor, he or she must flex the extremity excessively in the hip and lift the knee (cock gait). In the touchdown phase, the foot first rubs against the floor with the great toe or with the anterolateral edge before all of the sole of the foot steps down (steppage gait). Weakened dorsal flexion of the foot renders patients unable to walk on their heels as they cannot lift the tip of the foot on the affected side.

The involvement of the *posterior* group of crural muscles, especially of the triceps surae (separate or in combination with peroneal paresis), is characterized by weakened plantar flexion and leg adduction. While walking, the patient has problems rolling the sole of the foot off the floor and pushing off with the tip of the foot. Instead, the foot comes down flat like a flail (slapping gait, flail foot). In efforts to walk on tiptoe, the foot collapses on the affected side, or the patient is totally unable to assume the tiptoe position.

Gait Disorders with Widened Base

Widened-base with Directional Deviations (Veering Gait)

Balance disorders and other conditions that aggravate lateral stability force the patient to compensate by widening the base while standing or walking. Typically, the etiologies include disorders of the equilibrium system made up of the vestibular labyrinth in the inner ear, 8th cranial nerve, and its brainstem nuclei and connections. Deviations to one side may also be present in lesions of the nondominant parietal lobe associated with sensory neglect of the respective half of the space. Postural asymmetry and deviations in walking may also be due to unilateral leg weakness seen in peripheral or central paresis, except that in such cases base widening is not all that conspicuous.

The peripheral vestibular syndrome (reflecting disorders of the inner ear or 8th cranial nerve) is a typical cause of veering gait with patients feeling propelled in some direction and having the illusion that their body or the environment is in motion (vertigo). In extreme cases, attempts to stand up are immediately followed by a fall. In less severe cases, patients will stand on a widened base to make up for the lateral sway but lose their balance and fall sideways in the dark or upon closing the eyes. Sometimes the head is held stiff in an obvious effort to control vestibular input. While walking, patients show widened base, instability, staggering with pronounced lateral sway, or even falls. According to observations by Brandt et al. (35), lateral deviations affecting gait in the acute peripheral vestibular syndrome paradoxically abate while the person running. One possible explanation is that running requires the activation of spinal locomotor mechanisms, inhibiting vestibular information. In less severe cases, the lateral sway will only be revealed on closing the eyes (Romberg's sign) and in tandem gait. The sway to one side can likewise be brought out by stepping in place with the knees lifted high and with the eyes closed (Unterberger's sign). A typical sign of peripheral vestibular etiology is that after turning the head 90 degrees to one and then the other side, the deviations still follow the "affected ear," that is, swaying forward or backward. This can be explained by the unilateral functional preponderance of the vestibular apparatus forcing, as it were, the body and its segments in the direction of the relatively hypofunctional apparatus. This also accounts for the direction of tonic deviations of the arms outstretched horizontally in front of the body (Hautant's sign). There is often an obvious nystagmus with the fast component beating in the direction of the relatively hyperfunctional vestibular apparatus. Special examination may detect abnormalities in visually guided eye movements, saccades, and the vestibulo-ocular reflex.

In the *central vestibular syndrome* (reflecting affections of the brainstem vestibular nuclei and their projections) there is usually no typical vertigo, and body and extremity deviations show none of the consistent unilateral tendency typical of the peripheral syndrome. There is, however, instability and unsteadiness of posture and gait tending to deteriorate in proportion to increased motor demands or in visual input restriction.

Widened Base with Cadence Alterations (Ataxic, Tottering, Wobbling Gait)

Ataxic gait is marked by widened base and irregularities in the duration of steps and in planting the feet. The causative mechanism can be found either in sensory disorders responsible for spatial uncertainty, cerebellar dysmetria as a source of disordered motor coordination, or in abnormal involuntary movements unpredictably changing leg trajectory. Ataxic gait with the base widened or normal may also be part of a complex gait disorder in lesions of the cortex or white matter of frontal lobes (see section "Frontal Gait Disorder").

Disorders of Proprioception (Posterofunicular Spinal Ataxia, Tabes Gait)

Sensory ataxia accompanies disorders of deep sensation from lower extremities (as a rule, when posterior spinal funiculi are affected). The patient complains of feeling unsteady when placing the foot down, which can be likened to walking over moss-covered ground or on cushions. This unsteadiness is more pronounced in situations marked by decreased visual control while walking in darkness (e.g., to the toilet at night, or on closing the eyes while washing one's face). A fully developed picture of posterofunicular spinal ataxia is marked by wide-based gait, strides of irregular length and duration with the feet stepping down hard on the floor, and arms held in abduction. Patients have to keep watching their feet and the floor to avoid falling down. Apart from disordered vibration sensation and sense of position, there is, as a rule, areflexia of the lower extremities. The patients stand on a wide base; standing erect with the heels and toes close together (or in tandem gait) will increase unsteadiness. Romberg's sign is markedly positive, though without lateral fall predilection, and independent of head turns.

Cerebellar Ataxia ("Drunken Gait")

Ataxia is a major symptom of the *neocerebellar syndrome* in lesions of cerebellar hemispheres and their connections (34). In cases of unilateral involvement, ataxia and other symptoms of the cerebellar syndrome will become evident solely in the ipsilateral extremities. Cerebellar ataxia gait is marked by a wide base and irregular cadence of steps of unpredictable timing and site of foot contact with the floor. Patients fail to walk straight ahead, deviations follow an irregular pattern, usually without unilateral bias. In less serious cases, difficulties become recognized only in situations placing increased demands on motor coordination (arising from a chair, turning round, walking downstairs or in tandem). On examination, signs of the cerebellar syndrome predominate: dysmetria with overshoot of extremity movements, poor coordination, dyssynergy of muscles of the extremities and trunk, and rapid alternate movements irregularity (dysdiadochokinesia) (36). Equilibrium is unimpaired; pull-test responses are hypermetric but otherwise normal (37). Although gait is markedly disordered, falls are relatively rare.

Persons with *paleocerebellar syndrome* in lesions of the anterior vermis or floculonodular lobe have different symptoms, with severe postural and gait instability as a prominent sign, as well as a pronounced tendency toward toppling falls (explained hereinafter). As a rule, extremity ataxia or dysmetria remain unexpressed (34).

Choreic Gait ("Dancing Gait")

Lower limb chorea is superimposed on walking movements, thus giving rise to a peculiar ataxic gait pattern reminiscent of ballet dancing. Cadence is entirely irregular; the feet make accidental flat contact with the ground or, if turned, touch down with any of their parts; the feet purposelessly jump off the intended directions; and the strides or jumps are of irregular length. Where these involuntary movements simultaneously affect the trunk and upper extremities, there is a general impression of disorderliness and neglect. Although patients may at times assume highly unusual and unstable positions, falls are rare.

Stride Shortening with Cadence Changes and Disordered Gait Fluidity (Stiff Gait)

Stiff gait is marked by a general constriction of the range of movement affecting not only the legs but potentially also movements of the head, neck, upper limbs, and trunk. Possible causes include musculoskeletal involvement, spasticity, dystonia, akinetic-rigid syndrome, and other disturbances related to increased muscle tone (muscular rigidity). Characteristic patterns of stiff gait may also develop in some rare diseases, such as in stiff-man syndrome, dystrophic myotonia, and the like.

Musculoskeletal Disorders

Skeletal and articular disorders may perturb gait directly by mechanical curtailment of the range of movement in the affected body segment, or indirectly as a result of motion-induced pain. As a rule, this is later compounded by muscular weakness due to inactivity. Gait disorders differ according to which joint or body segment is affected. The general signs are stride shortening and irregularity with a limp and changed motor stereotype ("hobbling"). Postural compensations are common (e.g., the trunk partially bent forward owing to hip semiflexion).

Spastic Gait

Spastic gait is seen in the setting of diseases or dysfunctions of the motor cortex or corticospinal projections. Spastic hemiparesis and paraparesis lead to characteristic patterns of gait with reduced range of hip, knee, and ankle joint movements. Neurologic examination reveals common signs of upper motor neuron affection. *Spastic hemiparesis* typically produces Wernicke-Mann attitude characterized by upper limb flexion and lower limb extension. On walking, the stiff leg circumducts, possibly in association with contralateral trunk flexion. *Spastic paraparesis* usually shows spasticity of hip adductors, as a result of which gait is stiff and associated with thigh "scissoring."

Spasticity-based foot deformities later come to be fixed owing to the development of contractures and articular changes. Detailed classification comprises the following six patterns likely to occur separately or in diverse combinations (38). *Equinovarus deformity* is the most common pathologic position of the lower limb in central nervous system affections with the foot and ankle turned downward and inward mainly as a result of gastrocnemius and soleus hyperactivity. The foot touches down on the lateral edge where a tender bruise often develops. In the swing phase, the foot may rub against the floor and fail to provide stable support in the stance phase. *Valgus foot* is bent outward as a result of peroneal muscle group hyperactivity. The foot touches the floor with the medial edge. *Hyperextended great toe* tends to be a compensatory manifestation in paretically restricted dorsal flexion of the foot. *Flexed knee* persists in all phases of the walking cycle, forcing the patient to assume a compensatory position in the support phase, and thus curtailing the stride length due to insufficient extension in the swing phase. *Stiff (extended) knee* limits movement in the swing phase and leads to foot dragging which, in turn, is compensated by circumduction (see hemiparetic gait). *Adducted thigh* interferes, in particular, with the swing phase of gait, so that thigh scissoring curtails proper limb advancement (see spastic paraparesis). The base is narrow in the support phase and balance may be impaired. *Flexed hip* interferes with the support function of the extremity resulting in permanently flexed trunk and shortened stride.

Dystonic Gait

Dystonic gait may take the form of a simple limp, inadequate stepping down from high up, or foot dragging due to dystonic inversion or eversion. Dystonic postures and motions are constantly present or they may appear solely in some activities such as exactly in walking. As a rule, they will propagate from the lower extremities to other muscle groups. A typical feature of dystonic gait disorder is its abatement in response to a variety of "tricks" or maneuvers, such as walking backward, trotting, or dancing. Even sensory tricks, such as putting one's hands in the pockets, round the neck, or behind the back, may improve gait substantially. Bizarre pictures of dystonic gait are sometimes likened to animal gait. For instance, the so-called dromedary gait has been described in cases of progressive lordotic dysbasia (i.e., gradually growing lordoscoliosis of the lumbar spine in walking, inducing bizarre position of the trunk with the hip bulging backward and sideways and compensatory turning of the shoulders and neck with the head held vertically). A major gait disorder used to be described in *athetosis*, in today's terms classified as "mobile dystonia." Characteristic features of the complex gait patterns include climbing movement of the legs, or swinging flexion of the hips, often with contortion of the neck, trunk, and upper extremities sometimes simulating wing-like movements (2).

Akinetic-Rigid Syndrome

Parkinsonian syndromes are marked by characteristic gait disorders, which include stride shortening, increased cadence, decreased arm swing, and shuffling. Posture and gait are narrow based with characteristic flexion of the trunk and both upper and lower extremities. There may be impaired postural stability with a tendency to toppling falls. Stride shortening and postural unsteadiness are often more pronounced in change of direction and in turning (39). There may coincide disorders of gait initiation and maintenance that are described subsequently.

Disorders of Gait Initiation and Maintenance (Gait Freezing, Start Hesitation, Motor Blocks)

Depending on which gait phase is affected, distinction is made between disorders of gait initiation and maintenance. Problems at the start of walking and sudden freezing while locomotion is in progress occur either as an independent phenomenon or in combination with another disorder of the same patient's gait (e.g., with akinetic-rigid gait) (40). Patients suffering from *start hesitation* experience difficulties initiating locomotion, which may take the form of delayed start or of prolonged hesitation in place (41). A closer scrutiny will show that they are unable to shift weight and to unload the lower extremity so as to start walking. At times, they manage to walk by making minor swinging movements associated with weight shifts to the sides and forward, permitting nothing but short shuffling little steps rather then full-length strides (slipping clutch phenomenon) (42). At other times, in attempts to unload one extremity, the body shows exaggerated swaying with the heel coming up while the toes remain flexed and "glued" to the floor. Another characteristic of parkinsonian gait is a tendency to start running in an effort to catch up with displaced center of gravity (festination). Patients who suffer from *freezing gait* may experience this at any time while walking, as a rule, in changing direction, turning (turn hesitation), passing through constricted places (doorways), or

while clearing unexpected obstacles in their way (43). However, a mere visual stimulus, such as a stripe on the floor, a minor obstacle, or a narrow space, can impede gait and induce freezing. In contrast, freezing may occur while the patient is walking in an open space or in stressful situations requiring prompt locomotor reaction (doorbell or phone ringing, getting on or off a means of transport, crossing the street in response to a green light, and so forth). A block can also be induced by distraction when a competing simultaneous task is introduced while the patient is walking (speaking, counting, and the like) (44). Locomotion comes to a sudden halt with the feet as if frozen to the ground (motor block). This is usually followed by start hesitation when attempting to again initiate locomotion. A characteristic feature of a parkinsonian freeze is that visual and other sensory stimuli can facilitate gait initiation and help overcome freezing. Patients often take advantage of this *kinésie paradoxale* by employing different "tricks" that permit them to resume walking (stepping on stripes on the floor, stepping over the handle of an inverted L-shaped cane, responding to streaks of light, listening to rhythmic (marching) music or a metronome or military-style commands) (45–47). Start can at times be made easier from the squatting position. Parkinsonian patients who freeze often make the observation that freezing is much less likely to occur when they climb or descend stairs. These observations suggest that the motor program for gait is well preserved in patients with Parkinson's disease but that for some reason they cannot appropriately access it (48). Similar mechanisms have been implicated in apraxia (49). In addition, attention and processing of sensory information is critical to the execution of walking (50).

FALLS AND THEIR MECHANISMS

There are many reasons why patients with abnormal gaits experience frequent falling (4). Frequent falling in old age is due to the influence of many age-related changes, such as failing sight, proprioception, and vestibular functions, and/or articular changes in lower limbs, as well as muscle weakening (22). Orthostatic hypotension or cardiac arrhythmia may also contribute falling in the elderly. The principal mechanism of falls at old age is probably related to a reduced capacity for prompt postural adaptations to changing posture and walking conditions. Obviously, falls are also prominent manifestations of diseases such as stroke, Parkinson's disease and other parkinsonian syndromes, and other neurologic disorders that affect gait and balance. The following discussion is organized according to a phenomenologic classification of falls (33).

Collapsing Falls

In collapsing falls, the victim—either standing or walking—suddenly loses muscle tone and collapses or drops. The causes can be subdivided into cerebral (epilepsy, cataplexy, transient ischemic attack, sudden intracranial pressure increase) and extracerebral (orthostatic hypotension, cardiac syncope). This type of fall is also referred to as "drop attack," though the exact meaning of the term has yet to be precisely defined. In any case, it is necessary to look for potential causes. At times, the patient's history will reveal the etiology, at other times, continuous electroencephalography, electrocardiography, and blood pressure monitoring reveals the cause.

Toppling Falls

Toppling falls are due to severe disequilibrium, in which the patient topples over and falls "like a log," as a rule, without any reflex corrective effort, so that the fall often leads to injury. If this is only due to a transient state of disequilibrium, walking may be normal except that it is perturbed by falls. Falls of this type are observed in a number of pathologic states interfering with proprioception, such as in vestibular lesions and in cerebral affections leading to disordered integration of spatial information (ischemia and hemorrhage in the mesencephalon, putamen, and thalamus; lesions of frontal lobes and subcortical white matter; progressive supranuclear paralysis; and other extrapyramidal diseases).

Tripping Falls

Tripping falls are forward falls, usually onto the outstretched arms, resulting from catching the toe on the ground which the patient failed to clear in his or her forward locomotion. These falls may be due to distal weakness (peroneal paresis) or to spasticity of the foot, which is prevented from performing sufficient dorsiflexion in the ankle. A second group of causes are gait disorders marked by shuffling (Parkinson's disease, frontal apraxia of gait, etc.). As a result of little or no clearance of the support surface, the foot becomes arrested by the slightest irregularity.

Freezing Falls

Similar to tripping falls, freezing falls are forward falls caused by the extremity freezing in the middle of walking with the foot remaining "stuck" to the ground so that the body continues its advance without any compensatory stepping forward. Festination is a variant in which the patient with the lower extremity frozen sways forward to tiptoe at increased speed to catch up with the displaced center of the body mass and, unable to do so, ultimately falls.

Unpatterned Falls

In some cases it is impossible to classify falls phenomenologically for their atypical or nonconstant character. Their causes can be sought in simple neglect with failure to adapt gait to the conditions of terrain, or with the absence of insight, which is usual in persons with dementia or in those with focal lesions of frontal or parietal lobes. Added to this, there may be age-related deterioration of sensory functions and a poor state of the locomotor apparatus. As the disease and gait disorder progress, some of the typical patterns of fall may develop in due time.

ANATOMIC–CLINICAL CLASSIFICATION OF GAIT DISORDERS

A clinical disorder of gait is a combination of basic dysfunction and related compensatory changes. In the course of time and with the disease progression, the pattern of a particular patient's gait may evolve and change. The clinical classification and diagnosis of disorders of gait is difficult also because some diseases produce a combination of different abnormal gait patterns. The following classification is based on the categories defined by three basic anatomic levels of affection: frontal (top level), cortico-subcortical (medium level), and peripheral (lowest level) (14,24,51). Despite some overlap, these broad categories permit fairly accurate differentiation (Table 28.4). In addition, there are psychogenic disorders of gait with their distinctive features.

Frontal Gait Disorder

Frontal disorder of gait is a combination of disordered locomotion and balance. The mildest forms can be seen as manifestations of the "cautious gait," which is normal in clearing poorly negotiable terrain or in old age. The rest go beyond what is a rather fuzzy dividing line into the broad spectrum of "frontal apraxia of gait."

Cautious Gait

The term "cautious gait" refers to a careful gait that resembles a gait designed to prevent a fall on a slippery or unsteady surface, such as on ice, on board ship, or on a rickety footbridge. The characteristic features of this gait are widened base as well as slow, short steps, with a tendency of the subject to reach out with hands for support. This pattern may indicate a more or less adequate adaptation in the elderly who are aware of their age-related sensory weakening and locomotor apparatus fragility. Kinesiologic records of elderly healthy persons show slowed-down speed of walking, shortened strides, reduced synkinesias of the arms, flexed knees, and reduced toe lift (25,52). However, in some cases cautious gait evolves quite abruptly (e.g., as a result of a fall with or without injury). Following such a fall, which may be quite trivial, the patient loses confidence in his or her ability to walk and maintain balance and begin to walk on a wide base with the need to hold on to the walls or other persons (*postfall syndrome*) (53). Similarly, fear of moving in an open space may develop (*space phobia, pseudoagoraphobia*) (54), but with the ability to walk about

TABLE 28.4. ANATOMIC–CLINICAL–ETIOLOGIC CLASSIFICATION OF GAIT DISORDERS

Anatomic Classification (Previous Terminology)	Clinical Features	Pathology/Pathogenesis
FRONTAL GAIT DISORDERS [frontal disequilibrium, gait apraxia, frontal apraxia, frontal (Bruns') ataxia, parkinsonian ataxia, astasia-abasia, marche à petits pas, magnetic gait, senile gait, senile paraplegia, slipping clutch gait, arteriosclerotic parkinsonism, lower body parkinsonism]	A. *Pure* 1. short stride, 2. abnormal stance (wide > narrow base, variable, crossing of legs), 3. freezing (motor blocks), 4. loss of balance (disequilibrium in response to perturbation, unable to stand or sit unsupported), 5. inappropriate postural adjustments when arising from chair (extending instead of flexing trunk and legs) or turn in bed, 6. stiff trunk/legs (military gait), 7. leg apraxia (difficulty with stepping or bicycling movements), 8. minimal or no improvement with cues. B. *Associated Findings* 1. pseudobulbar palsy, 2. cognitive impairment, 3. pyramidal signs, 4. urinary disturbance, 5. foot grasp, 6. frontal release signs.	Bilateral frontal lobe white matter lesions, anterior cerebral artery infarction, periventricular multi-infarct state, Binswanger's disease, Pick's disease, frontal mass, normal pressure hydrocephalus. Disconnection between motor, pre-motor and supplementary motor cortex and subcortical motor areas such as the basal ganglia, brainstem, and cerebellum.
Cautious Gait [elderly gait, senile gait, sensory-deprivation gait, multi-sensory gait, walking-on-ice gait, post-fall syndrome, staso-basophobia, space phobia, pseudoagoraphobia]	1. short stride, 2. mildly widened base, 3. slow, 4. turns en bloc, 5. arms abducted and flexed (anticipating loss of balance, reaching for support), 6. improves with minimal support (light touch), 7. mild postural instability, 8. guarded or restrained gait, 9. associated anxiety and/or phobias, 10. no motor blocks (freezing) or shuffling.	Normal or exaggerated response to real or perceived disequilibrium, impaired postural responses due to abnormal sensory-motor-skeletal function, the most common abnormal gait pattern in the elderly and in patients with dementia
CORTICAL–SUBCORTICAL GAIT DISORDERS [isolated gait ignition failure, primary progressive freezing gait, motor blocks, lower body parkinsonism, pure akinesia, trepidant abasia, Petren's gait]	A. *Pure* 1. freezing (motor blocks), 2. start hesitation, 3. turn hesitation, 4. blocking in narrow spaces, 5. shuffling, 6. stride normal or lengthens with walking (no festination), 7. normal stepping or bicycling movements (in sitting or supine position), 8. normal postural responses, 9. normal arm swing, 10. improvement with cues. B. *Associated Findings* 1. cognitive impairment, 2. dysarthria, 3. loss of manual dexterity, 4. loss of balance and postural responses, 5. bradykinesia, 6. rigidity, 7. loss of associated movements.	Nonspecific cortical and subcortical white matter lesions, frontal cortical hypometabolism, early stages of progressive supranuclear palsy and other parkinsonian disorders. Cortical-brainstem disconnection.
Subcortical Hypokinetic Gait Disorders [parkinsonian gait]	A. *Pure* 1. short stride, 2. slow, 3. shuffling, 4. narrow base, 5. festination, 6. freezing (motor blocks), 7. start hesitation, 8. turns en bloc, 9. abnormal postural responses (retropulsion > propulsion) and falling, 10. motor blocks improve with cues. B. *Associated Findings* I. **Parkinson's Disease** 1. rest tremor, 2. body bradykinesia, 3. hypomimia, 4. dysarthria, 5. flexed posture and knees, 6. other parkinsonian features.	Vascular (or other) lesions in the thalamus, basal ganglia, brainstem (pedunculo-pontine nucleus), Parkinson's disease, progressive supranuclear palsy, multiple system atrophy.

Category	Features	Etiology / Examples
II. Parkinsonism Plus	1. parkinsonism-plus gait (stiff, knees extended, wide base, freezing, unsteady, frequent falls, crossing of feet and pivoting on turning, toe walking). 2. ocular palsy (vertical > horizontal), 3. neck extension/flexion, 4. pseudobulbar palsy, 5. dysautonomia.	
Subcortical Hyperkinetic Gait Disorders	I. **Choreic** (random brief movements, wide-based stance, variable stride and timing, disequilibrium in later stages)	Huntington's disease, primary and secondary dystonia, tardive dyskinesia, cerebral palsy, other hyperkinetic movement disorders
	II. **Dystonic** (inversion of foot or other foot/leg deformities, bizarre gait pattern, improved by walking backwards, "dystonic paraparesis" in dopa-responsive dystonia)	
	III. **Athetotic** (slow, often associated with dystonia and spasticity)	
	IV. **Stereotypic** (bizarre, but patterned gait)	
	V. **Myoclonic** (wide-based, bouncing stance, drop attacks)	
	VI. **Tremulous** (orthostatic tremor present while standing but disappears while walking)	
	VII. Other	
Subcortical Astasia [thalamic astasia, thalamic ataxia, subcortical disequilibrium]	1. marked disequilibrium (unable to stand or even sit, falls "like a falling log"), 2. normal strength and sensation.	Thalamotomy, thalamic strokes, thalamic arteriovenous malformation, putaminal or pallidal strokes
Pyramidal Gait [hemiparetic, hemiplegic, spastic gait]	1. shoulder adducted, 2. elbow flexed, 3. forearm pronated and wrist flexed, 4. hip slightly flexed and knee extended, 5. slow circumduction of affected leg with toe dragging. 6. wide stance, 7. spasticity on the affected side.	Cerebral hemisphere (internal capsule) stroke, demyelination, tumor, or other lesions
Cerebellar Gait [ataxic gait]	1. wide-based stance, 2. marked disequilibrium particularly rapid postural adjustments, 3. dyssenergia of leg movements (irregular and variable), 4. dysmetria (erratic foot placement), 5. titubation, 6. "bouncing" gait when combined with spasticity (spastic ataxia).	Strokes, demyelination, cerebellar degenerations, other cerebellar disorders
Brainstem Gait [spastic, myoclonic]	1. marked disequilibrium, 2. bouncing stance, 3. drop attacks (negative myoclonus), 4. hypertonia, 5. other brainstem signs.	Strokes, demyelination, other brainstem disorders
Myelopathic Gait [spastic, paraplegic]	1. stiff (spastic) legs, 2. narrow-base with adduction of legs (scissors gait), 3. slow and deliberate, dragging, 4. other myelopathic signs.	Cervical spondylosis with compressive myelopathy, multiple sclerosis, spinal cord injury, infarct, etc.
PERIPHERAL DISORDERS OF GAIT		
Neuromuscular-Skeletal Gait	A. **Myopathic** 1. waddling, 2. proximal weakness, 3. lordosis, 4. toe walking.	
	B. **Neuropathic** 1. steppage, 2. distal weakness, 3. distal sensory loss.	
	C. **Orthopedic** 1. associated with arthritis or other joint or skeletal abnormalities, 2. slow and stiff gait.	
Sensory-Deprivation Gait	A. **Sensory ataxia** (wide base, slow, "slapping," cautious, improves with visual guidance)	Peripheral neuropathy, posterior column degeneration (tabes dorsalis or subacute combined degeneration)
	B. **Vestibular ataxia**	
	C. **Visual ataxia**	
PSYCHOGENIC GAIT DISORDERS [astasia-abasia, acrobatic gait]	1. bizarre gait and stance, 2. widely lurching but without falls, 3. other positive criteria for hysteria.	Normal

Reprinted with permission from Jankovic J, Nutt JG, Sudarsky LR. Classification, diagnosis, and etiology of gait disorders. In: Růžička E, Hallett M, Jankovic J, eds. Gait disorders. Philadelphia: Lippincott Williams & Wilkins, 2001:119–133.

APPENDIX: GAIT AND BALANCE SCALE (GABS)

GAIT AND BALANCE SCALE (GABS)
PAGE 1 OF 4
©COPYRIGHT 2001
Parkinson's Disease Center and Movement Disorders Clinic
Baylor College of Medicine, Houston, Texas

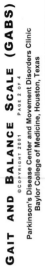

LAST NAME: ___ FIRST NAME: ___ DOB: ___

	DATE	A	B	C	D

HISTORICAL INFORMATION

1. Level of care (1)
- 0 = Entirely independent
- 1 = Requires minimal assistance in only a few activities
- 2 = Requires moderate assistance in several activities
- 3 = Requires assistance frequently with most activities
- 4 = Entirely dependent on nearly all ADL's, nursing care

2. Walking environment (2)
- 0 = Able to walk anywhere, able to negotiate any terrain
- 1 = Walks only in the immediate neighborhood, able to walk up and down gentle hills
- 2 = Walks only in the driveway; avoids uneven surface and hills
- 3 = Walks inside the house only
- 4 = Unable to walk even at home

3. Ambulation (3)
- 0 = Normal
- 1 = Mild difficulty, requires no assistance
- 2 = Independent with a cane or walker
- 3 = Severe limitation, requires assistance besides a cane or walker
- 4 = Unable to ambulate even with assistance, wheel-chair bound or bedridden

4. Falls (4)
- 0 = No falls
- 1 = Rare falls (< 1 per month)
- 2 = Falls ≥ 1 per month
- 3 = Falls ≥ 1 per week
- 4 = Falls ≥ 1 per day

5. Limitation of activity due to fear of falling (5)
- 0 = No limitation
- 1 = Able to ambulate independently, but with caution
- 2 = Usually holds on during walking, shower, or dressing
- 3 = Rarely ventures outside the house because of fear of falling
- 4 = Does not even attempt to stand or walk because of fear of falling

6. Freezing (Motor blocks) (6)
- 0 = No freezing
- 1 = Occasional start hesitation
- 2 = Freezes ≥ 1 per week
- 3 = Freezes ≥ 1 per day, occasionally falls
- 4 = Unable to ambulate due to freezing, frequent falls

7. Freezing (Motor blocks) – Modifying factors (7)
- 0 = No freezing
- 1 = Only occasionally when initiating gait, turning, walking through narrow passages, or reaching a destination
- 2 = More than 25% when initiating gait, turning, walking through narrow passages, or reaching a destination
- 3 = More than 50% when initiating gait, turning, walking through narrow passages, or reaching a destination
- 4 = Most of the time (more than 75%)

Subtotal (Items 1–7)

PHYSICAL EXAM

8. Rising from a chair (Patient attempts to arise from a straight-back wood or metal chair with arms folded across chest) (8)
- 0 = Normal
- 1 = Slow; may need more than one attempt
- 2 = Pushes self up from arms of seat
- 3 = Tends to fall back and may have to try more than once, but can get up without help
- 4 = Unable to arise without help

9. Posture (9)
- 0 = Normal
- 1 = Not quite erect, slightly stooped posture; could be normal for older person
- 2 = Moderately stooped posture, definitely abnormal; can be slightly leaning to one side
- 3 = Severely stooped posture with kyphosis; can be moderately leaning to one side
- 4 = Marked flexion with extreme abnormality of posture

10. Postural stability (Response to sudden posterior displacement produced by pull on shoulders while patient erect and prepared with eyes open and feet slightly apart) (10)
- 0 = Normal
- 1 = Retropulsion, but recovers unaided
- 2 = Absence of postural response, would fall if not caught by examiner
- 3 = Very unstable, tends to loose balance spontaneously
- 4 = Unable to stand without assistance

GAIT AND BALANCE SCALE (GABS)
PAGE 2 OF 4
©COPYRIGHT 2001
Parkinson's Disease Center and Movement Disorders Clinic
Baylor College of Medicine, Houston, Texas

LAST NAME: ___ FIRST NAME: ___ DOB: ___

	DATE	A	B	C	D

PHYSICAL EXAMINATION (CONT'D)

11. Balance during stance (Feet close together with eyes open) (11)
- 0 = No impairment
- 1 = Increased sway, but can stand with feet together
- 2 = Cannot stand with feet together, but able to stand with widened stance
- 3 = Balance is tenuous regardless of stance or foot position
- 4 = Cannot stand >10s without assistance or support

12. Romberg test (With eyes closed) (12)
- 0 = No difficulty, > 20s
- 1 = Mild difficulty, 10-20s
- 2 = Moderate difficulty, 5-10s
- 3 = Severe, < 5s
- 4 = Unable to stand without support

13. One limb stance (Best of two) (13)
- 0 = No difficulty, > 20s
- 1 = Mild difficulty, 10-20s
- 2 = Moderate difficulty, 5-10s
- 3 = Severe, < 5s
- 4 = Unable to do single stance

14. Tandem stance (One foot in front of the other) (14)
- 0 = No difficulty, > 20s
- 1 = Mild difficulty, 10-20s
- 2 = Moderate difficulty, 5-10s
- 3 = Severe, < 5s
- 4 = Unable to do single stance

15. Gait (Walking a distance of 5m) (15)
- 0 = Normal
- 1 = Walks slowly, may shuffle with short steps, decreased arm swing
- 2 = Walks with difficulty, but requires little or no assistance; may have some festination, short steps, or propulsion
- 3 = Severe disturbance of gait, requiring assistance
- 4 = Cannot walk at all, even with assistance

16. Turning 180 degrees after walking (16)
- 0 = Normal
- 1 = Takes an extra step or two to turn, but no freezing or problems with balance
- 2 = Turns en bloc, occasional freezing
- 3 = Able to turn but requires minimal assistance
- 4 = Unable to turn without full assistance

17. Turning 360 degrees (Turn completely around in a full circle, pause, and then turn a full circle in the other direction) (17)
- 0 = Able to turn 360 degrees in both directions, ≤ 4s per turn
- 1 = Able to turn 360 degrees safely only in one direction, ≤ 4s per turn
- 2 = Able to turn 360 degrees safely but slowly, > 4s per turn
- 3 = Needs close supervision or verbal cuing
- 4 = Needs assistance while turning

18. Walking on heels (18)
- 0 = Normal
- 1 = Impaired
- 2 = Unable

19. Walking on toes (19)
- 0 = Normal
- 1 = Impaired
- 2 = Unable

20. Walking in tandem (20)
- 0 = Normal
- 1 = Impaired
- 2 = Unable

21. Arm swing (Vertical wrist displacement) (21)
- 0 = Normal
- 1 = Reduced
- 2 = Absent

22. Provocative test for freezing, motor blocks (Rise from a chair and walk 5m, between two chairs spaced 24 inches apart, turn 180 degrees, walk back and sit down) (22)
- a) Start hesitation
  - 0 = No
  - 1 = Yes

GAIT AND BALANCE SCALE (GABS)

© COPYRIGHT 2001   PAGE 3 OF 4

Parkinson's Disease Center and Movement Disorders Clinic
Baylor College of Medicine, Houston, Texas

LAST NAME: FIRST NAME: DOB:

PHYSICAL EXAMINATION (CONT'D)

DATE	A	B	C	D

b) Sudden transient blocks interrupting gait — b
0 = No
1 = Yes

c) Motor blocks on turning — c
0 = No
1 = Yes

d) Motor blocks on reaching a target (chair) — d
0 = No
1 = Yes

e) Motor blocks when walking through narrow spaces (24 inches) — e
0 = No
1 = Yes

23. Functional reach *(Patient stands behind a line and is asked to reach as far forward as possible while maintaining balance. The distance of the forward reach is measured along a yardstick that is placed at the level of subject's acromion and secured to a wall. Functional reach is the distance from the starting point to the end of the reach.)* — 23
0 = Normal   (≥ 10 in)
1 = Impaired   (< 10 in)

24. Modified Tinetti Gait Evaluation *(Patient observed while walking a distance of 5m, total score 0–12)* — 24

a) Initiation of gait — a
0 = No hesitancy
1 = Any hesitancy or multiple attempts to start

b) Step length and height — b
   i) Right swing foot — i
   0 = Passes left stance foot
   1 = Does not pass left stance foot with step
   ii) Right foot — ii
   0 = Completely clears floor
   1 = Does not clear floor completely with step
   iii) Left swing foot — iii
   0 = Passes right stance foot
   1 = Does not pass right stance foot with step
   iv) Left foot — iv
   0 = Completely clears floor
   1 = Does not clear floor completely with step

c) Step symmetry — c
0 = Right and left step appear equal
1 = Right and left step length not equal (estimate)

d) Step continuity and rhythmicity — d
0 = Steps appear continuous
1 = Stopping or discontinuity between steps

e) Path *(Estimated in relation to floor tiles, 12-in. diameter; observe excursion of one foot over about 5m of the course)* — e
0 = Straight without walking aid
1 = Mild or moderate deviation or uses walking aid
2 = Marked deviation

f) Trunk — f
0 = No sway, no flexion, no use of arms, and no use of walking aid
1 = No sway but flexion of knees back or spreads arms
2 = Marked sway or uses walking aid

g) Walking distance — g
0 = Heels almost touching while walking
1 = Heels apart

25. Foam Posturography *(Stand barefooted with eyes closed on a 5 inch, medium density foam pad for 15 sec)* — 25
0 = Yes
1 = No

	A	B	C	D
Subtotal (Items 8 – 25)				
TOTAL SCORE (Items 1 – 25)				

GAIT AND BALANCE SCALE (GABS)

© COPYRIGHT 2001   PAGE 4 OF 4

Parkinson's Disease Center and Movement Disorders Clinic
Baylor College of Medicine, Houston, Texas

LAST NAME: FIRST NAME: DOB:

TIMED TASKS

DATE	A	B	C	D

26. Timed walking at usual speed (5m) — 26
   a) Time in seconds — a
   b) Number of steps — b
   c) Cadence (steps per minute) — c

27. Timed walking as fast as possible (5m, in sec) — 27

28. Stand-walk-sit time (total 10 m, in sec) — 28
(Rise from a chair and walk 5m, turn 180 degrees, walk back and sit down)

References for items in GABS: *(Note some items were modified from the original scale)*

1. Berg K, Maki B, Williams JI, et al. A comparison of clinical and laboratory measures of postural balance in an elderly population. Arch Phys Med Rehabil 1992;73:1073-1083.

    Items: 11,12,13,14,18,19,20,21,22,28.

2. Duncan PW, Studenski S, Chandler J, Prescott B. Functional reach: Predictive validity in a sample of elderly male veterans. J Gerontology Med Sci 1992;47:M93-98.

    Item: 23.

3. Fahn S, Elton RL, members of the UPDRS Development Committee. The Unified Parkinson's Disease Rating Scale. In Fahn S, Marsden CD, Calne DB, Goldstein M, eds. Recent developments in Parkinson's disease. Vol 2. Florham Park, New Jersey: Macmillan Healthcare Information. 1987:153-163, 293-304.

    Items: 4,6,8,9,10,15.

4. Tinetti ME. Performance-oriented assessment of mobility problems in elderly patients. J Am Geriatr Soc 1986;34: 119-126.

    Items: 11,12,13,14,17,24.

5. Webster, D. D. "Critical analysis of the disability in Parkinson's disease." Modern Treatment 1968;5(2): 257-82.

    Items: 22,28.

6. Weber PC, Cass SP. Clinical assessment of postural stability. Am J Otology 1993;14:566-569.

    Item: 25.

one's home remaining preserved. Some patients become totally incapable of walking due to exaggerated *fear of falling* (55), which is in no relation to the degree of their motor or sensory deficit. Patients with this "overcautious" gait thus become totally disabled, and only some of them can benefit from intensive gait training and anxiolytic medication.

Frontal Apraxia of Gait (Bruns Ataxia, Short-Stepped Gait, Magnetic Gait, Astasia-Abasia, Basophobia, Lower Body Parkinsonism, Arteriosclerotic or Vascular Parkinsonism, Lacunar Gait, Senile Gait)

It follows from the many different synonyms applied to this group of gait disorders that their classification poses some difficulties. Although the term "parkinsonism" is sometimes used in describing gait disorders from this group, the patients show few of the signs characteristic for Parkinson's disease such as tremor at rest, hypomimia, dysarthria, or upper limb bradykinesia (56). Nor does the term "senile gait" (57) seem to fit because young persons may display a similar gait pattern in the setting of frontal lobe dysfunction.

In reality, the clinical picture is, to a variable degree, characterized by a combination of features of a number of abnormal gait patterns—in particular, *disordered initiation*, *ataxia*, and *stiff gait*, with a *tendency to fall* (58). There is often abnormal body posture while standing, with the trunk held upright, sometimes in a hyperextension. The base is mostly widened, in walking almost excessively so, whether or not disequilibrium is present. As a rule, there is often disordered gait initiation with start hesitation, shortened stride, and shuffling feet stepping down with the full surface of the sole (59). The double-support phase is markedly prolonged in the walking cycle. Patients exhibit a marked tendency to retropulsion, leading to backward toppling falls (or so-called crescendo retropulsion, in which accelerating short-stepped backward locomotion ends up in a fall) (34). The upper limb synkinesis usually remain unaffected. If there is simultaneous gait freezing it may be accompanied by bizarre signs of an effort to initiate or maintain walking, with excessive arm swinging, with the trunk swaying from side to side, and the like. In marked contrast to this severe disorder of gait, leg motor function is well preserved when the patient is examined in the supine position, including the ability to perform stepping and pedaling movements. Hence, this group of disorders is sometimes referred to as "apraxia of gait" (60). Indeed, patients may exhibit apraxia while getting up or sitting down; attempts at changing position are marked by bizarre and purposeless movements. In addition, there are some other signs of frontal lobe involvement: disinhibition of behavior and primitive reflexes, cognitive disorders, and pseudobulbar palsy.

The disorder is often due to multiple ischemic lesions of the frontal lobe white matter corresponding to multi-infarct or subcortical encephalopathy (Binswanger's disease), or to circumscribed encephalomalacia in the area supplied by the anterior cerebral artery. This type of gait disorder is also present in normal pressure hydrocephalus, Alzheimer's disease, corticobasal degeneration, and in other bilateral affections of the frontal lobes (58,60,61). Treatment dispensed in accordance with the underlying cause will, as a rule, yield little success—except perhaps for shunt operations for normal-pressure hydrocephalus (62). Rehabilitation and gait training may offer at least temporary improvement and increased confidence. Support aids (walker, walking frame) remain largely without any great effect (63). Instruction for care providers, domestic environment rearrangements, or proper use of the wheelchair are important measures designed to improve quality of life and prevent fall-related injuries.

Cortico–Subcortical Disorders of Gait

Disordered Gait Initiation (Petrén's Gait, Trepidant Abasia, Gait Ignition Failure, Primary Progressive Gait Freezing, Motor Blocks, Pure Akinesia)

Disordered gait initiation and maintenance was described above as one of the basic patterns of gait disorder (see section, "Disorders of Gait Initiation and Maintenance") related to pathologic involvement of the circuits involving the basal ganglia together with the brainstem nuclei, thalamus, and frontal cortex. Apart from its crucial role in motor control, this system takes a share in triggering goal-directed activity and in the processes of attention. Damage to any component of the system may cause gait freezing and related disturbances. Hence, it is seen often in the context of Parkinson's disease, other neurodegenerative diseases (mainly in progressive supranuclear palsy), and secondary parkinsonian syndromes connected with multi-infarct encephalopathy, normal-pressure hydrocephalus, and focal lesions of frontal lobes (together with other manifestations of frontal gait disorder; see section, "Frontal Apraxia of Gait").

Disordered gait initiation is the principal sign of a nosologic entity known as *gait ignition failure* or *pure akinesia* (64,65). In addition to start hesitation, festination, and gait freezing, these patients may suffer from severe disequilibrium and falls. They may also have dysarthria and micrographia, but usually do not show rigidity, tremor, or dementia.

Treatment for disordered gait initiation and maintenance is no easy task, so that many patients find their only help in performing diverse sensory and motor "tricks" (45–47) (see section, "Disorders of Gait Initiation and Maintenance"). Dopaminergic medication may improve this symptom mainly in those cases of Parkinson's disease where start hesitation and freezing appear in the "off" state and disappear in the "on" state (66). However, freezing is often expressed also in the "on" state and fails to respond to dopaminergic therapy (66,67). Reports of favorable effects of the noradrenergic preparation L-*threo*-dihydroxyphenylserine (68) and selegiline (deprenyl) (69) have yet to be corroborated. Positive effects were also reported after botulinum toxin applied locally into the posterior tibialis and plantar muscles (70) where it might act by weakening the toe and foot flexors, which may "grasp" the floor and thus contribute to or cause freezing.

Subcortical Hypokinetic Gait (Akinetic-Rigid Gait, Parkinsonian Gait)

Patients with *Parkinson's disease* exhibit abnormal stiff gait marked by disordered physiologic posturo-locomotor synergies. Typical cases show narrow-based posture, with flexed trunk and extremities. Walking is slowed, short stepped, with poor clearance, shuffling, and *en bloc* turns. In addition, many patients with Parkinson's disease have disordered gait initiation. Walking cycle timing is considerably impaired, its variability being two to three times greater than in healthy persons (71). Dopaminergic medication tends to be quite efficacious in the early stages of the disease, even with respect to body posture and gait. In the later stages, and in the "postural instability gait disorder" (PIGD) type of involvement, where nondopaminergic systems lesions are thought to play an important role, the gait disorder shows little or no response to dopaminergic therapy. Deep brain stimulation (DBS) of the subthalamic nucleus affects solely those components of gait disorder that are responsive to dopaminergic medication (72). Unilateral thermolysis of the medial globus pallidus will, in some patients at least, also have a bearing on the nondopaminergic component of disordered posture and gait though improvement is seldom conspicuous or long lasting (73,74).

Whereas in Parkinson's disease serious postural changes due to disorders of balance and gait do not develop until after several years of duration, in *progressive supranuclear palsy (PSP)* they are usually present from the very early stages. That also accounts for frequent falls and injuries. Pronounced instability in PSP probably results from a combination of marked visuovestibular impairment, axial rigidity, and bradykinesia (75). Unlike in Parkinson's disease, there is a wider based posture as well as stiff gait with extended knees, trunk, and neck, with the arms in abduction, and often with motor blocks (freezing). Although gait may appear ataxic, no signs of cerebellar involvement are usually present. Spontaneous falls are of the "toppling" type; the pull test is markedly positive as even a slight stimulus will send the patient toppling (76). Loss of postural reflexes (mainly in connection with freezing during turns), together with patients' remarkable shortage of insight into

their own disordered stability (perhaps owing to frontal lobe dysfunction), is the source of frequent falls.

In the course of *multiple system atrophy* (MSA), the gait disorder develops as a result of parkinsonian as well as cerebellar involvement. In addition, falls may occur as a result of markedly impaired postural reflexes and orthostatic hypotension. Falls tend to occur earlier in MSA than in Parkinson's disease, but they are not quite so distinctive a feature as in PSP.

Disorders of Gait in Hyperkinetic Movement Disorders

Subcortical hyperkinetic disorders of gait comprise dystonic gait, choreic gait and posture and gait disorders underlying some other motor disorders such as orthostatic tremor and myoclonus.

Dystonic gait was described above (in section, "Stride Shortening with Cadence Changes and Disordered Gait Fluidity"). As a rule, gait disorder in generalized dystonia poses no diagnostic problems because it is accompanied by dystonic signs in other parts of the body. Less frequently seen is dystonic gait disorder temporarily or permanently isolated, such as in genetically linked cases of generalized dystonia and in dopa-responsive dystonia. Besides primary generalized dystonia and dopa-resposive dystonia, both of which frequently start with lower limb affections, disorders of gait may occur in secondary dystonias of different etiology, such as off-dystonia and levodopa-induced dystonia in Parkinson's disease, tardive dystonia, etc. Unless it is possible to eliminate the disorder by causal treatment of the underlying disease, local botulinum toxin chemodenervation of the hyperactive muscles is an option in focal and segmental types of dystonia (77).

Choreic gait typically occurs in patients with Huntington's disease. Its greatly irregular ataxic pattern is described as "stuttering" or "dancing" gait (see above, section "Gait Disorders with Widened Base"). A similar picture may develop in a number of causes of the choreic syndrome. Gait is markedly impaired, e.g., by choreic or even ballistic dyskinesias induced by levodopa in Parkinson's disease, or by neuroleptic-induced tardive dyskinesia, the stereotyped pattern of which is sometimes compared to goose-stepping.

Orthostatic tremor is a rapid (14 to 16 Hz) quivering that appears in the standing position on the lower extremities and trunk after a latency of several tens of seconds. It is associated with feelings of instability or even a tendency to falling; abating in the sitting and lying positions but mostly also while walking. Clonazepam finds good use in management of the disorder. Oddly, even patients with *essential tremor* were found to suffer from impaired stability shown in Romberg's test and in tandem gait (78).

Gait in *myoclonus* is perturbed by muscle twitching or loss of muscle tone (negative myoclonus) leading to buckling of the knees, collapses, and falls with posthypoxic myoclonus as the most typical cause (79). Gait and posture may also be perturbed by propriospinal myoclonus with axial twitches starting mostly in the abdominal muscles (80).

Subcortical Disequilibrium

Subcortical disequilibrium is essentially synonymous with the terms *thalamic astasia, abasia,* or *thalamic ataxia*. It is usually associated with pathologic involvement of the dorsolateral thalamus (nucleus ventrolateralis or nucleus posterior) including the dentatorubrothalamic projection, or basal ganglia–lentiform nuclei. Although as a rule patients are aware of their instability, they seem to ignore it and are unable to resist the lateral pull or falls ("toppling"). Some patients simultaneously develop motor neglect in the extremities contralateral to the lesion. Although they are able to control their limbs on command, they are not able to engage them spontaneously even in tasks that require bilateral coordination. As regards other signs of thalamic lesion, the situation is sometimes compounded by unilateral disorder of somatic sensation or asterixis. Subcortical disequilibrium usually improves within days or months of the onset of acute unilateral lesion, perhaps as a result of the bilaterality of the vestibulocerebellar projection to the medial ventrolateral thalamic nucleus (81). Disorder of gait and posture due to lesions of the pontomesencephalic junction with pedunculopontine nucleus involvement can be mentioned as another example of subcortical disequilibrium. Here an involvement of central vestibular projections may contribute to serious disequilibrium, associated with ataxia and gait initiation disorder (82).

Gait Disorder in Cerebellar Diseases

Cerebellar disorders of gait are associated with ataxia and/or other symptoms of the cerebellar syndrome. Their manifestations were described in the section, "Widened Base with Cadence Alterations." The cerebellar disorders most commonly responsible for posture and gait disorders include intoxication with ethyl alcohol and demyelinating and neurodegenerative diseases (spinocerebellar ataxias).

Gait Disorders in Upper Motor Neuron Affections

Depending on its localization and extent of the underlying lesion, gait disorder in cases of pyramidal (corticospinal) projection involvement may display a pattern of gait of the hemiparetic or paraparetic (spastic) type (see section, "Stride Shortening with Cadence Changes and Disordered Gait Fluidity"). Whereas cerebrovascular accident is the most common cause of hemiparesis, spastic paraparesis is often a sign of cerebral palsy, multiple sclerosis, or other spinal pathologic processes. Partial spinal compression, causing *cervical spondylotic myelopathy,* may cause spasticity combined with leg ataxia owing to a simultaneous lesion of

the lateral and posterior funiculi of spinal cord. Besides conventional rehabilitation procedures, therapy has of late been significantly enhanced with chemodenervation of muscles using botulinum toxin. This method proved to be convincingly efficacious in spastic hemiparesis (83), but in particular spastic paraparesis associated with cerebral palsy (84). Early chemodenervation in affected children forestalls the development of contractures and other lasting changes, and makes for continued gait development. Also, myorelaxation pharmacotherapy, phenol neurolysis (85), and surgical treatments, including implantation of baclofen pump and decompressive surgery, may be beneficial. Surgical correction may be necessary in fixed deformities of lower limb joints associated with permanent contractures (86).

Peripheral Disorders of Gait

Lower Motor Neuron and Musculoskeletal Affections

Muscular dystrophy, myopathy, and peripheral neuropathies affecting the lower extremities make up a relatively simple pattern of gait disorder, as described above within the scope of phenomenologic classification (waddling gait in myopathy, plexopathy, and proximal neuropathy; steppage and slapping gait in distal neuropathies and radiculopathies in the lower extremities).

Sensory Disorders (Vestibular Syndromes and Proprioceptive Affections)

Characteristic patterns of posture and gait disorders in the peripheral and central *vestibular syndromes* were described as part of the phenomenologic classification of the veering gait. Typical causes of the peripheral vestibular syndrome include otitis interna (often as a consequence of otitis media) and pathologic processes affecting 8th cranial nerve in the cerebellopontine angle. As a result, there is often unilateral hypacusia and/or tinnitus. Sudden postural and gait disorder of this type are part and parcel of Ménière's syndrome.

Ataxic gait, as described above, develops as a result of *impaired proprioception,* mostly due to lesions of the posterior funiculi of spinal cord. Typical causes include tabes dorsalis as part of quaternary syphilis, or funicular myelosis (neuroachylic syndrome) in disorders of vitamin B_{12} metabolism. Markedly disturbed sense of position, however, may also develop in neuropathies with less specific posterior funicular involvement. The combined picture of spinal ataxia, cerebellar and vestibular affections is often seen in Friedreich's disease, though this is also under the mechanical influence of a shortened and arched foot (pied-bôt).

Psychogenic Gait Disorders

Psychogenic disorders of gait (also called "hysterical" or "acrobatic" gaits) are marked by bizarre and inconsistent movements. In addition to dramatic lurching, patients often exhibit excessively slowed down movements or a tendency to knee buckling—mostly, however, without completing the fall and without self-injury. The symptoms are incongruent with any of the above-described organic gait disturbances. During medical examination, with the patient feeling in the limelight, there may be some typical adventitious manifestations such as "rope-walker's" gait (34), i.e., when the patient—asked to walk with eyes closed—paradoxically narrows the gait base or stages a fall in the direction of anticipated rescue. Asked to walk tandem, the patient sways inadequately to the sides, crossing the legs, assuming bizarre and poorly sustainable positions with balancing on one leg. Standing in Romberg's test, they assume an inadequate hyperextension of the body ("psychogenic Romberg's sign"). Frequently, there is a martyr face expression, often accompanied by panting and moaning. Normal gait may appear temporarily with distraction. Since one sign of a psychogenic gait is minute-to-minute and hour-to-hour fluctuation, it must be differentiated from organic intermittent or paroxysmal gait disorders such as seen occasionally in patients with periodic paralysis, episodic ataxia, or paroxysmal dystonia. The diagnosis of a psychogenic gait disorder should always be a positive one, not just established "per exclusionem." As a rule, the diagnosis is usually supported by the presence of other features indicative of psychogenic origin, such as abrupt onset or sudden resolution, false weakness, false sensory symptoms, multiform somatization, bizarre movements or pseudoseizures, inadequate indifference to the affection, abatement in the wake of psychotherapy, evident suggestibility, effects of placebo or physical therapy, and signs of psychological conflict or a positive psychiatric history and possible secondary benefit.

The presence of seemingly incongruous features does not necessarily prove that the gait is of psychogenic origin because apparent inconsistencies may be also encountered in some organic gait disorders. For instance, some patients with generalized dystonia, who are incapable of forward locomotion in any other than a grossly grotesque posture, can walk backwards without any major difficulties. This feature of dystonia, actually a type of sensory trick, sometimes leads to misdiagnosis of a psychogenic disorder. Another example may be cautious gait seen in patients with pseudoagoraphobia, in which individuals are able to walk only if they touch the wall, furniture, or other objects or people, not necessarily for physical support, but more for psychological support. Such conscious or subconscious support helps them regain confidence in their ability to walk. We do not necessarily regard this gait as "psychogenic" since even a light touch can serve as an important proprioceptive stimulus or a form of sensory trick.

REFERENCES

1. Dickson MH, Farley CT, Full RJ, et al. How animals move: an integrative view. *Science* 2000;288:100–106.
2. Švehla F. *Introduction to the neurology of gait* (in Czech). Prague: Zdravotnické nakladatelství (Health care publishers), 1950.
3. Sudarsky L. Clinical approach to gait disorders of aging: an overview. In: Masdeu JC, Sudarsky L, Wolfson L, eds. *Gait disorders of aging: falls and therapeutic strategies*. Philadelphia: Lippincott–Raven Publishers, 1997:147–158.
4. Tinetti ME, Speechley M, Ginter SF. Risk factors for falls among elderly persons living in the community. *N Engl J Med* 1988;319:1701–1707.
5. Burke RE. The central pattern generator for locomotion in mammals. In: Růžička E, Hallett M, Jankovic J, eds. *Gait disorders*. Philadelphia: Lippincott Williams & Wilkins, 2001:11–24.
6. Mori S, Matsuyama K, Mori F, et al. Supraspinal sites that induce locomotion in the vertebrate central nervous system. In: Růžička E, Hallett M, Jankovic J, eds. *Gait disorders*. Philadelphia: Lippincott Williams & Wilkins, 2001:25–40.
7. Berger W. Normal and impaired development of gait. In: Růžička E, Hallett M, Jankovic J, eds. *Gait disorders*. Philadelphia: Lippincott Williams & Wilkins, 2001:65–70.
8. Armstrong DM. The supraspinal control of mammalian locomotion. *J Physiol (Lond)* 1988;405:1–37.
9. Eidelberg E, Walden JG, Nguyen LH. Locomotor control in macaque monkeys. *Brain* 1981;104:647–663.
10. Pahapill PA, Lozano AM. The pedunculopontine nucleus and Parkinson's disease. *Brain* 2000;123:1767–1783.
11. Dietz V, Colombo G, Jensen L. Locomotor activity in spinal man. *Lancet* 1994;344:1260–1263.
12. Hanakawa T, Katsumi Y, Fukuyama H, et al. Mechanisms underlying gait disturbance in Parkinson's disease: a single photon emission computed tomography study. *Brain* 1999;122:1271–1282.
13. Schieppati M, Tacchini E, Nardone A, et al. Subjective perception of body sway. *J Neurol Neurosurg Psychiatry* 1999;66:313–322.
14. Nutt JG, Marsden CD, Thompson PD. Human walking and higher-level gait disorders, particularly in the elderly. *Neurology* 1993;43:268–279.
15. Forssberg H, Wallberg H. Infant locomotion: a preliminary movement and electromyographic study. In: Berg K, Eriksson BD, eds. *Children and exercise*. Baltimore: University Park Press, 1980:32–49.
16. Berger W, Altenmüller E, Dietz V. Normal and impaired development of children's gait. *Hum Neurobiol* 1984;34:163–170.
17. Berger W, Quintern J, Dietz V. Stance and gait perturbations in children: developmental aspects of compensatory mechanisms. *Electroenceph Vlin Neurophysiol* 1985;61:385–395.
18. Forssberg H, Dietz V. Neurobiology of normal and impaired locomotor development. In: Conolly KJ, Forssberg H, eds. *Neurophysiology and neuropsychology of motor development*. London: MacKeth Press, 1997:78–100.
19. Davis JW, Nevitt MC, Wasnich RD, et al. A cross-cultural comparison of neuromuscular performance, functional status, and falls between Japanese and white women. *J Gerontol A Biol Sci Med Sci* 1999;54:M288–M292.
20. Ebersbach G, Sojer M, Muller J, et al. Sociocultural differences in gait. *Mov Disord* 2000;15(6):1145–1147.
21. Sudarsky L. Geriatrics: gait disorders in the elderly. *N Engl J Med* 1990;322:1441–1446.
22. Tinetti ME, Baker DI, McAvay G, et al. A multifactorial intervention to reduce the risk of falling among elderly people living in the community. *N Engl J Med* 1994;331:821–827.
23. Tinetti ME. Performance-oriented assessment of mobility problems in elderly patients. *J Am Geriatr Soc* 1986;34:119–126.
24. Jankovic J, Nutt JG, Sudarsky LR. Classification, diagnosis, and etiology of gait disorders. In: Růžička E, Hallett M, Jankovic J, eds. *Gait disorders*. Philadelphia: Lippincott Williams & Wilkins, 2001:119–133.
25. Elble R. Changes in gait with normal aging. In: Masdeu JC, Sudarsky L, Wolfson L, eds. *Gait disorders of aging: falls and ther-*

apeutic strategies. Philadelphia: Lippincott–Raven Publishers, 1997:93–105.

26. Ebersbach J, Poewe W. Simple assessments of mobility: methodology and clinical application of kinetic gait analysis. In: Růžička E, Hallett M, Jankovic J, eds. *Gait disorders.* Philadelphia: Lippincott Williams & Wilkins, 2001:101–110.

27. Kempster PA, Frankel JP, Bovingdon M, et al. Levodopa peripheral pharmacokinetics and duration of motor response in Parkinson's disease. *J Neurol Neurosurg Psychiatry* 1989;51:745–752.

28. Kaufman KR, Shaughnessy WJ, Noseworthy JH. Use of motion analysis for quantifying movement disorders. In: Růžička E, Hallett M, Jankovic J, eds. *Gait disorders.* Philadelphia: Lippincott Williams & Wilkins, 2001:71–81.

29. Horak FB. Clinical measurement of postural control in adults. *Phys Ther* 1987;12:1881–1885.

30. Weber PC, Cass SP. Clinical assessment of postural stability. *Am J Otology* 1993;14:566–569.

31. VanSwearingen JM, Paschal KA, Bonino P, et al. The modified gait abnormality rating scale for recognizing the risk of recurrent falls in community-dwelling elderly adults. *Phys Ther* 1996;76:994–1002.

32. Fahn S, Elton RL, members of the UPDRS Development Committee. The Unified Parkinson's Disease Rating Scale. In: Fahn S, Marsden CD, Calne DB, et al., eds. *Recent developments in Parkinson's disease,* vol 2. Florham Park, NJ: Macmillan Healthcare Information, 1987:153–163, 293–304.

33. Nutt JG. Classification of gait and balance disorders. In: Růžička E, Hallett M, Jankovic J, eds. *Gait disorders.* Philadelphia: Lippincott Williams & Wilkins, 2001:135–141.

34. Henner K. *Special neurology* (in Czech). Prague: Státní zdravotnické nakladatelství (State health-care publishers), 1961.

35. Brandt T, Strupp M, Benson J. You are better off running than walking with acute vestibulopathy. *Lancet* 1999;354:746.

36. Hallett M. Cerebellar ataxic gait. In: Růžička E, Hallett M, Jankovic J, eds. *Gait disorders.* Philadelphia: Lippincott Williams & Wilkins, 2001:155–163.

37. Horak FB, Diener HC. Cerebellar control of postural scaling and central set in stance. *J Neurophysiol* 1994;72:479–493.

38. Mayer NH, Esquenazi A, Childers MK. Common patterns of clinical motor dysfunction. *Muscle Nerve* 1997;6:S21–S35.

39. Morris ME, Iansek R, Matyas TA, et al. Stride length regulation in Parkinson's disease: normalization strategies and underlying mechanisms. *Brain* 1996;119:551–568.

40. Giladi N. Freezing of gait: clinical Overview. In: Růžička E, Hallett M, Jankovic J, eds. *Gait disorders.* Philadelphia: Lippincott Williams & Wilkins, 2001:191–197.

41. Ambani LM, Van Woert MH. Start hesitation—a side effect of long-term levodopa therapy. *N Engl J Med* 1973;288:1113–1115.

42. Denny Brown D. The nature of apraxia. *J Nerv Ment Dis* 1958;126:9–31.

43. Achiron A, Ziv I, Goren M, et al. Primary progressive freezing gait. *Mov Disord* 1993;8:293–297.

44. Giladi N, McMahon D, Przedborski S, et al. Motor blocks in Parkinson's disease. *Neurology* 1992;42:333–339.

45. Stern GM, Lander CM, Lees AJ. Akinetic freezing and trick movements in Parkinson's disease. *J Neural Transm* 1980;[Suppl 16]:137–141.

46. Dietz MA, Goetz CG, Stebbins GT. Evaluation of a modified inverted walking stick as treatment for parkinsonian freezing episodes. *Mov Disord* 1990;5:243–247.

47. Marchese R, Diverio M, Zucchi F, et al. The role of sensory cues in the rehabilitation of parkinsonian patients: a comparison of two physical therapy protocols. *Mov Disord* 2001;15:879–883.

48. Yanagisawa N, Ueno E, Takami M. Frozen gait of Parkinson's disease and vascular parkinsonism—a study with floor reaction forces and EMG. In: Shimamura M, Grillner S, Edgerton VR, eds. *Neurobiological basis of human locomotion.* Tokyo: Scientific Societies Press, 1991:291–304.

49. Geschwind N. The apraxias: neural mechanisms of disorders of learned movement. *Am Scientist* 1975;63:188–195.

50. Ebersbach G, Dimitrijevic MR, Poewe W. Influence of concurrent tasks on gait: a dual task approach. *Percept Motor Skills* 1995;81:107–113.

51. Marsden CD, Thompson P. Towards a nosology of gait disorders: descriptive classification. In: Masdeu JC, Sudarsky L, Wolfson L, eds. *Gait disorders of aging: falls and therapeutic strategies.* Philadelphia: Lippincott–Raven Publishers, 1997:135–146.

52. Elble RJ, Sienko-Thomas S, Higgins C, et al. Stride-dependent changes in gait of older people. *J Neurol* 1991;238:1–5.

53. Murphy J, Isaacs B. The post-fall syndrome: a study of 36 elderly patients. *Gerontology* 1982;82:265–270.

54. Marks I. Space "phobia," a pseudo-agoraphobic syndrome. *J Neurol Neurosurg Psychiatry* 1981;44:387–391.

55. Overstall RW, Exton-Smith AN, Imms FJ, et al. Falls in the elderly related to postural imbalance. *Br Med J* 1977;1:261–264.

56. Winikates J, Jankovic J. Clinical correlates of vascular parkinsonism. *Arch Neurol* 1999;56:98–102.

57. Koller WC, Glatt SL, Fox JH. Senile gait: a distinct neurologic entity. *Clin Geriatr Med* 1985;1:661–669.

58. Thompson PD. Gait disorders accompanying diseases of the frontal lobes. In: Růžička E, Hallett M, Jankovic J, eds. *Gait disorders.* Philadelphia: Lippincott Williams & Wilkins, 2001:235–241.

59. Elble RJ, Cousins R, Leffler K, et al. Gait initiation by patients with lower-half parkinsonism. *Brain* 1996;119:1705–1716.

60. Estanol BV. Gait apraxia in communicating hydrocephalus. *J Neurol Neurosurg Psychiatry* 1981;44:305–308.

61. Fitzgerald PM, Jankovic J. Lower body parkinsonism: evidence for vascular etiology. *Mov Disord* 1989;4:249–260.

62. Krauss JK, Faist M, Schubert M, et al. Evaluation of gait in normal pressure hydrocephalus before and after shunting. In: Růžička E, Hallett M, Jankovic J, eds. *Gait disorders.* Philadelphia: Lippincott Williams & Wilkins, 2001:301–310.

63. Iansek R, Ismail NH, Bruce M, et al. Frontal gait apraxia: pathophysiological mechanisms and rehabilitation. In: Růžička E, Hallett M, Jankovic J, eds. *Gait disorders.* Philadelphia: Lippincott Williams & Wilkins, 2001:363–374.

64. Atchison PR, Thompson PD, Frackowiak SJ, et al. The syndrome of gait ignition failure: a report of six cases. *Mov Disord* 1993;8:285–292.

65. Riley DE, Fogt N, Leigh RJ. The syndrome of "pure akinesia" and its relationship to progressive supranuclear palsy. *Neurology* 1994;44:1025–1029.

66. Rascol O, Fabre A, Brefel-Courbon C, et al. The pharmacologic treatment of gait ignition failure. In: Růžička E, Hallett M, Jankovic J, eds. *Gait disorders.* Philadelphia: Lippincott Williams & Wilkins, 2001:255–264.

67. Kompoliti K, Goetz CG, Leurgans S, et al. "On" freezing in Parkinson's disease: resistance to visual cue walking devices. *Mov Disord* 2000;15:309–312.

68. Yamamoto M, Fuji S, Hatanaka Y. Result of long-term administration of L-threo-3,4-dihydroxyphenylserine in patients with pure akinesia as an early symptom of progressive supranuclear palsy. *Clin Neuropharmacol* 1997;20:371–373.

69. Giladi N, McDermott MP, Fahn S, et al. Freezing of gait in PD: prospective assessment of the DATATOP cohort. *Neurology* 2001;56:1712–1721.

70. Giladi A, Honigman S. Botulinum toxin injections to one leg alleviate freezing of gait in a patient with Parkinson's disease. *Mov Disord* 1997;12:1085.

71. Hausdorff JM, Cudkowicz ME, Firtion R, et al. Gait variability

and basal ganglia disorders: stride-to-stride variations of gait cycle timing in Parkinson's disease and Huntington's disease. *Mov Disord* 1998;13:428–437.

72. Limousin P, Krack P, Pollak P, et al. Electrical stimulation of the subthalamic nucleus in advanced Parkinson's disease. *N Engl J Med* 1998;339:1105–1111.

73. Roberts-Warrior D, Overby A, Jankovic J, et al. Postural control in Parkinson's disease after unilateral posteroventral pallidotomy. *Brain* 2000;123:2141–2149.

74. Jankovic J, Lai EC, Ondo WG, et al. Effects of pallidotomy on gait and balance. In: Růžička E, Hallett M, Jankovic J, eds. *Gait disorders.* Philadelphia: Lippincott Williams & Wilkins, 2001: 271–281.

75. Jankovic J, Friedman DI, Pirozzolo FJ, et al. Progressive supranuclear palsy: motor, neurobehavioral, and neuro-ophthalmic findings. *Adv Neurol* 1990;53:293–304.

76. Horak FB, Nutt JG, Nashner LM. Postural inflexibility in parkinsonian subjects. *J Neurol Sci* 1992;111:46–52.

77. O'Brien CF. Injection techniques for botulinum toxin using electromyography and electrical stimulation. *Muscle Nerve* 1997;6: S176–S180.

78. Singer C, Sanchez-Ramos J, Weiner WJ. Gait abnormality in essential tremor. *Mov Disord* 1994;9:193–196.

79. Werhahn KJ, Brown P, Thompson PD, et al. The clinical features and prognosis of chronic posthypoxic myoclonus. *Mov Disord* 1997;12:216–220.

80. Brown P, Rothwell JC, Thompson PD, et al. Propriospinal myoclonus: evidence for spinal "pattern" generators in humans. *Mov Disord* 1994;9:571–576.

81. Masdeu JC, Gorelick PB. Thalamic astasia: inability to stand after unilateral thalamic lesions. *Ann Neurol* 1988;23:596–603.

82. Masdeu JC, Alampur U, Cavaliere R, et al. Astasia and gait failure with damage of the pontomesencephalic locomotor region. *Ann Neurol* 1994;35:619–621.

83. Brin MF and the Spasticity Study Group. Dosing, administration, and a treatment algorithm for the use of botulinum toxin A for adult-onset spasticity. *Muscle Nerve* 1997;6:S208–S220.

84. Cosgrove AP, Corry IS, Graham HK. Botulinum toxin in the management of the lower limb in cerebral palsy. *Dev Med Child Neurol* 1994;36:386–396.

85. Gracies JM, Elovic E, McGuire J, et al. Traditional pharmacological treatment for spasticity. I. Local treatments. *Muscle Nerve* 1997;6:S61–S91.

86. Keanan MA, Esquenazi A, Mayer NH. Surgical treatment of common patterns of lower limb deformities resulting from upper motoneuron syndrome. In: Růžička E, Hallett M, Jankovic J, eds. *Gait disorders.* Philadelphia: Lippincott Williams & Wilkins, 2001:333–346.

PAROXYSMAL DYSKINESIAS

KAPIL D. SETHI

Paroxysmal dyskinesias are a heterogeneous group of disorders that have in common sudden abnormal involuntary movements out of a background of normal motor behavior. The abnormal movements may be choreic, ballistic, dystonic, or a combination of these (1). Frequently the attacks are unwitnessed by the physician, who must rely on the description given by the untrained onlooker. Misdiagnoses are common in this setting, and it is fairly common for the condition to be labeled "psychogenic." Because of the absence of videotape documentation in most of these patients, it is not useful to use precise terms such as parox-ysmal chorea or paroxysmal dystonia, and the term parox-ysmal *dyskinesia* is preferred.

HISTORY
Paroxysmal Kinesigenic Dyskinesia

Under the category of movement-induced seizures, Gowers described two patients. Both had atypical features, so it is unclear whether these were paroxysmal dyskinesias. Spiller described paroxysmal movements but called them striatal or subcortical epilepsy. Pitha (1938) described a case of involuntary movements induced by active and passive movements. However, it was Kertesz (1967) who first coined the term paroxysmal kinesigenic choreoathetosis (2).

Paroxysmal Nonkinesigenic Dyskinesia

Paroxysmal dyskinesia not precipitated by movement was first described by Sterling in 1924. A year later, short-lasting nonkinesigenic attacks were described by Wimmer as striatal epilepsy. Mount and Reback (1940) described a family with long-lasting attacks of dystonia and choreoathetosis (3). There were 28 affected members with an autosomal dominant mode of inheritance. These attacks were precipitated not by movement but by ingestion of alcohol or coffee. Lance reported idiopathic and secondary "tonic seizures." He subsequently recognized these to be paroxysmal dystonic choreoathetosis (4).

Paroxysmal Exertion-induced Dyskinesia

Under the category of intermediate form of attacks, Lance (1977) reported a family with attacks precipitated by prolonged exercise (4). Since then, several other families have been reported. Recently, sporadic forms of exertional dyskinesias have been reported (1).

Paroxysmal Hypnogenic Dyskinesia

The first report of attacks during sleep was that of a 31-year-old man with attacks of leg cramping with diplopia by Joynt

TABLE 29.1. PAROXYSMAL DYSKINESIAS: CLASSIFICATION

Kinesigenic
  Short (less than 5 min)
    Idiopathic, familial, sporadic
    Secondary
  Long (more than 5 min)
    Idiopathic, familial, sporadic
    Secondary
Nonkinesigenic
  Short
    Idiopathic, familial, sporadic
    Secondary
  Long
    Idiopathic, familial, sporadic
    Secondary
Exertion-induced
  Short
    Idiopathic, familial, sporadic
    Secondary
  Long
    Idiopathic, familial, sporadic
    Secondary
Hypnogenic
  Short
    Idiopathic, familial, sporadic
    Secondary
  Long
    Idiopathic, familial, sporadic
    Secondary

Reprinted with permission from Demirkiran M, Jankovic J. Paroxysmal dyskinesias: clinical features and classification. *Ann Neurol* 1995;38:571–579.

and Green (5). These were described as tonic seizures and were attributed to multiple sclerosis. Nine members of a family were described under the label *familial paroxysmal choreoathetosis* by Horner and Jackson in 1969. However, seven of these had only nocturnal attacks. The term *nocturnal* or *hypnogenic dystonia* was introduced by Lugaresi and Cirignotta (6). They divided the attacks into short-lasting and long-lasting attacks. The evidence indicates that the short-lasting hypnogenic attacks arise from frontal lobe seizures in most cases. For a more detailed review of the history of the paroxysmal dyskinesias, see the review by Fahn (5).

CLINICAL MANIFESTATIONS

The attacks of paroxysmal dyskinesia are often unwitnessed because of their brevity. The earlier classifications were inaccurate because they used terms like paroxysmal choreoathetosis or paroxysmal dystonic choreoathetosis, implying that in all attacks movements were easily characterized. However, there is an extreme variability in the type of dyskinesia observed. This has led to a new classification, proposed by Demirkiran and Jankovic, which will be used in this chapter (7) (Table 29.1).

Paroxysmal Kinesigenic Dyskinesia

Paroxysmal kinesigenic dyskinesia (PKD) is often inherited in an autosomal dominant fashion but some cases its incidence is sporadic. In a review of 111 idiopathic cases, 49 were familial. In the same review, 89 were male, giving a male/female ratio of 4:1, which is similar to an earlier review by Goodenough (8). The age of onset is 5 to 15 years in familial cases but varies in sporadic cases. The attacks are typically precipitated by startle or a sudden movement after a period of rest. There is a refractory period after an attack during which sudden movement may not provoke an attack. The attacks occur very frequently, up to 100 per day. The duration is short, usually a few seconds to a few minutes, although longer lasting attacks may occur rarely (7). Patients may only have an abnormal sensation in the limbs involved, or the sensation may precede motor manifestation. Most patients have dystonia, but some have a combination of chorea and dystonia and, rarely, ballism. The attacks may be limited to one side of the body or even one limb. In one review of 73 cases of PKD, 25 occurred on one side only, 12 occurred unilaterally on either side, 11 occurred unilaterally or bilaterally, and 22 were always bilateral (9). Frequency of the attacks decreases during adulthood (2). Irrespective of the duration, these patients respond well to anticonvulsants (see section, "Treatment").

Paroxysmal Nonkinesigenic Dyskinesia

Paroxysmal nonkinesigenic dyskinesia (PND) is usually inherited as an autosomal dominant trait. The attacks occur more often in male patients but not so consistently as seen in PKD. The age of onset can be in early childhood, but attacks may not start until the early twenties. The frequency varies from three per day to two per year. The usual precipitating factors are fatigue, alcohol, caffeine, and emotional excitement. The attack may start with involuntary movements of one limb but may spread to involve all extremities and the face. The usual duration is minutes to 3–4 hours. Traditionally, a major distinction between PND and PKD has been the longer duration in PND.

However, PND attacks may last only for seconds (7). During the attack the patient may be unable to communi-

TABLE 29.2. CLINICAL FEATURES OF PAROXYSMAL KINESIGENIC DYSKINESIA, PAROXYSMAL NONKINESIGENIC DYSKINESIA, PAROXYSMAL EXERTIONAL DYSKINESIA, AND PAROXYSMAL HYPNOGENIC DYSKINESIA

Feature	PKD	PND	PED	PHD
Inheritance	Autosomal dominant or sporadic	Autosomal dominant or sporadic	Autosomal dominant	Autosomal dominant or sporadic
Male/female	4:1	1.5:1	1:2	
Age at onset	<1–40 yr	<1–30 yr	2–20 yr	10–40 yr
Attacks				
Duration	<5 min	2 min–4 hr	5–30 min	Short, 20–50 sec long, 5–30 min
Frequency	100/d–1/mo	3/d–2/yr	1/d–2/mo	5/night to 2–3/yr
Trigger	Sudden movement, startle, hyperventilation	Nil	Prolonged exercise, vibration, passive movement, cold	Non-REM sleep
Precipitant	Stress	Alcohol, stress, caffeine, fatigue	Stress	Stress, menses
Treatment	Anticonvulsants, acetazolamide	Clonazepam, oxazepam	L-dopa	Anticonvulsants, acetazolamide

PKD, paroxysmal kinesigenic dyskinesia; PND, paroxysmal nonkinesigenic dyskinesia; PED, paroxysmal exertional dyskinesia; PHD, paroxysmal hypnogenic dyskinesia.

cate but continues to breathe normally, and consciousness is preserved. Some families have predominant dystonia, whereas others have predominant choreoathetosis (3). As already stated, most attacks are unwitnessed by a movement disorder specialist. The attacks are relieved by sleep and in some cases respond to pharmacologic intervention. PND has been reported in a patient with familial ataxia, and in one family PND was accompanied by myokymia (1). Some families also have exertional cramping, which may be a forme fruste of PND or may be paroxysmal exertional dyskinesia (discussed next).

Paroxysmal Exertional Dyskinesia

Paroxysmal exertional dyskinesia (PED) is usually inherited in an autosomal dominant fashion. Sporadic cases have been rarely described (1). The attacks are triggered by prolonged exercise (4). The frequency varies from one per day to two per month. The usual duration is 5 to 30 minutes. The clinical features may be indistinguishable from PND of the long-lasting type, but legs are usually more affected. However, exercise limited to an upper extremity may provoke an attack in the upper extremity only. The disorder may occur sporadically, and one reported patient had paroxysmal hemidystonia precipitated by prolonged running and cold (1).

Paroxysmal Hypnogenic Dyskinesia

Paroxysmal hypnogenic dyskinesia (PHD) is characterized by attacks of dystonia, chorea, or ballism during non-REM sleep (6). The frequency may be five times per year to five times per night. These attacks may be associated with electroencephalographic (EEG) signs of arousal, and the patient usually falls asleep after the attack. The usual duration of the attacks is 30 to 45 seconds but may be longer. Sometimes the patient has daytime attacks of dyskinesia. PHD is probably a heterogeneous condition comprising attacks of varying duration and clinical features. The longer lasting attacks may arise from a movement disorder, and short-lasting attacks in most cases are caused by a medial frontal lobe seizure (10). Some patients have PHD attacks preceding tonic-clonic seizures. The clinical features are summarized in Table 29.2.

Miscellaneous Conditions

Benign Paroxysmal Torticollis of Infancy

Benign paroxysmal torticollis of infancy, a familial condition, usually occurs in the first few months of life. The attacks occur once every 2 to 3 weeks and last for hours to days. The head and sometimes trunk tilts to one or the other side. The attacks cease at age 1 to 5 years. This condition is to be distinguished from head tilt in children with large hiatal hernias following a meal (Sandifer's syndrome).

CAUSATION

Most cases of PKD, PND, and PED are idiopathic. These conditions may be sporadic but are usually inherited in an autosomal dominant fashion. Rarely they are autosomal recessive in inheritance.

Secondary Paroxysmal Kinesigenic Dyskinesia

Demyelinating Disease

The most common cause of secondary PKD is demyelinating disease (11). Paroxysmal hemidystonia (tonic seizures) may be the presenting manifestation of multiple sclerosis or may occur in established disease (12). These attacks may be kinesigenic but are most consistently precipitated by hyperventilation and can be extremely painful. These typically involve one side of the body with or without the face but may occur bilaterally. Each attack lasts a few seconds to a few minutes, and multiple attacks may occur during the day. The attacks tend to subside spontaneously over many weeks in spite of continuing disease activity.

Cerebral Palsy

PKD has been described as a delayed manifestation after perinatal hypoxic encephalopathy (13). The age of onset was 12 years, and the attacks were precipitated by the patient's being bumped from behind rather than by a sudden movement. The attacks were short lasting (5 to 30 seconds) and occurred 5 to 20 times per day.

Metabolic Disorders

PKD has been reported with idiopathic hypoparathyroidism (1). A patient with features of both PKD and PND has been reported in association with familial idiopathic hypoparathyroidism (14). Basal ganglionic calcifications may be seen in these cases. Nonketotic hyperglycemia may cause PKD (15).

Head Injury

PKD may occur after head trauma, and there may be a lag period of several months between the head injury and onset of involuntary movements (16).

Cerebrovascular Disease

With advanced neuroimaging more cases of PKD are being attributed to cerebral infarcts, including putaminal and thalamic infarcts (17). Stimulus-sensitive and action-induced paroxysmal dyskinesia has been described in a patient with posterior thalamic infarct. A case of focal PKD involving the muscles supplied by the lower cranial nerves has been described (18). Magnetic resonance imaging (MRI) showed an area of old hemorrhage in the medulla.

Miscellaneous Conditions

PKD has been reported to occur in progressive supranuclear palsy and, in one case, after methylphenidate therapy. PKD has rarely been associated with a cervical spinal cord lesion. Peripheral trauma has been reported to cause PKD. For a detailed review of secondary paroxysmal dyskinesia, see ref. 19.

Secondary Paroxysmal Nonkinesigenic Dyskinesia

As in PKD, the most common cause of secondary PND is multiple sclerosis. Most disorders causing PKD have also been associated with PND, and in some reports it is not clear whether the patient had PKD or PND, and many individuals have a mixed type of dyskinesia (19). PND has been reported in hypoglycemia and in thyrotoxicosis (19). Both PKD and PND have been reported in association with familial idiopathic hypoparathyroidism (14). PND was reported to occur in inherited biopterin synthesis defect, but this was accompanied by other clinical problems (20).

Trauma both central and rarely peripheral may result in PND; the attacks have been reported to occur as early as 20 minutes after injury, and these attacks may be very brief (21). Transient ischemic attacks sometimes manifest as PND, and these attacks may herald a major stroke (22). Short-lasting (1 to 2 minutes) attacks of PND due to a solitary cervical cord lesion that was presumed to be demyelinating have been reported. Paroxysmal dyskinesias may present as a primary HIV-1-induced neurologic syndrome. Both PKD and PND have been reported in patients with HIV infection (23). A patient with PND and nonketotic hyperglycemia has been reported. Other reported causes include kernicterus, Chiari malformation, and cytomegalovirus encephalitis (19).

Secondary Paroxysmal Exertional Dyskinesia

Most reported cases are inherited in an autosomal dominant fashion, but there is one report of a posttraumatic PED (7).

Secondary Paroxysmal Hypnogenic Dyskinesia

Only three cases of secondary PHD have been described, two with multiple sclerosis (12,24) and one after trauma. Some patients with short-lasting PHD have frontal lobe seizures that may be attributable to a structural lesion.

PATHOPHYSIOLOGY

Paroxysmal dyskinesias are attributed to dysfunctional basal ganglia, but conclusive evidence is lacking. PKD has been thought to reflect striatal seizure discharge because of response to anticonvulsants, but electroencephalograms are usually normal in between the spells, and artifacts are present during the spells. However, some patients have abnormal baseline electroencephalograms consistent with seizures (25). Invasive monitoring of a girl with PKD was recently reported (26). This patient, who had attacks precipitated by movement, loud noise, and stress, had ictal discharges in the supplemental sensorimotor cortex and the caudate nucleus on the same side on depth recording. This suggests that in some patients with PKD an electrical discharge from the medial frontal lobe spreads to the caudate nucleus (25). Ictal single photon emission computed tomography (SPECT) using ^{99m}Tc-hexamethylpropyleneamineoxime revealed decrease of cerebral blood flow in the basal ganglia on the contralateral side of choreothetotic movements (27). The authors of that report hypothesized that the dysfunction of indirect pathway (negative feedback) may be the underlying mechanism of PKC.

The origin of PND is thought to be in the basal ganglia but there is a paucity of supporting evidence. In a patient with severe PND, an invasive video electrographic study demonstrated that the PND did not originate from the cortex, whereas a discharge was registered from the caudate nuclei (28). An ^{18}F-fluorodeoxyglucose positron emission tomography (PET) scan failed to show metabolic anomalies. An ^{18}F-DOPA and an ^{11}C-raclopride PET scans revealed a marked reduction in the density of presynaptic dopa decarboxylase activity in the striatum, together with an increased density of postsynaptic dopamine D2 receptors (27). These findings may suggest chronic up-regulation of postsynaptic dopa receptors, either because of an increase in the number or an increase in affinity. In another patient with PND, ^{11}C-dihydrotetrabenazine (DTBZ) PET scan showed no alteration, suggesting a normal dopamine terminal density in the striatum (29). Evidence implicating the basal ganglia in PND also comes from a patient with posttraumatic paroxysmal dystonia in whom PET revealed abnormalities in the basal ganglia metabolism (21).

In an animal model of paroxysmal dystonia there are predominant EEG changes in caudate, putamen, and globus pallidus, with a significant decrease in the high-frequency beta 2 range, and there was a tendency toward an increase in delta and theta activities. These changes were seen both before and after onset of dystonic attacks, indicating a permanent disturbance of neural activities in the basal ganglia of the dystonic animals (30). PHD, especially of short duration, is a form of frontal lobe epilepsy in most cases (10). In a patient with PHD, subtraction ictal SPECT coregistered to MRI indicated a bilateral significant hyperperfusion in the anterior part of the cingulate gyrus (31). This suggests that in some cases of PHD the epileptic focus may lie in the cingulate gyrus. The longer duration PHD may represent a true dystonic phenomenon.

Paroxysmal hemidystonia in demyelinating disease may reflect ephaptic transmission in the plaques (32). The site of the ephaptic transmission is unclear, but midbrain and thalamus have been suggested as possible locations (33). In some cases the demyelination is demonstrable exclusively or predominantly in the spinal cord.

NEUROCHEMISTRY

The neurochemistry of these disorders is largely unknown. The response to levodopa in one case of PKD suggests dopaminergic basal ganglionic dysfunction (34). Haloperidol gives inconsistent results (35). In a mutant hamster model of paroxysmal dystonia pharmacologic modulation of the GABAergic function affected the dystonia (36). In a genetically dystonic hamster with attacks of generalized dystonia there was an increased TBPS binding, implicating an abnormal function of a γ-aminobutyric acid (GABA)–gated chloride ion channel (37).

NEUROPATHOLOGY

There are only two autopsy reports in PKD. In one patient there was only a slight asymmetry of substantia nigra (38). The other reported some melanin pigment in macrophages of locus ceruleus suggestive of neuronal loss (2). In the animal model there have been no consistent pathologic changes in the brain and the spinal cord (39).

Two patients with HIV-associated dementia and PND had a progressive course to death. Autopsy of a patient with

PNDs revealed intense astrogliosis and loss of calbindin-positive neurons in the subcortical gray matter (23).

GENETICS

Familial dystonic choreoathetosis has been reported in a patient with familial ataxia (40). There is now evidence to suggest that paroxysmal dyskinesias may belong to a growing family of disorders similar to the inherited episodic ataxias, some which are known to be due to disorders of ion channels (channelopathies) (41,42) (Table 29.3). Several paroxysmal neurologic disorders are now being discovered to be due to gene mutations regulating ion channels that are intimately involved in maintaining normal neuronal excitability. Initially, episodic neuromuscular disorders, such as the periodic paralyses, were found to be caused by mutations in voltage-gated sodium and calcium channels (1). Subsequently, the two forms of inherited episodic ataxias (EA-1 and EA-2) were shown to be mutations of voltage-gated potassium (41) and calcium channels respectively (42,43).

There is a certain resemblance between PKD and EA-1 associated with continuous myokymia. Like PKD, the attacks of EA-1 are frequently provoked by sudden movement; the ataxic attacks are short lasting and can occur several times a day (44). Acetazolamide reduces the attacks in some kindreds and anticonvulsant drugs may reduce the myokymia and attacks in some patients (45). There are similarities between the two conditions with regard to the age of onset and improvement in adulthood (44). Some members of EA-1 families also have PKD suggesting similar pathophysiologic mechanism. The gene for PKD has been localized to chromosome 16 by different investigators (46–49).

TABLE 29.3. PAROXYSMAL DYSKINESIAS: GENETICS

Disorder	Gene Localization	Gene Function	Ref.
1) Paroxysmal kinesigenic dyskinesia	Chromosome 16P 11.2–q12.1	Unknown	Tomita, 1999 Bennett, 2000 Valente et al., 2000
Infantile convulsions, paroxysmal choreoathetosis syndrome	Chromosome 16q13–q22.1	Unknown	Szepetowski et al., 1997 Lee, 1998
2) Paroxysmal nonkinesigenic dyskinesia	FPD 1 on chromosome 2q	? Ion channel gene	Fouad et al., 1996 Jarman, 1997 Fink et al., 1996
3) Paroxysmal exertional dyskinesia	None known		
PED + migraine + writer's cramp	Chromosome 16 (overlaps with ICCA)	Unknown	Guerrini et al., 1999
4) ADNFLE	Chromosome 20q	Nicotinic ACh receptor	Philips et al., 1995
ADNFLE	Chromosome 15	Nicotinic ACh receptor	Philips et al., 1998
ADNFLE	Chromosome 1		Gambardella et al., 2000
5) Autosomal dominant paroxysmal choreoathetosis and spasticity	Chromosome 1P	Potassium channel	Auburger et al., 1996

PED, paroxysmal exertional dyskinesia; ADNFLE, autosomal dominant nocturnal frontal lobe epilepsy; ACh, acetylcholine.

Another evolving story is the relationship between infantile convulsions and PKD. Originally described as infantile convulsions and paroxysmal choreoathetosis (ICCA) syndrome (50,51) and linked to chromosome 16, the condition was thought to be uncommon. Subsequently, benign familial infantile convulsions were linked to the same area of chromosome 16p, suggesting allelism to the ICCA syndrome (52). Cosegregation of benign infantile convulsions and paroxysmal kinesigenic choreoathetosis was then demonstrated (53). It is now clear that the association between benign infantile convulsions and PKD is the rule rather than the exception (54).

The gene for familial PND has been linked to a locus on chromosome 2q (55–58). Although the exact gene remains to be discovered, the linkage area is in proximity to a cluster of ion channel genes including AE-3, which is an alkali extruder gene. This suggests that PND may be an ion channel disorder.

The exact locations of genes responsible for PED are unknown. However, a pedigree in which three members in the same generation are affected by rolandic epilepsy (RE), PED, and writer's cramp (WC) has been described (59). Both the seizures and paroxysmal dystonia had a strong age-related expression that peaked during childhood, whereas WC, also appearing in childhood, was stable. Genome-wide linkage analysis performed under the assumption of recessive inheritance mapped to chromosome 16. Although the syndrome is unique, its features inspire striking analogies with the autosomal dominant infantile convulsions and paroxysmal choreoathetosis (ICCA) syndrome, and the same gene may be responsible for both RE-PED-WC and ICCA, with specific mutations explaining each of these mendelian disorders.

Another gene for autosomal dominant paroxysmal choreoathetosis and spasticity has been mapped to chromosome 1 in the vicinity of potassium channel gene cluster (60).

The gene for ADNFLE has been localized to chromosome 20q and characterized as a mutation of the alpha 4 subunit of the neuronal acetylcholine receptor (CHRNA4) gene (61,62). However, this condition is genetically heterogeneous as shown by a family with ADNFLE that has been linked to chromosome 15 in the area of another nicotinic acetylcholine receptor gene (63) and another family where the locus maps to chromosome 1 (64).

One hopes the identification of distinct genetic loci will lead to a new genetic classification and to a better understanding of these disorders.

DIFFERENTIAL DIAGNOSIS

Paroxysmal dyskinesias must be differentiated from dopa-responsive dystonia, seizures, pseudoseizures, and tics. Dopa-responsive dystonia usually begins in childhood and may have marked diurnal fluctuations, with the patient improving with rest and worsening with exercise. However, discrete paroxysms do not occur. Seizures arising from the supplemental motor area may resemble dyskinesias and sometimes are precipitated by movement. The idiopathic paroxysmal dyskinesias have to be distinguished from symptomatic ones, as indicated in the section on clinical manifestation. Sometimes paroxysmal dyskinesia is psychogenic (7).

DIAGNOSTIC WORKUP

A detailed history and videotape documentation are most important in the differential diagnosis of paroxysmal dyskinesias. Detailed family history should be obtained. An interictal electroencephalogram may be helpful in ruling out seizures in doubtful cases. However, the electroencephalogram obtained during the episode is usually full of artifacts. Invasive electroencephalography is not recommended. If the attacks are precipitated by hyperventilation, MRI of the head should be done to provide evidence of demyelinating disease. This may be supplemented by evoked responses and a spinal tap looking for evidence for intrathecal immunoglobulin synthesis. If the attacks begin in an elderly person, vascular disease should be looked for. The blood sugar of every patient should be obtained during the attack to rule out hypoglycemia or hyperglycemia.

PROGNOSIS

Prognosis depends on the type of paroxysmal dyskinesia. PKD even of prolonged duration responds well to standard anticonvulsants, and the attacks tend to diminish during adulthood. PND and PED have a variable prognosis. Even with repeated attacks the neurologic function is normal between attacks. In symptomatic dyskinesias the prognosis depends on the underlying disease. In multiple sclerosis the attacks tend to run a self-limited course even with continued disease activity.

TREATMENT

Paroxysmal Kinesigenic Dyskinesia

PKD responds well to anticonvulsants, including phenytoin, valproate carbamazepine, and phenobarbital (1). The dose required is usually less than the standard anticonvulsant dosage. Other drugs that have been helpful are anticholinergics, levodopa, flunarizine, and tetrabenazine (7). Haloperidol has given inconsistent results.

Paroxysmal Nonkinesigenic Dyskinesia

Avoidance of precipitating factors, such as alcohol, caffeine, and stress, is important. Several drugs have been used, none with consistent success. These include clonazepam, haloperidol, alternate-day oxazepam, and anticholinergics (1). Anticonvulsants are ineffective in most cases.

Paroxysmal Exertional Dyskinesia

Avoidance of prolonged exercise may help diminish the frequency of attacks. Drug therapy is often ineffective. L-Dopa has been reported efficacious (1). In one severe case, posteroventral pallidotomy ameliorated attacks of paroxysmal dystonia induced by exercise (65).

Paroxysmal Hypnogenic Dyskinesia

Short-duration PHD may respond to anticonvulsants, including carbamazepine and phenytoin. The longer lasting attacks respond less well but may improve with haloperidol or acetazolamide.

Secondary Paroxysmal Dyskinesias

The paroxysmal dystonia associated with multiple sclerosis responds well to anticonvulsants. Acetazolamide is a useful alternative or adjunct to anticonvulsants (66). The choreoathetosis secondary to head injury may respond to anticonvulsants or a combination of anticonvulsants and trihexyphenidyl (21). In metabolic cases the underlying abnormality, including treatment for hypoglycemia or hyperglycemia and thyrotoxicosis, must be addressed. The PKD associated with hypoparathyroidism may resolve with management of hypocalcemia by vitamin D. Vascular risk factors must be addressed when the paroxysmal dyskinesia is thought to be due to transient ischemic attacks.

REFERENCES

1. Sethi KD. Paroxysmal dyskinesias. *The Neurologist* 2000;6(3): 77–85.
2. Kertesz A. Paroxysmal kinesigenic choreoathetosis: an entity within paroxysmal choreoathetosis syndrome: description of ten cases including one autopsied. *Neurology* 1967;17:680–690.
3. Mount LA, Reback S. Familial paroxysmal choreoathetosis: preliminary report on a hitherto undescribed clinical syndrome. *Arch Neurol Psychiatry* 1940;44:841–847.
4. Lance JW. Familial paroxysmal dystonic choreoathetosis and its differentiation from related syndromes. *Ann Neurol* 1977;2: 285–293.
5. Fahn S. The paroxysmal dyskinesias. In: Marsden CD, Fahn S, eds. *Movement disorders,* 3rd ed. Woburn, MA: Butterworth Heinemann, 1994:310–346.
6. Lugaresi E, Cirignotta F. Hypnogenic paroxysmal dystonia: epileptic seizure or a new syndrome? *Sleep* 1981;4:129–138.
7. Demirkiran M, Jankovic J. Paroxysmal dyskinesias: clinical features and classification. *Ann Neurol* 1995;38:571–579.
8. Marsden CD. Paroxysmal choreoathetosis. In: Luders HO, ed. *Supplementary sensorimotor area.* Advances in neurology, vol 70. Philadelphia: JB Lippincott, 1996:467–470.
9. Plant G. Focal paroxysmal kinesigenic choreoathetosis. *J Neurol Neurosurg Psychiatry* 1983;46:345–348.
10. Meierkord H, Fish DR, Smith SJM, et al. Is nocturnal paroxysmal dystonia a form of frontal lobe epilepsy? *Mov Disord* 1992;7: 38–42.
11. Tranchant C, Bhatia KP, Marsden CD. Movement disorders in multiple sclerosis. *Mov Disord* 1995;10:418–423.
12. Berger JR, Sheremata WA, Melamed E. Paroxysmal dystonia as the initial manifestation of multiple sclerosis. *Arch Neurol* 1984; 41:747–750.
13. Rosen JA. Paroxysmal choreoathetosis associated with perinatal hypoxic encephalopathy. *Arch Neurol* 1964;11:385–387.
14. Kato H, Kobayashi K, Kohari S, et al. Paroxysmal kinesigenic choreoathetosis and paroxysmal dystonic choreoathetosis in a patient with familial idiopathic hypoparathyroidism. *Tohoku J Exp Med* 1987;151:233–239.
15. Clark JD, Pahwa R, Koller WC. Diabetes mellitus presenting as paroxysmal kinesigenic dystonic choreoathetosis. *Mov Discord* 1995;10:354–355.
16. George MS, Pickett JB, Kohli H, et al. Paroxysmal dystonic reflex choreoathetosis after minor closed head injury. *Lancet* 1990;336:1134–1135.
17. Camac A, Greene P, Khandji A. Paroxysmal kinesigenic dystonic choreoathetosis associated with a thalamic infarct. *Mov Disord* 1990;5:235–238.
18. Riley DE. Paroxysmal kinesigenic dystonia associated with a medullary lesion. *Mov Disord* 1996;11:738–740.
19. Blakeley J, Jankovic J. In: Fahn, Hallett Frucht, eds. *Myoclonus, paroxysmal dyskinesias and related disorders.* Advances in neurology. Philadelphia: Lippincott Williams & Wilkins, 2002 (in press).
20. Factor SA, Coni RJ, Cowger M, et al. Paroxysmal tremor and orofacial dyskinesia secondary to biopterin synthesis defect. *Neurology* 1991;41:930–932.
21. Perlmutter JS, Raichle ME. Pure hemidystonia with basal ganglia abnormalities on positron emission tomography. *Ann Neurol* 1984;15:228–233.
22. Hess DC, Sethi KD, Nichols FT. Transient cerebral ischemia masquerading as paroxysmal dyskinesia. *Cerebrovasc Dis* 1991;1: 54–57.
23. Mirsattari SM, Berry ME, Holden JK, et al. Paroxysmal dyskinesias in patients with HIV infection. *Neurology* 1999;52(1):109–114.
24. Joynt RJ, Green D. Tonic seizures as a manifestation of multiple sclerosis. *Arch Neurol* 1962;6:293–299.
25. Goodenough DJ, Fariello RG, Annis BL, et al. Familial and acquired paroxysmal dyskinesias—a proposed classification with delineation of clinical features. *Arch Neurol* 1978;35:827–831.
26. Lombroso CT. Paroxysmal kinesigenic choreoathetosis: first report of an invasive EEG/video monitoring. *Neurology* 1996;46 [Suppl]:A259.
27. Kitagawa N, Hayashi M, Akiguchi I, et al. [Ictal 99mTC-HMPAO-SPECT in a case of paroxysmal kinesigenic choreoathetosis. *Rinsho Shinkeigaku Clin Neurol* 1998;38(8):767–770.
28. Lombroso CT, Fischman A. Paroxysmal non-kinesigenic dyskinesia: pathophysiological investigations. *Epileptic Disord* 1999;1 (3):187–193.
29. Bohnen NI, Albin RL, Frey KA, et al. (+)-alpha-[11C]Dihydrotetrabenazine PET imaging in familial paroxysmal dystonic choreoathetosis. *Neurology* 1999;52(5):1067–1069.
30. Gernert M, Richter A, Rundfeldt C, et al. Quantitative EEG analysis of depth electrode recordings from several brain regions of mutant hamsters with paroxysmal dystonia discloses frequency changes in the basal ganglia. *Mov Disord* 1998;13(3):509–521.

31. Schindler K, Gast H, Bassetti C, et al. Hyperperfusion of anterior cingulate gyrus in a case of paroxysmal nocturnal dystonia. *Neurology* 2001;57(5):917–920.
32. Osterman PO, Westerberg CE. Paroxysmal attacks in multiple sclerosis. *Brain* 1975;98:189–202.
33. Sethi KD. Paroxysmal hemidystonia: evidence of a midbrain lesion. *Neurology* 1993;43:329.
34. Loong SC, Ong YY. Paroxysmal kinesigenic choreoathetosis: report of a case relieved by L-dopa. *J Neurol Neurosurg Psychiatry* 1973;31:921–924.
35. Przuntek H, Monninger P. Therapeutic aspects of kinesigenic paroxysmal choreoathetosis and familial paroxysmal choreoathetosis of the Mount and Reback type. *J Neurol* 1983;230: 163–169.
36. Fredow G, Loscher W. Effects of pharmacological manipulation of GABAergic neurotransmission in a new mutant hamster model of paroxysmal dystonia. *Eur J Pharmacol* 1991;192: 207–219.
37. Nobrega JN, Richter A, Burnham WM, et al. Alterations in the brain: gaba/benzodiazepine receptor–chloride ionophore complex in a genetic model of paroxysmal dystonia: a quantitative autoradiographic analysis. *Neuroscience* 1995;64:229–239.
38. Stevens H. Paroxysmal choreoathetosis: a form of reflex epilepsy. *Arch Neurol* 1966;14:415–420.
39. Wahnschaffee U, Fredow G, Heintz P. Neuropathological studies in a mutant hamster model of paroxysmal dystonia. *Mov Disord* 1990;5:286–293.
40. Mayeux R, Fahn S. Paroxysmal dystonic choreoathetosis in a patient with familial ataxia. *Neurology* 1982;32:1184–1186.
41. Browne DL, Gancher ST, Nutt JG, et al. Episodic ataxia/myokymia syndrome is associated with point mutations in the human potassium channel gene, *KCNA1. Nat Genet* 1994;8:136–140.
42. Vehdi K, Joutel A, Van Bogaert P, et al. A gene for hereditary paroxysmal cerebellar ataxia maps to chromosome 19p. *Ann Neurol* 1995;37:289–293.
43. Ophoff RA, Terwindt GM, Vergouwe MN, et al. Familial hemiplegic migraine and episodic ataxia type-2 are caused by mutations in the Ca^{2+} channel gene *CACNLIA4. Cell* 1996;87: 543–552.
44. Brunt ERP, Van Weerden TW Familial paroxysmal kinesigenic ataxia and continuous myokymia. *Brain* 1990;113: 1361–1382.
45. Griggs RC, Moxley RT III, Lafralane RA, et al. Hereditary paroxysmal ataxia, response to acetazolamide. *Neurology* 1978;28: 1259–1264.
46. Bennett LB, Roach ES, Bowcock AM. A locus for paroxysmal kinesigenic dyskinesia maps to human chromosome 16. *Neurology* 2000;54:125–130.
47. Tomita Ha, Nagamitsu S, Wakui K, et al. Paroxysmal kinesigenic choreoathetosis locus maps to chromosome 16p11.2-q12.1. *Am J Hum Genet* 1999;65(6):1688–1697.
48. Valente EM, Spacey SD, Wali GM, et al. A second paroxysmal kinesigenic choreoathetosis locus (EKD2) mapping on 16q13-q22.1 indicates a family of genes which give rise to paroxysmal disorders on human chromosome 16. *Brain* 2000;123[Pt 10]: 2040–2045.
49. Bennett LB, Roach ES, Bowcock AM. A locus for paroxysmal kinesigenic dyskinesia maps to human chromosome 16. *Neurology* 2000;54(1):125–130.
50. Szepetowski P, Rochette J, Berquin P, et al. Familial infantile convulsions and paroxysmal choreoathetosis: a new neurological syndrome linked to the pericentromeric region of human chromosome 16. *Am J Hum Genet* 1997;61:889–898.
51. Lee W, Tay A, Long H, et al. Association of infantile convulsions with paroxysmal dyskinesias (ICCA syndrome): confirmation of linkage to human chromosome 16p12-q12 in a Chinese family. *Hum Genet* 1998;103:608–612.
52. Caraballo R, Pavek S, Lemainque A, et al. Linkage of benign familial infantile convulsions to chromosome 16p12-q12 suggests allelism to the infantile convulsions and choreoathetosis syndrome. *Am J Hum Genet* 2001;68(3):788–794.
53. Hattori H, Fujii T, Nigami H, et al. Co-segregation of benign infantile convulsions and paroxysmal kinesigenic choreoathetosis. *Brain Dev* 2000;22(7):432–435.
54. Swoboda KJ, Soong B, McKenna C, et al. Related Articles: Bennett LB, Bowcock AM, Roach ES, Gerson D, Matsuura T, Heydemann PT, Nespeca MP, Jankovic J, Leppert M, Ptacek LJ. Paroxysmal kinesigenic dyskinesia and infantile convulsions: clinical and linkage studies. *Neurology* 2000;55(2):224–230.
55. Fink JK, Hedera P, Mathay JG, et al. Paroxysmal dystonic choreoathetosis linked to chromosome 2q: clinical analysis and proposed pathophysiology. *Neurology* 1997;49:177–183.
56. Fink JK, Rainier S, Wilkowski J, et al. Paroxysmal dystonic choreoathetosis: tight linkage to chromosome 2q. *Am J Hum Genet* 1996;59:140–145.
57. Fouad GT, Sevidei S, Durcan S, et al. A gene for familial dyskinesia *(FPD1)* maps to chromosome 2q. *Am J Hum Genet* 1996; 59:135–139.
58. Jarman PR, Davis MB, Hogdson SV, et al. Paroxysmal dystonic choreoathetosis: genetic linkage in a British family. *Brain* 1997; 120:2125–2130.
59. Guerrini R, Bonanni P, Nardocci N, et al. Autosomal recessive rolandic epilepsy with paroxysmal exercise-induced dystonia and writer's cramp: delineation of the syndrome and gene mapping to chromosome 16p12-11.2. *Ann Neurol* 1999;45(3):344–352.
60. Auburger G, Ratzlaff T, Lunkes A, et al. A gene for autosomal dominant paroxysmal choreoathetosis/spasticity (CSE) maps to the vicinity of potassium channel gene cluster on chromosome 1p, probably within 2cM between D1S443 and D1S197. *Genomics* 1996;31(1):90–94.
61. Philips HA, Sceffer IE, Berkovic SF, et al. 20q Localisation of a gene for autosomal dominant nocturnal frontal lobe epilepsy to chromosome 13.2. *Nat Genet* 1995;10:117–118.
62. Steinlein OK, Mulley JC, Propping P, et al. A misense mutation in the neuronal acetylcholine receptor alpha-4 subunit is associated with autosomal dominant nocturnal frontal lobe epilepsy. *Nat Genet* 1995;11:201–202.
63. Phillips HA, Scheffer IE, Crossland KM, et al. Autosomal dominant nocturnal frontal-lobe epilepsy: genetic heterogeneity and evidence for a second locus at 15q24. *Am J Hum Genet* 1998;63: 1108–1116.
64. Gambardella A, Annesi G, De Fusco M, et al. Related Articles: Pasqua AA, Spadafora P, Oliveri RL, Valentino P, Zappia M, Ballabio A, Casari G, Quattrone A. A new locus for autosomal dominant nocturnal frontal lobe epilepsy maps to chromosome 1. *Neurology* 2000;55(10):1467–1471.
65. Bhatia KP, Marsden CD, Thomas DG. Posteroventral pallidotomy can ameliorate attacks of paroxysmal dystonia induced by exercise. *J Neurol Neurosurg Psychiatry* 1998;65(4):604–605.
66. Sethi KD, Hess DC, Huffnagle VH, et al. Acetazolamide treatment of paroxysmal dystonia in central demyelinating disease. *Neurology* 1992;42:4;919–923.

30

STEREOTYPY AND CATATONIA

JOSEPH H. FRIEDMAN

Stereotypy and catatonia are distinct syndromes with some overlap, and they are discussed separately in this chapter. Both are most commonly seen as parts of more severe behavioral disorders (1). Stereotypy is an "involuntary or unvoluntary [unvoluntary defined as a physical response to an inner force] . . . coordinated, patterned, repetitive, rhythmic, purposeless but seemingly purposeful or ritualistic movement, posture or utterance" (1). It occurs in response to external or inner stimuli and is often perceived as a self-stimulatory behavior. Stereotypy refers to both motor and mental behaviors, but this chapter focuses on motor stereotypy. Stereotypy was considered a core feature of schizophrenia until relatively recently. "The tendency to stereotype produces the inclination to cling to one idea to which the patient then returns again and again. This leads to repetitious motor and emotional behavior that is inescapable" (2). Catatonia is by definition a syndrome complex that includes motor and behavioral abnormalities (3). Catatonia includes stereotypic behaviors, but most stereotypies are not part of catatonic syndromes. Their inclusion in a book on movement disorders underscores the acknowledgment of the increasing overlap between neurologic and psychiatric disorders. Catatonia was redefined in the *Diagnostic and Statistical Manual of Mental Disorders*, 4th ed. (DSM-IV) (3) to be significantly different from earlier DSM definitions and is now thought to be considerably more prevalent than previously believed. Stereotypy has been suggested to be the most common motor manifestation of tardive dyskinesia (4).

CLINICAL ASPECTS OF STEREOTYPY

Phenomenology

Stereotypy is variably defined. The American Psychiatric Association defines a stereotypy as a repetitive, nonfunctional motor behavior (3). The movements are generally repeated in a monotonous fashion without apparent conscious control despite a normal level of consciousness. Although the definition given in the introduction includes an irresistible quality to the movement, this is not a universally accepted criterion. Tan et al. (5) qualify their definition of repeated purposeless movements by noting that a stereotypy is easily suppressible without the tension buildup that accompanies suppression of a tic. In addition, a stereotypy may simply be a habit or a self-stimulation in a manner that is not pathologic. For example, finger tapping, hair curling, and foot tapping are considered normal. All three are stereotypies, yet none is "pathologic" or involuntary. Twenty percent of normal children exhibit stereotypies (6,7) at some time and are also common in college students (8). Stereotypy also occurs in animals and has an agreed-on definition in farm animals as a repetitive action, fixed in form and orientation, that serves no obvious function.

Stereotypies may be simple or complex (1). Simple stereotypies are composed of a few simple maneuvers, such as rocking, tapping, clapping, clicking, hair twirling, and head banging. Complex stereotypies, such as running forward and backward with repeated gesticulations or vocalizations, repeated opening and closing of a door and then sitting down, and spitting into a hand then rubbing it in one's hair, are more clearly psychiatric and are not mistaken for tics, myoclonus, or other movement disorders. Either by the nature of the stereotypy or as a result of the repetitive nature of the act, self-mutilation may occur. Persistent hitting, rubbing, or licking, even lightly, may break down the skin. In other cases, the severity of each individual insult, such as hitting, biting, or scratching oneself, punching a wall, or head banging, may produce disfiguring wounds. Most cases of stereotypy are simple, with rocking, hugging, self-touching, patting, grunting, foot tapping, leg swinging, and hair pulling being the most common (1).

Differential Diagnosis

Distinguishing a stereotypy from other movements is important and often difficult (5). Mannerisms, akathisia, tics, compulsions, restless legs syndrome, paroxysmal dyskinesias, epilepsy, and perseveration may be included in the differential diagnostic list, with tics and mannerisms being the most

TABLE 30.1. DIFFERENTIAL DIAGNOSIS OF STEREOTYPIC MOVEMENTS

Akathisia
Automatisms
Compulsions
Drug-induced dyskinesias
Epileptic seizures
    Complex partial
    Focal tonic
    Petit mal
Mannerisms
Perseverations
Paroxysmal dyskinesias
Restless legs syndrome
Complex tics

likely to cause confusion (Table 30.1). Mannerisms are movements performed in a highly idiosyncratic manner, such as grasping a pen with both hands to write, or always holding a cup with the hand in a peculiar posture. "Mannerisms are a bizarre way of carrying out a purposeful act which usually occurs as the result of the incorporation of a stereotypy into a goal directed behavior" (9). On one end of the spectrum, the definition requires that these postures be grotesque and clearly abnormal to any untrained eye. On the other end of the spectrum, mannerisms may be simple gesticulations unique to that individual or a trait of a particular culture. For example, hand gesticulation is particularly common among the Haitians. Unusual rituals, such as ballplayers may exhibit before batting or making a free throw, are accepted as mannerisms by some authorities (1).

Complex tics may be repetitive and thus appear stereotypic. Simple tics are sudden, brief movements that occur in isolation or in brief bursts. The movements are generally repeated and typically involve eye blinking, grimacing, or head jerking. Complex tics are a more elaborate sequence of movements that may be repeated at regular or irregular intervals. Examples include repetitive head shaking, abnormal posturing, throwing oneself on the ground, and complex gesturing (see videotape in ref. 10). If the patient has Tourette's syndrome, these may be associated with vocalizations. Some authorities (11) distinguish between perseveration and stereotypy, with some authors limiting stereotypy to the motor and perseveration to the mental components of repetitive purposeless activities. However, some investigators consider perseverations to be motor acts. Ridley (11) proposed that perseveration refer to repetitive "but not excessive" actions, whereas stereotypy should refer to "excessive production of one type of motor act or mental state." Unlike a stereotypy, which is repeated endlessly, perseverations continue for a limited period. They do not become part of a fixed repertoire of movements. Perseverations generally occur at the end of a normal, purposeful movement and consist of repetitions of parts of the original movement, which fade out eventually. Neurologists often encounter

verbal perseverations in clinical practice, usually in demented, encephalopathic, or aphasic patients. The subject answers one question and then repeats this answer when asked further questions, no matter how unrelated the questions are. Motor perseverations are less common.

Restless legs syndrome is defined as a syndrome induced by a desire to move the legs (see Chapter 26). Limb restlessness is associated with sensory discomfort, improvement with movement and worsening with rest, worsening of symptoms at night, and absence of akathisia (no history of dopamine antagonists and no sign of whole-body restlessness). Over time the initially suppressible movements may become involuntary. The patients provide a history that clearly distinguishes this from stereotypy. The patients generally need to move their legs, and their movements appear normal. They stop frequently upon relieving their symptoms.

Compulsions are repetitive thoughts or activities, such as counting, touching, checking, tapping, gambling, risk taking, or avoiding (12). In contrast to obsessions, which are recurrent unwanted thoughts or ideas, compulsions ease anxiety, whereas obsessive thoughts increase them. Common compulsions are repeated hand washing, checking, tapping, arranging items on a desk so that everything is perfectly lined up, and stereotyped rituals. These may occur as part of a primary psychiatric disorder (obsessive-compulsive disorder), in association with Tourette's syndrome, as a result of encephalitis lethargica, or, rarely, in response to a focal brain lesion. The movements generally appear normal but rarely lead to a pattern of movements so restricted or odd in appearance that it becomes a stereotypy. For example, patients with obsessional slowness may move as if parkinsonian and get stuck attempting to walk or to sit, thereby adopting a relatively fixed posture; or they may move one step back and forth (13), as if caged.

Paroxysmal dyskinesias fall into two major categories: kinesogenic and nonkinesogenic (see Chapter 29). These are episodic, lasting for minutes or hours, during which the patient has normal mentation but displays chorea or dystonia. As the movements are odd, they may be misinterpreted as stereotypic, but the episodic nature and the patient's normal mentation should clearly distinguish these movements from stereotypies.

Akathisia is the inability to remain still because of an inner sense of restlessness. The afflicted person is unable to sit in one place, feeling compelled to stand up frequently, to march in place, or to shift weight from one foot to the other. The person may perform jumping jacks or other calisthenics or walk briskly up and down the corridor. When the activity is repetitive, it is in fact a stereotypy, an involuntary act that relieves an inner sense of tension. Most cases of akathisia are induced by both dopamine receptor–blocking drugs (neuroleptics) and by dopaminergic drugs (levodopa). The syndrome may occur in both untreated and treated patients with Parkinson's disease.

When a patient is noncommunicative, as is often the case in the psychotic or profoundly retarded, one cannot always categorize the movement pattern. For example, akathisia is a movement in response to an inner drive and can manifest in a variety of behaviors, including worsened psychosis or stereotypy, yet the patient may not be able to explain the problem. Simply observing a behavior without obtaining a complete history, such as changes of medication, will lead to an incorrect diagnosis.

Epileptic seizures of various types might also be misconstrued as stereotypic behaviors. Children with petit mal seizures will look dazed and blink, sometimes developing lip smacking if the spell lasts for several seconds. Complex partial seizures may induce stereotypic behaviors with an impaired consciousness, but if the patient has a mental impairment at baseline a change may not be evident. Finally, focal tonic seizures may produce a stereotypy.

Many cases of repetitive movements are not easy to delineate clearly as a stereotypy as opposed to another type of movement disorder. The clinical context in which the movement is seen must be taken into account, perhaps more than in the assessment of other movement disorders.

In rare cases the stereotypy is part of a neurodegenerative disorder, such as Rett's syndrome, Lesch-Nyhan syndrome, or neuroacanthocytosis.

Causation (Table 30.2)

Certain stereotypies are normal (6,7), and others are virtually diagnostic of a specific disorder, so that the complete

TABLE 30.2. CAUSES OF STEREOTYPIES

Autism
  Asperger's syndrome
  Infantile autism
  Kanner's syndrome
Drug induced
  Psychostimulants
  Tardive dyskinesia
Inborn errors of metabolism
  Lesch-Nyhan syndrome
  Neuroacanthocytosis
Infectious
  Encephalitis
Mental retardation (all types)
Neurodegenerative disorders
Physiologic disorders
Psychiatric disorders
  Catatonia
  Functional
  Obsessive-compulsive disorder
  Schizophrenia
Rett's syndrome
Sensory deprivation
  Caging, constraint
  Congenital blindness
  Congenital deafness
  Stroke

evaluation of the patient and the developmental history of the behavior are important. Thumb sucking is normal in children, and delayed onset or absence of this movement may indicate maturational dysfunction. Head banging, head rolling, and general rocking occurs in about 20% of normal children at some point (6,7) and usually resolves spontaneously, so that even a behavior as dramatically upsetting as a baby purposefully banging its head on the floor may be deemed normal. Certainly it is considered normal for adults to tap a foot or fingers, to pull on hair, and to cross and recross the legs, and thumb sucking in children is usually viewed as a normal and comforting stereotypy. The context of the movement and the culture of the patient help determine normality. Stress typically worsens stereotypies.

Stereotypy may be induced by alterations in perception. Probably the most common stereotypy is the self-stimulatory vacuous chewing of edentulous adults. This may be considered normal, as it arises so commonly in otherwise completely normal individuals.

Stereotypies most commonly occur in the autistic, retarded, psychotic, congenitally blind, and congenitally deaf (1,14). The age of onset of the movements depends on the syndrome. In genetically determined disorders the onset may be in late childhood. The incidence and phenomena of stereotypy vary to some degree with the syndrome and to a large degree with the severity of the underlying behavioral disorder. In studies of institutionalized nonhandicapped children, 59% exhibited one or more stereotypies (15). Thumb sucking declined and nail biting increased with age. In the retarded the prevalence of stereotypy is higher and the movements more sustained (19).

Autism is a childhood-onset syndrome characterized by abnormal socialization with poor attachment and interaction with people, disordered cognitive and language skills, abnormal responses to stimulation, necessity for sameness in the environment, repetitive behavior, and a normal physical appearance. Autism is considered distinct from retardation, and although it is often thought that acquisition of motor skills and motor function is normal in autistic children, about 50% of autistic children are motor delayed, and many are clumsy. Autistic patients most often display "facial grimacing, staring at flickering lights, waving objects in front of the eyes, producing repetitive sounds, arm flapping, rhythmic body rocking, repetitive touching, feeling and smelling objects, jumping, walking on toes and unusual hand and body gesturing" (1). Clapping and tapping are also common. There are several variants of autism, which, with the exception of Rett's syndrome, affects boys considerably more often than girls. Fragile X syndrome, Kanner's syndrome (the original describer of autism), and Asperger's syndrome are all causes or types of autism. Fragile X syndrome causes a wide variety of retardation syndromes and is the single most common cause of mental retardation in boys. Asperger's syndrome is a form of autism involving an isolated area of extreme, all-absorbing interest, such as astronomy or history. With good function in at least the one intellectual area, children with Asperger's syndrome have a mild form of autism. Those with Asperger's variant also have mild clumsiness, more so than those with the Kanner variant, but are otherwise more mildly affected.

Rett's syndrome (16), a disorder restricted to female patients, causes persistent hand wringing or hand washing, which usually points to the correct diagnosis. In addition to these typical stereotypies, patients with Rett's syndrome manifest a variety of other movement disorders, including dystonia and parkinsonism (17). Lesch-Nyhan syndrome is an X-linked disorder of boys that is attributable to a purine metabolism abnormality. Patients bite their lips, fingers, forearms, and nails. They may scratch their nose and mouth and draw blood. Unlike most other syndromes of self-injury, these children request restraints, an observation that contradicts the general hypothesis that stereotypy is a self-stimulatory behavior. The children also display a variety of movement disorders. They display aggressive behavior to other people and may hit objects, also sustaining injury. Neuroacanthocytosis is a constellation of disorders that include an increased percentage of acanthocytic red blood cells. One form of the syndrome includes tongue and lip biting.

Despite the different causes and ages of onset, the phenomena of most stereotypies tend to overlap, although certain ones tend to be more common in particular disorders. For example, the various sensory deprivation–induced stereotypies are relatively similar. Congenitally blind children rock, suck fingers, and display repetitive manipulation of objects (14). Blind adults rock and exhibit stereotypies as well, exemplified by the musician Stevie Wonder. Autistic and retarded children display eye poking as the most common stereotypy (14). Deaf children also have a high incidence of rocking behavior but do not seem to hit their ears as blind children hit their eyes. Generally, there is less self-injurious behavior (SIB) in these disorders than in the autistic and retarded (14). Intermittent stereotyped walking movements has been reported in a stuporous patient with medial frontoparietal cortical lesions in association with meningitis (18).

I once evaluated a rare case of focal stereotypy due to a parietal stroke. The patient developed right-sided numbness and a mild aphasia associated with a cortical infarct in the left parietal region seen on brain magnetic resonance imaging. Shortly after the stroke he noted persistent movements of his tongue, pushing against the right side of his upper denture, and constant rubbing of his right index finger across his right thumbnail. He denied any feeling of compulsion or inner release of tension achieved by the movements, and he could stop them if he focused his attention on it. The movements continued to the point where he broke down the skin on his fingers and his dentures had to be replaced. Use of a thick glove that reduced sensory stim-

ulation made it worse, but use of a thin silk glove made him feel better, although the movements persisted, suggesting that the loss of self-stimulation was bothersome despite his denial. Two other cases, both with more complex stereotypies, have been reported with strokes. One followed a series of brain insults in a child, including a right putaminal stroke, and the other followed a right lenticular infarction. I have also seen a stereotypy develop as part of an unknown neurodegenerative disorder manifested by progressive aphasia, right hemiparesis, dementia, and an eye movement disorder. The patient, while seated, bent over every few seconds to touch her left foot or stocking with her left hand.

Stereotypies can be induced in adult humans and animals by imprisonment in close quarters. These caging stereotypies may occur at any age. Ritualistic behavior and extreme slowness (13) are commonly seen in obsessive-compulsive disorder (OCD). The rituals may be simple or complex, and may be forms of stereotypy. Simple behaviors, such as repetitive touching, spitting, hair pulling, and hitting, are stereotypies. More complex behaviors, such as checking (repeated checks to confirm that the door is locked, the windows closed, the stove turned off, and so on) or persistent hand washing, may not be stereotypies in that the manner in which the repeated activity is carried out may vary and the behavior can be postponed. Obsessive slowness is a Parkinson-like bradykinesia that may accompany OCD (13). This may result in a manneristic approach to routine activities, such as sitting, in which the movement may be arrested for a period followed by extreme slowness in completion of the action. Alternatively, a patient may get stuck as if frozen (mental block) and attempt to move but be unable to do so, causing a motor activity to be repeated, shifting weight as if about to take a step, and repeating this for long periods. These movements may thus fall into a gray zone between mannerism and stereotypy. In a psychotic individual, whether the disorder is part of the primary diagnosis or neuroleptic induced, it occurs in adulthood, sometimes quite late. The stereotypies of autism, retardation, and developmental sensory deprivation occur in childhood. Psychotic patients display a primary form of stereotypy, more often rocking back and forth than any other stereotypy, but may be catatonic (discussed later). They also may have tardive stereotypy from their neuroleptic treatment (3).

Stereotypies as a central feature of tardive dyskinesia (TD) were highlighted in a study of patients with TD (4), most of whom were thought to have stereotypies as part of their syndrome. These affected the orolingual and facial regions most commonly, followed by the legs, arms, trunk, and pelvis, in that order. The orolingual movements were writhing with protrusion of the tongue, lip puckering, and chewing. Vocalization, with humming and belching most common, were also noted. Perhaps most typical of the stereotypies and least likely to cause disagreement over appropriate classification were leg crossing, leg swinging, finger or hand tapping, arm rubbing and grasping, picking, and thumb twiddling. These movements were described in patients already diagnosed as having TD, and the authors (4) believe that tardive stereotypy may occur in isolation without other signs of TD, such as facial akathisia. Clearly tardive stereotypy and tardive akathisia overlap, since akathisia frequently causes the patient to move about, rock, stand and sit, and fidget in general to relieve the urge to move.

Punding, a stereotypy typically induced by cocaine or amphetamines but also reported with levodopa (19), is a syndrome in which adults show intense fascination with repetitive handling of common objects or repeated picking to the point of self-injury. Cocaine and amphetamine may induce, under the spell of fascination, a desire to take apart (and rarely to rebuild) objects. In one Parkinson's patient anti-Parkinson drugs produced a need to tally strings of figures repetitively. This produced a feeling of great satisfaction in the patient despite his knowledge that the work produced was of little value. He could reflect on this as a peculiar behavior that he felt as foreign but that was satisfying at the time.

Self-injurious Behavior

SIB is viewed by some as a continuum on the spectrum of stereotypic behavior (20). It most often occurs in the setting of autism and retardation, but also with some genetic disorders. Body rocking has been associated with self-hitting (20) and other SIBs. Typical SIB includes nail biting, finger biting, punching objects and self, head banging, and lip biting. However, SIB is not specific for stereotypies and may be seen in Tourette's syndrome, neuroacanthocytosis, tuberous sclerosis, and in psychiatric conditions both psychotic and nonpsychotic. SIB in stereotypy tends to be the result of accumulated small injuries. While this may be the case in psychiatric patients, more commonly SIB in psychosis is a cataclysmic outpouring of emotion, perhaps as self-punishment or exorcism. Repeated self-inflicted cigarette burns and knife wounds are also seen in psychiatric patients but much less so in patients with retardation or autism. These injuries may occur in nonpsychotic states, such as personality disorder, or may represent disordered adjustment to an overwhelmingly bad social situation, as in the case of the physically abused wife who escapes beating by injuring herself first. Injuries in the psychiatric population may be a disguised plea for help. SIB occurs in 2% to 20% of the institutionalized retarded (20), depending on the study. SIB has been classified into two major categories: social and nonsocial. Social SIB creates greater social consequences, being more "blatant and dramatic" (20) to watch, suggesting that the caregiver's response is an important instigator for the action. Social SIB includes head banging, biting, scratching, gouging, pinching, and hair pulling. Nonsocial SIB includes stuffing orifices, mouthing and sucking, ruminative vomiting, coprophagy, aerophagy, and polydipsia (20).

Biological Basis

The basic mechanisms of stereotypy are unknown, although clear associations with causes, as discussed earlier, are known. There is a general belief that stereotypy in higher animals is a form of self-stimulation (11). Support for this is based in part on these behaviors in children born blind or deaf (14). It occurs in animals deprived of their mothers (21) and in autistic and retarded children, who generally interact little with their environment. It is a biologically fascinating phenomenon because many of the behaviors are shared across causation and species, although the causative mechanisms are very different (11,21). Animal data support the concept of deprivation as a cause for stereotypy. Animals raised alone develop deprivation stereotypy (11), which consists of repetitive movements, such as rocking, sucking, and head banging, that are seen in humans with impaired socialization (11). Once a critical period has passed, these behaviors are not reversible (11,21). An alternative theory holds that stereotypy reduces a state of chronic hyperarousal by channeling thought and action into the repeated movements, tempering environmental input rather than enhancing it. Stereotypies exist in animals as primitive as insects, which lack a brain. The foreleg and hindleg rubbing behavior of flies, or the stereotypic motor program by which some insects move their legs, indicates the genetic role for some repetitive motor programs that don't even require a brain.

The occurrence of particular stereotypies with certain drugs suggests common pharmacologic pathways for many of the behaviors. For example, both amphetamine and cocaine enhance catecholamine release and induce the same sniffing, picking, and repeated explorations in animals as in humans. Amphetamines given to rodents produce stereotypies that vary with the ratio of norepinephrine to dopamine. With a high ratio of norepinephrine to dopamine, amphetamine produces exploratory locomotor stereotypies, which are constrained by additional levodopa. Amphetamine-induced stereotypies are reduced when dopamine alone is depleted but are unaffected if both catecholamines are depleted. In rats there is a correlation between D2 receptor density and apomorphine-induced stereotypy, although not with altered spontaneous behavior, presumably because of decreased dopamine synthesis. Apomorphine and amphetamine given systemically or intrastriatally to rodents produce stereotypic licking, sniffing, gnawing behaviors that are blocked by D2 receptor–blocking drugs. Interestingly, apomorphine injected subcutaneously into humans produces yawning without sleepiness, yet the dopamine agonists bromocriptine, pergolide, and so forth do not. This implies that this one behavior is not specifically related to a pure dopamine effect or that the effect is extremely dependent on the ratio of the dopamine receptor activities of the drug, thus implying a need for caution in generalizing. Neuroleptics, which block dopamine receptors, cause TD and tardive stereotypy, possibly as the result of up-regulation of dopamine receptors. In Lesch-Nyhan syndrome a deficiency in hypoxanthine guanylribosyltransferase leads to dopamine deficiency in all basal ganglia structures except the substantia nigra, probably due to a reduction in terminal arborization of dopamine-secreting neurons. However, the importance of dopamine in the behavior is unknown. Dopamine-blocking and enhancing drugs both have been helpful in isolated cases.

Biochemical interpretations are helpful in understanding certain stereotypies but may be specific to the behavior under evaluation, generalizing to a limited degree only. Catecholamine treatments that induce stereotypy in rodents fail to do so in mice bred to lack D1 receptors, implying a necessity for D1 activity (22). Hypotheses to explain drug-induced stereotypy involve imbalances in distinct basal ganglia circuits as measured by gene expression (23) or by interruption of particular basal ganglia circuits (24).

Inherited disorders, such as Tourette's syndrome and Lesch-Nyhan syndrome, cause different types of stereotypies. In some cases, as in Tourette's syndrome, the particular stereotypy varies considerably even between affected individuals in the same family who presumably share the same genes, whereas the behavior in Lesch-Nyhan syndrome is relatively similar in all families.

In Rett's syndrome, an X-chromosome genetic abnormality, the girls begin to develop their movements in the first 2 years of life, and while hand wringing or "washing" is the major stereotypy, other self-mutilating behaviors occur (16). Some patients hit or bite themselves and, occasionally, others. Although the pathology is being defined, the explanation for this peculiar behavior remains a mystery.

Treatment

Patients with stereotypy may or may not require treatment. When stereotypy interferes with learning and socialization, treatment is necessary. SIB usually requires either treatment or restraint. This includes a very minor segment of all people who display stereotypy but a significant fraction of the institutionalized population.

Treatment obviously depends on causation. In most cases this means retardation and autism. Stereotypies in these conditions are most likely to interfere with education and socialization. Behavior modification using rewards or punishments, aversive therapy, or redirection to less intrusive behaviors is generally used. Results are mixed. Medications are sometimes effective. Neuroleptics may selectively reduce stereotypies but are not usually effective in SIB. Such high doses are required to reduce SIB that the drugs basically act as chemical restraints, reducing all behavior. It is possible that atypical antipsychotics may be more useful. Naltrexone, an opiate antagonist, has been found to be helpful in reducing SIB in some studies but not in others. Serotonin reuptake inhibitors also may be helpful.

Tardive stereotypy can be reduced with catecholamine-depleting drugs (3,25), such as tetrabenazine and reserpine. Using higher doses of the dopamine receptor–blocking drugs that caused the problems in the first place can mask the syndrome, but only temporarily, until the problem worsens.

Stereotypies associated with OCD respond to treatment for the OCD, usually with the selective serotonin reuptake–inhibiting antidepressant drugs (26).

CATATONIA

Catatonia is a syndrome that has undergone a change in conceptualization (27). It is not a diagnosis. No single definition exists, and its association with psychiatric disorders has been and continues to be rethought. In DSM-IV catatonia is considered a subtype of schizophrenia, a syndrome due to a systemic medical disorder, and a descriptor for affective disorders (3) (Table 30.3). Johnson (28) described catatonia as "a neuropsychiatric syndrome in which an abnormal mental state is associated with cataleptic phenomena, namely akinesia, posturing and mutism." *Catalepsy* is the term he reserved for akinesia, posturing, and mutism in the absence of "any psychiatric abnormality" (28). Bush et al. (29) described catatonia as "a neuropsychiatric syndrome in which the diagnosis does not depend

TABLE 30.3. DSM-IV SUBTYPES OF CATATONIA

Motor features
1. Motoric immobility
2. Excessive motor activity (purposeless and uninfluenced by external stimuli)
3. Extreme negativism or mutism
4. Peculiarities of voluntary movement
5. Echolalia or echopraxia

Catatonia due to a medical condition (293.89)
Motor features as above
Evidence of a general medical condition
No better psychiatric explanation
Disturbance not exclusively part of delirium

Catatonic schizophrenia (295.20)
Schizophrenia dominated by at least two of the five main motor features defined above

Catatonic features specifier
Major affective disorder with two of the five major motor features defined above

upon individual interpretation of mental status abnormalities but these are severe," thus using the term as a syndrome seen in psychosis but independent of a particular diagnosis. A syndrome of catatonia without psychosis has been described (28), and the term *medical catatonia* has been accepted for the catatonic syndrome, including mental abnormalities, that is due to an organic illness (30). The term also has been used to describe postural and tone abnormalities in animals (28) that lack other behavior problems, further complicating the literature.

Catalepsy, which was described at least as early as Galen's time, is derived from the Greek word meaning "a seizure of the body and soul." *Neuroleptic* derives from a term meaning "grips the nerves." Catalepsy describes the development of fixed postures, either self- or externally imposed. It was a phenomenon known for centuries and was associated with various mental disturbances. It could even be induced by psychosocial stressors, as occurred in epidemic fashion in response to religious preaching (28). *Catatonia*, however, was first coined in a famous monograph by Kahlbaum in 1874 (31). This term also is based on a Greek word, meaning "to stretch tight." Kahlbaum's manuscript refers to catatonia as the "tension insanity." The disorder was recognized as a brain disease with a remarkably diverse panoply of signs that cycled between a hypoactive state in which catalepsy and bizarre stereotypies predominated and a hyperactive physical and emotional state often associated with abnormal, nonsensical speech production.

"Catatonia" was then "hijacked" (28) by Kraepelin and subsumed into the entity dementia praecox. He interpreted the syndrome as a form of a mental blocking, in contrast to Kahlbaum's conceptualization of it as an organic brain disease. Bleuler (2) later reinforced this notion in his famous text on schizophrenia, in which 26 pages of his chapter on the symptoms of schizophrenia are devoted to "the catatonic symptoms" (Table 30.4). Catatonia remained a syndrome of schizophrenia until DSM-IV. After DSM-III-R failed to include catatonia as a manifestation of mania, critics noted the frequent association of catatonia with both affective and medical disorders. This association was noted early in the 20th century, and recent criticism resulted in a modification of the DSM definition. Increased interest in the catatonic syndrome coincided with this change. Several published studies examine phenomenology, epidemiology, and etiology (28–39). The associations among neuroleptic malignant syndrome, neuroleptic-induced catatonia, catatonia, and lethal catatonia have been explored in the literature as well (40,41). Small series of open-label treatment have been reported, generally with excellent outcomes. One hopes that over the next few years, as clinical information accumulates, refinement in definitions will allow for distinctions among the various symptoms of the catatonic syndrome and their relation to the various underlying diagnoses with which they are associated. The recognition of

TABLE 30.4. SIGNS OF CATATONIA

Bleuler, 1950
Catalepsy
Stupor
Hyperkinesis
Stereotypies, motor and behavioral, including speech
Mannerisms
Negativism
Command: automation and echopraxia
Automatisms, motor and speech
Impulsiveness

Johnson's cataleptic triad
Immobility
Maintenance of imposed postures
Mutism

Bush et al., 1996 (29)

Excitement	Grimacing
Immobility, stupor	Echophenomena
Mutism	Stereotypy
Staring	Verbigeration
Posturing	Rigidity
Withdrawal	Waxy flexibility
Impulsivity	Ambitendency
Automatic obedience	Grasp reflex
Mitgehen	Perseveration
Gegenhalten	Autonomic abnormality

Sadock and Sadock, 2000 (12)

Catalepsy	Posturing
Excitement	Waxy flexibility
Rigidity	

Rosebush et al., 1990

Immobility	Negativism
Staring	Waxy flexibility
Mutism	Echolalia/echopraxia
Rigidity	Stereotypy
Withdrawal	Verbigeration
Posturing, grimacing	

catatonic symptoms using DSM-IV criteria should lead to more accurate diagnoses and significantly better outcomes, given catatonia's purported high rate of response to appropriate interventions (often unrelated, seemingly, to the underlying psychiatric diagnosis) (42).

Clinical Signs

Signs considered part of the catatonic syndrome are wide ranging (2,28,29,32). The most important is catalepsy. At least 12 distinct but overlapping criteria have been proposed for the diagnosis of catatonia since 1976 (32). Presumably DSM-IV (3) represents the closest to a consensus opinion. In an attempt to objectively define likely diagnostic criteria, one study compared 32 catatonics to 155 noncatatonic psychiatric patients. Using receiver operating characteristic (ROC) analysis any cluster of 3 of 11 "classic" signs discriminated between the two groups, giving equal weight to each sign: immobility/stupor, mutism, negativism, oppositionalism, posturing, catalepsy, automatic obedience, echophenomena, rigidity, verbigeration, and withdrawal (32). Bleuler (2) described patients maintaining postures for months at a time and considered this situation "not at all rare." Bleuler believed that this rigidity was psychologically produced and did not constitute an organic rigidity, a hypothesis that contrasts with some modern authors (30). Bleuler noted that the patients exerted precise control over muscular contractions so that movements could be made "like a piece of wood" or "as a lever" with exact compensation of other parts of the body. More common than whole-body rigidity was waxy flexibility ("cerea flexibilities"). Patients were akinetic but would maintain a posture imposed on them, apparently completely indifferent to discomfort. These imposed postures would persist for several minutes before resolving into more comfortable, albeit still bizarre, postures. In having a posture altered by an examiner, patients often participated, responding easily to mildly applied pressures, or overresponded if moved quickly ("mitgehen"). At other times, however, displaying a negative approach the patient might also resist alteration of a posture. The waxy flexibility or fixed posture might apply only to one part of the body, while another limb performed a variety of maneuvers. The catalepsy could sometimes be provoked or aborted by environmental changes, so that patients might suddenly become hyperactive after being stuporous if a particular person entered the room, or would exhibit catalepsy only when observed and appear normal when thinking themselves unobserved.

"Catatonic stupor" is more difficult to define, as "stupor" has different meanings in the psychiatric and neurologic literature. Psychiatric stupor has been defined as "a temporary reduction or obliteration of both reactive and spontaneous relational functions" (33). Johnson (34) defined stupor as "a state of total psychomotor inhibition with retained normal or partial consciousness." This is obviously quite different from the standard neurologic definition. Yet it has been asserted that "stupor and catatonia have often been used interchangeably." Bleuler (2) considered it a form of "reduced psychic activity or of total blocking." He also merged states he considered "clouded" or "twilights" with conditions of complete alertness internally with external manifestations of stupor or coma. Examples would be the "comatose" patient who recalls complete details of events occurring during the apparent coma, or the patient who rouses from lethargy upon receiving the appropriate cue, then lapses back into the torpid state. Catatonic stupor has been reported with organic brain diseases, including brain tumors, metabolic derangements such as diabetic ketoacidosis, and hepatic encephalopathy, implying the existence of "neurologic" or true stupor, a condition in the continuum to coma, rather than a psychogenic stupor or pseudocoma. One report describes a patient with catatonia resembling nonconvulsive status epilepticus, thus presenting the appearance of a clouded consciousness. The issues of stupor, coma, and pseudocoma are discussed later, as they raise questions about the overlap between neurologic and psychiatric disorders.

Hyperkinetic states punctuate the akinetic, plastic, unresponsive baseline. This hyperactive phenomenon, along with the frequently more benign prognosis than is typical for schizophrenia, supported the association between catatonia and affective states, particularly manic depression (28). These opposite poles of the catatonic syndromes, which were termed "catatonic stupor" and "catatonic excitement," represented Kahlbaum's description of catatonia as having a cyclic alternating course (31). These hyperactive states involved outbursts of senseless activity such as running, jumping, exercising, and yelling.

Stereotypies of all types—motor, speech, and thought—were "one of the most striking external manifestations of schizophrenia" (2). The simple stereotypies, such as clapping, rocking, and tapping, appear similar to those seen in many other disorders. The complex behavioral routines, such as walking in a circle, bowing, and reciting a song, may be more diagnostic. Earlier authors (2) subsumed many of the features of catalepsy under the rubric of stereotypy, such as fixed bizarre postures, as well as features of immobility. Words, tunes, phrases, or rhymes may be repeated endlessly or for a precise number of times. In catatonia the stereotypy may be linked to an obvious conscious effort that differs from that seen in retardation, autism, and sensory deprivation but can be similar to the ritualistic behavior common in OCD. Some stereotypies, such as the rewriting of a phrase, are unlikely to be seen in organic disorders.

Mannerisms are a common feature of catatonia. Bleuler (2) noted that mannerisms may be always present but highly variable in certain individuals. For example, a patient may always grimace but may alter the facial expression each time or accompany it by a variety of body movements or sounds.

A core feature of catatonia is negativism, which can be divided into passive and active forms. In passive negativism the patient fails to perform the requested activity, and in the active form the patient performs the opposite. The rigid postural abnormality may be interpreted as a form of negativism, with the patient in some cases resisting the movement of a limb to a new position, in contrast to the patient with waxy flexibility, who may assist the examiner in the repositioning.

As with catatonic stupor and catatonic excitement, catatonic negativism has its polar opposite, command automatism. In this condition the patient obeys all commands like an automaton even when the request results in harm or in some other way goes against the patient's own externally perceived interest. Echopraxia describes the syndrome in which patients repeat activities that they see. Thus, one patient who displays a bizarre stereotypy may be emulated by another with echopraxia. Echolalia is the repetition of sounds and phrases. Communicating with such a patient is, of course, extremely difficult. Patients may be echolalic or echopractic or both.

Automatisms are activities carried out in response to inner commands. They are indistinguishable from activities displayed as part of a compulsion. The patient may in fact not want to perform the action and may find the impulse foreign, although it emerged from the patient's mind. Sometimes the automatism stands in contrast to other actions the patient is taking. For example, a patient may work at cleaning an area and then suddenly mess it up or break some object only to mend it.

The final category of the catatonic symptom complex Bleuler describes is impulsivity, which, he says, "often dominates the picture." The impulsivity, which may be explosive or less extreme, lasts from seconds to hours, rarely for days. The sudden discharge restores a sense of calm as if psychic tension has been temporarily relieved. The overlap among this form of impulse dyscontrol, automatic behavior responding to inner voices, and compulsive behavior in response perhaps to a perceived interruption of a mental or physical ritual can only be made in the context of the patient's diagnosis and other behavioral problems. Speech abnormalities, including echolalia (repetition of words and phrases), palilalia (repetition of syllables), and verbigeration (use of meaningless words and phrases), are sometimes present.

The presence of "neurologic" motor manifestations in catatonia raises questions, addressed later, regarding the diagnosis of catatonia in an organic disease. "Gegenhalten," a tone abnormality in which patients seemingly increase their resistance to passive movements, transiently producing a go-and-stop ratchety-type rigidity, is sometimes difficult to distinguish from the extrapyramidal rigidity of Parkinson's disease. Catatonia has been described as a rare feature of multiple sclerosis and central pontine myelinolysis. It has also been precipitated by psychotropic drugs.

Epidemiology

The prevalence of catatonia and its relation to various psychiatric disorders is still being determined. In part this is due to changing criteria for diagnosis (e.g., DSM-III versus DSM-IV). It is a function of both the diligence or lack of it in investigators, and the criteria used in terms of both the absolute criteria applied and how significant the sign must be to be counted. Bleuler (2) reported that more than half of institutionalized patients displayed "catatonic symptoms either transitorily or permanently." Mahendra (35) noted that the decreasing incidence of catatonia had been recognized for years and speculated that many of the cases described in the earlier literature may have had encephalitis lethargica, not primary schizophrenia. He also noted the association between catatonia and manic depression but

agreed that the syndrome had become less common. Gelenberg (30), considering catatonia a generic term describing a syndrome found in organic and functional disorders, including nonpsychotic neurotic conditions, wrote that it "is not a rare phenomenon." In my own university psychiatric hospital a review of discharge diagnostic codes between July 1991 and July 1996 yielded only three patients with a principal diagnosis of catatonia out of 20,545 admissions. This survey would have ignored all patients with catatonic features but a principal diagnosis of other types of schizophrenia, affective disorder, organic diseases, and many other disorders. The rarity of the diagnosis supports the observation that catatonic schizophrenia, a common entity in the 19th and early 20th centuries (2,31), has undergone a dramatic decline, akin, perhaps, to the decline in hebephrenic schizophrenia. Northoff (36) reported that the catatonia diagnosis constituted 2.5% of all admissions to a German psychiatric hospital.

Looking at catatonia as a syndrome, a collection of motor signs yields a vastly different result. In 140 consecutive admissions to an inpatient psychiatry service, 90% of which were emergency admissions, "catatonic syndrome" was diagnosed 15 times in 12 patients, constituting 9% of all admissions for the year. Four of these patients had an affective disorder, 2 had paranoid schizophrenia, 2 had atypical psychoses, 3 had organic causes (two of these due to cocaine), and 1 had a nonpsychotic personality disorder (37). In one year 65 patients admitted to a university hospital psychiatry service were catatonic, of whom 19 were schizophrenic, 16 depressed, and 30 "idiopathic." Other authors, using DSM-IV criteria, found "catatonic features," that is, any one of the five DSM-IV features of at least a moderate degree, in 49 (37.7%) of 130 consecutive drug-free patients admitted to a university psychiatric hospital. Only 5 patients (4%) were diagnosed with catatonic schizophrenia. Note the difference between this incidence and the incidence of catatonic schizophrenia cited earlier. There were no significant differences in psychiatric diagnoses between those admitted with catatonic features and those without; that is, catatonia did not cluster in one or two primary diagnostic categories. Patients with catatonic features suffered from various types of schizophrenia, affective disorder (depression and mania), OCD, and dementia. Bush et al. (29) found that 15 (7%) of 215 consecutive patients admitted to a university psychiatric hospital over a 6-month period met DSM-IV criteria for catatonia. In a review of 28 patients referred to a university psychiatric service meeting predetermined criteria for catatonia, regardless of underlying diagnosis, immobility or stupor was seen in all. Staring, mutism, and withdrawal were the next most common signs, present in more than 80%. Posturing and rigidity were present in more than 60%. Waxy flexibility was present in 40%, stereotypy in 30%, excitement and impulsivity in more than 40%. Grasp reflexes and gegenhalten were not present in any patients (29).

Some authors assert that catatonia can be readily distinguished from related syndromes (38). Starkstein et al. (38) used a modified Rogers scale to evaluate 79 consecutive outpatients referred to a psychiatric clinic for evaluation of depression and compared these with 41 consecutive nondepressed Parkinson's disease outpatients seen in routine follow-up. They found 16 depressed patients with catatonia. The Parkinson's disease patients (severity of illness not described) matched with the catatonics for rigidity, slowness, and immobility could be distinguished from the catatonia patients according to abnormal postures, persistence of imposed postures, mutism, underactivity, stereotypies, mannerisms, hyperactivity, and echolalia. Bush et al. (29) assert that using strict guidelines, catatonia patients are clearly distinguished from noncatatonic psychiatric patients, confirming another report. Although the underlying psychiatric diagnoses varied considerably, the catatonic syndrome appeared in a variety of primary and secondary psychiatric disorders (42).

Thus catatonic features, when looked for, are apparently quite common, even in unmedicated patients with a wide variety of psychiatric disorders. The term "catatonic syndrome," denoting the presence of two or more motor signs meeting DSM-IV criteria, is also common, probably in the 5% to 10% range of patients requiring psychiatric admission. The underlying psychiatric diagnoses in which the catatonic syndrome occurs fall into a broad spectrum, including schizophrenia, affective and organic psychoses, OCD, and, rarely, nonpsychiatric disorders. However, catatonic schizophrenia appears to be fairly rare, reflecting an epidemiologic change in schizophrenia, alterations in treatment, or alterations in diagnostic criteria as reflected in the revisions of the DSM.

Catatonia is rare in children and adolescents, with only 51 cases being reported as of 1999, the date of the most recent review (39). Only a single child younger than 10 years and four children younger than 13 years have been reported. The gender distribution favors males among children, whereas women are more commonly catatonic than men. Electroconvulsive therapy (ECT) may be the treatment of choice in catatonic children with an underlying psychotic depression (39).

Lethal Catatonia

One particular variant of catatonia, not yet identified with an underlying disease, is lethal catatonia or malignant catatonia (40,41). This syndrome, initially described in the preneuroleptic era, appears to be similar to neuroleptic malignant syndrome, with obtundation, extreme rigidity, and autonomic dysfunction leading to death but without exposure to any neuroleptic. The few autopsies of such patients have not found uniform abnormalities. Some authors suggested that neuroleptic malignant syndrome (NMS) is a drug-induced variant of lethal catatonia; however, another syndrome mimicking NMS occurs rarely when levodopa or amantadine is abruptly discontinued in patients with Parkinson's disease who have no history of psychiatric dysfunction. This suggests that psychiatric dysfunction need not be present for dopamine-blocking or depleting drugs to induce such a syndrome. The serotonin syndrome, which also resembles NMS, is another syndrome to consider in patients who are rigid, tremulous, and febrile; it is seen in patients typically taking serotonin-enhancing medications and a monoamine oxidase inhibitor.

As with catatonia in general, the response to ECT has been excellent (42).

Biological Basis

One can separate catatonia into organic and nonorganic categories. Using current terminology, the psychiatric, nonorganic, or functional catatonic disorders are schizophrenia or affective psychosis. The organic causes are numerous. Bush et al. (29) described cases brought on by neuroleptics (NMS and neuroleptic catatonia), anticholinergics, valproic acid, and risperidone in combination, as well as seizures and steroid-induced stupor. Encephalitis lethargica, which may induce both parkinsonism and psychiatric disorders, is one viral cause. While the virus has never been identified and has not been seen in epidemic form in 60 years, it may still be a causative factor in some cases. Other viral syndromes may rarely cause catatonia. Among other causes of catatonia are structural brain lesions, including tumors, infarcts, and hemorrhages in a variety of locations (30), such as thalamus, third ventricle, frontal lobes, and temporal lobes. Catatonia may be induced by metabolic conditions, including neuroleptic-induced disorders, aspirin intoxication, porphyria, hepatic encephalopathy, hypercalcemia, poisoning, and structural or metabolic disorders such as Wernicke's encephalopathy. Infectious causes include encephalitis lethargica, AIDS dementia complex, and typhoid fever. Certain uses of the term "catatonia," including as a replacement for "akinetic mutism," should be discouraged, as the two syndromes are quite different. It is unclear in many reports how the terms "stupor," "coma," and "immobility" are defined.

Perhaps the strongest support for a biological basis for catatonia comes from genetic advances. An identified missense mutation in a gene on chromosome 22 appears to cause an autosomal dominant form of schizophrenia with periodic catatonia (43). However, there appear to be other causes for familial schizophrenic syndromes with catatonia as well. The identified gene on chromosome 22 is thought to code for a protein involved in neuronal cation channels.

One author suggested that the medial frontal lobes may be important in catatonia based on rare case report material of lesions to this region causing gengenhalten, waxy flexibility, mutism, apathy, and loss of will (44). However, the rare physiologic imaging studies have not shown abnormalities in these areas and have not been consistent with each other either, consistent with the possible multiple etiologies for catatonia, the small number of subjects, and the still early stages in the development of these techniques (45).

Animal models of catatonia should be viewed with skepticism, as the psychiatric aspects of catatonia are crucial to a meaningful concept. Simply rendering an animal or person an akinetic mute via reserpine, neuroleptics, or a brainstem lesion would hardly advance insight into this condition. One report has found computed tomographic evidence of brainstem and cerebellar vermis atrophy in five cases of catatonia, but these findings are nonspecific and small. To attempt to localize a clinicopathologic correlation to midbrain pathology (28) is probably premature. Physiologic imaging will be more useful when applied to a large series of similar subjects.

If one looks at psychodynamic explanations for some of the "functional" cases, the concept of blocking figures quite large. When resistance to physical and emotional stimuli results in rigidity, negativism, muteness, and so on, leading to psychic tension, an eruption occurs (catatonic excitement), temporarily relieving the emotional pressure.

Treatment

Despite the apparent differences in causation, a significant number of reports indicate that catatonia, whether schizophrenic or affective, can be treated successfully with lorazepam or ECT (37,42). Reports on the successful treatment of neuroleptic malignant syndrome with ECT also have been published. Bush et al. (42) enrolled 28 catatonia patients in a trial of lorazepam for 5 days, followed by ECT if necessary. Of these, 5 patients experienced spontaneous remission, and 21 of 23 patients had a response to lorazepam. Improvements were seen in 16 of 21, with 11 having complete relief. Improvement varied inversely with the duration of signs prior to the treatment. ECT was successful in all four of the patients who were unresponsive to lorazepam. The fifth refused ECT. Success was defined as "catatonia no longer present." The authors noted that 2 of 3 patients with neuroleptic-induced catatonia responded to a single dose of intravenous lorazepam. Some 32% of patients were not psychotic upon completion of the treatment protocol. Patients primarily had the excited variant of catatonia.

Rosebush et al. (37) prospectively treated all patients suffering from catatonia with intravenous lorazepam, documenting that of 15 patients "12 responded completely or dramatically within 2 hours." Of these 12 patients, 8 had histories or evidence of coexisting neurologic disorders, such as old stroke, hydrocephalus, or alcohol abuse. One nonresponder had a personality disorder. Another responded to a ventricular peritoneal shunt. Four of the lorazepam responders took other benzodiazepines prior to

and during lorazepam treatment. Catatonia recurred if lorazepam was not maintained. Subjects in this series primarily had the depressed form of catatonia. Severity of the psychiatric disorder once the catatonia resolved was not discussed.

Ungvari et al. prospectively treated 18 catatonic patients, and those with the diagnosis of schizophrenia improved partially. The authors hypothesized that underlying diagnosis was important in outcome, unlike others (42) who noted no response differences among schizophrenic, affective, or organic patients. Several isolated reports also support the use of lorazepam and other benzodiazepines. One report describes a case of catatonia responsive within 50 minutes to one dose of oral lorazepam 2.5 mg, which reversed with a single dose of a benzodiazepine antagonist (see ref. 46 for a videotape demonstrating a catatonic patient's response to intravenous lorazepam). In the only placebo-controlled double-blind trial of lorazepam in catatonia, 12 patients with chronic schizophrenic catatonia were treated in a crossover trial. None had a beneficial response to lorazepam (47). Underlying diagnosis or duration of the catatonia may be pertinent to treatment responsiveness. Antipsychotics, including the atypicals, have been reported to be effective (48).

ECT has also been shown in several open studies, both retrospective and prospective (34,42), to cure the catatonic aspect of the psychosis. Ungvari et al. reported that 9 of 18 patients who failed lorazepam improved with ECT. Bush et al. (42) reported that 4 of 5 lorazepam failures responded promptly to ECT.

CONCLUSION

The existence of a syndrome, seen in a variety of primary psychiatric disorders as well as in organic disorders, all responsive by and large to lorazepam or ECT, raises the question as to whether these signs have a similar mechanism. The one report of reversal of improvement with a benzodiazepine antagonist supports the concept of a single pharmacologic mechanism responsive to benzodiazepines, possibly via a GABA mechanism. However, the case reports (37) of patients already on benzodiazepines (42) responding to lorazepam suggests either that lorazepam has a special action different from that of other benzodiazepines, or that these patients may have been only partially treated and required the extra boost of an intravenous infusion. More likely is the conclusion that catatonia is a heterogeneous syndrome. Some experts believe treatment must be designed with this in mind. Presumably further studies will determine whether catatonia has a single common pathway manifest in a variety of disorders or, like stereotypy, simply represents a common collection of behaviors that simply overlap among the various conditions.

The term "medical catatonia" should be reserved for catatonic syndromes in which a psychosis or other behavioral disorder is precipitated by a systemic medical condition such as dementia, encephalitis, lupus cerebritis, or toxic encephalopathy, in which an organic psychosis occurs.

SUMMARY

Stereotypy and catatonia are general terms for complex behavioral patterns that appear in a wide variety of disorders. It is clear that stereotypies arise from a multiple brain disorders with highly varied mechanisms, both structural and metabolic. It is unlikely that a unitary theory can be found to explain the variety of stereotypies. Catatonia, which can be conceived of in broad terms as a complex stereotypic disorder, with a fixed response to inner and external stimuli, also appears in a variety of syndromes: schizophrenia, affective psychoses, and medical diseases. The response of many of these patients to lorazepam suggests the possibility of a single shared biochemical lesion for the psychiatric cases. Further studies, especially those looking at biochemical and physiological changes will undoubtedly prove helpful.

REFERENCES

1. Jankovic J. Stereotypies. In: Marsden CD, Fahn S, eds. *Movement disorders 3.* London: Butterworth-Heinemann, 1994:503–517.
2. Bleuler E. *Dementia praecox.* New York: International University Press, 1950.
3. American Psychiatric Press. *Diagnostic and statistical manual of mental disorders (3),* 4th ed. Washington, DC: APA, 1994.
4. Stacey M, Cardoso F, Jankovic J. Tardive stereotypy and other movement disorders in tardive dyskinesia. *Neurology* 1993;43:937–941.
5. Tan A, Salgado M, Fahn S. The characterization and outcome of stereotypic movements in nonautistic children. *Mov Disord* 1997;12:47–52.
6. Kravitz H, Boehm JJ. Rhythmic and habit patterns of infancy: their sequence, age of onset and frequency. *Child Dev* 1971;42:399–413.
7. Sallustro A, Atwell CS. Body rocking, head banging, and head rolling in normal children. *J Pediatr* 1978;93:704–708.
8. Niehaus DJ, Emsley RA, Brink P, et al. Stereotypies: prevalence and association with compulsive and impulsive symptoms in college students. *Psychopathology* 2000;33:31–35.
9. Lees AJ. Facial mannerisms and tics. *Adv Neurol* 1988;49:255–261.
10. Jankovic J. Phenomenology of tics. *Mov Disord* 1986;1:17–26.
11. Ridley RM. The psychology of perseverative and stereotyped behavior. *Prog Neurobiol* 1994;44:221–231.
12. Sadock BJ, Sadock VA, eds. *Kaplan and Sadock's Comprehensive textbook of psychiatry,* 7th ed. Philadelphia: Lippincott Williams & Wilkins, 2000.
13. Hymas N, Lees A, Bolton D, et al. The neurology of obsessional slowness. *Brain* 1991;114:2203–2233.
14. Troster H, Brambring M, Beelmann A. Prevalence and situational causes of stereotyped behaviors in blind infants and preschoolers. *J Abnorm Child Psychol* 1991;19:569–590.
15. Troster H. Prevalence and functions of stereotyped behaviors in nonhandicapped children in residential care. *J Abnorm Child Psychol* 1994;22:79–97.
16. Shahbazian MD, Zoghbi HY. Molecular genetics of Rett syndrome and clinical spectrum of MECP2 mutations. *Curr Opin Neurol* 2001;14:171–176.
17. FitzGerald PM, Jankovic J, Percy AK. Rett syndrome and associated movement disorders. *Mov Disord* 1990;5:195–202.
18. Sato S, Hashimoto T, Nakamura A, et al. Stereotyped stepping associated with lesions in the bilateral frontoparietal cortices. *Neurology* 2001;57:711–713.
19. Fernandez HH, Friedman JH. Punding on L-dopa. *Mov Disord* 1999;14:836–838.
20. Rojahn J. Self injurious and stereotypic behavior of noninstitutionalized mentally retarded people: prevalence and classification. *Am J Ment Retard* 1986;91:268–276.
21. Cross HA, Harlow HF. Prolonged and progressive effects of partial isolation on the behavior of macaque monkeys. *J Exp Res Person* 1965;1:39–44.
22. Xu M, Moratalla R, Gold LH, et al. Dopamine D1 receptor mutant mice are deficient in striatal expression of dynorphin and in dopamine-mediated behavioral responses. *Cell* 1994;79:729–742.
23. Canales JJ, Graybiel AM. A measure of striatal function predicts motor stereotypy. *Nature Neurosci* 2000;3:377–383.
24. Canales JJ, Gilmour G, Iversen SD. The role of nigral and thalamic output pathways in the expression of oral stereotypies induced by amphetamine injections into the striatum. *Brain Res* 2000;856:176–183.
25. Jankovic J, Beach J. Long-term effects of tetrabenazine in hyperkinetic movement disorder. *Neurology* 1997;48:358–362.
26. Baldessarini RJ. Drugs and the treatment of psychiatric disorders: depression and mania. In: Hardman JG, Limbird LE, Molinoff PB, et al., eds. *Goodman and Gilman's Pharmacological basis of therapeutics,* 9th ed. New York: McGraw-Hill, 1996:431–460.
27. Fink M. Catatonia. In: Trimble MR, Cumming JL, eds. *Contemporary behavioral neurology.* Woburn, MA: Butterworth-Heinemann, 1997:289–310.
28. Johnson J. Catatonia: the tension insanity. *Br J Psychiatr* 1993;162:733–738.
29. Bush G, Fink M, Petrides G, et al. Catatonia: 1. Rating scale and standardized examination. *Acta Psychiatr Scand* 1996;93:129–136.
30. Gelenberg AJ. The catatonic syndrome. *Lancet* 1976;1:1339–1341.
31. Kahlbaum KL. *Catatonia* (translated by Levi Y, Pridon T). Baltimore: Johns Hopkins University Press, 1973.
32. Peralta V, Cuesta MJ. Motor features in psychotic disorders. II. Development of diagnostic criteria for catatonia. *Schizophr Res* 2001;47:117–126.
33. Berrios GE. Stupor revisited. *Comp Psychiatry* 1981;22:466–477.
34. Johnson J. Stupor: a review of 25 cases. *Acta Psychiatr Scand* 1984;70:370–377.
35. Mahendra B. Where have all the catatonics gone? *Psychol Med* 1981;11:669–671.
36. Northoff G, Koch A, Wenke J, et al. Catatonia as a psychomotor syndrome: a rating scale and extrapyramidal motor symptoms. *Mov Disord* 1999;14:404–416.
37. Rosebush P, Hildebrand AM, Furlong BG, et al. Catatonic syndrome in a general psychiatric inpatient population: frequency, clinical presentation, and response to lorazepam. *J Clin Psychiatr* 1990;51:357–362.
38. Starkstein S, Petracca G, Teson A, et al. Catatonia in depression: prevalence, clinical correlates, and validation of a scale. *J Neurol Neurosurg Psychiatry* 1996;60:326–332.

39. Cohen D, Flament M, Dubos PF, et al. Case series: catatonic syndrome in young people. *J Am Acad Child Adolesc Psychiatry* 1999; 38:1040–1046.

40. Stauder KH. Die todliche Katatonie. *Arch Psychiatr Nervenkr* 1934;102:614–634.

41. Philbrick KL, Rummans TA. Malignant catatonia. *J Neuropsychiatry Clin Neurosci* 1994;6:1–13.

42. Bush G, Fink M, Petrides G, et al. Catatonia: 2. Treatment with lorazepam and electroconvulsive therapy. *Acta Psychiatr Scand* 1996;93:137–143.

43. Meyer J, Huberth A, Ortega G, et al. A missense mutation in a novel gene encoding a putative cation channel is associated with catatonic schizophrenia in a large pedigree. *Mol Psychiatry* 2001; 6:302–306.

44. Joseph R. Frontal lobe psychopathology: mania, depression, confabulation, catatonia, perseveration, obsessive compulsions, and schizophrenia. *Psychiatry* 1999;62:138–172.

45. Escobar R, Rios A, Montoya ID, et al. Clinical and cerebral blood flow changes in catatonic patients treated with ECT. *J Psychosom Res* 2000;49:423–429.

46. Rosenfeld MJ, Friedman JH. Catatonia responsive to lorazepam: a case report. *Mov Disord* 1999:14:161–162.

47. Ungvari GS, Chiu HFK, Chow LY, et al. Lorazepam for chronic catatonia: a randomized, double-blind, placebo-controlled crossover study. *Psychopharmacology* 1999;142:393–398.

48. Valevski A, Loeb T, Keren T, et al. Response of catatonia to risperidone: two case reports. *Clin Neuropharmacol* 2001;24: 228–231.

MOVEMENT DISORDERS IN CHILDREN

HARVEY S. SINGER

Movement disorders in children provide diagnostic and therapeutic challenges that are similar to those seen in adults. Precise definitions of specific movements in children and adults overlap, and both are frequently classified either by the type of movement (e.g., dystonia, tremor, tic) or etiology (genetic, infection, vascular). In this chapter, the major focus will be on disorders that are more specific to children and less likely to appear elsewhere in this text. In order to avoid overlap and redundancy, movement disorders seen frequently in children, such as Tourette's syndrome (1a; see Chapter 22), dystonia (see Chapters 23 and 24), and chorea (see Chapter 15), will be dealt with in the respective chapters. Motor abnormalities seen in the pediatric population have several prominent differences from those occurring in adulthood, including (a) the presence of motor phenomena that are considered normal in early development; (b) the high prevalence of paroxysmal movement disorders (covered in other chapters); (c) the frequent association of extrapyramidal symptoms with hereditary/metabolic disorders; and (d) the residua of a static encephalopathy representing the primary etiology for chronic motor dysfunction in children. Each of these dissimilarities, in turn, provides an approach for classifying movement disorders and the basis for the four major sections within this chapter. In addition, since in the pediatric population it is often difficult to define an evolving, variable, progressive movement disorder as strictly chorea, dystonia, or other, and since multiple listing of disorders may cause further confusion, this author favors listings under the more generic term "extrapyramidal symptoms." As will readily be evident, the field of movement disorders within child neurology has rapidly evolved into an area of superspecialization.

GENERAL APPROACH TO THE CHILD WITH A MOVEMENT DISORDER

As a general rule, movement disorders are best diagnosed after being observed by a knowledgeable physician. Video-tapes are essential, especially when the problem is interspersed with periods of normalcy. An accurate description of the symptoms (including age of onset, type of movement, course, focality, timing, triggers, patient's ability to control, progression, effect on activities, associated difficulties, and others) is extremely important in defining the disorder. Historical details about the patient's gestation, delivery, early development, previous illnesses, drug history, exposure to potential toxins, as well as social and family history are often essential for proper classification. A critical feature is determining whether the presenting signs/symptoms are part of a static condition or are associated with loss of previously acquired skills (degenerative disorder). A comprehensive general examination is essential for properly defining the movement and identifying clues indicating a systemic problem. Since children with paroxysmal disorders often do not have attacks while in the physician's office, documentation of such attacks frequently requires the family to provide a videotaped recording. As will be discussed, especially with younger children, many unusual movements may be transient and do not represent pathologic disorders.

In approaching the child with a history of an episodic movement disorder, it is not uncommon for the clinician initially to consider the diagnosis of epilepsy. At times, separation of seizures from a dyskinetic movement disorder can be confusing because both attacks are paroxysmal, may have a preceding sensory phenomenon (e.g., complex partial seizures and paroxysmal choreoathetosis), and can respond to anticonvulsant medications. Factors helpful in separating dyskinetic disorders from epilepsy include the identification of certain specific movements (e.g., dystonic, choreoathetoid, tic-like, or stereotyped movements), maintenance of consciousness, a normal respiratory pattern, lack of a postictal state, and absence of an electroencephalographic (EEG) abnormality during attacks. Some conditions, such as supplementary motor area seizures and frontal lobe ictal discharges causing paroxysmal hypnogenic dyskinesia, clearly require EEG monitoring to clarify the diagnosis.

TRANSIENT DEVELOPMENTAL DISORDERS

Through experience the clinician learns that many newborns and infants manifest a variety of dyskinetic movements that tend to be brief in duration and of no apparent pathologic consequence (Table 31.1). Pursing and sucking of the lips, head and neck extensions, body and extremity twists, turns, and postures are but a few of the myriad of movements labeled as physiologic chorea or dystonia (1,2). Unfortunately, since little has been done to investigate these phenomena, their frequency and physiologic mechanisms remain undetermined. One speculation is that these movements may represent an interplay between the development of voluntary movements in an evolving nervous system and the presence of primitive reflexive responses. Difficulties with early coordination are routinely part of the maturational process. For example, a broad-based, uncoordinated, "ataxic" gait is the norm in infants beginning to walk independently. Brief myoclonic jerks are also common in early development. A more extreme example, with onset in the first month of life, is benign neonatal myoclonus. Head banging, body rocking, and hand flapping movements may occur in about one fourth of normal children (3). Shuddering and paroxysmal torticollis are benign movements that begin in infancy and resolve in childhood. Sandifer's syndrome (dyspeptic dystonia) represents an exaggerate posturing in young children due to the presence of gastrointestinal reflux.

Benign Neonatal Myoclonus

Movements are intermittent, repetitive, unilateral or bilateral, and largely confined to sleep (4). Onset is usually in the first month of life and myoclonus persists for several months, rarely into early childhood (5). Jerks may be triggered by noise and occur in brief clusters for several minutes before stopping spontaneously. They appear most frequently during quiet sleep and least often during REM sleep. In benign neonatal myoclonus, neurologic examina-

TABLE 31.1. TRANSIENT DEVELOPMENTAL DISORDERS

A. Chorea/dystonia
 Physiologic chorea or dystonia
B. Myoclonus
 Benign neonatal myoclonus
C. Torticollis
 Benign paroxysmal torticollis
 Sandifer's syndrome
 Spasmus nutans
D. Shuddering
 Shuddering (shivering) attacks
E. Head nodding
 Periodic head nodding
 Spasmus nutans

tion, EEG examination, and neuroimaging studies are normal, and there is no subsequent association with developmental delay or seizures (6,7).

Shuddering (Shivering) Attacks

Shuddering or shivering attacks are a benign movement disorder (8–10). Attacks are brief and may occur up to hundreds of times per day. Episodes start in infancy or early childhood, tend to become less frequent, and often spontaneously remit during the first decade. Three children studied with EEG monitoring during the attacks showed no alteration of the electrocerebral background (9). The cause of shuddering attacks is unknown. On the basis of a strong family history of essential tremor, it has been hypothesized that shuddering attacks may be a precursor for essential tremor. One patient has been successfully treated with beta blockade (10). Antiepileptic drugs do not suppress the movements.

Benign Paroxysmal Torticollis

Benign paroxysmal torticollis typically occurs within the first 8 months of life. Attacks comprising torticollis and slight head and neck movements may last from minutes to weeks (range 10 minutes to 14 days) (11,12). Some attacks may be preceded by agitation, crying, pallor, and vomiting, but no precipitating factor has been identified. Patients may have several attacks within a month and the torticollis may alternate from side to side. There is no diurnal fluctuation and torticollis is not affected by sleep. The attacks typically cease spontaneously by age 5 years, and no treatment is effective. Children with paroxysmal torticollis often later develop migraine with or without initially having benign paroxysmal vertigo. The latter is a disorder of otherwise healthy infants and young children who develop the sudden onset of severe vertigo.

Studies in children with paroxysmal torticollis including neuroimaging, cerebrospinal fluid (CSF) analysis, and EEG monitoring have been unremarkable. The precise etiology remains unknown, but some cases may be familial. A dysfunction of the vestibular apparatus has been hypothesized since some patients fail to develop nystagmus with ice water caloric testing or have an abnormal computerized sinusoidal rotation study (11,13). In contrast, an association with paroxysmal vertigo, the subsequent development of migraine, and a strong family history for migraine has suggested a migraine equivalent or disruption of blood flow to the brainstem (14).

Sandifer's Syndrome (Dyspeptic Dystonia)

This syndrome is one of gastroesophageal reflux, with or without a hiatal hernia, associated with dystonic movements of the head and neck and, at times, abnormal posturings of the body, including opisthotonos. Recurrent paroxysmal posturings are typically associated with feedings, although they may persist postprandially. Barium swallowing studies, esophagoscopy, and pH probes are used to document the reflux and hernia. Symptoms usually resolve after appropriate gastrointestinal intervention (15).

Head Nodding

Periodic head nodding, consisting of repetitive flexion of the neck, is seen in otherwise normal children. This entity needs to be differentiated from the more serious condition referred to as bobble-head doll syndrome. In the latter, infants and young children have intermittent jerky head movements, resembling those of a dolls's head perched atop a spring, with a frequency ranging from 2 to 3 cycles per second. Brief voluntary control is possible. Brain imaging studies typically identify an underlying structural abnormality, usually either a third ventricular cyst, tumor, or dilatation of the third ventricle secondary to either aqueductal stenosis or a suprasellar arachnoid cyst (16–18). Cases have also been described in individuals with normal third ventricles, including one with aqueductal and fourth ventricle enlargement (19). Surgical treatment usually corrects the abnormal movement.

PAROXYSMAL MOVEMENT DISORDERS

Paroxysmal movement disorders are the most common movement abnormalities encountered by child neurologists. The list of these nonepileptic paroxysmal movement disorders is extensive, and it is extremely helpful to separate the various conditions on the basis of the type of movement disorder observed, such as ataxia, choreoathetosis, dystonia, head bob, shudder, startle, stereotypy, tic, torticollis, and so forth (Table 31.2). The first step is to have a clear definition and understanding of these abnormalities of movement. The next step often requires seeing a videotape recording of the child's attack because patient/parent history may be vague and inconclusive. The diagnostic possibilities can then be considered and the likely disorder identified. Lastly, after fully assessing the child with an episodic atypical movement, the physician, in conjunction with the patient, family, and school personnel, must determine whether movements are having a negative functional or psychological impact. Medications should be targeted and reserved only for those problems that are disabling and not remediable by other interventions.

Associated with Ataxia

Several familial forms of episodic ataxia have been identified, each representing a different genetic disorder (see Chapter 37).

TABLE 31.2. PAROXYSMAL MOVEMENT DISORDERS

A. Ataxia
  Episodic ataxia without myokymia
  Episodic ataxia with myokymia
  Episodic ataxia with paroxysmal choreoathetosis
  Paroxysmal tonic upgaze with ataxia
  Familial metabolic periodic ataxias
  Other
B. Choreoathetosis or dystonia
  Paroxysmal dystonic choreoathetosis
  Paroxysmal kinesigenic choreoathetosis
  Intermediate or exertion induced
  Paroxysmal hypnogenic dyskinesia
  Secondary paroxysmal dyskinesias
C. Startle
  Hyperekplexia
  Startle epilepsy
  Brainstem reticular reflex myoclonus
  Others
D. Stereotypic movements
  Stereotypies (nonautistic and autistic types)
E. Tics
  Transient tics
  Chronic (motor/vocal) tic disorder
  Tourette's syndrome
  Tourette-like disorder
  Tardive tourettism

Associated with Choreoathetosis or Dystonia

One commonly used classification identifies four variants: paroxysmal kinesigenic dyskinesia (PKD), paroxysmal nonkinesigenic dyskinesia (PND), intermediate or exertional dyskinesia (PED), and paroxysmal hypnogenic dyskinesia (PHD) (19a; see Chapter 29). Secondary paroxysmal dyskinesias have been reported in association with a variety of calcium and metabolic problems, thyroid dysfunction, cerebral palsy (CP), post head trauma, medullary hemorrhage, and spinal cord lesions (19b).

Associated with Startle

A startle response is a brief motor response, usually a jerk, elicited by an unexpected auditory or, less commonly, tactile, visual, or vestibular stimulus. A normal startle response to auditory stimuli usually involves the upper half of the body and readily habituates. In contrast, in startle syndromes, movements are of greater amplitude, are more widely distributed, and habituate poorly. In most patients with startle disease (hyperekplexia), the startle is immediately followed by another movement abnormality. For example, several seconds after the initial startle, there may be a period of generalized stiffening lasting for seconds, termed *tonic spasms*. While these occur the patient is unable to respond voluntarily and, if standing, will fall rigidly to the ground without losing consciousness. If prevented from falling to the floor, the patient appears stiff despite a loss of muscle tone. In addition to tonic spasms, patients with familial or symptomatic hyperekplexia may experience excessive repetitive flexion of the limbs, especially the legs, during sleep, termed *nocturnal myoclonic jerks*. Despite its name, the movements are not myoclonic, and jerks may occur after an unexpected stimulus or as a spontaneous event.

Hyperekplexia (Hyperexplexia; Startle Disease)

Although it has been suggested that hyperexplexia and hyperekplexia are different, the general consensus is that they probably represent similar disorders, with hyperekplexia being the preferred and correct Greek term (20). Startle disease is inherited and, according to some investigators, may also occur secondary to acquired brainstem pathology (21). Clinically the two groups appear to be relatively indistinguishable except for family history and an abnormal gene located on the long arm of chromosome 5 in the former group.

Hyperekplexia is characterized by the presence of hypertonia in the neonatal period that disappears in sleep; a non-habituating, exaggerated startle response to auditory, visual, or tactile stimuli; hyperactive brainstem reflexes (e.g., head retraction, palmomental, snout); and, frequently, feeding difficulties and apnea (22). The startle response can be elicited by tapping the forehead, glabella, vertex, or nose, and is exaggerated by tension, cold, fatigue, and anxiety. Both tonic spasms and nocturnal myoclonic jerks may be part of hyperekplexia (23). Severe neonatal hypertonia may be associated with a marked reduction of spontaneous movements, and an increased incidence of congenitally dislocated hips and abdominal hernia (24). Unexpected stimuli, such as noises or handling, can precipitate massive generalized muscle spasms causing apnea, cyanosis, even death (25). Patients are often mistakenly given the diagnosis of spastic quadriplegia. Abnormal intrauterine movements, consisting of sudden forceful jerks lasting for seconds to minutes, may occur in response to external stimuli (26). As muscle tone diminishes during the first year of life, spontaneous activity increases. Cognitive capabilities are not affected. The course of the illness is variable, with some individuals improving and others showing some progression or remaining static. A milder familial form of hyperekplexia consisting of excess startle without any associated symptoms and an association with spastic paraparesis has been reported (27,28).

Hereditary hyperekplexia is a rare, highly penetrant autosomal dominant disorder. Linkage studies have localized the gene to the distal portion of the long arm of chromosome 5 (29). Subsequent studies identified several different mutations in *GLRA1*, the gene encoding the α_1 subunit of the glycine receptor in both hereditary and sporadic cases (30–32). It has been speculated that these muta-

tions alter agonist affinities, resulting in a change in conductance states and a partial loss of function. The mechanism for tonic spasms is unknown, although it has been suggested that it arises from altered glycinergic transmission mediating recurrent inhibition of pontomedullary reticular neurons and spinal motor neurons. The neuroanatomic site for nocturnal myoclonic jerks is unknown.

Hyperekplexia has been improved with clonazepam or diazepam (22,25). Other agents, such as valproic acid, 5-hydroxytryptophan (5-HTP), and piracetam, have also produced some benefit, but clobazam has not. In life-threatening situations, where prolonged stiffness impedes respiration and produces apnea and bradycardia, hypertonia can be manually relieved by forcible flexion of the head and legs toward the trunk (33).

Associated with Stereotypies

Although often inaccurately assumed to be strictly associated with mental retardation, autism, schizophrenia, tardive dyskinesia, or neurodegenerative diseases, stereotypic movements can occur in otherwise normal children (see Chapter 30).

Associated with Tics

Tic disorders represent the most common movement disorder seen by physicians caring for children. For example, in Monroe County, Rochester, New York, the weighted prevalence estimates for tics were 23.4% for students in special education and 18.5% in regular education classrooms (34) (see Chapter 22).

HEREDITARY/METABOLIC DISORDERS ASSOCIATED WITH EXTRAPYRAMIDAL SYMPTOMS

Movement abnormalities in children are frequently associated with hereditary metabolic disorders (Table 31.3). Because these entities are often typified by an evolving and variable pattern of signs and symptoms, they are commonly multilisted under headings of chorea, dystonia, and parkinsonism. For the clinician, this often leads to confusion, especially in the pediatric population where it may be difficult to define the dominating symptom or, in evolving disorders, to state which movement type dominates the disorder. With this in mind, this author believes that for progressive childhood disorders that have movement abnormalities as significant symptoms it is best to use the more generic term "extrapyramidal symptoms." In addition, the use of a broader heading enables a more comprehensible subdivision-based etiology. Predominating symptoms, if present, are given in the description of each disease.

TABLE 31.3. HEREDODEGENERATIVE CAUSES OF EXTRAPYRAMIDAL SYMPTOMS

A. Pediatric Neurotransmitter Disorders
  i. Tetrahydrobiopterin (BH4) metabolism
     a) BH4 defects *with* hyperphenylalaninemia
        AR form of GTP-1 cyclohydrolase deficiency
        6-Pyruvotetrahydropterin synthase deficiency
        Dihydropteridine reductase deficiency
     a) BH4 defects *without* hyperphenylalaninemia
        Dopa-responsive dystonia
        Dihydropteridin reductase deficiency without
           hyperphenylalaninemia
        Sepiapterin reductase deficiency
  ii. Primary defects of monoamine biosynthesis
     a) Tyrosine hydroxylase deficiency
     b) Aromatic L-amino acid cocarboxylase deficiency
  iii. Juvenile Parkinson's disease
B. Trinucleotide Repeat Diseases
  i. Juvenile Huntington's disease
  ii. Dentatorubropallidoluysian atrophy
  iii. Spinocerebellar atrophy type 7
        OPC type 1
        Spinocerebellar atrophy type 3 (Machado-Joseph)
C. Metabolic Disorders
  i. Mineral accumulation
     a) Wilson's disease
     b) Neurodegeneration with brain iron accumulation
        Pantothenate kinase associated neurodegeneration
        HARP syndrome
     c) Fahr's syndrome
  ii. Lysosomal disorders
     a) Neuronal storage diseases
        G_{M1} gangliosidosis
        G_{M2} gangliosidosis
        Gaucher's disease
        Niemann-Pick type C
          Fabry
          Mucolipidosis
          Siaidosis
     b) Neuronal ceroid lipofuscinosis
     c) White matter (dysmyelinating) disorders
        Krabbe's disease
        Metachromatic leukodystrophy

  iii. Amino acid and organic acid disorders
     a) Glutaric aciduria type 1
     b) Methylmalonic aciduria
     c) Homocystinuria
        Hartnup
        2-Hydroxyglutaric aciduria
        3-Methylglutaconic aciduria
        Nonketotic hyperglycinemia
        Propionic aciduria
  iv. Mitochondrial disorders
     a) Leigh's syndrome
     b) Leber's hereditary optic neuropathy
        Fumerase deficiency
  v. Other metabolic
     a) Succinic semialdehyde dehydrogenase deficiency
     b) Guanidinoacetate methyltransferase deficiency
     c) Molybdenum cofactor (sulfite oxidase) deficiency
        α-Ketoglutaric aciduria
        Biotinidase and biotin deficiency
        Carbohydrate-deficient glycoprotein deficiency
        Canavan's disease
        Congenital folate/B_{12} problems
        Familial glucocorticoid deficiency
        Glucose transport defects
        Triose phosphate isomerase deficiency
        Vitamin E deficiency
D. Other
  i. Lesch-Nyhan disease
  ii. Ataxia telangiectasia
  iii. Neuroacanthocytosis
  iv. Genetic (*DYT*) primary dystonia
     Pallidal degenerations
        Familial striatal necrosis, infantile bilateral striatal
           necrosis, progressive pallidal degeneration
     Pelizaeus-Merzbacher disease

HARP, hypoprebetalipoproteinemia, acanthocytosis, retinitis pigmentosa, and pallidal degeneration.

Pediatric Neurotransmitter Diseases

The term *pediatric neurotransmitter disease* has been applied to relatively uncommon genetic disorders that affect the synthesis, metabolism, and catabolism of neurotransmitters. The primary neurotransmitters involved in these diseases are the monoamines, which include serotonin and catecholamines (dopamine and norepinephrine), and γ-aminobutyric acid (GABA).

Monoamine-related neurotransmitter diseases can be divided into separate categories based on the site of abnormality affected in the metabolic pathway, such those affecting the cofactor tetrahydrobiopterin (BH$_4$), enzymes of monoamine biosynthesis, and enzymes involved in catabolism. However, despite their differing causes, they have many

common symptoms, including developmental delay, axial hypotonia, rigidity, movement abnormalities, speech problems, feeding difficulties, abnormal eye movements, and autonomic symptoms. Diagnostic studies include CSF for analysis of monoamines [dopamine, serotonin, norepinephrine], neurotransmitter metabolites [homovanillic acid (HVA), 5-hydroxyindoleacetic acid (5-HIAA), 3-methoxy-4-hydroxylphenylglycol (MHPG), and pterin (biopterin and neopterin)], quantitative plasma and urine catecholamines, and phenylalanine loading profiles with and without BH$_4$.

Tetrahydrobiopterin Metabolism

Tetrahydrobiopterin is an essential cofactor for the neurotransmitter-synthesizing enzymes tyrosine hydroxylase (which catalyzes the conversion of tyrosine to L-dopa) and tryptophan hydroxylase (which catalyzes the conversion of tryptophan to 5-HTP as well as for phenylalanine hydroxylase (which converts phenylalanine to tyrosine). BH_4 itself is synthesized in a multistep pathway starting from guanosine triphosphate (GTP) and, when formed, requires several enzymes to maintain it in its active state. Several enzymatic defects have been identified in BH_4 metabolism, such as deficiencies in the first and rate-limiting synthesizing enzyme GTP-1 cyclohydrolase (GCHI), in the second and third enzymatic steps, namely 6-pyruvotetrahydropterin synthase (6-PTS) and sepiapterin reductase, respectively, and in the maintenance enzyme dihydropteridine reductase (DHPR). Although one might expect that a defect in BH_4 metabolism would be readily detectable based on the presence of hyperphenylalaninemia, which occurs because of a deficiency of phenylalanine hydroxylase activity, this laboratory finding is not always present. Hence, classification of BH_4 metabolism defects can be based on presentations with or without hyperphenylalaninemia.

BH_4 Defects *with* Hyperphenylalaninemia

Individuals in this group have onset in the neonatal period and include those with *autosomal recessively inherited forms of GCHI deficiency, 6-PTS deficiency,* and *DHPR deficiency* (35,36). Since each produces hyperphenylalaninemia and reduced synthesis of monoamines, clinical signs and symptoms tend to overlap. In the neonatal period, presumably due to hyperphenylalaninemia, hypotonia, poor suck, diminished movements, and microcephaly may be present. Generally, beginning several months later, more monoaminergic symptoms appear including oculogyric crises, swallowing difficulties, hypersalivation, temperature instability, variable hypo- and hyperkinetic movements, seizures, and cognitive impairment (35,37). These patients can be detected by neonatal screening for phenylketonuria (PKU). In DHPR deficiency, a secondary reduction in central nervous system (CNS) folate has led to perivascular basal ganglia calcification and multifocal subcortical perivascular demyelination (38,39).

Management of the hyperphenylalaninemia BH_4 defects includes correction of phenylalanine metabolism, central monoamine deficits, and prevention of folate deficiency. Oral BH_4 will correct the peripheral metabolism of phenylalanine when the defect is not due to a DHPR deficiency. Since BH_4 does not readily cross the blood-brain barrier, management of central monoamine deficits is achieved by the use of levodopa and 5-hydroxytryptophan in combination with carbidopa. Therapy with folinic acid and monitoring of CSF folate is recommended.

BH_4 Defects *without* Hyperphenylalaninemia

The hallmark disorder of BH_4 metabolism without hyperphenylalaninemia is *dopa-responsive dystonia* (DRD) also known as Segawa's disease, hereditary progressive dystonia,

and DYT5. DRD is an autosomal dominantly inherited disorder caused by heterozygous mutations in the gene for GCHI located on chromosome 14 (40,41). New mutations are common, and there is an increased clinical penetrance in females. Although the spectrum of presentations is wide, patients typically present in mid-childhood (age 5 to 6 years) with dystonic posturing of leg or foot affecting the gait. Symptoms progressively worsen, and about one fourth of patients develop hyperreflexia and spasticity, leading some to be inappropriately diagnosed with CP. A diurnal variation has been emphasized, with progressive worsening throughout the day and improvement in the morning after sleep. However, cases without this variation have been reported. Other prominent symptoms include arm dystonia and features of parkinsonism (i.e., bradykinesia, rigidity, masked facies, hypophonic speech, and postural instability). An unusual case with myoclonus-dystonia syndrome (i.e., myoclonic jerks beginning in childhood) has been described (42). Since patients respond dramatically and in a sustained fashion to low-dose levodopa, it is important to diagnose this disorder. Some DRD patients have also shown a good response to anticholinergics such as trihexyphenidyl (43). DRD has been distinguished from juvenile parkinsonism by use of fluorodopa positron emission tomography (PET); there is no abnormality in DRD. Dopamine uptake sites in DRD, measured by single photon emission computed tomography (SPECT) with $[^{123}I]\beta$-CIT, are normal, but PET of D2 dopamine receptors suggests increased binding in both symptomatic and asymptomatic carriers (44,45). The phenylalanine loading test has been advocated as a sensitive and specific study for detection of both affected and nonmanifesting GCHI gene carriers (46,47). Since individuals with PKU would show similar abnormalities, DRD carriers are distinguished by correction of the loading test after administering biopterin.

Several cases of *DHPR deficiency without hyperphenylalaninemia* have been reported (48). Neurologic symptoms have included psychomotor retardation, microcephaly, spasticity, dystonia, oculomotor apraxia, and hypersomnolence. The oral phenylalanine loading test in these patients was abnormal, despite the lack of hyperphenylalaninemia. CSF measurements show reduced monoamines and their metabolites but normal BH_4 and neopterin levels. Treatment for this disorder includes the use of levodopa and 5-hydroxytryptophan in combination with carbidopa to correct central monoamine deficits.

Sepiapterin reductase (SR) deficiency is another inherited disorder of BH_4 metabolism characterized by the signs and symptoms related to monoamine neurotransmitter deficiency, but without hyperphenylalaninemia. SR catalyzes the final two-step reduction of the intermediate pyruvoyltetrahydropterin (PTP) to BH4. The deficiency is an autosomal recessive disorder that has been reported in a small number of patients with progressive psychomotor retardation, dystonia, severe dopamine and serotonin deficiencies, and high levels of biopterin and dihydrobiopterin (BH_2) in the CSF (49,50). Several mutations in the *SR* gene have been identified. It is speculated that alternative reductases, aldose reductase and carbonyl reductase, may be capable of replacing absent SR activity in peripheral tissues.

Nonhyperphenylalaninemia BH_4 deficiencies can be treated with low-dose levodopa.

Primary Defects of Monoamine Biosynthesis

Defects of monoamine biosynthesis have been defined at three sequential enzymatic steps: (a) tyrosine hydroxylase (TH), the rate-limiting step in the formation of dopamine and norepinephrine, which catalyzes the conversion of tyrosine to L-dopa; (b) aromatic L-amino acid decarboxylase (AADC), which converts L-dopa to dopamine, and (c) dopamine β-hydroxylase (DBH), the enzyme that converts dopamine to norepinephrine.

Tyrosine Hydroxylase Deficiency

Tyrosine hydroxylase deficiency comprises a group of autosomal recessive disorders localized to chromosome 11p11.5 that respond partially to levodopa treatment. At least eight different point mutations have been identified in the *TH* gene and, depending on the abnormality, syndromes have been extremely variable, ranging from severe presentations in infancy to milder juvenile DRD or juvenile parkinsonism (51–56). In cases with a severe reduction of TH activity, onset occurs in infancy with symptoms of psychomotor retardation, rigidity, hypokinesia, axial hypotonia, and paroxysmal eye movements. In other presentations, cases have included parkinsonism, gait disorder and stiffness after exercise, dystonia, and ataxia. Neuroradiographic scans are normal and electroencephalograms may show nonspecific background abnormalities (51,53). Diagnosis is confirmed by genetic analysis, but biochemical testing has been valuable (e.g., the presence of reduced levels of CSF dopamine, norepinephrine, HVA, and MHPG, normal 5-HIAA and pterins, and a normal phenylalanine load). Treatment involves the administration of low-dose levodopa.

Aromatic AADC Deficiency

AADC deficiency is an autosomal recessive disorder associated with a defect localized to chromosome 7p12.1-12.3 (57). Since AADC catalyzes both the formation of dopamine from L-dopa and serotonin from 5-HTP, a deficiency of this enzyme leads to a profound deficiency of CSF serotonin and catecholamines. Resultant clinical symptoms therefore tend to be more like a severe BH_4 deficiency. Problems include paroxysmal movements with arm and leg extension and rolling eyes, orofacial dystonia, irritability, myoclonus, temperature instability, autonomic dysfunction, disordered sleep and feeding, and a diurnal variation of symptoms (35,58,59). If untreated, affected children develop a characteristic phenotype of extrapyramidal movements often preceded by oculogyric crises and convergence spasms (35). Magnetic resonance images may show mild cortical atrophy, and electroencephalograms show spike or polyspike bursts (60). CSF monoamines and their metabolites are reduced, but levels of the L-dopa metabolite 3-*O*-methyldopa are elevated. A mild form of AADC deficiency has been reported (61). Treatment with monoamine oxidase (MAO) inhibitors and dopamine agonists has improved some symptoms but not signs of developmental delay. Although L-dopa would not be expected to be beneficial, one patient did experience improvement of symptoms, presumably because of decreased affinity for this substance (47), and a trial without carbidopa is felt prudent. Similarly, since B6 is a cofactor for AADC, high-dose pyridoxal phosphate is also recommended.

Juvenile Parkinson's Disease

Juvenile parkinsonism is a broad heterogeneous term representing multiple disorders that have the constellation of tremor, rigidity, bradykinesia, and loss of postural reflexes. In contrast, juvenile Parkinson's disease (JPD) is a specific autosomal recessive disorder associated with an abnormality in the *parkin* gene. This disorder has its onset before 21 years of age and often presents with dystonic features and occasionally hyperreflexia. JPD is therefore clinically similar to dopa-responsive dystonia. Distinguishing features of JPD include its requirement for larger levodopa doses, rapid appearance of motor fluctuations and dyskinesias, slower progression, and reduced fluorodopa uptake on PET scanning (61–63).

Pathologically, JPD is characterized by the degeneration of cells in the substantia nigra and locus ceruleus, but without the appearance of Lewy bodies. Nigral cell loss is more marked in the putamen and is demonstrable on PET analyses, which show a reduced number of striatal dopaminergic terminals (64). JPD is caused by mutations of a gene on chromosome 6q that encodes for the protein Parkin. A variety of Parkin mutations have been identified (65). How this mutation results in selective degeneration of nigral neurons is unknown. Parkin is associated with the axonal transport system and may be a phosphorylated protein associated with neuronal signaling. An additional pathologic mechanism may be altered protein handling, secondary to Parkin's interaction with the ubiquitin-conjugating enzyme E2 and its functionally linked role in the ubiquitin-proteasome pathway (62)

Trinucleotide Repeat Diseases

Trinucleotide repeat diseases have been divided into two types based on the site of the mutation within its respective gene. Type II disorders are those in which the expansions lie outside of the protein-coding region of the gene and the protein product is normal. Nevertheless, mutations in untranslated regions of the gene lead to abnormal transcription or RNA processing, resulting in altered levels of gene expression, such as fragile X syndrome and myotonic dystrophy. A type I disorder includes diseases in which an expanded repeat occurs in the coding region of the gene, which, in turn, produces an expanded amino acid stretch in the gene product. Examples are CAG repeat diseases, which encode an expanded polyglutamine tract in the disease protein, such as *spinocerebellar ataxia (SCA) 1–3, 6, and 7, Huntington's disease, dentatorubropallidoluysian atrophy (DRPLA), and spinobulbar muscular atrophy.* CAG/polyglutamine expansion diseases are further typified by their genetic inheritance, association with progressive neurologic signs and symptoms, highly variable phenotype within the same family, direct correlation between longer repeats and more severe disease, further expansion of repeats in successive generations (anticipation), and association with the formation of abnormal protein accumulations (66). Although most of the known CAG trinucleotide repeat disorders have their onset in adulthood, notable exceptions occur in childhood and can cause extrapyramidal manifestations.

Huntington's Disease

Although often considered an adult disorder, about 6% to 10% of patients with Huntington's disease (HD) present in childhood. Juvenile HD is defined as occurring before age 20 years; some cases have been reported in the first 2 years of life. Behavioral disturbances, declining school performance, and speech changes are often initial reasons for seeking medical attention. Seizures, rare in adults, are prominent in more than half of the children with HD. Diminished facial movements, oculomotor apraxia, and voluntary upgaze problems are common. Cerebellar ataxia can be prominent, and pyramidal findings of hyperreflexia and extensor plantar responses occur frequently. The duration of disease to death is shorter in children (5 to 10 years) than in adults.

Juvenile HD is an autosomal dominant condition, with most subjects inheriting this condition from their father. A careful family history is essential because cases are often concealed, misdiagnosed, or overlooked due to death before the onset of definitive symptoms. The genetic abnormality resides on the fourth chromosome and consists of an unstable expanded number of trinucleotide (CAG) repeats; repeats of more than 40 are found in HD patients. The number of repeats is inversely related to the age of onset, and repeat lengths greater than 60 are often found in the juvenile form (67). A tendency for CAG repeat length to increase during spermatogenesis accounts for the anticipation (further expansions in future generations) effect; that is, the juvenile form of HD occurs with male transmission. Predictive and prenatal testing in asymptomatic subjects is available, but ethical issues, informed consent, and confidentiality remain significant issues.

The function of the gene product, Huntington, remains unclear. Magnetic resonance imaging scanning may show atrophy of the caudate and prominent cortical sulci, although changes can be minimal in early stages. PET studies have shown reduced glucose metabolism in the caudate of patients with HD and in some subjects at risk for the disease. Pathophysiologic hypotheses include excitotoxicity and mitochondrial dysfunction. Management is strictly symptomatic, with the use of anticonvulsants for seizures, neuroleptic agents for behavioral difficulties and chorea, anticholinergics or dopamine agonists for rigidity, anxiolytics for anxiety, and selective serotonin reuptake inhibitors for affective disorders.

Dentatorubropallidoluysian Atrophy

DRPLA is a rare disorder, more common in Japan, characterized by the presence of progressive myoclonic epilepsy, ataxia, choreoathetosis, and dementia. The age of onset is broad, with most cases beginning in the third or fourth decade, but a juvenile form occurs in childhood. Neuroradiography shows atrophy of the cerebellum, midbrain tegmentum, and cerebral hemispheres with ex vacuo ventriculomegaly (68). The prominent pathologic features include extensive degeneration of the dentate nucleus, red nucleus, globus pallidus, and the subthalamic nucleus of Luys. DRPLA is a repeat expansion disorder mapped to chromosome 12p with an expansion of CAG repeats ranging from 49 to 84 (normal 6 to 36). Similar to HD, parental transmission leads to intergenerational instability. The product of the DRPLA is a protein named atrophin-1. Although it is distributed widely in neuronal cytoplasm, its function remains undetermined.

Spinocerebellar Atrophy Type 7

An additional expanded CAG trinucleotide repeat disorder, besides Huntington's disease, and DRPLA, that has presented early through the process of anticipation is spinocerebellar atrophy type 7. As with other spinocerebellar atrophies, type 7 is rare and is characterized by the presence of progressive neurologic symptoms, including cerebellar ataxia, pyramidal and extrapyramidal signs, ophthalmoplegia, and dementia. However, in contrast to the others spinocerebellar atrophies, type 7 is distinguished by the presence of retinal degeneration (69). Progressive loss of vision from pigmentary macular degeneration may precede the onset of other signs and has occurred in patients from 1 to 45 years of age. The defect is an expanded CAG repeat ranging from 34 to more than 200 repeats (normal 7 to 17) on chromosome 3. The encoded protein has been labeled ataxin-7 and to date its function is unknown.

Metabolic Disorders

Mineral Accumulation

Wilson's Disease (Hepatolenticular Degeneration)

Wilson's disease is inherited as an autosomal recessive trait; the gene, located on chromosome 13q14.3, encodes for an enzyme (copper-transporting P-type ATPase, ATP7B) that binds to copper and aids in its transport across the membrane (70). Mutations lead to failure to excrete copper in the bile and the subsequent accumulation in liver, brain, cornea, kidney, bones, and blood. Intestinal absorption of copper is normal and ceruloplasm, an α-globulin that binds and transports copper molecules, is frequently but not always reduced. Increased excretion of copper in the urine is insufficient to prevent copper accumulation.

In children, hepatic dysfunction (asymptomatic hepatomegaly, acute transient or fulminant hepatitis) is the most common clinical presentation; average age of onset is about 12 years (71). Since ceruloplasmin is an acute-phase reactant, its level may be increased in the presence of hepatitis, making this an unreliable diagnostic marker. The average age for the appearance of neurologic symptoms is about 19 years, although symptoms have been reported in a 6-year-old (72,73). Dysarthria or difficulties with gait are often an early manifestation. Several syndromes in this diagnosis have been described, including an akinetic-rigid and a generalized dystonic form (74). A resting, postural, or kinetic tremor occurs in about 50% of patients, and cerebellar symptoms ("pseudosclerotic") may also be present. Psychiatric symptoms precede the neurologic abnormalities in 20% of cases; ranging from subtle changes in personality and behavior to frank psychosis. The Kaiser-Fleischer ring, a yellow-brown deposition of copper in Descemet's membrane of the cornea, is best observed by slit-lamp examination. The diagnosis is made through the use of a combination of studies, including measurement of serum ceruloplasmin and 24-hour urine copper, slit-lamp examination, and most definitively by liver biopsy with histologic assessment and determination of copper content.

Treatment strategies are reviewed in detail elsewhere (71,75,76). In brief, approaches include dietary therapy (avoidance of foods high in copper), therapy to reduce copper absorption (potassium, zinc, tetrathiomolybdate), treatment to increase copper chelation and elimination (D-penicillamine, trientine [triethylene tetramine dihydrochloride], dimercaprol [British anti-Lewisite, BAL]) and liver transplantation.

Neurodegeneration with Brain Iron Accumulation

The nosology of neurodegenerative disorders associated with the accumulation of iron has undergone revision based on recent genetic advances and revelations about the personal history of Julius Hallervorden. More specifically, *pantothenate kinase–associated neurodegeneration (PKAN)* is the new suggested terminology for a group of disorders previously known as Hallervorden-Spatz syndrome (HSS). However, it is likely that a group of phenotypically similar cases may be defined without this specific gene abnormality.

PKAN is a rare autosomal recessive disorder pathologically associated with abnormal iron deposition and high concentrations of lipofuscin and neuromelanin in the substantia nigra pars reticulata and the internal segment of the globus pallidus. Mapped to chromosome 20p12.3-p13, investigators have identified a mutation in the gene for pantothenate kinase 2 (PANK2), a regulatory enzyme in the synthetic pathway for coenzyme A, which catalyzes the cytosolic phosphorylation of pantothenate (vitamin B_5), *N*-pantothenoylcysteine, and pantetheine (77). It has been hypothesized that the gene product results in an accumulation of cysteine, an iron chelator, and the combination, in turn, leads to oxidative stress and neurodegeneration.

HSS, which has variable presentations, has been divided into the more common early-onset form (diagnosis evident before age 10 years), a late-onset type (diagnosis evident between ages 10 and 18 years), and an adult variant (78). The classic presentation is characterized by onset between 5 and 8 years of age with progressive personality changes, cognitive decline, dysarthria, motor difficulties, and spasticity. Extrapyramidal dysfunction is usually present but may be delayed for several years. Dystonia is common but rigidity, choreoathetosis, and a resting or action tremor may also be present. Ophthalmologic abnormalities include retinitis pigmentosa and optic atrophy. Seizures can also occur.

The course of the disorder is variable. For example, the early-onset form is subdivided into rapidly and slowly progressive forms. The rapid-progressive early-onset type has a short transition from spasticity to severe movements with opisthotonos, and death within 1 to 2 years. In contrast, the more prevalent, slowly progressive, early-onset type can present with movement abnormalities but develop more slowly, with death occurring within 20 years. The late-onset childhood form is even slower in its progression than the early-onset types.

Diagnosis depends on the presence of obligate features: onset in the first two decades, progressive course, extrapyramidal symptoms, and classical magnetic resonance imaging (MRI) findings showing decreased T2-weighted and proton density signal in the globus pallidus and substantia nigra. Some patients also have a hyperintense area within the hypodense areas, named the "eye-of-the-tiger sign." Cranial MRI changes may predate the appearance of symptoms (79). Supportive diagnostic signs and symptoms include spasticity, extensor plantar signs, progressive intellectual impairment, ophthalmologic problems, abnormal cytosomes in lymphocytes, and sea-blue histiocytes in bone marrow (the latter findings being typical of ceroid-lipofuscin accumulation) (78). Cultured skin fibroblasts have been reported to accumulate ^{59}Fe-transferrin. There is no specific treatment for HSS, although theoretically the downstream delivery of products in the coenzyme A pathway may be therapeutic. Iron chelation therapy with desferrioxamine has not been effective. Therapy for movement disorders and spasticity is directed to symptoms.

The term *HARP syndrome* has been used to define a phenotype that includes *h*ypoprebetalipoproteinemia, *a*canthocytosis, *r*etinitis pigmentosa, and *p*allidal degeneration (80). The patient had orofacial dyskinesias and MRI findings similar to those found in HSS. Two other patients have been reported with symptoms of acanthocytosis, retinitis pigmentosa, faciobuccolingual dyskinesia, and the eye-of-the-tiger sign, but with normal serum lipoproteins (81). It has been suggested that HARP syndrome may be a variant of HSS.

Fahr's Syndrome

Based on a single case report of a man with calcification in the white matter and basal ganglia, Fahr's name has been widely but inaccurately associated with a variety of disorders presenting with bilateral calcifications involving the basal ganglia and cerebellum. Etiologically, calcifications in the basal ganglia can occur in a several metabolic disorders (e.g., mitochondrial, carbonic anhydrase deficiency, biopterin disorders, Cockayne's syndrome), but the most common cause is a parathyroid hormone abnormality. A familial/sporadic disorder named for the anatomic predilection of calcifications is bilateral striopallidodentate calcinosis (BSPDC (82,83). In an assessment of 99 subjects with this disorder, about two thirds were symptomatic (parkinsonism, cognitive impairment, cerebellar signs), and the mean age of the symptomatic group was significantly higher than that of the asymptomatic group. A locus in one large family with idiopathic basal ganglia calcification and genetic anticipation has been localized to chromosome 14q (84).

Lysosomal Disorders

Lysosomes are intracytoplasmic vesicles that contain a variety of degradative enzymes used to catabolize complex substrates, such as sphingolipids, gangliosides, cerebrosides, sulfatides, mucopolysaccharides, and glycoproteins. Levels of lysosomal enzyme activity are readily assayed in serum, white blood cells, or cultured fibroblasts. The inherited absence of a specific enzyme activity, in turn, results in the excessive deposition of the undegradable substance in the lysosome, with subsequent disruption of either neuronal or myelin function.

Neuronal Storage Diseases

Neuronal storage diseases, such as G_{M1} and G_{M2} gangliosidosis, Gaucher's disease, and Niemann-Pick disease, are generally characterized by the presence in infancy of progressive cognitive and motor deterioration, seizures, retino-pathy, and, in some cases, hepatosplenomegaly. In general, it is the more slowly progressive variants of these disorders, those that have only partial deficiencies of enzyme activity, that tend to have extrapyramidal signs. In *juvenile and adult forms of G_{M2} gangliosidosis* (deficiency of hexosaminidase A), dystonia and rigidity, primarily involving the lower extremities, may be the presenting symptom (85,86). In the *older (type 3) form of G_{M1} gangliosidosis* (deficiency of G_{M1} β-galactosidase), which presents at 2 to 27 years of age, patients may also have manifestations including dystonia and spinocerebellar deficits. In the typical *juvenile form of Niemann-Pick disease type C* (NPC, due to a defect in intracellular cholesterol transport), patients present with hepatosplenomegaly, cognitive deterioration, dysarthria, supranuclear vertical gaze palsy, gait problems, cataplexy, dystonia, and cerebellar ataxia (87,88). In Niemann-Pick disease type C, abnormal esterification of exogenous cholesterol in fibroblasts and the accumulation of unesterified cholesterol in lysosomes (seen with filipin staining) provide the basis for biochemical diagnosis. A mutated gene on chromosome 18q11-12 is responsible for most cases.

Neuronal Ceroid Lipofuscinoses

Neuronal ceroid lipofuscinoses (NCLs) are among the most common neurodegenerative diseases in children. In the pediatric population, they are autosomal recessive disorders characterized by the accumulation of autofluorescent ceroid lipopigment in brain tissue and various organs. Historically, classifications of NCL were based on age of onset, clinical symptoms, and ultrastructural aspects of inclusions. The three classical forms in children are *infantile (Santavuori-Haltia disease, INCL), late-infantile (Jansky-Bielschowsky disease, LINCL), and juvenile (Batten-Spielmeyer-Vogt disease, JNCL)* variants. INCL begins in the first year of life with regression of all psychomotor skills; LINCL begins between 2 and 4 years with acute seizures that increase rapidly in frequency, myoclonus, and, later, retinopathy; JNCL usually starts after age 5 years with visual failure due to pigmentary retinal degeneration and progresses to include behavioral, cerebellar, and extrapyramidal signs. A SPECT study in individuals with JNCL and extrapyramidal findings has demonstrated a significant reduction of striatal dopamine transporter density, more prominent in the putamen than the caudate (89).

More recently, clinicopathologic and genetic studies have shown that NCLs encompass a highly heterogeneous group with eight different forms, CLN1–8, based on mutations in specific genes (90,91). Currently, five genes associated with various childhood forms (CLN1, CLN2, CLN3, CLN5, and CLN8) have been characterized. CLN1 and CLN2 are caused by mutations in genes that code for the lysosomal enzymes palmitoyl protein thioesterase 1 and tripeptidyl peptidase 1, respectively. CLN3, CLN5, and CLN8 encode putative membrane proteins of unknown function (92). Although molecular advances are changing diagnostic classifications, the relationship among NCL types, lipopigment accumulation, and tissue damage remains unclear.

White Matter (Dysmyelinating) Disorders

White matter (dysmyelinating) disorders can also be associated with deficiencies of lysosomal enzymes: *Krabbe's disease* (has deficient galactocerebroside β-galactosidase); and *metachromatic leukodystrophy* (MLD, deficient arylsulfatase A). These disorders occur because both central and peripheral myelins contain cerebrosides and sulfatides, substances that require specific enzymes for degradation. Krabbe's disease and MLD typically present in infancy with symptoms and signs of progressive motor difficulties, spasticity, peripheral neuropathy, and optic atrophy. Extrapyramidal symptoms in these disorders are rare, although a dystonic phenotype has been reported in an individual with juvenile MLD (93).

Amino Acids and Organic Acid Disorders

Glutaric Aciduria Type 1

Glutaric aciduria type 1 is an autosomal recessive disorder caused by a defect in the gene that codes for glutaryl-CoA dehydrogenase (GCDH, involved in lysine, hydroxylysine, and tryptophan metabolism) (94). Biochemically, deficiency of this enzyme results in the accumulation and excretion of glutaric acid and 3-hydroxyglutaric acid, detectable in the urine, blood, and CSF. The diagnosis is confirmed by documentation of deficient glutaryl-CoA dehydrogenase activity in cultured skin fibroblasts. Clinically, there are several forms of presentation and phenotypic heterogeneity occurs within families (95,96). In about one fourth of patients, development tends to be normal until the latter part of the first year of life when progressive symptoms appear, including hypotonia, dystonia, choreoathetosis, and seizures. In the largest group, the patient is well for up to 2 years, until the abrupt onset of an acute deteriorating neurologic picture, typically associated with an infectious or encephalitic process. Residual symptoms include extrapyramidal movements and mental retardation. Repeated episodes of ketoacidosis, seizures, and loss of consciousness may occur throughout the course. A third form mimics the presentation of extrapyramidal CP. Clinical variability does not correlate with the extent of residual enzyme activity, more than 100 mutations in the *GCDH* gene have been identified, and no molecular basis differentiates the groups. Neuroradiographic studies show atrophy of the frontotemporal cortex and "bat-winged" dilatation of the sylvian fissures, hypodensity of the lenticular nuclei, and caudate degeneration. Bilateral temporal arachnoid cysts are common. The pathologic mechanism is unclear; hypotheses include an effect on glutamic acid decarboxylase, on glutamate reuptake, or interference with glutamatergic NMDA receptors. A low-protein diet, with riboflavin, and L-carni-

tine has been utilized, but appears to be of limited effect, especially in patients with striatal damage.

Methylmalonic Aciduria

In all genetic forms of methylmalonic aciduria (MMA), the conversion of methylmalonyl-CoA to succinyl-CoA is impaired secondary to impairment of methylmalonyl-CoA mutase due to a genetic defect in the mitochondrial apoenzyme, methylmalonyl-CoA mutase, or its adenosylcobalamin cofactor. Infants with absence of the apoenzyme (classical form) become symptomatic in the first week of life with hypotonia, lethargy, vomiting, metabolic acidosis, and ketosis. Survivors typically have severe residual neurologic impairments including dystonia. MRI studies show alterations in myelination and changes in the basal ganglia. The clinical phenotype is less severe in late-onset cases and those with cofactor deficiencies. Diagnosis is made by analysis of urine organic acids, and all patients should be tested for responsiveness to vitamin B_{12}.

Homocystinuria

In the most common form of homocystinuria, the metabolic defect involves the enzyme cystathionine synthase, which catalyzes the formation of cystathionine from homocysteine and serine. The primary pathologic alterations are intimal thickening and fibrosis in vessels of all calibers, which lead to arterial and venous thromboses occurring in multiple organs. Affected children have abnormalities of the skeleton, the eye, and vascular, and nervous systems. CNS dysfunction includes intellectual retardation, motor delays, and stroke syndromes. Extrapyramidal abnormalities, primarily dystonia, have occurred in both children and adolescents with homocystinuria (97–99). MRI studies have shown bilateral low-intensity basal ganglia lesions on T2-weighted imaging. It is likely that the dystonia is secondary to thromboembolic events, which occur frequently, although a defect in sulfur metabolism has also been postulated.

Mitochondrial Disorders

Leigh's Syndrome

Leigh's syndrome (subacute necrotizing encephalomyelopathy) is a complex of progressive neurodegenerative disorders caused by several defects of energy metabolism, including the pyruvate dehydrogenase complex, pyruvate carboxylase, and respiratory complexes I, II, IV, and V (100,101). The most common defect, affecting about one fourth of patients, involves cytochrome *c* oxidase deficiency (complex IV). In some cases the defect in cytochrome *c* oxidase-deficient Leigh's disease has been mapped to chromosome 9q34 with the putative candidate gene *(SURF-1)* shown to encode an assembly or maintenance factor (102). The disorder usually presents in infancy or early childhood with psychomotor delay and hypotonia. As the disease progresses, feeding and swallowing defects, nystagmus, ophthalmoplegia, optic atrophy, ataxia, pyramidal signs, and respiratory problems become apparent. Movement disorders, such as dystonia, choreoathetosis, and myoclonus, have been prominent in some cases and, at times, may be the initial sign (103–105). Pathologic findings include symmetric necrotic lesions (spongy degeneration) with demyelination, vascular proliferation, and gliosis affecting the basal ganglia, diencephalon, and brainstem. Diagnosis is based on the presence of elevated arterial or CSF lactate levels and on T2-weighted magnetic resonance images that show symmetric areas of increased signal in the putamen, or occasionally the caudate, globus pallidus, and substantia nigra (106).

Leber Hereditary Optic Neuropathy

Leber's hereditary optic neuropathy is an X-linked inherited disorder associated with a mitochondrial DNA point mutation. The disorder is dominated clinically by the sudden onset of visual loss in a young adult, although patients as young as 5 years have been reported. However, the spectrum of clinical findings is broad and includes individuals with dystonia and MRI lesions similar to those seen in Leigh's syndrome (107).

Other Metabolic Disorders

Succinic Semialdehyde Dehydrogenase Deficiency (4-Hydroxybutyric Aciduria; GABA-Related Neurotransmitter Disease)

Succinic semialdehyde dehydrogenase (SSADH) works in conjunction with GABA transaminase to convert 4-aminobutyric acid (GABA) to succinic acid. SSADH deficiency, localized to chromosome 6, results in increased concentrations of GABA and 4-hydroxybutyric acid (GHB). Diagnosis is based on the detection of massive increases of 4-hydroxybutyric acid in the urine, plasma, and CSF. CSF levels of GABA and a GABA peptide, homocarnosine, are elevated. Neurologic symptoms associated with this disease include developmental delay of speech, motor and cognitive function, ataxia, hypotonia, hyporeflexia, aggressive behavior, and occasionally choreoathetosis and seizures (108). Atrophy of the cerebellum may be present on MRI. Some patients have been improved by treatment with vigabatrin (γ-vinyl GABA), which blocks GABA transaminase.

Guanidinoacetate Methyltransferase Deficiency (Creatine Deficiency Syndrome)

Guanidinoacetate methyltransferase (GAMT) converts guanidinoacetate to creatine. A deficiency of this enzyme represents a newly recognized inborn error of creatine biosynthesis. The disorder presents in infancy with progressive dystonia and dyskinesias in addition to developmental delay and drug-resistant epilepsy (109–111). The neurologic manifestations are believed to reflect a combination of cerebral energy deficiency due to a depletion of brain crea-

tine/phosphocreatine and a neurotoxic effect of excess brain guanidinoacetate. The diagnosis is established by detection of creatine deficiency in the brain by magnetic resonance spectroscopy, the determination of guanidino compounds (decreased creatine and increased guanidinoacetate) in CSF and urine, low plasma and urine creatinine, and defective GAMT activity in fibroblasts or liver tissue. T2-weighted images have shown high signal in the globus pallidus bilaterally. Clinical and biochemical abnormalities have responded to treatment with oral creatine supplementation.

Molybdenum Cofactor (Sulfite Oxidase) Deficiency

Three mammalian enzymes require molybdenum as a cofactor for their function, including sulfite oxidase (essential for detoxifying sulfites), xanthine dehydrogenase (role in purine metabolism and formation of uric acid from xanthine and hypoxanthine), and aldehyde dehydrogenase (catalyzes conversion of aldehydes to acids) (112). Molybdenum cofactor deficiency is a rare, autosomal recessive, neurodegenerative disease that affects the CNS primarily through sulfite oxidase deficiency. The clinical manifestations are indistinguishable from those of isolated sulfite oxidase deficiency. The disorder often starts in the neonatal period with feeding difficulties and intractable seizures. Other manifestations include axial hypotonia, hypomotility, limb rigidity, dislocated lenses, and profound developmental delay. Dystonia and bilateral basal ganglia changes have been reported early in the presentation (113), and survivors may develop a variety of extrapyramidal movements. Diagnosis is suspected by low levels of uric acid in serum and urine and increased urinary sulfite (detectable by dipstick), thiosulfate, S-sulfocysteine (detectable by anion exchange chromatography), taurine, xanthine, and hypoxanthine levels. Brain imaging may show multiple cystic white matter cavities, loss of brain volume, and cessation of myelination. A short-term response to dietary methionine restriction with cysteine supplementation has been reported (114).

Other Inherited Disorders

Lesch-Nyhan Disease

Lesch-Nyhan disease (LND) is an X-linked recessive disorder associated with heterogeneous mutations in the gene for the enzyme hypoxanthine-guanine phosphoribosyltransferase (HPRT) located on chromosome Xq26-27 (115). The biochemical defect is a deficiency of HPRT that converts the free purine bases hypoxanthine and guanine to their respective nucleotides. Purines are important intermediaries in energy-dependent reactions and cofactor-requiring reactions, and inter- and intracellular signaling. In the absence of HPRT, hypoxanthine and guanine cannot be recycled and are degraded and excreted as uric acid.

Clinically the overproduction of uric acid leads to hyperuricemia and, if not treated, to renal stones and gouty arthritis. Since hyperuricemia is not present in all patients, measures of 24-hour urinary uric acid excretion and genetic testing may be required for diagnosis. Self-injurious behavior (e.g., self-biting, head banging, eye poking) is a hallmark, but nondiagnostic, feature of this disorder. These behaviors typically appear at about age 2 to 3 years, although they may not emerge until the late teenage years. Neurologic abnormalities have been variably described in the literature. In three older series, the cardinal features were either described as choreoathetosis and spasticity or dystonia with hypotonia (116–118). In a recent study of 17 patients (age range 8 to 38 years) with LND, performed with particular attention to neurological features (119), motor dysfunction was best described as severe dystonia superimposed on hypotonia. Dystonia, present in all subjects, was typically absent at rest and increased with excitement or attempted purposeful movements. Choreiform movements were present in about half the subjects, and ballismus of the upper extremity in about one fourth. Pyramidal signs were observed in a minority of cases. Ocular motility is grossly abnormal (fixation interrupted by unwanted saccades and voluntary saccades preceded by head movement or eye blink) in patients with severe enzyme deficiency (120).

Therapy includes generous hydration and allopurinol for hyperuricemia and protective measures, behavior modification therapy, and possibly pharmacotherapy (benzodiazepines, neuroleptics, gabapentin, carbamazepine) for self-injurious behavior. Although there have been no controlled trials, extrapyramidal signs have not been significantly improved by neuroleptics, tetrabenazine, or levodopa.

Ataxia Telangiectasia

Ataxia telangiectasia (A-T) is an autosomal recessive neurodegenerative disorder with associated immunodeficiency, endocrine and skin abnormalities, and a predisposition for lymphoreticular malignancies (121). The nonneurologic features are distinctive, with prominent ocular telangiectasia in more than 90% of patients over age 10 and more subtle lesions in exposed skin areas. Unfortunately, the characteristic conjunctival telangiectasias generally do not appear until after the appearance of neurologic findings. Progeric changes and vitiligo are common. Frequent sinopulmonary infections occur in less than half of cases. Most children with A-T have early ataxia, but the course may appear to be stable, leading to the misdiagnosis of ataxic CP. The ataxic gait, which begins in the first few years of life, may seem to be inappropriately narrow for the degree of instability. Children often have swaying movements of the trunk or head, at times to the extremes of postural stability, but without falling. Most develop abnormal eye movements characterized by an oculomotor apraxia with prominent head thrusts. Dysarthria with slow, hypophonic speech is common. Extrapyramidal manifestations are common. A multidimensional quantitative index of neurologic function has characterized disease progression and identified severe and mild forms of the disease (122). Most individuals die by the late teens or twenties, but some have reportedly survived into the sixth decade. Because of the enhanced susceptibility of A-T patients to ionizing radiation and the tendency for persistent abnormal DNA synthesis after irradiation, routine radiographs and radiotherapy doses should be reduced substantially.

Diagnostically, serum α-fetoprotein (AFP) levels are elevated in most affected children after the age of 1 year. and IgA and IgG are diminished in 80% of cases. Most patients have diminished cell-mediated responses to intradermal antigens and atrophy of the thymus. A-T is also confirmed by the finding of radiation-induced chromosomal breaks in lymphocytes. The large gene responsible for this disease, termed ataxia telangiectasia mutated *(ATM)*, comprises 9.3 kb of the genome and is located at 11q22-23. ATM appears to have a role in multiple physiologic processes as well as being a tumor suppressor.

Neuroacanthocytosis

Neuroacanthocytosis is a rare autosomal recessive disorder with linkage to chromosome 9 (123) characterized by the presence of orofacial dyskinesias, limb chorea, dystonia, motor and phonic tics, and an akinetic-rigid state. Acanthocytes (deformed erythrocytes with spicules of varying sizes) are seen in the peripheral smear. The disorder is associated with seizures, dementia, self-injurious behavior, psychiatric features, and an axonal neuropathy. The mean age of onset is about 30 years, but the disorder has been reported in children younger than 10 years.

An abnormality of membrane protein has been proposed, but the underlying mechanism is unknown. Pathologically the caudate and putamen are atrophic with depletion of medium-sized spiny neurons. PET studies have shown abnormalities in frontal-subcortical regions (124). Diagnosis depends on the presence of acanthocytes and neurologic abnormalities. Acanthocytes are also seen in other disorders, such as abetalipoproteinemia (Bassen-Kornzweig syndrome) and in the X-linked McLeod's syndrome.

Genetic (DYT) Primary Dystonia in Childhood

There are many genetic causes for the presence of dystonia and two broad categories, primary and secondary, are often used for classification. In primary dystonia, the only neurologic abnormality is the presence of dystonia, with the exception of a tremor that can resemble essential tremor. Hence, the presence of other symptoms (e.g., ataxia, reflex changes, dementia, retinopathy) would suggest that one is dealing with a secondary or heredodegenerative disorder. An additional requirement for a primary dystonia is that the diagnostic evaluation fails to identify an exogenous cause or other inherited or metabolic disease. Besides etiologic classifications, on the basis of advances in molecular biology, distinct genetic forms of dystonia have been classified by gene mapping and cloning (e.g., labeled as DYT or dystonia loci). Currently, as discussed elsewhere in this book (see Chapters 23 and 24), there are more than 12 separate genetic forms of dystonia (DYT1 to DYT12). Although a chromosomal location exists for all 12, only two have been shown to have mutated genes (DYT1 or early-onset generalized torsion dystonia, and DYT5 or dopa-responsive dystonia/Segawa's syndrome).

NONINHERITED SECONDARY CAUSES OF MOVEMENT DISORDERS

Noninherited secondary causes of movement disorders can be due to numerous instances of damage or injury to the nervous system (Table 31.4). In these cases, the movement disorder may occur at the time of the insult, while the

TABLE 31.4. SECONDARY NONINHERITED CAUSES OF EXTRAPYRAMIDAL SYMPTOMS IN CHILDHOOD

A. Perinatal cerebral injury
   Hypoxic-ischemic encephalopathy
   Kernicterus
B. Structural
   Tumors (mesencephalic)
   Trauma
   Burns
   Shunt failure
C. Vascular
   Stroke
   Intracranial hemorrhage
D. Infection/postinfectious/autoimmune
   Encephalitis: influenza, polio, mumps, measles, varicella,
      St. Louis, coxsackie, HIV, SSPE
   Poststreptococcal infections: Sydenham's chorea, PANDAS,
      acute disseminated encephalomyelitis
E. Hypoxic-ischemic encephalopathy
F. Drug/toxin
   Dopamine related: neuroleptics, metaclopramide,
      reserpine, α-methyldopa, L-dopa
   AEDs: valproate, phenytoin, vigabatrin
   Chemotherapy: vincristine, cytosine arabinoside, adriamycin
   Other: calcium channel blockers, captopril, lithium, selective
      serotonin uptake inhibitors, buspirone
   Toxins: MPTP, manganese, carbon monoxide, cyanide,
      methanol, disulfram
G. Hormonal disorders
   Thyroid
   Addison's disease
   Hypoparathyroidism
H. Associated with general medical conditions
   Systemic lupus erythematosus
   Polycythemia
   Antiphospholipid syndrome
   Paraneoplastic syndrome
I. Psychogenic

PANDAS, pediatric autoimmune neuropsychiatric disorder associated with streptococcal infection; MPTP, 1-methyl-4-phenyl-1,2,3,6-tetrahydropyridine.

patient is recovering from other neurologic deficits, or after a prolonged period of neurologic stability. Although a variety of brain insults can result in the delayed onset of symptoms, in infants and children they usually appear after prematurity, birth injury, encephalitis, trauma, and stroke. In some children, in whom the initial brain insult was at age 2 years or before, the onset of a progressive movement disorder (often dystonia) occurred more than 25 years later (125). Hence, static brain lesions can cause movement disorders after a long latency and even some have a progressive course. Since many of the etiologic factors listed in Table 31.4 are common to both pediatric and adult patients, the reader is referred to other chapters in this text for additional discussion. An important significant exception is the diagnosis and treatment of CP and movement disorders after streptococcal infections.

Perinatal Cerebral Injury

Cerebral Palsy

Cerebral palsy is not a single disease entity but rather a broad term used to describe a heterogeneous group of syndromes that cause a nonprogressive disorder of early onset, with abnormal control of movement and posture. Whether the age of onset should be before 2 or 5 years of age remains controversial. The spectrum of motor dysfunction in CP is broad (e.g., spasticity, plegias, choreoathetosis, dystonia, and ataxia) and, despite an underlying static lesion, movement problems may vary over time. The incidence of CP is about 1.5 to 2.5 per 1,000 live births, and the risk is higher in low-birth-weight infants and in twin pregnancies (126). In the United States, approximately 57,000 infants are born annually with a birth weight of less than 1,500 g. Of these, about 90% survive and about 10% to 15% exhibit motor effects. Premature and very-low-birth-weight infants are at greater risk for developing CP than are infants born at term. Major disability cannot be accurately predicted for individual survivors while in the newborn intensive care unit (127).

The etiology of CP is extensive, ranging from pre- and perinatal events (e.g., cerebral dysgenesis, hypoxia-ischemia), which account for about 85% of cases, to postnatal events (e.g., infection, trauma) (128,129). In the premature infant, periventricular leukomalacia (PVL), which affects the developing white matter, is the most common neuropathologic lesion associated with CP. The role of birth asphyxia as a prominent cause for CP has not been supported by current research, and elimination of this problem has not reduced its incidence (130,131). Potentially treatable causes, such as maternal infection and thyroid dysfunction, are currently being investigated. Lastly, although CP is defined by the presence of motor disabilities, individuals with CP have a variety of nonmovement problems, including mental retardation (>50%), strabismus (about

50%), epilepsy (about 30%), and disorders of vision or hearing (about 20%) (132).

The neurobiological mechanisms of perinatal brain injury are currently being actively investigated. Periventricular leukomalacia, the major neuropathology in the premature infant, is likely due to several interacting factors (133). Predisposing conditions for involvement of the cerebral white matter include the immature development of the vascular supply to this region and a maturation-dependent impairment of cerebral blood flow regulation. Another major factor is the vulnerability of the oligodendroglial precursor cell (pro-OL) to attack by free radicals and glutamate generated by ischemia-reperfusion. The pro-OL, in turn, undergoes an apoptotic death (134). Other factors besides ischemia-reperfusion and excitotoxic agents may also be involved in causing damage to the immature oligodendrocyte. For example, maternal or fetal infection, inflammation, and cytokines have been hypothesized to play important contributory roles through their effect on vascular hemodynamics, generation of reactive oxygen species, or direct toxicity. A recent study demonstrating distinct differences in inflammatory response and cytokine expression in postmortem neonatal brains with and without PVL provides support for involvement of the inflammation–cytokine mediation theory (135). An increased likelihood of PVL in the presence of intraventricular hemorrhage may be due to local increases in iron concentration. Neonatal hypoxic-ischemic injury, through the pathogenic process of energy depletion, release of excitatory amino acids, accumulation of reactive oxygen species, and initiation of apoptosis, also affects other brain regions in the prenatal and perinatal brain (136).

Cerebral palsy is divided into four major types based on the predominant motor disability: *spastic* (about 50%); *dyskinetic* (about 20%); *ataxic* (about 10%); and *mixed* (about 20%). In actuality, most CP patients are mixed in type to some degree, e.g., mild dyskinetic signs are present in subtypes of spastic CP. Serial neurodevelopmental evaluations, especially in young children, are required for proper classification of the subtype because findings on examination may be affected by the state of alertness, emotional stress, and irritability. Other contributors to the motor deficit include sensory deficits, and cognitive and perceptual impairments. Early indicators of significant motor disability include delay in the appearance of motor milestones and exaggerated or persistent primitive reflexes (137,138). MRI has demonstrated abnormal brain findings in more than three fourths of individuals with CP (139). The management of CP requires a comprehensive multidisciplinary team approach that can deal with the numerous psychological, behavioral, and physical needs of the child and family.

Spastic Type

The spastic type of CP is further divided into several subtypes, based on the distribution of impairment: *hemiplegia* with homolateral involvement of the arm and leg; *quadriplegia* with severe impairment of all four extremities, usually the lower more then the upper; *tetraplegia* with involvement of all four extremities, usually the upper greater then the lower; and *diplegia* with milder impairment of all four extremities, but with the arms relatively spared. All subtypes of spastic CP are associated with hypertonia, hyperreflexia, clonus, and abnormal plantar responses. Spastic hypertonia is defined by the presence of resistance to an externally imposed movement that (a) increases with increasing speed and varies with the direction of joint movement and (b) a "catch" occurs above a threshold velocity. However, many infants with CP pass through an initial hypotonic phase. In general, neurologic abnormalities indicating spasticity are present during quiet periods and sleep and do not change significantly with activity or emotional stress. Pseudobulbar palsy, indicated by expressionless facies, and clonus may be seen in both spastic and dyskinetic forms. The child with spastic CP is typically prone to develop earlier contractures and have more frequent orthopedic problems than a child with choreoathetotic CP.

The *hemiplegic* form is the most common subtype of spastic CP with findings localized to one extremity, usually with the upper extremity more involved then the lower. The appearance of hemiplegic CP in full-term infants is usually associated with prenatal circulatory disturbances or cerebral dysgenesis. The incidence of seizures approaches 70%, although cognitive capabilities are generally spared. The *diplegic* subtype has involvement of all four extremities, with the upper extremities being minimally impaired and maintaining good functional abilities. This form typically appears in premature infants and is associated with the presence of periventricular leukomalacia. The *quadriplegic* subtype is the most severe form, with all four limbs significantly involved and considerable compromise of motor function. Spastic quadriplegia in the full-term infant may be the result of prenatal insults or perinatal asphyxia. These children typically have severe mental retardation, epilepsy, dysarthria, microcephaly, and strabismus.

Medical management of spasticity includes the use of benzodiazepines, dantroline, baclofen, α_2-agonists, and neuromuscular blocking agents. In general, these approaches help to reduce spasticity but have little beneficial effect on signs of weakness and incoordination. Neuromuscular blocking agents, especially botulinum toxin type A, have been used to improve the balance between overly spastic agonist muscles and weakened antagonist muscles (140,141). Several studies in patients with CP have demonstrated the short-term value of botulinum toxin type A in facilitating posture/hygiene; as an alternative or augmenting agent for casting, bracing, and surgery; and as a means to improve ambulation or upper extremity function (140). Selective functional dorsal (posterior) rhizotomy has produced a significant impact on spasticity, changes in gait pattern, and improvement in the patient's ability to deal with the environment or tasks of daily care (142,143). However, since this procedure is a major operation, it remains controversial whether the functional outcomes outweigh potential intraoperative and postoperative complications.

Dyskinetic (Choreoathetoid; Extrapyramidal) Type

Dyskinetic CP syndromes are characterized by the presence of the involuntary movements of chorea, athetosis, and dystonia. These movements typically begin after age 2 years, may progress slowly for several years, and persist into adulthood. Abnormal movements usually involve all four extremities, with the upper usually being functionally more involved then the lower extremities. Dyskinetic CP is often misdiagnosed as a spastic form because of the misinterpretation of clinical signs (e.g., inaccurate separation of spastic, dystonic, and rigid hypertonias). Dystonic hypertonia is diagnosed by the return of the affected limb to a specific posture, the presence of muscle activity at rest in the absence of imposed movement, and a significant variation in tone in association with the child's position, movement, or behavioral state. In contrast, rigid hypertonia can be diagnosed by resistance to externally imposed movement at low speeds, the presence of the same resistance at any speed of stretch, and the lack of a consistent abnormal posture. Cogwheel rigidity is unusual in young children with CP. Oral motor dysfunction and tongue thrusting are common symptoms. Extrapyramidal movements show marked variability depending on the state of the individual; they are decreased during relaxation and sleep, and increased by anxiety and stress. Dyskinetic forms of CP, especially those associated with athetosis, tend to occur in term infants with severe perinatal asphyxia. Pathophysiologically, extrapyramidal CP has been localized within the basal ganglia (neostriatum and/or globus pallidus) and/or thalamus, although more precise localization is lacking (144). MRI studies in children with athetoid CP showed that 37% were normal and the rest had high-intensity lesions in the ventrolateral nucleus of the thalamus or the dorsal putamen (145).

The treatment of dyskinetic CP is complicated because most individuals have mixed degrees of chorea, athetosis, and dystonia. The general approach to therapy in the child with CP is to target the dyskinetic movement that is causing the greatest difficulty. Therapeutic trials are largely empiric and responses often individualized. When the symptom is primarily chorea or athetosis, benzodiazepines, valproate, and neuroleptics are often prescribed. In contrast, therapy for dystonic CP includes trials with anticholinergic medications (trihexyphenidyl), baclofen, anticonvulsants (carbamazepine, clonazepam), antiparkinsonian medications (levodopa/carbidopa), and botulinum toxin. Trihexyphenidyl in younger children improved fine-motor abilities and expressive language (146). Oral baclofen may be more effective as an antidystonic agent in children than in adults (147). Intrathecal baclofen has been successful in patients with severe generalized dystonia (148). In

three patients in whom dystonia was associated with CP, marked improvement was seen with continuous baclofen infusion (149). A test bolus of baclofen given via a lumbar puncture was not thought to predict accurately the ultimate response to infusion therapy (149). A therapeutic trial with levodopa is advised in all patients in whom dystonia has developed in childhood or early life (150). This recommendation is appropriate for several reasons, including a response to levodopa in children with symptomatic dystonia (150) and the presentation of dopa-responsive dystonia with clinical patterns simulating cerebral palsy (151).

Ataxic (Cerebellar) Form

The cerebellar or ataxic form represents a clinically and etiologically heterogeneous group (152). Classical associated findings include truncal titubation, dysmetria, and cerebellar eye movements. Children with ataxic syndromes usually have a prenatal etiology (e.g., developmental cerebellar abnormality) and are born after a full-term gestation. Neuroimaging may be normal or show either biparietal or infratentorial lesions (152).

Kernicterus

Kernicterus is a preventable neurologic syndrome caused by severe and untreated hyperbilirubinemia in the newborn period. High levels of bilirubin are toxic to the developing brain, especially the globus pallidus, subthalamic nucleus, cerebellum, and the auditory and vestibular pathways. In full-term infants, hyperbilirubinemia symptoms include severe jaundice, lethargy, and poor feeding. Features of kernicterus include dystonia, choreoathetosis, tremor, rigidity, mental retardation, sensorineural hearing loss, and gaze paresis. Pathologic findings include yellow staining of the subthalamic nucleus, Ammon's horn, globus pallidus, dentate nucleus, and inferior olives. MRI findings at the posteromedial border of the globus pallidus in patients with athetotic CP are suggestive evidence of brain damage caused by kernicterus (153).

Streptococcal Infections: Postinfectious Disorders

Group A β-hemolytic streptococcal (GABHS) infections are the primary etiology for several postinfectious movement disorders, including Sydenham's chorea (SC), pediatric autoimmune neuropsychiatric disorder associated with streptococcal infection (PANDAS), and acute disseminated encephalomyelitis.

Sydenham's Chorea

Sydenham's chorea is the prototype for an infectious agent (GABHS) triggering an autoimmune disorder that, in turn, causes a movement disorder. SC usually occurs between the ages 5 and 15 years, and a female predominance has been observed in all large studies. Chorea can range in severity, is usually generalized, but hemichorea can occurs in about 20% of individuals. Associated neurologic symptoms may include dysarthria (about one third), gait disturbances that correlate with severity of chorea, hypometric saccades, hypotonia, weakness, and hemiballismus (154,155). Most patients have concomitant psychological dysfunction presenting as personality changes, obsessive-compulsive symptoms, emotional irritability, distractibility, and age-regressed behaviors (156,157). Affected individuals may present with behavioral or emotional difficulties that predate the motoric abnormalities by weeks to months. Motor or vocal tics and oculogyric crises have also been reported in patients with SC (154,158). Rheumatic valvular cardiac disease is seen in about one third of patients, whereas arthritis is uncommon.

The outcome in SC is quite favorable, with most cases resolving in 1 to 6 months, although minor motor abnormalities (159), and neuropsychiatric problems may persist (156,157,160). About 20% to 60% of patients have recurrent episodes of chorea, usually within 1 to 2 years after the original event. An individual may have multiple attacks with reactivation precipitated by a streptococcal infection or some other factor (161). Berrios and colleagues (162) reported recurrences of pure chorea in 10 of 17 patients with SC, but in 4 subjects they were unable to identify any evidence of a streptococcal infection in the preceding 6 to 9 months. Pregnancy and oral contraceptives have stimulated the reappearance of chorea after many years of quiescence (163).

In an MRI volumetric study evaluating the size of the basal ganglia in 24 patients with SC and 48 matched controls, children with SC had a 10% increase in size of the caudate and a 7% increase in size of both putamen and globus pallidus (164). Neurochemically, SC has been postulated to be a dopaminergic dysfunction, primarily on the basis of measurements of CSF HVA, a dopamine metabolite. An autoimmune hypothesis has been proposed as the underlying mechanism in this disorder; that is, after a streptococcal infection in susceptible individuals, antibodies directed against bacterial antigens cross-react (molecular mimicry) with epitopes on neurons of the basal ganglia and possibly frontal lobes, causing choreiform movement abnormalities and behavioral disturbances. This hypothesis has been supported by documentation of autoreactive antibodies against human basal ganglia.

PANDAS (Pediatric Autoimmune Neuropsychiatric Disorder Associated with Streptococcal Infection)

In 1998, Swedo and colleagues (165) proposed that SC was not the only immune-mediated CNS manifestation of GABHS and described their diagnostic criteria for a new phenotype with tics and neuropsychiatric symptoms, called PANDAS. Based on 50 cases recruited from a nation-wide search, they established the following working criteria: (a) the presence of obsessive-compulsive disorder (OCD) and/or tic disorder; (b) prepubertal age at onset; (c) sudden, "explosive" onset of symptoms and a course of sudden exacerbations and remissions; (d) a temporal relationship between symptom onset and exacerbations and GABHS infections; and (e) the presence of neurologic abnormalities, including tics, hyperactivity, and choreiform movements during exacerbations. However, the existence of PANDAS is not free of controversy (166). One of several deficiencies includes the absence of a prospective epidemiologic study confirming that an antecedent GABHS infection is associated with either the onset or exacerbation of tic disorders (or OCD).

The majority of children with PANDAS have normal premorbid personalities, with few signs of hidden dysfunction. Symptom onset is acute and dramatic and occurs at an early age: tics 6.3 ± 2.7 years, OCD 7.4 ± 2.7 years (mean ± standard deviation). The disorder has a relapsing-remitting course, with dramatic and acute symptom exacerbations interspersed with periods of relative quiescence. Psychiatric comorbidity, including emotional lability, separation anxiety, night-time fears, cognitive deficits, oppositional behaviors, and motor hyperactivity, is common. Boys outnumber girls by a ratio of 2.6:1. In all subjects, recurrence of at least one symptom is preceded by a documented GABHS infection within the prior 6 weeks. In a study of first-degree relatives of children with PANDAS, the rates of tic disorders and OCD were higher than those in the general population, but similar to those published for tic disorders and OCD (167). MRI volumetric analyses in 34 children with PANDAS showed that the average size of the caudate, putamen, and globus pallidus, but not thalamus or total cerebrum, was significantly greater in the affected group than in 82 healthy children (168).

Similar to Sydenham's chorea, an immune-mediated mechanism involving molecular mimicry has been proposed for PANDAS. Indirect support for an immune hypothesis is derived from a single study showing that a small number of patients with PANDAS responded to immunotherapy with intravenous immunoglobulin and plasmapheresis (169). Studies of antineuronal antibodies by use of an enzyme-linked immunosorbent assay (ELISA) in children with Tourette's syndrome showed that, compared with control subjects, there is a significant increase in the mean and median optical density (OD) levels of serum antibodies against the putamen, but not the caudate or globus pallidus (170). However, preliminary ELISA data measuring serum antibodies against a variety of subcellular fractions (synaptosomes, synaptic membrane, and mitochondria) from human caudate and putamen do not show differences between patients with PANDAS and controls (171). Since the mere presence of autoantibodies in the serum of patients with SC and PANDAS does not imply causation, animal models have been developed for study of whether serum can induce stereotypies in rodents that may be analogous to tics in humans. Although there are conflicting results in the literature (172), in two studies infusions of serum from TS subjects into animals were followed by either increased motor (facial stereotypies) or vocal (episodic utterances) stereotypies (173,174). This concept of PANDAS generated broad interest from divergent groups and caused many physicians to become polarized on opposing sides of the issue. If true, identification of factors that convey susceptibility or render the host less susceptible would be major advances.

Acute Disseminated Encephalomyelitis

After a clinical pharyngitis with laboratory evidence of GABHS, 10 children with a mean age of 6.8 years developed behavioral changes (emotional lability, inappropriate laughter), somnolence, stupor or coma, and an extrapyramidal movement disorder (rigidity, dystonic posturing, or hemidystonia, but no tics or chorea) (175). CSF was abnormal in 7 of 10 (pleocytosis and/or elevated protein), MRI demonstrated T2 hyperintense lesions in the basal ganglia in 8 of 10, and all had elevated serum antibasal ganglia antibodies. Recovery was rapid and often complete, although two patients had relapses associated with further streptococcal infections.

REFERENCES

1. Rothfield K, Behr J, McBride M, et al. Developmental chorea and dystonia of infancy. *Neurology* 1987;37[Suppl 1]:37.
1a. Jankovic J. Tourette's syndrome. *N Engl J Med* 2001;345:1184–1192.
2. Willemse J. Benign idiopathic dystonia with onset in the first year of life. *Dev Med Child Neurol* 1986;28:355–363.
3. Pranzatelli MR. An approach to movement disorders of childhood. *Pediatr Ann* 1993;22:13–17.
4. Resnick TJ, Moshe SL, Perotta L, et al. Benign neonatal sleep myoclonus. *Arch Neurol* 1986;43:266–268.
5. DiCapua M, Fusco L, Ricco S, et al. Benign neonatal sleep myoclonus: clinical features and video-polygraphic recordings. *Mov Disord* 1993;8:191–194.
6. Coulter DL, Allen RJ. Benign neonatal sleep myoclonus. *Arch Neurol* 1982;39:191–192.
7. Daoust-Roy J, Seshia SS. Benign neonatal sleep myoclonus: a differential diagnosis of neonatal seizures. *Am J Dis Child* 1992;146:1236–1241.
8. Vanasse M, Bedard P, Andermann F. Shuddering attacks in children: an early clinical manifestation of essential tremor. *Neurology* 1976;26:1027–1030.
9. Holmes GL, Russman BS. Shuddering attacks: evaluation using electroencephalographic frequency modulation radiotelemetry and videotape monitoring. *Am J Dis Child* 1986;140:72–73.
10. Barron TF, Younkin DP. Propranolol therapy for shuddering attacks. *Neurology* 1992;42:258–259.
11. Snyder CH. Paroxysmal torticollis in infancy. *Am J Dis Child* 1969;117:458–460.
12. Cohen HA, Nussinovitch M, Ashkenasi A, et al. Benign paroxysmal torticollis in infancy. *Pediatr Neurol* 1993;9:488–490.
13. Eviatar L. Benign paroxysmal torticollis. *Pediatr Neurol* 1994;11:72.
14. Deonna T, Martin D. Benign paroxysmal torticollis in infancy. *Arch Dis Child* 1981;56:956–959.
15. Gorrotxategi P, Reguilon MJ, Arana J, et al. Gastroesophageal reflux in association with the Sandifer syndrome. *Eur J Pediatr Surg* 1995;5:203–205.
16. Wiese JA, Gentry LR, Menezes AH. Bobble-head doll syndrome: review of the pathophysiology and CSF dynamics. *Pediatr Neurol* 1985;1:361–366.
17. Nellhaus G. The bobble-head doll syndrome: a "tic" with a neuropathologic basis. *Pediatrics* 1967;40:250–253.
18. Pollack IF, Schor NF, Martinez AJ, et al. Bobble-head doll syndrome and drop attacks in a child with a cystic choroid plexus papilloma of the third ventricle. *J Neurosurg* 1995;83:729–732.
19. Coker S. Bobble-head doll syndrome due to a trapped fourth ventricle and aqueduct. *Pediatr Neurol* 1986;2:115–116.
19a. Demirkiran M, Jankovic J. Paroxysmal dyskinesias: clinical features and classification. *Ann Neurol* 1995;38:571–579.
19b. Blakeley J, Jankovic J. Secondary paroxysmal dyskinesias. *Mov Disord* 2002 (in press).
20. Andermann F, Keene DL, Andermann E, et al. Startle disease or hyperekplexia: further delineation of the syndrome. *Brain* 1980;103:985–997.
21. Brown P. Physiology of startle phenomena. *Adv Neurol* 1995;67:273–287.
22. Gordon N. Startle disease or hyperekplexia. *Dev Med Child Neurol* 1993;35:1015–1024.
23. Andermann F, Andermann E. Excessive startle syndromes: startle disease, jumping, and startle epilepsy. *Adv Neurol* 1986;43:321–338.
24. Morley DJ, Weaver DD, Garg BP, et al. Hyperexplexia: an inherited disorder of the startle response. *Clin Genet* 1982;21:388–396.
25. Nigro MA, Lim HC. Hyperekplexia and sudden neonatal death. *Pediatr Neurol* 1992;8:221–225.
26. Leventer RJ, Hopkins IJ, Shield LK. Hyperekplexia as cause of abnormal intrauterine movements. *Lancet* 1995;345:461.
27. Baxter P, Connolly S, Curtis A, et al. Co-dominant inheritance of hyperekplexia and spastic paraparesis. *Dev Med Child Neurol* 1996;38:736–743.
28. Crone C, Nielsen J, Petersen N, et al. Patients with the major and minor form of hyperekplexia differ with regards to disynaptic reciprocal inhibition between ankle flexor and extensor muscles. *Exp Brain Res* 2001;140:190–197.
29. Ryan SG, Sherman SL, Terry JC, et al. Startle disease, or hyperekplexia: response to clonazepam and assignment of the gene (STHE) to chromosome 5q by linkage analysis. *Ann Neurol* 1992;31:663–668.
30. Elmslie FV, Hutchings SM, Spencer V, et al. Analysis of GLRA1 in hereditary and sporatic hyperekplexia: a novel mutation in a family cosegregating for hyperekplexia and spastic paraparesis. *J Med Genet* 1996;33:435–436.
31. Rees MI, Lewis TM, Vafa B, et al. Compound heterozygosity and nonsense mutations in the alpha (1)-subunit of the inhibitory glycine receptor in hyperekplexia. *Hum Genet* 2001;109:267–270.
32. Kwok JB, Raskin S, Morgan G, et al. Mutations in the glycine receptor alpha subunit (GLRA1) gene in hereditary hyperekplexia pedigrees: evidence for non-penetrance of mutation Y279C. *J Med Genet* 2001;38:E17.
33. Pascotto A, Coppola G. Neonatal hyperekplexia: a case report. *Epilepsia* 1992;33:817–820.
34. Kurlan R, McDermott MP, Deeley C, et al. Prevalence of tics in

schoolchildren and association with placement in special education. *Neurology* 2001;57:1383–1388.

35. Hyland K. Presentation, diagnosis, and treatment of the disorders of monoamine neurotransmitter metabolism. *Semin Perinatol* 1999;23:194–203.

36. Blau N, Bonafé, Thöny B. Tetrahydrobiopterin deficiencies without hyperphenylalaninemia: diagnosis and genetics of dopa-responsive dystonia and sepiapterin deficiency. *Mol Genet Metab* 2001;74:172–185.

37. Hyland K. Abnormalities of biogenic amine metabolism. *J Inher Metab Dis* 1993;16:676–690.

38. Kaufman S, Holtzman, Milstein S. Phenyketonuria due to deficiency of dihydropteridine reductase. *N Engl J Med* 1975; 293:785–790.

39. Smith I, Hyland K, Kendall B, et al. Clinical role of pteridine therapy in tetrahydrobiopterin deficiency. *J Inher Metab Dis* 1985;8:39–45.

40. Ichinose H, Nagatsu T. Molecular genetics of dopa-responsive dystonia. *Adv Neurol* 1999;80:195–198.

41. Ichinose H, Inagaki H, Suzuki T, et al. Molecular mechanisms of hereditary progressive dystonia with marked diurnal fluctuation, Segawa's disease. *Brain Dev* 2000;22[Suppl 1]:107–110.

42. Leuzzi V, Cardona F, Carducci C, et al. Autosomal dominant guanosine triphosphate cyclohydrolase I deficiency presenting as inherited dopa-responsive myoclonus-dystonia syndrome (abst). *Ann Neurol Suppl* 2001;1:S116.

43. Jarman PR, Bandmann O, Marsden CD, et al. GTP cyclohydrolase 1 mutations in patients with dystonia responsive to anticholinergic drugs. *J Neurol Neurosurg Psychiatry* 1997;63: 304–308.

44. Naumann M, Pirker W, Reiners K, et al. [123]beta-CIT single photon emission tomography in dopa-responsive dystonia. *Mov Disord* 1997;12:448–451.

45. Kishore A, Nygaard TG, de la Fuente-Fernandez R, et al. Striatal D2 receptors in symptomatic and asymptomatic carriers of dopa-responsive dystonia measured with [^{11}C]-raclopride and positron emission tomography. *Neurology* 1998;50:1028–1032.

46. Hyland K, Fryburg JS, Wilson WG, et al. Oral phenylalanine loading in dopa-responsive dystonia: a possible diagnostic test. *Neurology* 1997;48:1290–1297.

47. Hyland K, Arnold LA, Trugman JM. Defects of biopterin metabolism and biogenic amine biosynthesis: clinical, diagnostic, and therapeutic aspects. *Adv Neurol* 1998;78:301–308.

48. Blau N, Thöny B, Renneberg A, et al. Dihydropteridine reductase deficiency localized to the central nervous system. *J Inher Metab Dis* 1998;21:433–434.

49. Bonafé L, Thöny B, Penzien JM, et al. Mutations in the sepiapterin reductase gene cause a novel tetrahydrobiopterin-dependent monoamine-neurotransmitter deficiency with hyperphenylalaninemia. *Am J Hum Genet* 2001;69:269–277.

50. Blau N, Thöny B, Cotton RGH, et al. Disorders of tetrahydrobiopterin and related biogenic amines. In: Scriver CR, Beaudet AL, Sly WS, et al., eds. *The metabolic and molecular basis of inherited disease*, 8th ed. New York: McGraw-Hill, 2001:1725–1776.

51. Ludecke B, Knappskog PM, Clayton PT, et al. Recessively inherited L-dopa-responsive parkinsonism in infancy caused by a point mutation (L205P) in the tyrosine hydroxylase gene. *Hum Mol Genet* 1996;5:1023–1028.

52. Knappskog PM, Flatmark T, Mallet J, et al. Recessively inherited L-dopa-responsive dystonia caused by a point mutation (Q381K) in the tyrosine hydroxylase gene. *Hum Mol Genet* 1995;4:1209–1212.

53. van den Heuvel LP, Luiten B, Smeitink JA, et al. A common point mutation in the tyrosine hydroxylase gene in autosomal recessive L-dopa-responsive dystonia in the Dutch population. *Hum Genet* 1998;102:644–646.

54. Swaans RJ, Rondot P, Renier WO, et al. Four novel mutations in the tyrosine hydroxylase gene in patients with infantile parkinsonism. *Ann Hum Genet* 2000;64:25–31.

55. Furukawa Y, Nygaard TG, Gutlich M, et al. Striatal biopterin and tyrosine hydroxylase protein reduction in dopa-responsive dystonia. *Neurology* 1999;53:1032–1041.

56. Furukawa Y, Graf WD, Wong H, et al. Dopa-responsive dystonia simulating spastic paraplegia due to tyrosine hydroxylase (TH) gene mutations. *Neurology* 2001;23:260–263.

57. Sumi-Ichinose C, Ishinose H, Takahashi E, et al. Molecular cloning of genomic DNA and chromosomal assignment of the gene for human aromatic L-amino acid decarboxylase, the enzyme for catecholamine and serotonin biosynthesis. *Biochemistry* 1992;31:2229–2238.

58. Maller A, Hyland K, Milstien S, et al. Aromatic L-amino acid decarboxylase deficiency: clinical features, diagnosis, and treatment of a second family. *J Child Neurol* 1997;12:349–354.

59. Korenke GC, Christen HJ, Hyland K, et al. Aromatic L-amino acid decarboxylase deficiency: an extrapyramidal movement disorder with oculogyric crises. *Eur J Paediatr Neurol* 1997;1: 67–71.

60. Hyland K, Surtees RA, Rodeck C, et al. Aromatic L-amino acid decarboxylase deficiency: clinical features, diagnosis, and treatment of a new inborn error of neurotransmitter amine synthesis. *Neurology* 1992;42:1980–1988.

61. Yokochi M. Development of the nosological analysis of juvenile parkinsonism. *Brain Dev* 2000;22[Suppl 1]:S81–S86.

62. Hattori N, Shimura H, Kubo S, et al. Autosomal recessive juvenile parkinsonism: a key to understanding nigral degeneration in sporatic Parkinson's disease. *Neuropathology* 2000;20[Suppl]: S85–S90.

63. Yamamura Y, Hattori N, Matsumine H, et al. Autosomal recessive early-onset parkinsonism with diurnal fluctuation: clinico-pathologic characteristics and molecular genetic identification. *Brain Dev* 2000;22[Suppl 1]:87–91.

64. Broussolle E, Lücking CB, Ginovart N, et al. The French Parkinson's Disease Genetics Study Group [^{18}F]-dopa PET study in patients with juvenile-onset PD and parkin gene mutations. *Neurology* 2000;55:877–879.

65. Shimizu N, Asakawa S, Minoshima S, et al. *PARKIN* as a pathogenic gene for autosomal recessive juvenile parkinsonism. *J Neural Transm* 2000[Suppl]58:19–30.

66. Paulson H, Ammache Z. Ataxia and hereditary disorders. *Neurol Clin* 2001;19:759–782.

67. Rasmussen A, Macias R, Yescas P, et al. Huntington disease in children: genotype–phenotype correlation. *Neuropediatrics* 2000;31:190–194.

68. Tsuji S. Dentatorubral-pallidoluysian atrophy (DRPLA): clinical features and molecular genetics. *Adv Neurol* 1999;79: 399–409.

69. Grattan-Smith PJ, Healey S, Grigg JG, et al. Spinocerebellar ataxia type 7: a distinctive form of autosomal dominant cerebellar ataxia with retinopathy and marked genetic anticipation. *J Paediatr Child Health* 2001;37:81–84.

70. Sarker B. Copper transport and its defect in Wilson disease: characterization of the copper-binding domain of Wilson disease ATPase. *J Inorg Biochem* 2000;79:187–191.

71. Brewer GJ. Recognition, diagnosis, and management of Wilson's disease. *Proc Soc Exp Biol Med* 2000;223:39–46.

72. Walshe JM. Wilson's disease (HLD). In: Viken PJ, Bruyn GW, eds. *Handbook of clinical neurology*, vol 27. Amsterdam: North-Holland, 1976:379–414.

73. Strickland GT, Leu ML. Wilson's disease: clinical and laboratory manifestations in 40 patients. *Medicine* 1975;54:113–137.

74. Svetel M, Kozic D, Stefanova E, et al. Dystonia in Wilson's disease. *Mov Disord* 2001;16:719–723.

75. Walshe JM. Penicillamine: the treatment of first choice for patients with Wilson's disease. *Mov Disord* 1999;14:545–550.

76. Brewer GJ, Dick RD, Johnson VD, et al. Treatment of Wilson's disease with zinc. XVI: Treatment during the pediatric years. *J Lab Clin Med* 2001;137:191–198.

77. Zhou B, Bae SK, Malone AC, et al. hGFR alpha-4: a new member of the GDNF receptor family and a candidate for NBIA. *Pediatr Neurol* 2001;25:156–161.

78. Swaiman KF. Hallervorden-Spatz syndrome. *Pediatr Neurol* 2001;25:102–108.

79. Hayflick SJ, Penzien JM, Michl W, et al. Cranial MRI changes may precede symptoms in Hallervorden-Spatz syndrome. *Pediatr Neurol* 2001;25:166–109.

80. Higgins JJ, Patterson MC, Papadopoulos NM, et al. Hypoprebetalipoproteinemia, acanthocytosis, retinitis pigmentosa, and pallidal degeneration (HARP syndrome). *Neurology* 1992;42:194–198.

81. Malandrini A, Cesaretti S, Mulinari M, et al. Acanthocytosis, retinitis pigmentosa, pallidal degeneration: report of two cases without serum lipid abnormalities. *J Neurol Sci* 1996;140:129–131.

82. Manyam BV, Bhatt MH, Moore WD, et al. Bilateral striopallidodentate calcinosis: cerebrospinal fluid, imaging, and electrophysiological studies. *Ann Neurol* 1992;31:379–384.

83. Manyam BV, Waters AS, Narla KR. Bilateral striopallidodentate calcinosis: clinical characteristics of patients seen in a registry. *Mov Disord* 2001;16:258–264.

84. Geschwind DH, Loginov M, Stern JM. Identification of a locus on chromosome 14q for idiopathic basal ganglia calcification (Fahr disease). *Am J Hum Genet* 1999;65:764–772.

85. Meek D, Wolfe LS, Andermann E, et al. Juvenile progressive dystonia: a new phenotype of GM2 gangliosidosis. *Ann Neurol* 1984;15:348–352.

86. Nardocci N, Bertagnolio B, Rumi V, et al. Progressive dystonia symptomatic of juvenile GM2 gangliosidosis. *Mov Disord* 1992;7:64–67.

87. Uc EY, Wenger DA, Jankovic J. Neimann-Pick disease type C: two cases and an update. *Mov Disord* 2000;15:1199–1203.

88. van den Vlasakker CJ, Gabreels FJ, Wijburg HC, et al. Clinical features of Niemann-Pick disease type C: an example of the delayed onset, slowly progressive phenotype and an overview of recent literature. *Clin Neurol Neurosurg* 1994;96:119–123.

89. Aberg L, Liewendahl K, Nikkinen P, et al. Decreased striatal dopamine transporter density in JNCL patients with parkinsonian symptoms. *Neurology* 2000;54:1069–1074.

90. Wisniewski KE, Kida E, Golabek AA, et al. Neuronal ceroid lipofuscinoses: classification and diagnosis. *Adv Genet* 2001;45:1–34.

91. Wheeler RB, Schlie M, Kominami E, et al. Neuronal ceroid lipofuscinosis: late infantile or Jansky Bielschowsky type—re-revisited. *Acta Neuropathol* 2001;102:485–488.

92. Mole SE, Zhong NA, Sarpong A, et al. New mutations in the neuronal ceroid lipofuscinosis genes. *Eur J Paediatr Neurol* 2001;5[Suppl A]:7–10.

93. Lang AE, Clarke JTR, Rosch L, et al. Progressive longstanding "pure" dystonia: a new phenotype of juvenile metachromatic leukodystrophy. *Neurology* 1985;35[Suppl 1]:194.

94. Hoffmann GF, Zschocke J. Glutaric aciduria type 1: from clinical, biochemical, and molecular diversity to successful therapy. *J Inherit Metab Dis* 1999;22:381–391.

95. Hauser SE, Peters H. Glutaric aciduria type 1: an under diagnosed cause of encephalopathy and dystonia-dyskinesia syndrome in children. *J Paediatr Child Health* 1998;34:302–304.

96. Zafeiriou DI, Zschocke J, Augoustidou-Savvopoulou P, et al. Atypical and variable clinical presentation of glutaric aciduria type 1. *Neuropediatrics* 2000;31:303–306.

97. Berardelli A, Thompson PD, Zaccagnini M, et al. Two sisters with generalized dystonia associated with homocystinuria. *Mov Disord* 1991;6:163–165.

98. Calne DB, Lang AE. Secondary dystonia. *Adv Neurol* 1988;50:9–33.

99. Kempster PA, Brenton DP, Gale AN, et al. Dystonia in homocystinuria. *J Neurol Neurosurg Psychiatry* 1988;51:859–862.

100. DiMauro S, DeVivo DC. Genetic heterogeneity in Leigh syndrome. *Ann Neurol* 1996;40:5–7.

101. De Vivo DC. Leigh syndrome: historical perspective and clinical variations. *Biofactors* 1998;7:269–271.

102. Zhu Z, Yao J, Johns T, et al. SURF1, encoding factor involved in the biogenesis of cytochrome c oxidase, is mutated in Leigh syndrome. *Nat Genet* 1998;20:337–343.

103. Macaya A, Munell F, Burke RE, et al. Disorders of movement in Leigh syndrome. *Neuropediatrics* 1993;24:60–67.

104. Campistol J, Cusi V, Vernet A, et al. Dystonia as the presenting sign of subacute necrotizing encephalomyelopathy in infancy. *Eur J Pediatr* 1986;144:589–591.

105. Cacic M, Wilichowski E, Mejaski-Bosnjak V, et al. Cytochrome c oxidase partial deficiency–associated Leigh disease presenting as an extrapyramidal syndrome. *J Child Neurol* 2001;16:616–619.

106. Barkovich AJ, et al. Mitochondrial disorders: analysis of their clinical and imaging characteristics. *Am J Neuroradiol* 1993;14:1119–1137.

107. Jun AS, Brown MD, Wallace DC. A mitochondrial DNA mutation at nucleotide pair 14459 of the NADH dehydrogenase subunit 6 gene associated with maternally inherited Leber hereditary optic neuropathy and dystonia. *Proc Natl Acad Sci USA* 1994;91:6206–6210.

108. Gibson KM, Christensen E, Jakobs C, et al. The clinical phenotype of succinic semialdehyde dehydrogenase deficiency (4-hydroxybutyric aciduria): case reports of 23 new patients. *Pediatrics* 1997;99:567–574.

109. Leuzzi V, Bianchi MC, Tosetti M, et al. Brain creatine depletion: guanidinoacetate methyltransferase deficiency (improving with creatine supplementation). *Neurology* 2000;55:1407–1409.

110. Ganesan V, Johnson A, Connelly A, et al. Guanidinoacetate methyltransferase deficiency: new clinical features. *Pediatr Neurol* 1997;17:155–157.

111. Stökler S, Holzbach U, Hanefeld F, et al. Creatine deficiency in the brain: a new treatable inborn error of metabolism. *Pediatr Res* 1994;36:409–413.

112. Johnson JL, Wadman SK. Molybdenum cofactor deficiency and isolated sulphite oxidase deficiency. In: Scriver CR, Beaudet AL, Sly WS, et al., eds. *The metabolic basis of inherited disease,* 7th ed. New York: McGraw-Hill, 1995:2271–2283.

113. Graf WD, Oleinik OE, Jack RM, et al. Ahomocysteinemia in molybdenum cofactor deficiency. *Neurology* 1998;51:668–670.

114. Boles RG, Ment LR, Meyn MS, et al. Short-term response to dietary therapy in molybdenum cofactor deficiency. *Ann Neurol* 1993;34:742–744.

115. Jinnah HA, DeGregorio L, Harris JC, et al. The spectrum of inherited mutations causing HPRT deficiency: 75 new cases and a review of 196 previously reported cases. *Mutat Res* 2000;463:309–326.

116. Christie R, Bay C, Kaufman IA, et al. Lesch-Nyhan disease: clinical experience with nineteen patients. *Dev Med Child Neurol* 1982;24:293–306.

117. Mizuno T. Long-term follow-up of ten patients with Lesch-Nyhan syndrome. *Neuropediatrics* 1986;17:158–161.

118. Watts RWE, Spellacy E, Gibbs DA, et al. Clinical, post-mortem, biochemical, and therapeutic observations on the Lesch-Nyhan syndrome with particular reference to the neurological manifestations. *Q J Med* 1982;201:43–78.

119. Jinnah HA, Harris JC, Reich SG, et al. The motor disorder of Lesch-Nyhan disease (abst.). *Mov Disord* 1998;13[Suppl 2]:98.

120. Jinnah HA, Lewis RF, Visser JE, et al. Ocular motor dysfunction in Lesch-Nyhan disease. *Pediatr Neurol* 2001;24:200–204.

121. Crawford TO. Ataxia telangiectasia. *Semin Pediatr Neurol* 1998; 5:287–294.

122. Crawford TO, Mandir AS, Lefton-Grief MA, et al. Quantitative neurologic assessment of ataxia-telangiectasia. *Neurology* 2000;54:1505–1509.

123. Rubio JP, Danek A, Stone C, et al. Chorea-acanthocytosis: genetic linkage to chromosome 9q21. *Am J Hum Genet* 1997; 61:899–908.

124. Brooks DJ, Ibanez V, Playford ED, et al. Presynaptic and postsynaptic striatal dopaminergic function in neuroacanthocytosis: a positron emission tomographic study. *Ann Neurol* 1991;30: 166–171.

125. Scott BL, Jankovic J. Delayed-onset progressive movement disorders after static brain lesions. *Neurology* 1996;46:68–74.

126. Kuban KCK, Leviton A. Cerebral palsy. *N Engl J Med* 1994; 330:188–195.

127. Lorenz JM. The outcome of extreme prematurity. *Semin Perinatol* 2001;25:348–359.

128. Mutch L, Alberman E, Hagberg B, et al. Cerebral palsy epidemiology: where are we now and where are we going. *Dev Med Child Neurol* 1992;34:547–555.

129. Nelson K. Epidemiology and etiology of cerebral palsy. In: Capute AJ, Accardo PJ, eds. *Development disabilities in infancy and childhood,* 2nd ed., vol 2. Baltimore: Paul Brooks, 1996: 73–79.

130. Bax M, Nelson KB. Birth asphyxia: a statement. *Dev Med Child Neurol* 1993;35:1022–1024.

131. Nelson KB, Emery ES. Birth asphyxia and the neonatal brain: what do we know and when do we know it? *Clin Perinatol* 1993;20:327–344.

132. Evans P, Elliot M, Alberman E, et al. Prevalence and disabilities in 4- to 8-year-olds with cerebral palsy. *Arch Dis Child* 1985;60: 940–945.

133. Volpe JJ. Neurobiology of periventricular leukomalacia in the premature infant. *Pediatr Res* 2001;50:553–562.

134. Ness JK, Romanko MJ, Rothstein RP, et al. Perinatal hypoxia-ischemia induces apoptotic and excitotoxic death of periventricular white matter oligodendrocyte progenitors. *Dev Neurosci* 2001;23:203–208.

135. Kadhim H, Tabarki Verellen G, DePrez C, et al. Inflammatory cytokines in the pathogenesis of periventricular leukomalacia. *Neurology* 2001;56:1278–1284.

136. Vexler ZS, Ferriero DM. Molecular and biochemical mechanisms of perinatal brain injury. *Semin Neonatol* 2001;6:99–108.

137. Capute AJ. Identifying cerebral palsy in infancy through study of primitive reflex profiles. *Pediatr Ann* 1979;8:589–595.

138. Capute AJ, Palmer FB, Shapiro BK, et al. Primative reflex profile: a quantitation of primitive reflexes in infancy. *Dev Med Child Neurol* 1984;25:375–383.

139. Candy EJ, Hoon AH, Capute AJ, et al. MRI in motor delay: important adjunct to classification in cerebral palsy. *Pediatr Neurol* 1993;9:421–429.

140. Koman LA, Mooney JF, Smith BP. Neuromuscular blockade in the management of cerebral palsy. *J Child Neurol* 1996;11 [Suppl 1]:S23–S28.

141. Korman LA, Brashear A, Rosenfeld S, et al. Botulinum toxin type a neuromuscular blockade in the treatment of equinus foot deformity in cerebral palsy: a multicenter, open-label clinical trial. *Pediatrics* 2001;108:1062–1071.

142. Kim DS, Choi JU, Yang KH, et al. Selective posterior rhizotomy in children with cerebral palsy: a 10-year experience. *Childs Nerv Syst* 2001;17:556–562.

143. von Koch CS, Park TS, Steinbok P, et al. Selective posterior rhizotomy and intrathecal baclofen for the treatment of spasticity. *Pediatr Neurosurg* 2001;35:57–65.

144. Filloux FM. Neuropathophysiology of movement disorders in cerebral palsy. *J Child Neurol* 1996;11[Suppl 1]:S5–S12.

145. Yokochi K, Aiba K, Fodama M, et al. Magnetic resonance imaging in athetoid cerebral palsied children. *Acta Paediatr Scand* 1991;80:818–823.

146. Hoon AH, Freese PO, Reinhardt EM, et al. Age-dependent effects of trihyxyphenidal in extrapyramidal cerebral palsy. *Pediatr Neurol* 2001;25:55–58.

147. Greene P. Review. Baclofen in the treatment of dystonia. *Clin Neuropharmacol* 1992;15:276–288.

148. Albright AL, Barry MJ, Shafton DH, et al. Intrathecal baclofen for generalized dystonia. *Dev Med Child Neurol* 2001;43: 652–657.

149. Albright AL. Intrathecal baclofen in cerebral palsy movement disorders. *J Child Neurol* 1996;11[Suppl 1]:S29–S35.

150. Fletcher NA, Thompson PD, Scadding JW, et al. Successful treatment of childhood onset symptomatic dystonia with levodopa. *J Neurol Neurosurg Psychiatry* 1993;56:865–867.

151. Nygaard TG, Waran SP, Levine RA, et al. Dopa-responsive dystonia simulating cerebral palsy. *Pediatr Neurol* 1994;11: 236–240.

152. Miller G, Cala LA. Ataxic cerebral palsy: clinico-radiologic correlations. *Neuropediatrics* 1989;20:84–89.

153. Sugama S, Soeda A, Eto Y. Magnetic resonance imaging in three children with kernicterus. *Pediatr Neurol* 2001;25:328–331.

154. Cardoso F, Eduardo C, Silva AP, et al. Chorea in fifty consecutive patients with rheumatic fever. *Mov Disord* 1997;12: 701–703.

155. Vidakovic A, Dragasevic N, Kostic VS. Hemiballism: report of 25 cases. *J Neurol Neurosurg Psychiatry* 1994;57:945–949.

156. Freeman JM, Aron AM, Collard JE, et al. The emotional correlates of Sydenham's chorea. *Pediatrics* 1965;35:42–49.

157. Swedo SE, Leonard HL, Schapiro MB, et al. Sydenham's chorea: physical and psychological symptoms of St. Vitus dance. *Pediatrics* 1993;91:706–713.

158. Mercadante MT, Campos MC, Marques-Dias MJ, et al. Vocal tics in Sydenham's chorea. *J Am Acad Child Adolesc Psychiatry* 1997;36:305–306.

159. Bird MT, Palkes H, Prensky AL. A follow-up study of Sydenham's chorea. *Neurology* 1976;26:601–606.

160. Swedo SE, Rapoport JL, Cheslow DL, et al. High prevalence of obsessive-compulsive symptoms in patients with Sydenham's chorea. *Am J Psychiatry* 1989;146:246–249.

161. Taranta A. Relation of isolated recurrences of Sydenham's chorea to preceding streptococci infections. *N Engl J Med* 1959;260:1204–1210.

162. Berrios X, Quesney F, Morales A, et al. Are all recurrence of "pure" Sydenham chorea true recurrences of acute rheumatic fever? *J Pediatr* 1985;107:867–872.

163. Nausieda PA, Koller WC, Weiner WJ, et al. Chorea induced by oral contraceptives. *Neurology* 1979;29:1605–1609.

164. Giedd JN, Rapoport JL, Kruesi MJ, et al. Sydenham's chorea: magnetic resonance imaging of the basal ganglia. *Neurology* 1995;45:2199–2202.

165. Swedo SE, Leonard HL, Garvey M, et al. Pediatric autoimmune neuropsychiatric disorders associated with streptococcal infections: clinical description of the first 50 cases. *Am J Psychiatry* 1998;155:264–271.

166. Kurlan R. Tourette's syndrome and "PANDAS": will the relation bear out? *Neurology* 1998;50:1530–1534.

167. Lougee L, Perlmutter SJ, Nicolson R, et al. Psychiatric disorders in first-degree relatives of children with pediatric autoimmune neuropsychiatric disorders associated with streptococcal infec-

tions (PANDAS). *J Am Acad Child Adolesc Psychiatry* 2000;39: 1120–1126.

168. Giedd JN, Rapoport JL, Garvey MA, et al. MRI assessment of children with obsessive-compulsive disorder or tics associated with streptococcal infection. *Am J Psychiatry* 2000;157: 281–283.

169. Perlmutter SJ, Leitman SF, Garvey MA, et al. Therapeutic plasma exchange and intravenous immunoglobulin for obsessive-compulsive disorder and tic disorders in childhood. *Lancet* 1999;354:1153–1158.

170. Singer HS, Giuliano JD, Hansen BH, et al. Antibodies against human putamen in children with Tourette syndrome. *Neurology* 1998;50:1618–1624.

171. Singer HS, Loiselle CL, Wendlandt J, et al. Antineuronal antibodies in Sydenham's chorea and PANDAS: an ELISA and Western blot analysis. *Neurology* 2002;58[Suppl3]: A372.

172. Singer HS, Loiselle CL, Kwak NG, et al. Effect of microinfused sera from children with PANDAS and Tourette syndrome and antibodies against streptococcal M5 protein into rodent striatum (abst.). *Ann Neurol* 2001;[Suppl 1]:S117.

173. Hallett JJ, Harling-Berg CJ, Knopf PM, et al. Anti-striatal antibodies in Tourette syndrome cause neuronal dysfunction. *J Neuroimmunol* 2000;111:195–202.

174. Taylor JR, Morshed SA, Parveen S, et al. An animal model of Tourette's syndrome. *Am J Psychiatry* 2002;159:657–660.

175. Dale RC, Church AJ, Cardoso F, et al. Poststreptococcal acute disseminated encephalomyelitis with basal ganglia involvement and auto-reactive antibasal ganglia antibodies. *Ann Neurol* 2001;50:588–595.

32

RIGIDITY AND SPASTICITY

VICTOR S. C. FUNG
PHILIP D. THOMPSON

The clinical assessment of muscle tone is an integral part of the neurologic evaluation of patients with movement disorders. *Rigidity* and *spasticity* are terms used to describe different patterns of increased muscle tone detected as an increase in resistance to passive limb movements about a joint (1). Rigidity implies pathology of the extrapyramidal system, and spasticity implies pathology of upper motor neurons or the corticospinal tracts (2). Increased resistance to passive movement of a limb can also arise from dystonia, peripheral nervous system disorders, and increased muscle activity due to failure to relax. Nonneural causes, such as joint stiffness or ankylosis, tendon shortening, and altered passive properties of muscle, such as muscle shortening due to fibrosis with contracture, also may contribute to a clinical impression of increased muscle tone.

RIGIDITY

Rigidity is a continuous and uniform increase in muscle tone, felt as a constant resistance throughout the range of passive movement. It is usually present in all directions of movement, such as during flexion and extension of the wrist and forearm. The relative uniformity of rigidity in all directions has given rise to the term *lead-pipe rigidity*. Where there is tremor superimposed on the background increase in tone, a ratchet like quality of resistance to limb manipulation, called *cogwheel rigidity*, is felt (1). This is commonly seen in Parkinson's disease, when the cogwheeling has a frequency of 5 to 8 Hz, corresponding to the frequency of postural tremor (6). However, it is not diagnostic and may be encountered in any condition with rigidity and tremor. Incomplete relaxation and background voluntary contraction in patients with a postural or action tremor may also produce cogwheeling.

Rigidity is commonly assessed in the upper limbs at the wrist and elbow, in the neck and trunk, and at the ankle. The patient is instructed to relax and not resist the passive movements. It is often useful to repeat this instruction during the course of the examination. In the upper limb, most examiners apply quasi-sinusoidal movements of around 0.5 to 2 cycles per second (3,4). Rigidity can be detected in axial, proximal, and distal muscle groups. Assessment of rigidity at the neck should be performed with the patient supine. Rigidity of the trunk and proximal muscles can be detected by assessing the ease of rotating the shoulders from side to side with the patient standing; at the same time, rigidity of the shoulders is assessed by the freedom with which the proximal upper limbs and arms swing during trunk rotation. Rigidity in the legs is often difficult to assess because of the weight of the lower limb. Wartenberg's pendulum test may be useful if there is doubt. With the patient seated on the examination table, the relaxed lower legs are raised to the horizontal in the sagittal plane and then released simultaneously. On the more affected side, the leg can be observed to drop at a slowed but uniform rate when compared with the opposite side (5).

Rigidity can be attenuated with drowsiness or relaxation, so that it may be absent or inconsistent at rest even in advanced Parkinson's disease (7), but is readily reinforced or activated by proximal voluntary movement of the opposite limb (Froment's maneuver). In basal ganglia ("extrapyramidal") disease rigidity is often more pronounced in proximal and axial muscles. Extensor rigidity of neck muscles is a striking feature of progressive supranuclear palsy, and neck rigidity with anterocollis suggests the diagnosis of multiple system atrophy (MSA).

SPASTICITY

The increase in muscle tone in mild-moderate spasticity is velocity dependent (8). Hypertonia may be detected only following the application of fast muscle stretches to the affected limb but is not detected during slow movements. This characteristic should be sought specifically in the examination. Spasticity is commonly assessed at the elbows, knees, and ankles. At the elbow, fast flexion or extension movements may elicit a sudden increase in tone whereas resistance to slow passive movements is normal. There may be a supinator catch if the forearm is suddenly rotated. With the patient supine, the whole of the lower limb should be quickly raised by lifting the thigh, while observing whether the heel is lifted from the bed, which suggests increased tone at the knee. Increased resistance to sinusoidal movements at the knee and ankle may be present, although this is often difficult to assess at the knee because of the weight of the lower leg. Wartenberg's pendulum test may demonstrate that the legs drop in a series of excursions with a "catch" between each movement, rotating about an axis instead of falling in a purely sagittal plane. A critical feature of the hypertonia of spasticity is the clasp-knife phenomenon (9,10), which is best seen in the lower limbs. As the knee is flexed from an extended posture, the resistance to passive movement is initially marked, but then suddenly gives way. The clasp-knife phenomenon has a directional preponderance, owing to the tendency of spasticity to affect the extensors more than the flexors in the lower limbs, and the flexors more than the extensors in the upper limbs.

The basic clinical characteristics of hypertonia following lesions of the descending motor pathways at the various sites from the cerebral hemispheres to the spinal cord are similar, with the exception of flexor spasms, which are a prominent feature of spinal lesions. Spasticity is usually accompanied by other signs that together comprise the upper motor neuron syndrome. Perhaps the most important of these is an increase in the tendon jerks, a phenomenon recognized by Charcot (11). Reflex threshold is lowered and the vibratory stimulus of the tendon tap is transmitted through muscle and bone leading to recruitment of distant muscle stretch reflexes and the irradiation of the tendon reflex throughout a limb or to the other limb as in the crossed adductor reflex. Other features include altered cutaneous reflexes with a Babinski or extensor plantar response, loss of superficial abdominal reflexes, spontaneous and stimulus-induced flexor spasms, clonus, and paresis. Clonus refers to the repetitive movements of a limb elicited by rapid muscle stretch following a tendon tap or during manipulation of the limb, and is caused by reverberating brisk spinal stretch reflexes. Paresis is usually in a "pyramidal" pattern, particularly affecting the extensors in the upper limbs and flexors in the lower limbs. Even in the absence of weakness, there may be loss of the capacity to perform fractionated movements of the digits, evident as a slowness or clumsiness of sequential touching of the fingertips with the thumb, or rapid movements of the distal limb such as foot tapping.

Spasticity typically evolves in the days and weeks after injury to upper motor neuron pathways. During the interval before the appearance of spasticity, muscle tone is often flaccid with depression of tendon reflexes. The duration of this interval varies according to the level of the lesion. For example, increased tone in the affected limbs may appear a few days after a capsular stroke, whereas flaccidity may persist after a spinal cord lesion for weeks or months. The changes responsible for the generation of spasticity are poorly understood. Once spasticity is established, the chronically shortened muscle may develop physical changes, such as shortening and contracture, that further contribute to the muscle stiffness (12).

DIFFERENTIATING RIGIDITY FROM SPASTICITY

Although the above discussion implies that differentiation of rigidity from spasticity is straightforward, the precise differences in the pathophysiology of *hypertonia* in the two conditions are poorly understood. The examination of tone is rarely undertaken without knowledge of the history or possible diagnosis, and this often influences the way in which muscle tone is evaluated. There are a number of other factors that potentially confound the distinction between rigidity and spasticity. Neither rigidity nor spasticity is associated with a single pathologic entity. The hypertonia accompanying cerebral infarction or spinal lesions is often described as spasticity, yet cerebral infarction may involve the pyramidal or extrapyramidal pathways. Conversely, the hypertonia of predominantly extrapyramidal pathologies in Steele-Richardson-Olszewski syndrome (progressive supranuclear palsy) (13) or multiple system atrophy (14) may have varying degrees of pyramidal system involvement.

To further complicate the issue, *dystonia* may also be associated with hypertonia. The term was first used by Oppenheim (15) to describe a motor disorder characterized by variable hyper- and hypotonia. Although dystonia is often present only with action in mild or early cases, in more advanced or secondary cases it can be associated with a sustained abnormality of resting posture with increased resistance to passive movement. Dystonia can be a prominent feature of juvenile or young-onset Parkinson's disease, and also advanced Parkinson's disease, especially as the effects of medication wear off (end-of-dose dystonia) (16). Separation of the rigid and dystonic components of hypertonia in parkinsonism is as much by convention as science. There are no objective studies that can separate the two, and accordingly the boundary between hypertonia in rigidity and dystonia is perhaps even more blurred than that between rigidity and spasticity.

OTHER CAUSES OF HYPERTONIA

Diseases of the frontal lobes and their connections may also produce a particular form of hypertonia. Frontal lobe hypertonia is characterized by increasing resistance to movement with increasing force of movement and is referred to as *gegenhalten* or *paratonia*. The examiner suspects that the patient is not fully relaxed or is opposing the movement, and contrary to instructions to relax, manipulation of the limb leads to a progressive increase in tone. If gegenhalten is marked and there are associated frontal lobe signs, such as grasp reflexes and mutism, or striatal signs, the distinction between hypertonia of frontal lobe origin and that associated with basal ganglia disease is straightforward. However, if the associated physical signs are minor, this distinction can be difficult. This raises the question of the mechanisms of hypertonia in different diseases whose primary pathologic change lies in the basal ganglia or the frontal lobes, or both, as in corticobasal degeneration. It is not known how the mechanisms responsible for hypertonia in each of these situations differ, and in view of the rich interconnections between frontal lobe motor areas and the basal ganglia, there may be some similarities.

Hypertonia may also be seen in patients with disease of the spinal cord in which unrestrained anterior horn cell discharge leads to "alpha rigidity." Isolation of the anterior horn cells from normal interneuron inhibitory control is the presumed mechanism. Other signs of spinal cord disease are invariably present. Continuous motor unit activity leading to stiffness of axial muscles, particularly the thoracolumbar paraspinal muscles and muscles of the anterior abdominal wall, presents a striking picture in the stiff-man syndrome. A robust feature that aids identification of this rare syndrome is the board-like stiffness of the anterior abdominal wall and an exaggerated lumbar lordosis resulting from continuous contraction of the abdominal and paraspinal muscles. Stimulus-sensitive muscle spasms are usually present. Continuous muscle discharge due to peripheral neuromuscular hyperexcitability in Isaacs' syndrome or acquired neuromyotonia is another cause of hypertonia. Clues to this include widespread fasciculations, myokymia, absent tendon reflexes, and, in some cases, other signs of a peripheral neuropathy. Finally, primary muscle disease can occasionally cause hypertonia. Myotonia may give rise to the complaint of stiffness or the appearance of hypertonia during voluntary movement, due to delayed muscle relaxation, although resistance to passive movement is normal. Rare congenital myopathies or muscular dystrophies with associated muscle contracture or hypertrophy also may limit the range of passive limb movement and be interpreted as hypertonia.

ANATOMICAL CORRELATES OF RIGIDITY AND SPASTICITY

Rigidity

Basal ganglia structures are clearly implicated in the pathophysiology of rigidity, since rigidity is a cardinal feature of nigrostriatal dopamine deficiency in Parkinson's disease. Moreover, rigidity is abolished following surgical lesions of the posteroventral globus pallidus, subthalamic nucleus, or ventrolateral thalamus in patients with Parkinson's disease. However, the changes in the basal ganglia are secondary rather than causal, since the above structures are structurally intact in Parkinson's disease and there are no reports of isolated rigidity following basal ganglia lesions. Bilateral lesions of the lentiform nucleus can cause parkinsonism, but this is rare and dystonia is more common (17). In contrast, unilateral lesions of the substantia nigra can cause typical parkinsonism with rigidity on the contralateral side. Rigidity with minimal other features of parkinsonism can develop in patients with a dopaminergic deficit due to exposure to neuroleptic medication or a metabolic defect in the production of dopamine. Therefore, the underlying basis of rigidity appears to be loss of dopaminergic modulation of basal ganglia function rather than loss of specific neural pathways.

Spasticity

Lesions of descending motor pathways at any level from the cerebral hemispheres to the spinal cord result in spasticity and the upper motor neuron syndrome. However, there is surprisingly little certainty as to which neural pathways are responsible for generating spasticity. It is worth noting John Hughlings Jackson's dictum that following a lesion of the nervous system, the *negative* features, or loss of function, inform us of the function of the structures that have been destroyed, whereas the *positive* abnormalities reflect the function of the structures that remain.

There are two striking and at first seemingly contradictory observations about spasticity that arise from lesion analysis:

1. *Spasticity does not develop following lesions restricted to primary motor cortex or lesions of the corticospinal (pyramidal) tracts at the level of the medulla, but it does develop with combined lesions of primary and premotor cortex or lesions of the corticospinal projections above the level of the medulla.* In subhuman primates selective damage to area 4, the origin of a significant portion of the pyramidal tract, results in a contralateral flaccid paralysis, greatest in distal and least in proximal muscle groups (18). With the passage of time strength recovers, though it does not return to normal, and fractionated movements of the digits remain significantly impaired. Increased muscle tone is not a prominent feature. Cortical lesions involving the premotor cortex, area 6 anterior to area 4, result in impaired postural control of the contralateral limbs, paresis, and spasticity. Whether these observations can be applied to humans has been the subject of debate over many years. The effects of selective lesions have rarely been reported in humans. Hemisphere lesions involving the corona radiata or internal capsule producing hemiplegia probably interrupt projections from both areas 4 and 6, since descending motor pathways lie in close proximity at these sites. Flaccid paresis with loss of skilled and dexterous finger movements has been described after pure lesions of the medullary pyramid (19) or selective lesions of the spinal cord (20), apparently without major changes in mus-

cle tone. In summary, loss of motor cortical input to structures rostral to the pyramidal tract in the medulla, most likely in the upper brainstem, lead to the development of spasticity but loss of the corticomotoneuronal projection to the spinal cord does not.

2. *Spasticity develops below the level of a spinal cord lesion.* This finding can be reconciled with that above as follows: The observation that loss of all descending inputs below the level of a spinal lesion also produces spasticity suggests that spinal projections from brainstem structures inhibit the development of spasticity. It follows that innervation from motor cortex facilitates activity in brainstem structures from which descending projections to the spinal cord, such as the reticulospinal pathways, maintain normal tone. It follows that spasticity may also result from loss of this facilitation, such as by interruption of cortical-brainstem pathways.

The typical flexed-limb posture after an upper motor neuron lesion is thought to reflect increased tone in flexor muscle groups and weakness of extensor muscles, although the latter has been questioned (21). This pattern of muscle activity does not appear to depend on reflexes driven by afferent feedback from sensory receptors in the affected limb, since dorsal root section has no effect on limb posture in the monkey (22). Voluntary mass movements of hemiplegic limbs and reflex mass movements, such as during yawning, indicate that descending inputs from brainstem motor centers still gain access to spinal motor neurons in upper motor neuron lesions. The origin of these inputs is not known. Residual corticospinal fibers, vestibulospinal (23) and reticulospinal (24) pathways are all capable of influencing the posture and degree of spasticity of hemiplegic limbs.

PHYSIOLOGIC CORRELATES OF RIGIDITY

There have been many studies of reflex activity in patients with rigidity. Many differ from the clinical assessment of rigidity in one or both of two crucial factors. First, rigidity is elicited by the application of relatively large-amplitude muscle stretches. Second, rigidity is assessed with the patient adopting a specific motor set, that of attempted relaxation of the limb or joint that is being manipulated. The relevance to the clinical phenomenon of rigidity of any abnormal reflex activity that is elicited under differing conditions must be questioned. With this caveat in mind, the physiology of rigidity will be reviewed.

Reflex Origin of Parkinsonian Rigidity

Rigidity can be abolished by dorsal root section (25) and by the intramuscular injection of nonparalytic doses of local anesthetic (26). These studies provide strong evidence of a reflex origin for rigidity, with the afferent limb originating in muscle.

Tonic Stretch Reflex Activity

During passive movements of the wrist or elbow, patients with parkinsonian rigidity develop muscle bursting at the frequency of the perturbation, indicating that rigidity is not simply due to unmodulated tonic muscle contraction (3,27). The timing of this bursting varies between subjects but it is primarily the stretch-related activity that is responsible for rigidity (28). Enhanced tonic stretch reflex activity has also been noted following linear muscle stretches (29,30).

Phasic Stretch Reflexes

The monosynaptic stretch reflex is not responsible for parkinsonian rigidity. Charcot recognized that tendon jerks are normal in Parkinson's disease. He wrote of the "essential distinction between rigidity and pyramidal or spinal hypertonicity—the absence of reflex accentuation in rigidity" (11). This dictum has subsequently been confirmed in quantitative studies (31,32). H reflexes have also generally been reported as being normal in Parkinson's disease.

Lee and Tatton (33,34) were the first to report enhanced long-latency stretch reflexes in Parkinson's disease and suggested that this abnormality might correlate with rigidity. Although these studies did not control for background levels of muscle contraction, Tatton et al. (35) later showed that heightened reflex responsiveness could not be attributed merely to inadequate relaxation or increased supraspinal drive to alpha motor neurons. However, the constancy of the relationship between long-latency stretch reflexes and rigidity has been questioned by a number of investigators (36–39).

One factor that has rarely been taken into account when interpreting studies of long-latency stretch reflexes in Parkinson's disease is that most recent studies have controlled for background electromyographic (EMG) activity by asking subjects to maintain a low-level tonic contraction. As noted above, clinical rigidity is tested with the subject attempting to relax the limb during passive movement. In normal subjects, long-latency stretch reflexes are modulated by alterations in motor set (40,41), and such modulation can be abnormal in Parkinson's disease (42). Therefore, the lack of a consistent correlation between long-latency stretch reflex amplitude and rigidity may merely be due to a failure to measure the two under comparable conditions.

Segmental and Supraspinal Influences

The tonic vibration reflex (TVR) is qualitatively normal in Parkinson's disease (43), although when the torque generated by this reflex is compared with controls, it is higher in patients and correlates with the degree of rigidity (32). However, it is unlikely to account for clinical rigidity, as the TVR is reduced following treatment with levodopa, even if rigidity persists (32). Inhibition of the H reflex by the TVR is normal in Parkinson's disease (44).

There are a number of segmental and supraspinal pathways that influence the excitability of the motor neuron pool. These can be studied by examining their effect on the amplitude of the H reflex. Following paired stimuli, the amplitude of the second H reflex varies in a characteristic fashion, showing periods of relative inhibition and excitation that depend on the interstimulus interval. In Parkinson's disease the period of late facilitation is increased (45). Recurrent Renshaw inhibition is normal (46,47), but reciprocal Ia inhibition is increased, at least in the lower limbs (48,49).

Reflexes mediated by large-diameter afferents are not the only spinal pathways altered in Parkinson's disease. Following non-nociceptive cutaneous stimulation, both excitatory and inhibitory modulation of tonic EMG activity in nearby muscles are observed (50). The first period of inhibition (I1), which is probably modulated at a spinal level, has been reported as being less marked in Parkinson's disease (51), although this has been disputed (52). It has subsequently been shown that I1 can be enhanced by the administration of apomorphine, which is a direct dopamine agonist (53).

One of the few reflex abnormalities demonstrated to correlate positively with parkinsonian rigidity is loss of short-latency autogenic Ib inhibition of the soleus H reflex (54). Corticospinal (55) and rubrospinal (56) projections augment Ib inhibition. However, the dorsal and noradrenergic reticulospinal tracts give rise to inhibitory inputs to Ib interneurons (54). Based on their findings and reports of increased Ia reciprocal inhibition in Parkinson's disease (48,49), Delwaide et al. (54) proposed that overactivity in the nucleus gigantocellularis of the dorsal reticulospinal system is responsible for rigidity in Parkinson's disease. This is consistent with previous suggestions that the Ib inhibitory system is concerned with the relation between muscle length and tension and therefore the control of muscle stiffness (57). Interestingly, inhibition in tonic activation of extensor digitorum communis by transcutaneous stimulation of Golgi tendon organ afferents is also less pronounced in Parkinson's disease (58), although the difference between patients and controls was more marked in patients with tremor rather than rigidity.

Finally, it has also been shown that alpha motor neuron and possibly cortical excitability is enhanced in Parkinson's disease as tested by measuring resting cortical thresholds to transcranial magnetic stimulation, the duration of the cortical silent period, and F-wave excitability (59). Each of these measures was found to correlate with clinical assessments of rigidity.

Voluntary Relaxation and Rigidity

Landau et al. (60) were the first to suggest that the primary abnormality in parkinsonian rigidity was "a continuous, excessive net excitatory drive to the final common path—a physiologically normal spinal cord," challenging the popular belief of the time that there was a fundamental abnormality in gamma drive. A decade later, Burke et al. (61) gave support to this hypothesis by reporting that direct recordings of human spindle afferents in parkinsonian and incompletely relaxed normal subjects showed similar characteristics. This led to the suggestion that "the most important cause of rigidity in Parkinson's disease is excessive and uncontrollable supraspinal drive to alpha motor neurons, evident in the patient's inability to relax" (62). This hypothesis is further supported by a correlation between clinical assessments of upper limb rigidity and the amount of surface EMG activity recorded during attempted voluntary relaxation of an intrinsic hand muscle (63).

However, it is unlikely that stretch reflex abnormalities in Parkinson's disease are entirely due to inadequate voluntary relaxation. Noth et al. (64) have shown that the short-latency stretch reflex recorded from the first dorsal interosseous muscle is attenuated following small stretches, but not when elicited by direct nerve stimulation in parkinsonian subjects when compared with controls. This was interpreted as consistent with enhanced static fusimotor drive in the patient group. Tatton et al. (35) demonstrated that long-latency stretch reflexes are enhanced in parkinsonian patients even when background levels of EMG activity and stretch velocity are matched with controls. These studies leave open the question of whether such changes are responsible for parkinsonian rigidity.

Shortening Reactions

Patients with Parkinson's disease can have a pronounced shortening reaction (Westphal's phenomenon). This is appreciated best in biceps of the arm and tibialis anterior in the leg. Passive shortening of the muscle leads to muscle contraction at latencies consistent with a reflex. This behavior is the opposite of a stretch reflex. The mechanism and significance of the shortening reaction are not known. The presence of the shortening reaction does not correlate with changes in muscle tone (65).

Altered Passive Properties of Muscle

Two studies have purported to show evidence of increased nonneural stiffness in parkinsonian patients, possibly as a result of altered passive properties of muscle. Dietz et al. (12) found that during the swing phase of gait, EMG activity in tibialis anterior was greater in parkinsonian patients when compared with controls, although similar angles of ankle dorsiflexion were present in the two groups. No evidence was found for increased co-contraction, or for alterations in joint properties or the EMG–force relationship, and the authors concluded that increased EMG activity was necessary to overcome increased nonneural stiffness in the triceps surae muscles. No attempt was made to correlate these changes with clinical measures of ankle rigidity. Watts et al. (66) measured nonneural elastic stiffness at the elbow using an objective technique that eliminated coexistent EMG activity, and found that it was increased in Parkinson's disease. However, no clear quantitative association with rigidity was demonstrated. These data suggest that Parkinson's disease can result in increased nonneural joint stiffness, possibly due to altered passive properties of muscle, but the contribution of these changes to clinical measures of rigidity remain uncertain.

PHYSIOLOGIC CORRELATES OF SPASTICITY

Reflex Origin of Spasticity

Like parkinsonian rigidity, spasticity can also be abolished by dorsal root section (25) and intramuscular injection of local anesthetic (30). These studies provide strong evidence that spasticity is also of reflex origin, with the afferent limb originating in muscle. At the doses of local anesthetic required to abolish hypertonia, muscle strength is preserved or occasionally augmented, although exceptions may occur (e.g., see Case 6 [30]).

Enhanced Stretch Reflex Activity

A widely but not universally accepted definition of spasticity is that of "a motor disorder characterized by a velocity-dependent increase in tonic stretch reflexes ('muscle tone') with exaggerated tendon jerks, resulting from hyperexcitability of the stretch reflex as one component of the upper motor neuron syndrome" (67).

Whereas rigidity is usually assessed with continuous sinusoidal stretches, spasticity is often assessed with a series of sudden, single movements corresponding to linear stretches. Short-latency reflex activity is elicited at much lower displacement velocities in spastic muscles than in muscles of normal subjects (68). This corresponds to the exaggerated tendon jerks. However, the critical abnormality that corresponds to spastic hypertonia is sustained stretch reflex activity following linear stretches. This sustained reflex activity does not occur in normal subjects. It persists as long as the muscle is undergoing an increase in length, ceases upon termination of movement (even if the muscle is maintained in the lengthened state), and increases linearly with the velocity of stretch (9,69). Similar stretch reflex abnormalities have been reported in patients with both spasticity of predominantly cerebral (69) and spinal (9) origin. The ease with which this late muscle activity is elicited increases in the first month of spasticity; following that, the threshold remains stable, then declines after a year (69). These observations led Thilmann et al. (69) to conclude that the increase in muscle tone of spasticity was the result of enhanced stretch reflexes that reached a stable threshold about a month after the onset of spasticity. The sustained late-onset stretch reflex activity in spasticity presumably arises from disinhibited segmental spinal pathways, since transcortical long-latency stretch reflexes can be abolished following lesions of the cortical and subcortical motor tracts that are associated with spasticity as well as following lesions of the dorsal columns in the spinal cord.

Spinal and Segmental Reflex Behavior in Spasticity

At the level of the spinal cord a number of alterations in reflex behavior have been described, some of which differ between spasticity of cerebral versus spinal origin. Subtle neurophysiologic changes in the excitability of motor neurons, interneuronal connections, and specific local reflex pathways have been demonstrated, though none can be held primarily responsible for the signs of spasticity. Many of these phenomena are secondary to changes in the descending control of the spinal circuits. These are discussed briefly.

1. *Alpha motor neuron* excitability. Enhanced H/M ratios (70) and F-wave amplitudes (71) suggest enhanced excitability of alpha motor neurons. These changes most likely reflect changes in descending control of segmental spinal networks as the result of the lesion upstream from the motor neurons.
2. *Alpha motor neuron* excitability. Fusimotor neurons innervate intrafusal muscle fibers and control primary spindle sensitivity. Hyperactivity of the fusimotor system increases spindle sensitivity to stretch, augmenting the Ia afferent response to stretch, and exaggerates the stretch reflex. This may contribute to decerebrate rigidity in the cat, but there is no evidence this is the case in humans. Local anesthetic injections into spastic muscles in humans can diminish spasticity by an effect on alpha motor neurons. This effect can be explained by reducing activity in the stretch reflex pathway without invoking a primary role in the mechanism of spasticity. Muscle spindle sensitivity is not enhanced in human spasticity as judged by recordings from Ia spindle afferents (72).
3. *Recurrent inhibition.* Recurrent collateral axons from motor neurons activate Renshaw cells, which inhibit alpha motor neurons. Renshaw cells receive inputs from descending motor pathways and therefore are subject to supraspinal control. Renshaw cell activity is not significantly reduced at rest in patients with cerebral spasticity (73), but may be increased in spinal spasticity (74).
4. *Reciprocal inhibition.* The reciprocal inhibition between antagonist muscles is mediated by the Ia inhibitory interneuron. Ia afferents make monosynaptic connections with homonymous motor neurons and project via the Ia inhibitory interneuron to antagonist muscles. The Ia inhibitory interneuron also receives synaptic input from descending pathways and other afferents. Altered activity in Ia inhibitory interneuronal pathways has been

shown in upper motor neuron lesions and spasticity (75,76). Loss of Ia inhibitory reciprocal inhibition may interfere with voluntary activation of an agonist muscle by allowing the antagonist to develop a stretch reflex during agonist contraction that opposes the agonist effect. These effects are of course most likely to be evident during movement rather than influencing resting muscle tone. Again, such changes are most likely secondary to alterations in descending control of spinal interneurons.

5. *Presynaptic inhibition.* Inhibitory effects on alpha motor neurons are also derived from inhibitory interneurons acting on primary afferent terminals of the alpha motor neuron. Vibration-induced inhibition of the tendon reflex is one example of presynaptic inhibition of Ia synapses onto motor neurons. Interneurons mediating presynaptic inhibition are also influenced by descending motor projections. Accordingly, alterations in the balance of this descending control may change spinal neuron behavior. Presynaptic inhibition has been reported as being reduced in spasticity of spinal origin but preserved in spasticity of cerebral origin (77).

6. *Plasticity within the central nervous system.* A new consideration in mechanisms of spasticity is the role of axonal sprouting and the formation of new synapses. Previously regeneration was not thought to occur within the central nervous system, and this is still the subject of debate. Nevertheless, the formation of new synapses and aberrant connections between motor neurons and interneurons is another theoretic explanation for some of the events in spasticity.

Clonus

Clonus, a common sign in spasticity, may be detected in any muscle group. It manifests as repetitive contraction and relaxation of an agonist–antagonist muscle pair. EMG recordings show alternating contraction of the muscle pairs. Clonus frequency varies inversely with reflex path length from the spinal cord, consistent with reexcitation within a peripheral reflex loop (78). Stretch of one muscle leads to an exaggerated reflex contraction, which in turn stretches the antagonist muscle, eliciting a further reflex contraction. Other authors have argued for oscillation within a central pacemaker because the rhythm of clonus may be difficult to entrain and the frequency of clonus may be similar at different sites (79).

Clasp-knife Phenomenon

In human spasticity the gradual increase in muscle tone with stretch of the knee extensor followed by an abrupt decline in resistance is called the clasp-knife phenomenon. Explanations for this reflex increase in muscle tone and its sudden abolition include activation of the Golgi tendon organ and autogenic inhibition of extensor motor neurons from group Ib afferents (9) and excitation of other muscle receptors and flexor reflex afferents. Nonspindle group II and III afferents from free endings in muscle also inhibit extensor and facilitate flexor muscles in spasticity. Flexor reflex afferents exhibit similar effects. The spinal interneurons mediating these effects are subject to descending inhibitory input, particularly from dorsal reticulospinal tracts. Lesions of these descending reticulospinal pathways enhance these reflex effects and are therefore considered an important factor in spasticity.

Flexor Spasms

One of the most dramatic manifestations of spasticity is flexor spasms of the legs and trunk after spinal cord injury. Bilateral interruption of the corticospinal and dorsal reticulospinal projections releases activity in flexor reflex afferent systems. Various "natural" stimuli ranging from cutaneous to bladder afferents also engage the flexor reflex system to produce uninhibited activity in flexor muscles.

Babinski's Sign and Flexor Reflexes

The Babinski response, consisting of extension of the great toe after stimulation of the sole of the foot, is one of the best-known signs of an upper motor neuron lesion. Stimulation of the outer plantar surface of the foot evokes extension of the great toe (the extensor plantar response), fanning of the lateral toes, and variable dorsiflexion of the ankle and flexion of the hip and knee. It is closely related to impairment of foot movement and therefore to interruption of corticospinal projections to motor neurons innervating muscles of the distal leg and foot (80). The relation of the extensor plantar response to the triple-flexion or withdrawal response of the leg has been the subject of much interest over the years. Walshe (81) emphasized that the Babinski response was one component of the flexion withdrawal response. Extension of the great toe was always accompanied by contraction of the proximal flexors of the leg and, in some cases, contraction of extensors of the contralateral leg: the crossed extensor response. This complex synergy added weight to the notion that the Babinski sign was one part of a flexion withdrawal response of the lower limb in response to a noxious stimulus. In a recent study van Gijn (80) also noted that flexor reflex activity frequently accompanied the Babinski's sign, though this was not necessarily increased.

Nonneural Stiffness in Spasticity

The notion that hypertonia in spasticity is predominantly due to enhanced reflex activity has been challenged. Reduced ankle dorsiflexion was observed during walking in patients with lower limb spasticity despite enhanced activity in the ankle dorsiflexors and in the absence of co-contraction in antagonist muscles (12). Hypertonia at the elbow measured with mechanically driven, passive, low-amplitude, sinusoidal movements was found to correlate not with stretch reflex activity in biceps but with the degree of contracture (82). These observations have led to the suggestion that a significant contribution to hypertonia in spasticity arises from alterations in the intrinsic properties of muscle.

TREATMENT

A variety of strategies are available to reduce the muscle tone of spasticity and to lessen flexor spasms in patients who have upper motor neuron lesions. An important initial consideration is the indication for treatment and the expectations from such treatment. For example, loss of manual dexterity or weakness is not improved by treatments that reduce muscle tone. In the patient who can walk, a reduction of leg muscle tone may be detrimental to mobility if tone compensates for leg weakness and allows the patient to stand. Accordingly, treatment for spasticity may not lead to an improvement in function. Physiotherapy is useful in maintaining limb mobility and preventing muscle contracture, in addition to maximizing functional capacity from residual movement. In patients with spinal cord lesions, management of cutaneous or bladder infections, maintenance of bladder function, and reduction of noxious stimuli may reduce painful flexor spasms and associated polysynaptic reflex activity. Pharmacologic approaches entail the use of drugs that interfere with transmission in spinal reflexes and muscle contraction. Baclofen and diazepam increase presynaptic (GABAergic) inhibition of Ia afferents, depressing monosynaptic reflex activity. Baclofen also inhibits polysynaptic reflex activity. Gabapentin has also been effective. Tizanidine and clonidine block α_2-adrenergic receptors in excitatory interneuronal pathways. Spasms can also be lessened by inducing weakness of peripheral muscle by dantrolene, which reduces calcium release from sarcoplasmic reticulum, or injections of botulinum toxin, which creates a presynaptic neuromuscular blockade.

REFERENCES

1. Holmes G. *Introduction to clinical neurology,* 2nd ed. Edinburgh: E & S Livingstone, 1952.
2. Rothwell JC. *Control of human voluntary movement,* 2nd ed. London: Chapman and Hall, 1994.
3. Meara RJ, Cody FW. Relationship between electromyographic activity and clinically assessed rigidity studied at the wrist joint in Parkinson's disease. *Brain* 1992;115:1167–1180.
4. Prochazka A, Bennett DJ, Stephens MJ, et al. Measurement of rigidity in Parkinson's disease. *Mov Disord* 1997;12:24–32.
5. Wartenberg R. *Diagnostic tests in neurology.* Chicago: Year Book Publishers, 1953.
6. Lance J, Schwab R, Peterson E. Action tremor and the cogwheel phenomenon in Parkinson's disease. *Brain* 1963;86:95–110.
7. Webster DD. Dynamic measurement of rigidity, strength, and tremor in Parkinson patients before and after destruction of mesial globus pallidus. *Neurology* 1960;10:157–163.
8. Burke D, Lance JW. Studies of the reflex effects of primary and secondary spindle endings in spasticity. In: Desmedt J, ed. *New developments in electromyography and clinical neurophysiology.* Basel: Karger, 1973:475–495.
9. Burke D, Gillies JD, Lance JW. The quadriceps stretch reflex in human spasticity. *J Neurol Neurosurg Psychiatry* 1970;33:216–223.
10. Lance JW. The control of muscle tone, reflexes, and movement. *Neurology* 1980;30:1303–1313.
11. Charcot J-M. *Charcot, the clinician: the Tuesday lessons.* New York: Raven Press, 1987.
12. Dietz V, Quintern J, Berger W. Electrophysiological studies of gait in spasticity and rigidity: evidence that altered mechanical properties of muscle contribute to hypertonia. *Brain* 1981;104:431–449.
13. Steele J, Richardson J, Olszewski J. Progressive supranuclear palsy. *Arch Neurol* 1964;10:333–359.
14. Wenning GK, Ben Shlomo Y, Magalhaes M, et al. Clinical features and natural history of multiple system atrophy: an analysis of 100 cases. *Brain* 1994;117:835–845.
15. Oppenheim H. Über eine eigenartige Krampfkrankheit des kindlichen und jugendlichen Alters (Dysbasia lordotica progressiva, Dystonia musculorum deformans). *Neurologie Centralblatt* 1911;30:1090–1107.
16. Marsden CD. Parkinson's disease. *J Neurol Neurosurg Psychiatry* 1994;57:672–681.
17. Bhatia KP, Marsden CD. The behavioural and motor consequences of focal lesions of the basal ganglia in man. *Brain* 1994;117:859–876.
18. Tower S. Pyramidal lesions in the monkey. *Brain* 1940;63:36–90.
19. Chokroverty S, Rubino FA, Haller C. Pure motor hemiplegia due to pyramidal infarction. *Arch Neurol* 1975;32:647–648.
20. Nathan PW. Effects on movement of surgical incisions into the human spinal cord. *Brain* 1994;117:337–346.
21. Colebatch JG, Gandevia SC. The distribution of muscular weakness in upper motor neuron lesions affecting the arm. *Brain* 1989;112:749–763.
22. Denny-Brown D. *The cerebral control of movement.* Liverpool: Liverpool University Press, 1966.
23. Walshe FMR. On the variations in the form of reflex movements, notably the Babinski plantar response, under different degrees of spasticity and under the influence of the Magnus and de Kleijn's tonic neck reflex. *Brain* 1923;46:281–300.
24. Burke D, Knowles L, Andrews C, et al. Spasticity, decerebrate rigidity and the clasp-knife phenomenon: an experimental study in the cat. *Brain* 1972;95:31–48.
25. Foerster O. Analyse und Pathophysiologie der striaren Bewegungsstorungen. *Z Ges Neurol Psychiat* 1921;73:1–169.
26. Walshe FMR. Observations on the nature of the muscular rigidity of paralysis agitans and its relationship to tremor. *Brain* 1924;47:159–177.
27. Meyer M, Adorjani C. Quantification of the effects of muscle relaxant drugs in man by tonic stretch reflex. *Adv Neurol* 1983;39:997–1011.
28. Fung VS, Burne JA, Morris JG. Objective measurement of parkinsonian rigidity II: Relationship with simultaneously acquired EMG activity. *Mov Disord* 1998;13[Suppl]:48.
29. Andrews CJ, Burke D, Lance JW. The response to muscle stretch and shortening in parkinsonian rigidity. *Brain* 1972;95:795–812.

30. Rushworth G. Spasticity and rigidity: an experimental study and review. *J Neurol Neurosurg Psychiatry* 1960;23:99–118.

31. Dietrichson P. Phasic ankle reflex in spasticity and parkinsonian rigidity: the role of the fusimotor system. *Acta Neurol Scand* 1971;47:22–51.

32. McLellan DL. Dynamic spindle reflexes and the rigidity of parkinsonism. *J Neurol Neurosurg Psychiatry* 1973;36:342–349.

33. Tatton WG, Lee RG. Evidence for abnormal long-loop reflexes in rigid Parkinsonian patients. *Brain Res* 1975;100:671–676.

34. Lee RG, Tatton WG. Motor responses to sudden limb displacements in primates with specific CNS lesions and in human patients with motor system disorders. *Can J Neurol Sci* 1975;2:285–293.

35. Tatton WG, Bedingham W, Verrier MC, et al. Characteristic alterations in responses to imposed wrist displacements in parkinsonian rigidity and dystonia musculorum deformans. *Can J Neurol Sci* 1984;11:281–287.

36. Cody FW, MacDermott N, Matthews PB, et al. Observations on the genesis of the stretch reflex in Parkinson's disease. *Brain* 1986;109:229–249.

37. Marsden CD, Merton PA, Morton HB, et al. Automatic and voluntary responses to muscle stretch in man. In: Desmedt JE, ed. *Cerebral motor control in man: long loop mechanisms.* Progress in clinical neurophysiology, vol 4. Basel: Karger, 1978:334–341.

38. Meara RJ, Cody FW. Stretch reflexes of individual parkinsonian patients studied during changes in clinical rigidity following medication. *Electroencephalogr Clin Neurophysiol* 1993;89:261–268.

39. Rothwell JC, Obeso JA, Traub MM, et al. The behaviour of the long-latency stretch reflex in patients with Parkinson's disease. *J Neurol Neurosurg Psychiatry* 1983;46:35–44.

40. Bonnet M, Requin J, Stelmach GE. Changes in electromyographic responses to muscle stretch related to the programming of movement parameters. *Electroencephalogr Clin Neurophysiol* 1991;81:135–151.

41. Dietz V, Discher M, Trippel M. Task-dependent modulation of short- and long-latency electromyographic responses in upper limb muscles. *Electroencephalogr Clin Neurophysiol* 1994;93:49–56.

42. Johnson MT, Kipnis AN, Lee MC, et al. Modulation of the stretch reflex during volitional sinusoidal tracking in Parkinson's disease. *Brain* 1991;114:443–460.

43. Lance JW, De Gail P, Neilson PD. Tonic and phasic spinal cord mechanisms in man. *J Neurol Neurosurg Psychiatry* 1966;29:535–544.

44. Delwaide P, Gonce M. Pathophysiology of Parkinson's signs. In: Jankovic J, Tolosa E, eds. *Parkinson's disease and movement disorders.* Baltimore: Williams & Wilkins, 1993:77–92.

45. Sax DS, Johnson TL, Cooper IS. Reflex activity in extrapyramidal disorders. *Adv Neurol* 1976;14:285–296.

46. Delwaide PJ, Schoenen J. Clinical neurophysiology in the evaluation and physiopathology of Parkinson's disease. *Rev Neurol (Paris)* 1985;141:759–773.

47. Lelli S, Panizza M, Hallett M. Spinal cord inhibitory mechanisms in Parkinson's disease. *Neurology* 1991;41:553–556.

48. Bathien N, Rondot P. Reciprocal continuous inhibition in rigidity of parkinsonism. *J Neurol Neurosurg Psychiatry* 1977;40:20–24.

49. Day BL, Marsden CD, Obeso JA, et al. Peripheral and central mechanisms of reciprocal inhibition in the human forearm. *J Physiol (Lond)* 1981;317:59–60.

50. Caccia MR, McComas AJ, Upton ARM, et al. Cutaneous reflexes in small muscles of the hand. *J Neurol Neurosurg Psychiatry* 1973;36:960–967.

51. Fuhr P, Zeffiro T, Hallett M. Cutaneous reflexes in Parkinson's disease. *Muscle Nerve* 1992;15:733–739.

52. Chen R, Ashby P, Lang AE. Stimulus-sensitive myoclonus in akinetic-rigid syndromes. *Brain* 1992;115:1875–1888.

53. Clouston PD, Lim CL, Sue C, et al. Apomorphine can increase cutaneous inhibition of motor activity in Parkinson's disease. *Electroencephalogr Clin Neurophysiol* 1996;101:8–15.

54. Delwaide PJ, Pepin JL, Maertens de Noordhout A. Short-latency autogenic inhibition in patients with Parkinsonian rigidity. *Ann Neurol* 1991;30:83–89.

55. Illert M, Lundberg A, Tanaka R. Integration in descending motor pathways controlling the forelimb in the cat. 2. Convergence on neurones mediating disynaptic cortico-motoneuronal excitation. *Exp Brain Res* 1976;26:521–540.

56. Hongo T, Jankowska E, Lundberg A. The rubrospinal tract. II. Facilitation of interneuronal transmission in reflex paths to motoneurones. *Exp Brain Res* 1969;7:365–391.

57. Houk J, Rymer WZ. Neural control of muscle length and tension. In: Brooks VB, ed. *Handbook of physiology.* Bethesda: American Physiological Society, 1981:257–323.

58. Burne JA, Lippold OC. Loss of tendon organ inhibition in Parkinson's disease. *Brain* 1996;119:1115–1121.

59. Cantello R, Gianelli M, Bettucci D, et al. Parkinson's disease rigidity: magnetic motor evoked potentials in a small hand muscle. *Neurology* 1991;41:1449–1456.

60. Landau WM, Struppler A, Mehls O. A comparative electromyographic study of the reactions to passive movement in parkinsonism and in normal subjects. *Neurology* 1966;16:34–48.

61. Burke D, Hagbarth KE, Wallin BG. Reflex mechanisms in parkinsonian rigidity. *Scand J Rehabil Med* 1977;9:15–23.

62. Marsden CD. The mysterious motor function of the basal ganglia: the Robert Wartenberg Lecture. *Neurology* 1982;32:514–539.

63. Cantello R, Gianelli M, Civardi C, et al. Parkinson's disease rigidity: EMG in a small hand muscle at "rest." *Electroencephalogr Clin Neurophysiol* 1995;97:215–222.

64. Noth J, Schurmann M, Podoll K, et al. Reconsideration of the concept of enhanced static fusimotor drive in rigidity in patients with Parkinson's disease. *Neurosci Lett* 1988;84:239–243.

65. Berardelli A, Hallett M. Shortening reaction of human tibialis anterior. *Neurology* 1984;34:242–245.

66. Watts RL, Wiegner AW, Young RR. Elastic properties of muscles measured at the elbow in man: II. Patients with parkinsonian rigidity. *J Neurol Neurosurg Psychiatry* 1986;49:1177–1181.

67. Lance JW. Symposium synopsis. In: Feldman R, Young RR, Koella W, eds. *Spasticity: disordered motor control.* Chicago: Year Book Medical, 1980:485–494.

68. Thilmann AF, Fellows SJ, Garms E. Pathological stretch reflexes on the "good" side of hemiparetic patients. *J Neurol Neurosurg Psychiatry* 1990;53:208–214.

69. Thilmann AF, Fellows SJ, Garms E. The mechanism of spastic muscle hypertonus: variation in reflex gain over the time course of spasticity. *Brain* 1991;114:233–244.

70. Angel RW. Muscular contractions elicited by passive shortening. *Adv Neurol* 1983;39:555–563.

71. Eisen A, Odusote K. Amplitude of the F wave: a potential means of documenting spasticity. *Neurology* 1979;29:1306–1309.

72. Hagbarth KE, Wallin G, Lofstedt L. Muscle spindle responses to stretch in normal and spastic subjects. *Scand J Rehab Med* 1973;5:156–159.

73. Katz R, Pierrot-Deseilligny E. Recurrent inhibition of alpha-motoneurons in patients with upper motor neuron lesions. *Brain* 1982;105:103–124.

74. Shefner JM, Berman SA, Sarkarati M, et al. Recurrent inhibition is increased in patients with spinal cord injury. *Neurology* 1992;42:2162–2168.

75. Nakashima K, Rothwell JC, Day BL, et al. Reciprocal inhibition between forearm muscles in patients with writer's cramp and other occupational cramps, symptomatic hemidystonia and hemiparesis due to stroke. *Brain* 1989;112:681–697.

76. Ashby P, Wiens M. Reciprocal inhibition following lesions of the spinal cord in man. *J Physiol* 1989;414:145–157.

77. Faist M, Mazevet D, Dietz V, et al. A quantitative assessment of presynaptic inhibition of Ia afferents in spastics: differences in hemiplegics and paraplegics. *Brain* 1994;117:1449–1455.

78. Iansek R. The effects of reflex path length on clonus frequency in spastic muscles. *J Neurol Neurosurg Psychiatry* 1984;47:1122–1124.

79. Walsh EG, Wright GW. Patellar clonus: an autonomous central generator. *J Neurol Neurosurg Psychiatry* 1987;50:1225–1227.

80. van Gijn J. The Babinski sign and the pyramidal syndrome. *J Neurol Neurosurg Psychiatry* 1978;41:865–873.

81. Walshe FMR. The physiological significance of the reflex phenomena in spastic paralysis of the lower limbs. *Brain* 1914;37:269–336.

82. O'Dwyer NJ, Ada L, Neilson PD. Spasticity and muscle contracture following stroke. *Brain* 1996;119:1737–1749.

33

MUSCLE CRAMPS, STIFFNESS, AND MYALGIA

YADOLLAH HARATI
OPAS NAWASIRIPONG

Muscle cramps, stiffness, and myalgia are among the most common medical ailments (1,2). Many of the conditions causing these symptoms are benign, self-limited, and unlikely to cause confusion with typical movement disorders. Yet many uncommon disorders can result in postural abnormalities that simulate movement disorders. The main diagnostic confusion may be with the dystonic disorders (see Chapter 23). Also, the profuse fasciculation or myokymia associated with several of these conditions may cause small-amplitude joint movements superficially resembling segmental myoclonus or choreiform movements. This chapter discusses these disorders in detail and briefly reviews other conditions associated with muscle cramps, stiffness, or myalgia. It focuses on recent advances that have helped to reveal the causation of specific cramp syndromes and attempts to classify these disorders according to their site of pathogenesis: (a) muscle, (b) motor neurons or peripheral nerves, or (c) central nervous system (CNS). When evaluating patients, applying this classification is useful in distinguishing among the various causes and provides the focus on recognizing specific disorders underlying the symptoms of muscle cramps (3).

MYOGENIC DISORDERS CAUSING MUSCLE CRAMP AND/OR CONTRACTURE

Muscle contraction is a complex process by which an electrical current, carried by the muscle membrane along T tubules, evokes calcium release with subsequent contractile protein interaction and fiber shortening. This ATP- and calcium-dependent process is disrupted in several disorders with exercise-related cramps or muscle pain. The myopathic conditions causing cramps are listed in Table 33.1.

Although many patients refer to the muscle discomfort caused by myogenic disorders as cramp or muscle ache,

some simply have myalgia, and others have cramps, which should be differentiated, in a strict sense, from muscle contracture and myotonia (Table 33.2). Myogenic causes are often suspected for otherwise unexplained general myalgia. Muscle biopsies in various series have shown abnormalities, although not necessarily diagnostic, in up to 50% of such cases (4). Patients with persistent isolated myalgia and normal neurologic examination are among the most difficult to diagnose, and muscle biopsy identified a specific muscle disease (polymyositis in 2, McArdle's disease in 2, mitochondrial myopathy in 1) in 5 of 100 patients reported by Pourmand (4). The disorders to be discussed in this section include cramp, contracture, or myotonia with or without associated myalgia. A typical cramp may be defined as an involuntary, irregular, painful, usually brief skeletal muscle contraction in which muscle action potentials are recorded on an electromyogram during the cramp. Stretching or massaging the affected muscle often brings relief. In contrast, a contracture is an involuntary muscle shortening that usually lasts for seconds to minutes.

Electrical activity is not present on electromyogram during the contracture, and stretching or massaging the contracted muscle will not relieve the symptoms. Conditions known to cause such electrically silent contracture are listed in Table 33.1. Contracture is also defined in a different sense as a painless fixed limitation of joint movement, although this definition is not relevant to this chapter. Myotonia does not involve involuntary muscle contractions; rather, forceful muscle contraction is followed by delayed relaxation (action myotonia) caused by prolonged excitation of the muscle membrane. Myotonia can also be elicited by direct percussion of the muscle (percussion myotonia). Prolonged waxing and waning electrical discharges with gradually declining amplitude and the characteristic "dive bomber's sound" are induced by the insertion and subsequent manipulation of an electromyography needle (electrical myotonia).

TABLE 33.1. MYOGENIC DISORDERS CAUSING COMPLAINTS OF MUSCLE CRAMP AND PAIN

Disorders resulting from deficient muscle fuel use
  "Muscle cramp" resulting from glycogen metabolism abnormalities
    Myophosphorylase deficiency (type V glycogenosis)[a]
    Phosphofructokinase deficiency (type VII glycogenosis)[a]
    Phosphorylase b kinase deficiency (type VIII glycogenosis)[a]
    Phosphoglycerate kinase deficiency (type IX glycogenosis)[a]
    Muscle phosphoglycerate mutase deficiency (type X glycogenosis)[a]
    Lactate dehydrogenase deficiency (type XI glycogenosis)
  "Muscle cramp" resulting from lipid metabolism abnormalities
    Carnitine palmitoyltransferase II deficiency
  Myalgia resulting from purine nucleotide metabolism
    Myoadenylate deaminase deficiency
Disorders resulting from other muscle dysfunctions
  "Muscle cramp" resulting from dysfunction of sarcoplasmic reticulum
    Brody or Lambert-Brody syndrome
  Myalgia associated with other muscle dysfunctions
    Myalgia associated with tubular aggregates
    Myalgia with abnormal structure or function of mitochondria
    Myalgia with intracellular acidosis
    Myalgia with low myosin ATPase and phosphocreatine content
    Myalgia with type 2 muscle fiber predominance
Myotonic disorders
  Chloride channel diseases
    Myotonia congenita
      Thomsen's disease (autosomal dominant)
      Becker's disease (autosomal recessive)
    Sodium channel diseases
      Paramyotonia congenita (autosomal dominant)
        Normokalemic or hyperkalemic (adynamia episodica, autosomal dominant)
        Other sodium channel myotonias
          ■ Acetazolamide-responsive myotonia
          ■ Myotonia fluctuans
          ■ Myotonia permanens
  Calcium channel diseases
    Hypokalemic periodic paralysis (autosomal dominant)
  Nondystrophic myotonias with unknown defect
    Myotonia congenita with painful cramps (autosomal dominant)
  Dystrophic myotonias (autosomal dominant)
    Myotonic dystrophy
    Proximal myotonic myopathy
  Schwartz-Jampel syndrome (autosomal recessive)
  Acquired myotonia
    Drug induced
    Associated with malignancy

[a]Disorders with documented electrically silent contracture.

Disorders of Muscle Fuel Use

Disorders of Glycogen Metabolism

Muscle Phosphorylase Deficiency (McArdle's Disease, Type V Glycogenosis)

Muscle phosphorylase (myophosphorylase) deficiency was described by McArdle (1951), who correctly postulated that the illness resulted from an enzyme defect along the glycolytic pathway. Eight years later the deficient enzyme was shown to be a muscle-specific phosphorylase, an enzyme responsible for breaking down glycogen (Fig. 33.1) (5,6). This defect causes a deficiency in "energy" production that leads to exercise intolerance secondary to muscle fatigue, stiffness, and pain. Indirect effects of this defect, such as impaired oxidative metabolism (7), sarcolemmal function with reduced sodium-potassium pump (8), or muscle tissue perfusion with exercise (9), may also contribute to symptoms. Moderate activities are well tolerated, even for long periods, and many affected patients learn their exercise threshold. However, with vigorous activity symptoms usually develop within minutes and resolve with rest over minutes to hours. Exercise may involve intensive, brief isometric contraction (pushing an object or carrying a heavy load) or sustained repetitive use of any muscle group (riding a

TABLE 33.2. CRAMP, CONTRACTURE, AND MYOTONIA

Clinical Findings, Observations	Cramp	Contracture	Myotonia	Dystonia
EMG	Normal action potentials	Silent	Myotonic discharges	Normal action potentials
Duration	Minutes	Seconds to minutes	Seconds	500 ms, sustained
Physical activity at onset of symptoms	Rest (exacerbated by exercise)	Forceful exercise	Forceful exercise, direct muscle percussion	Often action task specific at onset; later occurs at rest
Pain	+	+/–[a]	–	+/–
Warm-up phenomenon	–	–	+	–
Second-wind phenomenon	–	+/–[a]	–	–
Alleviation by muscle massage	+	–	–	–
Effect of focal curare injection	+	–	–	+
Pathophysiology	Neurogenic diseases	Muscle metabolic abnormality	Muscle membrane ion conductance abnormality	Basal ganglia or brainstem dysfunction

[a]Present in glycogen metabolism defects.
+, present; –, absent; +/–, variable.

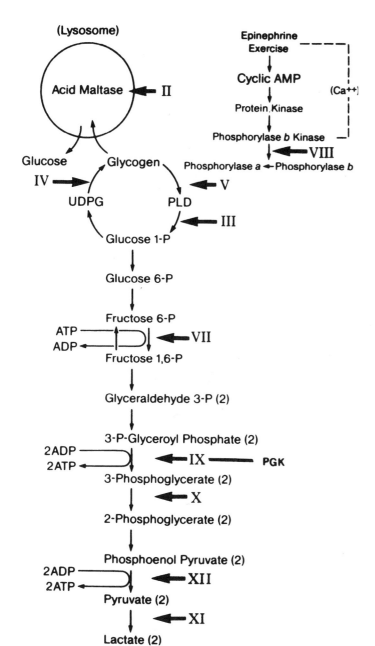

FIG. 33.1. Glycogen metabolism and glycolysis. *Arrows*, enzyme defects that produce disease in the human; *II*, acid maltase; *III*, debranching enzyme; *IV*, branching enzyme; *V*, phosphorylase; *VII*, phosphofructokinase; *VIII*, phosphorylase *b* kinase; *IX*, phosphoglycerate kinase; *X*, phosphoglycerate mutase; *XI*, lactate dehydrogenase, and XII, β-enolase. *UDPG*, uridine diphosphate glucose; *PLD*, phosphorylase limit dextrin. (Courtesy Dr. S. DiMauro, College of Physicians and Surgeons, Columbia University, New York, NY.)

bicycle, swimming, climbing stairs). Any skeletal muscle group can be affected, including the jaw and oropharynx (10). Patients often complain that they cannot fully extend the fingers after sustained gripping movements. Attempts to open the "clawed" fingers may result in increasing pain. This hand posture may superficially resemble that of myotonia or dystonia (Fig. 33.2). Severe spasms of large muscles may be followed by muscle necrosis, myoglobinuria, and renal failure. Most patients' performance improves after a "warm-up" period of nonstrenuous exercise. This "second wind phenomenon" is attributed to two main factors: mobilization of plasma free fatty acids with the use of amino acids as alternative energy sources and increased blood flow to the exercising muscles (11,12). Fasting patients often demonstrate improved exercise capacity, a marked fall in creatine kinase (CK), and low serum free fatty acids at the end of the fast (13), again suggesting increased dependence on free fatty acids.

Most patients have normal neurologic findings between attacks. Thus, their complaints may be considered psychogenic or indicative of malingering. A history of elevated CK levels or myoglobinuria ("Coca-Cola urine") distinguishes most cases. Forced exercise can precipitate severe myoglobinuria and renal failure. About one third of patients develop a mild and permanent myopathy with weakness, rarely asymmetric (14), and atrophy as a late consequence of recurrent attacks (15).

McArdle's disease most commonly begins during the second decade of life, although milder unrecognized symp-toms of easy fatigability without cramp or myalgia typically occur during childhood. Rarely do severe symptoms of cramps and myoglobinuria begin in childhood (16). Atypical presentations (15,17) include (a) very mild forms with exercise fatigue; (b) fatal infantile form (18); (c) mild congenital myopathy in childhood (19); and (d) late onset (fifth decade or later) of typical syndrome or pure myopathy (20,21). Patients with McArdle's syndrome, as well as patients with phosphofructokinase (PFK) deficiency, may have myogenic hyperuricemia (22).

The best-substantiated mode of inheritance is autosomal recessive. Reports of autosomal dominant inheritance (23) have yet to be supported by biochemical data. Heterozygotes demonstrate partial decrease in enzyme activity (24) and are usually asymptomatic, although they may show a propensity to "cramp," especially during forearm exercise tests (25). Rarely, heterozygotes manifest overt symptoms when their enzyme activity falls below a critical threshold (26,27). This may explain the occasional reports of "autosomal dominant" inheritance as it may be a pseudoautosomal dominant inheritance. Male patients are affected 2.5 times as commonly as female ones (28). Gender-related differences in strenuous physical activity or metabolic control are probably responsible, but a sex-linked, sex-limited pattern of inheritance has not been excluded. The disorder is molecularly and genetically heterogeneous. Bartram et al. (29) summarizes the molecular phenotypes, which include absent myophosphorylase protein (great majority of patients) with absent, normal, decreased, or truncated mes-

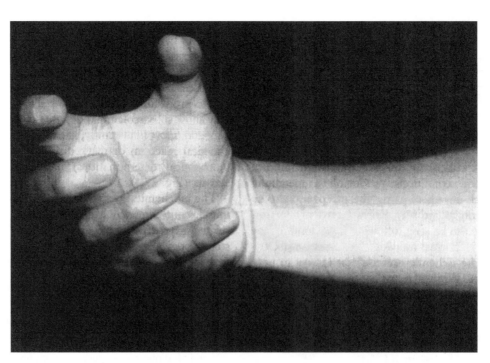

FIG. 33.2. Forearm exercise test in McArdle's disease. Characteristic cramping posture developed after forearm exercise.

senger RNA; decreased protein with normal messenger RNA; and rarely, normal levels of inactive protein.

In mammals, besides the muscle form, liver and brain isozymes of glycogen phosphorylase under the control of different genes are present in other tissues and are not clinically involved in McArdle's disease. In humans the liver isozyme predominates in most nonmuscular tissues, whereas the brain isozyme is the predominant form in brain and cardiac muscle (15) and is also probably the fetal form (28). The "fetal" isozyme is present in fetal and regenerating muscle cultures of patients with McArdle's disease (29), suggesting that the expression of this isozyme differs from that of the mature enzyme. The synthesis of the fetal form is repressed by the time of birth (30,31) and replaced during skeletal muscle maturation by the muscle isozyme (32).

Genetic studies have focused on the defect in the myophosphorylase q13 locus identified on chromosome 11 (33). DNA analysis revealed a point mutation or other small event, and several mutations causing myophosphorylase deficiency have been described (34–36). The most common among American and European patients appears to be a nonsense mutation (CGA to TGA) at arginine codon 49 (37), while a single codon 708/709 deletion is most common in Japanese patients (38). No clear genotype–phenotype correlation has emerged (34).

Phosphorylase itself exists in two forms. The less active dimer, phosphorylase *b,* is converted to a more active tetramer, phosphorylase a, by phosphorylase *b* kinase (PBK). PBK is controlled by hormonal and neural factors via protein kinase and calcium-mediated activation. Epinephrine, by stimulating adenylate cyclase, increases cyclic adenosine monophosphate production, which activates protein kinase. This enzyme in turn activates PBK by phosphorylation. Neural control occurs through the events of muscle excitation. Calcium released from the sarcoplasmic reticulum activates PBK by binding to its calmodulin subunit. Thus, a defect in any of these cascade reactions theoretically should prevent phosphorylase activity.

PBK is composed of four subunits: α, β, γ, and δ. The distinct genetic control of these subunits (39) and the existence of tissue-specific isoforms contribute to the clinical and genetic heterogeneity of PBK deficiency (type VIII glycogenosis). The clinical spectrum includes isolated involvement of liver and cardiac and skeletal muscle (15, 40,41), combined clinical involvement of liver and muscle, and possibly liver and renal diseases. Most myopathic cases have clinical features similar to those of McArdle's disease, including age of onset and symptoms of exercise intolerance, cramps, and myalgias (42–44). However, the forearm exercise test (discussion to follow) is less sensitive in this disorder. Other myopathic variants include infantile hypotonia (42,45–47) and possibly one infantile case of fatal arthrogryposis (48). Two cases of infantile hypotonia demonstrated a deficiency in one additional enzyme in glycogen metabolism: PFK in one (46) and debranching

enzyme in another (42). Another variant was described in one patient with progressive distal weakness beginning at age 46 (49).

Classically, a simple provocative test, the forearm exercise test for lactate production (50), is used to diagnose McArdle's disease (Figs. 33.2 and 33.3A, B). In McArdle's disease, lactic acid and pyruvate production are decreased. This test is not specific and may indicate any of several conditions producing a metabolic block along the glycogenolytic or glycolytic pathway. Failed lactate production may also be seen following ingestion of alcohol in normal individuals and alcoholics.

The forearm exercise test is easy to perform, but reliable results require preparation, cooperation of the patient, and good laboratory support. While the patient is at rest, blood is drawn for baseline levels of ammonia and lactate. The patient immediately begins repetitive rapid grip exercises. With strong encouragement normal subjects are able to tolerate forearm exercise for 90 to 180 seconds before pain and fatigue force discontinuation of the test. Patients with disorders of glycogen metabolism seldom exercise for more than 60 seconds. When the patient fatigues, the exercise is terminated and immediately blood ammonia and lactate levels are drawn from the arm that has exercised. Similar samples are drawn again at 1, 2, 4, 6, and 10 minutes following the end of exercise. A flexible intravenous catheter (heparin lock) for phlebotomy and prelabeling of the test tubes enhances the ease of the test performance. Normal subjects exhibit a threefold to fivefold increase in lactate level within 5 minutes after the end of exercise, with a full return to baseline level in about 30 minutes. Suboptimal exercise also results in an inadequate rise in venous lactate. The venous level of ammonia also rises during forearm exercise; failure of the two to rise together suggests an inadequate test. Normal lactate but impaired ammonia production suggests myoadenylate deaminase deficiency or a related disorder of purine nucleotide metabolism. Rarely, however, these two enzyme deficiencies coexist (51). In disorders of glycogenolysis ammonia production during exercise may be excessive.

Muscle biopsy is the most definitive diagnostic procedure for McArdle's disease. It may show subsarcolemmal deposits of glycogen and, most important, absence (by histochemical reaction) or marked reduction (by biochemical determinations) of phosphorylase activity in most fibers (52) (Fig. 33.4). However, genetic analysis of blood may obviate muscle biopsy in most cases, since DNA isolated from leukocytes can be diagnostic for McArdle's disease in up to 90% of patients (53).

The biochemical basis of electrically silent muscle contractures in McArdle's disease and related glycolytic disorders is not understood. Logically, the unavailability of glycogen for anaerobic work should rapidly deplete adenosine triphosphate (ATP) stores in actively contracted muscles. Low ATP levels should in turn retard ATP-dependent cal-

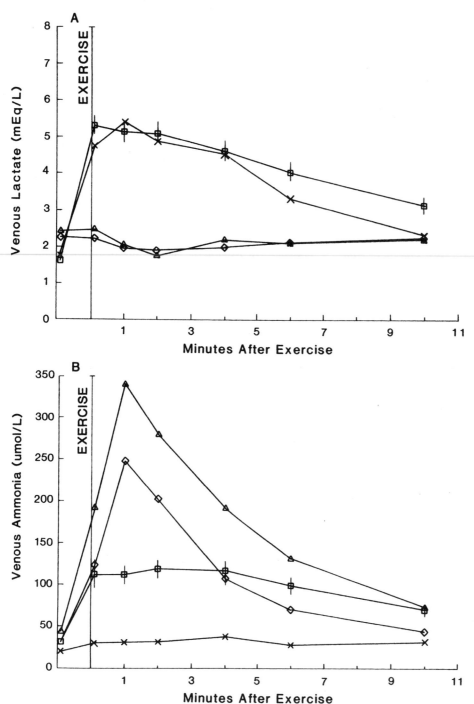

FIG. 33.3. Forearm exercise test in McArdle's disease. Lactate and ammonia production after exercise. A venous blood sample was obtained from the antecubital vein at rest before the ischemic exercise. Then the patient was asked to repeat full extension and flexion of the fingers until muscle contracture developed. The venous blood samples were obtained 0, 1, 2, 4, 6, and 10 minutes later. **A:** Venous lactate levels. **B:** Venous ammonia levels. *Box line*, controls with a bar of standard error of mean (*n* = 21). *Diamond* and *triangle lines*, patients with McArdle's disease; *x line*, patient with myoadenylate deaminase deficiency. In McArdle's disease lactate production is deficient, but ammonia production shows a compensatory increase (Brooke et al., 1983). In myoadenylate deaminase deficiency lactate production is normal but ammonia production is deficient (Fishbein et al., 1978).

cium uptake by the sarcoplasmic reticulum, and the muscle should therefore shorten. However, neither biochemical studies of muscle biopsies (54) nor in vivo ^{31}P-nuclear magnetic resonance (NMR) spectroscopy (55,56) has shown any drop of ATP levels in whole muscle. Whether ATP reduction affects only a specific subcellular component or involves a relatively small percentage of muscle fibers is not known. Besides retarded energy-dependent calcium uptake, increased sarcoplasmic calcium may result if the sarcoplas-

mic reticulum calcium transport system itself is directly damaged. It has been hypothesized that such damage is mediated by the products of lipid peroxidation produced by increased reliance on fatty acid oxidation in this disorder (57).

The treatment of McArdle's disease begins with counseling the patient regarding the risks of exercise-induced rhabdomyolysis. Patients should be instructed to adjust their lifestyle to avoid strenuous exercise and excessive weight

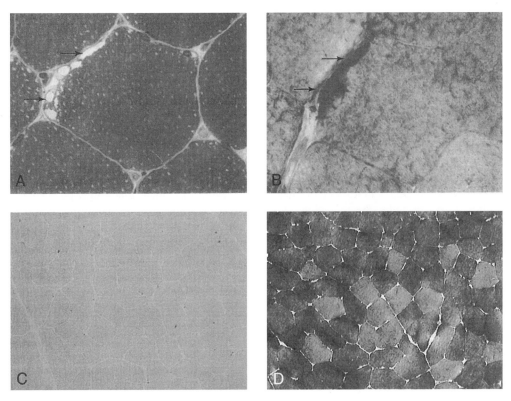

FIG. 33.4. Muscle histopathology in McArdle's disease. Note subsarcolemmal blebs (**A,** hematoxylin and eosin) (*arrows*), which contain PAS-positive material (**B,** *arrows*). Phosphorylase activity is absent in muscle fibers (**C**) in contrast to the control (**D**).

and to seek prompt medical attention and treatment if myoglobinuria develops. Minor adjustments in lifestyle can prevent attacks in some patients. Treatments aimed at bypassing the biochemical block by supplying the muscle with a glycolytic intermediate (i.e., glucose, fructose) or increasing alternative energy sources (e.g., plasma free fatty acids) improve exercise endurance in some patients (11). However, long-term oral glucose or fructose or high-fat diets usually show disappointing results and have potential deleterious health effects, including weight gain (58). Injection of D-ribose did not benefit the patients (59). Injection of glucagon to promote hepatic glycogenolysis and to increase blood glucose concentration had inconsistent results, and its repeated injection is objectionable for prolonged treatment. However, a, high-protein diet may be beneficial (60,61). Which amino acid contributes to this improvement is uncertain. In vivo ^{31}P-NMR spectroscopy and exercise performance were partially normalized by a high-protein diet but were unaffected by intravenous amino acid infusion (61). Despite expectation, branched chain amino acids have not proven to be beneficial (62) although their oxoacid analogs, which delay ammonia production, may have short-term benefit (63). These findings suggest that intramuscular protein stores are providing an alternative energy substrate and partially correcting the metabolic deficits. Harati treated a female patient experiencing mild

proximal weakness secondary to late-onset McArdle's syndrome with a high-protein, low-carbohydrate diet, with nearly complete resolution of weakness within 3 months.

A derivative of vitamin B_6 is bound to myophosphorylase and constitutes the body's major pool of this vitamin. Therefore, vitamin B_6 is deficient in patients with McArdle's disease who lack phosphorylase protein. Preliminary data with oral vitamin B_6 suggests benefit in reducing muscle fatigue, possibly by enhancing any one of a number of vitamin B_6-dependent processes that increase energy production or use (64,65). Recently the beneficial effect of daily creatine intake has been reported (66).

The potential of gene therapy has been shown by studies with recombinant adenovirus capable of introducing myophosphorylase into differentiating myoblasts and especially mature myotubes (67). Sustained functional enzyme activity, which is also regulable, was demonstrated in myotubes. This offers the hope of restoring glycogenolytic function in McArdle's disease patients by direct adenovirus-mediated enzyme delivery into skeletal muscle (68).

Phosphofructokinase Deficiency (Tarui's Disease, Type VII Glycogenosis)

Phosphofructokinase deficiency, described by Tarui in 1965 (69), is a rare familial disorder with clinical characteristics closely mimicking those of McArdle's disease. It is distinguished by histochemical and biochemical evidence of deficiency (usually absence) of PFK in muscle, resulting in blockage of glycolysis. The forearm exercise test and muscle biopsy results are otherwise similar to those of McArdle's disease. The diagnosis may be suggested by a mild anemia and elevated reticulocyte count resulting from a partial defect of the erythrocyte PFK enzyme with a resultant impaired erythrocyte Ca^{2+} homeostasis (70) leading to hemolytic tendency (71). Additional inconsistent features include more significant hemolysis, gouty arthritis, and possibly recurrent gastric ulcers (72). Clinical heterogeneity similar to McArdle's disease includes the following: late-onset myopathy with (73,74) or without (75) preceding symptoms of exercise intolerance; (b) infantile or childhood severe myopathy without hemolysis with multiple contractures and/or progressive weakness and respiratory failure (15), rare association with cerebral and cerebellar abnormalities (76), or intrauterine fetal akinesia (77); and (c) isolated hemolysis.

PFK is a tetrameric enzyme composed of three subunits: muscle (M), liver (L), and platelets (P), which are variably expressed in tissues. Human skeletal muscle PFK consists only of M subunits, which are usually absent in this disorder (78). Tissues that express both M subunit and another, such as the L subunit in erythrocytes, demonstrate partial PFK deficiency. Demonstrating a partial deficiency in red blood cells may be useful in diagnosing cases in which histochemical or biochemical studies of muscle are not feasible (79). Muscle study is still needed in infantile variants, since their erythrocyte PFK activity is usually normal.

With ^{11}P-NMR spectroscopy, disorders of glycolysis, such as PFK deficiency, can be differentiated from those of glycogenolysis, such as McArdle's syndrome (80,81). Only in the former do glycolytic intermediates with exercise accumulate as phosphorylated sugars whose dephosphorylation during recovery results in a slow return to normal of orthophosphate (Pi). Also, in PFK deficiency, ^{11}P-NMR spectroscopy has shown decreased ATP levels at rest that continue to decline during exercise, a finding not present in McArdle's syndrome (80,82). The exact reason for this difference is unknown.

The inheritance pattern in most cases of PFK deficiency is autosomal recessive, and reduced erythrocyte PFK activity may be demonstrated in otherwise asymptomatic parents. Genetic studies have revealed several mutations in the PFK M-subunit gene on chromosome 12q13. Two common mutations involving a splicing defect and nucleotide deletion with frameshift mutation have been recognized in Ashkenazi Jews (83). Several mutations of these types and missense mutations have been identified in patients from at least six other ethnic backgrounds (84,85).

No specific treatment for PFK deficiency is available. Since the metabolic block affects glycolysis rather than glycogenolysis, there is no rationale for giving glucose or hyperglycemic agents in this condition. In fact, glucose may induce exertional fatigue by inhibiting lipolysis and depriving the muscle of these fuel sources (86). However, dietary supplementation with ketone bodies or fatty acids may be beneficial, and in theory, a high-protein diet may be helpful.

Phosphoglycerate Kinase Deficiency (Type IX Glycogenosis)

Phosphoglycerate kinase (PGK) deficiency is an X-linked recessive disorder of the second stage of glycolysis. Since the enzyme is a single ubiquitous polypeptide without tissue-specific isozymes, one might expect multisystem involvement. Nevertheless, primary muscle disorder with exercise-induced painful muscle cramps, myoglobinuria, and impaired lactate production (87–90) and one case with retinitis pigmentosa (91) have been reported. Besides muscle and myoblast cultures, PGK activity in these cases has also been reduced in red blood cells, leukocytes, platelets, and fibroblasts. Cases of PGK deficiency without muscle symptoms are associated with hemolytic anemia, mental retardation, behavioral abnormalities, tremor, and seizure. Combinations of myopathy with hemolytic anemia (92) or with mental retardation (93,94) have also been reported. The gene of PGK, a monomeric enzyme, is located on chromosome Xq13. Molecular genetics studies have shown most errors to be missense mutations with single amino acid substitutions and one splice-junction mutation. The genetic heterogeneity continues to expand (95), although explanation for clinical heterogeneity remains uncertain. The only effective treatment is avoidance of intense exercise.

Phosphoglycerate Mutase Deficiency (Type X Glycogenosis)

Phosphoglycerate mutase (PGAM) deficiency, which also affects the second stage of glycolysis, has been recognized as a cause of recurrent episodes of exercise-induced muscle cramp and myoglobinuria in adults of African ancestry with no known family history of neuromuscular disorders (96–100) and in two siblings of an Italian family (101). In most of these studies the rise of venous lactate after forearm exercise was found to be abnormally low, and muscle biopsy showed increased glycogen content. PGAM activity was reduced markedly, and the residual activity represented by the brain (BB) isoenzyme suggested a genetic defect of the M subunit, which predominates in normal muscle. However, the cultured muscle displayed normal PGAM activity, which is explained by the predominant or exclusive presence of PGAM-BB at earlier stages of muscle development. ^{11}P-NMR spectroscopy findings have been described (102,103). The gene encoding PGAM-M subunit has been mapped to chromosome 7 (104). So far a common missense mutation at codon 78 has been identified in African-Americans and another at codon 90 in the Italian kindred

(101). No specific therapy other than exercise avoidance is available. In one patient with both PGAM deficiency and tubular aggregation, dantrolene was effective (105). This raises the possibility that cramps in muscle PGAM deficiency are caused by high calcium release from the sarcoplasmic reticulum relative to calcium reuptake capacity.

Lactate Dehydrogenase Deficiency (Type XI Glycogenosis)

Reduced levels of lactate dehydrogenase (LDH), the last enzyme involved in the second stage of glycolysis, were thought to cause exercise-induced pigmenturia, easy fatigability, and contracture during forearm exercise tests in an 18-year-old Japanese man. Lack of this enzyme retarded conversion of pyruvate to lactate, and the patient showed no rise in lactate despite a marked increase in venous pyruvate level (106). Since this original report, the same author and others have identified similarly affected Japanese families (107) and, rarely, Caucasian patients (108). One Japanese woman who was otherwise asymptomatic had skin lesions and childbirth difficulties with uterine stiffness (109). The significance of the typical scaly erythematous patches on extensor surfaces of extremities that worsens in the summer in these patients was later recognized (110), and nearly absent LDH activity in the skin lesions has been shown (111).

LDH is a tetrameric enzyme with subunits M (or A) and H (or B) and five isozymes. The M subunit is deficient in type XI glycogenosis. This subunit predominates in skeletal muscle and is also abundant in other tissues, including skin and uterus. The biochemical mechanism that leads to marked reduction in muscle ATP and the presumed basis for symptoms has been demonstrated (112). Genetic analysis has shown a 20 base pair (bp) deletion in exon 6 of chromosome 11 (107,113), and additional mutations have been reported (108,114).

β-Enolase Deficiency (Type XII Glycogenosis)

β-Enolase is an enzyme that catalyses the step interconverting 2-phosphoglycerate and phosphoenolpyruvate. Deficiency of this enzyme has recently been reported to cause episodic exercise intolerance, myalgia, and elevated creatine phosphokinase in a single adult patient (115).

Disorders of Lipid Metabolism

Use of free fatty acids is essential in prolonged exercise; 1 to 4 hours after uninterrupted exercise, muscle uptake of free fatty acid rises by 70% and the relative contribution of fatty acids to total oxygen use becomes twice that of carbohydrates. The free fatty acids taken up by muscle are actively transported across the muscle mitochondrial membrane by a carrier, carnitine, with the help of the enzymes carnitine

palmitoyltransferase (CPT) I and II (Fig. 33.5) located on separate mitochondrial membranes, CPT I on the outer and CPT II on the inner (116,117). They are distinct enzymes (118), with tissue-specific isoforms for CPT I but not CPT II (119).

Initially it was believed that both CPT enzymes could cause a disorder of lipid muscle metabolism. It is now recognized that CPT I deficiency causes hepatic disease and CPT II deficiency is heterogeneous in its expression, with muscle presentation being most common (120). This presentation, in contrast to carnitine deficiency, results in muscle ache and fatigability, and affected patients, mostly male, have a subjective feeling of muscle stiffness with observable contracture, followed by swelling, elevation of serum muscle enzymes, and sometimes progression to pigmenturia. These features develop usually after sustained, prolonged exertion, especially if exercise occurs during caloric deprivation (fasting), exposure to cold, or mild infection (121). Occasionally, symptoms are precipitated even without exercise by these and other factors, including general anesthesia, which has also been associated with rhabdomyolysis (122). Most patients develop symptoms in their first or second decade, although later onset is reported. Symptoms can persist for hours to days, and the frequency of attacks during one's life can vary from a few to many. Any muscle group can be affected, including respiratory. Progression to persistent muscle weakness is uncommon (123).

Useful signs accompanying these symptoms are elevations in serum CK and myoglobinuria. In their review of the metabolic causes of myoglobinuria, Tonin et al. (124) found CPT deficiency to be the most common cause. Between attacks, as well as during short-term exercise, patients usually are normal. Fasting at rest for 30 to 72 hours can increase the CK, triglyceride, and cholesterol levels or delay the rise of serum ketone bodies. The forearm exercise test is normal. Muscle biopsy between attacks is usually normal but may show variable lipid excess, especially in type 1 muscle fibers. During attacks, foci of muscle necrosis have been described; one report emphasized associated vascular lesions (125). Although CPT can be reduced in liver, leukocytes, platelets, and fibroblasts, biochemical determination of muscle CPT has been the standard for definitive diagnosis. However, a new biochemical technique using peripheral blood cells and fibroblasts may simplify diagnosis in the future (126).

CPT II deficiency is an autosomal recessive disorder (127), although autosomal dominant cases have been suggested, such as in a family with affected members over four generations (128). The gene encoding CPT II has been localized to chromosome 1p32 (129). The most common mutation in muscle CPT deficiency is a serine-to-leucine substitution at codon 113 (130). Additional point mutations causing this disorder have been identified. These mutations have been shown to result in reduced catalytic activity and levels of the CPT II protein, the latter because

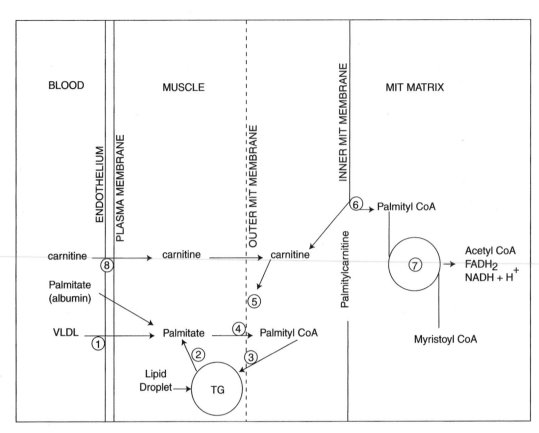

FIG. 33.5. Lipid metabolism. Fatty acid (exemplified by palmitate) arrives in the blood either bound to albumin or as triglycerides in the very low density lipoproteins (VLDLs). *TG*, endogenous lipid stores (triglycerides). The fatty acids pass through the mitochondrial membrane to the mitochondrial matrix, where they undergo β oxidation. Numbers indicate the enzymes or enzyme complexes involved in the process: *1,* lipoprotein; *2,* triglyceride, diglyceride, and monoglyceride lipase; *3,* synthesis of triglycerides from long-chain acyl-CoA involving glycerol-1-phosphate and the three enzyme glycerol phosphate acetyltransferase, phosphatidate phosphatase, and diglyceride acyltransferase; *4,* palmitoyl-CoA synthetase; *5,* carnitine palmitoyltransferase I; *6,* carnitine palmitoyltransferase II; *7,* modified β oxidation; *8,* active transport system of carnitine into muscle. (Courtesy Dr. D. C. DeVivo, Neurological Institute, New York, NY.)

of decreased stability. Zierz et al. (131) provide possible biochemical explanations for how various provocative factors cause intermittent symptoms in patients whose CPT II enzyme shows impaired regulation. Also, since ATP depletion does not fully explain rhabdomyolysis, other mechanisms proposed include effects of increased substrates found in muscle (e.g., long-chain fatty acylcarnitine) on sarcolemmal Na^+,K^+-ATPase and phospholipid membranes (132) and on calcium release channel of muscle sarcoplasmic reticulum (133). There is poor phenotype–genotype correlation with CPT II deficiency (134,135).

Treatment includes informing the patient of the situations likely to precipitate muscle damage (fasting, prolonged exercise, extreme cold) and encouraging moderation in exercise and consumption of a high-carbohydrate, high-protein diet with frequent snacks (136). Since CPT catalyzes the transport of long-chain fatty acids into the mitochondria, a diet low in long-chain and high in

medium-chain triglycerides (MCTs) may be beneficial (137). However, the benefit of MCTs may be limited, since recent evidence indicates that CPT is more involved in MCT transport than previously assumed (126).

Unusual nonmuscular presentations of CPT II deficiency involving liver, heart, brain, and kidney have been described. Rarely, muscular CPT deficiency has been associated with CNS manifestations, including seizures, infantile spasms (138,139), and athetotic quadriplegia (139). This latter report involving an 18-month-old Japanese boy is worth noting. At age 2 months he developed hypertonicity that gradually progressed to rigospastic quadriplegia; dystonic posture; athetotic movements of neck, trunk, and extremities; and signs of mental retardation. At approximately 1 year he developed recurrent rhabdomyolysis provoked by mild viral infections. Ketone body production was delayed following long-chain triglyceride loading. Muscle histochemistry and biochemistry were consistent with CPT

II deficiency. Treatment with a high-carbohydrate, low-fat (predominantly MCT) diet was successful in preventing myoglobinuria. Hypertonicity responded to diazepam and trihexyphenidyl, but the involuntary movements did not respond to any treatment, including levodopa.

Although true cramps are unusual in CPT deficiency, other defects of muscle lipid metabolism may be associated with repeated episodes of cramps and myalgia (140). They are probably responsible for many of the 51% of cases of myoglobinuria in which no enzyme deficiency is identified (124). In some cases a defect in long-chain acyl-coenzyme A dehydrogenase (LCAD) enzyme has been identified. However, the defect remains unknown in other cases, such as in a report by Engel et al. (141) of 18-year-old identical twin women who, following several hours of exercise, prolonged standing, or long car trips, developed myalgia and cramps, often accompanied by myoglobinuria. Fasting or a low-carbohydrate, high-fat diet precipitated attacks and was associated with sharply increased serum CK and no ketone body production. No CPT deficiency was identified in the muscle biopsy of one of the two patients. Administration of MCT resulted in normal ketone production, suggesting defective use of long-chain fatty acids. Besides MCT, oral carnitine has improved myopathic features in similar patients, and prednisone has reduced cramping and muscle membrane irritability (142).

Harati has studied a similar case in an 18-year-old man who had two episodes of myoglobinuria following prolonged exercise while fasting. During the 25th hour of a diagnostic fast he developed mild rhabdomyolysis, episodic vomiting without ketosis, and postfast urine and serum elevations of medium- and long-chain acylcarnitines suggesting a deficiency in LCAD. Typically patients with LCAD deficiency have fasting-induced infantile metabolic attacks (hypoketotic hypoglycemia with dicarboxylic aciduria) often resulting in coma. However, some who survive to adulthood develop a clinical picture with muscle involvement, as in the case just described. The human LCAD gene has been localized to chromosome Iq34-35 (143), and the molecular defects underlying LCAD deficiency are under investigation.

Another syndrome similar to CPT II deficiency, but associated with peripheral neuropathy, has been linked to a deficiency of the mitochondrial trifunctional enzyme of β oxidation (144).

OTHER MUSCLE DYSFUNCTIONS

Disorders with Contracture

Brody or Lambert-Brody Syndrome

Lambert and Goldstein (145) described a patient who exhibited impaired muscle relaxation that clinically, but not by electromyography, resembled myotonia ("silent myoto-

nia"). Brody (146) described a similar patient and demonstrated that calcium ion (Ca^{2+}) uptake by isolated sarcoplasmic reticulum was reduced markedly. Lambert-Brody syndrome develops during the first or second decade of life and consists of progressive exercise-induced pain, stiffness, and cramping in arm and leg muscles. After only 30 to 60 seconds of rapidly clenching and unclenching the fist there is a transient, painless slowing of movements; when the fist is forcefully clenched for 10 seconds, the hand can be opened slowly only with initial flexion of the wrist; with excessive activity, pain develops. Similar but less severe impairment of relaxation is sometimes observed in craniobulbar (e.g., frontalis muscle during eye opening) or trunk muscles. The absence of impaired muscle relaxation in some cases (147) and the rare association with recurrent exertional rhabdomyolysis (148) challenge physicians to consider this diagnosis in the broader spectrum of patients with exercise-induced pain, stiffness, and myoglobinuria. There is no percussion or electrical myotonia, and immersion of the forearm in cold water does not influence the stiffness in typical cases. Electromyography shows no abnormalities, and during the phase of delayed relaxation of strongly contracted muscles there is electrical silence. Muscle biopsy usually shows mild, nonspecific, type 2 fiber atrophy and a normal ultrastructural appearance, although mild myopathic histology and swollen mitochondria with crystals were described in one atypical case (148). Although in vitro muscle response to halothane is normal, there is excessive sensitivity to caffeine, suggesting that precautionary anesthesia for malignant hyperthermia syndrome might be appropriate.

Sarcoplasmic reticulum calcium ATPase (SERCA) has been shown to be defective in this disorder. This enzyme exists in mammals as fiber type–specific isoforms (149) and is responsible for calcium reuptake, which allows for muscle relaxation. Cultured muscle cells of patients showing delayed restoration of calcium concentration following depolarization (150) and the distinct pattern of abnormal metabolic response to exercise with ^{11}P-NMR spectroscopy (147) are both consistent with a defect that affects calcium homeostasis. Sarcoplasmic reticulum calcium ATPase is found in much higher concentrations in type 2 (fast-twitch) fibers (151), which helps explain why impaired relaxation is noted only after phasic exercise, when primarily type 2 motor units are recruited. Earlier immunocytochemical analysis revealed severe reduction in both calcium ATPase content (152) and biologic activity (147). More recent studies on whole-muscle homogenates and muscle cultures using various methods to confirm their results (including monoclonal antibodies to fast-twitch muscle calcium ATPase isozyme) have shown a specific reduction in enzyme activity by about 50% but with normal enzyme concentration (150). This evidence supports the conclusion that this syndrome is due to a reduction in molecular activity of the type 2 muscle fiber sarcoplasmic reticulum calcium-ATPase isozyme, which Benders et al. (150) speculate is due to a structural modification of the protein.

Karpati et al. (152) reported four male patients who inherited the condition through an autosomal recessive or X-linked recessive mode. Harati has seen a female patient with this syndrome whose brother was similarly affected, supporting an autosomal recessive inheritance. Autosomal dominant inheritance has been suggested in one family (153). In about 59% of families with Brody's disease, different mutations of sarcoplasmic reticulum Ca^{2+} ATPase create stop codons that delete all or part of the Ca^{2+} binding and translocation domain, resulting in loss of SERCA1 function (154,155).

Studies on cultured muscle cells of patients showed that dantrolene sodium and calcium channel–blocking drugs improved calcium homeostasis (150). Despite such in vitro evidence of benefit, treatment with these drugs has been unsuccessful in some patients (152). However, other patients with less pronounced impairment of muscle relaxation had improvement of exertional myalgia with verapamil (147) or improvement of exercise intolerance with dantrolene sodium (148).

Rippling Muscle Disease

This rare disorder characterized by rippling movement in muscles suddenly stretched by voluntary contraction or percussion has been described in families with autosomal dominant inheritance (156–159). There may be substantial phenotypic variability among members of families affected with this disease (160). Sporadic cases have also been reported (161–163). Patients develop painful muscle stiffness, often with initiation of physical activity after a period of rest, painless or painful localized muscle mounding or myoedema produced by percussion, and elevated serum muscle enzyme levels. The rippling movements and myoedema, which are electrically silent, usually occur in limb muscles, although involvement of extraocular muscles may be possible (162). Mild nonspecific myopathic features have been reported on muscle histology and electron microscopy (157,161), including abnormalities of sarcolemma and sarcoplasmic reticulum. The pathophysiology remains speculative. In vitro muscle studies show sarcolemmal excitability and findings consistent with abnormal sensitivity of sarcoplasmic reticulum (calcium channel) to muscle distortion (158). An autoimmune mechanism has been hypothesized in sporadic cases associated with myasthenia gravis and thymoma (163,164). The genetic and molecular bases are unknown, although genetic heterogeneity is suggested by strong linkage to chromosome region 1q41 (159). Recently, a de novo missense mutation of caveoline-3 gene on chromosome 3p25 has been described in a sporadic case of rippling muscle disease (165).

Myotonia Congenita with Painful Cramps

Myotonia congenita with painful cramps is another rare muscle disorder with contracture, although it is more frequently included in discussions of autosomal dominant myotonic disorders (166–168). As opposed to most myotonic disorders, myotonia congenita has muscle contractions that are painful and are electrically silent after an initial period of electrical myotonia. Often prolonged, the contractions follow exercise. It is unclear whether this disease is a variant of typical autosomal dominant myotonia congenita (Thomsen's disease). A sporadic case resembling the recessive type (Becker's disease) has also been reported (169). Thomsen's and Becker's myotonia congenita are now known to be caused by mutations of the gene *7q32* encoding the skeletal muscle chloride channel protein (170,171). In familial myotonic disorder with painful myotonia and cramps, the symptom may be aggravated by injection of potassium (potassium-aggravated myotonia) (172). This condition was previously known as myotonia fluctuans, myotonia permanens, and acetazolamide-sensitive myotonia. This disease, like others in the adynamia–paramyotonia complex (173), is now known to be due to mutations of the skeletal muscle sodium channel gene *(17q23)* (174,175).

Hypothyroidism

Neuromuscular dysfunction is common in hypothyroidism (176,177). Three overlapping syndromes of hypothyroid myopathy have been identified. In infants and children, hypothyroidism often results in generalized muscular stiffness and hypertrophy, often most remarkable in the calf muscles, a condition known as Kocher-Debré-Sémélaigne syndrome. Adults with hypothyroid myopathy typically have mild shoulder and pelvic girdle weakness, with three fourths of patients complaining of muscle pain, cramps, or stiffness (178). Muscular hypertrophy occasionally accompanies these symptoms in a constellation known as Hoffman's syndrome. Uncommonly, patients have exercise-induced myalgia with histologic (179) and clinical evidence of rhabdomyolysis (180). Myalgia and cramps with elevated serum CK may also accompany rapid reduction of serum thyroid hormone levels toward normal during treatment of hyperthyroidism, perhaps reflecting a relative hypothyroid state within muscle tissue (181).

Common to all forms of hypothyroid myopathy is slowness of muscle contraction and relaxation. When severe, this may result in muscle stiffness with slowed movements that suggest parkinsonism or dystonia. This is true especially of the intense stiffness that can accompany Kocher-Debré-Sémélaigne syndrome, and affected infants initially may be suspected of having tetany, dystonia, or spasticity. Hypothyroid-related prolongation of muscle contraction and relaxation is worsened by cold and can be detected clinically by the slowed return phase of the Achilles' reflex and by myoedema following muscle percussion.

In all three conditions serum CK levels may be elevated, and the electromyogram may reveal myopathic and polyphasic potentials, as well as hyperirritability with complex repetitive discharges (178,182). The delayed relaxation of grip combined with the "pseudomyotonia" that may be seen on electromyogram may produce diagnostic confusion with the myotonic disorders. However, the myotonia is not present except in patients believed to have an associated inherited myotonia (183), which may be unmasked by the hypothyroidism (184). Confusion may also arise between inflammatory myopathies and hypothyroid myopathy. Serum thyroid function tests reveal the proper diagnosis in most cases, although an associated inflammatory myopathy should be considered in patients with evidence of autoimmune thyroid disease, particularly in those who do not respond to treatment.

Muscle pathology has revealed a host of nonspecific or inconsistent findings, including focal necrosis, variation in fiber size, vacuoles, increased numbers of central nuclei, type I fiber predominance, type II fiber atrophy, and central changes (178,185,186); it also reveals ultrastructural evidence of polysaccharide and glycogen accumulation, mitochondrial abnormalities and lipid droplets, dilated sarcoplasmic reticulum, and T-tubule proliferation (186). We have also observed muscle fibrosis and multiple ring fibers in a severely hypothyroid patient with a serum CK level 40 times normal. The mechanisms of hypothyroid-induced muscle pain, stiffness, cramps, hypertrophy, and delayed contraction and relaxation are uncertain. It is speculated that metabolic changes, particularly those affecting carbohydrate metabolism and mitochondrial function, may explain myalgias, cramps, and exercise intolerance (187). Forearm muscle exercise testing may reveal impaired lactate production, and ^{11}P-NMR spectroscopy has shown delayed glycogen breakdown in muscle with exercise (188). Impaired muscle lysosomal acid maltase activity has been implicated (178,189). Glycogenolysis may also be diminished on the basis of decreased muscle β-adrenergic receptor density (190). Reduced mitochondrial oxidative capacity may be especially important (187). The delay in muscle contraction and relaxation may be related to the effects of reduced myosin ATPase activity (191) and decreased calcium uptake by the sarcoplasmic reticulum (192). Other abnormalities in muscle function include decreased muscle protein synthesis and diminished sodium-potassium pump activity.

The management of muscle dysfunction associated with hypothyroidism has not been studied objectively. In most cases, all signs and symptoms as well as many pathologic and metabolic changes (180,189) resolve within 6 months of adequate thyroid hormone replacement. However, temporary worsening of the muscle pain and stiffness with the initiation of treatment has been reported (193).

Hyperparathyroidism

Muscle pain and cramps are common in hyperparathyroidism (194,195). The exact mechanisms responsible are unknown, and several explanations have been put forward. Elevated intracellular calcium concentrations, which result in prolonged muscle contraction, have been reported (196,197). Other researchers have demonstrated reductions in muscle energy production, transfer, and use induced by parathyroid hormone (198). The finding that the calcium channel blocker verapamil experimentally reverses most of these abnormalities suggests that calcium homeostasis plays a central role in hyperparathyroid-induced muscle dysfunction.

Myotonic Disorders

Myotonia is not difficult to diagnose once symptoms have been reported. However, except for unusual myotonic disorders discussed previously (see section "Myotonia Congenita with Painful Cramps"), this condition is painless, and many patients do not voluntarily complain of stiffness. It is usually relatively simple to differentiate the transient muscle stiffness of myotonia from muscle cramp and contracture (Table 33.2).

The myotonic disorders listed in Table 33.1 have been reviewed in detail elsewhere (199). We also direct interested readers to reviews of the advances in the understanding of the nondystrophic myotonias and periodic paralyses (200).

One condition in which muscle cramp and stiffness are prominent is Schwartz-Jampel syndrome (chondrodystrophic myotonia). This autosomal recessive illness [autosomal dominant inheritance has also been reported by Ferrannini et al. (201) and Pascuzzi et al. (202)] usually begins in infancy with myotonia, continuous muscle discharges, osteochondrodysplasia, respiratory distress, feeding difficulties, growth retardation, hypertrophic musculature, and a characteristic facies with blepharophimosis, micrognathia, pursed lips, and low-set ears (203; reviewed in 202) (Fig. 33.6). Patients are at risk for malignant hyperthermia (204). Cognitive impairment, estimated to occur in 25% of cases, may take the form of a developmental language disorder (205). Obstructive sleep apnea with hypoxia has been reported (206). Patients with normal osteochondral development (207), including some without significant skeletal alterations (208), have been reported. It has been suggested that these patients develop mild skeletal dysplasia only as a consequence of myotonia and are distinct from the larger group of patients with heterogeneous forms of primary bone dysplasia (209). Muscle stiffness and osteochondrodysplasia often limit joint mobility, resulting in a rigid gait. This, combined with the mask-like facies and paucity of movements observed in some cases, may suggest a movement disorder. Almost all patients have prominent action

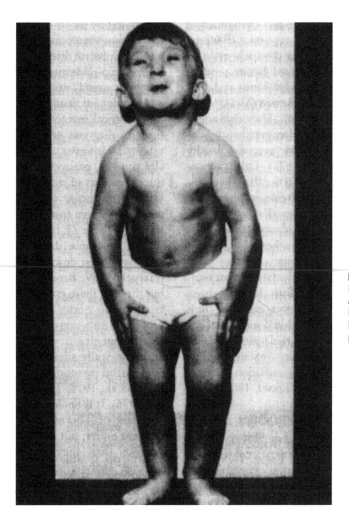

FIG. 33.6. Schwartz-Jampel syndrome. Note blepharophimosis, low-set ears, hypertrophic muscles, and muscle stiffness with abnormal arm posture. (Reprinted with permission from Scriban N, Ionasescu V. Schwartz-Jampel syndrome: a case report—stimulatory effect of calcium and A 23187 calcium ionophore for propane synthesis in muscle cell cultures. *Eur Neurol* 1981;20:46–61.)

and percussion myotonia, and fine myokymic movements frequently are seen in resting muscle. On electromyogram, although true myotonic discharges have been noted, the electrical discharges often lack a waxing and waning pattern, and at rest there may be continuous bizarre high-frequency discharges. Although these discharges are not blocked by peripheral nerve block, the effect of curare has varied from one report to another (210). Thus, the origin of the discharges may be within the muscle in some cases but may be in the distal terminal of the nerve as well. In vitro studies of skeletal muscle fibers from a single patient revealed an unstable resting membrane potential, decreased chloride conductance, and delayed sodium channel opening (211). These abnormalities were partially normalized by in vitro addition of the sodium channel blocker procainamide, which also resulted in reduced clinical myotonia and increased mobility. Further confirmation is needed regarding the efficacy of this treatment as well as carbamazepine, which has been used successfully in improving myotonia, blepharospasm, stair climbing, height (212), and respiratory status. Early treatment may prevent features of skeletal dysplasia (213). The pathophysiology is probably distinct from known skeletal muscle channelopathies (211). This is supported by genetic studies that found linkage to chromosome 1p34-36.1 in several families with varying ethnicity (214), although there are reports that another locus may be responsible for the severe form (215).

Other Myogenic Conditions and Drug-induced Myalgia and Cramps

A complete discussion of drug-induced myalgia and cramps and other myogenic conditions is beyond the scope of this chapter. For further information, see the recent reviews by Roy and Gutmann (216) and Simchak and Pascuzzi (217). Sufit and Peters (218) have reported exercise-induced myalgias in two patients with associated proximal muscle weakness of uncertain origin that responded to treatment with nifedipine. Other cases have been associated with abnormal components of skeletal muscle structure or function, such as mitochondrial alterations (219), intracellular acidosis (220), low myosin ATPase and phosphocreatine content (221), type 2 muscle fiber predominance (222), abnormal dystrophin (223,224), vascularized muscle fibers (225,

226), and muscle tubular aggregates (227,228). Muscle pain and cramps may also be caused by local and diffuse myositis, polymyalgia rheumatica, endocrine myopathies, uremia, cirrhosis, gastrectomy, dehydration, and drugs. These drugs include clofibrate and other cholesterol-lowering agents, diuretics, ε-aminocaproic acid, vincristine, captopril, phencyclidine, ketoconazole, lithium, salbutamol, isoetharine, emetine, danazol, amphetamine, cimetidine, methoxyprogesterone, alcohol, amphotericin B, nifedipine, nicotinic acid, and cyclosporine (229,235). Muscle cramps have also been reported in cases of Becker's muscular dystrophy of later onset (223,224) and as an early manifestation of mild disease (236). Cramps also occur in the rare syndrome of insulin resistance, acanthosis nigricans, and acral hypertrophy (237). Sometimes myalgia and cramps occur with drug treatments or conditions in which there are overlapping myogenic and neurogenic causation. In adults, the neuromuscular depolarizing blocking agent succinylcholine has a high association with postoperative myalgia and muscle damage. This is possibly due to the shearing forces of fasciculating muscle fibers induced by the drug's effect on neuromuscular junction and muscle spindles (238–240). Severe painful cramp is a major symptom of a rare probably autoimmune disease affecting local areas of muscle (interstitial myositis), skin, and subcutaneous fat (lipoatrophy) (241,242). This myogenic disorder has features, discussed in the next section, more commonly associated with neurogenic cramps, including their occurrence at rest and association with fasciculations.

Muscle pain and cramp should also be differentiated from disorders that affect bones, joints, and periarticular structures. Intermittent claudication secondary to atherosclerotic occlusion of leg arteries or vascular aneurysms should be considered in individuals with lower extremity myalgia or cramp induced by effort. However, such ischemic pain typically subsides quickly with rest and does not cause residual muscle soreness unless the ischemia is severe.

NEUROGENIC CAUSES OF MUSCLE CRAMPS

Most, but not all, disorders discussed in this section produce cramp at rest, which may worsen with exercise or repetitive use of the muscle. These conditions are thought to cause cramps or similar symptoms through a mechanism involving the portions of the motor unit proximal to the neuromuscular junction. Neurogenic cramps are common, affecting the majority of patients evaluated by the neurologist.

Common and Nocturnal Cramps

Approximately one third of the population suffers at least one spontaneous cramp in a given year (243). Common muscle cramps typically entail a sudden involuntary and painful muscle shortening, induced by movement, with visible and palpable contraction confined to one muscle or part of the muscle. Such cramps usually affect the gastrocnemius or the small intrinsic muscles of the soles of the feet, and they may cause abnormal posture of the affected joint. The individual may be aware of twitching (fasciculation) of the muscle before onset or at the end of the cramp; in some cases, fasciculations are widespread and continuous (244–246). The cramp usually is terminated by passive stretching of the affected muscle or by active contraction of antagonist muscles, but there may be residual soreness and swelling. Passive stretching before and after exercise tends to prevent such cramping during exercise.

The cause of common muscle cramps is unknown. Cramps occur frequently in two common circumstances, acute fluid or salt loss, such as with prolonged physical activity, and when muscles are maintained in shortened position, such as the feet and calves of swimmers (247). This suggests that electrolyte imbalance and muscle length may be important (248). In a comparison between marathon runners who had a cramp during a marathon (18%) and those who were without cramps, there were no significant differences in degree of pretraining, performance, plasma electrolyte or bicarbonate concentrations, or changes in plasma volume (249). In a similar study, under conditions of more profuse sweating, magnesium loss correlated with cramping (250). Further studies of this common problem are needed, perhaps using ^{31}P-NMR techniques to monitor intracellular electrolyte and pH changes.

Nocturnal leg cramps are extremely common, especially among the elderly (1,247). Exactly why this symptom is prevalent among the elderly is not known; speculation about such causal phenomena as progressive age-related loss of upper motor neurons, local tissue abnormalities of the leg, varicose veins, and muscle dehydration have remained unsubstantiated. Analysis of questionnaires completed by outpatients with general medical problems at a Veterans Affairs medical center revealed that nocturnal cramps were significantly associated with peripheral vascular disease, hypokalemia, and coronary artery disease (1). A significant association with peripheral neurologic deficits was found in a retrospective study of male veterans (251). Evidence best supports a neurogenic origin for ordinary and nocturnal muscle cramps, and factors that cause cramp may have in common a hyperexcitable effect on intramuscular motor nerve terminals (252).

Prevention of ordinary and nocturnal muscle cramps is often difficult, as evidenced by the large number of proposed treatments (217). Patients should avoid the use of caffeine and adrenergic agonist medications. A simple set of exercises designed to gently stretch the gastrocnemius muscles should be discussed with all patients. The patient stands with feet flat on the floor, an arm's length away from and facing a wall, using the arms to support the body in a "standing push-up" as the upper torso is moved slowly toward the wall while the legs are held straight. This may result in a mild "burning" pain in the area behind the knees. The position is maintained for 10 seconds and repeated nine times twice daily (253). Other stretching exercises may also be beneficial.

Nocturnal leg cramps can also be avoided by minimizing passive plantar flexion of the feet during sleep. Individuals who habitually sleep in a supine position should be advised to keep the bed covers loose or to use a foot cradle to keep the weight of the covers from exaggerating passive plantar flexion. Patients can also place a pillow against the sole of the feet as a footboard, a technique also used to prevent foot drop in unconscious or paralyzed patients. Prone sleepers can let their feet hang over the end of the mattress to maintain a more neutral foot position.

For patients whose symptoms do not respond to physical maneuvers, various medications have been found to be effective in the treatment of cramps, although most lack confirmation in well-designed studies. Quinine sulfate or its derivatives has been used for more than 50 years since its effectiveness in nocturnal leg cramps was initially reported (254). We and other physicians can attest to patient satisfaction with quinine. However, the U.S. Food and Drug Administration in August 1994 issued regulations that led to the removal of quinine from over-the-counter (OTC) use, and in early 1995 prescription quinine products could no longer be labeled for use in nocturnal leg cramps (255). Stopping OTC availability was mainly driven by potentially serious, although rare, idiosyncratic side effects of hypersensitivity reactions and thrombocytopenia or pancytopenia. Other side effects include cinchonism (nausea, vomiting, tinnitus, and deafness), visual toxicity, and cardiac effects (256), which occur at toxic drug levels not expected to result from usual low doses of quinine used in patients with common or nocturnal cramps. However, this may not be true in patients with hepatic or renal disease or those using drugs that decrease either clearance (cimetidine) or urinary excretion (alkalinizing agents) of quinine. The controversy over quinine's efficacy stems from placebo-controlled studies showing conflicting negative (257–259) and positive results (260,261) that have been questioned because of design flaws and/or small numbers of patients. The largest blinded placebo-controlled studies to date have clearly demonstrated in 4-week trials the efficacy with mild side effects of quinine sulfate 500 mg (262) and hydroquinine hydrobromide 300 mg (263) in reducing the frequency of ordinary muscle cramps. The latter study showed an almost threefold benefit over placebo. These studies support the short-term use of low-dose quinine products in the prevention of frequent common muscle cramps in otherwise healthy adults who are informed and monitored for adverse reactions. Since benefit from quinine can last weeks to months after discontinuation of treatment (264), short periods of treatment followed by "drug holidays" may be advisable and effective (263). Questions for future studies include long-term safety, dose-related responses, and value of monitoring drug levels.

Since quinine is contraindicated in pregnancy, other treatments are needed. Under the guidance of the obstetrician, pregnancy-related cramps can often be relieved by an increase in dietary calcium and magnesium. Other medications that anecdotally or in uncontrolled studies have been found useful in managing neurogenic cramps include other "membrane-stabilizing" agents, such as phenytoin and carbamazepine; baclofen and clonazepam; verapamil 120 mg at bedtime (265); carisoprodol 350 mg four times daily (266); and nifedipine (218), which can also cause cramp (267). We have effectively used oral dantrolene sodium or mexiletine in patients with some forms of severe neurogenic cramps. Vitamin E has been reported effective in nocturnal leg cramps; however, in the only controlled study for this condition, benefit was not demonstrated (262).

Peripheral Nerve Injury, Nerve Root Compression, Radiculopathy, and Anterior Horn Cell Disease

Muscle cramps commonly are caused by dysfunction of peripheral nerves, nerve roots, and anterior horn cells. They are responsible for the majority of cramps in which a specific cause is determined. In a prospective study of 50 cancer patients referred for new complaints of muscle cramps, the problem originated in the peripheral nerve in 44%, in spinal roots in 26%, and in the plexus in 8%; no cause was found in 16% (268). Muscle cramps were the first symptom in 64% of these patients, emphasizing the importance of a thorough diagnostic workup in patients with the new onset of cramps.

Localized motor unit hyperactivity, including myokymia and cramp, sometimes follows individual nerve or plexus injury (269,270), diffuse peripheral neuropathy (271), focal demyelinating neuropathy (272), and motor neuropathy with multifocal conduction block (273,274). It may also occur as a late effect of poliomyelitis (275). The persistent motor conduction block in many of these conditions except the last may be important to the pathogenesis of myokymia and cramp (273,276). The alpha motor neuron itself also has been proposed as the site of origin of cramp and myokymia, perhaps reflecting the "bistable" property of its membrane, which can switch from a low- to high-equilibrium potential capable of generating self-sustaining rhythmic firing (275). Central influences may affect these neural discharges, since in some patients these symptoms disappear during sleep and spinal anesthesia. In one case, back averaging of the electroencephalogram revealed that severe cramps were preceded by a cortical potential (277).

Compression of a nerve root may cause fasciculation, myokymia, or cramp, with or without persistent muscle spasm, in muscles supplied by that root. Rish (278) estimated a 20% to 30% incidence of cramps in lumbar radiculopathy and noted that symptoms may persist after surgery. However, this may reflect the chronicity of the radiculopathy, since myokymia has been shown to cease immediately after decompression of a more acute nerve root lesion (279). On electromyogram, regular, rhythmic, and in some cases continuous discharges of motor unit potentials are often seen. Stretching the nerve increases spasm and muscle discharges (280).

A pseudomyotonic phenomenon consisting of difficulty opening the hand after holding an object has been reported in patients with chronic radiculopathy at the level of the seventh cervical nerve root (281). Electromyographic (EMG) examination revealed coactivation of finger flexors and finger extensors during voluntary contraction of the latter group of muscles. No electrical or percussion myotonia was present. This phenomenon is caused by misdirected reinnervation of the flexor muscles by nerve root fibers belonging to the extensor muscles. Local anesthetic block of the median nerve at the elbow level eliminates flexor muscle activity and temporarily abolishes the pseudomyotonic phenomena.

Muscle cramps are known to occur in motor neuron disease, and in the hereditary spinal muscular atrophies it can be the only clinical manifestation of early disease (282). It is a common, though seldom obtrusive, feature of amyotrophic lateral sclerosis (ALS) (283). As with fasciculation, it has been suspected that the cramps of ALS originate from dysfunction of the terminal branches of intramuscular nerves (284,285). The identification of antibodies to voltage-gated calcium channels on nerve terminals and muscle fibers (286,287) suggests that some aspects of the pathogenesis of ALS are similar to those reported by Sinha et al. (288) in Isaacs' syndrome. Recommended treatments for the cramps of ALS include stretching exercises, baclofen, phenytoin, carbamazepine, and quinine (289).

Many patients who have had poliomyelitis have cramps and fasciculation (246). Following anterior horn cell damage, extensive sprouting of the remaining motor neurons allows for reinnervation of the muscle. These terminal nerve sprouts are less stable electrically and may discharge spontaneously or degenerate, presumably leading to fasciculation and cramps. Similar mechanisms may be active in ALS, chronic spinal muscular atrophies, and other disorders of motor neurons. Central mechanisms of cramp may also play a role in some of these disorders. Peripheral nerve stimulation distal to a nerve block could not induce cramps in a patient with ALS or bulbospinal neuronopathy (290). Cramps were suppressed selectively by γ-aminobutyric acid (GABA) receptor agonists (diazepam and baclofen), suggesting that impairment of inhibitory GABAergic interneurons was involved in the pathogenesis of cramps in these patients.

Heat Cramps

Prolonged exertion in high temperatures can cause heat cramps. They are an occupational hazard among skilled mill workers, furnace stokers, boiler room workers, miners, and others who face high temperatures (291,292). They are more common among "acclimatized" workers, perhaps because of the increased volume and salt concentration of their sweat. Cramps are also a feature of the more severe syndrome of heat exhaustion; in both, the cause is probably sweat-induced hyponatremia or fluid replacement–induced osmotic shifts. However, a recent study has deemphasized the role of hyponatremia and indicated dehydration as the main pathogenic factor (293). The cramps may be delayed up to 24 hours following heat exposure. Although heat cramps have not been studied extensively, their clinical similarities to common and exertion-related cramps suggest that they are neurogenic and may share a common mechanism. The treatment of heat cramps consists of cessation of exertion, rest in a cool environment, and electrolyte and fluid replacement. A high-sodium diet or salt supplements along with fluid intake may be helpful in preventing attacks. Combination of vitamin E and C has also been reported to be effective (294).

Hemodialysis Cramps

Muscle cramp is prevalent in patients on hemodialysis, and it is the most common reason for early termination of treatment (295). They frequently appear toward the end of the dialysis sessions (associated with loss of 2 to 4 L of body water), although they can occur earlier in dialysis when high rates of ultrafiltration are used (256). Hemodialysis-induced muscle cramps (296) are accompanied by high-voltage EMG activity and are considered to be neurogenic (297). Dialysis cramps are comparable with cramps induced by diuretics, diarrhea, vomiting, and profuse perspiration. Plasma volume contraction through an unknown mechanism is the most common explanation given for muscle cramps (298). Hypertonic solutions of dextrose, saline, and mannitol used to correct this volume change were all found to be equally safe and effective in relieving these muscle cramps (299). Plasma volume contraction leads to increased catecholamines, which may play a role in hemodialysis-induced muscle cramp (300). Medication that attenuates this sympathetic activation (low-dose prazosin) reduced cramp frequency, but it is limited for practical use because of hypotensive effects (301). Nifedipine, a vasodilator and calcium channel blocker, produced prompt relief of cramps and was three times as effective as placebo (302). Other treatments include quinine sulfate 325 mg and vitamin E 400 IU at bedtime, which proved to be equally effective in reducing cramp frequency and severity of pain in dialysis patients (303). Hemodialysis-induced cramps may be alleviated by oral quinine sulfate 300 mg given just before dialysis (304); and L-carnitine intravenous supplementation at the end of the dialysis session decreased cramp incidence (305).

Generalized Motor Unit Hyperactivity of Peripheral Nerve Origin

Motor unit hyperactivity arising in the peripheral nerves is a heterogeneous group of acquired and hereditary disorders that all have in common sustained, diffuse motor unit activity probably of peripheral nerve origin with or without associated evidence of peripheral neuropathy; see the review and classification in Auger (306). In Isaacs' (307) report of this syndrome he used the term *continuous muscle fiber activity* (CMFA). A number of terms have been used to describe related syndromes, including Isaacs-Mertens syndrome, neuromyotonia, generalized myokymia, pseudomyotonia, continuous motor unit activity, normocalcemic tetany, quantal squander, armadillo disease, and Morvan's chorea. Broadly classified, these terms have limitations for accurate description of the spectrum of clinical and EMG findings in this group of disorders. Perhaps the most descriptive, although cumbersome, is sustained muscle activity of peripheral nerve origin (308); even then the word "general" must be added to lend distinction from local conditions (see section "Peripheral Nerve Injury, Nerve Root Compression, Radiculopathy, and Anterior Horn Cell Disease"). *Neuromyotonia,* favored by many (309), emphasizes the neurogenic origin of the myotonic-like clinical features. It also describes the most common EMG finding in Isaacs' form of this disorder, spontaneous (also induced by needle movement or voluntary contraction), irregularly occurring trains (usually few seconds) of variably formed motor unit potentials firing at a frequency of 150 to 300 Hz (neuromyotonic discharge). *Generalized myokymia* emphasizes clinical myokymia (visible rippling movements from continuous muscle contractions) and one of its EMG correlates, the spontaneous, more regularly occurring grouped discharges (often brief bursts) of motor unit potentials (myokymic discharge). Other EMG findings include fasciculation or individual motor unit potentials spontaneously firing at fixed intervals of less than 20 ms, such as doublets, triplets, and multiplets (Fig. 33.7, which shows two doublets, triplets, and fasciculation). Cramp discharges with motor unit potentials firing at high frequency (up to 150 Hz) may occur in a probably related disorder at the mild end of the spectrum as well as a major feature in some hereditary conditions. These EMG patterns often occur in combination and do not provide a clear basis for pathogenic distinction. Since the predominant discharges are motor unit potentials, the term *continuous motor unit activity* (CMUA) (271) is more informative than *CMFA* because CMFA may imply spontaneous activity of individual muscle fibers. In this chapter CMUA is used as an abbreviated term when referring to this syndrome in general. Finally, the word *continuous* is relative, variably applying to overall clinical muscle activity or EMG discharges, and does not apply to lesser degrees of motor unit hyperactivity.

This section discusses generalized motor unit hyperactivity of peripheral nerve origin under the following main categories: idiopathic or autoimmune syndrome not associated with peripheral neuropathy, other acquired conditions, and hereditary disorders.

Idiopathic or Autoimmune (Isaacs') Syndrome Not Associated with Peripheral Neuropathy

The eponym *Isaacs' syndrome* is probably best applied to idiopathic cases without peripheral neuropathy. Current evidence indicates that at least some of these have an autoimmune basis. The onset is typically during the second or third decade of life, although onset up to the sixth decade also occurs (310). The sexes are affected equally. Complaints include muscle stiffness, intermittent cramping, and difficulty chewing, speaking, and even breathing. Ocular muscles and sphincters function normally, and sensation is not affected.

The most remarkable feature of Isaacs' syndrome is myokymia affecting limb (especially distally), trunk, jaw, face, and abdominal muscles. These widespread continuous twitching movements resemble but usually are slower than fasciculation and have been described as having the appearance of a bag of worms. Repetitive passive limb movement leads to increasing resistance and pain. Voluntary movements are slow, resulting in gait difficulty, and fatigue sets in rapidly. However, repetitive voluntary activity tends to increase muscle mobility, although temporarily. There is no percussion or electrical myotonia. The cramps and myokymic movements persist during sleep. Some patients display marked hyperhidrosis, muscle hypertrophy, or elevated CK. Limited forms of the disease with facial myokymia and elevated voltage-gated potassium channel (VGKC) antibody (311) has also been reported. Some cases may be associated with thymoma (312). One case associated with malignant hyperthermia has been reported (313). Detailed

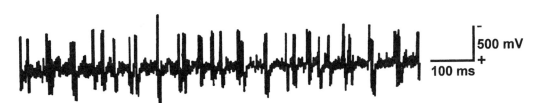

FIG. 33.7. Continuous motor unit activity.

laboratory and cerebrospinal fluid evaluations are usually normal, although cerebrospinal fluid oligoclonal bands were found in all three patients tested in one report (310), and mild elevations in cerebrospinal fluid total protein can occur (314).

EMG studies typically show neuromyotonic and myokymic discharges; fasciculations, doublets, and multiplets are also seen. These discharges are abolished by curare, distinguishing them from myotonia, but persist during spinal and general anesthesia and sleep, indicating that they arise in the peripheral nerves. The site of origin along the nerve can be proximal or distal, as shown by variable response to nerve block. These discharges frequently persist after nerve block, and in some cases there is evidence that this activity arose quite distally and perhaps even in nerve terminals (315). Others have found that nerve block abolished these spontaneous discharges, indicating their source in proximal parts of nerves (316,317). In an isolated case, epidural block reduced the spontaneous discharges and led to a silent period after the H response, suggesting that the discharges arose in the ventral roots or spinal cord (318). The long trains of discharges can be difficult to distinguish from those of tetany. The clinical and electrophysiologic similarities of Isaacs' syndrome to hyperventilation-induced tetany (described in more detail in the section "Tetany") raised some doubt about the authenticity of some reports (54). It is essential that all patients suspected of having Isaacs' syndrome have calcium, phosphorus, and blood gas studies as well as investigations of clinical and electrophysiologic effects of hyperventilation.

The cause of Isaacs' syndrome remains unknown, although evidence of autoimmunity is accumulating (319–322). Sinha et al. (288) reported an antibody-mediated mechanism in a man with a 7-year history of severe symptoms, serum thyroid microsomal antibodies, a poor clinical response to phenytoin and carbamazepine, but otherwise typical Isaacs' syndrome. Treatment with plasma exchange (PE) (5 to 10 exchanges) resulted in a transient but nearly complete subjective and objective improvement. Improvement was maximal at 7 to 14 days after the last exchange, and symptoms returned over the following few weeks. Attempts to transfer electrophysiologic or clinical signs of the disease passively to mice were unsuccessful. However, a phrenic nerve diaphragm preparation from mice pretreated with patient's plasma or gamma immunoglobulin (Ig) showed increased neuromuscular resistance to the effects of *d*-tubocurarine without altering postsynaptic ionic currents. These findings suggest that this patient's syndrome was caused by an IgG directed against a presynaptic ion channel that increases nerve terminal excitability, possibly a potassium channel. Since then, more similar patients, with no or partial control of symptoms from anticonvulsants, have responded to PE. Shillito et al. (323) studied three patients with Isaacs' syndrome and three patients with CMUA associated with peripheral neu-

ropathy. Increased quantal release of acetylcholine (quantal content) was shown using a similar mouse nerve–muscle preparation, and the patient's IgG also caused increased repetitive electrical activity when applied to cultured dorsal root ganglion cells. Immunoglobulins from patients with Isaacs' syndrome suppress voltage-gated potassium currents but do not alter gating kinetics or significantly affect sodium currents (324). Antibodies against VGKCs were detected in half the patients, with highest titers in two patients with classic Isaacs' syndrome and low titers in one patient with anti-G_{M1}-associated neuropathy. All three patients with Isaacs' syndrome and the one mentioned earlier with neuropathy responded to PE. This response did not fully correlate with presence of VGKC antibodies, although decline in titers following therapy was demonstrated. Direct evidence that a humoral factor in patients with Isaacs' syndrome is indeed suppressing potassium channels from a neuronal cell line (PC12) was recently demonstrated (325). Immune staining showed that these antibodies, particularly IgM, reacted to VGKC and/or a closely associated protein (confirmed by cross-linking studies) as well as human intramuscular nerve axons (326). Recent studies employing newer molecular immunohistochemical assay may increase the detection rate of VGKC antibodies (322).

Successful symptomatic treatment with phenytoin 300 to 400 mg/day or carbamazepine 200 mg three or four times a day has been reported frequently. In one patient with increased GABA in the cerebrospinal fluid, dantrolene sodium was as effective as phenytoin or carbamazepine (318). Combined oral steroids and azathioprine (310) or azathioprine alone (327) has been effective for longer term treatment and has given additional benefit to those showing response to PE. High-dose intravenous immunoglobulin (IVIG) has been reported both to improve (328) and to exacerbate symptoms (329), the latter possibly because of a direct effect of IVIG on muscle or nerve terminal (330). Patients often remain well on symptomatic therapy alone over many years, leading normal lives, as demonstrated by Isaacs' own 10-year follow-up report of his original cases (331). Diazepam, clonazepam, and baclofen usually offer no benefit, although partial response has been rarely noted (310,332).

Other Acquired Conditions

Other acquired conditions include those possibly related to or responsible for CMUA clinically similar to that of Isaacs' syndrome. Those associated with tumor or other autoimmune disorders may prove to be indistinguishable from Isaacs' syndrome and may share an immune-mediated mechanism (312,320). A paraneoplastic syndrome has been implicated in those associated with bronchogenic carcinoma, with (333) and without (334,335) peripheral neuropathy; Hodgkin's lymphoma with resolution of cancer and CMUA following chemotherapy (336); and thymoma with (337,338) and without (337) peripheral neuropathy. The same association has occurred in patients who also had myasthenia gravis and peripheral neuropathy (338), and these two disorders with the CMUA all dramatically improved with PE (339), implicating autoimmunity as a common pathogenetic factor. Patients with CMUA have been reported in association with immune-mediated neuropathy, including Guillain-Barré syndrome (342,343) and chronic inflammatory demyelinating polyneuropathy (CIDP) (340,341), including a nerve biopsy–proven case in which remission of the CIDP and motor unit hyperactivity followed treatment with prednisone and azathioprine (344,345). Le Gars et al. described a patient with antinuclear and anti-G$_m$ antibodies and motor conduction block who responded to PE. Other autoimmune diseases associated with CMUA include juvenile rheumatoid arthritis (346).

An autoimmune pathogenesis may even play a role in some cases associated with drugs or toxins, such as penicillamine (347), which is also a known cause of myasthenia gravis. CMUA has been associated with exposure to other toxins—some with peripheral neuropathy, such as insecticides (348), and others without peripheral neuropathy, including gold therapy (349) and mercury (350). Some cases of mercury or gold intoxication may be the cause of Morvan's fibrillary chorea. This syndrome, mostly reported in the French literature, causes profuse fasciculations and can resemble Isaacs' syndrome, although it differs in the absence of muscle stiffness, presence of acrodynia, and signs of central disorder (337,351–354). It is now recognized that some cases of Morvan's syndrome may be of paraneoplastic origin or associated with other autoimmune disorders and increased VGKC antibody titers (355). There are some patients with CMUA whose symptoms may be exacerbated by other types of exposure, such as alcohol consumption, heat, and metrizamide myelography (the latter in one patient we observed). This syndrome also has been reported in association with peripheral neuropathy of known causation, such as diabetes (356) and nutritional (340) as well as idiopathic peripheral neuropathy (271,310,357,358). In a review of patients with CMUA and peripheral neuropathy, no significant difference from Isaacs' syndrome was found other than differences due to signs of neuropathy; splitting these disorders on this or any other basis has been questioned (359). However, there may be differences in pathogenesis. The electrophysiology may be more complicated in patients with peripheral neuropathy. For example, it has been suggested that the generator site for spontaneous activity in a patient with CMUA and an axonal motor neuropathy varies among discharges, perhaps affected by the location of conduction block within an axon (360). In addition, response to treatment may differ, although more studies are needed before conclusions can be drawn. According to rare reports, immunosuppression and PE have been used without success in patients with this syndrome and idiopathic

peripheral neuropathy (310), including a patient whose disease was refractory to multiple symptomatic medicines and oral steroids but who responded dramatically to valproic acid 200 mg three times a day (361). The only patients with peripheral neuropathy responding to immunotherapy have been those previously discussed who probably had immune-mediated neuropathy, suggesting that these patients have a disease closely related to Isaacs' syndrome and that patients with other acquired or idiopathic peripheral neuropathy may have had different pathogenetic factors.

Within the spectrum of this syndrome not associated with peripheral neuropathy are two disorders with mild and intermediate degrees of motor unit hyperactivity. Several similar cases of a mild phenotype of Isaacs' syndrome were characterized by cramps (whose discharges may also be captured on electromyograms) and occasionally myokymia, but with fasciculations as the only predominant EMG abnormality. This has been described by Tahmoush et al. (362) as the "cramp-fasciculation syndrome," which is effectively managed with carbamazepine. A similar syndrome has been reported as "muscular pain-fasciculation syndrome" (243,245), which Harati has managed successfully with oral mexiletine. Intermediate in this spectrum is myokymia-cramp syndrome, which has both clinical and EMG evidence of myokymia (363). Symptomatic treatment is similar to that for Isaacs' syndrome; quinine sulfate may also be effective. Some of these cases may also have an autoimmune or paraneoplastic basis.

Hereditary Disorders

CMUA has been found in association with hereditary disorders with or without peripheral neuropathy. Those with peripheral neuropathy include hereditary motor neuropathy (364,365); hereditary motor sensory neuropathy (HMSN) type 2 (366,367); an interesting case of HMSN 1 whose predominant manifestation was incapacitating muscle cramps (368); and a case of autosomal dominant spinocerebellar ataxia type 1 (SCA2 linked) (369). Recently, the new type of hereditary motor and sensory neuropathy linked to chromosome 3 associated with painful muscle cramps and fasciculation has been reported from Japan (370). Those not associated with peripheral neuropathy are also commonly autosomal dominant. What follows is a brief review of these families, whose main features include (a) stiffness and continuous motor unit discharges or myokymia with cramps; (b) myokymia with paroxysmal movement disorders; and (c) persistent muscle cramps.

Persistent muscle twitching and episodic stiffness since early childhood were the predominant symptoms in an African-American family with the autosomal dominant form of CMUA (371). The continuous discharges appear to originate in the intrathecal portion of the nerve roots or motor neuron somata. Families with continuous discharges generated from distal portions of nerves have also been described (372). Generalized myokymia and mild calf cramps were the major manifestations in hereditary myokymia reported by Sheaff (373). Clinical variation within the same family can be seen with some of these inherited forms of CMUA. Harati examined a patient with Isaacs' syndrome phenotype whose daughter had myalgia, cramps, exercise intolerance, fasciculation, and electrical evidence of mild, distal denervation. Unlike her mother, she did not have myokymia and responded poorly to phenytoin and carbamazepine treatment. Rippling muscle disease, discussed previously, superficially resembles this group of hereditary disorders associated with CMUA. Schwartz-Jampel syndrome, described previously in the section on myotonic disorders, also can be classified under this section because its electrical discharges have muscle or neurogenic origin.

Myokymia is present in several rare familial paroxysmal movement disorders. These conditions display intrafamilial and interfamilial variations that often overlap and are traditionally named after the predominant clinical features. Several families with an autosomal dominant illness with paroxysmal (or episodic) ataxia (PA) and persistent myokymia (PA type 1, or PA-1) have been reported (374–377). Affected patients have attacks of sudden onset of stiffness or limpness, incoordination, trembling, and dysarthria that typically last for seconds to as long as 15 minutes. Associated congenital contractures of the distal extremities have also been described (375). The attacks are commonly precipitated by sudden, forceful movements (kinesigenic type) or by physical or emotional stress. Myokymia, present on the electromyogram and often clinically, helps distinguish these families from those with the more common illness, PA with interictal nystagmus (PA-2). PA-2 usually responds to treatment with carbonic anhydrase inhibitors, possibly because of normalization of intracellular pH with stabilization of neuronal membranes, normalization of transmitter release or ion channel function, or restoration of enzyme function (378). In contrast, it is usually stated that this treatment is ineffective in PA-1 (376,379). However, others have reported reduction in attacks, although the myokymia may actually worsen (377,380). Phenytoin may give partial control of symptoms, including myokymia. Potassium channels have been implicated, as in Isaacs' syndrome, in the pathogenesis of this disorder. Several point mutations in the *VGKC* gene have been reported (381,382).

Possibly related to PA-1 are some phenotypes of paroxysmal dyskinesia that rarely have been associated with myokymia. This is supported by some members of families with clinical and genetic features of PA-1 who also display clinical features of paroxysmal kinesigenic choreoathetosis (380,382). An even rarer disorder, paroxysmal dystonic choreoathetosis (PDC) with myokymia, has been reported affecting five generations in a single family whose members suffered from minute- to hour-long episodes of paroxysmal muscle stiffness, dystonic posturing, and choreoathetosis

from childhood. These episodes were relieved rapidly by rest or sleep (383). Two of the seven affected family members had prominent myokymia. It remains to be seen whether this form is a variant of PDC without myokymia linked to chromosome 2q (384).

Finally, a hereditary form of CMUA has been reported with persistent widespread or local cramps. Two families have been described with a dominantly inherited cramp syndrome affecting almost any muscle (especially thorax, abdomen, and neck) except those of the head (385,386). It begins in adolescence or young adulthood, is not associated with other neurologic abnormalities, and is neurogenic. A more localized dominantly inherited syndrome with persistent distal cramps also has been described (387,388). This syndrome is characterized by painful distal cramps resulting in flexion or extension of toes, flexion of wrists and metacarpophalangeal joints, and extension of interphalangeal joints. The symptoms usually begin in childhood, initially only after exertion but later occurring at rest, especially after strenuous activity. Cramps also occur during sleep and are aggravated by exposure to cold. Episodes of muscle pain in the neck, chest, low back, and legs can be precipitated by infections, but alcohol ingestion, fasting, or excitement does not provoke cramping. Exercise-induced twitching of calf muscles without evidence of weakness and atrophy is sometimes present. The symptoms persist throughout life. Nerve conduction studies do not indicate a peripheral neuropathy, although mild abnormalities were noted in one case (388). Electromyogram shows signs of mild denervation with normal motor unit potentials during cramps and electrical silence afterward. Neither spinal anesthesia nor nerve block modifies the cramp, but local infiltration of the hand muscles with lidocaine halts contraction, indicating a peripheral nerve origin. Carbamazepine, phenytoin, quinine, and various muscle relaxants offer no benefit.

Tetany

Tetany, commonly associated with hypocalcemia, is broadly characterized by distal nerve paresthesia, muscle cramps, involuntary carpopedal spasms, attacks of laryngeal stridor, and convulsions. Overt or subclinical hyperventilation with respiratory alkalosis and compression-induced ischemia are well-known triggering factors that can reveal "latent" tetany (389,390). The peripheral nerves of susceptible individuals also display hyperirritability to mechanical (Chvostek's sign) or electrical stimulation. Latent tetany has also been termed *spasmophilia* by French and German authors.

In tetany paresthetic symptoms almost always precede spasm and cramp. In the hands the intrinsic muscles are affected earliest, causing tonic adduction of the thumb and fingers, flexion of metacarpophalangeal joints, extension of interphalangeal joints, and flexion of wrist and elbow (Fig. 33.8). In susceptible individuals these symptoms can be

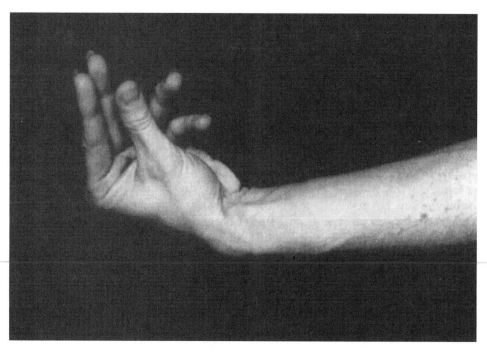

FIG. 33.8. Tetany.

reproduced easily by application and inflation of a blood pressure cuff above the elbow (Trousseau's sign). If the sensory symptoms or signs appear within 3 minutes of ischemia, the test is interpreted as positive. In the feet there is plantar flexion of the foot and toes followed by foot inversion. Rarely, trunk spasm occurs and causes opisthotonic posture. On EMG tetanic spasms characteristically are accompanied by irregular repetitive action potentials resembling motor unit potentials. As the disorder progresses, pairs or groups of potentials (double spikes, doublets, or multiplets), repeated at 5- to 15-ms intervals, appear. In well-developed spasm large, higher frequency motor unit potentials, indistinguishable from one another, predominate (391,392). Tetanic potentials abate with infusion of curare but not with peripheral nerve block, suggesting that the spontaneous discharges occur at some point along the length of the peripheral nerve. Application of a blood pressure cuff below the nerve block induces carpopedal spasm. If the plasma level of ionized calcium is reduced (e.g., hypoparathyroidism, hyperventilation-induced alkalosis), decreased extracellular calcium results in increased sodium conductance, membrane depolarization, and spontaneous rhythmic action potentials (393). The largest nerves have the lowest thresholds, sensory nerves more than motor, and the proximal parts of nerves are more susceptible than distal portions to the effects of ischemia and hypocalcemia. If a subject hyperventilates with an inflated blood pressure cuff on one arm, the spasm occurs first in the free hand, implying that the alkalotic blood must reach the periphery to trigger the symptom. Ischemia of one arm leaves that hand more susceptible to spasm from hyperventilation.

Other electrolyte abnormalities can cause tetany and carpopedal spasm. Hypocalcemia was probably the primary cause for tetany also associated with hyperphosphatemia resulting from routine bowel preparation with an oral phosphate–based laxative (394). Magnesium deficiency has also been associated with tetany (395), although levels of plasma-ionized calcium are seldom reported in these cases. Tetany has also been associated with drugs such as diltiazem (396) and alendronate (Fosamax) (397), and has occurred during thyroid surgery postoperative course (397,398). Even in patients diagnosed with panic disorder, concomitant latent tetany due to decreased intracellular magnesium responsive to magnesium salts can occur; therefore, it has been suggested that evaluation of such patients should include red blood cell magnesium levels (399). The alterations in potassium that can lead to tetany appear to be more complicated. While potassium administration in hypocalcemic patients can exacerbate tetany, isolated hypokalemia also can paradoxically provoke tetany through an unknown mechanism (400). Occasional reports of "normocalcemic tetany" (401,402) are difficult to explain but emphasize that neuronal hyperirritability may be related to any mechanism that brings the membrane potential nearer the firing threshold or delays repolarization.

Tetany is managed by correcting the underlying metabolic disorder or hyperventilation syndrome. In hyperventilation or anxiety states, patients usually are not aware of their overbreathing, although they sometimes admit to periods of sighing. It is therefore important to reproduce the tetanic symptom by encouraging the patient to overbreathe spontaneously, and demonstrate that they can hold their breath for a considerable period, even during an attack. An attack sometimes can be terminated by having the patient breathe in and out of a paper bag or inhale a 5% carbon dioxide mixture. However, attention to the underlying anxiety state is of utmost importance.

Other Mineral and Electrolyte Disorders

In addition to calcium, several other mineral and electrolyte disorders can induce cramps (403,404). Hypokalemia, commonly resulting from diuretic use, laxative abuse, diarrhea, hyperaldosteronism, or metabolic acidosis, is often associated with cramps. Cramps and fasciculation frequently are seen in acute hyponatremia. Hypomagnesemia—commonly resulting from inadequate dietary intake associated with alcoholism and malnutrition; malabsorption and increased intestinal losses associated with vomiting, diarrhea, or laxative abuse; or increased urinary excretion associated with renal dysfunction and diuretic use—can cause weakness, cramps, fasciculation, and tetany. A detailed history and appropriate laboratory studies readily reveal these reversible conditions.

Eosinophilia-Myalgia Syndrome

In 1989 and 1990 a transient epidemic known as eosinophilia-myalgia syndrome (EMS) affected more than 1,500 users of L-tryptophan, with estimates of at least twice that number ultimately affected in the United States (405,406). The epidemic has been linked with the use of a single manufacturer's product containing several contaminants that appear to be chemically related to L-tryptophan. The exact toxin and its mechanism of action remain undefined. Theories include direct toxic effect from one or more contaminants, eosinophil products, or L-tryptophan metabolites as well as effects mediated by activated T cells, macrophages, and fibroblasts, all possibly influenced by host factors such as genetic susceptibility (405). EMS shares many features with the Spanish toxic oil syndrome, including recent identification of a chemical link (407), and both appear to be chronic contaminant-induced immune-mediated disorders.

EMS is a clinically heterogeneous syndrome characterized by myalgia and fatigue with associated symptoms and signs that include eosinophilia, eosinophilic pneumonia, edema, fasciitis, alopecia, sclerodermatous skin changes, myopathy, arthralgia, and neuropathy (408,409). Severe disabling cramps and spasms, usually in axial muscles, can occur as a late sequela. Postural tremor and myokymia of suspected peripheral origin and myoclonus have also been reported as uncommon delayed manifestations of EMS (406). Although overall most signs and symptoms of EMS improve with time (410), it is common for patients to suffer from chronic myalgia and fatigue with variable presence of cardiac, neurologic, hematologic, dermatologic, and pulmonary complications (411,412). Some patients may show delayed neurocognitive deficits and have abnormalities of brain white matters (413). Muscle cramps are a common complaint among EMS patients. Among 19 EMS patients followed by Harati, severe cramps were noted by four; moderate cramps, by six; and mild cramps, by five. The cramps typically have sudden onset precipitated by activity. They can occur in any muscle group, with the jaw, thorax, and legs particularly affected. The clinical features of the cramps suggest a neuropathic origin, but cramps can also occur in patients who do not have clinical or electrodiagnostic evidence of a neuropathy. When the cramps and spasms are severe and result in distortion of body posture, they bear some resemblance to those in Satoyoshi's syndrome (see section, "Central Nervous System Causes of Cramps and Myalgia," below). In muscle biopsy specimens inflammatory cells frequently surround the muscle spindles and small intramuscular nerves, and we suspect that immune-mediated damage to these structures leads to cramps. Most of the commonly used treatments for cramps are ineffective in EMS. Some patients have been treated successfully with oral dantrolene sodium.

Toxic Envenomation

Severe muscle spasm may accompany a variety of toxic envenomations and ingestions (414). In these conditions the history and associated clinical findings are paramount in making the correct diagnosis. Muscle cramps are a significant clinical feature of stings by the stingray, scorpion, catfish's spike, and jellyfish. Timber rattlesnake venom can induce myokymia, and South American rattlesnake venom can cause myalgia, myonecrosis, and myoglobinuria. Cramps that follow the bite of the black widow spider can be relieved with intravenous calcium gluconate and intramuscular antivenin.

CNS CAUSES OF CRAMPS AND MYALGIA

Satoyoshi's Syndrome (Progressive Muscle Spasm, Alopecia, and Diarrhea)

This distinctive progressive syndrome, first described by Satoyoshi and Yamada (415), has been mainly reported in several unrelated Japanese patients under the name *komuragaeri* (calf spasm) disease. Although also seen in three Chinese patients, individual non-Asian cases have also occurred in a Briton, a Russian, an Amerindian from Argentina, and a European-American (416). It usually begins in childhood or adolescence and is marked by intermittent painful muscle spasms that are so severe that the limb, trunk, or other affected body part is twisted into a sustained abnormal posture (Fig. 33.9A, B). Non-stimulus-sensitive myoclonus may be present at rest, giving the patient a twitchy appearance. Characteristically patients are completely normal before the onset of cramps. Most patients are simultane-

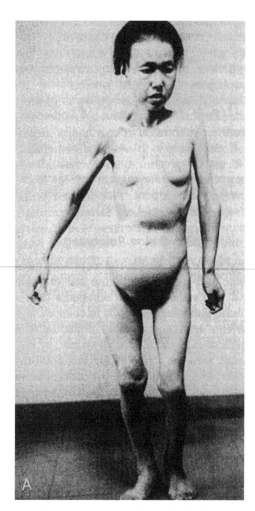
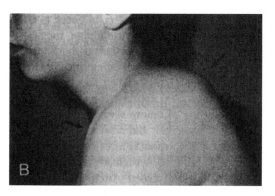

FIG. 33.9. A: Satoyoshi's syndrome. Note the extreme emaciation, with distended abdomen; loss of scalp hair, eyebrows, and body hair; deformities of both knee joints and left elbow; and atrophy of the left biceps, deltoid, and triceps muscles. Muscle cramps continue to occur in the right arm and thigh muscles. Some muscles were hypertrophic when the subject was younger. **B:** Satoyoshi's syndrome. Note the severe pectoralis and trapezius cramps *(arrows)* induced by an attempt to lift the arm over the head. Severe neck extensor weakness is also present. **(A:** courtesy of E. Satoyoshi, National Center of Neurology and Psychiatry, Kodaira-shi, Tokyo.)

ously or subsequently affected by additional abnormalities, including alopecia universalis, intestinal malabsorption with diarrhea, endocrinopathy with amenorrhea, and multiple secondary skeletal abnormalities mimicking metaphysial dysplasia (416). Patients are at risk for skeletal deformities, growth retardation, and general emaciation, which to some degree are preventable with early diagnosis and treatment.

In almost all cases the initial symptom is muscle cramping. Alopecia appears simultaneously in about half of patients. Muscle spasms become progressively more severe and frequent; each painful spasm lasts up to a few minutes but may recur immediately with movement or stimulation of the affected area. The frequency of muscle spasms varies from several to hundreds per day. The spasms are precipitated readily by voluntary contraction and generally do not

occur during rest or sleep. Factors such as exposure to cold, fever, dehydration, and emotional stress tend to lower the threshold for spasm. The spasms often displace and fix the limb (Fig. 33.9A), and with sustained contraction the muscle becomes board-like to palpation and bulges prominently (Fig. 33.9B). The frequency, severity, and chronic course of cramps in this syndrome are far beyond the usual muscle spasm, may require emergency care for pain control, and are appropriately described as myospasm gravis (417). The recurrent and severe nature of the cramps is probably responsible for traumatic injury to skeletal structures leading to the various skeletal abnormalities described in this syndrome (418).

During spasms, EMG recordings reveal synchronized motor unit discharges of 40 to 60 per second and of 4- to 10-mV amplitudes, similar to the rate of discharges in maximal voluntary contraction. Spasms also can be induced by repetitive nerve stimulation. There may be an afterdischarge following H reflex, suggesting an interruption of the inhibitory effect of Renshaw cells on motor neurons (417). This evidence, with the alleviation of cramp during sleep and general anesthesia and its elimination by nerve block and curare, supports a central origin for the cramp, presumably resulting from hyperexcitability of the anterior horn cells. Autopsy studies have not revealed structural abnormalities of the CNS. The pathogenesis of this syndrome remains unknown. Indirect evidence for autoimmune mechanism includes beneficial response of muscle spasm, amenorrhea, and alopecia to glucocorticoids (416,419); association with other autoimmune disorders, such as myasthenia gravis (420), systemic lupus erythematosus, and idiopathic thrombocytopenia, (421); and evidence of IgG production in the cerebrospinal fluid (422). Malabsorption-related mechanisms, such as metabolic derangement, have also been suggested (417). However, with the exception of mild iron deficiency, a flat response to oral glucose loading, and mild hyperphosphatemia, metabolic measurements usually are normal.

Harati is following a white patient with Satoyoshi's syndrome (Fig. 33.9B) in whom colonoscopy, esophagogastroduodenoscopy, intestinal biopsies, and laboratory tests for malabsorption are all normal. These findings make it unlikely that malabsorption is responsible for the syndrome. The patient, while keeping a daily log of cramp severity, was first treated with oral dantrolene sodium 200 mg/day, and later oral prednisone 1 mg/kg per day was added. Two months after starting prednisone, a significant, sustained reduction in cramp severity was noted. Attempts to taper prednisone below 0.5 mg/kg per day have resulted in worsening of cramps. Multiple studies of immune function were normal before treatment, including cerebrospinal fluid (with oligoclonal banding), sedimentation rate, serum immunoelectrophoresis, C-reactive protein, C3, C4, CH100, antinuclear antibodies, rheumatoid factor, and antithyroid antibodies. A Raji cell assay for circulating immune complexes was elevated, and mild eosinophilia was present. The beneficial response to prednisone and the generally normal immunologic workup are consistent with reports from other investigators, although abnormalities in lymphocyte subpopulation studies have been noted (416). A similar patient from Thailand (423) was also treated successfully with corticosteroid.

The need for adequate management of muscle spasms is particularly important when they are life threatening. Patients with severe and frequent spasm are at risk for death from respiratory arrest, and feeding difficulties from masticatory muscle spasm can lead to severe wasting. Some patients respond to calcium gluconate, quinine sulfate, procainamide, or phenytoin. Botulinum toxin may prove to be useful in the management of severe masticatory spasm (424). Dantrolene sodium 100 to 200 mg orally decreases

or abolishes attacks of cramping but neither controls spasms completely nor prevents muscle spasms precipitated by voluntary effort or by electrical stimulation. With dantrolene therapy the long-term prognosis has improved, with patients surviving into adulthood and occasional remission of the illness. Immunosuppression shows promise in improving treatment, not only for the muscle spasms but also for other associated features. IVIG with frequent pulse therapy was effective in reducing muscle spasms and titers of serum autoantibodies in one patient and may prove to be a safer alternative to immunosuppressive agents in these young patients (421).

Strychnine Poisoning

Strychnine was previously used in rodent poisons and in some tonics and cathartics. Since it was removed from commercial use and from all medicinal products in the United States, strychnine poisoning has become rare (425). However, accidental and intentional poisonings continue as a result of its use as an adulterant for illicit drugs, presence in stored rodenticides and in products from other countries, and use in home remedies. It acts by interfering with postsynaptic inhibition at all levels of the CNS via competition with the action of glycine. Its rapid absorption and distribution to neuronal tissues allow symptoms to develop within an hour after ingestion. The patient experiences heightened irritability and muscle twitching, followed by leg rigidity, facial tetanus, and apnea caused by spasm of the respiratory muscles. Opisthotonos and general convulsions develop, but the patient remains alert. Excessive muscle activity may cause muscle injury and myoglobinuria; severe respiratory muscle involvement can result in anoxia and death. The clinical picture sometimes resembles that of tetanus or of stiff-man syndrome (SMS). Intravenous diazepam or short-acting barbiturates can control spasms quite effectively. Supportive care and close observation are essential. Gastric lavage should be performed only after the airway is secure and seizures controlled.

Tetanus

Tetanus is an acute fulminant disease with an improved but still significant mortality rate. It is caused by an exotoxin produced in a wound by *Clostridium tetani* (426). Worldwide there are probably 300,000 to 500,000 cases of tetanus each year; improvement of treatment with intensive care has reduced mortality from 44% to 15% (427,428). In the United States fewer than 100 cases per year are reported. Rarely, tetanus occurs in the fully immunized person (429).

The typical first symptom of tetanus, muscle stiffness and pain, can begin 2 to 56 (usually 4 to 14) days after injury. Reflex spasm of the masseters on touching the posterior pharyngeal wall (spatula test) is highly specific for tetanus and can be useful in the evaluation of patients presenting during early stages of illness (430). A short incubation period indicates severe disease. Jaw stiffness progressing to lockjaw (trismus), dysphagia, and rigidity of the back (opisthotonos), abdomen, and eventually all muscles are the cardinal symptoms of generalized tetanus. The intensity and severity of muscle involvement are variable. Within 24 to 72 hours of the first symptoms, reflex spasms (sudden intensification of a spasm triggered by sensory stimuli, emotion, or movement) develop. These severe spasms can be quite painful and can cause respiratory difficulties or muscle injury; they result from disinhibition of usual motor neuron dampening mechanisms. Patients are almost invariably conscious and mentally alert. After about 10 days, spasms become less frequent. A hypersympathetic state often supervenes but disappears by the end of 2 weeks. A few patients have prolonged residual stiffness. Rare cases of chronic tetanus can closely resemble stiff-man syndrome, described in the next section (431); a primary differentiating factor is trismus, which is never seen in stiff-man syndrome, and the spasms seen in tetanus typically are more violent than in stiff-man syndrome.

A small proportion of patients develop yet another variety of tetanus—local tetanus—in which signs and symptoms develop only in the region of the injury. This disease is often mild and may persist for months. The symptoms of local tetanus usually resolve spontaneously but may develop into the general form. Rarely, local tetanus affects the facial and lower cranial musculature (cephalic tetanus), with a very poor prognosis.

Electromyographic examination in tetanus reveals continuous motor unit discharges that disappear during sleep and general or spinal anesthesia and after peripheral nerve block. Masseter muscle reactions are usually abnormal in generalized tetanus. Specifically, there is no silent period following the elicitation of the masseter reflex by a jaw tap. Normally, this silent period lasts 50 to 100 ms and is mainly the result of recurrent inhibition of motor neuron excitability. The shortened or absent silent period in tetanus (431) probably results from failed Renshaw cell inhibition. This characteristic electrodiagnostic feature seldom occurs in other disorders of motor unit hyperactivity, including stiff-man syndrome.

The tetanus toxin is known to bypass retrograde axoplasmic transport to the CNS and to enter the presynaptic nerve terminal of inhibitory interneurons, blocking release of the inhibitory transmitter glycine and GABA (432). This results in the release of motor neurons from inhibitory controls, increasing motor neuron activity.

Strychnine poisoning and, superficially, the dystonic reactions resulting from phenothiazines and metoclopramide resemble tetanus. Doubt about the diagnosis usually is clarified by clinical observation over several hours. Treatment of tetanus is discussed in detail in standard textbooks and reviews (426,433). Spasms and rigidity are best treated with GABA agonists. A long-acting benzodiazepine

(lorazepam) is recommended, but whenever high doses fail to control spasm, neuromuscular blocking agents should be used. Intravenous magnesium sulfate has also been used successfully in severe cases (434).

Stiff-Man Syndrome (Moersch-Woltman Syndrome)

Stiff-man syndrome, described by Moersch and Woltman (435) and critically reviewed by Gordon et al. (436), Whiteley et al. (437), Lorish et al. (438), McEvoy (439), and Pleitez and Harati (440), is characterized by the insidious onset of intermittent, usually symmetric, stiffness, particularly of the axial muscles (thoracolumbar, abdominal, and neck) and those of proximal limbs (Fig. 33.10). This syndrome usually occurs in adults, although it is seen in a wide range of ages, is slightly more common in women (441), and is usually sporadic. A congenital form also has been reported (442-444). As the disease slowly worsens, the fluctuating stiffness becomes persistent, and many patients develop painful and often violent spasms evoked by noise, fright, initiation of speech, strain at voiding, and other external stimuli. Active or passive movement aggravates the pain, and the extremities may be immobilized in unnatural positions, with simultaneous contractions of agonist and antagonist muscles. A lumbar hyperlordosis is common, and the neck may be held against the chest in a tonic posture of the fixed shrug. Paraspinal hypertrophy can be seen in later stages of disease. Stiffness produces a characteristic slow, stiff-legged gait with difficulties accentuated by attempts to turn. Generalized spasms show a pattern of opisthotonos and if the patient is standing, can cause him or her to fall forward suddenly "like a wooden soldier" (439). The facial muscles usually are spared, although muscles of swallowing are occasionally affected (435). Attacks of muscle spasms have been associated with autonomic instability, which may explain some cases of sudden death (445). A focal form of SMS limited to one limb, with no or slow progression to other limbs, has been described (441,446, 447).

Other than findings related to muscle rigidity, neurologic examination is normal, although there can be exaggeration of deep tendon reflexes and atrophy and weakness related to disuse. Myokymia or fasciculations are absent. In rare cases an unusual type of reflex myoclonus (spontaneous or triggered by muscle stretch or other sensory stimuli), can be superimposed on the rigidity in jerking SMS (448,449). SMS is typically a slowly progressive disease, but some cases remain stable for many years. Others may progress to total disability in a few years, and rare cases remit spontaneously.

The EMG in SMS shows continuous motor unit discharges (sustained interference pattern) similar to normal voluntary contractions, with simultaneous contractions in antagonist muscles despite the patient's attempts to relax. These findings are not pathognomonic for SMS, and it is

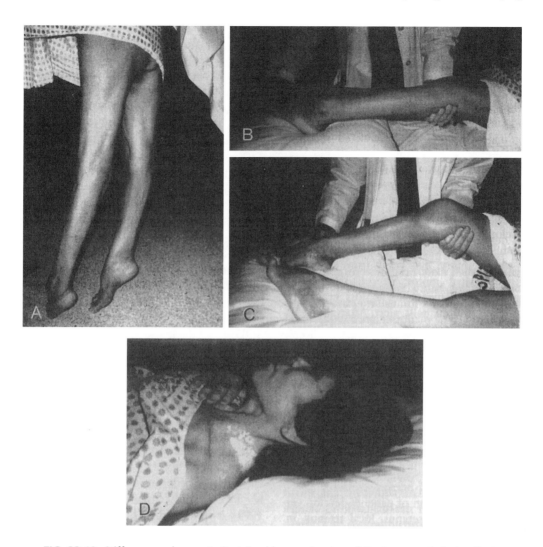

FIG. 33.10. Stiff-man syndrome. **A:** Sustained hyperextension of the knees and plantar flexion of the feet. **B:** An examiner unsuccessfully attempts to flex the knees. **C:** After spinal anesthesia the knees can be flexed. **D:** Vitiligo in a patient with stiff-man syndrome. (Courtesy of J. Jankovic, MD, Baylor College of Medicine, Houston, TX.)

the clinical setting that allows distinction from activity of unrelaxed muscles in otherwise normal patients or from abnormal muscle tone in patients with pyramidal or extrapyramidal disease. As expected from the clinical features, the motor unit discharges are more intense in axial and proximal limb muscles. Superimposed spontaneous and stimulus-evoked worsening of these discharges can be recorded in most patients. The clinical and electrical muscle activity disappears or decreases markedly during sleep, especially during rapid eye movement (REM) sleep; sedation; general anesthesia; nerve or ventral root block; or with administration of curare or diazepam. The silent period following elicitation of a stretch reflex (H reflex) has a normal duration, indicating no impairment of Renshaw cell inhibition. Meinck et al. (450), in a study of patients similar to those previously reported as having jerking SMS, described

spasmodic reflex myoclonus and the unique characteristics of its burst potentials.

Routine laboratory testing and cerebrospinal fluid analysis usually are normal. Nearly one-third of patients have evidence of insulin-dependent diabetes (IDDM); rare patients have oligoclonal bands in the cerebrospinal fluid; and approximately 40% have organ-specific autoantibodies (439) related to associated autoimmune diseases (Hashimoto's thyroiditis, Graves' disease, myasthenia gravis vitiligo, pernicious anemia, and others). Autoantibodies to glutamic acid decarboxylase (GAD) (discussed in subsequent paragraphs) were found in the serum in up to 60% of patients (451) and in the cerebrospinal fluid in 68% of patients from pooled data (440). A new immunoprecipitation assay is reported to make such autoantibody testing simpler and more readily available (452). Magnetic resonance imaging (MRI) of the brain in one patient revealed inflammatory type of lesions that were first detected years after the onset of stiffness (439). Involvement of thoracic muscles results in a restrictive pattern on pulmonary function tests. Skeletal muscles are usually normal, although mild nonspecific changes of atrophic fibers, nuclear clumps, internal nuclei, and slight fibrosis (possibly due to spasm-induced prolonged ischemia) have been reported (453,454). In two cases perimysial and perivascular inflammatory changes were observed (456).

Specific diagnostic criteria for SMS have been proposed by Gordon (436) and updated by Lorish et al. (438). They include (a) a prodrome of axial aching and stiffness; (b) slow progression of stiffness to include proximal limb muscles, with resultant difficulties in walking and other volitional movement; (c) a fixed lumbar lordosis or, less commonly, a permanent shrug of the shoulders; (d) superimposed episodic spasms precipitated by emotional or external stimuli; (e) abolition of rigidity during sleep; (f) normal findings on motor and sensory examinations; (g) normal intellect; and (h) typical EMG findings of continuous motor unit activity that is abolished or reduced by intravenous or oral diazepam. Meinck et al. (455) expanded the clinical features to include (a) spasmodic myoclonus with opisthotonos and stereotypic motor response in legs and feet, often preceded by (b) aura-like feeling of an impending attack; and (c) phobia associated with unaccompanied walking in open space. Supportive evidence includes the presence of anti-GAD antibodies (Abs) in the serum.

Since the spasms and rigidity of SMS abate or lessen during sleep and general anesthesia, abnormalities of the brain and/or spinal cord were investigated. In one autopsy case a detailed count of neural perikarya in the spinal ventral horn confirmed that the disease selectively destroyed small and medium-sized neurons, most of which were spinal internuncial neurons. Damage to these inhibitory neurons theoretically allows for excessive and abnormal discharges by the motor neurons, producing stiffness and spasms (437). Pharmacologic "correction" of this deficient inhibition with diazepam has proved effective and provides support for this hypothesis. Several other autopsy studies have revealed normal or inconclusive findings (439). Histopathologic examinations of the CNS in SMS have shown in individual cases no pathologic changes (453); slightly decreased motor neurons in the lateral nuclei of the central horn in the cervical cord without gliosis (456); spinal neuronal atrophy, gliosis, and fibrosis, with a slight pallor of the dorsal columns (454); and cell loss in the medial motor nuclei of anterior horns that innervate the muscle attached to the axial skeleton (457,458).

Guilleminault et al. (459) suggested that a relative neurotransmitter imbalance, leading to a decreased GABA-mediated neuronal inhibition, was responsible for SMS. In this imbalance either there is overactivity of the facilatory descending catecholaminergic influences and/or underac-

tivity of the inhibitory GABAergic influences. Drugs that increase the former (amine uptake inhibitors and levodopa) exacerbated stiffness and spasms, and drugs that either decreased the former (central adrenergic blockers such as clonidine) or increased the latter (diazepam or baclofen) improved these symptoms (459,460). Catecholamine overactivity in SMS was supported in two case reports demonstrating increased urinary excretion of 3-methoxy-4-hydroxyphenylglycol (MHPG), which correlated with clinical status (461,462).

A deficiency of GABA, the main inhibitory neurotransmitter in the CNS, subsequently has become the focus of SMS research. Work by Solimena, De Camilli, and colleagues provided a link with the hypothesis of GABA deficiency and support for an autoimmune mechanism in SMS (449,463,464). Coexistence of other autoimmune diseases and other autoantibodies with SMS, as already discussed, was the first indication that SMS may be an autoimmune disorder. In accordance with the association of SMS with IDDM and the knowledge that pancreatic β cells contain a high concentration of the enzyme GAD, which is responsible for the formation of GABA, they investigated the possibility that SMS was an autoimmune disease caused by autoantibodies directed against GAD (anti-GAD Abs). They postulated that anti-GAD Abs would result in a decrease in CNS GABA with resultant stiffness and spasms. Their initial report of a single SMS patient (who also had epilepsy, IDDM, oligoclonal IgG bands in the cerebrospinal fluid, and serum antibodies to pancreatic β cells, parietal cells, thyroglobulin, and thyroid microsomes) provided support for this hypothesis. Antibodies in both the serum and cerebrospinal fluid of this patient were immunocytochemically reactive to brain and pancreatic β cells in a pattern suggesting anti-GAD activity. The antibodies also reacted to a single protein that Western blot analysis revealed to be the same protein labeled by GAD antiserum. In subsequent studies, Western blot analysis and immunoprecipitation showed that 20 of 33 patients with SMS had anti-GAD Abs. Patients with anti-GAD activity had a much higher rate of associated autoimmune disease and serum autoantibodies to other antigens than did those without anti-GAD activity but were otherwise clinically similar. This work subsequently has been confirmed by others, with Lennon and colleagues reporting anti-GAD antibodies in 10 of 10 patients diagnosed with SMS (439).

Interestingly, four patients without SMS who were studied by Solimena and colleagues also had anti-GAD Abs, and all had IDDM. This work has provided an exciting speculation that GAD may be the antigen in many cases of IDDM. Up to 80% of patients with newly diagnosed IDDM have serum antibodies to a 64-kd protein shown to be GAD (465). The degree of humoral response and the difference in target antigens are among the suggested explanations for few patients with IDDM developing SMS. Although anti-GAD Abs may arise as a secondary reaction to cellular destruction from other mechanisms, an autoimmune cause for many cases of SMS and IDDM appears likely (466).

More recent support for autoimmunity in SMS comes from human leukocyte antigen (HLA) studies that showed a twofold greater incidence in affected subjects than in controls of carrying a known susceptibility allele (DQB1*0201) for IDDM and other autoimmune diseases (467). SMS patients have an even greater frequency (61%) of circulating autoantibodies if non-organ-specific types, such as antimitochondrial and anti-smooth muscle Abs, are included (468). Multiple organ-specific polyendocrine autoantibodies were reported in a patient with SMS and IDDM, and anti-GAD Abs were found to recognize a cerebellar protein when she later developed a pancerebellar syndrome (469). Additional organ-specific autoantibodies recognize antigens with similar tissue distribution as GAD. They include SMS cases that are anti-GAD Ab negative (470,471). Current research is focusing on the clues provided by the presence of anti-GAD Abs in SMS, IDDM, and other autoimmune diseases, which may help determine what pathogenic role, if any, this autoantibody has in SMS. In these diseases antibodies to one of the two GAD isozymes (GAD65) appears to be most selective. Although there is overlap in the humoral response against GAD in SMS and IDDM, Daw et al. (472) found the titers 100- to 500-fold higher in SMS and, expounding on earlier studies (473), demonstrated that there were GAD65 epitopes uniquely recognized by SMS but not IDDM sera. However, the data also indicate that such disease-specific antibody differences probably do not solely determine whether SMS or IDDM develops. Differences in host factors and autoimmune response may also be important. Other factors, such as hormones, though not causative may have a role in pathophysiology. For instance, stiffness in a patient who also had deficiency of adrenocorticotropic hormone (ACTH), prolactin, and growth hormone, as well as SMS, was resolved with administration of ACTH (474). Stiffness of another patient with hyperthyroidism also decreased after the thyroid abnormality was corrected (475).

Several disorders may be confused with SMS. Tetanus, strychnine poisoning, and the tonic spasms of multiple sclerosis are discussed in other sections of this chapter. During early stages of this disease, when motor disturbances are intermittent and neurologic examination is entirely normal, it may be difficult to distinguish from psychogenic disorder. Trojaborg et al. (476) reported a patient whose spinal rigidity was later attributed to ankylosing spondylitis, and Drake (477) reported a patient with "SMS and dementia," which in our opinion was the result of a cerebral multi-infarct state.

The rare congenital myopathy known as rigid-spine syndrome is characterized by infantile or childhood onset of proximal limb weakness followed by painless progressive severe limitations in spine flexion with associated myopathy of paraspinal muscles. Intramedullary spinal cord tumors, primarily cervical, have been associated with continuous motor unit discharges (alpha rigidity) (478). However, most of these patients have additional neurologic, laboratory, or imaging abnormalities.

Several disorders are closely related to SMS. A familial congenital form was mentioned in early discussions of this topic. An anti-GAD Ab negative stiff-man-like syndrome confined to the legs (stiff-leg syndrome) has been postulated to be due to a chronic spinal interneuronitis (479). A rapidly progressive stiff-man-like syndrome has been reported in some cases of encephalomyelitis (437, 480–483). It is distinguished from SMS by its clinical course and abnormal neurologic findings, but idiopathic cases may be associated with anti-GAD Abs (484). Neuropathologic studies have shown findings of diffuse encephalomyelitis with perivascular inflammation (445, 485) as well as dense mononuclear infiltrates with surrounding astrocytosis in the anterior horns of the lumbar greater than cervical cord with relative preservation of large motor neurons and axons (485). Several patients with SMS and malignancy, including some with signs of encephalomyelitis, have been reported (439). These paraneoplastic cases of SMS have Abs directed against a synaptic vesicle–associated protein (amphiphysin) rather than GAD and may be pathogenically distinct from idiopathic SMS (440). The paraneoplastic SMS occurs most often with breast cancer (486), and SMS may precede the discovery of cancer (487).

The most effective symptomatic treatment for SMS is incremental high-dose diazepam or clonazepam. If these drugs have an unsatisfactory response or are not tolerated, other medications that potentiate the effect of GABA, such as baclofen or sodium valproate (488), and vigabatrin or tiagabine (489–491), may prove beneficial. Baclofen may be used intrathecally in severe cases (492). Phenytoin and carbamazepine are ineffective. Immunosuppression, including a dramatic response to corticosteroids, PE (440), and IVIG (493), has been reported in uncontrolled and controlled (494) studies. The role of anti-GAD Ab measurement in predicting response to immunosuppressive treatment is not known. In paraneoplastic SMS, management of underlying cancer may improve the symptoms.

Familial Nocturnal Cramps

In this unique familial condition, sleep-associated myoclonus is accompanied by sustained painful cramping of the legs, abdomen, and face. The severity of cramps often awakens the patient and causes children to cry (495). All-night polysomnographic recordings show nearly continuous or intermittent muscle EMG activity during sleep, abolished by peripheral nerve block. However, waking electromyography shows no evidence of peripheral neuropathy or radiculopathy. While sleep normally attenuates muscle activity of central origin, the fact that the activity occurs only during sleep implicates a disturbance of sleep-related inhibitory influences on the lower motor neuron. These findings suggest a central origin (brainstem or spinal) for this syndrome. Treatment with clonazepam produces sustained improvement of symptoms. A similar autosomal dominant syndrome with cramps occurring during both exertion and at rest and during sleep has been reported in four generations of a Japanese family (496).

Tonic Spasm of Multiple Sclerosis

Paroxysmal dystonia, tonic spasm, or tonic seizures, first described by Matthews (497), involve brief, recurrent, often painful abnormal posturing of one or more extremities without alteration of consciousness, loss of sphincter control, or clonic movements. Episodes can occur at any time during the course of multiple sclerosis but can also be the initial symptoms of the disease (498–500). Episodes may be precipitated by voluntary movement, spinal flexion, tactile stimulation, hyperventilation, sudden noise, ingestion of alcohol, or sudden exposure to cold (501). Facial grimacing and paroxysmal dysarthria may be associated with dystonic posturing of an extremity. A few patients may have transient (only a few seconds) sensory or autonomic disturbances in the involved limb preceding or during the attack. The entire phenomenon is brief, generally 30 to 45 seconds, and rarely longer than a few minutes in duration, but can recur as often as 30 times daily (502). The absence of electroencephalographic abnormalities and the high frequency of spinal cord abnormalities in these patients suggests that these paroxysms originate from the brainstem or spinal cord (503,504) and, in particular, within the corticospinal tract. This is supported by the findings of exacerbated upper motor neuron signs on the side of the tonic spasm immediately following an attack and by MRI evidence of demyelinating lesions affecting the contralateral corticospinal tract, which also shows electrophysiologic evidence of impairment (505). The most effective treatment is carbamazepine, although phenytoin occasionally is useful. The value of antispasmodic medications is uncertain, and future studies await newer and potentially more effective treatments for spasticity such as tizanidine (506) and intrathecal baclofen (507).

REFERENCES

1. Oboler SK, Prochazka AV, Meyer TJ. Leg symptoms in outpatient veterans. *West J Med* 1991;155:256–259.
2. Riley JD, Antony SJ. Leg cramps: differential diagnosis and management. *Am Fam Physician* 1995;52:1794–1798.
3. Jansen PH, Joosten EM, Vingerhoets HM. Muscle cramp as a feature of neuromuscular disease: five neuromuscular disorders, accompanied by frequent muscle cramps. *Acta Neurol Belg* 1992;92:138–147.
4. Pourmand R. The value of muscle biopsy in myalgia. *Neurologist* 1997;3:173–177.
5. Mommaerts WFHM, Illingworth B, Pearson CM, et al. A functional disorder of muscle associated with the absence of phosphorylase. *Proc Natl Acad Sci USA* 1959;45:791–797.
6. Schmid R, Mahler R. Chronic progressive myopathy with myoglobinuria: demonstration of a glycogenolytic defect in the muscle. *J Clin Invest* 1959;38:2044–2058.
7. De Stefano N, Argov Z, Matthews PM, et al. Impairment of muscle mitochondrial oxidative metabolism in McArdle's disease. *Muscle Nerve* 1996;19:764–769.
8. Haller RG, Clausen T, Vissing J. Reduced levels of skeletal muscle Na$^+$-K$^+$-ATPase in McArdle disease. *Neurology* 1998;50:37–40.
9. Jehenson P, Leroy-Willig A, de Kerviler E, et al. Impairment of the exercise-induced increase in muscle perfusion in McArdle's disease. *Eur J Nucl Med* 1995;22:1256–1260.
10. Thornhill MH. Masticatory muscle symptoms in a patient with McArdle's disease. *Oral Surg Oral Med Oral Pathol Oral Radiol Endodont* 1996;81:544–546.
11. Porte D, Crawford DW, Jennings DB, et al. Cardiovascular and metabolic response to exercise in a patient with McArdle's syndrome. *N Engl J Med* 1966;275:406–412.
12. Pernow BB, Havel RJ, Jennings DB. The second wind phenomenon in McArdle's syndrome. *Acta Med Scand* 1967;472 [Suppl]:294–307.
13. Carroll JE, DeVivo DC, Brooke MH, et al. Fasting as a provocative test in neuromuscular diseases. *Metabolism* 1979;28:683–687.
14. Wolfe GI, Baker NS, Haller RG, et al. McArdle's disease presenting with asymmetric, late-onset arm weakness. *Muscle Nerve* 2000;23:641–645.
15. DiMauro S, Tsujino S. Nonlysosomal glycogenoses. In: Engel AG, Franzini-Armstrong C, eds. *Myology.* New York: McGraw-Hill, 1994:1554–1576.
16. Kristjcinsson K, Tsujino S, DiMauro S. Myophosphorylase deficiency: an unusually severe form with myoglobinuria. *J Pediatr* 1994;125:409–410.
17. Chiadò-Piat L, Mongini T, Doriguzzi C, et al. Clinical spectrum of McArdle disease: three cases with unusual expression. *Eur Neurol* 1993;33:208–211.
18. DiMauro S, Hartlage PL. Fatal infantile form of muscle phosphorylase deficiency. *Neurology* 1978;28:1124–1129.
19. Cornelio F, Bresolin N, DiMauro S, et al. Congenital myopathy due to phosphorylase deficiency. *Neurology* 1983;33:1383–1385.
20. Engel WK, Eyerman EL, Williams HE. Late-onset type of skeletal muscle phosphorylase deficiency: a new familial variety with completely and partially affected subjects. *N Engl J Med* 1963;268:135–137.
21. Felice KI, Schneebaum AB, Jones HR. McArdle's disease with late-onset symptoms: case report and review of the literature. *J Neurol Neurosurg Psychiatry* 1992;55:407–408.
22. Mineo I, Kono N, Hara N, et al. Myogenic hyperuricemia: a common pathophysiologic feature of glycogenosis types III, V, and VII. *N Engl J Med* 1987;317:75–80.
23. Chui LA, Munsat TL. Dominant inheritance of McArdle syndrome. *Arch Neurol* 1976;33:636–644.
24. Servidei S, Shanske S, Zeviani M, et al. McArdle's disease: biochemical and molecular genetic studies. *Ann Neurol* 1988;24:774–781.
25. Dawson DM, Spong LF, Harrington JF. McArdle's disease: lack of muscle phosphorylase. *Ann Intern Med* 1968;69:229–235.
26. Schmidt B, Servidei S, Gabbai AA, et al. McArdle's disease in two generations: autosomal recessive transmission with manifesting heterozygote. *Neurology* 1987;37:1558–1561.

27. Manfredi G, Silvestri G, Servidei S, et al. Manifesting heterozygotes in McArdle's disease: clinical, morphological, and biochemical studies in a family. *J Neurol Sci* 1993;115:91–94.

28. Bartram C, Edwards RH, Beynon RJ. McArdle's disease: muscle glycogen phosphorylase deficiency. *Biochim Biophys Acta* 1995;1272:1–13.

29. Roelofs RI, Engel WK, Chauvin PB. Histochemical phosphorylase activity in regenerating muscle fibers from myophosphorylase-deficient patients. *Science* 1972;177:795–797.

30. Sato K, Imai F, Hatayama I, et al. Characterization of glycogen phosphorylase isoenzymes present in cultured skeletal muscle from patients with McArdle's disease. *Biochem Biophys Res Commun* 1977;78:663–668.

31. DiMauro S, Arnold S, Miranda AF, et al. McArdle disease: the mystery of reappearing phosphorylase activity in muscle culture: a fetal isoenzyme. *Ann Neurol* 1978;3:60–66.

32. Lockyer JM, McCracken JB. Identification of a tissue-specific regulatory element within the human muscle glycogen phosphorylase gene. *J Biol Chem* 1991;266:20262–20269.

33. Lebo RV, Gorin F, Fletterick RJ, et al. High-resolution chromosome sorting and DNA spot-blot analysis assign McArdle's syndrome to chromosome 11. *Science* 1984;225:57–59.

34. Martin MA, Rubio JC, Buchbinder J, et al. Molecular heterogeneity of myophosphorylase deficiency (McArdle's disease): a genotype–phenotype correlation study. *Ann Neurol* 2001;50:574–581.

35. Martin MA, Rubio JC, Campos Y, et al. Two homozygous mutations (R193W and 794/795 delAA) in the myophosphorylase gene in a patient with McArdle's disease. *Hum Mutat* 2000;15:294.

36. Martin MA, Rubio JC, Garcia A, et al. Resolution of a mispaired secondary structure intermediate could account for a novel microinsertion/deletion (387 insA/del 8 bp) in the *PYGM* gene causing McArdle's disease. *Clin Genet* 2001;59:48–51.

37. Tsujino S, Shanske S, DiMauro S. Molecular genetic heterogeneity of myophosphorylase deficiency (McArdle's disease). *N Engl J Med* 1993;329:241–245.

38. Sugie H, Sugie Y, Ito M, et al. Genetic analysis of Japanese patients with myophosphorylase deficiency (McArdle's disease): single-codon deletion in exon 17 is the predominant mutation. *Clin Chim Acta* 1995;236:81–86f.

39. Van den Berg IE, Berger R. Phosphorylase b kinase deficiency in man: a review. *J Inher Metab Dis* 1990;13:442–451.

40. Elleder M, Shin YS, Zuntova A, et al. Fatal infantile hypertrophic cardiomyopathy secondary to deficiency of heart specific phosphorylase b kinase. *Virchows Arch A Pathol Anat Histopathol* 1993;423:303–307.

41. Kagalwalla AF, Kagalwalla YA, al Ajaj S, et al. Phosphorylase b kinase deficiency glycogenosis with cirrhosis of the liver. *J Pediatr* 1995;127:602–605.

42. Iwamasa T, Fukuda S, Tokumitsu S, et al. Myopathy due to glycogen storage disease. *Exp Mol Pathol* 1983;38:405–420.

43. Abarbanel JM, Bashan N, Potashnik R, et al. Adult muscle phosphorylase "b" kinase deficiency. *Neurology* 1986;36:560–562.

44. Wilkinson DA, Tonin P, Shanske S, et al. Clinical and biochemical features of 10 adult patients with muscle phosphorylase kinase deficiency. *Neurology* 1994;44:461–466.

45. Strugalska-Cynowska M. Disturbances in the activity of phosphorylase b kinase in a case of McArdle myopathy. *Folia Histochem Cytochem (Krakow)* 1967;5:151–156.

46. Danon MJ, Carpenter S, Manaligod JR, et al. Fatal infantile glycogen storage disease: deficiency of phosphofructokinase and phosphorylase b kinase. *Neurology* 1981;31:1303–1307.

47. Ohtani Y, Matsuda I, Iwamasa T, et al. Infantile glycogen storage myopathy in a girl with phosphorylase kinase deficiency. *Neurology* 1982;32:833–838.

48. Shin YS, Plochl E, Podskarbi T, et al. Fatal arthrogryposis with respiratory insufficiency: a possible case of muscle phosphorylase b-kinase deficiency. *J Inherit Metab Dis* 1994;17:153–155.

49. Clemens PR, Yamamoto M, Engel AG. Adult phosphorylase b kinase deficiency. *Ann Neurol* 1990;28:529–538.

50. Coleman RA, Stajich JM, Pact VW, et al. The ischemic exercise test in normal adults and in patients with weakness and cramps. *Muscle Nerve* 1986;9:216–221.

51. Heller SL, Kaiser KK, Planer GJ, et al. McArdle's disease with myoadenylate deaminase deficiency: observations in a combined enzyme deficiency. *Neurology* 1987;37:1039–1042.

52. Martinuzzi A, Schievano G, Nascimbeni A, et al. McArdle's disease: the unsolved mystery of the reappearing enzyme. *Am J Pathol* 1999;154:1893–1897.

53. El-Schahawi M, Tsujino S, Shanske S, et al. Diagnosis of McArdle's disease by molecular genetic analysis of blood. *Neurology* 1996;47:579–580.

54. Rowland LP, Araki S, Carmel P. Contracture in McArdle's disease. *Arch Neurol* 1965;13:541–544.

55. Ross BD, Radda GK, Gadian DG, et al. Examination of a case of suspected McArdle's syndrome by 11P nuclear magnetic resonance. *N Engl J Med* 1981;304:1338–1342.

56. Argov Z, Bank WJ, Maris J, et al. Muscle energy metabolism in McArdle's syndrome by in vivo phosphorus magnetic resonance spectroscopy (^{31}P NMR). *Neurology* 1987;37:1720–1724.

57. Russo PJ, Phillips JW, Seidler NW. The role of lipid peroxidation in McArdle's disease: applications for treatment of other myopathies. *Med Hypotheses* 1992;39:147–151.

58. Cochrane PR, Hughes R, Buxton PH, et al. Myophosphorylase deficiency (McArdle's disease) in two interrelated families. *J Neurol Neurosurg Psychiatry* 1973;36:217–224.

59. Steele IC, Patterson VH, Nicholls DP. A double-blind, placebo controlled, crossover trial of D-ribose in McArdle's disease. *J Neurolog Sci* 1996;136(1–2):174–177.

60. Slonim AE, Goans PJ. Myopathy in McArdle's syndrome: improvement with a high-protein diet. *N Engl J Med* 1985;312:355–359.

61. Jansen PHP, Joosten EMG, Vingerhoots HM. Muscle cramp: main theories as to aetiology. *Eur Arch Psychiatr Neurol Sci* 1990;239:337–342.

62. MacLean D, Vissing J, Vissing SF, et al. Oral branched-chain amino acids do not improve exercise capacity in McArdle disease. *Neurology* 1998;51:1456–1459.

63. Coakley JH, Wagenmakers AJ, Edwards RH. Relationship between ammonia, heart rate, and exertion in McArdle's disease. *Am J Physiol* 1992;262:E167–E172.

64. Beynon RJ, Bartram C, Hopkins P, et al. McArdle's disease: molecular genetics and metabolic consequences of the phenotype. *Muscle Nerve* 1995;[Suppl 3]:S18–S22.

65. Phoenix J, Hopkins P, Bartram C, et al. Effect of vitamin B6 supplementation in McArdle's disease: a strategic case study. *Neuromuscular Disord* 1998;8:210–212.

66. Vorgerd M, Grehl T, Jager M, et al. Creatine therapy in myophosphorylase deficiency (McArdle disease): a placebo-controlled crossover trial. *Arch Neurol* 2000;57:956–963.

67. Baqué S, Newgard CB, Gerard RD, et al. Adenovirus-mediated delivery into myocytes of muscle glycogen phosphorylase, the enzyme deficient in patients with glycogen-storage disease type V. *Biochem J* 1994;304:1009–1014.

68. Pari G, Crerar MM, Nalbantoglu J, et al. Myophosphorylase gene transfer in McArdle's disease myoblasts in vitro. *Neurology* 1999;53:1352–1354.

69. Tarui S, Okuno G, Ikura Y, et al. Phosphofructokinase deficiency in skeletal muscle: a new type of glycogenosis. *Biochem Biophys Res Commun* 1965;19:517–520.

70. Ronquist G, Rudolphi O, Engstrom I, et al. Familial phospho-

fructokinase deficiency is associated with a disturbed calcium homeostasis in erythrocytes. *J Intern Med* 2001;249:85–95.

71. Rowland LP, DiMauro S, Lazer RB. Phosphofructokinase deficiency. In: Engel AG, Banker BQ, eds. *Myology.* New York: McGraw-Hill, 1986:1603–1617.

72. Nakagawa C, Mineo I, Kaido M, et al. A new variant case of muscle phosphofructokinase deficiency, coexisting with gastric ulcer, gouty arthritis, and increased hemolysis. *Muscle Nerve* 1995;[Suppl 3]:S39–S44.

73. Argov Z, Barash V, Soffer D, et al. Late-onset muscular weakness in phosphofructokinase deficiency due to exon 5/intron 5 junction point mutation: a unique disorder or the natural course of this glycolytic disorder? *Neurology* 1994;44:1097–1100.

74. Sivakumar K, Vasconcelos O, Goldfarb L, et al. Late-onset muscle weakness in partial phosphofructokinase deficiency: a unique myopathy with vacuoles, abnormal mitochondria, and absence of the common exon 5/intron 5 junction point mutation. *Neurology* 1996;46:1337–1342.

75. Massa R, Lodi R, Barbiroli B, et al. Partial block of glycolysis in late-onset phosphofructokinase deficiency myopathy. *Acta Neuropathol* 1996;91:322–329.

76. Pastoris O, Dossena M, Vercesi L, et al. Muscle phosphofructokinase deficiency in a myopathic child with severe mental retardation and aplasia of cerebellar vermis. *Childs Nerv Syst* 1992;8:237–241.

77. Moerman P, Lammens M, Fryns JP, et al. Fetal akinesia sequence caused by glycogenosis type VII. *Genet Couns* 1995;6:15–20.

78. Vora S, DiMauro S, Spear D, et al. Characterisation of enzymatic defect in late onset muscle phosphofructokinase deficiency: new subtype of glycogen storage disease type VII. *J Clin Invest* 1987;80:1479–1485.

79. Buetler E. *Red cell metabolism: a manual of biochemical methods,* 3rd ed. New York: Grune & Stratton, 1984.

80. Argov Z, Bank WJ, Maris J, et al. Muscle energy metabolism in human phosphofructokinase deficiency as recorded by ^{31}P nuclear magnetic resonance spectroscopy. *Ann Neurol* 1987;22:46–51.

81. Grehl T, Muller K, Vorgerd M, et al. Impaired aerobic glycolysis in muscle phosphofructokinase deficiency results in biphasic post-exercise phosphocreatine recovery in ^{31}P magnetic resonance spectroscopy. *Neuromuscular Disord* 1998;8:480–488.

82. Bertocci LA, Haller RG, Lewis SF, et al. Abnormal high-energy phosphate metabolism in human muscle phosphofructokinase deficiency. *J Appl Physiol* 1991;70:1201–1207.

83. Raben N, Sherman JB, Adams E, et al. Various classes of mutations in patients with phosphofructokinase deficiency (Tarui's disease). *Muscle Nerve* 1995;3:S35–S38.

84. Nakajima H, Hamaguchi T, Yamasaki T, et al. Phosphofructokinase deficiency: recent advances in molecular biology. *Muscle Nerve* 1995;[Suppl 3]:S28–S34.

85. Nichols RC, Rudolphi O, Ek B, et al. Glycogenosis type VII (Tarui disease) in a Swedish family: two novel mutations in muscle phosphofructokinase gene (PFK-M) resulting in intron retentions. *Am J Hum Genet* 1996;59:59–65.

86. Haller RG, Lewis SF. Glucose-induced exertional fatigue in muscle phosphofructokinase deficiency. *N Engl J Med* 1991;324:364–369.

87. DiMauro S, Dalakas M, Miranda AF. Phosphoglycerate kinase (PGK) deficiency: another cause of recurrent myoglobinuria. *Ann Neurol* 1983;13:11–19.

88. Rosa R, George C, Fardeau M, et al. A new case of phosphoglycerate kinase deficiency: PGK Creteil associated with rhabdomyolysis and lacking hemolytic anemia. *Blood* 1982;60(1):84–91.

89. Cohen-Solal M, Valentin C, Plassa F, et al. Identification of new mutations in two phosphoglycerate kinase (PGK) variants expressing different clinical syndromes: PGK Creteil and PGK Amiens. *Blood* 1994;84:898–903.

90. Ookawara T, Dave V, Willems P, et al. Retarded and aberrant splicings caused by single exon mutation in a phosphoglycerate kinase variant. *Arch Biochem Biophys* 1996;327:35–40.

91. Tonin P, Shanske S, Miranda AF, et al. Phosphoglycerate kinase deficiency: biochemical and molecular genetic studies in a new myopathic variant (PGK Alberta). *Neurology* 1993;43:387–391.

92. Fujii H, Kanno H, Hirono A, et al. A single amino acid substitution (157 Gly to Val) in a phosphoglycerate kinase variant (PGK Shizuoka) associated with chronic hemolysis and myoglobinuria. *Blood* 1992;79:1582–1585.

93. Sugie H, Sugie Y, Nishida M, et al. Recurrent myoglobinuria in a child with mental retardation: phosphoglycerate kinase deficiency. *J Child Neurol* 1989;4:95–99.

94. Tsujino S, Tonin P, Shanske S, et al. A splice junction mutation in a new myopathic variant of phosphoglycerate kinase deficiency (PGK North Carolina). *Ann Neurol* 1994;35:349–353.

95. Tsujino S, Nonaka I, Dimauro S. Glycogen storage myopathies. *Neurol Clin* 2000;18:125–150.

96. DiMauro S, Miranda AF, Khan S, et al. Human muscle phosphoglycerate mutase deficiency: a newly discovered metabolic myopathy. *Science* 1981;212:1277–1279.

97. DiMauro S, Miranda AF, Olarte M, et al. Muscle phosphoglycerate mutase deficiency. *Neurology* 1982;32:584–592.

98. Bresolin N, Ro YI, Reyes M, et al. Muscle phosphoglycerate mutase (PGAM) deficiency: a second case. *Neurology* 1983;33:1049–1053.

99. Kissel JT, Beam W, Bresolin N, et al. Physiologic assessment of phosphoglycerate mutase deficiency: incremental exercise test. *Neurology* 1985;35:828–833.

100. Tsujino S, Shanske S, Sakoda S, et al. The molecular genetic basis of muscle phosphoglycerate mutase (PGAM) deficiency. *Am J Hum Genet* 1993;52:472–477.

101. Toscano A, Tsujino S, Vita G, et al. Molecular basis of muscle phosphoglycerate mutase (PGAM-M) deficiency in the Italian kindred. *Muscle Nerve* 1996;19:1134–1137.

102. Argov Z, Bank WJ. Phosphorus magnetic resonance spectroscopy (^{31}P-MRS) in neuromuscular disorders. *Ann Neurol* 1991;30:90–97.

103. Vita G, Toscano A, Bresolin N, et al. Muscle phosphoglycerate mutase (PGAM) deficiency in the first Caucasian patient: biochemistry, muscle culture, and P-MR spectroscopy. *J Neurol* 1994;241:289–294.

104. Edwards YH, Sakoda S, Schon E, et al. The gene for human muscle-specific phosphoglycerate mutase, *PGAM2,* mapped to chromosome 7 by polymerase chain reaction. *Genomics* 1989;5:948–951.

105. Vissing J, Schmalbruch H, Haller RG, et al. Muscle phosphoglycerate mutase deficiency with tubular aggregates: effect of dantrolene. *Ann Neurol* 1999;46:274–277.

106. Kanno T, Sudo K, Takeuchi I, et al. Hereditary deficiency of lactate dehydrogenase M subunit. *Clin Chim Acta* 1980;108:267–276.

107. Miyajima H, Takahashi Y, Suzuki M, et al. Molecular characterization of gene expression in human lactate dehydrogenase-A deficiency. *Neurology* 1993;43:1414–1419.

108. Tsujino S, Shanske S, Brownell AK, et al. Molecular genetic studies of muscle lactate dehydrogenase deficiency in white patients. *Ann Neurol* 1994;36:661–665.

109. Maekawa M, Kanda S, Sudo K, et al. Estimation of the gene frequency of lactate dehydrogenase subunit deficiencies. *Am J Hum Genet* 1984;36:1204–1214.

110. Yoshikuni K, Tagami H, Yamada M, et al. Erythematosquamous skin lesions in hereditary lactate dehydrogenase M-subunit deficiency. *Arch Dermatol* 1986;122:1420–1424.

111. Takayasu S, Fujiwara S, Waki T. Hereditary lactate dehydrogenase M-subunit deficiency: lactate dehydrogenase activity in skin lesions and in hair follicles. *J Am Acad Dermatol* 1991; 24:339–342.

112. Kanno T, Maekawa M. Lactate dehydrogenase M-subunit deficiencies: clinical features, metabolic background, and genetic heterogeneities. *Muscle Nerve* 1995;[Suppl 3]:S54–S60.

113. Maekawa M, Sudo K, Li SSL, et al. Genotypic analysis of families with lactate dehydrogenase A(M) deficiency by selective DNA amplification. *Hum Genet* 1991;88:34–38.

114. Maekawa M, Sudo K, Li SSL, et al. Analysis of genetic mutations in human lactate dehydrogenase-A(M) deficiency using DNA conformation polymorphism in combination with polyacrylamide gradient gel and silver staining. *Biochem Biophys Res Commun* 1991;180:1083–1090.

115. Comi GP, et al. Beta-enolase deficiency: a new metabolic myopathy of distal glycolysis. *Annals of Neurology* 2001;50: 202–207.

116. Murthy MS, Pande SV. Some differences in the properties of carnitine palmitoyltransferase activities of the mitochondrial outer and inner membranes. *Biochem J* 1987;248:727–733.

117. McGarry JD, Brown NF. The mitochondrial carnitine palmitoyltransferase system: from concept to molecular analysis. *Eur J Biochem* 1997;244:1–14.

118. Murthy MS, Pande SV. Characterization of a solubilized malonyl-CoA-sensitive carnitine palmitoyltransferase from the mitochondrial outer membrane as a protein distinct from the malonyl-CoA-insensitive carnitine palmitoyltransferase of the inner membrane. *Biochem J* 1990;268:599–604.

119. Woeltje KF, Esser V, Weis BC, et al. Inter-tissue and interspecies characteristics of the mitochondrial carnitine palmitoyltransferase enzyme system. *J Biol Chem* 1990;265: 10714–10719.

120. Demaugre F, Bonnefont JP, Mitchell G, et al. Hepatic and muscular presentations of carnitine palmitoyl transferase deficiency: two distinct entities. *Pediatr Res* 1988;24:308–311.

121. Villard J, Fischer A, Mandon G, et al. Recurrent myoglobinuria due to carnitine palmitoyltransferase II deficiency: expression of the molecular phenotype in cultured muscle cells. *J Neurolog Sci* 1996;136:178–181.

122. Katsuya H, Misumi M, Ohtani Y, et al. Postanesthetic acute renal failure due to carnitine palmityl transferase deficiency. *Anesthesiology* 1988;68:945–948.

123. Kieval RI, Sotrel A, Weinblatt ME. Chronic myopathy with a partial deficiency of the carnitine palmitoyltransferase enzyme. *Arch Neurol* 1989;46:575–576.

124. Tonin P, Lewis P, Servidei S, et al. Metabolic causes of myoglobinuria. *Ann Neurol* 1990;27:181–185.

125. Mantz J, Hindelang C, Mantz JM, et al. Vascular and myofibrillar lesions in acute myoglobinuria associated with carnitine-palmityl-transferase deficiency. *Virchows Arch A Pathol Anat Histopathol* 1992;421:57–64.

126. Schaefer J, Jackson S, Taroni F, et al. Characterization of carnitine palmitoyltransferases in patients with a carnitine palmitoyltransferase deficiency: implications for diagnosis and therapy. *J Neurol Neurosurg Psychiatry* 1997;62:169–176.

127. Angelini C, Freddo L, Battistella P, et al. Carnitine palmityl transferase deficiency: clinical variability, carrier detection, and autosomal recessive inheritance. *Neurology* 1981;31:883–886.

128. Lonasescu V, Hug G, Hoppel C. Combined partial deficiency of muscle carnitine palmitoyltransferase and carnitine with autosomal dominant inheritance. *J Neurol Neurosurg Psychiatry* 1980;43:679–682.

129. Van der Leij FR, Huijkman NC, Boomsma C, et al. Genomics of the human carnitine acyltransferase genes. *Mol Genet Metab* 2000;71:139–153.

130. Taroni F, Verderio E. Willems PJ, et al. Identification of a common mutation in the carnitine palmitoyltransferase 11 gene in familial recurrent myoglobinuria patients. *Nat Genet* 1993;4: 314–320.

131. Zierz S, Neumann-Schmidt S, Jerusalem F. Inhibition of carnitine palmitoyltransferase in normal human skeletal muscle and in muscle of patients with carnitine palmitoyltransferase deficiency by long- and short-chain acylcarnitine and acyl-coenzyme A. *Clin Invest* 1993;71:763–769.

132. Zierz S. Carnitine palmitoyltransferase deficiency. In: Engel AG, Franzini-Armstrong C, eds. *Mycology.* New York: McGraw-Hill, 1994:1577–1586.

133. El-Hayek R, Valdivia C, Valdivia HH, et al. Activation of the Ca^{2+} release channel of skeletal muscle sarcoplasmic reticulum by palmitoyl carnitine. *Biophys J* 1993;65:779–789.

134. Vladutiu GD, Bennett MJ, Smail D, et al. A variable myopathy associated with heterozygosity for the R503C mutation in the carnitine palmitoyltransferase II gene. *Mol Genet Metab* 2000;70:134–141.

135. Handig I, Dams E, Taroni F, et al. Inheritance of the S113L mutation within an inbred family with carnitine palmitoyltransferase enzyme deficiency. *Hum Genet* 1996;97:291–293.

136. Carroll JE. Myopathies caused by disorders of lipid metabolism. *Neurol Clin* 1988;6:563–574.

137. Przyrembel H. Therapy of mitochondrial disorders. *J Inherit Metab Dis* 1987;10:129–146.

138. Shintani S, Shiigai T, Sugiyama N. Atypical presentation of carnitine palmitoyltransferase (CPT) deficiency as status epilepticus. *J Neurol Sci* 1995;129:6973.

139. Ohtani Y, Tomoda A, Miike T, et al. Central nervous system disorders and possible brain type carnitine palmitoyltransferase 11 deficiency. *Brain Dev* 1994;16:139–145.

140. Stanley CA. New genetic defects in mitochondrial fatty acid oxidation and carnitine deficiency. *Adv Pediatr* 1987;34:59–88.

141. Engel WK, Vick NA, Glueck J, et al. A skeletal muscle disorder associated with intermittent symptoms and a possible defect in lipid metabolism. *N Engl J Med* 1970;282:697–704.

142. Snyder TM, Little BW, Roman-Campos G, et al. Successful treatment of familial idiopathic lipid storage myopathy with L-carnitine and modified lipid diet. *Neurology* 1982;32: 1106–1115.

143. Indo Y, Yang-Feng T, Glassberg R, et al. Molecular cloning and nucleotide sequence of cDNAs encoding human long-chain acyl-CoA dehydrogenase and assignment of the location of its gene (ACADL) to chromosome 2. *Genomics* 1991;11:609–620.

144. Schaefer J, Jackson S, Dick DJ, et al. Trifunctional enzyme deficiency: adult presentation of a usually fatal beta-oxidation defect. *Ann Neurol* 1996;40:597–602.

145. Lambert EH, Goldstein NP. Unusual form of "myotonia" (abst). *Physiologist* 1957;1:51.

146. Brody I. Muscle contracture induced by exercise: a syndrome attributable to decreased relaxing factor. *N Engl J Med* 1969;281:187–192.

147. Taylor DJ, Brosnan MJ, Arnold DL, et al. Ca^{2+}-ATPase deficiency in a patient with an exertional muscle pain syndrome. *J Neurol Neurosurg Psychiatry* 1988;51:1425–1433.

148. Poels PJ, Wevers RA, Braakhekke JP, et al. Exertional rhabdomyolysis in a patient with calcium adenosine triphosphatase deficiency. *J Neurol Neurosurg Psychiatry* 1993;56:823–826.

149. Brandl CJ, Green NM, Korczak B, et al. Two Ca^{2+} ATPase genes: homologies and mechanistic implications of deduced amino acid sequences. *Cell* 1986;44:597–607.

150. Benders AA, Veerkamp JH, Oosterhof A, et al. Ca^{++} homeosta-

sis in Brody's disease: a study in skeletal muscle and cultured muscle cells and the effects of dantrolene an verapamil. *J Clin Invest* 1994;94:741–748.

151. Benders AG, Van Kuppevelt TH, Oosterhof A, et al. Adenosine triphosphatases during maturation of cultured human muscle cells and in human muscle. *Biochim Biophys Acta* 1992; 1112:89–98.

152. Karpati G, Charuk J, Carpenter S, et al. Myopathy caused by a deficiency of Ca⁺⁺-adenosine triphosphatase in sarcoplasmic reticulum (Brody's disease). *Ann Neurol* 1986;20:38–49.

153. Danon MJ, Karpati G, Charuk J, et al. Sarcoplasmic reticulum adenosine triphosphatase deficiency with probably autosomal dominant inheritance. *Neurology* 1988;38:812–815.

154. Odermatt A, Barton K, Khanna VK, et al. The mutation of Pro789 to Leu reduces the activity of the fast-twitch skeletal muscle sarco(endo)plasmic reticulum Ca²⁺ ATPase (SERCA1) and is associated with Brody disease. *Hum Genet* 2000;106: 482–491.

155. MacLennan DH, Rice WJ, Odermatt A, et al. Structure–function relationships in the Ca(2+)-binding and translocation domain of SERCA1: physiological correlates in Brody disease. *Acta Physiol Scand* 1998[Suppl];643:55–67.

156. Torbergsen T. A family with dominant hereditary myotonia, muscular hypertrophy, and increased muscular irritability, distinct from myotonia congenita (Thomsen). *Acta Neurol Scand* 1975;51:225–232.

157. Ricker K, Moxley RT, Rohkamm R. Rippling muscle disease. *Arch Neurol* 1989;46:405–408.

158. Bums RJ, Bretag AH, Blumbergs PC, et al. Benign familial disease with muscle mounding and rippling. *J Neurol Neurosurg Psychiatry* 1994;57:344–347.

159. Stephan DA, Buist NR, Chittenden AB, et al. A rippling muscle disease gene is localized to 1q41: evidence for multiple genes. *Neurology* 1994;44:1915–1920.

160. Vorgerd M, Bolz H, Patzold T, et al. Phenotypic variability in rippling muscle disease. *Neurology* 1999;52:1453–1459.

161. Alberca R, Rafel E, Castilla JM, et al. Increased mechanical muscle irritability syndrome. *Acta Neurol Scand* 1980;62: 250–256.

162. Kosmorsky GS, Mehta N, Mitsumoto H, et al. Intermittent esotropia associated with rippling muscle disease. *J Neuroophthalmol* 1995;15:147–151.

163. Ansevin CF, Agamanolis DP. Rippling muscles and myasthenia gravis with rippling muscles. *Arch Neurol* 1996;53:197–199.

164. Vernino S, Auger RG, Emslie-Smith AM, et al. Myasthenia, thymoma, presynaptic antibodies, and a continuum of neuromuscular hyperexcitability. *Neurology* 1999;53:1233–1239.

165. Vorgerd M, Ricker K, Ziemssen F, et al. A sporadic case of rippling muscle disease caused by a de novo caveolin-3 mutation. *Neurology* 2001;57:2273–2277.

166. Stohr M, Schlote W, Bundschu HD, et al. Myopathia myotonica. *J Neurol* 1975;210:41–46.

167. Sanders DB. Myotonia congenita with painful muscle contractions. *Arch Neurol* 1976;33:580–582.

168. Becker PE. Syndromes associated with myotonia. In: Rowland LP, ed. *Pathogenesis of the human muscular dystrophies.* Amsterdam: Excerpta Medica, 1977:699–703.

169. Sunohara N, Tomi H, Nakamura A, et al. Myotonia congenita with painful muscle cramps. *Intern Med* 1996;35:507–511.

170. Koch MC, Steinmeyer K, Lorenz C, et al. The skeletal muscle chloride channel in dominant and recessive human myotonia. *Science* 1992;257:797–800.

171. George AL Jr, Crackower MA, Abdalla JA, et al. Molecular basis of Thomsen's disease (autosomal dominant myotonia congenita). *Nat Genet* 1993;3:305–310.

172. Davies NP, Hanna MG. The skeletal muscle channelopathies:

basic science, clinical genetics, and treatment. *Curr Opin Neurol* 2001;14:539–551.

173. Rüdel R, Ricker K, Lehmann-Horn F. Genotype–phenotype correlations in human skeletal muscle sodium channel diseases. *Arch Neurol* 1993;50:1241–1248.

174. Ptáček LJ, Tawil R, Griggs RC, et al. Linkage of atypical myotonia congenita to a sodium channel locus. *Neurology* 1992; 42:431–433.

175. Ptáček LJ, Tawil R, Griggs RC, et al. Sodium channel mutations in acetazolamide-responsive myotonia congenita, paramyotonia congenita, and hyperkalemic periodic paralysis. *Neurology* 1994;44:1500–1503.

176. Laycock MA, Pascuzzi RM. The neuromuscular effects of hypothyroidism. *Semin Neurol* 1991;11:288–294.

177. Duyff RF, Van den Bosch J, Laman DM, et al. Neuromuscular findings in thyroid dysfunction: a prospective clinical and electrodiagnostic study. *J Neurol Neurosurg Psychiatry* 2000;68: 750–755.

178. Ramsey I. *Thyroid disease and muscle dysfunction.* Chicago: Year Book Medical, 1974.

179. Lochmiller H, Reimers CD, Fischer P, et al. Exercise-induced myalgia in hypothyroidism. *Clin Invest* 1993;71:999–1001.

180. Riggs JE. Acute exertional rhabdomyolysis in hypothyroidism: the result of a reversible defect in glycogenolysis? *Milit Med* 1990;155:171–172.

181. Suzuki S, Ichikawa K, Nagai M, et al. Elevation of serum creatine kinase during treatment with antithyroid drugs in patients with hyperthyroidism due to Graves' disease: a novel side effect of antithyroid drugs. *Arch Intern Med* 1997;157:693–696.

182. Pearce I, Aziz H. The neuromyopathy of hypothyroidism: some new observations. *J Neurol Sci* 1969;9:243–253.

183. Ruff RL. Endocrine myopathies (hyper- and hypofunction of adrenal, thyroid, pituitary, and parathyroid glands and iatrogenic steroid myopathy). In: Engel AG, Banker BQ, eds. *Myology.* New York: McGraw-Hill, 1986:1871–1906.

184. Klostermann W, Wessel K, Moser A. Unmasking congenital myotonia by hypothyroidism (in German). *Nervenarzt* 1993; 64:266–268.

185. Ho K. Basophilic degeneration of skeletal muscle in hypothyroid myopathy. *Arch Pathol Lab Med* 1984;108:239–245.

186. Evans RM, Watanabe I, Singer PA. Central changes in hypothyroid myopathy: a case report. *Muscle Nerve* 1990;13:952–956.

187. Kaminsky P, Klein M, Duc M. La myopathie hypothyroidienne: approche physiopathologyique. *Ann Endocrinol (Paris)* 1992;53:125–132.

188. Taylor D, Rajagopalan B, Radda G. Cellular energetics in hypothyroid muscle. *Eur J Clin Invest* 1992;22:358–365.

189. McDaniel HG, Pittman CS, Oh SJ, et al. Carbohydrate metabolism in hypothyroid myopathy. *Metabolism* 1977;26:867–873.

190. Sharma VK, Banerjee SP. (β-Adrenergic receptors in rat skeletal muscle: effect of thyroidectomy. *Biochem Biophys Acta* 1978; 539:538–542.

191. Wiles CM, Young A, Jones DA, et al. Muscle relaxation rate, fibre-type composition, and energy turnover in hyper- and hypo-thyroid patients. *Clin Sci* 1979;57:375–384.

192. Fanburg BL. Calcium transport by skeletal muscle sarcoplasmic reticulum in the hypothyroid rat. *J Clin Invest* 1968;47: 2499–2506.

193. Fessel WJ. Myopathy of hypothyroidism. *Ann Rheum Dis* 1968; 27:590–595.

194. Stern LZ, Fagan JM. The endocrine myopathies. In: Vinken PJ, Bruyn GW, eds. *Handbook of clinical neurology,* vol 41. Amsterdam: Elsevier Science, 1979:235–258.

195. Turken SA, Cafferty M, Silverberg SJ, et al. Neuromuscular involvement in mild, asymptomatic primary hyperparathyroidism. *Am J Med* 1989;87:553–557.

196. Ritz E, Boland R, Krevsser W. Effects of vitamin D and parathormone on muscle. *Am J Clin Nutr* 19890;33:1522–1529.

197. Matthews C, Heimberg KW, Ritz E, et al. Effect on impaired calcium transport by the sarcoplasmic reticulum in experimental uremia. *Kidney Int* 1977;11:227–235.

198. Baczynski R, Massry SG, Magott M, et al. Effect of parathyroid hormone on energy metabolism of skeletal muscle. *Kidney Int* 1985;28:722–727.

199. Nagamitsu S, Ashizawa T. Myotonic dystrophies. *Neuromuscular disorders.* Advances in neurology, vol 88. Philadelphia: Lippincott Williams & Wilkins, 2002.

200. Renner DR, Ptacek LL. Periodic paralyses and nondystrophic myotonias. *Neuromuscular disorders.* Advances in neurology, vol 88. Philadelphia: Lippincott Williams & Wilkins, 2002.

201. Ferrannini E, Perniola T, Krajewska G, et al. Schwartz-Jampel syndrome with autosomal-dominant inheritance. *Eur Neurol* 1982;21:137–146.

202. Pascuzzi RM, Gratianne R, Azzarelli B, et al. Schwartz-Jampel syndrome with dominant inheritance. *Muscle Nerve* 1990;13:1152–1163.

203. Schwartz O, Jampel RS. Congenital blepharophimosis associated with a unique generalized myopathy. *Arch Ophthalmol* 1962;68:52–57.

204. Viljoen D, Beighton P. Schwartz-Jampel syndrome (chondrodystrophic myotonia). *J Med Genet* 1992;29:58–62.

205. Paradis CM, Gironda F, Bennett M. Cognitive impairment in Schwartz-Jampel syndrome: a case study. *Brain Lang* 1997;56:301–305.

206. Cook SP. Borkowski WJ. Obstructive sleep apnea in Schwartz-Jampel syndrome. *Archives of Otolaryngology—Head & Neck Surg* 1997;123:1348–1350.

207. Spaans F, Theunissen P, Reekers AD, et al. Schwartz-Jampel syndrome: 1. Clinical, electromyographic, and histologic studies. *Muscle Nerve* 1990;13:516–527.

208. Figuera LE, Jimenez-Gil FJ, Garcia-Cruz MO, et al. Schwartz-Jampel syndrome: an atypical form? *Am J Med Genet* 1993;47:526–528.

209. Giedion A, Boltshauser E, Briner J, et al. Heterogeneity in Schwartz-Jampel chondrodystrophic myotonia. *Eur J Pediatr* 1997;156:214–223.

210. Cao A, Cianchetti C, Calisti L, et al. Schwartz-Jampel syndrome: clinical, electrophysiological, and histopathological study of a severe variant. *J Neurol Sci* 1978;35:175–187.

211. Lehmann-Horn F, Iaizzo PA, Franke C, et al. Schwartz-Jampel syndrome: 2. Na⁺ channel defect causes myotonia. *Muscle Nerve* 1990;13:528–535.

212. Topaloglu H, Serdaroglu A, Okan M, et al. Improvement of myotonia with carbamazepine in three cases with the Schwartz-Jampel syndrome. *Neuropediatrics* 1993;24:232–234.

213. Squires LA, Prangley J. Neonatal diagnosis of Schwartz-Jampel syndrome with dramatic response to carbamazepine. *Pediatr Neurol* 1996;15:172–174.

214. Nicole S, Ben Hamida C, Beighton P, et al. Localization of the Schwartz-Jampel syndrome (SJS) locus to chromosome 1p34-p36.1 by homozygosity mapping. *Hum Mol Genet* 1995;4:1633–1636.

215. Brown KA, al-Gazali LI, Moynihan LM, et al. Genetic heterogeneity in Schwartz-Jampel syndrome: two families with neonatal Schwartz-Jampel syndrome do not map to human chromosome 1p34-p36.1. *J Med Genet* 1997;34:685–687.

216. Roy EP, Gutmann L. Myalgia. *Neurol Clin North Am* 1988;6:621–636.

217. Simchak AC, Pascuzzi RM. Muscle cramps. *Semin Neurol* 1991;11:281–287.

218. Sufit RL, Peters HA. Nifedipine relieves exercise-exacerbated myalgias. *Muscle Nerve* 1984;7:647–649.

219. Morgan-Hughes JA. Defects of the energy pathways of skeletal muscle. In: Matthews WB, Glaser GH, eds. *Recent advances in clinical neurology,* vol 3. Edinburgh: Churchill-Livingstone, 1982:1–46.

220. Arnold DL, Radda GK, Bore PJ, et al. Excessive intracellular acidosis of skeletal muscle on exercise in a patient with a postviral fatigue syndrome. *Lancet* 1984;1:1367–1369.

221. Sreter FA, Banman ML, Gergelo J, et al. Changes in muscle chemistry associated with stiffness and pain. *Neurology* 1972;22:1172–1175.

222. Telerman-Toppet N, Bac QM, Khoubesserian P, et al. Type 2 fiber predominance in muscle cramp and exertional myalgia. *Muscle Nerve* 1985;8:563–567.

223. Gospe SM, Lazaro RP, Lava NS, et al. Familial X-linked myalgia and cramps: a nonprogressive myopathy associated with a deletion in the dystrophin gene (abst). *Ann Neurol* 1989;26:466.

224. Kuhn E, Fiehn W, Schroder M, et al. Early myocardial disease and cramping myalgia in Becker-type muscular dystrophy: a kindred. *Neurology* 1979;29:1144–1149.

225. Sulaiman AR, Kinder DS. Vascularized muscle fibers: etiopathogenesis and clinical significance. *J Neurol Sci* 1989;82:37–54.

226. Isaacs H, Badenhorst ME. Internalized capillaries, neuromyopathy and myalgia. *J Neurol Neurosurg Psychiatry* 1992;55:921–924.

227. Niakan E, Harati Y, Danon MJ. Tubular aggregates: their association with myalgia. *J Neurol Neurosurg Psychiatry* 1985;48:882–886.

228. Brumback RA, Staton RD, Susaq ME. Exercise-induced pain, stiffness, and tubular aggregates in skeletal muscle. *J Neurol Neurosurg Psychiatry* 1981;44:250–254.

229. Eaton JM. Is this really a muscle cramp? *Postgrad Med* 1989;86:227–232.

230. Arellano F, Krupp O. Muscle disorders associated with cyclosporine. *Lancet* 1991;337:915.

231. Litin SC, Anderson CF. Nicotinic acid–associated myopathy: a report of three cases. *Am J Med* 1989;86:481–483.

232. Argov Z, Mastaglia FL. Drug-induced neuromuscular disorders in man. In: Walton SJ, ed. *Disorders of voluntary muscle.* Edinburgh: Churchill-Livingstone, 1988:981–1014.

233. Baker PCH. Drug-induced and toxic myopathies. *Semin Neurol* 1983;3:265–274.

234. Lane RJM, Mastaglia FL. Drug-induced myopathies in man. *Lancet* 1978;2:562–565.

235. Kunci RW, Wiggins WW. Toxic myopathies. *Neurol Clin North Am* 1988;6:593–619.

236. Ishigaki C, Patria SY, Wishio H, et al. A Japanese boy with myalgia and cramps has a novel in-frame deletion of the dystrophin gene. *Neurology* 1996;46:1347–1350.

237. Minaker KL, Flier JS, Landsberg L, et al. Phenytoin-induced improvement in muscle cramping and insulin action in three patients with the syndrome of insulin resistance, acanthosis nigricans, and acral hypertrophy. *Arch Neurol* 1989;46:981–985.

238. Waters DJ, Mapleson WW. Suxamethonium pains: hypothesis and observation. *Anaesthesia* 1971;26:127–141.

239. McLoughlin C, Leslie K, Caldwell JE. Influence of dose on suxamethonium-induced muscle damage. *Br J Anaesth* 1994;73:194–198.

240. Poon PW, Lui PW, Chow LH, et al. EMG spike trains of succinylcholine-induced fasciculations in myalgic patients. *Electroencephalogr Clin Neurophysiol* 1996;101:206–210.

241. Palliyath S, Garcia CA. Multifocal interstitial myositis associated with localized lipoatrophy: a benign course. *Arch Neurol* 1982;39:722–724.

242. Créange A, Renard JL, Millet P, et al. A patient with one limb interstitial myositis with localised lipoatrophy presenting with severe cramps and fasciculations. *J Neurol Neurosurg Psychiatry* 1994;57:1541–1543.

243. Jansen PHP, VanDijck JAAM, Verbeck ALM, et al. Estimation of the frequency of the muscular pain-fasciculation syndrome and the muscular cramp-fasciculation syndrome in the adult population. *Eur Arch Psychiatry Clin Neurosci* 1991;241: 102–104.

244. Denny-Brown D, Foley JM. Myokymia and the benign fasciculation of muscle cramp. *Trans Assoc Am Physicians* 1948;61: 88–96.

245. Hudson AJ, Brown WF, Gilbert JJ. The muscular pain-fasciculation syndrome. *Neurology* 1978;28:1105–1109.

246. Fetell MR, Smallberg G, Lewis LD, et al. A benign motor neuron disorder: delayed cramps and fasciculation after poliomyelitis or myelitis. *Ann Neurol* 1982;11:423–427.

247. Weiner IH, Weiner HL. Nocturnal leg muscle cramps. *JAMA* 1980;244:2332–2333.

248. Miles MP, Clarkson PM. Exercise-induced muscle pain, soreness, and cramps. *J Sports Med Phys Fitness* 1994;34:203–216.

249. Maughan RJ. Exercise-induced muscle cramp: a prospective biochemical study in marathon runners. *J Sports Sci* 1986;4: 31–34.

250. Williamson SL, Johnson RW, Hudkins PG, et al. Exertional cramps: a prospective study of biochemical and anthropometric variables in bicycle riders. *Cycling Sci* 1993;[Spring]:15–20.

251. Haskell SG, Fiebach NH. Clinical epidemiology of nocturnal leg cramps in male veterans. *Am J Med Sci* 1997;313:210–214.

252. Layzer RB. The origin of muscle fasciculations and cramps. *Muscle Nerve* 1994;17:1243–1249.

253. Daniel HW. Simple cure for nocturnal leg cramps. *N Engl J Med* 1979;301:216.

254. Moss HK, Herrmann LG. Use of quinine for relief of "night cramps" in the extremities. *JAMA* 1940;115:1358–1359.

255. Nightingale SL. Quinine for nocturnal leg cramps (letter). *ACP J Club* 1995;123:86–87.

256. Mandal AK, Abernathy T, Nelluri SN, et al. Is quinine effective and safe in leg cramps? *J Clin Pharmacol* 1995;35:588–593.

257. Lim SH. Randomised double-blind trial of quinine sulphate for nocturnal leg cramp. *Br J Clin Pract* 1986;40:462.

258. Warburton A, Royston JP, O'Neill Q, et al. A quinine a day keeps the leg cramps away? *Br J Clin Pharmacol* 1987;23:459–465.

259. Sidorov J. Quinine sulfate for leg cramps: does it work? *J Am Geriatr Soc* 1993;41:498–500.

260. Jones K, Castleden CM. A double-blind comparison of quinine sulphate and placebo in muscle cramps. *Age Ageing* 1983;12: 155–158.

261. Fung MC, Holbrook JH. Placebo-controlled trial of quinine therapy for nocturnal leg cramps. *West J Med* 1989;151:42–44.

262. Connolly PS, Shirley DA, Wasson JH, et al. Treatment of nocturnal leg cramps: a crossover trial of quinine vs. vitamin E. *Arch Intern Med* 1992;152:1877–1880.

263. Jansen PH, Veenhuizen KC, Wesseling AI, et al. Randomized controlled trial of hydroquinine in muscle cramps. *Lancet* 1997; 349:528–532.

264. Jansen PH, Veenhuizen KC, Verbeek AL, et al. Efficacy of hydroquinine in preventing frequent ordinary muscle cramp outlasts actual administration. *J Neurol Sci* 1994;122:157–161.

265. Baltodano N, Gallo BV, Weidler DJ. Verapamil vs quinine in recumbent nocturnal leg cramps in the elderly. *Arch Intern Med* 1988;148:1969–1970.

266. Stern FH. Value of carisoprodol (Soma) in relieving leg cramps. *J Am Geriatr Soc* 1963;11:1008–1013.

267. Keidar S, Binenboim C, Palant A. Muscle cramps during treatment with nifedipine. *Br Med J* 1982;85:1241–1242.

268. Steiner I, Siegal T. Muscle cramps in cancer patients. *Cancer* 1989;63:574–577.

269. Medina JL, Chokroverty S, Reyes M. Localized myokymia caused by peripheral nerve injury. *Arch Neurol* 1976;33: 587–588.

270. Albers JW, Allen AA II, Bastron JA, et al. Limb myokymia. *Muscle Nerve* 1981;4:494–504.

271. Welch LK, Appenzeller O, Bicknell JM. Peripheral neuropathy with myokymia, sustained muscular contraction, and continuous motor unit activity. *Neurology* 1972;22:161–169.

272. Thomas PK, Claus D, Workman JM, et al. Focal upper limb demyelinating neuropathy. *Brain* 1996;119:765–774.

273. Roth G, Magistris MR. Neuropathies with prolonged conduction block, single and grouped fasciculation, localized limb myokymia. *Electroencephalogr Clin Neurophysiol* 1987;67: 428–438.

274. O'Leary CP, Mann AC, Lough J, et al. Muscle hypertrophy in multifocal motor neuropathy is associated with continuous motor unit activity. *Muscle Nerve* 1997;20:479–485.

275. Baldissera F, Cavallari P, Dworzak F. Motor neuron "bistability": a pathogenetic mechanism for cramps and myokymia. *Brain* 1994;117:929–939.

276. Esteban A, Traba A. Fasciculation-myokymic activity and prolonged nerve conduction block: a physiopathologic relationship in radiation-induced brachial plexopathy. *Electroencephalogr Clin Neurophysiol* 1993;89:382–391.

277. Robberecht W, VanHees J, Adriaensen H, et al. Painful muscle spasms complicating algodystrophy: central or peripheral disease? *J Neurol Neurosurg Psychiatry* 1988;51:563–567.

278. Rish BL. Nerve root compression and night cramps. *JAMA* 1985;254:361.

279. Calancie B, Ayyar DR, Eismont FJ. Myokymic discharges: prompt cessation following nerve root decompression during spine surgery. *Electromyogr Clin Neurophysiol* 1992;32:443–447.

280. Denny-Brown D. Clinical problems in neuromuscular physiology. *Am J Med* 1953;15:368–390.

281. Satoyoshi E, Doi Y, Kinoshita M. Pseudomyotonia in cervical root lesions with myelopathy: a sign of the misdirection of regenerating nerve. *Arch Neurol* 1972;27:307–313.

282. Bussaglia E, Tizzano EF, Illa I, et al. Cramps and minimal EMG abnormalities as preclinical manifestations of spinal muscular atrophy patients with homozygous deletions of the SMN gene. *Neurology* 1997;48:1443–1445.

283. Mulder DW, Espinosa RE. Amyotrophic lateral sclerosis: comparison of the clinical syndrome in Guam and the United States. In: Norris NH Jr, Kurland LT, eds. *Motor neuron diseases: research on amyotrophic lateral sclerosis and related disorders.* New York: Grune & Stratton, 1969:12–19.

284. Roth G. The origin of fasciculations. *Ann Neurol* 1982;12: 542–547.

285. Conradi S, Grimby L, Lundemo G. Pathophysiology of fasciculations in ALS as studied by electromyography of single motor units. *Muscle Nerve* 1982;5:202–208.

286. Smith RG, Hamilton S, Hofman F, et al. Serum antibodies to L-type calcium channels in patients with amyotrophic lateral sclerosis. *N Engl J Med* 1992;327:172–178.

286. Smith RG, Kimura F, McKinley K, et al. Alterations in dihydropyridine receptor binding kinetics in amyotrophic lateral sclerosis (ALS) skeletal muscle. *Soc Neurosci Abstr* 1991;17: 1451.

288. Sinha S, Newsome-Davis J, Mills K, et al. Autoimmune aetiology for acquired neuromyotonia (Isaacs' syndrome). *Lancet* 1991;338:75–77.

289. Stewart SS, Appel SH. The treatment of amyotrophic lateral sclerosis. In: Appel SH, ed. *Current neurology,* vol 7. Chicago: Year Book Medical, 1987:51–90.

290. Obi T, Mizoguchi K, Matsuoka H, et al. Muscle cramp as the result of impaired GABA function: an electrophysiological and pharmacological observation. *Muscle Nerve* 1993;16: 1228–1231.

291. Talbott JH. Heat cramps. *Medicine* 1935;14:323–376.

292. Knochell JP. Environmental heat illness. *Arch Intern Med* 1974;133:841–864.

293. Donoghue AM, Sinclair MJ, Bates GP. Heat exhaustion in a deep underground metalliferous mine. *Occup Environ Med* 2000;57:165–174.

294. Khajehdehi P, Mojerlou M, Behzadi S, et al. A randomized, double-blind, placebo-controlled trial of supplementary vitamins E, C, and their combination for treatment of haemodialysis cramps. *Nephrology Dialysis Transplantation* 2001;16: 1448–1451.

295. Rocco MV, Burkart JM. Prevalence of missed treatments and early sign-offs in hemodialysis patients. *J Am Soc Nephrol* 1993;4:1178–1183.

296. Neal CR, Resnikoff E, Unger AM. Treatment of dialysis-related muscle cramp with hypertonic dextrose. *Arch Intern Med* 1981; 141:171–173.

297. Howe RC, Wombolt DG, Michil DD. Analysis of tonic muscle activity and muscle cramps during hemodialysis. *J Dialysis* 1978;2:85–99.

298. Mujais SK. Muscle cramps during hemodialysis (editorial). *Int J Artif Organs* 1994;17:570–572.

299. Canzanello VI, Hylander-Rossner B, Sands RE, et al. Comparison of 50% dextrose water, 25% mannitol, and 23.5% saline for the treatment of hemodialysis-associated muscle cramps. *ASAIO Trans* 1991;37:649–652.

300. Kaplan B, Wang T, Rammohan M, et al. Response to head-up tilt in cramping and noncramping hemodialysis patients. *Int J Clin Pharmacol Ther Toxicol* 1992;30:173–180.

301. Sidhom OA, Odoh YK, Krumlovsky FA, et al. Lowdose prazosin in patients with muscle cramps during hemodialysis. *Clin Pharmacol Ther* 1994;56:445–451.

302. Peer G, Blum M, Aviram A. Relief of hemodialysis-induced muscular cramps by nifedipine. *Dialysis Transplant* 1983;12: 180–181.

303. Roca AO, Jarjoura D, Blend D, et al. Dialysis leg cramps: efficacy of quinine versus vitamin E. *ASAIO J* 1992;38:M481–M485.

304. Panadero Sandoval J, Perez Garcia A, Martin Abad L, et al. Action of quinine sulphate on the incidence of muscle cramps during hemodialysis. *Med Clin* 1980;75:247–249.

305. Ahmad S, Robertson HT, Golper TA, et al. Multicenter trial of L-carnitine in maintenance hemodialysis patients: 2. Clinical and biochemical effects. *Kidney Int* 1990;38:912–918.

306. Auger RG. AAEM Mini-Monograph 44: Diseases associated with excess motor unit activity. *Muscle Nerve* 1994;17:1250–1263.

307. Isaacs H. A syndrome of continuous muscle-fiber activity. *J Neurol Neurosurg Psychiatry* 1961;24:319–325.

308. Auger RG, Daube JR, Gomez MR, et al. Hereditary form of sustained muscle activity of peripheral nerve origin causing generalized myokymia and muscle stiffness. *Ann Neurol* 1984;15: 13–21.

309. Layzer RB. Neuromyotonia: a new autoimmune disease. *Ann Neurol* 1995;38:701–702.

310. Newsom-Davis J, Mills KR. Immunological associations of acquired neuromyotonia (Isaacs' syndrome). *Brain* 1993;116: 453–469.

311. Gutmann L, Tellers JG, Vernino S. Persistent facial myokymia associated with K(+) channel antibodies. *Neurology* 2001;57: 1707–1708.

312. Mygland A, Vincent A, Newsom-Davis J, et al. Autoantibodies in thymoma-associated myasthenia gravis with myositis or neuromyotonia. *Arch Neurol* 2000;57:527–531.

313. Griffiths TD, Connolly S, Newman PK, et al. Neuromyotonia in association with malignant hyperpyrexia. *J Neurol Neurosurg Psychiatry* 1995;59:556–557.

314. Horikawa M, Yamaguchi Y, Katafuchi Y, et al. A case of Isaacs syndrome with high CSF protein and a large cisterna magna. *Brain Dev* 1993;15:129–132.

315. Kiernan MC, Hart IK, Bostock H. Excitability properties of motor axons in patients with spontaneous motor unit activity. *J Neurol Neurosurg Psychiatry* 2001;70:56–64.

316. Irani PF, Porhout AV, Wadia NH. The syndrome of continuous muscle fiber activity: evidence to suggest proximal neurogenic causation. *Acta Neurol Scand* 1977;55:273–288.

317. Ochoa JJ, Castilla JM, Bautista J, et al. Neuromiotonia: origen periferico proximal de la actividad muscular continuua. *Arch Neurobiol (Madr)* 1979;42:309–320.

318. Sakai T, Hosokawa S, Shibisaki H, et al. Syndrome of continuous muscle fiber activity: increased C.S.F. GABA and effect of dantrolene. *Neurology* 1983;33:495–498.

319. Hart IK. Acquired neuromyotonia: a new autoantibody-mediated neuronal potassium channelopathy. *Am J Med Sci* 2000; 319:209–216.

320. Vernino S, Auger RG, Emslie-Smith AM, et al. Myasthenia, thymoma, presynaptic antibodies, and a continuum of neuromuscular hyperexcitability. *Neurology* 1999;53:1233–1239.

321. Heidenreich F, Vincent A. Antibodies to ion-channel proteins in thymoma with myasthenia, neuromyotonia, and peripheral neuropathy. *Neurology* 1998;50:1483–1485.

322. Hart IK, Waters C, Vincent A, et al. Autoantibodies detected to expressed K+ channels are implicated in neuromyotonia. *Ann Neurol* 1997;41:238–246.

323. Shillito P, Molenaar PC, Vincent A, et al. Acquired neuromyotonia: evidence for autoantibodies directed against K+ channels of peripheral nerves. *Ann Neurol* 1995;38:714–722.

324. Nagado T, Arimura K, Sonada Y, et al. Potassium current suppression in patients with peripheral nerve hyperexcitibility. *Brain* 1999;122:2056–2066.

325. Sonoda Y, Arimura K, Kurono A, et al. Serum of Isaacs' syndrome suppresses potassium channels in PC12 cell lines. *Muscle Nerve* 1996;19:1439–1446.

326. Arimura K, Watanabe O, Kitajima I, et al. Antibodies to potassium channels of PC12 in serum of Isaacs' syndrome: western blot and immunohistochemical studies. *Muscle Nerve* 1997;20: 299–305.

327. Riche G, Trouillas P, Bady B. Improvement of Isaacs' syndrome after treatment with azathioprine. *J Neurol Neurosurg Psychiatry* 1995;59:448.

328. Hayashi A, Ishii A, Ohkoshi N, et al. Reply (letter). *J Neurol Neurosurg Psychiatry* 1995;58:393.

329. Ishii A, Hayashi A, Ohkoshi N, et al. Clinical evaluation of plasma exchange and high dose intravenous immunoglobulin in a patient with Isaacs' syndrome. *J Neurol Neurosurg Psychiatry* 1994;57:840–842.

330. Van Engelen BG, Benders AA, Gabreels FJ, et al. Are muscle cramps in Isaacs' syndrome triggered by human immunoglobulin? *J Neurol Neurosurg Psychiatry* 1995;58:393.

331. Isaacs H, Heffron JJA. The syndrome of continuous muscle fibre activity cured: further studies. *J Neurol Neurosurg Psychiatry* 1974;37:1231–1235.

332. Koley KC, Roy AK, Sinho G. Neuromyotonia. *J Ind Med Assoc* 1992;90:131–132.

333. Waerness E. Neuromyotonia and bronchial carcinoma. *Electromyogr Clin Neurophysiol* 1974;14:527–535.

334. Walsh JC. Neuromyotonia: an unusual presentation of intrathoracic malignancy. *J Neurol Neurosurg Psychiatry* 1976; 39:1086–1091.

335. Partanen VSJ, Soinen H, Saksa M, et al. Electromyographic and

nerve conduction findings in a patient with neuromyotonia, normocalcemic tetany and small-cell lung cancer. *Acta Neurol Scand* 1980;61:216–226.

336. Caress J, Preston DC, Abend WK, et al. A case of Hodgkin's lymphoma producing neuromyotonia (abst). *Neurology* 1997;48[Suppl 2]:A147.

337. Halbach M, Homberg V, Freund HJ. Neuromuscular autonomic and central cholinergic hyperactivity associated with thymoma and acetylcholine receptor antibody. *J Neurol* 1987;234:433–436.

338. Garcia R, Boudene C, Cinsbourg M. Choree fibrillaire de Morvan et polyradiculonevrite d'etiologie mercurielle probable. *Rev Neurol* 1971;125:322–326.

339. Martinelli P, Patuelli A, Minardi C, et al. Neuromyotonia, peripheral neuropathy, and myasthenia gravis. *Muscle Nerve* 1996;19:505–510.

340. Vasilescu C, Florescu A. Peripheral neuropathy with a syndrome of continuous motor activity. *J Neurol* 1982;226:275–282.

341. Preston DC, Kelly JJ. "Pseudospasticity" in Guillain-Barré syndrome. *Neurology* 1991;41:131–134.

342. Valenstein E, Watson RT, Parker JL. Myokymial muscle hypertrophy and percussion "myotonia" in chronic recurrent polyneuropathy. *Neurology* 1978;28:1130–1134.

343. Joy JL, Allen RF, Sunwool N, et al. Isaacs' syndrome associated with chronic inflammatory demyelinating polyneuropathy. *Muscle Nerve* 1990;13:868.

344. Odabasi Z, Joy JL, Claussen GC, et al. Isaacs' syndrome associated with chronic inflammatory demyelinating polyneuropathy. *Muscle Nerve* 1996;19:210–215.

345. Bady B, Chauplannaz G, Vial C. Autoimmune aetiology for acquired neuromyotonia (letter). *Lancet* 1991;338:1330.

346. Le Gars L, Clerc D, Cariou D, et al. Systemic juvenile rheumatoid arthritis and associated Isaacs' syndrome. *J Rheumatol* 1997;24:178–180.

347. Reeback J, Benton JS, Swash M, et al. Penicillamine-induced neuromyotonia. *Br Med J* 1979;1:1464–1465.

348. Black JT, Garcia-Mullin R, Good E, et al. Muscle rigidity in a newborn due to continuous peripheral nerve hyperactivity. *Arch Neurol* 1972;27:413–425.

349. Mitsumoto H, Wilbourn AJ, Subramony SH. Generalized myokymia and gold therapy. *Arch Neurol* 1982;39:449–450.

350. Fraisse P, Sutter B, Tritschler JL, et al. Morvan's fibrillary chorea after gold therapy (letter). *Presse Med* 1985;14:1097.

351. Morvan A. De la choree fibrillaire. *Gaz Heb Med Chirurg* 1890;27:173–202.

352. Garcia-Merino A, Cabello A, Mora JS, et al. Continuous muscle fiber activity, peripheral neuropathy, and thymoma. *Ann Neurol* 1991;29:215–218.

353. Gil R, Lefevre JP, Neau JPH, et al. Choree fibrillaire de Morvan et syndrome acrodynique apres un troutement mercuriel. *Rev Neurol (Paris)* 1984;140:728–733.

354. Serratrice G, Azulay JP. What is left of Morvan's fibrillary chorea? (in French). *Rev Neurol* 1994;150:257–265.

355. Lee EK, Maselli RA, Ellis WG, et al. Morvan's fibrillary chorea: a paraneoplastic manifestation of thymoma. *J Neurol Neurosurg Psychiatry* 1998;65:857–862.

356. Hosokawa S, Shinoda H, Sakai T, et al. Electrophysiological study on limb myokymia in three women. *J Neurol Neurosurg Psychiatry* 1987;50:877–881.

357. Lublin FD, Tsairis P, Streletz LJ, et al. Myokymia and impaired muscular relaxation with continuous motor unit activity. *J Neurol Neurosurg Psychiatry* 1979;42:557–562.

358. Grassa C, Figa-Talamanca L, Lo Russo F, et al. Syndrome of continuous muscle fiber activity: case report. *Ital J Neurol Sci* 1981;4:415–418.

359. Jamieson PW, Katirji MB. Idiopathic generalized myokymia. *Muscle Nerve* 1994;17:42–51.

360. Torbergsen T, Stalberg E, Brautaset N. Generator sites for spontaneous activity: an EMG study. *Electroencephalogr Clin Neurophysiol* 1996;101:69–78.

361. O'Brien TJ, Gates P. Isaac's syndrome: report of a case responding to valproic acid. *Clin Exp Neurol* 1994;31:52–60.

362. Tahmoush AJ, Alonso RJ, Tahmoush GP, et al. Cramp-fasciculation syndrome: a treatable hyperexcitable peripheral nerve disorder. *Neurology* 1991;41:1021–1024.

363. Smith KK, Claussen G, Fesenmeier JT, et al. Myokymia-cramp syndrome: evidence of hyperexcitable peripheral nerve. *Muscle Nerve* 1994;17:1065–1067.

364. Lance JW, Burke D, Pollard J. Neuromyotonia in the spinal form of Charcot-Marie-Tooth disease. *Clin Exp Neurol* 1979; 16:49–56.

365. Hahn AF, Parkes AW, Bolton CF, et al. Neuromyotonia in hereditary motor neuropathy. *J Neurol Neurosurg Psychiatry* 1991;54:230–235.

366. Lance JW, Burke D, Pollard J. Hyperexcitability of motor and sensory neurons in neuromyotonia. *Ann Neurol* 1979;5: 523–532.

367. Vasilescu C, Alexianu M, Dan A. Neuronal type of Charcot-Marie-Tooth disease with a syndrome of continuous motor activity. *J Neurol Sci* 1984;63:11–25.

368. Thomas PK, Marques W Jr, Davis MB, et al. The phenotypic manifestations of chromosome 17p11.2 duplication. *Brain* 1997;120:465–478.

369. Burk K, Stevanin G, Didierjean O, et al. Clinical and genetic analysis of three German kindreds with autosomal dominant cerebellar ataxia type I linked to the SCA2 locus. *J Neurol* 1997;244:256–261.

370. Takashima H, Nakagawa M, Nakahara K, et al. A new type of hereditary motor and sensory neuropathy linked to chromosome 3. *Ann Neurol* 1997;41:771–780.

371. Ashizawa T, Butler IJ, Harati Y, et al. A dominantly inherited syndrome with continuous motor discharges. *Ann Neurol* 1983; 13:285–290.

372. McGuire SA, Tomasovic FF, Ackerman NJ R. Hereditary continuous muscle fiber activity. *Arch Neurol* 1984;41:395–396.

373. Sheaff HM. Hereditary myokymia. *Arch Neurol Psychiatry* 1952;68:236–247.

374. Van Dyke DH, Griggs RC, Murphy MJ, et al. Hereditary myokymia and periodic ataxia. *J Neurol Sci* 1975;25:109–118.

375. Hanson PA, Martinez LB, Cassidy R. Contractures, continuous muscle discharges, and titubation. *Ann Neurol* 1977;1:120–124.

376. Gancher ST, Nutt JG. Autosomal dominant episodic ataxia: a heterogeneous syndrome. *Mov Disord* 1986;1:239–253.

377. Brunt ER, VanWeerden W. Familial paroxysmal kinesigenic ataxia and continuous myokymia. *Brain* 1990;113:1361–1382.

378. Bain PG, O'Brien MD, Keevil SF, et al. Familial periodic cerebellar ataxia: a problem of cerebellar intracellular pH homeostasis. *Ann Neurol* 1992;31:147–154.

379. Vaamonde J, Artieda J, Obeso JA. Hereditary paroxysmal ataxia with neuromyotonia. *Mov Discord* 1991;6:180–182.

380. Lubbers WJ, Brunt ER, Scheffer H, et al. Hereditary myokymia and paroxysmal ataxia linked to chromosome 12 is responsive to acetazolamide. *J Neurol Neurosurg Psychiatry* 1995;59:400–405.

381. Browne DL, Gancher ST, Nutt JG, et al. Episodic ataxia / myokymia syndrome is associated with point mutations in the human potassium channel gene, *KCNA1*. *Nat Genet* 1994; 8:136–140.

382. Browne DL, Brunt ER, Griggs RC, et al. Identification of two new *KCNA1* mutations in episodic ataxia/myokymia families. *Hum Mol Genet* 1995;4:1671–1672.

383. Byme E, White O, Cook M. Familial dystonic choreoathetosis with myokymia: a sleep responsive disorder. *J Neurol Neurosurg Psychiatry* 1991;54:1090–1092.

384. Fink JK, Rainer S, Wilkowski J, et al. Paroxysmal dystonic choreoathetosis: tight linkage to chromosome 2q. *Am J Hum Genet* 1996;59:140–145.

385. Van den Bergh P, Bulcke JA, Dom R. Familial muscle cramps with autosomal dominant transmission. *Eur Neurol* 1980;19: 207–212.

386. Ricker K, Moxley RT III. Autosomal dominant cramping disease. *Arch Neurol* 1990;47:810–812.

387. Jusic A, Dogan S, Stojanovic V. Hereditary persistent distal cramps. *J Neurol Neurosurg Psychiatry* 1972;35:379–384.

388. Lazaro PR, Rollinson RD, Fenichel GM. Familial cramps and muscle pain. *Arch Neurol* 1981;38:22–24.

389. Lun LC. Hyperventilation and anxiety state. *J Soc Med* 1981; 74:1–4.

390. Magarian GJ. Hyperventilation syndromes: infrequently recognized common expressions of anxiety and stress. *Medicine* 1982; 61:219–236.

391. Kugelberg E. Activation of human nerves by ischemia. Trousseau's phenomenon in tetany. *Arch Neurol Psychiatry* 1948; 60:140–152.

392. Kugelberg E. Activation of human nerve by hyperventilation and hypocalcemia: neurologic mechanism of symptoms of irritation in tetany. *Arch Neurol Psychiatry* 1948;60:153–164.

393. Stein RB. *Nerve and muscles: membranes, cells, and systems.* New York: Plenum Press, 1980:56–59.

394. Vukasin P, Weston LA, Beart RW. Oral Fleet "Phospho-Soda" laxative-induced hyperphosphatemia and hypocalcemic tetany in an adult: report of a case. *Dis Colon Rectum* 1997;40: 497–499.

395. Ramage IJ, Ray M, Paton RD, et al. Hypomagnesaemic tetany. *J Clin Pathol* 1996;49:343–344.

396. Shuster J. Methylprednisolone as a cause of anaphylaxis; diltiazem-induced tetany; NSAID-induced colonic stricture with ulceration and NSAID-induced erythema multiforme; lamotrigine and Tourette symptoms; anaphylactic reaction after dermal exposure to cephalexin. *Hosp Pharmacy* 2000;35: 137,138,140,143.

397. Campisi P, Badhwar V, Morin S, et al. Postoperative hypocalcemic tetany caused by Fleet Phospho-Soda preparation in a patient taking alendronate sodium: report of a case. *Dis Colon Rectum* 1999;42:1499–1501.

398. Yamashita H, Noguchi S, Tahara K, et al. Postoperative tetany in patients with Graves' disease: a risk factor analysis. *Clin Endocrinol* 1997;47:71–77.

399. Taborska V. Incidence of latent tetany in patients with panic disorder. *Cesk Psychiatr* 1995;91:183–190.

400. Ault MJ, Geiderman J. Hypokalemia as a cause of tetany. *West J Med* 1992;1–57:65–67.

401. Isgreen WP. Normocalcemic tetany. *Neurology* 1976;26:825–834.

402. Day JW, Parry GJ. Normocalcemic tetany abolished by calcium infusion. *Ann Neurol* 1990;27:438–440.

403. Knochell JP. Neuromuscular manifestation of electrolyte disorders. *Am J Med* 1982;72:521–535.

404. Corbett AJ. Electrolyte disorders affecting muscle. *Semin Neurol* 1983;3:248–257.

405. Harati Y. Eosinophilia-myalgia syndrome and its relation to toxic oil syndrome. In: de Wolff FA, ed. *Handbook of clinical neurology: intoxications of the nervous system,* Part 1, Vol 20. Amsterdam: Elsevier Science, 1994:249–271.

406. Kaufman LD, Kaufman MA, Krupp LB. Movement disorders in the eosinophilia-myalgia syndrome: tremor, myoclonus, and myokymia. *J Rheumatol* 1995;22:157–160.

407. Mayeno AN, Benson LM, Naylor S, et al. Biotransformation of 3-(phenylamino)-1,2-propanediol to 3(phenylamino)alanine: a chemical link between toxic oil syndrome and eosinophilia-myalgia syndrome. *Chem Res Toxicol* 1995;8:911–916.

408. Martin RW, Duffy J, Engel AG, et al. The clinical spectrum of the eosinophilia-myalgia syndrome associated with L-tryptophan ingestion. *Ann Intern Med* 1990;113:124–134.

409. Hertzman PA, Clauw DJ, Duffy JM, et al. Rigorous new approach to constructing a gold standard for validating new diagnostic criteria, as exemplified by the eosinophilia-myalgia syndrome. *Arch Intern Med* 2001;161:2301–2306.

410. Hertzman PA, Clauw DJ, Kaufman LD, et al. The eosinophilia-myalgia syndrome: status of 205 patients and results of treatment 2 years after onset. *Ann Intern Med* 1995;122:851–855.

411. Eosinophilia-myalgia syndrome: follow-up survey of patients—New York, 1990–1991. *MMWR* 1991;40:401–403.

412. Kaufman LD. Chronicity of the eosinophilia-myalgia syndrome: a reassessment after three years. *Arthritis Rheum* 1994; 37:84–87.

413. Armstrong C, Lewis T, D'Esposito M, et al. Eosinophilia-myalgia syndrome: selective cognitive impairment, longitudinal effects, and neuroimaging findings. *J Neurol Neurosurg Psychiatry* 1997;63:633–641.

414. White J. Bites and stings from venomous animals: a global overview. *Ther Drug Monit* 2000;22:65–68.

415. Satoyoshi E, Yamada K. Recurrent muscle spasms of central origin. *Arch Neurol* 1967;16:254–263.

416. Ehlayel MS, Lacassie Y. Satoyoshi syndrome: an unusual postnatal multisystemic disorder. *Am J Med Genet* 1995;57: 620–625.

417. Satoyoshi E. A syndrome of progressive muscle spasms, alopecia, and diarrhea. *Neurology* 1978;28:458–461.

418. Ikegawa S, Nagano A, Satoyoshi E. Skeletal abnormalities in Satoyoshi's syndrome: a radiographic study of eight cases. *Skel Radiol* 1993;22:321–324.

419. Yamagata T, Miyao M, Momoi M, et al. A case of generalized komuragaeri disease (Satoyoshi disease) treated with glucocorticoid. *Rinsho Shinkeigaku* 1991;31:79–83.

420. Satoh AI, Tsujihata M, Yashimura T, et al. Myasthenia gravis associated with Satoyoshi syndrome: muscle cramps, alopecia, and diarrhea. *Neurology* 1983;33:1209–1211.

421. Arita J, Hamano S, Nara T, et al. Intravenous gamma-globulin therapy of Satoyoshi syndrome. *Brain Dev* 1996;18:409–411.

422. Takahashi J, Takahashi S, Kikuchi T, et al. The siblings of painful muscle cramps (generalized muscle cramp disease) with alopecia and endocrinological disorders (in Japanese). *Rinsho Shinkeigaku* 1994;34:152–156.

423. Wisuthsarewong W, Likitmaskul S, Manonukul J. Satoyoshi syndrome. *Pediatric Dermatol* 2001;18:406–410.

424. Merello M, Garcia H, Nogues M, et al. Masticatory muscle spasm in a non-Japanese patient with Satoyoshi syndrome successfully treated with botulinum toxin. *Mov Disord* 1994; 9:104–105.

425. Katz J, Prescott K, Woolf AD. Strychnine poisoning from a Cambodian traditional remedy. *Am J Emerg Med* 1996;14:475–477.

426. Roos KL. Tetanus. *Semin Neurol* 1991;11:206–214.

427. Trujillo MJ, Castillo A, Espana JV, et al. Tetanus in the adult: intensive care and management experience with 233 cases. *Crit Care Med* 1980;8:419–423.

428. Trujillo MJ, Castillo A, Espana J, et al. Impact of intensive care management on the prognosis of tetanus: analysis of 641 cases. *Chest* 1987;92:63–65.

429. Crone NE, Reder AT. Severe tetanus in immunized patients with high anti-tetanus titers. *Neurology* 1992;42:761–764.

430. Apte NM, Kamad DR. Short report: the spatula test—a simple bedside test to diagnose tetanus. *Am J Trop Med Hyg* 1995; 53:386–387.

431. Risk WS, Bosch EP, Kimura J, et al. Chronic tetanus: clinical report and histochemistry of muscle. *Muscle Nerve* 1981;4: 363–366.

432. Melanby J, Green J. How does tetanus toxin act? *Neuroscience* 1981;6:281–300.

433. Bleck TP. Pharmacology of tetanus (review). *Clin Neuropharmacol* 1986;9:103–120.

434. Attygalle D, Rodrigo N. Magnesium sulphate for control of spasms in severe tetanus: can we avoid sedation and artificial ventilation? *Anaesthesia* 1997;52:956–962.

435. Moersch FP, Woltman HW. Progressive fluctuating muscular rigidity and spasm (stiffman syndrome): report of a case with some observations in 13 other cases. *Proc Staff Meet Mayo Clin* 1956;31:421–427.

436. Gordon EE, Janusko DM, Kaufman L. A critical survey of stiff-man syndrome. *Am J Med* 1967;42:589–599.

437. Whiteley AM, Swash M, Urish H. Progressive encephalomyelitis with rigidity: its relation to "subacute myoclonic spinal neuronitis" and to the "stiff-man syndrome." *Brain* 1976;99: 27–42.

438. Lorish TR, Thorsteinsson G, Howard FM Jr. Stiff-man syndrome updated. *Mayo Clin Proc* 1989;64:629–636.

439. McEvoy KM. Stiff-man syndrome. *Semin Neurol* 1991;11: 197–204.

440. Pleitez MY, Harati Y. Stiff-person syndrome. In: Rolak LA, Harati Y, eds. *Neuroimmunology for the clinician.* Boston: Butterworth, 1997:253–262.

441. Dalakas MC, Fujii M, Li M, et al. The clinical spectrum of anti-GAD antibody-positive patients with stiff-person syndrome. *Neurology* 2000;55:1531–1535.

442. Klein R, Haddow JE, DeLuca C. Familial congenital disorder resembling stiff-man syndrome. *Am J Dis Child* 1972;124: 730–731.

443. Sander JE, Layzer RB, Goldsobel AB. Congenital stiffman syndrome. *Ann Neurol* 1980;8:195–197.

444. Lingam S, Wilson J, Hart EW. Hereditary stiff-baby syndrome. *Am J Dis Child* 1981;135:909–911.

445. Schwartzman MJ, Mitsumoto H, Chou M, et al. Sudden death in stiff-man syndrome with autonomic instability (abst). *Ann Neurol* 1989;26:166.

446. Barker RA, Revesz T, Thom M, et al. Review of 23 patients affected by the stiff man syndrome: clinical subdivision into stiff trunk (man) syndrome, stiff limb syndrome, and progressive encephalomyelitis with rigidity. *J Neurol Neurosurg Psychiatry* 1998;65:633–640.

447. Saiz A, Graus F, Valldeoriola F, et al. Stiff-leg syndrome: a focal form of stiff-man syndrome. *Ann Neurol* 1998;43:400–403.

448. Leigh PN, Rothwell JC, Traub M, et al. A patient with reflex myoclonus and muscle rigidity: "jerking stiffman syndrome." *J Neurol Neurosurg Psychiatry* 1980;43:1125–1131.

449. Alberca R, Romero M, Chaparro J. Jerking-stiff-man syndrome. *J Neurol Neurosurg Psychiatry* 1982;45:1159–1160.

450. Meinck HM, Ricker K, Hulser PJ, et al. Stiff man syndrome: neurophysiological findings in eight patients. *J Neurol* 1995; 242:134–142.

451. Solimena M, Folli F, Aparisi R, et al. Autoantibodies to GABAergic neurons and pancreatic beta cells in stiff-man syndrome. *N Engl J Med* 1990;322:1555–1560.

452. Vincent A, Grimaldi LME, Martino G, et al. Antibodies to ^{125}I-glutamic acid decarboxylase in patients with stiff man syndrome. *J Neurol Neurosurg Psychiatry* 1997;62:395–397.

453. Asher R. A woman with the stiff-man syndrome. *Br Med J* 1958;1:265–266.

454. Trethowan WH, Allsop JL, Turner B. The "stiff-man" syndrome: a report of two further cases. *Arch Neurol* 1960;3: 448–456.

455. Meinck HM, Ricker K, Solimena M. Stiff-man syndrome: clinical and laboratory findings in eight patients. *J Neurol* 1994; 241:157–166.

456. Martinelli P, Pazzaglia P, Montagna P, et al. Stiff-man syndrome associated with nocturnal myoclonus and epilepsy. *J Neurol Neurosurg Psychiatry* 1978;41:463–465.

457. Fujiya S, Yahara O, Kawakami Y, et al. A case of stiffman syndrome with pathological changes in the spinal cord. *Nippon Naika Gakkai Zasshi* 1982;71:1154–1163.

458. Nakamura N, Fujiya S, Yahara O, et al. Stiff-man syndrome with spinal cord lesion. *Clin Neuropathol* 1986;5:40–46.

459. Guilleminault C, Sigwald J, Castaigne P. Sleep studies and therapeutic trial with L-dopa in a case of stiffman syndrome. *Eur Neurol* 1973;10:89–96.

460. Meinck HM, Ricker K, Conrad B. The stiff-man syndrome: new pathophysiologic aspects from abnormal exteroceptive reflexes and the response to clomipramine, clonidine, and tizanidine. *J Neurol Neurosurg Psychiatry* 1984;47:280–287.

461. Schmidt RT, Stahl SM, Spehlmann R. A pharmacologic study of the stiff-man syndrome: correlation of clinical symptoms with urinary 3-methoxy-4-hydroxyphenyl glycol excretion. *Neurology* 1975;25:622–626.

462. Isaacs H. Stiffman syndrome in a black girl. *J Neurol Neurosurg Psychiatry* 1979;42:988–994.

463. Solimena M, Folli F, Denis-Donini S, et al. Autoantibodies to glutamic acid decarboxylase in a patient with stiff-man syndrome, epilepsy, and type I diabetes mellitus. *N Engl J Med* 1988;318:1012–1020.

464. Solimena M, DeCamilli P. Autoimmunity to glutamic acid decarboxylase (GAD) in stiff-man syndrome and insulin-dependent diabetes mellitus. *Trends Neurosci* 1991;14:452–457.

465. Baekkeskov S, Aanstoot HJ, Chistgau S, et al. Identification of the 64K autoantigen in insulin-dependent diabetes as the GABA-synthesizing enzyme glutamic acid decarboxylase. *Nature* 1990;347:151–156.

466. Lohmann T, Hawa M, Leslie RD, et al. Immune reactivity to glutamic acid decarboxylase 65 in stiffman syndrome and type 1 diabetes mellitus. *Lancet* 2000;356:31–35.

467. Pugliese A, Solimena M, Awdeh ZL, et al. Association of HLA-DQBI*0201 with stiff-man syndrome. *J Clin Endocrinol Metab* 1993;77:1550–1553.

468. Grimaldi LM, Martino G, Braghi S, et al. Heterogeneity of autoantibodies in stiff-man syndrome. *Ann Neurol* 1993;34: 57–64.

469. Giometto B, Miotto D, Faresin F, et al. Anti-gabaergic neuron autoantibodies in a patient with stiff-man syndrome and ataxia. *J Neurol Sci* 1996;143:57–59.

470. Bjork E, Velloso LA, Kampe O, et al. GAD autoantibodies in IDDM, stiff-man syndrome, and autoimmune polyendocrine syndrome type I recognize different epitopes. *Diabetes* 1994; 43:161–165.

471. Martino G, Grimaldi LM, Bazzigaluppi E, et al. The insulin-dependent diabetes mellitus–associated ICA 105 autoantigen in stiff-man syndrome patients. *J Immunol* 1996;156:818–825.

472. Daw K, Ujihara N, Atkinson M, et al. Glutamic acid decarboxylase autoantibodies in stiff-man syndrome and insulin-dependent diabetes mellitus exhibit similarities and differences in epitope recognition. *J Immunol* 1996;156:818–825.

473. Kim J, Namchuk M, Bugawan T, et al. Higher autoantibody levels and recognition of a linear NH_2-terminal epitope in the autoantigen GAD65, distinguish stiff-man syndrome from insulin-dependent diabetes mellitus. *J Exp Med* 1994;180: 595–606.

474. George TM, Burke JM, Sobotka PA, et al. Resolution of stiffman syndrome with cortisol replacement in a patient with deficiencies of ACTH, growth hormone, and prolactin. *N Engl J Med* 1984;310:1511–1513.

475. Werk EE Jr, Sholiton LJ, Mamell RT. The "stiff-man" syndrome and hyperthyroidism. *Am J Med* 1961;31:647–653.

476. Trojaborg W, Rowland LP, Katz RI, et al. Stiff muscles and bony tendons. *Trans Am Neurol Assoc* 1970;95:169–171.

477. Drake ME Jr. Stiff-man syndrome and dementia. *Am J Med* 1983;74:1085–1987.

478. Rushworth G, Lishman WA, Hughes JT, et al. Intensive rigidity of the arms due to isolation of motoneurons by spinal tumor. *J Neurol Psychiatry* 1961;24:132–142.

479. Brown P, Rothwell JC, Marsden CD. The stiff leg syndrome. *J Neurol Neurosurg Psychiatry* 1997;62:31–37.

480. Kasperek S, Zebrowski S. Stiff-man syndrome and encephalomyelitis: report of a case. *Arch Neurol* 1971;24:22–30.

481. Lhermitte F, Chain F, Escouvolle R, et al. Un nouveau cas de contracture tetaniforme distinct du "stiffman syndrome." *Rev Neurol* 1973;128:321.

482. Howell DA, Lees AJ, Toghill PJ. Spinal internuncial neurones in progressive encephalomyelitis with rigidity. *J Neurol Neurosurg Psychiatry* 1979;42:773–785.

483. Watanabe K, Shimizu T, Mannen T, et al. An autopsy case with unusual muscle rigidity resembling the stiff-man syndrome. *Clin Neurol (Tokyo)* 1984;24:839–847.

484. Bum DJ, Ball J, Lees AJ, et al. A case of progressive encephalomyelitis with rigidity and positive antiglutamic acid decarboxylase antibodies. *J Neurol Neurosurg Psychiatry* 1991;54:449–451.

485. Armon C, Swanson JW, McLean JM, et al. Subacute encephalomyelitis presenting as stiff-person syndrome: clinical, polygraphic, and pathologic correlations. *Mov Disord* 1996;11:701–709.

486. Antoine JC, Absi L, Honnorat J, et al. Antiamphiphysin antibodies are associated with various paraneoplastic neurological syndromes and tumors. *Arch Neurol* 1999;56:172–177.

487. Schmierer K, Grosse P, De Camilli P, et al. Paraneoplastic stiff-person syndrome: no tumor progression over 5 years. *Neurology* 2002;58:148.

488. Miller F, Korsvik H. Baclofen in the treatment of stiffman syndrome. *Ann Neurol* 1981;9:511–512.

489. Vermeij FH, van Doom PA, Busch HF. Improvement of stiff-man syndrome with vigabatrin. *Lancet* 1996;348:612.

490. Prevett MC, Brown P, Duncan JS. Improvement of stiffman syndrome with vigabatrin. *Neurology* 1997;48:1133–1134.

491. Murinson BB, Rizzo M. Improvement of stiff-person syndrome with tiagabine. *Neurology* 2001;57:366.

492. Stayer C, Tronnier V, Dressnandt J, et al. Intrathecal baclofen therapy for stiff-man syndrome and progressive encephalomyelopathy with rigidity and myoclonus. *Neurology* 1997;49:1591–1597.

493. Barker RA, Marsden CD. Successful treatment of stiff man syndrome with intravenous immunoglobulin (letter). *J Neurol Neurosurg Psychiatry* 1997;62:426–427.

494. Dalakas MC, Fujii M, Li M, et al. High-dose intravenous immune globulin for stiff-person syndrome. *N Engl J Med* 2001;345:1870–1876.

495. Jacobsen JH, Rosenberg RS, Huttenlocher PR, et al. Familial nocturnal cramping. *Sleep* 1986;9:54–60.

496. Chiba S, Saitoh M, Hatanaka Y, et al. Autosomal dominant muscle cramp syndrome in a Japanese family. *J Neurol Neurosurg Psychiatry* 1999;67:116–119.

497. Matthews WB. Tonic seizures in multiple sclerosis. *Brain* 1958;81:193–206.

498. Twomey JA, Espir MLE. Paroxysmal symptoms as the first manifestation of multiple sclerosis. *J Neurol Neurosurg Psychiatry* 1980;43:296–304.

499. Heath PD, Nightingale S. Clusters of tonic spasms as an initial manifestation of multiple sclerosis. *Ann Neurol* 1982;12:494–495.

500. Berger JR, Sheremata WA, Melamed G. Paroxysmal dystonia as the initial manifestation of multiple sclerosis. *Arch Neurol* 1984;41:747–750.

501. Shibasaki H, Kuroiwa Y. Painful tonic seizure in multiple sclerosis. *Arch Neurol* 1974;30:47–51.

502. Matthews WB. Paroxysmal symptoms in multiple sclerosis. *J Neurol Neurosurg Psychiatry* 1975;38:617–623.

503. Osterman PO, Westberg CE. Paroxysmal attacks in multiple sclerosis. *Brain* 1975;98:198–202.

504. Watson CP, Chiu M. Painful tonic seizures in multiple sclerosis: localization of a lesion. *Can J Neurol Sci* 1979;6:359–361.

505. Rose MR, Ball JA, Thompson PD. Magnetic resonance imaging in tonic spasms of multiple sclerosis. *J Neurol* 1993;241:115–117.

506. Lataste X, Emre M, Davis C, et al. Comparative profile of tizanidine in the management of spasticity. *Neurology* 1994;44 [Suppl 9]:S53–S59.

507. Penn RD. Intrathecal baclofen for spasticity of spinal origin: seven years of experience. *J Neurosurg* 1992;77:236–240.

FRONTOTEMPORAL DEMENTIA AND OTHER TAUOPATHIES

HUW R. MORRIS

Two aspects of frontotemporal dementia and parkinsonism linked to chromosome 17 (FTDP-17) are of particular interest to movement disorders physicians. First, FTDP-17 should be considered in the differential diagnosis of young-onset or autosomal dominant neurodegenerative conditions with extrapyramidal and/or cognitive features. Second, the pathologic processes involved in FTDP-17 may elucidate the pathogenesis of more common sporadic tau deposition neurodegenerative diseases (tauopathies), such as progressive supranuclear palsy (PSP) and corticobasal degeneration (CBD), which commonly present as Parkinson's-plus syndromes. The biochemical classification of tauopathies, together with the genetic information derived from the study of FTDP-17, provides a framework for understanding and classifying this group of diseases. This chapter describes FTDP-17, its genetic basis, and its relationship to other tauopathies. In addition, recent data on its clinical features and the types of movement disorders that may be seen in FTDP-17 are reviewed.

FTDP-17

The identification of linkage to chromosome 17q21 in the dementia–disinhibition——parkinsonism–amyotrophy complex family (DDPAC, family Mo) led to a series of reports of further families with FTD linked to this region, summarized in a 1996 workshop report on FTDP-17 (1,2). Subsequent reports of the clinical features of chromosome 17–linked families described broadly similar syndromes although each was given a distinct name. These families included pallidopontinonigral degeneration (PPND) (3), progressive subcortical gliosis (PSG) (4), and familial multisystem tauopathy with presenile dementia (FMSTD) (5). In addition, three Dutch families were described with hereditary frontotemporal dementia linked to chromosome 17 (6). Affected individuals in these families presented between the ages of 40 and 50 with early personality change and disinhibition, later followed by withdrawal and apathy. Many of the families had extrapyramidal syndromes (2).

The pathologic topography of these families was similar. Frontal and temporal atrophy was a consistent finding, together with involvement of the substantia nigra, amygdala, and caudate/putamen/globus pallidus (2). Initially, there was more heterogeneity in the description of the immunohistochemical pathology of these diseases. The report of the 1996 workshop concluded that the FTDP-17 families could be pathologically divided into four groups: tau pathology with ballooned neurons; tau pathology without ballooned neurons; ballooned neurons alone; and dementia without specific pathologic features (2). The majority of these families have subsequently been shown to have significant tau deposition pathology (7) and mutations in the *tau* gene (8).

FTDP-17 AND TAU MUTATIONS

Tau protein has been intensively studied because tau neurofibrillary tangles are a prominent part of the pathology of Alzheimer's disease (9). The normal function of tau protein is to bind to tubulin, to promote its polymerization into microtubules, and to maintain microtubular stability. Tau is a small molecule that has a number of microtubule binding domains located at its carboxy terminus. The *tau* gene is alternatively spliced to form six different protein isoforms in adult human brain, which vary in the presence or absence of a fourth microtubule binding domain encoded by exon 10, and an amino terminus insert encoded by exons 2 and 3 (9). The four potential microtubule binding domains consist of imperfectly repeated sequences, so that tau protein containing the exon 10 domain is referred to as four-repeat tau, and tau lacking exon 10 is known as three-repeat tau. Tau is deposited as neurofibrillary tangles in Alzheimer's disease and also deposited in a number of other neurodegenerative conditions, sometimes referred to as tauopathies. These conditions are diverse and include Alzheimer's disease, PSP, and CBD, but also the Guam parkinsonism-dementia complex, postencephalitic parkinsonism, familial British dementia, posttraumatic parkinsonism, subacute sclerosing panencephalitis, and Niemann-Pick disease type C. The *tau* gene is encoded on chromosome 17q and was a strong candidate gene for FTDP-17. Three reports in 1998 described pathogenic *tau* mutations in FTDP-17 families. The *tau* exon 12 coding change V337M was described in the FTDP-17 family Seattle family A (10). This sequence change was reported together with a number of polymorphic variants in *tau*. Three supportive criteria for the definition of a pathogenic mutation were met: (a) cosegregation of the mutant allele with the disease phenotype; (b) evolutionary conservation of the wild-type residue; (c) absence of the mutant allele in a series of control chromosomes. Hutton and co-workers were able to conclusively demonstrate that *tau* was the causative gene for FTDP-17 by describing six separate coding and intronic mutations in *tau*, and by providing an explanation for the mechanism of action of the intronic mutations (11). The coding mutations described were G272V, P301L, and R406W. G272V and P301L disrupt the microtubule binding domains of exons 9 and 10, respectively. The exon 13 mutation R406W occurs adjacent to two serine residues, Ser396 and Ser404, which may act as sites for phosphorylation by Ser/Thr-Pro–directed protein kinases (11). The intronic mutations seem capable of causing neurodegeneration and tau deposition without altering the tau protein coding sequence. The splicing mutations that occur at the *tau* exon 10 intron–exon junction, exon 10 +13, +14 and +16, were proposed to alter the splicing of exon 10 and the normal ratio between four-repeat and three-repeat tau. This hypothesis has been supported by both in vitro evidence, demonstrating the effect of this sequence variation on exon 10 splicing in an exon-trapping system, and in vivo evidence, using RNA and protein analysis from postmortem

tissue (11,12). It appears that in these autosomal dominant families, alteration of the normal tau four-repeat/three-repeat protein ratio can lead to neurodegeneration with parkinsonism and dementia. The original chromosome 17–linked family DDPAC was shown to have a *tau* exon 10 +14 mutation. An additional *tau* splice site mutation, exon 10 +3, was described in the FTDP-17 family FMSTD by Spillantini and colleagues (12). The *tau* splicing hypothesis was supported in this publication by protein analysis of tau in the family and demonstration of an abnormal tau protein isoform ratio (12).

Since the original description of *tau* mutations in 1998, a number of other mutations have been described together with molecular pathologic data and in vitro data on their possible functional effects (Table 34.1). There are three main groups of tau mutations—exon 10 splicing mutations, exon 10 coding mutations, and non–exon 10 coding mutations—and each has a separate molecular pathologic profile. As described, intronic mutations are believed to affect the alternative splicing of *tau* through disruption of a stem loop structure (13). In addition to the exon–intron boundary splicing mutations, exonic mutations have been described that affect the splicing of tau exon 10. These mutations, some of which do not lead to an amino acid substitution, are postulated to either increase the efficiency of an exon splice enhancer element (e.g., N279K) or decrease the efficiency of an exonic splice inhibitor (e.g., L284L) (13). Support for this hypothesis of the effect of exon 10 splicing mutations comes both from postmortem tau RNA analysis and from in vitro analysis of the exon 10 region with containing the described sequence changes (13). Exon 10 coding mutations lead to a deposition of tau containing neurofibrillary tangles with predominantly four-

TABLE 34.1. TAU MUTATIONS AND THEIR EFFECTS

Tau Mutation	Microtubule Interaction (Either Binding or Stabilization)	Filament Formation	4R:3R Tau RNA Isoform Ratio	Ref.
G272V	↓	↑	NA	11,14,15
N279K	↔	—	↑	49,50
ΔK280	↓	—	↓	13,32
L284L	↔	↔	↑	13
P301L	↓	↑	↔	15
P301S	↓	↑	NA	11,14
S305N	↔	↔	↑	14,37,50
S305S	↔	↔	↑	43
Exon 10 +3	—	—	↑	41
Exon 10 +12	—	—	↑	51
Exon 10 +13	—	—	↑	11
Exon 10 +14	—	—	↑	11
Exon 10 +16	—	—	↑	11
V337M	↓	↑	—	14,15
G389R	↓	NA	NA	19
R406W	↓	↔	NA	11,14,15

"Effect" refers to the pure mutation containing protein or RNA. The alteration in the 4R:3R ratio may have secondary effects on microtubule interaction or filament formation.

TABLE 34.2. BIOCHEMICAL AND GENETIC CLASSIFICATION OF TAUOPATHIES

Tau Isoforms	Three- and Four-Repeat Tau		Four-Repeat Tau		Three-Repeat Tau	
Hyperphosphorylated tau Western blot	Triplet (59,64,68)		Doublet (64,68)		Doublet (59,64)	
Inheritance	Familial	Sporadic	Familial	Sporadic	Familial	Sporadic
Filament ultrastructure	Paired helical	Paired helical		Straight		
Diseases	Alzheimer's disease	Exon 10 FTDP-17	PSP	Myotonic dystrophy	Pick's disease	Pick's disease
	Non-exon 10 FTDP-17	PDC	PSP	CBD	FTDP-17: G389R ΔK280 (?) K257T	
	PDC (?)	PEP				

FTDP-17, frontotemporal dementia with parkinsonism linked to chromosome 17; PDC, Guam parkinsonism-dementia complex; PEP, postencephalitic parkinsonism; CBD, corticobasal degeneration; PSP, progressive supranuclear palsy.

repeat tau isoforms, without a concomitant change in RNA splicing (11). Non–exon 10 coding mutations lead to a deposition of both four-repeat and three-repeat tau, like Alzheimer's disease (Table 34.2) (7).

Experimental evidence has been gathered for two different effects of the tau coding mutations: first, an acceleration of filament formation, and second, loss of binding to and alteration in the stabilization of microtubules (Table 34.1) (14–17). Both mechanisms may be important and contribute to neural toxicity, and the balance between these two mechanisms is difficult to determine. However, perhaps significantly, the mutation P301S has a more marked effect on acceleration of filament formation than P301L, whereas for microtubule destabilization the situation is reversed. Given the very early age of disease onset in families with P301S, and the more aggressive neurodegeneration associated with this mutation, the clinicogenetic correlation suggests that acceleration of filament formation may be a more important factor than microtubule destabilization in disease pathogenesis.

CLASSIFICATION OF TAUOPATHIES

Sporadic and familial tauopathies can be classified according to the type of tau protein deposited. Alzheimer's disease involves deposition of all six isoforms of the alternatively spliced *tau* gene to produce a major triplet of abnormal hyperphosphorylated protein bands on Western blotting (59, 64, and 68 kd) (7,18). PSP involves the preferential deposition of four-repeat tau and the formation of a doublet of protein bands (64 and 68 kd). Pick's disease involves the predominant deposition of three-repeat tau with a smaller doublet of protein bands (59 and 64 kd). Familial and sporadic tauopathies can be classified according to this system, and the type of tau mutation correlates with the pattern of tau deposition (Table 34.2). Most non–exon 10 coding mutations lead to the deposition of all six isoforms of tau as

a major triplet of tau protein bands. Some non–exon 10 tau mutations, such as K257T and G389R, lead to a Pick's disease-like pathologic phenotype, with the formation of dense round tau immunoreactive inclusions, very similar to Pick bodies (19,20). The tau deposited in these Pick's disease-like kindreds forms a smaller doublet of hyperphosphorylated tau bands on Western blotting, like sporadic Pick's disease. Exon 10 coding and exon 10 splicing mutations lead to the deposition of predominantly four repeat tau similarly to PSP and CBD (Table 34.2). Rarer tau deposition disorders such as postencephalitic parkinsonism and Guam parkinsonism-dementia complex can also be classified according to this scheme, following biochemical analysis of the tau profiles in these diseases (21,22).

Thus, for each of the sporadic tauopathies a familial genetic form exists that provides a model for understanding the disease pathogenesis and for developing new treatments. The relationship between PSP/CBD and FTDP-17 is of particular interest. Sporadic forms of PSP and CBD are associated with a common population wide variant in *tau*—the A0 allele of the *tau* intronic dinucleotide polymorphism, which lies on the *tau* H1 haplotype (23–26). Possession of this disease-associated haplotype is not in itself sufficient to cause PSP or CBD, but it is overrepresented in the PSP/CBD population indicating a positive disease association. This *tau* haplotype association does not apply to Pick's disease (27,28). If PSP is regarded as a sporadic version of exon 10 mutation FTDP-17, then this is likely to be one of a few conditions in which a common variant (*tau* H1) and rare mutations (*tau* exon 10) of the same gene can lead to related conditions. In other words, there are very low penetrance and high penetrance changes present in the same gene.

Some individual mutations in *tau* have been described that have clinical or pathologic features that are particularly similar to those expressed in PSP, and these are discussed in the following section. However, although there may be close clinical and pathologic similarities between PSP and

FTDP-17, the vast majority of sporadic and familial cases of PSP do not involve mutations in *tau* (24,29,30).

CLINICAL ASPECTS

Reed and colleagues have recently published a comprehensive review of the clinical features of FTDP-17 (8). The prevalence of tau mutations in clinically ascertained families with FTD has been described as 43% and 50% in European studies, and 9.4% and 10.5% in North American studies (31–34). These differences in the estimates of *tau* gene mutation frequency may relate to the presence of founder effects in the European population or to the type of family history required for inclusion in these studies. In general, the age of onset for the majority of FTDP-17 cases is between 40 and 60 years of age, with a disease duration of around 8 to 13 years (35). There are some kindreds that differ from that pattern. Two mutations seem to manifest at a particularly early age and may have a rapidly progressive course. The P301S mutation families have a usual age of onset in the twenties with a disease duration of around 8 years, and the Japanese S305N kindred has an average age of onset of 35 with disease duration of 6 years in one individual (36,37). Conversely, the R406W kindred has a later age of onset, in the late fifties or sixties, and an indolent clinical course with an average disease duration of 26 years in one family (38).

The DDPAC kindred has typical clinical features. In the DDPAC kindred insidious personality change with disinhibition begins at an average age of 45. This is often accompanied by hypersexuality and hyperphagia. DDPAC patients become increasingly withdrawn, apathetic, and emotionally blunted (39). L-Dopa-unresponsive parkinsonism is a feature of each DDPAC case. One patient (case III-39) also developed clinical amyotrophy with electromyographic evidence of widespread denervation. Despite the name given to this kindred, the clinical features of anterior horn cell disease are not present in other members, and this has included normal electromyographic examination in two further cases.

Many of the kindreds are described as having L-dopa-unresponsive parkinsonism, and this is particularly common in the exon 10 (coding and splicing) mutations that lead to the deposition of four-repeat tau (8). This correlation may be of relevance to sporadic neurodegeneration given that PSP and CBD also involve the deposition of four-repeat tau. The parkinsonism is usually described as involving symmetric bradykinesia and rigidity without tremor. In Janssen and colleagues' series of FTDP-17 families with *tau* exon 10 +16 mutations, one of the more common extrapyramidal presentations was an adverse response to neuroleptic medication (40). Some kindreds have a specifically PSP-like presentation. The clinical features of the exon 10 +3 mutation, originally described in the

FMSTD kindred, are particularly striking. Members of this family present with disequilibrium and go on to develop axial rigidity, dysphagia, and vertical gaze palsy (5). However, the extent and type of neuronal and glial tau deposition in this kindred is far more extensive than that seen in PSP (41). This mutation has also been described in a British family in which, remarkably, in the later stages of the disease chorea was described (42). This seems to be a family-specific feature since other members of this family had been initially diagnosed as having Huntington's disease although this was not genetically confirmed. In general, chorea is not a feature of FTDP-17. Several families have been described to have pathologic and/or clinical features reminiscent of PSP. These families possess the autosomal dominant mutations *tau* exon 10 +3, S305S, N279K, and R406W (12,38, 43,44). Interestingly, a PSP-like phenotype has recently been described in a family with a homozygous deletion of codon 296 of tau (ΔK296) (45). In addition to exon 10 +3, families that have been described as having a supranuclear gaze palsy include DDPAC (exon 10 +14), PPND (N279K), and S305S (39,43,44). Although several families have been described as having pathologic CBD-like features, typical asymmetric apraxia, dystonia, and cortical sensory loss has occurred most clearly in the exon 10–coding mutation family, P301S (46). Reports of clinical and pathologic CBD-like features in some but not all individuals in this family and in the exon 10 +16 progressive subcortical gliosis family suggest that there are genetic or environmental cofactors that govern the expression of a CBD phenotype within individual kindreds (46,47). This may also be of relevance to sporadic disease given that CBD and PSP may both be related to a common underlying genetic risk factor, the *tau* H1 haplotype, and perhaps factors governing phenotypic heterogeneity within families are also important in sporadic cases. Further non-extrapyramidal phenotypic heterogeneity is present in that the young-onset aggressive FTD caused by the P301S mutation may involve a seizure disorder—all three individuals studied in detail by Sperfeld and colleagues developed clinical and electroencephalographic evidence of a partial and secondary generalized seizure disorder (36).

A recent publication from Wszolek and colleagues described in detail the longitudinal progression of FTDP-17 in individuals with PPND due to the N279K mutation (48). The individual described initially developed asymmetric mild tremor, stiffness, and rigidity together with other parkinsonian features. Within a year of the onset of his motor symptoms he developed cognitive impairment leading to problems with work, and an initial favorable response to L-dopa seemed to diminish. Two years after the disease onset frontal release signs were apparent, together with a supranuclear gaze palsy. The patient died 6 years after disease onset, having become anarthric and developed extensive dystonia/spasticity. The authors describe the distinction between parkinsonism and cognitive predominant form of

FTDP-17 (8,48). The patient described could have been diagnosed to have idiopathic Parkinson's disease in the earliest stage of the illness, but the subsequent course illustrates the emergence of both cognitive and atypical parkinsonian features, pointing to FTDP-17. Some cases of FTDP-17 have been described in which tau mutation neurodegeneration occurred as an apparently sporadic phenomenon presumably due to low-penetrance mutations or to nonpaternity. However, it should be emphasized that despite the clinical and pathologic similarities between FTDP-17, PSP, CBD, and Pick's disease, the vast majority of patients with PSP, CBD, and Pick's disease do not have mutations in *tau*, including familial forms of these diseases (24,27,30). It could be argued that *tau* mutations define a disease as being FTDP-17, and thus by exclusion not PSP, CBD, or Pick's.

Tau mutation screening should be reserved for those with a positive family history of an FTDP-17-like disorder or atypical neurodegenerative disease cases with a young age at onset. The highest yield from *tau* mutation screening comes from sequencing *tau* in families in which there is an autosomal dominant history of FTD with a pathologically confirmed diagnosis of tau-related FTD (34). The presence of extensive glial pathology should direct the *tau* analysis to sequencing exon 10 of *tau*, which seems to be particularly correlated with glial and neuronal tau deposition.

CONCLUSION

The initial descriptions of the mutations in *tau* in FTDP-17 led immediately to a wealth of information on further mutations, proposed pathogenic mechanisms, and molecular pathologic correlation. The clinical data on these conditions is being reevaluated and categorized, and although there is phenotypic heterogeneity between FTDP-17 families, broad patterns are emerging, particularly in the similarities between exon 10 mutation FTDP-17 and PSP and CBD. While the pathologic mechanisms underlying these disease are clearly of central importance, accurate clinicopathologic description and classification of these families provides a crucial framework for understanding these diseases. The genetics of FTD is likely to move on to the analysis of the genes responsible for other kindreds with FTD, such as motor neuron disease inclusion dementia and chromosome 3–linked FTD, and the clinicopathologic correlation in these "new" diseases with different pathologies and genetic causes will become of even greater interest (34).

REFERENCES

1. Wilhelmsen KC, Lynch T, Pavlou E, et al. Localization of disinhibition-dementia-parkinsonism-amyotrophy complex to 17q21-22. *Am J Hum Genet* 1994;55(6):1159–1165.
2. Foster NL, Wilhelmsen K, Sima AA, et al. Frontotemporal dementia and parkinsonism linked to chromosome 17: a consensus conference. *Ann Neurol* 1997;41(6):706–715.
3. Wijker M, Wszolek ZK, Wolters EC, et al. Localization of the gene for rapidly progressive autosomal dominant parkinsonism and dementia with pallido-ponto-nigral degeneration to chromosome 17q21. *Hum Mol Genet* 1996;5(1):151–154.
4. Petersen RB, Tabaton M, Chen SG, et al. Familial progressive subcortical gliosis: presence of prions and linkage to chromosome 17. *Neurology* 1995;45(6):1062–1067.
5. Murrell JR, Koller D, Foroud T, et al. Familial multiple-system tauopathy with presenile dementia is localized to chromosome 17. *Am J Hum Genet* 1997;61(5):1131–1138.
6. Heutink P, Stevens M, Rizzu P, et al. Hereditary frontotemporal dementia is linked to chromosome 17q21-q22: a genetic and clinicopathological study of three Dutch families. *Ann Neurol* 1997;41(2):150–159.
7. Spillantini MG, Bird TD, Ghetti B. Frontotemporal dementia and parkinsonism linked to chromosome 17: a new group of tauopathies. *Brain Pathol* 1998;8(2):387–402.
8. Reed LA, Wszolek ZK, Hutton M. Phenotypic correlations in FTDP-17. *Neurobiol Aging* 2001;22(1):89–107.
9. Goedert M. Tau protein and the neurofibrillary pathology of Alzheimer's disease. *Trends Neurosci* 1993;16:460–465.
10. Poorkaj P, Bird TD, Wijsman E, et al. Tau is a candidate gene for chromosome 17 frontotemporal dementia. *Ann Neurol* 1998;43 (6):815–825.
11. Hutton M, Lendon CL, Rizzu P, et al. Association of missense and 5′-splice-site mutations in tau with the inherited dementia FTDP-17. *Nature* 1998;393(6686):702–705.
12. Spillantini MG, Murrell JR, Goedert M, et al. Mutation in the tau gene in familial multiple system tauopathy with presenile dementia. *Proc Natl Acad Sci USA* 1998;95(13):7737–7741.
13. D'Souza I, Poorkaj P, Hong M, et al. Missense and silent tau gene mutations cause frontotemporal dementia with parkinsonism-chromosome 17 type, by affecting multiple alternative RNA splicing regulatory elements. *Proc Natl Acad Sci USA* 1999;96 (10):5598–5603.
14. Goedert M, Jakes R, Crowther RA. Effects of frontotemporal dementia FTDP-17 mutations on heparin-induced assembly of tau filaments. *FEBS Lett* 1999;450(3):306–311.
15. Hasegawa M, Smith MJ, Goedert M. Tau proteins with FTDP-17 mutations have a reduced ability to promote microtubule assembly. *FEBS Lett* 1998;437(3):207–210.
16. DeTure M, Ko LW, Yen S, et al. Missense tau mutations identified in FTDP-17 have a small effect on tau–microtubule interactions. *Brain Res* 2000;853(1):5–14.
17. Nacharaju P, Lewis J, Easson C, et al. Accelerated filament formation from tau protein with specific FTDP-17 missense mutations. *FEBS Lett* 1999;447(2-3):195–199.
18. Spillantini MG, Goedert M. Tau protein pathology in neurodegenerative diseases. *Trends Neurosci* 1998;21(10):428–433.
19. Murrell JR, Spillantini MG, Zolo P, et al. Tau gene mutation G389R causes a tauopathy with abundant pick body-like inclusions and axonal deposits. *J Neuropathol Exp Neurol* 1999;58(12): 1207–1226.
20. Rizzini C, Goedert M, Hodges JR, et al. Tau gene mutation K257T causes a tauopathy similar to Pick's disease. *J Neuropathol Exp Neurol* 2000;59(11):990–1001.
21. Buee-Scherrer V, Buee L, Leveugle B, et al. Pathological tau proteins in postencephalitic parkinsonism: comparison with Alzheimer's disease and other neurodegenerative disorders. *Ann Neurol* 1997;42(3):356–359.
22. Perez-Tur J, Buee L, Morris HR, et al. Neurodegenerative diseases of Guam: analysis of TAU. *Neurology* 1999;53(2):411–413.
23. Houlden H, Baker M, Morris HR, et al. Corticobasal degenera-

tion and progressive supranuclear palsy share a common tau haplotype. *Neurology* 2001;56(12):1702–1706.

24. Baker M, Litvan I, Houlden H, et al. Association of an extended haplotype in the tau gene with progressive supranuclear palsy. *Hum Mol Genet* 1999;8(4):711–715.

25. Conrad C, Andreadis A, Trojanowski JQ, et al. Genetic evidence for the involvement of tau in progressive supranuclear palsy. *Ann Neurol* 1997;41:277–281.

26. Morris HR, Janssen JC, Bandmann O, et al. The tau gene A0 polymorphism in progressive supranuclear palsy and related neurodegenerative diseases. *J Neurol Neurosurg Psychiatry* 1999; 66(5):665–667.

27. Morris HR, Baker M, Yasojima K, et al. Analysis of tau haplotypes in Pick's disease. *Neurology* (submitted).

28. Russ C, Lovestone S, Baker M, et al. The extended haplotype of the microtubule associated protein tau gene is not associated with Pick's disease. *Neurosci Lett* 2001;299(1–2):156–158.

29. Hoenicka J, Perez M, Perez-Tur J, et al. The tau gene A0 allele and progressive supranuclear palsy. *Neurology* 1999;53(6): 1219–1225.

30. Morris HR, Katzenschlager R, Janssen JC, et al. Sequence analysis of tau in familial and sporadic progressive supranuclear palsy. *J Neurol Neurosurg Psychiatry* 2002;72:388–390.

31. Houlden H, Baker M, Adamson J, et al. Frequency of tau mutations in three series of non-Alzheimer's degenerative dementia. *Ann Neurol* 1999;46(2):243–248.

32. Rizzu P, Van Swieten JC, Joosse M, et al. High prevalence of mutations in the microtubule-associated protein tau in a population study of frontotemporal dementia in the Netherlands. *Am J Hum Genet* 1999;64(2):414–421.

33. Poorkaj P, Grossman M, Steinbart E, et al. Frequency of tau gene mutations in familial and sporadic cases of non-Alzheimer dementia. *Arch Neurol* 2001;58(3):383–387.

34. Morris HR, Khan MN, Janssen JC, et al. The genetic and pathological classification of familial frontotemporal dementia. *Arch Neurol* 2001;58:1813–1816.

35. van Swieten JC, Stevens M, Rosso SM, et al. Phenotypic variation in hereditary frontotemporal dementia with tau mutations. *Ann Neurol* 1999;46(4):617–626.

36. Sperfeld AD, Collatz MB, Baier H, et al. FTDP-17: an early-onset phenotype with parkinsonism and epileptic seizures caused by a novel mutation. *Ann Neurol* 1999;46(5):708–715.

37. Iijima M, Tabira T, Poorkaj P, et al. A distinct familial presenile dementia with a novel missense mutation in the tau gene. *Neuroreport* 1999;10(3):497–501.

38. Reed LA, Grabowski TJ, Schmidt ML, et al. Autosomal dominant dementia with widespread neurofibrillary tangles. *Ann Neurol* 1997;42(4):564–572.

39. Lynch T, Sano M, Marder KS, et al. Clinical characteristics of a family with chromosome 17-linked disinhibition-dementia-parkinsonism-amyotrophy complex. *Neurology* 1994;44(10): 1878–1884.

40. Janssen JC, Warrington EK, Morris HR, et al. Clinical features of frontotemporal dementia due to the intronic tau 10 +16 mutation. *Neurology* 2002;58:1161–1168.

41. Spillantini MG, Goedert M, Crowther RA, et al. Familial multiple system tauopathy with presenile dementia: a disease with abundant neuronal and glial tau filaments. *Proc Natl Acad Sci USA* 1997;94:4113–4118.

42. Tolnay M, Grazia Spillantini M, Rizzini C, et al. A new case of frontotemporal dementia and parkinsonism resulting from an intron 10 +3-splice site mutation in the tau gene: clinical and pathological features. *Neuropathol Appl Neurobiol* 2000;26(4): 368–378.

43. Stanford PM, Halliday GM, Brooks WS, et al. Progressive supranuclear palsy pathology caused by a novel silent mutation in exon 10 of the tau gene: expansion of the disease phenotype caused by tau gene mutations. *Brain* 2000;123(Pt 5):880–893.

44. Delisle MB, Murrell JR, Richardson R, et al. A mutation at codon 279 (N279K) in exon 10 of the Tau gene causes a tauopathy with dementia and supranuclear palsy. *Acta Neuropathol (Berl)* 1999;98(1):62–77.

45. Pastor P, Pastor E, Carnero C, et al. Familial atypical progressive supranuclear palsy associated with homozygosity for the delN296 mutation in the tau gene. *Ann Neurol* 2001;49(2):263–267.

46. Bugiani O, Murrell JR, Giaccone G, et al. Frontotemporal dementia and corticobasal degeneration in a family with a P301S mutation in tau. *J Neuropathol Exp Neurol* 1999;58(6):667–677.

47. Goedert M, Spillantini MG, Crowther RA, et al. Tau gene mutation in familial progressive subcortical gliosis. *Nat Med* 1999; 5(4):454–457.

48. Wszolek ZK, Kardon RH, Wolters EC, et al. Frontotemporal dementia and parkinsonism linked to chromosome 17 (FTDP-17): PPND family: a longitudinal videotape demonstration. *Mov Disord* 2001;16(4):756–760.

49. Clark LN, Poorkaj P, Wszolek Z, et al. Pathogenic implications of mutations in the tau gene in pallido-ponto-nigral degeneration and related neurodegenerative disorders linked to chromosome 17. *Proc Natl Acad Sci USA* 1998;95(22):13103–13107.

50. Hasegawa M, Smith MJ, Iijima M, et al. FTDP-17 mutations N279K and S305N in tau produce increased splicing of exon 10. *FEBS Lett* 1999;443(2):93–96.

51. Yasuda M, Takamatsu J, D'Souza I, et al. A novel mutation at position +12 in the intron following exon 10 of the tau gene in familial frontotemporal dementia (FTD-Kumamoto). *Ann Neurol* 2000;47(4):422–429.

COGNITIVE AND BEHAVIORAL ASPECTS OF BASAL GANGLIA DISEASES

BRUNO DUBOIS
BERNARD PILLON

The basal ganglia have been implicated in cognitive processes and behavioral regulation on the basis of two main arguments. First, experimental studies in primates have shown that limited lesions of the striatum induce deficits in working memory, rule acquisition, and behavioral control. Second, cognitive changes have long been observed in patients with degenerative diseases that involve primarily the basal ganglia, such as Parkinson's disease (PD), Huntington's disease (HD), or progressive supranuclear palsy (PSP). From the clinical picture of these neurodegenerative disorders, the main changes postulated to result from basal ganglia dysfunction are slowing of information processing (1), dysexecutive syndrome (2), impaired memory retrieval (3), and personality changes such as inertia (4) and depressed mood (5). These symptoms have been brought together under the term *subcortical dementia* (6) in order to highlight the influence of deep gray matter structures on cognition and behavior. However, the term is debatable for at least two reasons. The clinical criteria commonly accepted by the American Psychiatric Association to define dementia do not fit well with patients whose global cognitive deficiency is mild or moderate and whose loss of autonomy can be largely attributed to associated movement disorders. Moreover, it cannot be firmly demonstrated that these deficits result from dysfunction of subcortical structures alone since associated lesions have been described in the cerebral cortex, as in Parkinson's disease dementia (7) or in PSP (8). For that reason, the cognitive and behavioral functions of the basal ganglia can be further drawn from observation of patients suffering from focal and isolated lesions within these structures (9,10). Such lesions induce changes that resemble the consequences of frontal lobe damage and, to a lesser extent, some features of neuropsychiatric disorders (11), raising the question of the underlying neuronal circuits that mediate these functions and of the specific contribution of the basal ganglia to cognitive processes and behavioral control.

This chapter will review the cognitive and behavioral changes observed in degenerative diseases, such as PD, diffuse Lewy body disease (DLBD), multiple system atrophy, PSP, HD, corticobasal degeneration (CBD), and in focal lesions of the basal ganglia.

PARKINSON'S DISEASE

Parkinson's disease is clinically and neuropathologically heterogeneous. It is therefore not surprising that the cognitive profiles of PD patients may vary. Complaints of patients and their families usually include forgetfulness, deficits of concentration, and decreased ability to follow conversations involving several persons. If one uses appropriate neuropsychological tests, it appears that cognitive deficits (a) may be found in up to 93% of patients; (b) mainly affect visuospatial, memory, and executive functions; and (c) are observed even at the early stages of the disease, when the lesions are considered to be restricted to the nigrostriatal dopaminergic pathway, strongly suggesting therefore that they may be related to the subcortical pathology of the disease (12). In contrast, a more global impairment is far less common.

Specific Changes in Nondemented Parkinson's Disease Patients

Visuospatial Dysfunction

Systematic neuropsychological testing has provided evidence of a visuospatial dysfunction in PD, even when tests require few motor components, leading some authors to claim that there may be a genuine visuospatial deficit in the disease. However, most attribute the impaired performance to the high cognitive demand of visuospatial paradigms that generally require set shifting, set maintaining, self-elaboration of the response, or forward planning capacity. Moreover, Bondi et al. (13) showed that visuospatial deficits disappeared once performance on frontal lobe–related tasks was statistically covaried. These data suggest that visuospatial disorders in PD result from a decrease in control of central processing resources rather than from a specific visu-

TABLE 35.1. BASAL GANGLIA DISEASES IMPAIR SPECIFIC ASPECTS OF MEMORY

"Frontal" and "basal ganglia" components are impaired
Working memory
    In PD [Fournet et al. (14)], PSP [Litvan et al. (15)], and HD [Moss et al. (16)]
Strategic aspects of encoding and recall
    In PD [Buytenhuijs et al. (17)], PSP [Sommer et al. (18)], HD [Kramer et al. (19)], CBD [Massman et al. (20)], and focal lesions
    [Bhatia and Marsden (9)]
Procedural learning
    In PD [Doyon et al. (21)], PSP [Grafman et al. (22)], HD [Knopman and Nissen (23)], and focal lesions [Dubois et al. (10)]
"Medial temporal" components are preserved
Recognition
    In PD [Vriezen and Moscovitch (24)], PSP [Litvan et al. (15)], HD [Butters (25)], and focal lesions [Mendez et al. (26)]
Cued recall
    In PD, PSP, HD, CBD [Pillon et al. (3,27,28)], and focal lesions [Dubois et al. (10)]

PD, Parkinson's disease; PSP, progressive supranuclear palsy; HD, Huntington's disease; CBD,
corticobasal degeneration; SND, striatonigral degeneration.

ospatial dysfunction. However, preattentive visual processing has been found impaired in patients with PD and might also interfere with visuospatial deficits.

Memory Disorders

Several memory processes are impaired in PD (Table 35.1). *Working memory* capacity is decreased, as shown by defective short-term recall on tasks requiring the inhibition of interfering stimuli; sequential digit ordering; spatial organization; or capacity to generate information randomly. *Long-term memory* is impaired as well. In fact, storage abilities that are under the control of the temporal lobes are preserved in the disease insofar as we consider the slopes of learning curves and maintenance of information after a delay. In contrast, PD patients are impaired in tasks involving (a) organization of the material to be remembered; (b) temporal ordering; or (c) conditional associative learning. In other words, a deficit of internal control of attention disrupts the performance of PD patients in tasks requiring the spontaneous generation of efficient encoding and retrieval strategies (29). There is evidence that *procedural learning* is also impaired to some extent. For example, nondemented

PD patients show less procedural learning than control subjects in rotor pursuit, serial reaction time task, mirror reading, and Tower of Toronto task. However, the results depend on the severity of the dysexecutive syndrome. A difficulty in the maintenance of attention might, therefore, explain these procedural deficits.

Dysexecutive Syndrome

The cognitive domain of executive functions refers to the mental processes involved in the elaboration and control of the execution of cognitive and behavioral responses to challenging situations, including the processing of relevant information, the elaboration of new mental sets, and cognitive flexibility. All these processes can be investigated with several tasks all of which require internally guided behavior: (a) Wisconsin Card Sorting Test and delayed response tasks for concept formation and rule finding; (b) Trail-Making and Odd Man Out tests for set shifting; (c) verbal fluency and Stroop test for set maintenance and inhibition of interference; (d) tower tasks for problem solving. All of these tasks, considered as specifically sensitive regarding frontal lobe–like lesions, are disturbed in patients with PD (Table 35.2).

TABLE 35.2. BASAL GANGLIA DISEASES IMPAIR TESTS OF EXECUTIVE FUNCTIONS

Wisconsin Card Sorting Test
    In PD [Taylor et al. (2)], SND [Soliveri et al. (30)], PSP [Dubois et al. (1)], HD [Brandt (31)], CBD [Pillon et al. (28)], and focal lesions
    [Eslinger and Grattan (32)]
Verbal fluency
    In PD [Cools et al. (33)], SND [Pillon et al. (34)], PSP [Cambier et al. (35)], HD [Butters et al. (36)], CBD [Massman et al. (20)], and
    focal lesions [Habib and Poncet (37)]
Trail Making Test
    In PD [Pirozzolo et al. (38)], SND [Pillon et al. (34)], PSP [Grafman et al. (22)], and HD [Bamford et al. (39)]
Stroop Test
    In PD [Brown and Marsden (40)], SND [Meco et al. (41)], PSP [Grafman et al. (22)], HD [Fisher et al. (42)], and focal lesions [Strub (43)]

PD, Parkinson's disease; PSP, progressive supranuclear palsy; HD, Huntington's disease; CBD,
corticobasal degeneration; SND, striatonigral degeneration.

Underlying Neuropsychological Mechanisms of Cognitive Changes in Parkinson's Disease

Despite the apparent diversity of cognitive disorders in non-demented patients, there is some evidence that they result from a more fundamental dysfunction, such as (a) a deficit in behavioral control and regulation, which would explain the difficulty in maintaining or shifting mental sets; (b) an inability to elaborate internally guided behavior, accounting for problem solving and learning deficits; or (c) a decrease in processing resources and internal control of attention, penalizing PD patients in tasks that are heavily loaded in cognitive demand (12). Interestingly, recent studies have indicated that the basal ganglia and the prefrontal cortex interfere with these functions in a complementary manner. For instance, if both patients with frontal lobe lesions and those with PD have difficulty in achieving criteria on the Wisconsin Card Sorting Test, the number of perseverative responses is only increased in patients with frontal lobe lesions. In contrast, PD patients have more difficulty in maintaining a response set for a new relevant dimension than in disengaging their attention from a previously reinforced category (44). Here again, the role of the striatum in the maintenance of a mental set, already suggested from procedural learning studies, is highlighted.

Other cognitive changes have been reported in PD patients, extending the number of cognitive domains in which the basal ganglia may play a role: (a) the discrimination of two sensory stimuli, suggesting that the striatum would interfere with the ability to focus attention on a single event while "suppressing" all others; and (b) the ability to process concurrent stimulations, implicating the basal ganglia in the parallel processing of sensorimotor information.

Underlying Pathophysiologic Mechanisms of Cognitive Changes in Parkinson's Disease

Degeneration of nigrostriatal dopaminergic neurons is the major neuropathologic feature of PD, as shown both postmortem and in vivo by positron emission tomography (PET) studies with ^{18}F-6-Fluoro-L-dopa. Clinical and experimental observations implicate impaired dopaminergic transmission in some cognitive deficits in patients, particularly in frontal lobe–related functions. First, intoxication by 1-methyl-4-phenyl-1,2,3,6-tetrahydropyridine (MPTP), a drug that selectively destroys the nigrostriatal dopaminergic neurons, interferes with planning and internal control both in animals after experimental injection, and humans after accidental administration. Second, problems in cognition have been observed in newly diagnosed and untreated "de novo" PD patients, particularly in tasks requiring internal control of attention and recent memory. Third, a beneficial effect of levodopa therapy on cognition has been observed in nondemented PD patients, particularly in the modulation of information processing, time reproduction, simultaneous

processing of cognitive information, verbal and visuospatial working memory, and psychomotor speed—processes that are sensitive to internal control of attentional resources and frontal lobe functions (12).

How might nigrostriatal dysfunction interfere with frontal lobe functions? The most promising approach is to analyze corticostriatal connections, even though they have been described in different ways: (a) parallel to segregated frontostriatal circuits; (b) massively convergent on pallidal dendritic disks of striatal neurons; or (c) mixed with separate corticostriatal projections and reconvergence of information on both pallidal segments. Whatever the nature of information processing in the basal ganglia, it is unanimously accepted that output is via the thalamus to specific prefrontal areas: dorsolateral, orbitofrontal, and anterior cingulate. Given their cortical targets, it is reasonable to assume that these striatofrontal projections are involved in complex cognitive, behavioral, or motivational functions. Thus, the frontal dysfunction observed in nondemented PD patients may result from disruption of specific striatofrontal connections, either at the level of the striatum, resulting from a lesion of the nigrostriatal dopaminergic pathway, or at the level of their cortical target, as a consequence of the additional lesion of the mesocortical dopaminergic system. Furthermore, cognitive changes are mediated, at least in part, by lesions of nondopaminergic neuronal systems, such as the ascending cholinergic, noradrenergic, and serotoninergic neurons, that have been detected postmortem (45).

Influence of Therapy on Cognitive Changes in Parkinson's Disease

If the cognitive functions that deteriorate in PD are mediated by a dopaminergic mechanism, levodopa would improve cognitive changes in the same way that it reverses dopamine-dependent motor signs. Unfortunately, the role of levodopa on cognition is much more limited, even in the early stages, as indicated in the previous paragraph. By contrast with motor or mood disorders, there is no evidence that cognitive performance fluctuates in response to levodopa in patients with on–off phenomena. In fact, the influence of L-dopa on cognition is debated, since it has been reported to either improve, impair, or not affect cognitive performance of parkinsonian patients. These discrepancies are contingent on the tests used for assessing cognition and on the patients selected.

Other drugs interfere with cognitive functions of PD patients. For example, blocking cholinergic transmission with anticholinergic drugs consistently results in learning and frontal lobe–like deficits in patients with PD. These results indicate that dopaminergic and cholinergic neuronal systems, both damaged in PD, have little influence on information storage, but modify the level of active attentional control, affecting acquisition and retrieval. Attentional control is increased by naphtoxazine (SD NVI-085), a selective noradrenergic α_1 agonist that partially reverses attentional deficits, whereas the α_2 agonist clonidine improves spatial working memory performance in PD.

The failure of dopaminergic therapy to achieve long-term motor symptom relief in patients with PD and advances in stereotactic techniques have led to renewed interest in surgical treatments, through pallidotomy and chronic high-frequency deep brain stimulation (DBS). Posteroventral pallidotomy improves the cardinal symptoms of PD and levodopa-induced dyskinesias, particularly on the side contralateral to the surgical lesion. Although pallidotomy targets motor symptoms, lesioning the posterior third of the internal globus pallidus may disrupt basal ganglia–thalamocortical circuits needed for processing cognitive information. The literature on the effects of the surgical procedure on cognitive functioning is in fact contradictory to reports showing cognitive decline, no overall cognitive change, or even cognitive improvement after unilateral pallidotomy. These conflicting results may be due to the small size of the groups of patients in most of the studies. More consistent cognitive failures are found with larger groups of patients. The risks of adverse cognitive effects may be increased after bilateral lesioning of the pallidum. Chronic DBS, a reversible nonlesioning surgical treatment, is an exciting alternative to pallidotomy. It can be applied to the internal globus pallidus (GPi) or subthalamic nucleus (STN), with a significant bilateral reduction in parkinsonian disability. The first study reported on nine patients with unilateral pallidal stimulation (46). Semantic verbal fluency and visuoconstructional test scores declined significantly after stereotaxy. However, there were no significant changes in memory or executive functions 3 to 6 months after surgery in a large series of 62 PD patients treated by bilateral STN or GPi stimulation (47). The specific effect of DBS was analyzed in a new study comparing patients with the stimulator turned on or off. The results showed a mild but significant improvement, when "on" for tests of psychomotor speed and working memory, previously shown to be sensitive to L-dopa therapy (48). Thus, the direct effects of DBS mimic the action of L-dopa treatment in the cognitive as in the motor domain. Behavioral disorders have been found, however, after DBS in STN patients older than 69 years. These behavioral disorders concerned executive dysfunction and apathy and were not related to mood. Therefore, old age might be a contraindication for DBS. Psychiatric changes are observed in some cases and consist mainly of amplification or decompensation of previous disorders, such as depressive episodes, generalized anxiety, or drug dependence (49). Personality changes, such as lack of initiative, lack of persistence, apathy, or vulnerability to pressure, might be related to subthalamic nucleus stimulation and depend on the electrode location. Bilateral subthalamic or pallidal DBS can also induce depressive reaction, bipolar mood swings, and laughter (50).

Mood and Behavioral Changes in Parkinson's Disease

Patients are described as introverted, cautious, less novelty seeking, hypercontrolled, repressing aggressive behaviors and emotions. An obsessive-compulsive-like personality has been suggested in PD, but this is not unanimously accepted. Depression is encountered in about 40% of patients and has been the focus of a large number of studies (Table 35.3). It is sometimes a presenting symptom, before the handicap is significant, suggesting endogenous constituents. However, it is not related to the severity of motor dysfunction, as psychosocial determinants can also intervene. Diagnosis of depression is important because it induces attention and memory disorders and, if sufficiently severe, impairs cognitive functions, especially those of the executive system in relation to a significant decrease in frontal metabolism evidenced on PET studies. More recently, attention has been drawn to apathy and its relation to basal ganglia disorders. Apathy has been defined as a lack of motivation and responsiveness to both positive and negative events, in the absence of emotional distress or negative thoughts. It can be clinically distinguished from depression using new scales, such as the Neuropsychiatric Inventory. It

TABLE 35.3. BASAL GANGLIA DISEASES IMPAIR BEHAVIOR

Depressed mood
  In PD [Mayeux et al. (5)], SND [Ghika et al. (50)], CBD [Cummings and Litvan (51)], and focal lesions [Danel et al. (52)]
Apathy
  In PD [Starkstein et al. (53)], PSP [Litvan et al. (54)], HD [Caine et al. (55)], and focal lesions [Bhatia and Marsden (9)]
Autoactivation deficit
  In HD [Fedio et al. (56)], and focal lesions [Laplane et al. (11)]
Environmental dependency syndrome
  In PSP [Pillon et al. (28)]
Disinhibition
  In HD [Fedio et al. (56)], CBD [Litvan et al. (51)], and focal lesions [Richfield et al. (57)]
Delusions and hallucinations
  In PD [Aarsland et al. (58)], and HD [McHugh and Folstein (59)]

PD, Parkinson's disease; PSP, progressive supranuclear palsy; HD, Huntington's disease; CBD, corticobasal degeneration; SND, striatonigral degeneration.

is not uncommon in PD: 12% of a consecutive series of 50 patients showed apathy as their primary psychiatric problem, whereas 30% were both apathetic and depressed, and 26% had depression but no apathy (53). Apathy was associated with impairment in neuropsychological tests with time constraints and on verbal memory tasks. These results were confirmed by an epidemiologic survey from a large community sample: apathy was observed in 16.5% of 139 patients and associated with executive dysfunction (60). The neurobiological substrate of apathy may be the limbic ventral striatopallidal system, suggested as the key to the translation of motivation into action. The ventral tegmental area has a fundamental role in the motivational aspects of behavioral responses by regulating this circuit via the mesolimbic and mesocortical dopaminergic systems. Unfortunately, pharmacologic agents that directly act on central dopaminergic neurons, such as amphetamine, methylphenidate, and bromocriptine, show no significant clinical effect on apathy in patients with PD. Alternatively, neuronal depletion in the locus ceruleus and dysfunction of the noradrenergic system may also intervene in apathy. Unlike depression, anxiety symptoms almost always begin after the onset of the motor symptoms and are related to medication-induced on–off fluctuations in most cases. Indeed, drug-induced psychiatric disorders are frequently found in PD. They mainly consist of hallucinations and delusions. In contrast with hallucinosis, in which patients remain aware of the illusory character of their experience, in psychosis there is congruence between the sensory distortion and the patients beliefs. These disorders are much more common in PD with dementia or DLBD where they would be related to central cholinergic deficiency (58).

Parkinsonism and Dementia

It is important to consider dementia in PD because it affects the prognosis of the disease and has repercussions on the caregivers' burden. In a survey of caregivers, the most frequently cited reason for patients being institutionalized was the triple association of dementia, incontinence, and sleep disorders. Managing dementia in PD is not easy because it is generally assumed to be due to nondopaminergic lesions of the brain and, consequently, not responsive to dopaminergic drugs. Dementia may also be difficult to recognize. First, it is noteworthy that current test batteries do not always include the assessment of executive functions, although such an evaluation is crucial to the evaluation of subcortical dementia. Second, an overestimation of the severity of cognitive impairment may result from nonspecific factors, which interfere with the evaluation of cognitive functions. When in the "off" condition (i.e., when the effect of levodopa treatment is minimal), patients are severely akinetic with motor and cognitive slowing, hypophonic with slurred speech, and anxious—all factors that affect the cognitive evaluation. When in the "on" condition

(i.e., when the effect of levodopa treatment is maximal), patients are inattentive and hampered by uncontrolled dyskinesias. Depression needs to be taken into account, as it has been shown to induce executive dysfunction (see above). Treatment can also interfere with the cognitive status of the patients. Anticholinergics provoke acute confusional states or a permanent cognitive decline, especially when patients are older and have memory disorders, conditions in which the risk of severe damage to the ascending cholinergic system is increased. Administration of anticholinergics to patients older than 70 years should therefore be avoided, at least when a memory disorder is present.

Despite these limitations, dementia was estimated to occur in about 15% to 20% of patients. In an epidemiologic study of 339 consecutive patients, the overall prevalence was 10.9% (61). This is likely an underestimate due to the shorter life expectancy of PD patients with dementia, as shown by survival analysis. The risk of dementia in PD was found to be almost twice and even almost sixfold that of age-matched nondemented elderly controls. Dementia in PD occurs after a certain period of evolution and, typically, in the late-onset form of the disease. The delay between the onset of parkinsonian symptoms and the occurrence of intellectual decline characterizes the dementia in PD and usually distinguishes it from the dementia of the Lewy body type, where the cognitive dysfunction appears very early (less than 2 years) or even precedes the appearance of parkinsonism, when it is present.

If one refers to *Diagnostic and Statistical Manual of Mental Disorders*, 4th ed. (DSM-IV) criteria, dementia in PD may be described as a progressive dysexecutive syndrome with memory deficits, in the absence of aphasia, apraxia, or agnosia. In patients with dementia of the subcorticofrontal type, the loss of intellectual ability is better evaluated with the Mattis Dementia Rating Scale than with the Mini-Mental State Examination of Folstein et al., because it includes tests assessing attention and executive functions. Such tools provide cutoff scores that permit a psychometric definition of dementia and help to distinguish between demented and nondemented patients.

A deficit in the learning of new information, the hallmark for the diagnosis of dementia, is regularly reported in demented PD patients, although it is less severe than in Alzheimer's disease (AD). The nature of the memory deficit may be specified using the Grober and Buschke procedure, designed to control for the effective encoding of the verbal items to be retrieved. Despite a marked deficit in free recall, the performance of demented PD patients was dramatically improved by using the same semantic cues as at encoding, which triggered efficient retrieval processes (3). Therefore, the recall deficit is not primarily due to a memory disruption, since the ability to register, store, and consolidate information is preserved, but rather to difficulties in activating the neuronal processes involved in the functional use of memory stores. Correlation analysis showed that the memory scores in this task were strongly related to performance in tests of executive functions, favoring the role of frontal lobe dysfunction in the defective activation of memory processes. The existence of a dysexecutive syndrome in PD patients with dementia, though less severe than in those with PSP, is in agreement with this interpretation.

If this dysexecutive syndrome is the main characteristic of dementia in PD, instrumental activities are on the whole preserved. However, linguistic difficulties have been described in these patients. They include word-finding difficulties, decreased information content of spontaneous speech, diminished word list generation, and impaired strategies in sentence comprehension (12). Moreover, poor performance in tests of verbal fluency are predictive of dementia in PD. Praxic disorders have also been reported, although their nature is still a matter of debate. In any case, these instrumental deficits are far less severe than in AD and have been related to frontal lobe dysfunction. As underlined by Girotti et al. (62), cognitive deficits are more severe and widespread in demented than in nondemented PD patients, but affect particularly those tests that already distinguished nondemented patients from controls.

Apathy, delusions, and hallucinations are more severe in demented than in nondemented PD patients and in patients with DLBD than in PD patients (58). The diagnosis of DLBD, or dementia with Lewy bodies, can be suspected clinically on the basis of the early occurrence of a cognitive decline resembling a chronic confusional state with fluctuating cognitive signs and visual and/or auditive hallucinations in a patient with mild parkinsonism (63). The rapidly progressive dementia is accompanied by aphasia, dyspraxia, or spatial disorientation, suggestive of temporoparietal dysfunction. The neuropsychological profile differs from that of patients with AD: cognitive deficits are more acute, attentional fluctuations more intense, and psychotic features more precocious. Moreover, patients with DLBD present more severe dysexecutive impairment but less severe memory deficits than patients with AD. The neuropsychological pattern of DLBD can also be distinguished from the subcortical dementia of PD on the basis of the early occurrence of cognitive deficits and psychotic features, and the presence of linguistic and particularly visuospatial disorders.

Pathologic studies of DLBD indicate that the neurodegenerative process is not limited to specific neuronal systems (64). Therefore, it can be proposed that the impairment of instrumental functions results from cortical Lewy bodies, the subacute confusional state with attentional fluctuations from severe cell loss in the nucleus basalis of Meynert, and psychotic features from limbic involvement.

Underlying Pathophysiologic Mechanisms of Dementia in Parkinsonism

If one considers that dementia in PD mainly results from subcortical lesions, this implies that it occurs when damage

of both the basal ganglia and several ascending neuronal pathways reaches the necessary threshold required for the expression of severe cognitive impairment (45). These dopaminergic, cholinergic, noradrenergic, and serotoninergic neuronal systems contribute in parallel or by mutual interaction to the expression of integrated behaviors, as demonstrated in experimental studies. For example, the simultaneous disruption of the nigrostriatal and mesocorticolimbic dopaminergic systems causes marked impairment of the conditioned avoidance response in rats, whereas the selective disruption of one or the other of these systems has no effect. It has also been shown that destruction of the ascending cholinergic system increases the behavioral consequences of damage to serotonergic neurons.

Cortical changes must also be taken into account to explain the occurrence of dementia in PD. In addition to subcortical lesions, cortical neuronal loss, Alzheimer-like histologic changes, and neuronal Lewy bodies in the cerebral cortex may have a crucial role in the intellectual deterioration seen in PD. This observation leads some authors to conclude that dementia in PD could result from the coexistence of AD. In favor of this hypothesis, there is (a) a high frequency of Alzheimer-like changes in the cerebral cortex of PD patients, although it is not correlated with dementia; (b) a high level of abnormal Tau protein in temporal and prefrontal cortices of demented PD patients, although the pattern and intensity of immunostaining differ from that observed in AD; and (c) a marked hypoperfusion in single photon emission computed tomography (SPECT) studies in posterior cortical regions of demented PD patients, which resembles the pattern observed in AD, although the perfusion defect is greater and more extensive in the later disease. We should not forget that the cognitive pattern in demented PD patients is markedly different from that of patients with AD, with respect to mnemonic deficits, the intensity of the dysexecutive syndrome, and the absence of true aphasia, apraxia, or agnosia (see above). Moreover, some cases of dementia have been reported in PD in the absence of apparent cortical lesions, suggesting that subcortical lesions may be sufficiently severe to cause overt dementia, at least in some patients. Thus, the respective role of the two contingents of lesions (cortical and subcortical) remains to be determined. The subcortical lesions alone may be responsible for the frontal lobe–like dysfunction and the inefficient activation of memory processes observed in PD patients, even in those who are demented.

Lewy bodies are intracytoplasmic eosinophilic inclusions that are most often observed in the perikarya of nonpyramidal neurons in the deep cortical layers V and VI, with a predilection for paralimbic (the cingulate and insular cortex), temporal and frontal areas of the neocortex. When dementia is associated with Lewy body disease, the Lewy bodies are often found in these neocortical regions. However, there is no definite consensus about the density of limbic and neocortical Lewy bodies that are associated with dementia, or even sufficient to confirm the diagnosis of diffuse Lewy body disease. The problem is even more complex if we take into account the frequent association of AD pathology, which may itself contribute to clinical dementia. This led to divide Lewy body disease into (a) "DLBD pure form," with numerous neocortical Lewy bodies in the predilection sites but without AD pathology; and (b) "DLBD common form," with fewer neocortical Lewy bodies associated with senile plaques and, sometimes, neurofibrillary tangles. How the distribution and density of Lewy bodies and concomitant AD pathology determine the symptoms and signs in individual patients is still unknown.

In accordance with Gibb et al. (64), we suggest that the neuropathology of demented parkinsonian patients emphasizes the interaction of subcortical and cortical lesions. Furthermore, age of onset of the disease can influence the threshold at which neuronal lesions become symptomatic, explaining the high frequency of dementia in older PD patients.

STRIATONIGRAL DEGENERATION

The first attempt to isolate the neuropsychological pattern of striatonigral degeneration (SND) was made by Sullivan et al. (65), who reported, in one patient, subtle difficulties limited to serial arm movement programming, letter fluency, and working memory, whereas overall cognitive and affective status was within normal range. Performance was normal in other frontal lobe–related tests, such as the Wisconsin Card Sorting Test, design fluency, self-ordering, and Trail-Making Test. In contrast, a subsequent study reported a more diffuse frontal lobe dysfunction similar to that observed in patients with PD or PSP, at least at first glance (66).

To clarify this matter, 14 consecutive patients with probable SND were evaluated with an extensive neuropsychological battery (34), which revealed a selective pattern of subcorticofrontal dysfunction, qualitatively different from that of PD and PSP: the patients were impaired in some frontal lobe–related tasks (category and phonemic fluency, Trail-Making Test A and B, free recall of the Grober and Buschke test, and presence of abnormal behaviors of prehension and imitation), and normal in the Wisconsin Card Sorting Test, the Stroop interference condition, and in explicit memory tests such as the Wechsler Memory Scale and the California Verbal Learning Test. In other words, the neuropsychological pattern of SND was characterized by a normal overall cognitive and affective status with a mild impairment of memory and executive functions. This pattern was recently confirmed in a longitudinal study (30). However, performance on the Stroop test was found to be impaired, with another version of the test requiring a longer maintenance of attention and inhibition of interference (41). The subcorticofrontal syndrome is far less severe than in PSP and helps to differentiate the two diseases.

Psychiatric disorders have been poorly studied in SND. Depression, anxiety, and emotional lability have been described, but not psychosis (50).

Underlying Pathophysiologic Mechanisms of Cognitive Changes in Striatonigral Degeneration

As far as we know, the distribution of lesions in SND is mainly subcortical: (a) severe degeneration of the substantia nigra, inducing an equal loss in the dopaminergic efferents to the putamen and the caudate nucleus; (b) severe loss of large and small striatal neurons; and (c) partial degeneration of the dopaminergic and cholinergic systems (67). Cortical involvement is limited to a laminar astrocytosis in layer V of the motor cortex. It can, therefore, be postulated that the dysexecutive syndrome of SND results from the combined degeneration of the dopaminergic nigrostriatal system and of the striatum, which may alter the neuronal activity within the striatofrontal loops.

PROGRESSIVE SUPRANUCLEAR PALSY

The first symptoms of PSP are postural instability and falls. In fact, cognitive slowing and inertia are also precocious and occur in the first year in 52% of cases. Patients with PSP typically have cognitive deficits and personality changes suggestive of frontal lobe dysfunction. As the disease progresses, these changes worsen. Of 24 patients who underwent two or more neuropsychological evaluations over time, 38% showed a global impairment at their first examination, and 70% 15 months later (68). The changes may become severe enough to warrant the diagnosis of dementia, but the deficits still conform to the pattern of subcorticofrontal dementia described more than 20 years ago by Albert and collaborators (6). The dysexecutive syndrome of PSP is much more severe than that observed in any other subcortical disorders, and the memory deficit is dramatically improved, or normalized, in conditions that facilitate retrieval processing such as cueing and recognition.

Cognitive Slowing

Cognitive slowing appears evident in patients with PSP, who answer questions and solve even the simplest problems with delay. It is not merely a subjective interpretation of the examiner faced with akinesia, slurred speech, depression, and frontal inertia in the patient. There is a genuine slowing of central processing time unrelated to motor or affective disorders, as demonstrated experimentally using reaction time (RT) tasks (1). The paradigm was designed to investigate central processing time by comparing RT in different conditions that required increasingly complex cognitive operations but with the same motor response. A significant increase of central processing time was noticed in PSP patients compared with control subjects and patients with PD, and was correlated with the performance of the PSP patients in frontal lobe tests. This result suggests that cognitive slowing is a byproduct of frontal deafferentation and that it is important in PSP because of the severity of the frontal lobe dysfunction in the disease. Slowed information processing was also shown by several investigators using event-related brain potentials.

Dysexecutive Syndrome

Cognitive slowing may account for poor performance in tasks used to investigate executive functions. For instance, it might contribute to decreased lexical fluency because the time allotted for response is limited. Lexical fluency is more severely impaired in patients with PSP than in patients with PD or AD, although naming is more affected in the latter. The deficit is observed in different types of fluency, including semantic fluency, where patients have to list animal names or objects that can be found in a supermarket; phonemic fluency, where patients are required to produce words beginning with a given letter; and design fluency, where patients must produce abstract designs.

A tendency to perseverate may also account for some of the deficits, particularly in tasks involving concept formation and shifting ability (Table 35.2). In the Wisconsin Card Sorting Test, PSP patients completed a smaller number of categories than patients with PD or SND. This lack of flexibility affects both categorical and motor sequencing, as shown by the poor performance of patients with PSP in the Trail-Making Test and in the motor series of Luria. Patients with PSP also experience difficulty in conceptualization and problem solving ability, which may account for their performance in similarities, interpretation of proverbs, comprehension of abstract concepts, arithmetic and lineage problems, tower tasks, and picture arrangement. A bedside short battery was recently created for the evaluation of frontal lobe–like symptoms [the Frontal Assessment Battery, or FAB (69)]. It consists of six subtests for a total duration of less than 10 minutes. Performance on the FAB has been found significantly more impaired in patients with PSP than in those with PD or SND, and the FAB scores were significantly correlated with the Mattis Dementia Rating Scale ($\rho = 0.82$, $p < 0.01$) and Wisconsin Card Sorting Test ($\rho = 0.77$, $p < 0.01$) scores in these patients.

Memory Disorders

This severe dysexecutive syndrome contributes to the memory deficits and instrumental disorders observed in PSP (Table 35.1). *Short-term memory* was found to be impaired using the Brown-Peterson paradigm, a working memory task in which the patients were more sensitive than controls to interference. *Long-term memory* is also disturbed in PSP, as shown by immediate and delayed recall of the subtests of the Wechsler Memory Scale, the Rey Auditory Verbal Learning Test, and the California Verbal Learning Test. However, when encoding was controlled by using semantic category cues and when recall was performed with the same cues, as in the Grober and Buschke procedure, recall performance of the patients improved dramatically because their total recall score was similar to that of an age-matched control group (27). *Procedural learning* was also investigated in PSP. Eyeblink classical conditioning was found to be impaired. In the serial reaction time task (SRTT), no significant learning was observed in response to a repeated sequence, in contrast to AD patients. As PSP patients were able to press the correct key in only 50% of the trials, their impaired performance on the SRTT might result from the task being too complex as well as from impaired procedural learning ability. Nevertheless, skill learning deficits were found in other tasks, such as the mirror reading procedure, where they cannot be explained by sensorimotor factors alone because patients had normal learning curves for the repeated word triplets. By contrast, impaired learning curves for word triplets presented only once indicate an inability to acquire the new procedure of reading from right to left that resembles the shifting deficit observed in tests of executive functions. Unlike procedural learning, *priming abilities* were shown to be normal in patients with PSP in a perceptual identification task involving words with a masking procedure, in agreement with the preservation of the temporo-occipital cortex in the disease.

Instrumental Disorders

Various speech disorders have been described in PSP. A severe reduction of spontaneous speech resembling dynamic aphasia is usually observed (35), but abnormal loquacity has also been reported. Word finding difficulty may occur, but it is generally less severe than in AD patients. Semantic or syntactic comprehension disorders are absent or mild (70). Dynamic apraxia may be found (28). Bilateral apraxic errors for transitive and intransitive movements have been reported, but they are much less severe than in CBD (71). Visual and auditory perception may be disturbed, but there is no evidence of object agnosia or alexia. Therefore, instrumental disorders of patients with PSP, when present, are rather considered to be a consequence of impaired executive and perceptual-motor functions or attentional disorders.

Behavioral Disorders

Administering the Neuropsychiatric Inventory to patients' informants showed that patients with PSP exhibited apathy almost as a rule as it was observed in 91% of the cases (54). Apathy was also more frequent in PSP than in PD or HD.

Moreover, patients with PSP show severe difficulty in self-guided behavior and are abnormally dependent on stimuli from the environment. They involuntarily grasp all the objects presented in front of them; they imitate the examiner's gestures passively and use objects in the absence of any explicit verbal orders (68). Such uncontrolled behaviors are never observed in normal control subjects in the absence of explicit demands and are considered to result from a lack of the inhibitory control normally exerted by the frontal lobes. PSP patients also have difficulty in inhibiting an automatic motor program once it is initiated. This can easily be evaluated with the "signe de l'applaudissement" [or "clapping sign" (10)]: when asked to clap their hands three times consecutively, as quickly as possible, these patients have a tendency to clap more (four or five times), sometimes initiating an automatic program of clapping that they are unable to stop, as if they had difficulty in programming voluntary acts that compete with overlearned motor skills. This sign seems to be specific to striatal dysfunction occurring in PSP. Changes in mood, emotion, and personality have also been described: most frequently bluntness of affective expression and lack of concern about personal behavior or the behavior of others, but sometimes obsessive disorders or disinhibition with bulimia, inappropriate sexual behavior, or aggressiveness. These changes are difficult to investigate, given the lack of insight and the transient nature of the emotions expressed. The testimony of the attendants is therefore required.

Underlying Pathophysiologic Mechanisms of Cognitive and Behavioral Changes in Progressive Supranuclear Palsy

The concept of subcortical dementia was first formulated by Albert et al. (6) on the basis of the neuropsychological pattern of five patients with PSP. The authors postulated that the cognitive changes resulted from a deactivation of the cerebral cortex due to the damage to subcortical structures. Indeed, severe lesions are observed in the basal ganglia (substantia nigra pars compacta, internal pallidum, subthalamic nucleus), brainstem nuclei (locus ceruleus, pontomedullary reticular formation, pontomesencephalic tegmentum, periaqueductal gray and pretectal region), and cerebellum (cerebellar dentate nucleus), which project for the most part to the prefrontal cortex [for review, see Jellinger and Banchet (72)]. In addition to these massive lesions of subcortical structures, a mild cortical involvement has been reported (8), consisting of neocortical neurofibrillary tangles in the precentral cortex (Brodmann's area 4) and to a lesser extent in cingulate (area 23), frontal (area 9), and temporal (area 22) cortices. Despite these cortical changes, there is no doubt that the severe frontal lobe–like symptomatology of the disease is mainly the consequence of the loss of the specific afferents to the prefrontal cortex

from subcortical regions: internal pallidum and thalamus, brainstem reticular nuclei, and neocerebellum.

Influence of Therapy on Cognitive or Behavioral Changes in Progressive Supranuclear Palsy

Current treatments for PSP are ineffective as a result of the widespread involvement of dopaminergic and nondopaminergic neurotransmitter systems (73). Thus far, neurotransmitter replacement therapeutic approaches have failed. Clinical experience shows no significant improvement with levodopa. Physostigmine (a cholinesterase inhibitor) induced only mild improvement of specific cognitive functions. Donepezil improved memory performance, but the motor scores worsened. Antidepressants and support therapy may improve depression or apathy. Amitriptyline has been reported to improve emotional incontinence.

HUNTINGTON'S DISEASE

Huntington's disease is characterized by an insidious onset of symptoms, associating choreic movements, affective disorders, behavioral changes, and cognitive impairment. The diagnosis is based on the presence of an excessive number of CAG repeats in the IT 15 gene of chromosome 4. Affective and cognitive changes may occur early in the course of the disease, even before the choreic movements, as shown in recent studies on "asymptomatic" gene carriers (74). They are consistently found after a certain period of evolution, even in sporadic cases (75), and slowly worsen with the evolution of the disease (76). The cognitive changes have been considered to be characteristic of a "subcortical dementia" (59) and mainly consist of disorders of visuospatial, memory, and executive functions.

Visuospatial Disorders

Severe impairments have been found in visuospatial tasks, with or without prominent motor components. A double dissociation has been observed between egocentric spatial perception (right–left personal orientation in a road-map test), impaired in HD and normal in AD, and extrapersonal spatial perception (constructional skills), impaired in AD and normal in HD (77). It may be proposed, therefore, that the caudate nucleus, damaged in HD, has a role in updating perceived position in space to compensate for self-initiated movements, a function similar to that of the corollary discharge considered to be related to the frontal lobes.

Memory Deficits

Memory deficits are an early-appearing feature of HD (Table 35.1). *Working memory* is impaired even in presymptomatic HD, particularly in depressed gene carriers (78). Working memory for words is more preserved in HD than in AD, whereas working memory for colors, patterns, faces and spatial positions is as or more severely impaired in HD. Visual object working memory is, however, better preserved than spatial working memory in the early stages of the disease. *Long-term memory* is disturbed. Patients with HD display immediate recall and learning scores comparable to those of patients with AD in the California Verbal Learning Test, where encoding is free, although retention over time, resistance to interference, and recognition are better preserved. In contrast, their performance is not significantly different from that of control subjects in Grober and Buschke's test, where encoding and recall are controlled by the same semantic cues (3). Patients with HD also differ from those with amnesic syndromes in *remote memory*. Although patients with Korsakoff's disease display a marked temporal gradient of retrograde amnesia affecting more severely events in the recent past, patients with HD are equally impaired in remembering public events from all periods of time (79). These findings suggest that the retrograde memory deficit of patients with HD is due to retrieval failures rather than to decreasing storage efficiency as the disease progresses. *Procedural learning* seems to be more severely impaired than explicit memory. HD patients show marked skill learning difficulties in rotor pursuit, mirror reading, maze or tower learning, and in the serial reaction paradigm. Although impairments have been reported in all of these tasks, there is considerable variability within the HD population. Moreover, difficulty in allocating sufficient attentional resources to the task might explain the failure of patients on procedural tasks with cognitive components. *Perceptual and conceptual implicit memory* are also impaired.

Executive Dysfunction

More than motor disability, executive dysfunction severely impairs daily functioning (Table 35.2). The patients or their caregivers often cite difficulty in planning, organizing, and scheduling activities. Objective testing shows an inability to shift mental sets and perseverative tendencies—less severe than in patients with PSP—and a low frequency of pathologic behaviors of prehension, utilization, and imitation.

Speech planning, initiation, and production are impaired in HD because the caudate nucleus has a major role in controlling the timing of speech movements. Linguistic difficulties are observed as well, and can be displayed in visual confrontation naming, lexical fluency, proverb definitions, syntax production, and narrative language (80). Language informativeness and comprehension are highly correlated with the severity of overall dementia. This is, however, a general tendency for all cognitive functions, and patients tested after several years of evolution display a low-

ering of performance on all tests of intellectual and mnemonic functioning. Nevertheless, despite an overall intellectual decline, their cognitive pattern differs from that of patients with AD or other movement disorders in the predominance of attentional disturbances.

Mood and Behavioral Changes in Huntington's Disease

Patients usually present with inertia and loss of interest toward their environment that resembles the loss of autoactivation described in patients with focal lesions of the basal ganglia (Table 35.3). This behavioral syndrome is characterized by a marked reduction in spontaneous activity that can be temporarily reversed by external stimulation. Indeed, apathy of HD patients has been considered to result from difficulty in initiating activities, since it is not usually observed in externally guided tasks or situations. As noted by Folstein et al. (81), "many patients are willing to participate in activities initiated and sustained by others but revert to inertia as soon as outside stimulation is withdrawn." Psychiatric symptoms are also characteristic of the disease and may be present before the appearance of chorea. They occur in 98% of the patients and consist of dysphoria, agitation, irritability, apathy, anxiety, peculiarities of thought, and interpersonal difficulties. Disorders of impulse control are also frequent. These symptoms range from mild to severe and are unrelated to dementia and chorea. They are also unrelated to CAG repeats in neurologically asymptomatic carriers. Schizophreniform disorders with persecutory delusions and auditory or visual hallucinations have been described, but estimates of their frequency vary considerably.

Underlying Pathophysiologic Mechanisms of Cognitive and Behavioral Changes in Huntington's Disease

Several arguments specifically implicate dysfunction of the caudate nucleus in the cognitive and behavioral changes of HD: (a) severe damage to the caudate nucleus is a rule in all immunochemical and neuropathologic studies; (b) scores on several cognitive tests correlate significantly with caudate atrophy measured on computed tomography scans; (c) hypometabolism is found in the caudate nucleus of HD patients, and the rate of glucose metabolism correlates significantly with verbal and total memory scores; (d) the caudate nucleus subserves those functions that are disturbed in HD (i.e., working memory, attention, and planning); (e) systematic neuropsychological evaluation reveals subtle cognitive changes in asymptomatic gene carriers (i.e., at a stage of the disease where the lesions are supposed to be restricted to the caudate nucleus). This recent finding may be of importance given the controversy over the role of additional cortical lesions that have been described postmortem.

Influence of Therapy on Cognitive or Behavioral Changes in Huntington's Disease

Riluzole improves chorea, but whether it would also improve cognition or behavior is still under investigation. Another promising perspective might be fetal neural allografts associated with cognitive improvement in some patients with HD. New antipsychiatric drugs such as olanzapine or risperidone would be more appropriate for reducing psychotic symptoms than the classic neuroleptics because they have fewer side effects involving cognition.

CORTICOBASAL DEGENERATION

Corticobasal degeneration was first described by Rebeiz et al. (82). This disease is typically defined by unilateral rigidity of one arm with apraxic disorders, accounting for the proposition of the new term "progressive asymmetric rigidity and apraxia syndrome" (83). However, the cognitive syndrome is not limited to motor and praxic disorders. Besides these main features, dysarthric disorders, speech apraxia, frontal lobe signs, and a moderate cognitive deterioration can also be observed, even in early stages of the disease. Furthermore, recent pathologic studies have shown clinical heterogeneity, explaining that the inclusion criteria generally used in most of the studies have a good specificity but low sensitivity (84,85).

Instrumental Disorders

Gesture disorders are so characteristic of the disease that the diagnosis can be suspected on the simple analysis of the motor disturbances. They consist, at first, of the patient experiencing difficulty or showing perplexity in the performance of delicate and fine movements of the fingers of one hand. At this stage, patients complain of clumsiness and loss of manual dexterity, reminiscent of "limb apraxia," variously described as "kinesthetic" in patients with lesions of the parietal cortex or "kinetic" in patients with lesions of the premotor cortex. Systematic evaluation shows disorders of dynamic motor execution (impaired bimanual coordination, temporal organization, control, and inhibition). Asymmetric praxis disorders (difficulty in posture imitation, symbolic gesture execution, and object utilization) are also regularly observed, even at this stage. Ideomotor apraxia is common, especially in patients who have initial symptoms in the right limb, in agreement with the hypothesis of a predominant storage of "movement formulae" in the left hemisphere (86). In contrast with the involvement of all aspects of gesture execution, gesture identification is preserved, suggesting that mental representations or conceptual aspects of gestures are not involved. This finding is in agreement with the fact that conceptual apraxia is not reported in the absence of a severe cognitive impairment

(i.e., in the absence of more diffuse lesions of the cerebral cortex). In advanced cases, dystonia, rigidity, and bradykinesia may be sufficiently severe to prevent the interpretation of gesture disorders at least for the more impaired limb.

Other signs of cortical involvement have been observed in CBD. Buccofacial apraxia is generally milder than limb apraxia, except in patients with progressive loss of speech output. Constructive apraxia is observed in patients with predominant right hemisphere lesions, in relation to the well-known influence of this hemisphere on visuospatial function. Reflexive horizontal saccade latency is markedly increased, as in focal lesions affecting the posterior parietal cortex, and this slowing has been correlated with the severity of apraxia. Alien-limb phenomenon, in which a limb behaves in an uncooperative or foreign fashion, occurs in CBD, although its frequency is highly variable among studies. Its occurrence, in the absence of a known callosal lesion, is highly suggestive of the diagnosis of CBD. Linguistic disturbances may be found, consisting of transcortical motor aphasia, progressive phonetic disintegration, decreased lexical fluency, and word finding difficulties (87). Primary progressive nonfluent aphasia can even be an initial symptom of CBD. Neglect and visuospatial deficits have also been reported.

Memory Deficits

Temporospatial orientation and remote or recent memories are preserved at least in the early stages of the disease. However, the encoding and recall strategic processes are dysfunctioning, as shown by the impaired performance of patients with CBD on more demanding tasks, such as the Logical Memory, Associate Learning, and Visual Retention subtests of the Wechsler Memory Scale (Table 35.1). The impairment is not as severe as that observed in patients with AD at the same level of global intellectual deterioration. For example, the percent of information retained from the Logical Memory stories over a 30-minute delay was 61.6% on average in CBD versus only 23.3% in AD (20). In the Grober and Buschke test, the performance of patients with CBD was lower than that of control subjects in free recall, but did not differ from that of control subjects at total recall. Their memory performance did not differ from that of patients with PSP, either at free or cued recall, but was better than that of patients with AD, particularly at cued recall, either immediate or delayed (28).

Dysexecutive Syndrome

In subcorticofrontal degenerative diseases there are strong relationships between memory performance and executive functions (3). The similarity of memory patterns in CBD and PSP would imply the existence of a dysexecutive syndrome as severe in CBD as in PSP. This hypothesis was effectively confirmed (Table 35.2). Utilization behavior, related to a release of the inhibition normally exerted by the frontal lobes on the activity of the parietal lobes, was less common in CBD, probably because of the parietal lobe dysfunction in this disease.

Mood and Behavioral Changes in Corticobasal Degeneration

Besides frontal lobe–type behavioral alterations, patients with CBD may present with neuropsychiatric disorders (Table 35.3). The stereotyped movements described include repeated touching of clothing and objects in the environment in one patient, and excessive eating and drinking in another. These stereotyped movements have been interpreted as possibly consistent with obsessive-compulsive behavior. In a series of CBD patients, the Neuropsychiatric Inventory showed that depression, apathy, irritability, and agitation were the most common symptoms (51). The depression and irritability of patients with CBD were more common and severe than those of patients with PSP, whereas patients with PSP exhibited more apathy.

Dementia in Corticobasal Degeneration

In most of the clinical studies performed in CBD patients, the level of intellectual deterioration was mild or moderate until an advanced stage of the disease. For example, the mean verbal IQ on the Revised Wechsler Intelligence Scale was 95.6 (SD = 16.7) in a group of 21 patients with an educational level of 13.2 (SD = 2.6) years (20). In some cases, however, patients with a severe dysexecutive syndrome associated with memory disorders and impaired instrumental activities may reach the threshold of dementia in which both cortical and subcorticofrontal components have a role. Thus, dementia is not uncommon in CBD. In 10 of 13 cases with pathologically proven CBD, dementia was noticed within 3 years of onset of symptoms (88). It is interesting to note that the clinical pattern of dementia in this study was relatively homogeneous, since most of the cases presented with early behavioral changes, whereas only one case was misdiagnosed as AD. Dementia may also be observed from the onset in unusual clinical presentations of CBD.

No longitudinal study of the cognitive evolution of CBD has been reported to date, but it greatly differs from one patient to another. Some patients present only limb clumsiness and gesture disorders at the first examination, with few or no cognitive or behavioral symptoms. Others begin with a subcorticofrontal cognitive and behavioral syndrome similar to that of PSP patients and their gesture disorders become manifest only after several years of evolution. Clinically, such a neuropsychological picture may be difficult to distinguish from frontotemporal dementia (87). Early subcorticofrontal syndrome in CBD predicts a shorter survival.

Underlying Pathophysiologic Mechanisms of Cognitive Changes in Corticobasal Degeneration

The performance of complex gestures (posture reproduction, evocation and imitation of symbolic gestures, object use) can easily be related to the parietal lesions observed both in postmortem (82) and in metabolic studies (89). Severe neuronal loss with gliosis has been found in parietal regions, but it is currently more widespread and can be observed in frontal regions as well, probably accounting for intellectual decline. This frontal involvement, particularly in premotor areas, may also be responsible for the precocious disturbances of motor programming (bimanual coordination, temporal organization of segmental movements, inhibition of interfering motor activities) and for an alien-limb syndrome that was recently related to hypometabolism in the medial frontal cortex (Brodmann's area 24). Severe pathology in subcortical areas may also affect motor control and execution of movements. A subgroup of patients with CBD may have a more global cognitive impairment that reflects a more diffuse cortical degeneration, affecting the anterior frontal lobe, amygdala and entorhinal cortex, or more rarely the hippocampus (84,85). Furthermore, a damage of large-scale networks between cortical regions would lead to disconnection contributing to the disturbance of complex cortical functions in CBD with a subsequent atrophy of the corpus callosum.

In conclusion, appropriate neuropsychological tests may help to differentiate between degenerative diseases associated with extrapyramidal motor disorders (90). Most patients with PD or SND share a mild to moderate subcorticofrontal pattern of impairment. More dramatic planning, monitoring, and recall deficits are observed in PSP and HD, associated with a severe environmental dependency syndrome (prehension, utilization, and imitation behaviors) in PSP and more severe attentional disorders in HD. Signs of cortical involvement are found early in CBD and DLBD, with asymmetric instrumental disorders in CBD (praxic and linguistic or visuospatial deficits) and more severe dementia in DLBD. Therefore, the neuropsychological picture of patients with movement disorders may vary from subtle behavioral abnormalities to florid dementia with delusions and hallucinations. The nature and severity of cognitive disorders, the type of impaired memory processes, the presence of instrumental deficits, the precocity of a dysexecutive syndrome, and the frequency of psychosis depend on the underlying neuronal lesions, which in most cases remain to be discovered.

FOCAL LESIONS OF THE BASAL GANGLIA

The basal ganglia may also be damaged by nondegenerative disorders. The lesions result from various etiologies: (a) toxic, mainly due to a carbon monoxide intoxication, less frequently to intoxication with potassium cyanide, manganese, carbon disulfide, or disulfiram; (b) vascular, due to ischemia or hemorrhage. Even though some of these lesions are not strictly limited to the basal ganglia, the careful analysis of the associated changes may explain the functions of these structures in cognition and behavior (9,10).

Cognitive Deficits in Focal Lesions of the Basal Ganglia

Global intellectual efficiency is preserved. However, the autoactivation deficit, described in the next paragraph, may slightly reduce the performance. A mild dysexecutive syndrome is observed, but not in all cases (91). When present, it affects problem solving ability, conceptualization, interference inhibition, or lexical fluency (Table 35.2). The strategic aspects of explicit memory are deficient, particularly when the caudate nucleus is involved. The deficit of free recall contrasts with the preservation of cued recall and recognition (Table 35.1). Procedural learning has been poorly studied in focal lesions of the basal ganglia. A deficit in mirror reading and the serial reaction time task has been observed in patients with lesions of the caudate nucleus, whereas motor learning in the rotor pursuit task was only disturbed in a patient with a lesion restricted to the putamen (10). Aphasic disorders have been described in connection with focal damage of the thalamus or when lesions extend outside the caudate nucleus of the dominant hemisphere to the adjacent white matter, whereas the neostriatum is only involved in modulation of speech parameters and initiation of spoken output. Hemispatial neglect is encountered only when the thalamus or the internal capsule is involved.

Behavioral Changes in Focal Lesions of the Basal Ganglia

Inertia and blunted affect are frequently encountered in patients with basal ganglia lesions. Their occurrence depends on etiology, precise location of the lesion, and time of examination. These changes may appear only several months after the occurrence of the lesion, but they tend to remain stable over time (92). They are part of a syndrome recently termed *autoactivation deficit* (93). The syndrome is characterized by a deficit in spontaneous activation of mental processing, observed in behavioral, cognitive, or affective domains, that can be totally reversed by external stimulation that activates normal patterns of response. This dramatic influence of external stimulation allows one to distinguish the autoactivation deficit from inertia or aboulia observed in patients with frontal lobe lesions. For instance, Trillet et al. (94) described a patient who spent 45 minutes with his hands on a lawn mower, totally unable to initiate the act of mowing. This "kinetic blockade" disappeared instantaneously when his son told him to move. This lack of spontaneity is also observed in mental life. "My mind is empty, it's like a blank," said a patient, who was otherwise able to participate in complex cognitive and behavioral activities when stimulated by the environment. Finally, affectivity is also subject to a similar disruption of autoactivation. Affect appears flattened and emotional responses are blunted. Patients with autoactivation deficit generally react to good or bad news, but their reaction is short-lived and they rapidly return to their usual "neutral" state. Although they admit that they have become a burden to their family, they are not subject to self-depreciation. However, some patients also suffer from true depression (Table 35.3). Despite their overall decreased activity, some patients with autoactivation deficit engage in repetitive and stereotyped activities, which may be either motor (snapping or sucking the fingers) or mental (arithmomania). Hyperactivity, impulsiveness, or violent outbursts have been described in patients with lesions mainly involving the ventromedial region of the caudate nucleus, a region known to project to the orbitofrontal part of the prefrontal cortex (57).

Underlying Pathophysiologic Mechanisms of Behavioral Disorders in Focal Lesions of the Basal Ganglia

Autoactivation deficit has been reported in lesions involving mainly the globus pallidus (11) or the caudate nucleus (37). It has also been noticed in a bilateral lesion of the thalamus, following thalamopeduncular paramedian infarction (95). These findings suggest that both the striatopallidal complex and the thalamus may be part of a neuronal network implicated in cognitive, affective, and behavioral activation. The relationship between autoactivation deficit and the striatopallidal complex was recently confirmed by a meta-analysis of behavioral changes following lesions of the basal ganglia. Six of the seven patients with pallidal lesions were reported to have aboulia, and the seventh patient had an obsessive-compulsive disorder; in addition, half of those with caudate lesions (17 of 33) had behavioral inertia. However, none of the patients with lesions of the putamen presented such behavioral changes (9). The interpretation of the mechanisms by which the basal ganglia interfere with behavior depends on the anatomofunctional model to which we refer. One model relies on the description of five discrete parallel circuits in the monkey, each of which links a specific prefrontal cortical area to a discrete zone in the striatum (96). According to this model, the pathways linking the ventral striatum to the anterior cingulate cortex and the ventral part of the caudate nucleus to the orbitofrontal cortex may be good candidates to have a role in psychic autoactivation because (a) neuronal activity in the ventral striatum and caudate nucleus is increased by anticipation of a subsequent positive event (97) and (b) recordings of orbitofrontal neurons in monkeys indicate that they provide motivational components for the control of goal-directed behavior (98). However, the model of parallel and independent circuits does not take into account the massive convergence of the striatal efferents onto the pallidum, which certainly has an influence (99). The pallidum is not just a relay but a structure that filters, selects, and integrates pieces of information, whatever the domain of the information (i.e., motor, cognitive, behavioral, and affective). The consequence of a pallidal dysfunction might therefore be an activation deficit affecting various brain functions.

In conclusion, these data confirm the implication of striatofrontal loops in cognitive, affective, and behavioral regulation. At a first glance, the basal ganglia and the prefrontal cortex participate in the same executive and behavioral functions. In fact, recent studies suggest that they have complementary rather than similar roles. For example, studies based on a delayed-response paradigm may help to explain their respective intervention. In one such study, both patients with frontal lobe lesions (100) and patients with basal ganglia lesions (44) were impaired in set elaboration, but their deficit resulted from the impairment of different processes. Patients with frontal lobe lesions could not suppress previously acquired routine behaviors, whereas patients with basal ganglia lesions were impaired in maintaining the new behavior. It may be suggested, therefore, that the frontal lobes are required by inhibition of routine schemas and elaboration of new ones by constant interaction with the environment, permitting adaptation to new situations, whereas the basal ganglia intervene to transform the new program into a procedure and free the attentional resources needed by the prefrontal cortex for the elaboration of new programs. This interpretation fits well with the role attributed to the basal ganglia in the automatic maintenance of attention and procedural learning (12). Such a model might explain the differences between the effects of frontal lobe lesions, mainly impairing the voluntary control of attention and motivation, and those of basal ganglia lesions, mainly disturbing their automatic components.

ACKNOWLEDGMENTS

The work was supported by INSERM. Thanks to Nikki Horne for assistance with the English language.

REFERENCES

1. Dubois B, Pillon B, Legault F, et al. Slowing of cognitive processing in progressive supranuclear palsy: a comparison with Parkinson's disease. *Arch Neurol* 1988;45:1194–1199.
2. Taylor AE, Saint-Cyr JA, Lang AE. Frontal lobe dysfunction in Parkinson's disease—the cortical focus of neostriatal outflow. *Brain* 1986;109:845–883.
3. Pillon B, Deweer B, Agid Y, et al. Explicit memory in Alzheimer's, Huntington's, and Parkinson's diseases. *Arch Neurol* 1993;50:374–379.
4. Cummings JL. Frontal-subcortical circuits and human behavior. *Arch Neurol* 1993;50:873–880.
5. Mayeux R, Stern Y, Rosen J, et al. Depression, intellectual impairment, and Parkinson's disease. *Neurology* 1981;31:645–650.
6. Albert ML, Feldman RG, Willis AL. The subcortical dementia of progressive supranuclear palsy. *J Neurol Neurosurg Psychiatry* 1974;37:121–130.
7. Vermersch P, Delacourte A, Javoy-Agid F, et al. Dementia in Parkinson's disease. *Ann Neurol* 1993;33:445–450.
8. Hauw JJ, Verny M, Delaere P, et al. Constant neurofibrillary changes in the neocortex in progressive nuclear palsy: basic differences with Alzheimer's disease and aging. *Neurosci Lett* 1990;119:182–186.
9. Bhatia KP, Marsden CD. The behavioural and motor consequences of focal lesions of the basal ganglia in man. *Brain* 1994;117:859–876.
10. Dubois B, Défontaines B, Deweer B, et al. Cognitive and behavioral changes in patients with focal lesions of the basal ganglia. In: Weiner WJ, Lang AE, eds. *Behavioral neurology of movement disorders.* Advances in neurology, vol 65. New York: Raven Press, 1995:29–41.
11. Laplane D, Levasseur M, Pillon B, et al. Obsessive-compulsive and other behavioral changes with bilateral basal ganglia lesions: a neuropsychological, magnetic resonance imaging and positron tomography study. *Brain* 1989;112:699–725.
12. Pillon B, Boller F, Levy R, et al. Cognitive deficits and dementia in Parkinson's disease. In: Boller F, Cappa SF, eds. *Handbook of neuropsychology,* 2nd ed, vol 6. Amsterdam: Elsevier Science, 2001:311–371.
13. Bondi MW, Kaszniak AW, Bayles KA, et al. Contribution of frontal system dysfunction to memory and perceptual abilities in Parkinson's disease. *Neuropsychology* 1993;7:89–102.
14. Fournet N, Moreaud O, Roulin JL, et al. Working memory in medicated patients with Parkinson's disease: the central executive seems to work. *J Neurol Neurosurg Psychiatry* 1996;60: 313–317.
15. Litvan I, Grafman J, Gomez C, et al. Memory impairment in patients with progressive supranuclear palsy. *Arch Neurol* 1989;46:765–767.
16. Moss MB, Albert MS, Butters N, et al. Differential pattern of memory loss among patients with Alzheimer's disease, Huntington's disease, and alcoholic Korsakoff's syndrome. *Arch Neurol* 1986;43:239–246.
17. Buytenhuijs EL, Berger HJ, Van Spaendonck KP, et al. Memory and learning strategies in patients with Parkinson's disease. *Neuropsychologia* 1994;32:335–342.
18. Sommer M, Grafman J, Litvan I, et al. Impairment of eyeblink classical conditioning in progressive supranuclear palsy. *Mov Disord* 2001;16:240–251.
19. Kramer JH, Delis DC, Blusewicz MJ, et al. Verbal memory in Alzheimer's and Huntington's dementias. *Dev Neuropsychol* 1988;4:1–15.
20. Massman PJ, Kreiter KT, Jankovic J, et al. Neuropsychological functioning in cortical-basal ganglionic degeneration: differentiation from Alzheimer's disease. *Neurology* 1996;46:720–726.
21. Doyon J, Gaudreau D, Laforce R, et al. Role of the striatum, cerebellum, and frontal lobes in the learning of a visuomotor sequence. *Brain Cognition* 1997;34:218–245.
22. Grafman J, Litvan I, Gomez C, et al. Frontal lobe function in progressive supranuclear palsy. *Arch Neurol* 1990;47:553–558.
23. Knopman DS, Nissen MJ. Procedural learning is impaired in Huntington's disease: evidence from the serial reaction time task. *Neuropsychologia* 1991;29:245–254.
24. Vriezen ER, Moscovitch M. Memory for temporal order and conditional associative learning in patients with Parkinson's disease. *Neuropsychologia* 1990;28:1283–1293.

25. Butters N. The clinical aspects of memory disorders: contribution from experimental studies of amnesia and dementia. *J Clin Neuropsychol* 1984;6:17–36.

26. Mendez MF, Adams NL, Lewandowski KS. Neurobehavioral changes associated with caudate lesions. *Neurology* 1989;39:349–354.

27. Pillon B, Deweer B, Michon A, et al. Are explicit memory disorders of progressive supranuclear palsy related to damage of striato-frontal circuits? Comparison with Alzheimer's, Parkinson's, and Huntington's diseases. *Neurology* 1994;44:1264–1270.

28. Pillon B, Blin J, Vidailhet M, et al. The neuropsychological pattern of corticobasal degeneration: comparison with progressive supranuclear palsy and Alzheimer's disease. *Neurology* 1995;45:1477–1483.

29. Pillon B, Deweer B, Vidailhet M, et al. Is impaired memory for spatial location in Parkinson's disease domain specific or dependent on "strategic" processes? *Neuropsychologia* 1998;36:1–9.

30. Soliveri P, Monza D, Paridi D, et al. Neuropsychological follow-up in patients with Parkinson's disease, striatonigral degeneration-type multisystem atrophy, and progressive supranuclear palsy. *J Neurol Neurosurg Psychiatry* 2000;69:313–318.

31. Brandt J. Cognitive impairment in Huntington's disease: insights into the neuropsychology of the striatum. In: Boller F, Grafman J, eds. *Handbook of neuropsychology*, vol 5. Amsterdam: Elsevier Science, 1991:241–264.

32. Eslinger PJ, Grattan LM. Frontal lobe and frontal-striatal substrates for different forms of human cognitive flexibility. *Neuropsychologia* 1993;31:17–28.

33. Cools AR, Van Der Bercken JH, Horstinsk MW, et al. Cognitive and motor shifting aptitude disorder in Parkinson's disease. *J Neurol Neurosurg Psychiatry* 1984;47:443–453.

34. Pillon B, Gouider-Khouja N, Deweer B, et al. The neuropsychological pattern of striatonigral degeneration: comparison with Parkinson's disease and progressive supranuclear palsy. *J Neurol Neurosurg Psychiatry* 1995;58:174–179.

35. Cambier J, Masson M, Viader F, et al. Le syndrome frontal de la paralysie supranucléaire progressive. *Revue Neurologique* 1985;141:528–536.

36. Butters N, Sax D, Montgomery K, et al. Comparison of the neuropsychological deficits associated with early and advanced Huntington's disease. *Arch Neurol* 1978;35:585–589.

37. Habib M, Poncet M. Perte de l'élan vital, de l'intérêt et de l'activité (syndrome athymhormique) au cours de lésions lacunaires des corps striés. *Revue Neurologique* 1988;144:571–577.

38. Pirozzolo FJ, Hansch EC, Mortimer JA, et al. Dementia in Parkinson's disease: a neuropsychological analysis. *Brain Cognition* 1982;1:71–83.

39. Bamford KA, Caine ED, Kido DK, et al. Clinical-pathological correlation in Huntington's disease: a neuropsychological and computed tomography study. *Neurology* 1989;39:796–801.

40. Brown RG, Marsden CD. Internal versus external cues and the control of attention in Parkinson's disease. *Brain* 1988;111:323–345.

41. Meco G, Gasparini M, Doricchi F. Attentional functions in multiple system atrophy and Parkinson's disease. *J Neurol Neurosurg Psychiatry* 1996;60:393–398.

42. Fisher JM, Kennedy JL, Caine ED, et al. Dementia in Huntington's disease: a cross-sectional analysis of intellectual decline. In: Mayeux R, Rosen WG, eds. *The dementias*. New York: Raven Press, 1983:229–238.

43. Strub RL. Frontal lobe syndrome in a patient with bilateral globus pallidus lesions. *Arch Neurol* 1989;46:1024–1027.

44. Partiot A, Vérin M, Pillon B, et al. Delayed response task in basal ganglia lesions in man. Further evidence for a striato-frontal cooperation in behavioral adaptation. *Neuropsychologia* 1996;34:709–721.

45. Dubois B, Pillon B. Biochemical correlates of cognitive changes and dementia in Parkinson's disease. In: Huber SJ, Cummings JL, eds. *Parkinson's disease: neurobehavioral aspects.* Oxford: Oxford University Press, 1992:178–198.

46. Tröster AI, Fields JA, Wilkinson SB, et al. Unilateral pallidal stimulation for Parkinson's disease: neurobehavioral functioning before and 3 months after electrode implantation. *Neurology* 1997;49:1078–1083.

47. Ardouin C, Pillon B, Peiffer E, et al. Bilateral subthalamic or pallidal stimulation for Parkinson's disease affects neither memory nor executive functions: a consecutive series of 62 patients. *Ann Neurol* 1999;46:217–223.

48. Pillon B, Ardouin C, Damier Ph, et al. Neuropsychological changes between "off" and "on" STN or GPi stimulation in Parkinson's disease. *Neurology* 2000;55:411–418.

49. Houeto JL, Mesnage V, Mallet L, et al. Behavioural disorders, Parkinson's disease, and subthalamic stimulation. *J Neurol Neurosurg Psychiatry* 2002;72:701–707.

50. Ghika J. Mood and behavior in disorders of the basal ganglia. In: Bogousslavsky J, Cummings JL, eds. *Behavior and mood disorders in focal brain lesions.* Cambridge, UK: Cambridge University Press, 2000:122–200.

51. Cummings JL, Litvan I. Neuropsychiatric aspects of corticobasal degeneration. In: Litvan I, Goetz CG, Lang AE, eds. *Corticobasal degeneration.* Advances in neurology, vol 82. Philadelphia: Lippincott Williams & Wilkins, 2000:147–152.

52. Danel TH, Goudemand M, Ghawche F, et al. Mélancolie délirante et lacunes multiples des noyaux gris centraux. *Revue Neurologique* 1991;147:60–62.

53. Starkstein SE, Mayberg HS, Preziosi TJ, et al. Reliability, validity, and clinical correlates of apathy in Parkinson's disease *J Neuropsychiatry Clin Neurosci* 1992;4:134–139.

54. Litvan I, Mega MS, Cummings JL, et al. Neuropsychiatric aspects of progressive supranuclear palsy. *Neurology* 1996;47:1184–1189.

55. Caine ED, Hunt RD, Weingartner H, et al. Huntington's dementia: clinical and neuropsychological features. *Arch Gen Psychiatry* 1978;35:378–384.

56. Fedio P, Cox CS, Neophytides A, et al. Neuropsychological profiles in Huntington's disease: patients and those at risk. In: Chase TN, Wexler NS, Barbeau A, eds. *Huntington's disease.* Advances in neurology, vol 23. New York: Raven Press, 1979:239–255.

57. Richfield EK, Twyman R, Berent S. Neurological syndrome following bilateral damage to the head of the caudate nuclei. *Ann Neurol* 1987;22:768–771.

58. Aarsland D, Ballard C, Larsen JP, et al. A comparative study of psychiatric symptoms in dementia with Lewy bodies and Parkinson's disease with and without dementia. *Int J Geriatr Psychiatry* 2001;16:528–536.

59. McHugh PR, Folstein MF. Psychiatric symptoms of Huntington's chorea: a clinical and phenomenological study. In: Benson DF, Blumer D, eds. *Psychiatric aspects of neurological disease.* New York: Raven Press, 1975:267–285.

60. Aarsland D, Larsen JP, Lim NG, et al. Range of neuropsychiatric disturbances in patients with Parkinson's disease. *J Neurol Neurosurg Psychiatry* 1999;67:492–496.

61. Mayeux R, Stern Y, Rosenstein R, et al. An estimate of the prevalence of dementia in idiopathic Parkinson's disease. *Arch Neurol* 1988;45:260–262.

62. Girotti F, Soliveri P, Carella F, et al. Dementia and cognitive impairment in Parkinson's disease. *J Neurol Neurosurg Psychiatry* 1988;51:1498–1502.

63. McKeith IG, Perry EK, Perry RH. Report of the second dementia with Lewy body international workshop: diagnosis and treatment. *Neurology* 1999;53:902–905.

64. Gibb WR, Luthert PJ, Janota I, et al. Cortical Lewy body dementia: clinical features and classification. *J Neurol Neurosurg Psychiatry* 1989;52:185–192.

65. Sullivan EV, De La Paz R, Zipursky RB, et al. Neuropsychological deficits accompanying striatonigral degeneration. *J Clin Exp Neuropsychol* 1991;13:773–788.

66. Robbins TW, James M, Lange KW, et al. Cognitive performance in multiple system atrophy. *Brain* 1992;115:271–291.

67. Adams RD, Salam-Adams S. Striatonigral degeneration. In: Viken PJ, Bruyn GW, Klawans HL, eds. *Handbook of clinical neurology*, vol 5. Amsterdam: Elsevier Science, 1986:205–212.

68. Pillon B, Dubois B. Cognitive and behavioral impairments. In: Litvan I, Agid Y, eds. *Progressive supranuclear palsy.* Oxford: Oxford University Press, 1992:223–239.

69. Dubois B, Slachevsky A, Litvan I, et al. The FAB: a frontal assessment battery at bedside. *Neurology* 2000;55:1621–1626.

70. Podoll K, Schwartz M, Noth J. Language function in progressive supranuclear palsy. *Brain* 1991;114:1457–1472.

71. Pharr V, Uttl B, Stark M, et al. Comparison of apraxia in corticobasal degeneration and progressive supranuclear palsy. *Neurology* 2001;56:957–963.

72. Jellinger KA, Bancher C. Neuropathology. In: Litvan I, Agid Y, eds. *Progressive supranuclear palsy: clinical and research approaches.* Oxford: Oxford University Press, 1992:44–88.

73. Litvan I, Dickson DW, Buttner-Enever JA, et al. Research goals in progressive supranuclear palsy: conference report. *Mov Disord* 2000;15:446–458.

74. Hahn V, Deweer B, Dürr A, et al. Are cognitive changes the first symptoms of Huntington's disease? A study of gene carriers. *J Neurol Neurosurg Psychiatry* 1998;64:172–177.

75. Durr A, Dodé C, Hahn V, et al. Diagnosis of "sporadic" Huntington's disease. *J Neurol Sci* 1995;129:51–55.

76. Bachoud-Levi AC, Maison P, Bartolomeo P, et al. Retest effects and cognitive decline in longitudinal follow-up of patients with early HD. *Neurology* 2001;56:1052–1058.

77. Brouwers P, Cox C, Martin A et al. Differential perceptual-spatial impairment in Huntington's and Alzheimer's dementia. *Arch Neurol* 1984;41:1073–1076.

78. Nehl C, Ready RE, Hamilton J, et al. Effects of depression on working memory in presymptomatic Huntington's disease. *J Neuropsychiatry Clin Neurosci* 2001;13:342–346.

79. Beatty WW, Salmon DC, Butters N, et al. Retrograde amnesia in patients with Alzheimer's disease and Huntington's disease. *Neurobiol Aging* 1988;9:181–186.

80. Murray LL. Spoken language production in Huntington's and Parkinson's disease. *J Speech Language Hear Res* 2000;43:1350–1366.

81. Folstein SE, Brandt J, Folstein MF. The subcortical dementia of Huntington's disease. In: Cummings J, ed. *Subcortical dementia.* Oxford: Oxford University Press, 1990.

82. Rebeiz JJ, Kolodny EH, Richarson EP. Corticodentatonigral degeneration with neuronal achromasia. *Arch Neurol* 1968;18:20–33.

83. Lang AE, Maragonore D, Marsden CD, et al. Movement Disorder Society Symposium on cortico-basal ganglionic degeneration (CBGD) and its relationship to other asymmetrical cortical degeneration syndromes. *Mov Disord* 1996;11:346–357.

84. Bergeron C, Davis A, Lang AE. Corticobasal ganglionic degeneration and progressive supranuclear palsy presenting with cognitive decline. *Brain Pathol* 1998;8:355–365.

85. Schneider JA, Watts RL, Gearing M. Corticobasal degeneration: neuropathologic and clinical heterogeneity. *Neurology* 1997;48:959–989.

86. Leiguarda R, Lees AJ, Merello M, et al. The nature of apraxia in corticobasal degeneration. *J Neurol Neurosurg Psychiatry* 1994;57:455–459.

87. Kertez A, Martinez-Lage P, Davidson W, et al. The corticobasal degeneration syndrome overlaps progressive aphasia and frontotemporal dementia. *Neurology* 2000;55:1368–1375.

88. Grimes DA, Lang AE, Bergeron C. Dementia is the most common presentation of corticobasal ganglionic degeneration. *Neurology* 1999;53:1969–1974.

89. Blin J, Vidailhet MJ, Pillon B, et al. Cortico-basal degeneration: decreased and asymmetrical glucose consumption as studied with PET. *Mov Disord* 1992;7:348–354.

90. Pillon B, Dubois B, Agid Y. Testing cognition may contribute to the diagnosis of movement disorders. *Neurology* 1996;46:329–333.

91. Godefroy O, Rousseaux M, Leys D, et al. Frontal lobe dysfunction in unilateral lenticulo-striate infarcts. *Arch Neurol* 1992;49:1285–1289.

92. Laplane D, Widlocher D, Pillon B, et al. Comportement compulsif d'allure obsessionnelle par nécrose circonscrite bilatérale pallido-striatale: encéphalopathie par piqûre de guêpe. *Revue Neurologique* 1981;137:269–276.

93. Laplane D, Dubois D. Auto-activation deficit: a basal ganglia related syndrome. *Mov Disord* 2002 (in press).

94. Trillet M, Croisile B, Tourniaire D, et al. Perturbation de l'activité motrice volontaire et lésions des noyaux caudés. *Revue Neurologique* 1990;146:338–344.

95. Bogousslavsky J, Regli F, Delaloye B, et al. Loss of psychic self-activation with bithalamic infarction: neurobehavioral, CT, MRI, and SPECT correlates. *Acta Neurol Scand* 1991;83:309–316.

96. Alexander GE, De Long MR, Strick PL. Parallel organization of functionally segregated circuits linking basal ganglia and cortex. *Annu Rev Neurosci* 1986;9:357–381.

97. Schultz W, Apicella P, Scarnati E, et al. Neuronal activity in monkey ventral striatum related to the expectation of reward. *J Neurosci* 1992;12:4595–4610.

98. Rolls ET. *The brain and emotion.* Oxford: Oxford University Press, 1999.

99. Yelnik J, Percheron G, François C. A Golgi analysis of the primate globus pallidus. III. Quantitative morphology and spatial orientation of dendritic arborizations. *J Comp Neurol* 1984;227:200–213.

100. Vérin M, Partiot A, Pillon B, et al. Delayed response tasks and prefrontal lesions in man: evidence for self-generated patterns of behavior with poor environmental modulation. *Neuropsychologia* 1993;31:1379–1396.

PSYCHOGENIC MOVEMENT DISORDERS

WILLIAM C. KOLLER
JILL MARJAMA-LYONS
ALEXANDER I. TROSTER

Neurologic dysfunction of psychogenic origin is common (1–3). Abnormal movements and motor disorders are among the most common psychogenic symptoms (1,2,4). Toone (5) noted motor symptoms to be cited with greater consistency across studies than sensory symptoms or amnesia. Movement disorders described as psychogenic include dystonia (6), tremor (7), myoclonus (8,9), tics (10), hemiballismus (11), chorea (12), parkinsonism (9), and a host of bizarre gait and stance disturbances (13,14). We will discuss general principles and diagnostic strategies common to all psychogenic movement disorders (PMDs). We reviewed this material in an earlier report (15).

DIAGNOSIS

One difficulty in the literature on psychogenic disorders is the inconsistent use of the terminology over time and among authors (1). *Hysterical functional conversion disorder* and *psychogenic disorder* (most frequently used in the current neurology literature) are terms implying that no organic basis can be found for the patient's symptoms and the symptoms are a manifestation of an underlying psychiatric illness.

Another difficulty in using these terms is that a significant number of patients are misdiagnosed: between 6% and 30% of patients with psychogenic disorders eventually are found to have a physical illness that accounts for their symptoms (16). This is true especially in cases of idiopathic dystonia, in which 25% to 52% of patients were initially diagnosed as having a psychiatric illness (17,18). Kulisevsky (19) describes four patients with psychiatric diagnoses who were referred for evaluation of psychogenic tremor and found to have unrecognized Tourette's syndrome. The majority of idiopathic movement disorders are diagnosed by history and physical examination and lack a specific diagnostic laboratory test or neuroimaging finding; this allows for greater error in diagnosis. To complicate matters further, organic neurologic disease has been reported in as many as 28% of

patients with psychogenic disorders. In the vast majority of these the organic disease is unrelated to the psychogenic symptoms. However, Ranawaya et al. (20) described six cases of psychogenic dyskinesias complicating a preexisting organic movement disorder, and they estimate that 10% to 15% of all patients with psychogenic dyskinesia have an organic movement disorder. Likewise, Factor (4) reported 7 of 28 (25%) of patients with a documented or clinically established psychogenic movement disorder to have a coexisting organic movement disorder. This is similar to the reports of 10% to 37% of patients with pseudoseizures having true seizures (10,21).

Finally, the use of the term *psychogenic* is vague. That is, the psychiatric syndrome of which the symptom is a part remains unspecified. It is crucial that the investigating neurologist attempt to establish an accurate psychiatric diagnosis with the aid of a consulting neuropsychologist or psychiatrist to facilitate proper treatment. The various psychiatric diagnoses reported in patients with psychogenic neurologic disorders are described later in the chapter.

When a diagnosis of PMD is considered, the correct psychiatric diagnosis may fall under a number of categories listed in the *Diagnostic and Statistical Manual of Mental Disorders*, 4th ed. (DSM-IV) (22). These include somatoform disorders, factitious disorders, malingering, depression, anxiety disorders, and, less frequently, histrionic personality disorder. The first three categories are readily thought of when encountering a patient complaining of physical pain with no apparent organic basis. In somatoform disorders, in contrast to malingering and factitious disorders, symptoms are *not* consciously produced and are linked to psychological factors. Five disorders are subsumed under this category: body dysmorphic disorder, conversion disorder, hypochondriasis, somatization disorder (also called hysteria or Briquet's syndrome), and somatoform pain disorder. *Conversion disorder* is a loss or change in physical functioning that is temporally linked to a psychosocial stressor and related to a psychological need or conflict. *Hypochondriasis* is characterized by an excessive preoccupation with physical signs that the patient believes to be manifestations of serious illness despite contradictory medical evidence. *Somatization disorder*, which involves a history of numerous physical complaints (DSM-IV), requires at least 13 such symptoms from a list of 35, of which 12 are neurologic and have an onset prior to age 30 years. Complaints should be several years in duration and should be so severe that the patient has taken medication, consulted a physician, or altered his or her lifestyle because of them. Both *factitious disorder* and *malingering* entail the intentional production of symptoms. Factitious disorder, unlike malingering, is a psychological need to assume the sick role. Munchausen's syndrome falls under this category. Malingering, not considered to be a psychiatric illness, is the production of physical symptoms solely for some external gain, such as financial compensation or avoidance of work or imprisonment.

Aside from somatoform disorder, factitious disorder, and malingering, other psychiatric disorders may complicate the symptoms of movement disorders. Depression may manifest as somatic complaints rather than the classic vegetative signs. In fact, the most recent reports of PMD (7,8) list depression as the most common psychiatric diagnosis. This is in agreement with the report of Lempert et al. (2) that 38% of patients with psychogenic neurologic disorders suffer from depression. Depression may be the cause of the motor symptoms in some cases. This is supported by the observation that treatment with psychotherapy and antidepressant medication in some of these patients resulted in a remission of their movement disorder (6). Depression may also occur in reaction to or simply coexist with the psychogenic motor disorder. In any case, given the high incidence of this highly treatable psychiatric illness, it behooves the neurologist to search carefully for depression in a patient with possible psychogenic movement disorder. As with depression, anxiety has been reported as a common symptom in patients with PMD, although to a lesser degree (2,7,8). These reports are flawed in that they fail to define whether the patient suffers from one of the specific anxiety disorders listed in DSM-IV (22), simply reports feelings of anxiety, or is judged to be anxious by the examiner. Finally, histrionic personality disorder, previously called hysterical personality, which is coded in DSM-IV on Axis II, was found in only 9% of 390 patients with psychogenic neurologic illness in the review of Lempert et al. (2). The more recent reports of PMD had virtually no patients with this diagnosis (7,8).

Clearly, when a patient presents with symptoms of likely psychological origin, several possibilities exist:

1. The symptoms are exclusively a function of somatoform disorder, factitious disorder, or malingering.

2. The symptoms are part of some other form of psychological disorder (e.g., depression, panic attacks) unrelated to a physical illness.

3. The symptoms are part of a psychological disease that is linked to an organic disorder. Examples are somatization symptoms, common in depression, which in turn frequently occurs in Parkinson's and Huntington's diseases, and the high association of pseudodyskinesias with organic movement disorders.

4. The symptoms are a manifestation of an unusual clinical presentation of a physical disorder.

5. A combination of these possibilities (e.g., temporal lobe abnormalities, multiple sclerosis, and head injury have been suggested to predispose to conversion symptoms) (23).

Finally, in some cases, despite a high suspicion for psychogenicity of the motor symptoms, a psychiatric diagnosis may not be found (2,6,7). This does not necessarily preclude a diagnosis of psychogenic illness.

DIAGNOSTIC CRITERIA FOR PSYCHOGENIC MOVEMENT DISORDERS

Although psychiatric assessment is essential, the diagnosis of PMD must be made by the neurologist and based on neurologic observations. The presence of a psychiatric illness does not prove that the movement disorder is psychogenic. A comprehensive neurologic history, including a detailed review of current and prior medications, and examination as well as appropriate diagnostic studies (e.g., magnetic resonance imaging of the brain and spinal cord, serum copper and ceruloplasmin levels, thyroid functions, cerebrospinal fluid analysis) should be performed in an attempt to exclude an organic basis for the neurologic symptoms and an unrelated neurologic disorder. Once this has been accomplished, certain clues suggesting psychogenicity should be sought. Fahn and Williams (6) defined four levels of certainty for the diagnosis of psychogenic dystonia that can be applied to all types of movement disorders:

1. *Documented PMD.* The movements are relieved by psychotherapy, psychological suggestion (including physical therapy), or the administration of placebos, or the patient is seen to be free of symptoms when supposedly unobserved.

2. *Clinically established PMD.* The movements are inconsistent over time or incongruent with the classical symptoms (e.g., a patient complaining of posturing of the limb resists passive and active movement but easily grooms himself or herself daily). In addition, one or more of the following are present: other neurologic signs that are definitely psychogenic (false weakness or sensory

findings and self-inflicted injuries), multiple somatizations, or a documented psychiatric illness.

3. *Probable PMD.* The movements are inconsistent or incongruent with the classical disorder, but other features in support of psychogenicity are lacking.

4. *Possible PMD.* A suspicion of a psychogenic basis for the movements is based only on the presence of an obvious emotional disturbance.

These definitions, although not flawless, do allow for a common language for diagnosis and further study of PMD, which until recently had been lacking.

Specific clinical features of PMD are listed next. This list was compiled from studies of patients who were diagnosed with a documented or clinically established psychogenic movement disorder based on the aforementioned definitions (6–8).

1. Acute onset
2. Static course
3. Spontaneous remissions
4. Inconsistent character of movements (amplitude, frequency, distribution, selective disability)
5. Unresponsiveness to appropriate medications
6. Response to placebo
7. Movements increasing with attention
8. Movements decreasing with distraction
9. Remission with psychotherapy
10. Diagnosed psychopathology

Other factors suggesting psychogenicity but with less diagnostic importance include the following:

1. Multiple somatizations
2. Multiple undiagnosed conditions
3. False sensory complaints
4. False weakness
5. Deliberate slowness of movement
6. Employment in a health profession
7. Pending litigation or compensation
8. Secondary gain
9. Unwitnessed paroxysmal disorders
10. Negative family history

The diagnosis of PMD may appear obvious in patients fulfilling many of these criteria. However, this is often not the case. The use of placebo and suggestion in an inpatient setting has been extremely useful in documenting psychogenicity (6,8). Monday and Jankovic (8) noted no untoward effects in nine patients after disclosing the nature of the injection (placebo) and the diagnosis. In fact, it may be argued that such an objective method may assist the patient in more readily accepting the diagnosis of a psychogenic illness and facilitate appropriate therapy earlier. The use of placebo may be particularly helpful in the diagnosis of complex movement disorders and in those that coexist with an organic neurologic disease.

Despite the common guidelines for diagnosis of all PMD, some features of the motor symptoms and diagnosis are unique to the particular movement disorder. Findings of the most comprehensive studies of psychogenic dystonia (6), tremor (7), myoclonus (8), and parkinsonism (24) are summarized in Table 36.1.

Psychogenic Dystonia

Dystonia is a syndrome characterized by sustained muscle contractions commonly causing repetitive twisting and abnormal postures (25). Approximately two thirds of these patients suffer from the idiopathic form, for which no identifiable neuropathologic lesion has been found (25). Therefore, the diagnosis of psychogenic dystonia may be very difficult, as no diagnostic test for organic dystonia exists. Clinical aspects of idiopathic dystonia that might aid the clinician in avoiding an incorrect diagnosis of psychogenic dystonia are listed below (25):

1. Dystonia may occur anywhere in the body and may fluctuate and spread over time to involve other parts of the body.
2. Childhood-onset idiopathic dystonia usually begins in the foot, which is almost never the case in adult-onset idiopathic dystonia.
3. Generalized dystonia develops gradually over years, and the majority of patients have a history of childhood onset. Generalized dystonia developed in 85% of cases with onset before age 11 years in a series of 72 patients (26).
4. The dystonic movements may accompany movement (action dystonia) or occur when the patient is at rest, although typically idiopathic dystonia begins with a specific action.
5. A unique feature of idiopathic dystonia is the use of sensory tricks to reduce dystonic postures. For example, a patient with torticollis may get relief by lightly touching the chin or the back of the head.
6. Occupational or task-specific dystonias, once thought to be psychiatric, are now considered to be organic dystonic disorders (27). For example, a person may have overcontraction and posturing of the hand muscles while writing (writer's cramp) but have no difficulty typing or sewing.
7. Dystonic movements usually worsen with the use of the affected part and remit with relaxation, hypnosis, and sleep.
8. Dystonic movements or postures can occur as bursts, with return to normal function between attacks (so-called paroxysmal dystonia).
9. Dystonic movements may have a diurnal variation, with the symptoms markedly worse in the evening.
10. A rare form of childhood-onset dystonia, dopa-responsive dystonia, is characterized by gait dystonia, bizarre

TABLE 36.1. PSYCHOGENIC MOVEMENT DISORDERS

	Psychogenic Dystonia (Fahn and William, 1988)	Psychogenic Tremor (Koller et al., 1989)	Psychogenic Myoclonus (Monday and Jankovic, 1993)	Psychogenic Parkinsonism (Lang et al., 1994)
N	21	24	18	14
Female/male	19:2	15:9	13:5	7:7
Age ranges (yr)	8–58	15–78	22–75	21–63
Time from symptom onset to diagnosis	1 mo–15 yr	1 mo–10 yr	1 mo–9 yr	4 mo–13 yr
Unphysiologic weakness, gait sensation	19	+	5	10
Multiple somatizations	8	+	—	+
Psychiatric diagnosis				
Depression	+	8	4	4
Anxiety	+	4	2	0
Conversion prescription	+	8	0	4
Malinger factitious	+	2	0	+
Personality disorder	—	0	2	0
Other	+	0	2	1
No psychiatric diagnosis	+	6	7	5
Organic neurologic disorder	+	5	14	1
Decrease with distraction	+	24	14	12
+ Placebo response	10	—	9	3
Spontaneous remission	+	+	6	2
Moderate response or remission with psychotherapy	9/12	+	7/12	1
History of trauma reported as precipitant of motor symptom	+	5	6	6

−, not reported; +, present but not quantified.

gait, or unexplained falls and is highly responsive to low doses of levodopa.

11. Dystonia rarely remits (28).

Familiarity with these clinical features of organic dystonia is essential when attempting to make a diagnosis of psychogenic dystonia. Out of a total of 814 patients, Fahn and Williams (6) were able to diagnose 21 patients with documented or clinically established psychogenic dystonia and 793 with idiopathic dystonia. They are quick to point out that the clinician should be careful not to overdiagnose psychogenic dystonia, as this number constitutes only 2.6% of all cases of dystonia.

The diagnoses were made according to many of the criteria discussed in the section on diagnostic criteria for PMD. From the study of these 21 patients they found that involvement of the foot or leg was common in adults (6 of 21), which is not true for adult-onset idiopathic dystonia. They also noted 11 of 15 patients with continual dystonia to report the onset of symptoms with rest, in contrast to idiopathic dystonia, which usually begins with action. Paroxysmal dystonia occurred in 7 of the 21 patients, mak-

ing up 26% of *all* cases of paroxysmal dystonia (7 psychogenic plus 20 idiopathic).

Other observations were that 12 patients were diagnosed initially with an organic movement disorder, and 5 of these had undergone invasive diagnostic and surgical (thalamotomy) procedures. The time from the onset of symptoms until diagnosis of psychogenic dystonia varied from 1 month to 15 years. The ages ranged from 8 to 58 years, and 19 of the 21 patients were female. A complete description of the psychiatric diagnoses was not given. Of 21 patients, 9 were reported to have had complete remission of symptoms, although the duration of follow-up was not specified.

Psychogenic Tremor

Tremor is rhythmic, bidirectional, oscillating movements due to contraction of antagonistic muscles. It may occur at rest, with posture, or with movement (kinetic tremor) (29). It may be physiologic, associated with a neurologic disorder (e.g., Parkinson's disease, essential tremor, tumor, trauma, stroke, multiple sclerosis, Wilson's disease, peripheral neuropathy), or be due to any of several toxins (lead, mercury, arsenic) or drugs (lithium, valproic acid, theophylline, caffeine, alcohol withdrawal) (29).

Although a variety of organic tremors exist, certain principles, outlined next, help distinguish this group of disorders from psychogenic tremor.

1. Organic tremor usually begins gradually and rarely (except in cases of a vascular insult or trauma) has an abrupt onset (7).
2. Organic tremor typically begins on one side, increases in severity over time, and later involves the other side. (This is not the case with drug- or toxin-induced tremors, which tend to be bilateral, as they are an exacerbation of physiologic tremor) (30).
3. Organic tremor is usually more pronounced with rest (Parkinson's disease), posture (essential tremor), or movement (essential tremor or cerebellar disease). It is unusual to have a tremor in all three states, although this does occur with midbrain rubral tremor (29,30). However, in midbrain tremor the amplitude is greatest with movement, less with posture, and least at rest.
4. Task-specific tremor is a rare form that occurs only with a specific activity, usually writing (29). Many of these patients also have a mild postural tremor or tremor evident with slow active pronation and supination of the forearm.
5. Tremor, as with most movement disorders, increases with anxiety and distraction (e.g., having the patient perform a mental task or a complex motor task, such as walking backward on the heels, increases the tremor) (7).
6. Tremor frequency rarely has a significant change in organic tremor (7). Tremor amplitude but not frequency may decrease with drug therapy (31).
7. Tremor associated with neurologic disease almost never remits spontaneously, although a mild reduction in severity has been reported with placebo (32).

Koller et al. (7) diagnosed 24 patients with documented or clinically established psychogenic tremor. They found 21 patients who had an abrupt onset of tremor, and in 3 the onset was undetermined. Tremor varied in frequency and amplitude in all 24 patients. Some patients had tremor in one position during one clinic visit and absence of tremor in the same position with the next visit. Psychogenic tremor was commonly complex, occurring with rest, posture, and action and with amplitudes unlike that of midbrain tremor. Tremor lessened with distraction in all 24 cases and commonly increased when attention was drawn to it. Some patients displayed selective dysfunction; for example, they could write normally but drew a tremulous spiral. Many patients exhibited entrainment of the tremor to the frequency of repetitive movements of another limb. Psychiatric diagnoses included 8 patients with depression, 8 with conversion disorder, 4 with anxiety, and 2 with

malingering. Also, 4 patients had more than one psychiatric diagnosis, and in 6 patients no psychiatric diagnosis could be found.

Additional characteristics of the patients was the greater number of female patients (15 female and 9 male), which is a consistent finding in most studies of psychogenic disorders (33); an age range of 15 to 78 years; and a range of time from onset until diagnosis of 1 month to 10 years. There was no mention of the number of patients who underwent treatment or had remission of their symptoms.

Psychogenic Myoclonus

Myoclonus is brief, shock-like movements caused either by muscle contraction (positive myoclonus) or by lapses in posture (negative myoclonus, such as asterixis) (34). Organic myoclonus may be physiologic (sleep jerks, anxiety or exercise induced, hiccups) or it may be a symptom of a variety of disorders affecting the central nervous system (essential myoclonus, epileptic myoclonus, neurodegenerative diseases, encephalitis, metabolic and toxic encephalopathies, vascular insults, tumors, trauma, and sequela of hypoxia) (34).

The frequency, amplitude, body distribution, symmetry, and course of myoclonus vary with the different causes. Common features of most organic types of myoclonus are as follows:

1. The frequency and amplitude vary little over time (8).
2. Typically the myoclonus remains in one body region (8). An exception to these first two points is essential myoclonus, which can vary in intensity, frequency, and distribution (35).
3. Organic myoclonus usually decreases with rest, is absent with sleep, and worsens with movements and distraction (34).
4. Organic myoclonus that is not associated with treatable transient disorders (infectious, toxic, metabolic) rarely remits (8).

Monday and Jankovic (8) diagnosed 18 patients with documented or clinically established psychogenic myoclonus. Myoclonus occurred at rest in all 18 patients, was increased with movement in 14, and decreased in amplitude during distraction in 14. Also, 6 patients had spontaneous remissions that lasted up to 10 hours, and 9 had reduction of myoclonus with placebo; 5 patients had nonphysiologic weakness or sensory loss.

Patients were observed with various types of myoclonus, including 10 patients with predominantly segmental myoclonus, 7 with generalized myoclonus, and 1 with focal involvement. Patients reported the myoclonus to vary in frequency, amplitude, and pattern of distribution, although the exact numbers of patients with these changes were not stated.

Psychiatric diagnoses, which were made prior to the development of myoclonus in 10 patients, included 4 patients with depression, 2 with panic attacks, 2 with personality disorder, 1 with adjustment disorder, and 1 with bipolar disorder. After neuropsychological testing, only 1 additional patient was found to have evidence of psychopathology, leaving 7 patients with no psychiatric diagnosis. Of the 12 patients who had follow-up, 7 reported marked improvement (2 with complete remission), 3 noted a worsening of their symptoms, and 2 believed no change had occurred.

Psychogenic Parkinsonism

Parkinsonism is a symptom complex consisting of resting tremor, rigidity, bradykinesia, and impaired postural reflexes (36). Parkinsonism may be classified as either primary idiopathic disease, the cause of which remains unknown, or secondary, resulting from a variety of possible causes including infection (encephalitis lethargica), stroke, tumor, head trauma, toxins (manganese, 1-methyl-4-phenyl-1,2,3,6-tetrahydropyridine [MPTP], cyanide, carbon monoxide) and drugs (neuroleptics, lithium, reserpine, α-methyldopa) (36). A number of neurodegenerative diseases may also have clinical features of parkinsonism (multiple system atrophy, Alzheimer's disease, idiopathic dystonia, Creutzfeldt-Jakob disease, and Guam parkinsonism-dementia complex) (36).

The clinical presentation of parkinsonism varies considerably and, as with the aforementioned movement disorders, no definitive diagnostic test exists, which makes diagnosis of organic and psychogenic parkinsonism difficult. Lang et al. (24) described 14 patients with documented and clinically established psychogenic parkinsonism. Of these, 11 had been previously diagnosed with organic parkinsonism; 12 had tremor at rest that, unlike tremor of organic parkinsonism, persisted with the same amplitude with posture and action. Tremor also commonly varied in frequency and rhythmicity, changed to the frequency of other movements, and remitted with distraction. Rigidity, observed in 6 patients, consisted of voluntary resistance without cogwheeling and lessened with distraction. All 14 patients demonstrated bradykinesia that lacked the fatiguing component (decreasing amplitude and frequency) seen in organic parkinsonism. Gait was atypical, with the affected arm held tightly to the trunk; postural instability was extreme or bizarre in reaction to minimal displacement. The symptoms were maximal at the onset, as was early disability, in marked contrast to organic parkinsonism, which begins with mild symptoms that gradually worsen over years. Also, 3 patients had normal fluorodopa striatal uptake with positron emission tomography, and 1 patient who had a placebo response to psychotherapy and haloperidol (Haldol) had decreased fluorodopa uptake on one side, pointing out that psychogenic parkinsonism may coexist with organic parkinsonism.

The most common psychiatric diagnoses were depression and conversion disorder. A few patients were involved in litigation and compensation, and 5 had no identified psychiatric diagnosis.

Additional characteristics included multiple somatizations, functional weakness or sensory changes, spontaneous remission, and a positive placebo response. Half of the patients were women and half were men, with ages ranging from 21 to 63 years. The time of onset of symptoms until diagnosis of psychogenicity varied between 1 month and 9 years.

TREATMENT

Treatment of patients with PMDs demands a strong alliance of the neurologist with the patient to assure proper follow-up of therapeutic recommendations. Assistance is required to help the patient gain insight into the psychological causes of the movement disorder. A primary psychologist or psychiatrist may be needed. However, many patients resist a psychiatric referral. The manner in which the physician discusses the suspected diagnosis of a psychogenic disorder and the need for such a referral is critical. It is important that the patient not be confronted in a way that suggests "there is nothing I can find wrong with you." Such a statement is likely to be interpreted as "the physician thinks I'm crazy and doesn't take my symptoms seriously." It may be preferable to phrase the diagnosis along the lines: "We've run numerous tests and I'm relieved to be able to tell you that your symptoms are not due to a serious neurologic disease. Unfortunately, the tests do not tell us what is causing the problems. Nonetheless, because the symptoms are very distressing and disruptive to you, I feel it may be helpful to get the opinion of a consultant about how we can proceed and minimize the difficulties these symptoms are causing you." If the patient gets angry, it may be beneficial to inquire about the grounds for this anger; this may also provide a useful illustration to the patient about how distressing the symptoms are. Some patients more readily accept that psychological factors may underlie their motor symptoms, and it may be helpful to say, "The mind and body work closely together, and emotional stress, anxiety, and even depression may actually cause physical symptoms. Because these are treatable with counseling and certain medications, I think it is important to have a specialist assess whether you are suffering from anxiety or depression that you may not be aware of." It may also help to give an example of a more acceptable physical illness, such as a peptic ulcer, developing as a result of stress.

Patients are also more likely to go along with psychological consults if a psychologist or psychiatrist is involved in their evaluation from the beginning (e.g., if psychological tests are scheduled over the period when physical tests are performed). It is also important that the patient not perceive himself or herself as being "shunted around" the medical system or "dumped." Many patients have already seen several specialists over a long period without ever being informed properly about the psychological nature of their illness. It is imperative that the neurologist schedule a follow-up appointment to restate physical test results and integrate psychological test results. In some patients, despite the lack of an organic neurologic illness, periodic neurologic evaluation with the same neurologist in conjunction with psychotherapy may be necessary to alleviate excessive concern about the possibility of having an organic illness and to maintain a reduction or remission of motor symptoms.

Insight-oriented psychotherapy in combination with positive reinforcement and physical therapy has resulted in a reduction or cessation of symptoms in many patients (6–8). Positive statements, such as "I expect your movements to decrease over the next several weeks and then to stop," may act as a template for the patient to follow. Suggesting physical therapy to help retrain the muscles to move normally may likewise be beneficial.

The use of placebo for diagnosis and therapy is debatable. Some patients interpret this as confrontational and become more resistant to the diagnosis and psychiatric treatment. Fahn and Williams (6) and Monday and Jankovic (8) advocate the use of placebo when the diagnosis of psychogenicity is difficult. They recommend admitting the patient to the hospital and explaining the results in a supportive manner with immediate inpatient treatment with the aforementioned modalities. Finally, the use of medications, such as mild anxiolytics and antidepressants, is recommended for short-term management of anxiety, which is common in these patients, or for long-term management of a primary anxiety disorder or depression. As concerns prognosis, acute onset, short duration of symptoms, healthy premorbid functioning, absence of coexisting organic and psychogenic disease, and presence of an identifiable stressor are related to a relatively good prognosis (37).

REFERENCES

1. Marsden CS. Hysteria: a neurologist's view. *Psychol Med* 1986;16: 277–288.
2. Lempert T, Dietrich M, Huppert D, et al. Psychogenic disorders in neurology: frequency and clinical spectrum. *Acta Neurol Scand* 1990;82:335–340.
3. Shaibani A, Sabbagh MN. Pseudoneurologic syndromes: recognition and diagnosis. *Am Fam Physician* 1998;58:1970–1972.
4. Factor SA, Podskalny GD, Molho ES. Psychogenic movement disorders: frequency, clinical profile, and characteristics. *J Neurol Neurosurg Psychiatry* 1995;59:406–412.
5. Toone BK. *Disorders of hysterical conversion.* Oxford: Blackwell Scientific, 1990:207–234.
6. Fahn S, Williams D. Psychogenic dystonia. *Adv Neurol* 1988;50: 431–455.
7. Koller W, Lang A, Vetere-Overfield B, et al. Psychogenic tremors. *Neurology* 1989;39:1094–1099.
8. Monday K, Jankovic J. Psychogenic myoclonus. *Neurology* 1993; 43:349–352.
9. Walters AS, Boudwin J, Wright D, et al. Three hysterical movement disorders. *Psychol Rep* 1988;62:979–985.
10. Kurlan R, Deeley C, Corno P. Psychogenic movement disorder (pseudo-tics) in a patient with Tourette's syndrome. *J Neuropsychiatry Clin Neurosci* 1992;4:347–349.
11. Hoogdvin CA. Therapy of a female patient with hemiballismus: a case report. *Exp Klin Hypnose* 1990;6:57–64.
12. Woolsey RM. Hysteria 1875–1975. *Dis Nerv Syst* 1976;37: 379–386.
13. Keane J. Hysterical gait disorders. *Neurology* 1989;39:586–589.
14. Hayes MW, et al. A video review of the diagnosis of psychogenic gait: appendix and commentary. *Mov Disord* 1999;14:914–921.
15. Marjama J, Troster A, Koller WC. Psychogenic movement disorders. *Neurol Clin* 1995;13:283–297.
16. Putnam FW. *Conversion symptoms: movement disorders in neurology and neuropsychiatry.* Boston: Blackwell Scientific, 1992: 430–437.
17. Cooper IS, Cullinan T, Riklan M. The natural history of dystonia. *Adv Neurol* 1976;14:157–169.
18. Eldridge R, Riklan M, Cooper IS. The limited role of psychotherapy in torsion dystonia: experience with 44 cases. *JAMA* 1969;210:705–708.
19. Kulisevsky J, et al. Unrecognized Tourette syndrome in adult patients referred for psychogenic tremor. *Arch Neurol* 1998;55: 409–414.
20. Ranawaya R, Riley D, Lang A. Psychogenic dyskinesias with organic movement disorders. *Mov Disord* 1990;5:127–133.
21. Krumholz A, Niedermeyer E. Psychogenic seizures: a clinical study with follow-up data. *Neurology* 1983;33:498–502.
22. American Psychiatric Association. *Diagnostic and statistical manual of mental disorders,* 4th ed. Washington, DC: 1996:21.
23. Pincus J. *Hysteria.* New York: John Wiley & Sons, 1982.
24. Lang AE, Koller WC, Fahn S. Psychogenic parkinsonism. *Arch Neurol* 1995;52:802–810.
25. Weiner W, Lang A. Idiopathic torsion dystonia. In: Weiner W, Lang A, eds. *Movement disorders: a comprehensive survey.* New York: Futura, 1989:347–418.
26. Marsden CD, Harrison M, Bundey S. Natural history of idiopathic torsion dystonia. *Adv Neurol* 1976;14:177–187.
27. Sheehy MP, Marsden CD. Writer's cramp: a focal dystonia. *Brain* 1982;105:461–480.
28. Friedman A, Fahn S. Spontaneous remissions in spasmodic torticollis. *Neurology* 1986;36:398–400.
29. Weiner WJ, Lang AE. Tremor. In: Weiner WJ, Lang AE, eds. *Movement disorders: a comprehensive survey.* New York: Futura, 1989b:221–256.
30. Holmes G. On certain tremors in organic cerebral lesions. *Brain* 1904;27:327–375.
31. Koller WC. Diagnosis and treatment of tremors. *Neurol Clin* 1984;2:449–514.
32. Koller WC. Treatment of essential tremor. In: Marsden CD, Conrad B, Benecke R, eds. *Motor disorders.* London: Academic Press, 1987:55–67.
33. Kaplan H, Sadock B. Synopsis on psychiatry. In: Fisher MC, ed. Baltimore: Williams & Wilkins, 1991:332–333.
34. Weiner WJ, Lang A. Myoclonus and related syndromes. In: Weiner WJ, Lang A, eds. *Movement disorders: a comprehensive survey.* New York: Futura, 1989:457–461.
35. Korten JJ, Notermans SL, Frenken CW, et al. Familial essential myoclonus. *Brain* 1974;97:131–138.
36. Koller W, ed. *Classification of parkinsonism. Handbook of Parkinson's disease.* New York: Marcel Dekker, 1987:51–80.
37. Lazare A. Current concepts in psychiatry: conversion symptoms. *N Engl J Med* 1981;305:745–748.

HEREDITARY ATAXIAS

THOMAS KLOCKGETHER

The hereditary ataxias comprise a wide spectrum of genetically determined disorders with progressive ataxia as the prominent symptom. In most of these disorders, ataxia is due to degeneration of the cerebellar cortex and the spinal cord. The underlying gene mutations have been identified in most hereditary ataxias. Knowledge of the causative mutations allows a rational classification of hereditary ataxias (Table 37.1). Principally, it is distinguished between autosomal recessive and autosomal dominant ataxias. The autosomal dominant ataxias can be further subdivided into the progressive spinocerebellar ataxias (SCA) and the episodic ataxias (EA), which are characterized by paroxysmal occurrence of ataxia.

AUTOSOMAL RECESSIVE ATAXIAS

Overview

Until now the gene mutations of eight autosomal recessively inherited ataxias [Friedreich's ataxia (FRDA), ataxia

TABLE 37.1. CLASSIFICATION OF HEREDITARY ATAXIAS

Autosomal recessive ataxias
  with known gene mutation
    Friedreich's ataxia
    Ataxia telangiectasia
    Autosomal recessive spastic ataxia of Charlevoix-Saguenay
    Abetalipoproteinemia
    Ataxia with isolated vitamin E deficiency
    Refsum's disease
    Cerebrotendinous xanthomatosis
    Autosomal recessive ataxia with oculomotor apraxia
  with known gene locus
    Autosomal recessive ataxia linked to chromosome 9q
    Autosomal recessive ataxia with hearing impairment and optic atrophy
    Infantile-onset spinocerebellar ataxia
  gene locus and mutation unknown
    Early-onset cerebellar ataxia
Autosomal dominant ataxias
  Spinocerebellar ataxias
  Episodic ataxias

telangiectasia (A-T), autosomal recessive spastic ataxia of Charlevoix-Saguenay (ARSACS), abetalipoproteinemia, ataxia with isolated vitamin E deficiency (AVED), Refsum's disease, cerebrotendinous xanthomatosis ataxias, autosomal recessive ataxia with oculomotor apraxia (AOA)] have been identified. In three other autosomal recessive ataxias [recessive ataxia linked to chromosome 9q, autosomal recessive ataxia with hearing impairment and optic atrophy, infantile-onset spinocerebellar ataxia (IOSCA)], linkage to chromosomal regions has been established. In a heterogeneous group of ataxias with early disease onset, recessive inheritance is assumed, but the gene loci and mutations are unknown. These disorders have been named early-onset cerebellar ataxias (EOCAs).

Friedreich's Ataxia

Etiology and Pathogenesis

FRDA is the most common autosomal recessively inherited ataxia. In most cases of FRDA, the causative mutation is a homozygous, intronic GAA repeat expansion in a gene coding for a mitochondrial protein named frataxin. Less than 4% of FRDA patients are compound heterozygotes with one allele carrying the GAA repeat expansion and the other a point mutation (1,2). Recently, a second FRDA locus was mapped to chromosome 9p (3).

Due to the GAA repeat expansion, tissue levels of frataxin are severely reduced. Studies in yeast show that frataxin binds iron in a high molecular weight form and keeps it in a reduced form. Loss of frataxin consequently leads to mitochondrial iron overload, increased production of free radicals, and impaired utilization of iron for synthesis of iron-sulfur clusters resulting in decline of mitochondrial respiratory activity (4).

Neuropathology

The first pathologic changes in FRDA are thought to occur in the dorsal root ganglia with loss of large sensory neurons. In advanced cases, the neuropathologic abnormalities comprise axonal sensory and motor neuropathy, degeneration of spinal tracts (spinocerebellar tracts, posterior columns, pyramidal tract), and concentric hypertrophic cardiomyopathy affecting both chambers and the septum. There is only occasional involvement of the cerebellum with loss of Purkinje cells and moderate cerebellar atrophy.

Epidemiology

The prevalence of FRDA is estimated at 2 to 3 per 100,000.

Clinical Presentation

The prominent sign of FRDA is progressive ataxia, initially affecting gait and stance, and later also arm movements. Muscle reflexes of the legs are absent in about 90% of the patients. Approximately 80% of the patients have extensor plantar responses. With progression of the disease, distal wasting of the lower and upper extremities develops. Due to pyramidal involvement and muscle wasting, FRDA patients may have considerable weakness. Approximately half of the patients have skeletal deformities (scoliosis, pes cavus), which are due to muscle wasting starting early in life. Almost all patients have sensory disturbances with reduced vibration and position sense (5).

All FRDA patients develop an ataxic speech disorder, usually within the first 5 years of their disease. Disorders of ocular motility are part of the clinical spectrum of FRDA. Oculomotor disorders include square-wave jerks during fixation and reduced gain of vestibulo-ocular reflex. Oculomotor disturbances pointing to cerebellar dysfunction, such as gaze-evoked nystagmus or saccadic hypermetria, are usually absent in FRDA. Physical examination reveals pale disks in many FRDA patients. However, a loss of visual acuity is encountered in only 10% to 20% of patients. Similarly, 10% to 20% develop sensorineural hearing problems.

In approximately 60% of FRDA patients, echocardiography reveals a hypertrophic cardiomyopathy. Diabetes mellitus is present in 10% to 30% of patients (5).

Natural Course

Mean age at onset is 15 years ranging from 2 to 51 years (5). FRDA is a progressive disease leading to disability and premature death. Median latency to become wheelchair bound after disease onset is 11 years. Life expectancy after disease onset is estimated 35 to 40 years (6). Age of onset and progression rate are partly determined by the GAA repeat length of the shorter allele: in patients with longer expansions, disease onset is earlier and progression faster (5).

Diagnosis

A genetic test demonstrating the GAA repeat expansion is widely available and can be used to confirm a clinical diagnosis of FRDA. Genetic testing is particularly useful in atypical cases with preserved muscle reflexes and late disease onset. If the genetic test is negative, serum levels of vitamin E should be determined because the clinical phenotype of FRDA can be mimicked by AVED. To distinguish FRDA from hereditary motor and sensory neuropathies, nerve conduction studies are useful. Magnetic resonance imaging (MRI) typically shows cervical spinal cord atrophy without major cerebellar atrophy. Nerve conduction studies reveal an axonal form of sensory neuropathy. Most patients have repolarization changes of the electrocardiogram. Hypertrophic cardiomyopathy is demonstrated by echocardiography.

Management

Since frataxin deficiency leads to increased production of free radicals, free-radical scavengers are currently investigated in FRDA. Rustin et al. recently reported that idebenone (5 mg/kg per day), a short-chain quinone analog acting as a free-radical scavenger given over 4 to 9 months, decreased the left ventricular mass index in three FRDA patients (7). Randomized, controlled trials with this compound have not been completed. Antiataxic drugs, such as 5-hydroxytryptophan, buspirone, and amantadine, are ineffective or only marginally effective in FRDA. Physiotherapy and speech therapy are generally recommended. Patients with clinically relevant cardiomyopathy and diabetes mellitus should receive standard medical treatment.

Ataxia Telangiectasia

Etiology and Pathogenesis

Ataxia telangiectasia is an autosomal recessively inherited multisystem disorder caused by mutations of the *ATM* gene. The *ATM* gene encodes a member of the phosphoinositol 3-kinase family involved in cell cycle checkpoint control and DNA repair (8). More than 200 distinct mutations distributed over the entire gene have been reported. Very rarely, a disorder similar to A-T is caused by mutations in the double-strand break repair gene *hMRE11* (9).

Neuropathology

There is atrophy of the cerebellum mainly affecting the cerebellar cortex of the vermis. The number of cerebellar Purkinje cells is reduced, and Purkinje cells show abnormal arborization and ectopic localization. In addition, there are degenerative changes of the spinal cord including degeneration of the posterior and lateral columns and atrophy of the anterior horn. The peripheral nervous system may be involved with a demyelinating neuropathy.

Epidemiology

The incidence of A-T has been estimated at 0.3 per 100,000 live births.

Clinical Presentation

A-T is clinically characterized by a combination of neurologic and nonneurologic symptoms. Cerebellar ataxia is the clinical hallmark of A-T. Ataxia of gait and stance usually become apparent when the child has learned to walk. Other cerebellar symptoms, including dysarthria and ataxia of the upper extremities, develop later. In addition, many patients have choreoathetosis and dystonia. Muscle reflexes are usually weak or absent. A-T patients have a peculiar difficulty initiating saccades (oculomotor apraxia). In contrast to ophthalmoplegia, eye movements can be completed in the full range when given sufficient time. When A-T patients intend gaze shifts, they move their head into the desired direction causing a reflectory, tonic drift of the eyes away from the target. The target is then refixated with considerable delay. Intellectual abilities are normal in the beginning of the disease. Later, there may be mild impairments that are partly secondary to the physical disability. In late disease stages, patients develop sensory disturbances with impaired vibration and positional sense and distal muscle wasting.

Telangiectasias are the second hallmark of A-T. They develop after the onset of ataxia and are most frequently found in the lateral angles of the conjunctivae and the external earlobes. Approximately 60% of A-T patients have immunodeficiency. The most common clinical manifestations are recurrent sinopulmonary infections. A-T patients have a considerably increased risk of malignancies. Overall, one third of A-T patients develop a malignant disease during their lives. Before the age of 20 years, malignancies are mainly lymphoid. In older patients, solid tumors are more common.

Natural Course

A-T usually begins at the age of 2 to 4 years after the child has learned to walk. In those cases, A-T begins after the age of 20 years. Most patients need wheelchairs at the age of 10 years. Life expectancy is severely reduced due to recurrent infections and neoplasia. Most patients die in their third decade.

Diagnosis

A diagnosis of A-T is probable in patients with a typical clinical phenotype and elevated serum levels of α-fetoprotein. In vitro demonstration of radiosensitivity of lymphocytes is used as a laboratory test to confirm the diagnosis. Genetic testing is not used routinely due to the diversity of mutations causing A-T.

Management

Although the gene defect causing A-T has been found and the cellular pathogenesis is partly understood, effective therapies are not available. In particular, there is no way to improve ataxia.

Management of infections should be initiated early and maintained over a prolonged time. Usually, infections require intravenous or oral application of wide-spectrum antibiotics. Administration of immunoglobulins can be considered in patients with repeated infections. However, standard immunoglobulin preparations are often poorly tolerated by A-T patients owing to IgA deficiency. In these patients, a switch to preparations with low or absent IgA levels is required.

Management of malignant neoplasias is a particular problem because A-T patients have increased sensitivity to radiation and chemotherapy. Therefore, conventional radiotherapy should be avoided, and chemotherapy should be administered only on an individual basis.

Autosomal Recessive Spastic Ataxia of Charlevoix-Saguenay

Etiology and Pathogenesis

ARSACS is an autosomal recessive ataxia with a distinctive phenotype that is prevalent in a restricted area in Quebec, Canada. ARSACS is due to mutations in a large, single-exon gene encoding a novel protein named sacsin. The most common mutation accounting for more than 90% of all mutations is a deletion leading to protein truncation. Sacsin contains a heat-shock domain, suggesting that it subserves chaperone function (10).

Neuropathology

Autopsies of ARSACS patients showed cortical atrophy, pyramidal degeneration, atrophy of the upper cerebellar vermis, and loss of motor neurons. Immunocytochemical studies revealed abnormal accumulations of neurofilaments (Y. Robitaille, personal communication, 2001). The central nervous system abnormalities are accompanied by a mixed sensorimotor neuropathy.

Epidemiology

The prevalence of ARSACS in the founder population in Quebec is estimated 50 per 100,000. Outside Quebec families have been ascertained in Tunisia, Turkey and France.

Clinical Presentation

ARSACS is characterized by the combination of progressive cerebellar ataxia and spasticity. Muscle reflexes are exaggerated and plantar responses are extensor. With progression of the disease, the ankle jerks disappear, and distal wasting of foot muscles develops. A highly characteristic ocular sign is the presence of prominent myelinated fibers radiating from the optic disk at fundoscopy.

Natural Course

ARSACS typically starts at the age of 1 to 2 years. On average, patients become wheelchair bound around the age of 40 years.

Diagnosis

A genetic test for ARSACS has been established at the Genetic Service of the St. Justine Hospital in Montreal (A. Richter, personal communication, 2001).

Management

There is no effective therapy for ARSACS. A minority of patients with pronounced spasticity may benefit from anti-spasticity drugs.

Abetalipoproteinemia

Abetalipoproteinemia is a rare, autosomal recessively inherited disorder characterized by onset of diarrhea soon after birth and slow development of a neurologic syndrome thereafter. The neurologic syndrome consists of ataxia, weakness of the limbs with loss of tendon reflexes, disturbed sensation, and retinal degeneration. Abetalipoproteinemia is caused by mutations in the gene encoding a subunit of a microsomal triglyceride transfer protein (11). As a consequence, circulating apoprotein B–containing lipoproteins are almost completely missing, and the patients are unable to absorb and transport fat and fat-soluble vitamins. The neurologic symptoms are due to vitamin E deficiency. Management of abetalipoproteinemia consists of a diet with reduced fat intake and oral vitamin E supplementation (50 to 100 mg/kg per day).

Ataxia with Isolated Vitamin E Deficiency

AVED is a rare, autosomal recessively inherited disorder with a phenotype resembling that of FRDA. AVED patients carry homozygous mutations of the gene encoding the α-tocopherol transport protein, a liver-specific protein that incorporates vitamin E into very-low-density lipoproteins (12). As a consequence, vitamin E is rapidly eliminated. AVED is a common cause of recessive ataxia in North African countries but is rarely encountered in other parts of the world. Since there is no absorption deficit, oral supplementation of vitamin E at a dose of 800 to 2,000 mg/day is recommended.

Refsum's Disease

Refsum's disease is a rare, autosomal recessively inherited disorder caused by mutations in the gene encoding phytanoyl-coenzyme A (CoA) hydroxylase that is involved in the α-oxidation of phytanic acid (13). The clinical phenotype of Refsum's disease is caused by accumulation of phytanic acid in body tissues. Clinically, Refsum's disease is characterized by ataxia, demyelinating sensorimotor neuropathy, pigmentary retinal degeneration, deafness, cardiac arrhythmias, and ichthyosis-like skin changes. Whereas ocular and hearing problems are usually slowly progressive, there may be acute exacerbations that are precipitated by low caloric intake and mobilization of phytanic acid from adipose tissue.

Management of Refsum's disease is by dietary restriction of phytanic acid from 50–100 mg contained in a normal Western diet to less than 10 mg/day. With good dietary supervision, ataxia and neuropathy may improve. In contrast, the progressive loss of vision and hearing cannot be prevented. In acute exacerbations, plasma exchange is effective in lowering phytanic acid levels and improving neurologic and cardiac function.

Cerebrotendinous Xanthomatosis

Cerebrotendinous xanthomatosis is a rare, autosomal recessively inherited lipid storage disorder with accumulation of cholestanol and cholesterin in various tissues. The disorder is due to mutations of the gene encoding 27-hydroxylase (14). The clinical syndrome includes xanthomatous swelling of the tendons, cataracts, and slowly progressive neurologic symptoms including ataxia, pyramidal signs, and cognitive decline. Cerebrotendinous xanthomatosis is managed by oral administration of chenodeoxycholate (750 mg/day). Treatment can be further improved by addition of 3-hydroxy-3-methylglutaryl-CoA reductase inhibitors, such as simvastatin or lovastatin.

Autosomal Recessive Ataxia with Oculomotor Apraxia

AOA is a rare, autosomal recessively inherited ataxia caused by mutations in gene coding for a novel protein named aprataxin. The neurologic presentation of AOA is variable. The gene has been simultaneously found by two research groups, one studying Portuguese families with an A-T-like phenotype including progressive ataxia, oculomotor apraxia, and peripheral neuropathy, and another studying Japanese families with ataxia and hypoalbuminemia (M. Koenig, personal communication, 2001). In contrast to A-T, telangiectasias, neoplasias, and immunodeficiency are always absent. Disease onset ranges from early childhood to adolescence. Patients survive into middle or late adulthood albeit in a severely disabled state (15).

Autosomal Recessive Ataxia Linked to Chromosome 9q

Recently, linkage to chromosome 9q was demonstrated in a consanguineous Japanese family with ataxia associated with elevated levels of serum creatine kinase, γ-globulin, and α-fetoprotein (16). Another family with the clinical phenotype of ataxia with oculomotor apraxia was mapped to the same chromosomal region (17).

Autosomal Recessive Ataxia with Hearing Impairment and Optic Atrophy

Linkage to chromosome 6p was demonstrated in an Israeli family with early-onset recessive ataxia. Patients subsequently developed hearing impairment and optic atrophy (16).

Infantile-onset Spinocerebellar Ataxia

IOSCA is an early-onset recessive ataxia linked to a locus on chromosome 10q that has been described in Finnish families. The disease manifests around the age of 1 year as acute or subacute clumsiness, athetoid movements in hands and face, hypotonia, and loss of deep tendon reflexes in the legs. Ophthalmoplegia and a sensorineural hearing deficit are found by school age, sensory neuropathy, and optic atrophy by the age of 10 to 15 years, and female hypogonadism and epilepsy by the age of 15 to 20 years. Most patients are wheelchair bound by the age of 20 years (18).

Early-onset Cerebellar Ataxia

EOCA denotes those ataxias with an onset before the age of 20 years in which the etiology is unknown. It is assumed that most EOCAs are autosomal recessive disorders. The most common form of EOCA, EOCA with retained tendon reflexes, is clinically distinguished from typical FRDA by the preservation of muscle reflexes. On MRI, these patients have cerebellar atrophy, and disease progression is slower than in FRDA (19). Other EOCA patients may present with a variety of additional symptoms including retinal degeneration (Hallgren's syndrome), hypogonadism (Holmes' syndrome), cataracts and mental retardation (Marinesco-Sjögren syndrome), and myoclonus (Ramsay Hunt syndrome).

AUTOSOMAL DOMINANT ATAXIAS

Spinocerebellar Ataxias

Genetics

The SCAs are a genetically heterogeneous group of autosomal dominantly inherited progressive ataxia disorders. Up to now, 15 different gene loci (SCA1–8, 10–14, 16, 17) have been found in association with SCA. SCA9 and 15 have been reserved for new loci that have not been published yet.

All mutations that have been identified so far (SCA1–3, 6, 8, 10, 12, 17) are expanded repeats. In six of them (SCA1–3, 6, 7, 17), the mutation is a translated CAG repeat expansion coding for an elongated polyglutamine tract within the respective proteins (Table 37.2). These disorders belong to larger group of polyglutamine disorders that also includes Huntington's disease, dentatorubropallidoluysian atrophy, and spinobulbar muscular atrophy. It is assumed that the polyglutamine disorders share important pathogenetic features. In other SCAs, the repeat expansion

TABLE 37.2. MUTATIONS AND CLINICAL PHENOTYPES OF SPINOCEREBELLAR ATAXIAS

Disorder	Mutation	Gene Product	Clinical Phenotype
SCA1	Translated CAG repeat expansion	Ataxin-1	Ataxia, pyramidal signs, neuropathy, dysphagia, restless legs syndrome
SCA2	Translated CAG repeat expansion	Ataxin-2	Ataxia, slow saccades, neuropathy, restless legs syndrome
SCA3 (Machado-Joseph disease)	Translated CAG repeat expansion	Ataxin-3	Ataxia, pyramidal signs, ophthalmoplegia, neuropathy, dystonia, restless legs syndrome
SCA4	Unknown	Unknown	Ataxia, neuropathy
SCA5	Unknown	Unknown	Almost pure cerebellar ataxia
SCA6	Translated CAG repeat expansion	Calcium channel subunit (CACNA1A)	Almost pure cerebellar ataxia
SCA7	Translated CAG repeat expansion	Ataxin-7	Ataxia, ophthalmoplegia, visual loss
SCA8	Untranslated CTG repeat expansion	Unknown	Almost pure cerebellar ataxia
SCA10	Intronic ATTCT repeat expansion	Unknown	Ataxia, epilepsy
SCA11	Unknown	Unknown	Almost pure cerebellar ataxia
SCA12	Untranslated CAG repeat expansion	Phosphatase subunit (PP2A-PR55β)	Ataxia, tremor
SCA13	Unknown	Unknown	Ataxia, mental retardation
SCA14	Unknown	Unknown	Ataxia, myoclonus
SCA16	Unknown	Unknown	Almost pure cerebellar ataxia
SCA17	Translated CAG repeat expansion	TATA-binding protein	Ataxia, dystonia

SCA, spinocerebellar ataxia.

is found in the 5′ untranslated region (SCA12), in an intron (SCA10), and in the 3′ untranslated region (SCA8).

Clinical Features

Although ataxia is the prominent symptom in all SCAs, their clinical presentation is diverse. Most SCAs are multisystemic disorders with a clinical syndrome suggesting widespread involvement of the central and peripheral nervous system going far beyond the cerebellum and spinal cord. In particular, the most common forms SCA1–3 usually present with progressive ataxia accompanied by a variety of additional symptoms. Correspondingly, neuropathologic studies show neurodegeneration not only in the spinocerebellar system but also in the cortex, basal ganglia, and brainstem. Only a few mutations are characterized by an almost pure cerebellar syndrome and isolated degeneration of the cerebellar cortex. The most common disorder of this group is SCA6.

Epidemiology

The prevalence of all the dominantly inherited progressive ataxias is estimated 0.9 to 1.3 per 100,000. Epidemiologic data of specific SCA mutations are not available. However, there is some information on the distribution of specific SCA mutations among all dominant ataxias in different populations.

Management

Studies of the molecular pathogenesis of the SCAs have not yet resulted in development of therapies that are available for use in humans. It has been repeatedly claimed that drugs that increase neurotransmission at central 5-hydroxytryptamine (5-HT, serotonin) receptors improve cerebellar ataxia. Three recent studies investigated the antiataxic effect of the anxiolytic 5-HT$_{1A}$ receptor agonist buspirone. Results of an open-label study of 20 patients with different forms of degenerative cerebellar ataxia suggested an antiataxic action of buspirone at a dose of 30 to 60 mg/day (20). Efficacy of buspirone was confirmed in a randomized, placebo-controlled study of 19 patients with ataxia due to cerebellar cortical atrophy (21). In contrast, another study did not report a favorable effect of buspirone in ataxia (22). All patients should receive physiotherapy and speech therapy, if necessary.

Spinocerebellar Ataxia Type 1 (SCA1)

Etiology and Pathogenesis

The mutation causing SCA1 is a translated CAG repeat expansion in a gene coding for ataxin-1. While the repeat length in normals varies between 6 and 39 trinucleotides, SCA1 patients have one allele within a range of 40 to 81 repeat units (23). Normal alleles have a midstream CAT interruption and are stably transmitted to the next generation. In contrast, mutated SCA1 alleles contain uninterrupted CAG stretches and are unstable with a tendency to further expansion during meiosis.

Ataxin-1 is expressed ubiquitously within the central nervous system. Its physiologic function is poorly understood. SCA1 knockout mice have mild learning disturbances but are otherwise normal. This observation makes it highly improbable that SCA1 is caused by a loss of ataxin-1 function. Rather, it is assumed that the pathogenesis of SCA1 is due to a novel deleterious function of the elongated ataxin-1 protein. To study the pathogenesis of SCA1, transgenic mouse models have been created. Mice carrying an expanded ataxin-1 allele whose expression is directed specifically to Purkinje cells develop Purkinje cell pathology and an associated ataxia (24). A highly characteristic feature of SCA1 transgenic mice is the occurrence of neuronal intranuclear inclusions in Purkinje cells containing aggregated ataxin-1. However, these inclusions do not appear to be a prerequisite for neurodegeneration (25).

Numerous observations suggest that abnormal folding and aggregation of mutated ataxin-1 are essential for the pathogenesis of SCA1. The most persuasive evidence comes from experiments showing that overexpression of chaperones, intracellular proteins that serve to refold proteins and prevent aggregation, prevents the development of neuropathology in SCA1 transgenic mice. The abnormally folded ataxin-1 is thought to interact with a variety of proteins, among them transcription factors resulting in transcriptional dysregulation.

Epidemiology

The proportion of SCA1 among all dominant ataxias varies widely from population to population. In Germany, 27% of all families with dominant ataxia harbor the SCA1 mutation. In contrast, the proportion of SCA1 is much lower among Japanese and American families.

Neuropathology

Neuropathologic abnormalities involve degenerative changes with neuronal cell loss and gliosis in the cerebellar cortex, pontine nuclei, and inferior olives compatible with a neuropathologic diagnosis of olivopontocerebellar atrophy. Often, there is additional cell loss in the caudal cranial nerve nuclei. Degeneration within the basal ganglia, thalamus, and cerebral cortex has been found less frequently. In the spinal cord, axonal loss and pallor of myelin is observed in the dorsal column pathways, the spinocerebellar tracts, and, less frequently, the pyramidal tracts (26). Recently, the presence of ubiquitin-positive nuclear inclusions containing ataxin-1 has been demonstrated in surviving neurons of the nucleus centralis pontis.

Clinical Presentation

All SCA1 patients suffer from a progressive cerebellar syndrome with ataxia of gait and stance, ataxia of limb movements, dysarthria, and cerebellar oculomotor abnormalities. The oculomotor abnormalities include gaze-evoked nystagmus, saccade hypermetria, broken-up smooth pursuit, reduced optokinetic nystagmus, and impaired suppression of vestibulo-ocular reflex by fixation. In the majority of patients, there are additional noncerebellar symptoms. About half of the patients have supranuclear gaze paresis and/or saccade slowing. Pyramidal tract signs with spasticity, extensor plantar responses, and hyperreflexia are found in more than 50% of SCA1 patients. Decreased vibration sense is found in up to 80% of the SCA1 patients. Dysphagia is a common complaint of SCA1 patients and is a particular clinical problem in late-state disease. Disturbances of sphincter control, mainly bladder dysfunction, occur less frequently and are encountered in about 20% of patients. Basal ganglia symptoms with parkinsonism or dystonia are observed only occasionally. Mental disturbances are encountered in less than 10% of SCA1 patients (27,28).

Natural Course

Disease onset in SCA1 varies between adolescence and late adulthood with an average around the age of 35 years. As in other polyglutamine disorders, there is an inverse correlation between CAG repeat length and age of onset. Anticipation has been observed in many SCA1 families. Median latency to become wheelchair bound after disease onset is 14 years, median survival after onset of symptoms 21 years, and median age at death 56 years (6).

Diagnosis

A genetic test demonstrating the CAG repeat expansion of the *SCA1* gene is widely available. MRI typically shows cerebellar, brainstem, and spinal cord atrophy (29). Electrophysiologic tests often provide evidence of both axonal polyneuropathy and pyramidal dysfunction.

Spinocerebellar Ataxia Type 2 (SCA2)

Etiology and Pathogenesis

The mutation causing SCA2 is a translated CAG repeat expansion in a gene coding for ataxin-2. The repeat length in normals varies between 6 and 31 trinucleotides, with more than 90% of control alleles having 22 or 23 repeats. SCA2 patients have one allele within a range of 36 to 63 repeat units. Alleles with a length of 30 to 34 repeats represent an intermediate range that may give rise to expansion in the offspring. Normal alleles have CAA interruptions. Expanded alleles are unstable with a tendency to further expansion, particularly in father-to-child transmission (30).

Recently, transgenic mice overexpressing an expanded SCA2 allele in cerebellar Purkinje cells have been generated. These mice show progressive incoordination and morphologic alterations of Purkinje cells. In contrast to SCA1, nuclear localization of the abnormal protein is not necessary for the development of the disease (31).

Neuropathology

Autopsy studies of SCA2 patients consistently show olivopontocerebellar atrophy with marked reduction of Purkinje cells, as well as degeneration of the inferior olives, pontine nuclei, and pontocerebellar fibers. In most cases, there is additional degeneration of posterior columns and spinocerebellar pathways, and cell loss in the substantia nigra. Ubiquitinated nuclear inclusions have not been observed in SCA2.

Epidemiology

The proportion of SCA2 among all dominant ataxias varies from 4% to 40%. In the Holguin province of Cuba, the prevalence of SCA2 is as high as 100 per 100,000 due to a founder effect.

Clinical Presentation

All SCA2 patients suffer from a progressive cerebellar syndrome with ataxia of gait and stance, ataxia of limb movements, and dysarthria. Saccade slowing is a highly characteristic feature that is observed in the majority of SCA2 patients. About half of the patients have vertical or horizontal gaze palsy. Cerebellar oculomotor abnormalities are rarely found in SCA2. Typically, tendon reflexes are absent or decreased. Pyramidal tract signs are present in less than 20% of the patients. Vibration sense is decreased in most patients, whereas sensation is otherwise normal (28,32). Atypical SCA2 phenotypes with prominent dementia, an amyotrophic lateral sclerosis-like presentation, and parkinsonism have been described.

Natural Course

Disease onset in SCA2 varies between childhood and adulthood, with an average around age 30 years. As in other polyglutamine disorders, there is an inverse correlation between CAG repeat length and age of onset. Anticipation is present in many SCA2 families, in particular if the disease is inherited from the father. Median latency to become wheelchair bound after disease onset is 15 years, median survival after onset of symptoms 21 years, and median age at death 68 years (6).

Diagnosis

A genetic test demonstrating the CAG repeat expansion of the *SCA2* gene is widely available. MRI typically shows cerebellar and brainstem atrophy suggestive of olivoponto-cerebellar atrophy (29). In addition, there is atrophy of the spinal cord. Electrophysiologic tests often provide evidence of axonal polyneuropathy.

Spinocerebellar Ataxia Type 3 (SCA3)

Etiology and Pathogenesis

The mutation causing SCA3 is a translated CAG repeat expansion in a gene coding for ataxin-3 (33). The SCA3 mutation was initially found in families with the Machado-Joseph disease phenotype. Machado-Joseph disease is a historical term used to denote a dominantly inherited ataxic disorder with large phenotypic variation that was first described in patients of Azorean descent (34). After discovery of the gene mutation it was found that this mutation is frequently found in ataxic families of non-Azorean origin.

While the repeat length of the *SCA3* gene in normals varies between 14 and 37 trinucleotides, SCA3 patients have one allele within a range of 55 to 84 repeat units. Both the normal and mutated *SCA3* genes contain uninterrupted CAG stretches. Expanded SCA3 alleles display intergenerational instability with a tendency to further expansion. As shown by a worldwide haplotype analysis, the majority of abnormal alleles are derived from two founder mutations that originated in Portuguese families settling in the Azores (35).

As in SCA1, abnormal folding and aggregation of the expanded disease protein appear to be of importance for the pathogenesis. Overexpression of a chaperone in a *Drosophila* model of SCA3 prevents neurodegeneration (36). Expanded ataxin-3 has been shown to interact with a variety of transcription factors resulting in transcriptional dysregulation (37).

Neuropathology

SCA3 is a multisystemic disorder characterized by degeneration of spinocerebellar tracts, dentate nucleus, pontine and other brainstem nuclei, substantia nigra, and pallidum. In contrast to most other SCAs, the cerebellar cortex and the inferior olives are widely spared. Nuclear inclusions containing expanded ataxin-3 have been found in neurons of affected brain regions.

Epidemiology

SCA3 is the most common mutation causing dominant ataxia worldwide. Among German families with dominant ataxia, the proportion of SCA3 is almost 40%. The corresponding figure for American families is 21%. Due to a founder effect, SCA3 is endemic on the Azorean islands Flores and San Miguel with a prevalence of 700 per 100,000.

Clinical Presentation

The clinical picture of SCA3/Machado-Joseph disease is characterized by a wide range of clinical manifestations, the precise nature of which partly depends on repeat length. All SCA3 patients suffer from a progressive syndrome with ataxia of gait and stance, ataxia of limb movements, and dysarthria. Vertical or horizontal gaze palsy is a common additional finding that occurs independently of age of onset. At least 40% of SCA3 patients have L-dopa-responsive restless legs syndrome. Saccade velocity is usually normal. Patients with a repeat length of more than 74 have an early disease onset as well as clinical features of pyramidal tract and basal ganglia involvement. Most of these patients have increased tendon reflexes, extensor plantar responses, spasticity, and dystonia. Patients with an intermediate repeat length of 71 to 74 units have a disease onset in middle age and show mainly ataxia and gaze palsy. Patients with a repeat length of less than 71 have a later disease onset and show signs of peripheral neuropathy with loss of tendon reflexes, amyotrophy, and decreased vibration sense. However, the boundaries between these clinical syndromes are vague, and the clinical phenotype of an individual may change with progression of the disease (38).

Natural Course

Disease onset in SCA3 varies between adolescence and late adulthood, with an average around age 42 years. As in other polyglutamine disorders, there is an inverse correlation between CAG repeat length and age of onset. Median latency to become wheelchair bound after disease onset is 15 years, median survival after onset of symptoms 25 years, and median age at death 72 years (6).

Diagnosis

A genetic test demonstrating the CAG repeat expansion of the *SCA3* gene is widely available. MRI typically shows brainstem and spinal cord atrophy. In contrast to other SCAs, cerebellar atrophy is mild (29). Nerve conduction studies show axonal polyneuropathy, the severity of which increases with age (39).

Spinocerebellar Ataxia Type 4 (SCA4)

SCA4 is a rare, autosomal dominantly inherited ataxia characterized by the combination of progressive ataxia and sensory axonal neuropathy. Families with a similar phenotype have been described earlier by Biemond and found to have mainly spinal pathology. The gene locus of SCA4 has been mapped to chromosome 16q, but the gene mutation has not yet been found (40). Recently, Japanese families linked to the same chromosomal region were reported. Surprisingly, these families had cerebellar ataxia and cerebellar pathology (41).

Spinocerebellar Ataxia Type 5 (SCA5)

SCA5 is a rare, autosomal dominantly inherited ataxia characterized by a pure cerebellar phenotype. Linkage with the *SCA5* gene locus on chromosome 11cen was established in a family descended from the grandparents of U.S. President Abraham Lincoln (42).

Spinocerebellar Ataxia Type 6 (SCA6)

Etiology and Pathogenesis

The mutation causing SCA6 is a CAG repeat expansion in the 3' translated region of the *CACNA1A* gene coding for the α_{1A} voltage-dependent calcium channel subunit (43). Calcium channels containing the α_{1A} subunit mediate P- and Q-type currents. The α_{1A} subunit is expressed throughout the brain with highest expression levels in cerebellar Purkinje cells. In contrast to other CAG repeat mutations, the expansions causing SCA6 are relatively short, ranging between 21 and 27, and do not undergo intergenerational length changes (44).

The pathogenesis of SCA6 is not completely understood. One hypothesis says that SCA6 is due to a gain of function mechanism resembling that of other polyglutamine disorders. On the other hand, there is evidence for altered calcium channel function in SCA6 resulting in excessive entry of calcium ions into cerebellar Purkinje cells (45). The view that altered calcium channel function may be sufficient to cause progressive ataxia is supported by the observation that a missense mutation in the *CACNA1A* gene may cause progressive ataxia without episodic features (46). The pathogenetic mechanisms—polyglutamine-induced gain of function and altered calcium channel function—do not appear to be mutually exclusive.

Neuropathology

Autopsy studies of SCA6 patients consistently show pure cerebellar degeneration with prominent loss of cerebellar Purkinje neurons. In contrast to other polyglutamine disease, neurons do not contain ubiquitinated nuclear inclusions, but rather cytoplasmic inclusions containing channel protein (47).

Epidemiology

The proportion of SCA6 among all dominant ataxias varies from 1% to 30% in different populations. SCA6 is the most common cause of dominant ataxias with a pure cerebellar presentation.

Clinical Presentation

SCA6 patients suffer from a progressive cerebellar syndrome with ataxia of gait and stance, ataxia of limb move-

ments, and dysarthria. Horizontal gaze-evoked nystagmus is almost universally present, and downbeat nystagmus is found in more than half of SCA6 patients. Other cerebellar oculomotor findings are also common, such as impaired smooth pursuit and dysmetric saccades. With disease progression, some SCA6 patients have clinical evidence of noncerebellar involvement, including pyramidal signs and mild sensory disturbances (48).

Natural Course

Disease onset in SCA6 is later than in other SCAs and varies between 30 and 75 years. Most patients become ataxic in their fifties. As in other polyglutamine disorders, there is an inverse correlation between CAG repeat length and age of onset. Disease progression in SCA6 is slower than in other SCA. Although SCA6 is associated with considerable disability, life expectancy is almost normal.

Diagnosis

A genetic test demonstrating the CAG repeat expansion of the *SCA6* gene is widely available. MRI typically shows pure cerebellar atrophy without involvement of the brainstem. Electrophysiologic tests only occasionally reveal abnormalities.

Spinocerebellar Ataxia Type 7 (SCA7)

Etiology and Pathogenesis

SCA7 is a rare, autosomal dominantly inherited ataxia that is distinct from all other SCAs in having the constant additional feature of retinal degeneration. The causative gene mutation is a translated CAG repeat expansion in a gene coding for ataxin-7. The normal range is 7 to 19 repeats, and the pathogenic alleles range from 37 to more than 300 repeats (49). Expanded alleles are unstable with a strong tendency to further expansion, particularly in father-to-child transmission. SCA7 patients with childhood onset have almost always inherited the disease from their father.

Ataxin-7 is widely expressed through the brain and localized in the cytoplasm of neurons. In patients, ataxin-7 is redistributed to the nucleus to form ubiquitinated intranuclear inclusions. A transgenic mouse model of SCA7 has been created that replicates important features of the disease (50).

Neuropathology

Neuropathologic examinations of SCA7 patients consistently reveal olivopontocerebellar atrophy. All patients have primarily macular degeneration, which then spreads to involve the retina. There is often secondary atrophy of the optic nerve.

Clinical Presentation

The clinical picture of SCA7 partly depends on the age of onset. In patients with late disease onset after the age of 40 years, cerebellar ataxia is always the first symptom. There are some exceptional patients who never develop visual problems. In most patients, however, ataxia is followed by progressive loss of vision. In about half of the patients with late disease onset, there is no evidence of retinal degeneration or optic atrophy, suggesting that retinopathy only affects the macula. All patients with earlier disease onset before the age of 40 years have visual problems, starting either prior to or at the same time as cerebellar ataxia. The majority of these patients have retinal degeneration, some of them also optic atrophy. Tendon reflexes are usually absent. There are a number of additional symptoms that occur in less than half of the patients and that tend be more common in patients with long disease duration. These symptoms include gaze palsy, dysphagia, hearing loss, and muscle weakness. Dementia and basal ganglia symptoms are not typical features of SCA7 (51).

Natural Course

Mean age of disease onset of SCA7 is 30 years, with a wide variation from 3 months to 70 years. As in other polyglutamine disorders, there is an inverse correlation between CAG repeat length and age of onset. Disease progression is more rapid in patients with early disease onset. On average, patients with juvenile disease onset die 5 years after onset, whereas patients with adult onset survive for about 15 years.

Spinocerebellar Ataxia Type 8 (SCA8)

SCA8 is a rare, autosomal dominantly inherited disorder associated with an untranslated CTG repeat expansion in the 3′ untranslated region of a novel gene located on chromosome 13q (52). In the general population, the CTG expansion is polymorphic, with allele sizes ranging from 16 to 91 units. However, more than 99% of the normal alleles have 16 to 37 repeats. The allele sizes of SCA8 patients ranged from 107 to 127 repeats. Expanded CTG repeats of the *SCA8* gene were also found in unaffected members of SCA8 families and in individuals with neuropsychiatric disorders other than ataxia, raising some doubt about whether the CTG repeat expansion is sufficient to cause ataxia.

SCA8 patients have an almost pure cerebellar phenotype with marked cerebellar atrophy on MRI. In some patients, pyramidal signs and cognitive impairment is seen. Compared with other SCAs, disease progression is rather slow.

Spinocerebellar Ataxia Type 10 (SCA10)

SCA10 is a rare, autosomal dominantly inherited disorder caused by an intronic ATTCT pentanucleotide repeat in a novel gene located on chromosome 22q. Whereas normal repeats range from 10 to 22 units, the expanded repeats may have a length of up to 22.5 kb (53). Clinically, SCA10 is distinct from all other SCAs in that ataxia is frequently associated with epilepsy.

Spinocerebellar Ataxia Type 11 (SCA11)

SCA11 is a rare, autosomal dominantly inherited disorder clinically characterized by an almost pure cerebellar syndrome. SCA11 has been mapped to chromosome 15q (54).

Spinocerebellar Ataxia Type 12 (SCA12)

SCA12 is a rare, autosomal dominantly inherited disorder caused by a CAG repeat expansion in the 5′ untranslated region of a gene encoding a regulatory subunit of a phosphatase expressed in the brain (55). The prominent clinical features of SCA12 are ataxia and tremor.

Spinocerebellar Ataxia Type 13 (SCA13)

SCA13 is a rare, autosomal dominantly inherited disorder characterized by ataxia and mental retardation. SCA13 has been mapped to chromosome 19q (56).

Spinocerebellar Ataxia Type 14 (SCA14)

SCA14 is a rare, autosomal dominantly inherited disorder clinically characterized by ataxia and axial myoclonus. SCA14 has been mapped to chromosome 19q (57).

Spinocerebellar Ataxia Type 16 (SCA16)

The SCA16 locus was recently described in a four-generation Japanese family with an almost pure cerebellar phenotype. The locus was mapped to chromosome 8q (58).

Spinocerebellar Ataxia Type 17 (SCA17)

SCA17 is a rare, autosomal dominant disorder resulting from a CAG repeat expansion in the gene encoding the TATA binding protein (59). Clinically, SCA17 is characterized by ataxia, dystonia, and intellectual decline (60).

Episodic Ataxia Type 1 (EA-1)

Etiology and Pathogenesis

EA-1 is a rare disorder caused by point mutations in the *KCNA1* gene encoding the pore-forming α subunit of the voltage-gated potassium channels Kv1.1 (61). Voltage-gated potassium channels consisting of Kv1.1 give rise to delayed-rectifier potassium currents. Mutations causing EA-1 are found in highly conserved regions of the protein.

Clinical Presentation

Clinically, EA-1 is characterized by brief attacks of ataxia and dysarthria. The attacks last for seconds to minutes and may occur several times per day. They are often provoked by movements and startle. Apart from ataxia, the attacks may have dystonic or choreic features. EA-1 is associated with interictal myokymia (twitching of small muscles around the eyes or in the hands). Ataxia and gaze-evoked nystagmus are absent between attacks.

Natural Course

EA-1 starts in early childhood. It has a favorable prognosis because it does not result in permanent disability. In most patients attacks become milder with increasing age.

Diagnosis

Since a genetic test for EA-1 is not routinely available, the diagnosis is based on a carefully taken history and clinical examination. In EA-1, interictal electromyogram of muscles displaying myokymia shows spontaneous repetitive discharges that subside after nerve blockade. Imaging studies give normal results.

Management

Some patients learn to prevent attacks by avoiding sudden abrupt movements. If medical treatment is required, acetazolamide (500 to 700 mg/day) is used to prevent attacks (62). However, the action of acetazolamide is less reliable than in EA-2. As a second-line treatment carbamazepine and phenytoin can be tried.

Episodic Ataxia Type 2 (EA-2)

Etiology and Pathogenesis

EA-2 is a rare disorder caused by nonsense mutations causing truncation of the *CACNA1A* gene coding for the α_{1A} voltage-dependent calcium channel subunit (63). Missense mutations of the same gene are associated with familial hemiplegic migraine, whereas a CAG repeat expansion in the 3' end of the gene causes SCA6 (43,63).

Clinical Presentation

Compared with EA-1, attacks in EA-2 last longer and are precipitated by emotional stress and exercise but not by startle. The episodes vary from pure ataxia to combinations of symptoms suggesting involvement of the cerebellum and brainstem and, occasionally, the cortex. Vertigo, nausea, and vomiting are the most common associated symptoms, being present in more than 50% of patients. About half of the patients report headaches that meet criteria for migraine. Between attacks many EA-2 patients have a gaze-evoked nystagmus. With increasing age, some patients develop mild ataxia of gait and stance.

Natural Course

The age of onset in EA-2 varies from 2 to 30 years. Although EA-2 is principally an episodic disorder, some patients develop a persistent or slowly progressive ataxia.

Diagnosis

Since a genetic test for EA-2 is not routinely available, the diagnosis is based on a carefully taken history and clinical examination. EA-2 patients may have mild cerebellar atrophy. In addition, magnetic resonance spectroscopy shows an elevated cerebellar pH in these patients (64).

Management

Acetazolamide (500 to 700 mg/day) is the treatment of choice.

REFERENCES

1. Campuzano V, Montermini L, Moltò MD, et al. Friedreich's ataxia: autosomal recessive disease caused by an intronic GAA triplet repeat expansion. *Science* 1996;271:1423–1427.
2. Cossee M, Dürr A, Schmitt M, et al. Friedreich's ataxia: point mutations and clinical presentation of compound heterozygotes. *Ann Neurol* 1999;45:200–206.
3. Christodoulou K, Deymeer F, Serdaroglu P, et al. Mapping of the second Friedreich's ataxia (FRDA2) locus to chromosome 9p23-p11: evidence for further locus heterogeneity. *Neurogenetics* 2001;3:127–132.
4. Puccio H, Simon D, Cossee M, et al. Mouse models for Friedreich ataxia exhibit cardiomyopathy, sensory nerve defect, and Fe-S enzyme deficiency followed by intramitochondrial iron deposits. *Nat Genet* 2001;27:181–186.
5. Dürr A, Cossee M, Agid Y, et al. Clinical and genetic abnormalities in patients with Friedreich's ataxia. *N Engl J Med* 1996;335:1169–1175.
6. Klockgether T, Lüdtke R, Kramer B, et al. The natural history of degenerative ataxia: a retrospective study in 466 patients. *Brain* 1998;121:589–600.
7. Rustin P, von Kleist-Retzow JC, Chantrel-Groussard K, et al. Effect of idebenone on cardiomyopathy in Friedreich's ataxia: a preliminary study. *Lancet* 1999;354:477–479.
8. Savitsky K, Bar-Shira A, Gilad S, et al. A single ataxia telangiectasia gene with a product similar to PI-3 kinase. *Science* 1995;268:1749–1753.
9. Stewart GS, Maser RS, Stankovic T, et al. The DNA double-strand break repair gene *hMRE11* is mutated in individuals with an ataxia-telangiectasia-like disorder. *Cell* 1999;99:577–587.
10. Engert JC, Berube P, Mercier J, et al. ARSACS, a spastic ataxia common in northeastern Quebec, is caused by mutations in a new gene encoding an 11.5-kb ORF. *Nat Genet* 2000;24:120–125.
11. Sharp D, Blinderman L, Combs KA, et al. Cloning and gene defects in microsomal triglyceride transfer protein associated with abetalipoproteinaemia. *Nature* 1993;365:65–69.

12. Ouahchi K, Arita M, Kayden H, et al. Ataxia with isolated vitamin E deficiency is caused by mutations in the α-tocopherol transfer protein. *Nat Genet* 1995;9:141–145.
13. Jansen GA, Ofman R, Ferdinandusse S, et al. Refsum disease is caused by mutations in the phytanoyl-CoA hydroxylase gene. *Nat Genet* 1997;17:190–193.
14. Leitersdorf E, Reshef A, Meiner V, et al. Frameshift and splice-junction mutations in the sterol 27-hydroxylase gene cause cerebrotendinous xanthomatosis in Jews or Moroccan origin. *J Clin Invest* 1993;91:2488–2496.
15. Barbot C, Coutinho P, Chorao R, et al. Recessive ataxia with ocular apraxia—review of 22 Portuguese patients. *Arch Neurol* 2001;58:201–205.
16. Bomont P, Watanabe M, Gershoni-Barush R, et al. Homozygosity mapping of spinocerebellar ataxia with cerebellar atrophy and peripheral neuropathy to 9q33-34, and with hearing impairment and optic atrophy to 6p21-23. *Eur J Hum Genet* 2000;8:986–990.
17. Nemeth AH, Bochukova E, Dunne E, et al. Autosomal recessive cerebellar ataxia with oculomotor apraxia (Ataxia-telangiectasia-like syndrome) is linked to chromosome 9q34. *Am J Hum Genet* 2000;67:1320–1326.
18. Lonnqvist T, Paetau A, Nikali K, et al. Infantile onset spinocerebellar ataxia with sensory neuropathy (IOSCA): neuropathological features. *J Neurol Sci* 1998;161:57–65.
19. Klockgether T, Petersen D, Grodd W, et al. Early onset cerebellar ataxia with retained tendon reflexes: clinical, electrophysiological, and MRI observations in comparison with Friedreich's ataxia. *Brain* 1991;114:1559–1573.
20. Lou JS, Goldfarb L, McShane L, et al. Use of buspirone for treatment of cerebellar ataxia—an open-label study. *Arch Neurol* 1995;52:982–988.
21. Trouillas P, Xie J, Adeleine P, et al. Buspirone, a 5-hydroxytryptamine$_{1A}$ agonist, is active in cerebellar ataxia—results of a double-blind drug placebo study in patients with cerebellar cortical atrophy. *Arch Neurol* 1997;54:749–752.
22. Hassin-Baer S, Korczyn AD, Giladi N. An open trial of amantadine and buspirone for cerebellar ataxia: a disappointment. *J Neural Transm* 2000;107:1187–1189.
23. Orr HT, Chung MY, Banfi S, et al. Expansion of an unstable trinucleotide CAG repeat in spinocerebellar ataxia type 1. *Nat Genet* 1993;4:221–226.
24. Burright EN, Clark HB, Servadio A, et al. SCA1 transgenic mice: a model for neurodegeneration caused by an expanded CAG trinucleotide repeat. *Cell* 1995;82:937–948.
25. Klement IA, Skinner PJ, Kaytor MD, et al. Ataxin-1 nuclear localization and aggregation: role in polyglutamine-induced disease in SCA1 transgenic mice. *Cell* 1998;95:41–53.
26. Genis D, Matilla T, Volpini V, et al. Clinical, neuropathologic, and genetic studies of a large spinocerebellar ataxia type 1 (SCA1) kindred: (CAG)n expansion and early premonitory signs and symptoms. *Neurology* 1995;45:24–30.
27. Dubourg O, Dürr A, Cancel G, et al. Analysis of the SCA1 CAG repeat in a large number of families with dominant ataxia: clinical and molecular correlations. *Ann Neurol* 1995;37:176–180.
28. Bürk K, Abele M, Fetter M, et al. Autosomal dominant cerebellar ataxia type I—clinical features and MRI in families with SCA1, SCA2, and SCA3. *Brain* 1996;119:1497–1505.
29. Klockgether T, Skalej M, Wedekind D, et al. Autosomal dominant cerebellar ataxia type I: MRI-based volumetry of posterior fossa structures and basal ganglia in spinocerebellar ataxia types 1, 2, and 3. *Brain* 1998;121:1687–1693.
30. Pulst SM, Nechiporuk A, Nechiporuk T, et al. Moderate expansion of a normally biallelic trinucleotide repeat in spinocerebellar ataxia type 2. *Nat Genet* 1996;14:269–276.
31. Huynh DP, Figueroa K, Hoang N, et al. Nuclear localization or inclusion body formation of ataxin-2 are not necessary for SCA2 pathogenesis in mouse or human. *Nat Genet* 2000;26:44–50.
32. Schöls L, Gispert S, Vorgerd M, et al. Spinocerebellar ataxia type 2—genotype and phenotype in German kindreds. *Arch Neurol* 1997;54:1073–1080.
33. Kawaguchi Y, Okamoto T, Taniwaki M, et al. CAG expansions in a novel gene for Machado-Joseph disease at chromosome 14q32.1. *Nat Genet* 1994;8:221–228.
34. Rosenberg RN. Machado-Joseph disease: an autosomal dominant motor system degeneration. *Mov Disord* 1992;7:193–203.
35. Gaspar C, Lopes-Cendes I, Hayes S, et al. Ancestral origins of the Machado-Joseph disease mutation: a worldwide haplotype study. *Am J Hum Genet* 2001;68:523–528.
36. Warrick JM, Chan HY, Gray-Board GL, et al. Suppression of polyglutamine-mediated neurodegeneration in *Drosophila* by the molecular chaperone HSP70. *Nat Genet* 1999;23:425–428.
37. Evert BO, Vogt IR, Kindermann C, et al. Inflammatory genes are upregulated in expanded ataxin-3-expressing cell lines and spinocerebellar ataxia type 3 brains. *J Neurosci* 2001;21:5389–5396.
38. Maciel P, Gaspar C, DeStefano AL, et al. Correlation between CAG repeat length and clinical features in Machado-Joseph disease. *Am J Hum Genet* 1995;57:54–61.
39. Klockgether T, Schols L, Abele M, et al. Age related axonal neuropathy in spinocerebellar ataxia type 3/Machado-Joseph disease (SCA3/MJD). *J Neurol Neurosurg Psychiatry* 1999;66:222–224.
40. Flanigan K, Gardner K, Alderson K, et al. Autosomal dominant spinocerebellar ataxia with sensory axonal neuropathy (SCA4): clinical description and genetic localization to chromosome 16q22.1. *Am J Hum Genet* 1996;59:392–399.
41. Takashima M, Ishikawa K, Nagaoka U, et al. A linkage disequilibrium at the candidate gene locus for 16q-linked autosomal dominant cerebellar ataxia type III in Japan. *J Hum Genet* 2001; 46:167–171.
42. Ranum LP, Schut LJ, Lundgren JK, et al. Spinocerebellar ataxia type 5 in a family descended from the grandparents of President Lincoln maps to chromosome 11. *Nat Genet* 1994;8:280–284.
43. Zhuchenko O, Bailey J, Bonnen P, et al. Autosomal dominant cerebellar ataxia (SCA6) associated with small polyglutamine expansions in the α$_{1A}$ voltage–dependent calcium channel. *Nature Genet* 1997;15:62–69.
44. Matsuyama Z, Kawakami H, Maruyama H, et al. Molecular features of the CAG repeats of spinocerebellar ataxia 6 (SCA6). *Hum Mol Genet* 1997;6:1283–1287.
45. Restituito S, Thompson RM, Eliet J, et al. The polyglutamine expansion in spinocerebellar ataxia type 6 causes a beta subunit-specific enhanced activation of P/Q-type calcium channels in *Xenopus* oocytes. *J Neurosci* 2000;20:6394–6403.
46. Yue Q, Jen JC, Nelson SF, et al. Progressive ataxia due to a missense mutation in a calcium-channel gene. *Am J Hum Genet* 1997;61:1078–1087.
47. Ishikawa K, Fujigasaki H, Saegusa H, et al. Abundant expression and cytoplasmic aggregations of α$_{1A}$ voltage–dependent calcium channel protein associated with neurodegeneration in spinocerebellar ataxia type 6. *Hum Mol Genet* 1999;8:1185–1193.
48. Geschwind DH, Perlman S, Figueroa KP, et al. Spinocerebellar ataxia type 6—frequency of the mutation and genotype–phenotype correlations. *Neurology* 1997;49:1247–1251.
49. David G, Abbas N, Stevanin G, et al. Cloning of the SCA7 gene reveals a highly unstable CAG repeat expansion. *Nat Genet* 1997; 17:65–70.
50. Yvert G, Lindenberg KS, Picaud S, et al. Expanded polyglutamines induce neurodegeneration and trans-neuronal alterations in cerebellum and retina of SCA7 transgenic mice. *Hum Mol Genet* 2000;9:2491–2506.
51. Enevoldson TP, Sanders MD, Harding AE. Autosomal dominant

cerebellar ataxia with pigmentary macular dystrophy: a clinical and genetic study of eight families. *Brain* 1994;117:445–460.

52. Koob MD, Moseley ML, Schut LJ, et al. An untranslated CTG expansion causes a novel form of spinocerebellar ataxia (SCA8). *Nat Genet* 1999;21:379–384.

53. Matsuura T, Yamagata T, Burgess DL, et al. Large expansion of the ATTCT pentanucleotide repeat in spinocerebellar ataxia type 10. *Nat Genet* 2000;26:191–194.

54. Worth PF, Giunti P, Gardner TC, et al. Autosomal dominant cerebellar ataxia type III: linkage in a large British family to a 7.6-cM region on chromosome 15q14-21.3. *Am J Hum Genet* 1999;65:420–426.

55. Holmes SE, O'Hearn EE, McInnis MG, et al. Expansion of a novel CAG trinucleotide repeat in the 5+ region of PPP2R2B is associated with SCA12. *Nat Genet* 1999;23:391–392.

56. Herman-Bert A, Stevanin G, Netter JC, et al. Mapping of spinocerebellar ataxia 13 to chromosome 19q13.3-q13.4 in a family with autosomal dominant cerebellar ataxia and mental retardation. *Am J Hum Genet* 2000;67:229–235.

57. Yamashita I, Sasaki H, Yabe I, et al. A novel locus for dominant cerebellar ataxia (SCA14) maps to a 10.2-cM interval flanked by D19S206 and D19S605 on chromosome 19q13.4-qter. *Ann Neurol* 2000;48:156–163.

58. Miyoshi Y, Yamada T, Tanimura M, et al. A novel autosomal dominant spinocerebellar ataxia (SCA16) linked to chromosome 8q22.1-24.1. *Neurology* 2001;57:96–100.

59. Nakamura K, Jeong SY, Uchihara T, et al. SCA17, a novel autosomal dominant cerebellar ataxia caused by an expanded polyglutamine in TATA-binding protein. *Hum Mol Genet* 2001;10:1441–1448.

60. Zühlke C, Hellenbroich Y, Dalski A, et al. Different types of repeat expansion in the TATA-binding protein gene are associated with a new form of inherited ataxia. *Eur J Hum Genet* 2001;9:160–164.

61. Browne DL, Gancher ST, Nutt JG, et al. Episodic ataxia/myokymia syndrome is associated with point mutations in the human potassium channel gene, *KCNA1*. *Nature Genet* 1994;8:136–140.

62. Griggs RC, Moxley RT, Lafrance RA, et al. Hereditary paroxysmal ataxia: response to acetazolamide. *Neurology* 1978;28:1259–1264.

63. Ophoff RA, Terwindt GM, Vergouwe MN, et al. Familial hemiplegic migraine and episodic ataxia type 2 are caused by mutations in the Ca^{2+} channel gene *CACNL1A4*. *Cell* 1996;87:543–552.

64. Sappey-Marinier D, Vighetto A, Peyron R, et al. Phosphorus and proton magnetic resonance spectroscopy in episodic ataxia type 2. *Ann Neurol* 1999;46:256–259.

38

GENETICS OF PARKINSONISM

THOMAS GASSER

ABSTRACT

Over the last few years, several genes for monogenically inherited forms of Parkinson's disease (PD) have been mapped and/or cloned. In a small number of families with autosomal dominant inheritance and typical Lewy body pathology, mutations have been identified in the gene for α-synuclein. Aggregation of this protein in Lewy bodies may be a crucial step in the molecular pathogenesis of familial and sporadic PD. Mutations in the *parkin* gene cause autosomal recessive parkinsonism of early onset. In this form of PD, nigral degeneration is not accompanied by Lewy body formation. *Parkin* mutations appear to be a common cause of parkinsonism in patients with very early onset. Parkin has been implicated in the cellular protein degradation pathways, functioning as a ubiquitin ligase. The potential importance of this pathway is also highlighted by the finding of a mutation in the gene for ubiquitin C-terminal hydrolase L1 in another small family with PD. Other loci have been mapped to chromosomes 2p, 4p, and 1p, respectively, but the genes have not yet been identified. These findings prove that there are several genetically distinct forms of PD that can be caused by mutations in single genes.

There is at present no direct evidence that any of these genes has a direct role in the etiology of the common sporadic form of PD. Epidemiologic, case-control, and twin studies, although supporting a genetic contribution to the development of PD, all suggest a clear familial clustering only in a minority of cases. It is therefore widely believed that a combination of interacting genetic and environmental causes may be responsible in the majority of PD cases. However, studies of gene–environment interactions have not yet produced any convincing results. Nevertheless, elucidation of the molecular sequence of events leading to nigral degeneration in clearly inherited cases is likely to shed light also on the molecular pathogenesis of the common sporadic form of this disorder.

INTRODUCTION

Parkinsonism is a clinically defined syndrome, characterized by variable combinations of akinesia, rigidity, tremor and postural instability, which may occur in the context of a number of different neurodegenerative diseases. The most common cause of parkinsonism is PD. In PD, parkinsonism is caused by a degeneration of dopaminergic neurons of the substantia nigra, leading to a deficiency of dopamine in the striatal projection areas of these neurons. Characteristic eosinophilic inclusions, the Lewy bodies, are found in surviving dopaminergic neurons but also, though less abundantly, in other parts of the brain, and have been considered to be essential for the pathologic diagnosis of PD.

However, degeneration of dopaminergic neurons with ensuing dopamine deficiency is not limited to pathologically typical PD. Patients with a large number of other neurodegenerative disorders may present with, or develop during the course of their disease, signs and symptoms of parkinsonism. In some cases, the pathogenic process may be closely related to that of idiopathic PD (as probably in diffuse Lewy body disease, which shares with PD the typical inclusion bodies); in other cases, pathology (and presumably the pathogenic process) may be clearly different (as in tauopathies associated with parkinsonism); and in still other cases, the relationship in terms of pathogenesis is unknown (as in recessive parkinsonism caused by *parkin* mutations).

A major breakthrough in recent years was the mapping and cloning of an increasing number of genes that cause monogenically inherited forms parkinsonism with different associated pathologies and a variable, but overlapping, spectrum of clinical signs and symptoms. However, all of the mutations and loci identified so far appear to be responsible in only a small number of families, and their relevance for the vast majority of patients with PD and other parkinsonian syndromes, who do not show a mendelian mode of inheritance, is still unknown. Nevertheless, there is considerable promise that elucidation of the molecular pathways leading to monogenically inherited forms of parkinsonism will also allow important insight into the common sporadic disorders, and eventually lead to the development of novel protective and therapeutic strategies.

MONOGENIC FORMS OF PARKINSON'S DISEASE

A minority of patients with the typical clinical picture of PD have a positive family history compatible with a mendelian (autosomal dominant or autosomal recessive) inheritance. As a rule, age at onset in most of these cases is younger than that of patients with sporadic disease, but no other specific clinical signs or symptoms distinguish familial from sporadic cases. Pathologically, all forms have in common a predominant degeneration of dopaminergic neurons of the substantia nigra, although in some forms the pathologic process appears to be highly selective (as in parkin-associated parkinsonism, PARK2), whereas in others the degenerative process is more widespread (e.g., PARK4). In some families there is typical Lewy body pathology (PARK1, PARK3), whereas in others, there are atypical ubiquitin-positive inclusions (PARK4) or no Lewy bodies (PARK2). This observation indicates, that different pathogenic processes are likely to lead to nigral cell death. Whether all those pathogenic processes are connected to a single cellular metabolic pathway [possibly the ubiquitin-dependent proteasomal protein degradation pathway (1); see below] remains to be determined.

AUTOSOMAL DOMINANT FORMS OF PARKINSONISM

Five genetic loci have been identified by linkage studies to cosegregate with parkinsonism in families with dominant inheritance (Table 38.1). To date, only one of these genes, that for α-synuclein, has been identified, but this discovery has proven to be extremely important as it focused researchers on the role of α-synuclein aggregation in Lewy bodies as a probable major step in the molecular pathogenesis of PD.

PARK1: Parkinson's Disease Caused by Mutations in the Gene for α-Synuclein (PARK1)

The first "PD gene" to be recognized was mapped to the long arm of chromosome 4 in a large family with dominant inheritance and relatively early age at onset (mean 44 years), but otherwise typical PD with Lewy body pathology, and identified as the gene for α-synuclein (2). Two point mutations were recognized (2,3). α-Synuclein is a relatively small protein that is abundantly expressed in many parts of the brain and localized mostly to presynaptic nerve terminals. Many aspects of the normal function of α-synuclein are still unknown. The protein has been shown to bind to brain vesicles and other cellular components (4) and may be functionally involved in brain plasticity (song learning in birds). However, knockout mice for α-synuclein show only very subtle alterations in dopamine release under certain experimental conditions, but no other phenotype (5).

Mutations in the α-synuclein gene clearly appear to be a very rare cause of the disease and have been excluded in a large number of patients with sporadic or familial PD (6–8). The mutation that was found in the original Contursi family (Ala53Thr) has also been identified in several Greek kindreds (2,9). Haplotype analyses support the hypothesis that this is due to a founder effect (9). The only other mutation has been found in a small German pedigree (3).

The clinical picture in the affected subjects from these pedigrees is compatible with idiopathic PD, although age at onset is lower (mean of about 45 years) and progression appears to be more rapid than in sporadic cases (9,10). There is still only limited information available on the neuropathology in this pedigree, but Lewy bodies have been described (10). The close resemblance, both on a clinical and a neuropathologic level, to typical sporadic PD increases the likelihood that the exploration of the molecular pathogenesis of this rare form of familial PD will also be pertinent to the more common sporadic form of the disease.

The identification of α-synuclein as a "PD gene" lead to the discovery that the encoded protein is one of the principle components of the Lewy body (11), which has always been considered to be the pathologic hallmark of PD in both familial and sporadic cases. α-Synuclein may therefore play a crucial role in the development of the disease, and α-synuclein staining has replaced staining for ubiquitin as the most sensitive tool in the detection of Lewy bodies.

TABLE 38.1. GENETICALLY DEFINED FORMS OF PARKINSON'S DISEASE AND PARKINSONISM

Locus	Inheritance	Onset	Pathology	Map Position	Gene	Ref.
PARK1	Dominant	40s	Nigral degeneration with Lewy bodies	4q21	α-synuclein	2
PARK2	Recessive	20s	Nigral degeneration without Lewy bodies	6q25	*parkin*	37
PARK3	Dominant	60s	Nigral degeneration with Lewy bodies. Plaques and tangles in some	2p13	?	22
PARK4	Dominant	30s	Nigral degeneration with Lewy bodies, vacuoles in neurons of the hippocampus	4p16	?	30
PARK5	Dominant	~50	No pathology	4p14	Ubiquitin C-terminal hydrolase L1	31
PARK6	Recessive	~40	No pathology	1p35–37	?	47
PARK7	Recessive	~40	No pathology	1p38	?	48
PARK8	Dominant	~50	Nigral degeneration without Lewy bodies	12p	?	101

The currently favored hypothesis states that the amino acid changes in the α-synuclein protein associated with PD may favor the β-pleated sheet conformation, which in turn may lead to an increased tendency to form aggregates (12). This has been demonstrated in vitro (13). However, the precise relationship between the formation of aggregates and cell death is unknown. One could hypothesize that a failure of proteasomal degradation of α-synuclein and other proteins may lead to an accumulation of toxic compounds, ultimately leading to cell death (1). Formation of α-synuclein-containing aggregates would then be a secondary effect.

However, other mechanisms of pathogenesis may also be important. Known α-synuclein mutations appear to alter the vesicle binding properties of the protein (14), and the functional homology of α-synuclein to the 14-3-3 protein, a ubiquitously expressed chaperone, may indicate a more profound role for this protein in cellular metabolism and suggests still other possible pathogenic mechanisms.

There is still no good explanation for the striking selectivity of neuronal damage, which is largely restricted to dopaminergic cells whereas α-synuclein is abundantly expressed in many areas of the brain. The identification of proteins that specifically bind α-synuclein, like synphilin (15), may shed new light on this important question. In addition, several animal models have recently been described. Transgenic mice overexpressing α-synuclein, both the normal and the mutated human sequence, under different promoters show either no (16) or very mild degenerative changes (17) and, despite accumulation of α-synuclein, no fibrillar aggregates comparable to Lewy bodies. A transgenic *Drosophila* model may be more true to the human disease on the cellular level, but needs to be characterized in more detail (18).

The elucidation of the molecular pathways leading to α-synuclein aggregation and dopaminergic degeneration will undoubtedly generate novel candidate genes for evaluation in as yet unlinked families with PD. However, attempts to identify mutations in homologous genes, such as β-synuclein (19) and persyn (20), or in genes encoding proteins interacting in these pathways, such as synphilin (21), have so far been unsuccessful.

PARK3: Parkinson's Disease Linked to Chromosome 2

Another dominant locus has been described (PARK3), located on chromosome 2p13, in a subset of families with autosomal dominant inheritance and typical Lewy body pathology (22). Clinical features relatively closely resemble those of sporadic PD (23), including a similar mean age of onset (59 years in these families). Two of the families supporting linkage to this locus (families B and C) originated from a relatively small area in northern Germany and southern Denmark, and share a common haplotype within the linked region, suggesting the existence of a possible founder effect. Based on the relatively common occurrence of the affected haplotype in clinically asymptomatic members in two of the linked families, the penetrance of the mutation was estimated to be 40%, suggesting that it might also play a role in apparently sporadic cases. So far, however, the founder haplotype has not been identified in other German patients with familial and sporadic PD (24,25), arguing against a recent and prevalent founder effect in Germany.

At present, based on the observed haplotype, the disease gene should reside in a region encompassing a genetic distance of less than 3 cM (26). A large number of genes in this region, among them potential candidate genes such as the gene for transforming growth factor α (27), or for sepiapterine reductase, dynactin, and semaphorine, have already been fully sequenced, but no mutation has been detected (26).

Follow-up examination of these families over the years showed that in addition to parkinsonism, several members of chromosome 2–linked families showed signs of dementia, and neuropathology revealed, in addition to neuronal loss in the substantia nigra and typical brainstem Lewy bodies, the presence of neurofibrillary tangles and Alzheimer plaques (28). Therefore, the underlying mutation may be associated with a range of phenotypes, that includes varying degrees of dementia and Alzheimer's disease pathology, as is also known for a subset of patients with idiopathic PD.

PARK4: Parkinsonism-Dementia Linked to Chromosome 4p

In a family with parkinsonism with autosomal dominant inheritance, originally described by Muenter et al. (29), evidence for linkage was found on the short arm of chromosome 4 (30). Affected individuals in this family have L-dopa-responsive parkinsonism, but age at onset is considerably younger (mean 33.6 years), and several atypical features are present, such as early weight loss, dysautonomia, and dementia. Neuropathologic changes include, in addition to nigral degeneration and Lewy body formation, conspicuous vacuoles in the hippocampus and several other brain areas.

Despite the very striking phenotype (uniform onset in the mid-thirties, rapid progression, and early death), there have been no other families described that conform to this clinical picture. Interestingly, several members of this family presented with isolated postural tremor only. They had not been scored as affecteds in the initial linkage analysis, but were later found to carry the affected haplotype (30). At present, this observation has to be interpreted with caution, but eventually it may shed new light on the old question of whether postural tremor can be a forme fruste of PD.

PARK5: Parkinsonism Associated with a Mutation in the Gene for Ubiquitin Hydrolase L1

A missense mutation in the gene for ubiquitin carboxy-terminal hydrolase L1 gene *(UCHL1)*, which is located on chromosome 4p (but outside the region supporting linkage in the Spellman-Muenter kindred; see below), has been identified in affecteds in one family of German ancestry (31). This mutation was shown to reduce the enzymatic activity of ubiquitin hydrolase in vitro. The fact that this mutation again points to the importance of the proteasomal ubiquitination–protein degradation pathway is intriguing (see also discussion of α-synuclein- and parkin-related parkinsonism below). To date, however, no other potentially pathogenic mutations of this gene have been identified (32). In fact, another rare variant has been found in a family with PD, which did not segregate with the disease, raising doubts as to the pathogenic role (33).

The observation of a polymorphism in the *UCHL1* gene and its possible protective role in patients with sporadic PD (34) has not been confirmed in another study (35).

AUTOSOMAL RECESSIVE FORMS OF PARKINSONISM

One of the surprising developments of recent years was the recognition of the relatively high proportion of patients with early-onset parkinsonism caused by recessive mutations in a number of genes (Table 38.1). So far, one of them, *parkin (PARK2)* has been cloned and extensively studied. Two others *(PARK6* and *PARK7)* have been mapped. The study of parkin-associated parkinsonism and parkin function has provided valuable insight into the molecular mechanisms of dopaminergic degeneration, particularly on the role of the cellular ubiquitination/protein degradation mechanisms in the disease process.

PARK8: Autosomal Dominant Parkinsonism Linked to Chromosome 12

A novel locus has been recently mapped in a large Japanese family to the pericentromeric region of chromosome 12. Affecteds in this family showed typical L-dopa responsive parkinsonism with onset in their fifties. Pathologically, nigral degeneration was found without distinctive inclusions (101).

PARK2: Autosomal Recessive Juvenile Parkinsonism (AR-JP) Caused by Mutations in the Gene for Parkin

Juvenile cases of parkinsonism with recessive inheritance (families with affected siblings, but no transmission from one generation to the next) were first recognized in Japan (36). Clinically, these patients suffer from L-dopa-responsive parkinsonism and some show diurnal fluctuations, with symptoms becoming worse later in the day. Dystonia at onset of the disease is quite common. In contrast to patients with dopa-responsive dystonia, which is caused by mutations in the gene for guanosine triphosphate cyclohydrolase (one of the genes involved in dopamine biosynthesis), patients with recessive parkinsonism often develop early and severe levodopa-induced motor fluctuations and dyskinesias (36).

The genetic locus for AR-JP has been mapped to chromosome 6 in the Japanese population, and mutations have been identified in a large gene in that region that was called *parkin* (37), a novel gene of, at that time, unknown function.

Parkin mutations turned out to be a common cause of parkinsonism with early onset, particularly in individuals with evidence of recessive inheritance. Nearly 50% of families from a population of sibling pairs collected by the European Consortium on Genetic Susceptibility in PD showed *parkin* mutations (38). In addition to the exon deletions described in the original Japanese study, a large number of smaller deletions, point mutations, and even exon duplications and triplications have been described. The study population was restricted to those families suggestive of recessive inheritance (two affected siblings), and it was required that at least one of the siblings had disease onset before 45 years of age. As this study used stringent diagnostic criteria for "typical" L-dopa-responsive PD, it is not surprising that the clinical picture was frequently indistinguishable from that of sporadic disease, with the exception, of course, of an earlier mean age at onset (38 ± 12 years). However, the latest onset age of the disease in this series was 58 years, emphasizing that parkinsonism associated with *parkin* mutations is not necessarily "juvenile." More *parkin*-positive cases with late disease onset have been reported in the literature (39), but overall, *parkin* mutations are still very rare in sporadic late-onset PD. Although they seem to be responsible for the majority of sporadic cases with onset before age 20, and are still somewhat common (25%) when onset is between 20 and 30, prevalence in older patients is almost certainly well below 5% (38).

The European study population allowed the characterization of the clinical spectrum of *parkin*-associated parkinsonism. Mean age at onset in a European population was 32 years; progression of the disease was usually relatively slow, but L-dopa-associated fluctuations and dyskinesias occurred frequently. Dystonia (usually in a lower extremity) at disease onset was found in about 40% of patients, and brisk reflexes of the lower limbs were present in 44% (38). There was no discernible difference in the clinical phenotype between patients with missense mutations, truncating point mutations, or deletions, suggesting that a complete loss of *parkin* function is associated with all of these mutations and with the full phenotype of early-onset parkinsonism.

The question of whether heterozygous mutations in the *parkin* gene can cause parkinsonism or can confer an increased susceptibility for typical late-onset PD is still unsettled. There is evidence from imaging studies (40) that heterozygotes may have mildly reduced uptake of fluorodopa in the basal ganglia. Furthermore, occasional families with heterozygous mutation carriers manifesting symptoms of PD have been described (39,41). However, in these cases it is difficult to prove the causal relationship between genotype and phenotype. The obvious study to answer this question, the systematic examination of (heterozygous) parents of patients with *parkin* mutations, has not been performed. So far, from the European population, there is no evidence of an increased frequency of parkinsonism in the parents of *parkin* gene patients.

The observation of heterozygous mutation carriers becoming symptomatic may also be explained by as yet undetected mutations in regulatory or intronic regions of the gene, which might affect splicing or transcription. It is likely that some 10% to 20% of pathogenic mutations remain undetected using current techniques of sequence analysis and exon dosage (38).

There is still relatively little information available on the neuropathology of molecularly confirmed cases of AR-JP. Severe and very selective degeneration of dopaminergic neurons and gliosis in the substantia nigra, usually with absence of Lewy bodies, has been described (42). The fact that Lewy bodies do not appear to be necessary for the selective degeneration of nigral neurons raises the interesting question of whether this neuropathologic feature should be regarded as an essential component of the disease process. The recent observation of typical ubiquitin-positive Lewy bodies in a patient with a compound heterozygous *parkin* mutation (41) may point to a closer relationship between Lewy body–positive and Lewy body–negative parkinsonism, but is still difficult to reconcile with present concepts of the molecular pathogenesis of the disorder (see below).

As mutations in *parkin* cause parkinsonism, in all likelihood by a loss-of-function mechanism, the study of the normal function of parkin should provide insight into the molecular pathogenesis of the disorder. Several groups have now shown that parkin, a protein found in the cytosol but also associated with membranes, functions in the cellular ubiquitination/protein degradation pathway as a ubiquitin ligase (43). It is therefore conceivable that the loss of *parkin* function may lead to the accumulation of a nonubiquitinated substrate that is deleterious to the dopaminergic cell but, due to its nonubiquitinated nature, does not accumulate in typical Lewy bodies. Several proteins have been shown to interact with parkin and could possibly be its crucial partner with regard to neurodegeneration: an O-glycosylated form of α-synuclein (44), a protein associated with synaptic vesicles named CDCrel-1 (45), and a transmembrane protein called the pael receptor (46). The possible interaction with α-synuclein is intriguing, as it may provide the link between parkin-associated juvenile parkinsonism and typical late-onset PD (44). However, as both parkin and α-synuclein are widely expressed in the brain, this does not explain the striking selectivity of the degenerative process for dopaminergic neurons. The pael receptor, on the other hand, shows preferential expression in tyrosine hydroxylase–positive neurons (46). However, regional selectivity may well be caused by other factors, such as the high burden of oxidative stress in dopaminergic neurons, or by the lack of some, as yet undefined, compensatory mechanisms.

RECESSIVE EARLY-ONSET PARKINSONISM LINKED TO CHROMOSOME 1 (PARK6 AND PARK7)

Recently, two other recessive loci have been linked in families with early-onset L-dopa-responsive parkinsonism, both to chromosome 1: one in a large Sicilian family with four definitely affected members (the Marsala kindred). The phenotype was characterized by early-onset (range 32 to 48 years) parkinsonism, with slow progression and sustained response to levodopa (47), which is similar to *parkin*-associated parkinsonism. Preliminary analyses suggest that this gene may also be responsible in more than a limited number of patients and families.

A second novel recessive locus, *PARK7*, has been mapped by van Duijn and co-workers (48), also in a consanguineous Italian family. Again, the clinical picture is that of early-onset, L-dopa-responsive parkinsonism, but little else is known.

GENETIC CONTRIBUTION TO SPORADIC PARKINSON'S DISEASE

Although molecular genetic analysis has produced significant progress in families with parkinsonian phenotypes with mendelian inheritance, it must be remembered that in the great majority of cases PD is a sporadic disorder. There is a subset of about 5% to 15% of families with more than one affected family member. Secondary cases are found more frequently among relatives of patients with PD than in unaffected control populations (49–51), but a clear mode of inheritance cannot be established. The type and the extent of a genetic contribution to nonmendelian PD are still controversial. A population-based case-control study indicates that the relative risk for first-degree family members of PD patients is increased only in the order of 2 to 3 (52). A segregation analysis was best compatible with an inherited component to the age of onset of the disease, and not to the development of the disease itself (53), and a second study of this kind performed in Finland confirmed a genetic factor in PD but was unable to distinguish between autosomal dominant and autosomal recessive inheritance (54).

A very large twin study indicates that genetic causes may be particularly important in young-onset cases (onset before age 50 years) but appeared negligible in those with onset

TABLE 38.2. ASSOCIATION STUDIES IN PARKINSON'S DISEASE[a]

Candidate Gene	Locus	Positive (or Negative) Association	No Association
Dopaminergic transmission:			
Dopamine D2 receptor	11q22–23	83	84
Dopamine D3 receptor	3q13.3		84
Dopamine D4 receptor	11p15.5		84
Dopamine transporter	5p15.3	85	83
Tyrosine hydroxylase	11p15.5		83
Catechol *O*-methyltransferase	22q12.1	86	87
Monoamine oxidase A	X		88
Monoamine oxidase B	Xp11.3	89,90	91
Heme oxigenase-1	22q12		92
Xenobiotic metabolism:			
Debrisoquine-4-hydroxylase	22q13	93,58	94
Cytochrome P450$_{1A1}$	5q22–24		95
Paraoxonase 1	7q21.3	60	96
N-Acetyltransferase 2	8p23.1	59	97
Protein aggregation:			
Apolipoprotein E	19q13.2	98	99
α-Synuclein	4q21.3–22	98	100
UCH-L1	4p15	34	35

[a]Only a few studies are cited as representative examples.

above age 50 (55), a distinction that was also evident in one of the segregation studies (54).

Most attempts to identify the susceptibility genes that are operative in these populations have followed a candidate gene approach. Based on pathologic, pathobiochemical, and epidemiologic findings, hypotheses on the etiology of PD can be generated and genetic polymorphisms within, or closely linked to, genes that are thought to be involved in these pathways have been examined (Table 38.2). Unfortunately, no consistent findings have emerged so far.

Studied genes include those identified in monogenic forms of PD, such as those for α-synuclein and parkin (34,56,57); genes encoding enzymes involved in the detoxification of xenobiotic compounds, such as debrisoquine hydroxylase (58), *N*-acetyltransferase (59), and paraoxonase (60); as well as genes involved in dopamine metabolism and neurotransmission. Despite a large number of initial positive results, findings have not been confirmed beyond doubt in any of these cases (Table 38.2), indicating that studies with improved methodology (e.g., transmission disequilibrium testing, examination of haplotypes instead of single polymorphisms) may be necessary.

A second approach to identification of putative genetic risk factors for PD is the genome-wide analysis of a large population of small PD families (affected sib-pairs or affected pedigree members) with polymorphic DNA markers. The results of three of these studies have now become available (61,62,102). Several genomic regions with moderately positive lod scores (1 to 1.5) have been identified in these studies, but only a few regions appeared in more than one study. However, one of the methodologic limitations of this type of study is that the identified regions are too large to be useful for the identification of specific candidate genes. Nevertheless, this approach will be valuable in the future because it will be expanded to encompass larger patient populations and denser marker maps using single nucleotide polymorphisms (SNPs) instead of the microsatellite markers commonly used today.

OTHER GENETIC DISORDERS PRESENTING WITH SIGNS AND SYMPTOMS OF PARKINSONISM

Recently, it has become apparent that a number of inherited neurodegenerative conditions that are neuropathologically (and usually also clinically) clearly distinct from PD can present with signs and symptoms of parkinsonism. These disorders may sometimes, at least in the initial stages, mimic idiopathic PD.

Tau-related Disorders

An increasing number of neurodegenerative disorders are found to be related to the abnormal deposition of the microtubule-associated protein tau (MAPTau). A detailed discussion of this complex group of disorders is beyond the scope of this chapter. Excellent reviews on the clinical (63) and molecular aspects (64) of tauopathies have been published. The brief discussion here will be restricted to aspects directly related to parkinsonian syndromes.

Inherited Tauopathies with Mutations in the MAPTau Gene

The term "frontotemporal dementia with parkinsonism linked to chromosome 17," or FTDP-17, has been adopted to characterize a familial disorder characterized by behavioral and cognitive disturbances, progressing to dementia, and a variable degree of extrapyramidal, pyramidal, and lower motor neuron signs, all genetically linked to a locus on the long arm of chromosome 17 (17q21-22) (65). Mutations in the gene for MAPTau have been identified (66), located in exons 9, 10, 12, and 13, or in adjacent intronic sequences, affecting the microtubule-binding repeat domain, encoded by this part of the gene. In most families, behavioral disturbances and dementia are the most prominent symptom, with parkinsonism and other neurologic disturbances, such as supranuclear gaze palsy, pyramidal tract dysfunction, and urinary incontinence, appearing to a variable degree during the later course of the disease (63). In a few families, particularly the one described by Wszolek et al. clinically and pathologically as pontopallidonigral degeneration (67), rapidly progressive L-dopa-unresponsive parkinsonism with supranuclear gaze palsy is the leading symptom, with dementia, frontal lobe release signs, and perseverative vocalizations developing later. This family was found to harbor a tau mutation (N279K) (68), which appears to be usually associated with a parkinsonism-predominant variety of the disease (69). However, other mutations, such as the most common mutation P301L, have been found to be associated with a variety of clinical phenotypes, resembling Pick's disease, progressive supranuclear palsy, or corticobasal degeneration in different families as well as within single families (70).

The variability of the clinical phenotype is accounted for, at least in part, by the fact that tau mutations probably lead to pathology by different mechanisms. Intronic and some exonic mutations affect alternative splicing of exon 10, and as a consequence alter the relative abundance of three-repeat and four-repeat tau, the two major classes of the protein present in the brain. Other mutations seem to impair the ability of tau to bind microtubules or to promote microtubule assembly (71).

Other Tauopathies

Progressive supranuclear palsy (PSP) and corticobasal ganglionic degeneration (CBGD) are two other distinct entities with some overlapping clinical features, which are pathologically characterized by the deposition of abnormally phosphorylated tau protein.

With very few notable exceptions, these disorders are sporadic, and no mutations in the coding region or in the splice sites of the *tau* gene have been identified in most patients.

As noted above, in a very small number of patients a phenotype resembling typical PSP or CBGD is in fact associated with *tau* gene mutations. One interesting mutation has been identified in a family with a PSP-like phenotype (72). The mutation (S305S) is located in exon 10 of the *tau* gene and forms part of a stem-loop structure at the 5′ splice donor site. Although the mutation does not give rise to an amino acid change in the tau protein, functional exon-trapping experiments show that it results in a significant (4.8-fold) increase in the splicing of exon 10, resulting in the overproduction of tau containing four microtubule-binding repeats.

Although no coding region or splice site mutations can be identified in the majority of patients with PSP or CBGD, there appears to be a genetic susceptibility to the disease related to a particular haplotype of DNA markers surrounding the *tau* gene. Initially, Conrad and co-workers observed that the "A0" allele of a dinucleotide repeat marker within the *tau* gene is highly associated, in homozygous form, with PSP (73). This allele was later found to be part of an extended haplotype (H1 haplotype) of more than 100 kb, which is usually inherited en bloc (74). The same genetic background is found in patients with CBGD, supporting the close relationship between these two disorders (75). As the H1 haplotype is common in the general population (approximately 60% of chromosomes), it does not, per se, carry a high risk for the development of a tau-related disorder. It is possible that either a more recent mutation that occurred on the background of this haplotype is responsible for the development of the disease, or that H1 haplotype is "permissive" for the action of some other disease-causing factors.

Huntington's Disease

Huntington's disease (HD) is an autosomal dominantly inherited disorder, usually characterized by a hyperkinetic movement disorder, personality changes, and dementia. It is caused by the pathologic expansion of a CAG trinucleotide repeat sequence in the gene for Huntingtin on chromosome 4. The fact that cases of early onset frequently present with dystonia and parkinsonism, rather than with chorea, has long been recognized.

Widespread use of molecular diagnosis for HD has shown that the phenotypic spectrum may even include late-onset levodopa-responsive parkinsonism (76) and atypical parkinsonian syndromes (77).

Spinocerebellar Ataxias

Like HD, the spinocerebellar ataxias (SCAs) are caused by expansions of CAG repeat sequences. The core syndrome is usually that of a progressive cerebellar ataxia with or without additional neurologic features. Particularly in SCA1, 2, and 3, extrapyramidal symptoms are relatively common, having been described in 10% to 50% of patients. Patients with SCA3 have occasionally been found to present with dopa-responsive parkinsonism (78). This has recently been confirmed in another family (79) and extended to a family with SCA2 (80). It is, therefore, not unlikely that other forms of SCA might also occasionally mimic PD. The reason for the variable expressivity of the genes with expanded CAG repeat expansion is still largely unknown.

Dopa-responsive Dystonia

A rare variant of primary dystonia, *dopa-responsive dystonia*, is caused by point mutations in the gene for guanosine triphosphate cyclohydrolase I in the majority of cases (81). The phenotype is usually characterized by a childhood-onset dystonia, affecting the extremities first, but rarely craniocervical dystonia may be the only manifestation. Mild parkinsonism of adult onset has long been recognized as one clinical feature of the disease and may be the sole manifestation in some gene carriers. The positive family history of more typical childhood-onset dopa-responsive dystonia usually indicates the correct diagnosis. However, early-onset parkinsonism not uncommonly presents with dystonia as a first symptom, making it difficult to distinguish from dopa-responsive dystonia in some cases. In fact, 3 of 22 cases with a phenotype of dopa-responsive dystonia proved to be due to mutations in the *parkin* gene (82).

CONCLUSION

The genetic findings in rare inherited forms of PD have contributed to our understanding of the clinical, neuropathologic, and genetic heterogeneity of PD. The variability of clinical features, such as age at onset, occurrence of dementia, or other associated features found within single families, suggests that a single genetic cause (the pathogenic mutation in a given family) can lead to a spectrum of clinical manifestations. On the other hand, individuals with different genetic defects and different neuropathology may be clinically indistinguishable from each other and fulfill all presently accepted criteria of idiopathic PD. It is therefore apparent that a new genetic classification of PD that is only partially congruent with the classic clinical-pathologic classification is about to emerge.

At present, there is convincing evidence that genetic factors have an important role in the etiology of at least a subset of patients with PD. Probably only a small percentage of cases with dominant or recessive inheritance can be explained by mutations in the genes that have been identified so far (the genes for α-synuclein, ubiquitin carboxy-terminal hydrolase L1, and parkin) or by mutations in the as-yet-unidentified genes on chromosome 1p, 2p, 4p, and 12p. The study of wild-type and mutated gene products will provide important insight into the molecular pathogenesis of nigral degeneration. However, it appears that intense efforts are still needed to unravel the full spectrum of etiologic factors leading to the sporadic form of this common neurodegenerative disorder.

REFERENCES

1. McNaught KS, Olanow CW, Halliwell B, et al. Failure of the ubiquitin-proteasome system in Parkinson's disease. *Nat Rev Neurosci* 2001;2(8):589–594.
2. Polymeropoulos MH, Lavedan C, Leroy E, et al. Mutation in the α-synuclein gene identified in families with Parkinson's disease. *Science* 1997;276:2045–2047.
3. Krüger R, Kuhn W, Müller T, et al. Ala39Pro mutation in the gene encoding α-synuclein in Parkinson's disease. *Nat Genet* 1998;18:106–108.
4. Jensen PH, Gai WP. Alpha-synuclein: axonal transport, ligand interaction, and neurodegeneration. *Adv Exp Med Biol* 2001; 487:129–134.
5. Abeliovich A, Schmitz Y, Farinas I, et al. Mice lacking alpha-synuclein display functional deficits in the nigrostriatal dopamine system. *Neuron* 2000;25(1):239–252.
6. Gasser T, Müller-Myhsok B, Wszolek Z, et al. Genetic complexity and Parkinson's disease. *Science* 1997;277:388–389.
7. Scott WK, Stajich JM, Yamaoka L-H, et al. Genetic complexity in Parkinson's disease. *Science* 1997;277:387–388.
8. Vaughan JR, Durr A, Gasser T, et al. The α-synuclein Ala53Thr mutation is not a common cause of familial Parkinson's disease: a study of 230 European cases. *Ann Neurol* 1998;44(2):270–273.
9. Papadimitriou A, Veletza V, Hadjigeorgiou GM, et al. Mutated alpha-synuclein gene in two Greek kindreds with familial PD: incomplete penetrance? *Neurology* 1999;52(3):651–654.
10. Golbe LI, Di Iorio G, Bonavita V, et al. A large kindred with autosomal dominant Parkinson's disease. *Ann Neurol* 1990;27 (3):276–282.
11. Spillantini MG, Schmidt ML, Lee VM, et al. Alpha-synuclein in Lewy bodies. *Nature* 1997;388(6645):839–840.
12. Goedert M, Spillantini MG, Davies SW. Filamentous nerve cell inclusions in neurodegenerative diseases. *Curr Opin Neurobiol* 1998;8(5):619–632.
13. Biere AL, Wood SJ, Wypych J, et al. Parkinson's disease associated α-synuclein is more fibrillogenic than β- and γ-synuclein and cannot cross-seed its homologs. *J Biol Chem* 2000;274(14):9843.
14. Jensen PH, Nielsen MS, Jakes R, et al. Binding of alpha-synuclein to brain vesicles is abolished by familial Parkinson's disease mutation. *J Biol Chem* 1998;273(41):26292–26294.
15. Engelender S, Kaminsky Z, Guo X, et al. Synphilin-1 associates with alpha-synuclein and promotes the formation of cytosolic inclusions. *Nat Genet* 1999;22(1):110–114.
16. Kahle PJ, Neumann M, Ozmen L, et al. Subcellular localization of wild-type and Parkinson's disease-associated mutant alpha-synuclein in human and transgenic mouse brain. *J Neurosci* 2000;20(17):6365–6373.
17. Masliah E, Rockenstein E, Veinbergs I, et al. Dopaminergic loss and inclusion body formation in alpha-synuclein mice: implications for neurodegenerative disorders. *Science* 2000;287(5456): 1265–1269.
18. Feany MB, Bender WW. A *Drosophila* model of Parkinson's disease. *Nature* 2000;404(6776):394–398.
19. Lavedan C, Buchholtz S, Auburger G, et al. Absence of mutation in the beta- and gamma-synuclein genes in familial autosomal dominant Parkinson's disease. *DNA Res* 1998;5(6):401–402.
20. Lincoln S, Gwinn-Hardy K, Goudreau J, et al. No pathogenic mutations in the persyn gene in Parkinson's disease. *Neurosci Lett* 1999;259(1):65–66.

21. Farrer M, Destee A, Levecque C, et al. Genetic analysis of synphilin-1 in familial parkinson's disease. *Neurobiol Dis* 2001;8(2):317–323.

22. Gasser T, Müller-Myhsok B, Wszolek ZK, et al. A susceptibility locus for Parkinson's disease maps to chromosome 2p13. *Nat Genet* 1998;18:262–265.

23. Wszolek ZK, Cordes M, Calne DB, et al. Hereditary Parkinson disease: report of 3 families with dominant autosomal inheritance. *Nervenarzt* 1993;64(5):331–335.

24. Gasser T, Bereznai B, Wieditz G, et al. Evaluation of a Danish/German founder haplotype at the PARK3-locus on chromosome 2p13. *Mov Disord* 1999;13[Suppl 2]:103.

25. Klein C, Vieregge P, Hagenah J, et al. Search for the PARK3 founder haplotype in a large cohort of patients with Parkinson's disease from northern Germany. *Ann Hum Genet* 1999;63(Pt 4):285–291.

26. West AB, Zimprich A, Lockhart PJ, et al. Refinement of the PARK3 locus on chromosome 2p13 and the analysis of 14 candidate genes. *Eur J Hum Genet* 2001;9(9):659–666.

27. Zink M, Grimm L, Wszolek ZK, et al. Autosomal-dominant Parkinson's disease linked to 2p13 is not caused by mutations in transforming growth factor alpha (TGF alpha). *J Neural Transm* 2001;108(8-9):1029–1034.

28. Wszolek ZK, Gwinn-Hardy K, Wszolek EK, et al. Family C (German-American) with late onset parkinsonism: longitudinal observations including autopsy. *Neurology* 1999;52.

29. Muenter MD, Forno LS, Hornykiewicz O, et al. Hereditary form of parkinsonism-dementia. *Ann Neurol* 1998;43(6):768–781.

30. Farrer M, Gwinn-Hardy K, Muenter M, et al. A chromosome 4p haplotype segregating with Parkinson's disease and postural tremor. *Hum Mol Genet* 1999;8(1):81–85.

31. Leroy E, Boyer R, Auburger G, et al. The ubiquitin pathway in Parkinson's disease [letter]. *Nature* 1998;395(6701):451–452.

32. Harhangi BS, Farrer MJ, Lincoln S, et al. The Ile93Met mutation in the ubiquitin carboxy-terminal-hydrolase-L1 gene is not observed in European cases with familial Parkinson's disease. *Neurosci Lett* 1999;270(1):1–4.

33. Farrer M, Destee T, Becquet E, et al. Linkage exclusion in French families with probable Parkinson's disease. *Mov Disord* 2000;15(6):1075–1083.

34. Maraganore DM, Farrer MJ, Hardy JA, et al. Case-control study of the ubiquitin carboxy-terminal hydrolase L1 gene in Parkinson's disease. *Neurology* 1999;53(8):1858–1860.

35. Mellick GD, Silburn PA. The ubiquitin carboxy-terminal hydrolase-L1 gene S18Y polymorphism does not confer protection against idiopathic Parkinson's disease. *Neurosci Lett* 2000;293(2):127–130.

36. Ishikawa A, Tsuji S. Clinical analysis of 17 patients in 12 Japanese families with autosomal-recessive type juvenile parkinsonism. *Neurology* 1996;47(1):160–166.

37. Kitada T, Asakawa S, Hattori N, et al. Mutations in the *parkin* gene cause autosomal recessive juvenile parkinsonism. *Nature* 1998;392:605–608.

38. Lücking CB, Dürr A, Bonifati V, et al. Association between early-onset Parkinson's disease and mutations in the *parkin* gene. *N Engl J Med* 2000;342(21):1560–1567.

39. Klein C, Pramstaller PP, Kis B, et al. Parkin deletions in a family with adult-onset, tremor-dominant parkinsonism: expanding the phenotype. *Ann Neurol* 2000;48(1):65–71.

40. Hilker R, Klein C, Ghaemi M, et al. Positron emission tomographic analysis of the nigrostriatal dopaminergic system in familial parkinsonism associated with mutations in the *parkin* gene. *Ann Neurol* 2001;49(3):367–376.

41. Farrer M, Chan P, Chen R, et al. Lewy bodies and parkinsonism in families with *parkin* mutations. *Ann Neurol* 2001;50(3):293–300.

42. van De Warrenburg BP, Lammens M, Lucking CB, et al. Clinical and pathologic abnormalities in a family with parkinsonism and *parkin* gene mutations. *Neurology* 2001;56(4):555–557.

43. Shimura H, Hattori N, Kubo S, et al. Familial parkinson disease gene product, parkin, is a ubiquitin-protein ligase [in process citation]. *Nat Genet* 2000;25(3):302–305.

44. Shimura H, Schlossmacher MG, Hattori N, et al. Ubiquitination of a new form of alpha-synuclein by parkin from human brain: implications for Parkinson's disease. *Science* 2001;293(5528):263–269.

45. Zhang Y, Gao J, Chung KK, et al. Parkin functions as an E2-dependent ubiquitin- protein ligase and promotes the degradation of the synaptic vesicle–associated protein, CDCrel-1. *Proc Natl Acad Sci USA* 2000;97(24):13354–13359.

46. Imai Y, Soda M, Inoue H, et al. An unfolded putative transmembrane polypeptide, which can lead to endoplasmic reticulum stress, is a substrate of Parkin. *Cell* 2001;105(7):891–902.

47. Valente EM, Bentivoglio AR, Dixon PH, et al. Localization of a novel locus for autosomal recessive early-onset parkinsonism, park6, on human chromosome 1p35-p36. *Am J Hum Genet* 2001;68(4):895–900.

48. van Duijn CM, Dekker MC, Bonifati V, et al. Park7, a novel locus for autosomal recessive early-onset parkinsonism, on chromosome 1p36. *Am J Hum Genet* 2001;69(3):629–634.

49. Bonifati V, Fabrizio E, Vanacore N, et al. Familial Parkinson's disease: a clinical genetic analysis. *Can J Neurol Sci* 1995;22(4):272–279.

50. Lazzarini AM, Myers RH, Zimmerman TR, Jr. et al. A clinical genetic study of Parkinson's disease: evidence for dominant transmission. *Neurology* 1994;44(3 Pt 1):499–506.

51. De Michele G, Filla A, Volpe G, et al. Environmental and genetic risk factors in Parkinson's disease: a case-control study in southern Italy. *Mov Disord* 1996;11(1):17–23.

52. Marder K, Tang MX, Mejia H, et al. Risk of Parkinson's disease among first-degree relatives: a community-based study. *Neurology* 1996;47(1):155–160.

53. Zareparsi S, Taylor TD, Harris EL, et al. Segregation analysis of Parkinson disease. *Am J Med Genet* 1998;80(4):410–417.

54. Moilanen JS, Autere JM, Myllyla VV, et al. Complex segregation analysis of Parkinson's disease in the Finnish population. *Hum Genet* 2001;108(3):184–189.

55. Tanner CM, Ottman R, Goldman SM, et al. Parkinson disease in twins: an etiologic study. *JAMA* 1999;281(4):341–346.

56. Scott WK, Yamaoka LH, Stajich JM, et al. The alpha-synuclein gene is not a major risk factor in familial Parkinson disease. *Neurogenetics* 1999;2(3):191–192.

57. Klein C, Schumacher K, Jacobs H, et al. Association studies of Parkinson's disease and parkin polymorphisms. *Ann Neurol* 2000;48(1):126–127.

58. Armstrong M, Daly AK, Cholerton S, et al. Mutant debrisoquine hydroxylation genes in Parkinson's disease. *Lancet* 1992;339(8800):1017–1018.

59. Bandmann O, Vaughan JR, Holmans P, et al. Association of slow acetylator genotype for *N*-acetyltransferase 2 with familial Parkinson's disease. *Lancet* 1998;350:1136–1139.

60. Akhmedova SN, Yakimovsky AK, Schwartz EI. Paraoxonase 1 Met–Leu 54 polymorphism is associated with Parkinson's disease. *J Neurol Sci* 2001;184(2):179–182.

61. DeStefano AL, Golbe LI, Mark MH, et al. Genome-wide scan for Parkinson's disease: the Gene PD Study. *Neurology* 2001;57(6):1124–1126.

62. Scott WK, Nance MA, Watts RL, et al. Complete genomic screen in Parkinson disease: evidence for multiple genes. *JAMA* 2001;286(18):2239–2244.

63. Reed LA, Wszolek ZK, Hutton M. Phenotypic correlations in FTDP-17. *Neurobiol Aging* 2001;22(1):89–107.

64. Lee VM, Goedert M, Trojanowski JQ. Neurodegenerative tauopathies. *Annu Rev Neurosci* 2001;24:1121–1159.

65. Foster NL, Wilhelmsen K, Sima AA, et al. Frontotemporal dementia and parkinsonism linked to chromosome 17: a consensus conference. *Ann Neurol* 1997; 41(6):706–715.

66. Hutton M, Lendon CL, Rizzu P, et al. Association of missense and 5′-splice-site mutations in tau with the inherited dementia FTDP-17. *Nature* 1998;393(6686):702–705.

67. Wszolek ZK, Pfeiffer RF, Bhatt MH, et al. Rapidly progressive autosomal dominant parkinsonism and dementia with pallido-ponto-nigral degeneration. *Ann Neurol* 1992;32(3):312–320.

68. Clark LN, Poorkaj P, Wszolek Z, et al. Pathogenic implications of mutations in the tau gene in pallido-ponto-nigral degeneration and related neurodegenerative disorders linked to chromosome 17. *Proc Natl Acad Sci USA* 1998;95(22):13103–13107.

69. Yasuda M, Takamatsu J, D'Souza I, et al. A novel mutation at position +12 in the intron following exon 10 of the tau gene in familial frontotemporal dementia (FTD-Kumamoto). *Ann Neurol* 2000;47(4):422–429.

70. Mirra SS, Murrell JR, Gearing M, et al. Tau pathology in a family with dementia and a P301L mutation in tau. *J Neuropathol Exp Neurol* 1999;58(4):335–345.

71. Spillantini MG, Goedert M. Tau gene mutations and tau pathology in frontotemporal dementia and parkinsonism linked to chromosome 17. *Adv Exp Med Biol* 2001;487:21–37.

72. Stanford PM, Halliday GM, Brooks WS, et al. Progressive supranuclear palsy pathology caused by a novel silent mutation in exon 10 of the tau gene: expansion of the disease phenotype caused by tau gene mutations. *Brain* 2000;123(Pt 5):880–893.

73. Conrad C, Andreadis A, Trojanowski JQ, et al. Genetic evidence for the involvement of tau in progressive supranuclear palsy. *Ann Neurol* 1997;41(2):277–281.

74. Baker M, Litvan I, Houlden H, et al. Association of an extended haplotype in the tau gene with progressive supranuclear palsy. *Hum Mol Genet* 1999;8(4):711–715.

75. Houlden H, Baker M, Morris HR, et al. Corticobasal degeneration and progressive supranuclear palsy share a common tau haplotype. *Neurology* 2001;56(12):1702–1706.

76. Racette BA, Perlmutter JS. Levodopa responsive parkinsonism in an adult with Huntington's disease. *J Neurol Neurosurg Psychiatry* 1998;65(4):577–579.

77. Reuter I, Hu MT, Andrews TC, et al. Late onset levodopa responsive Huntington's disease with minimal chorea masquerading as Parkinson plus syndrome. *J Neurol Neurosurg Psychiatry* 2000;68(2):238–241.

78. Tuite PJ, Rogaeva EA, St George Hyslop PH, et al. Dopa-responsive parkinsonism phenotype of Machado-Joseph disease: confirmation of 14q CAG expansion. *Ann Neurol* 1995;38(4):684–687.

79. Gwinn-Hardy K, Singleton A, O'Suilleabhain P, et al. Spinocerebellar ataxia type 3 phenotypically resembling Parkinson disease in a black family. *Arch Neurol* 2001;58(2):296–299.

80. Gwinn-Hardy K, Chen JY, Liu HC, et al. Spinocerebellar ataxia type 2 with parkinsonism in ethnic Chinese. *Neurology* 2000;55(6):800–805.

81. Ichinose H, Ohye T, Takahashi E, et al. Hereditary progressive dystonia with marked diurnal fluctuation caused by mutations in the GTP cyclohydrolase I gene. *Nat Genet* 1994;8(3):236–242.

82. Tassin J, Durr A, Bonnet AM, et al. Levodopa-responsive dystonia: GTP cyclohydrolase I or parkin mutations? *Brain* 2000;123(Pt 6):1112–1121.

83. Plante Bordeneuve V, Taussig D, Thomas F, et al. Evaluation of four candidate genes encoding proteins of the dopamine pathway in familial and sporadic Parkinson's disease: evidence for association of a DRD2 allele. *Neurology* 1997;48:1589–1593.

84. Nanko S, Ueki A, Hattori M, et al. No allelic association between Parkinson's disease and dopamine D2, D3, and D4 receptor gene polymorphisms. *Am J Med Genet* 1994;54(4):361–364.

85. Le Couteur DG, Leighton PW, McCann SJ, et al. Association of a polymorphism in the dopamine-transporter gene with Parkinson's disease. *Mov Disord* 1997;12(5):760–763.

86. Yoritaka A, Hattori N, Yoshino H, et al. Catechol-O-methyl-transferase genotype and susceptibility to Parkinson's disease in Japan [in process citation]. *J Neural Transm* 1997;104(11-12):1313–1317.

87. Xie T, Ho SL, Li LS, et al. G/A1947 polymorphism in catechol-O-methyltransferase (COMT) gene in Parkinson's disease. *Mov Disord* 1997;12(3):426–427.

88. Hotamisligil GS, Girmen AS, Fink JS, et al. Hereditary variations in monoamine oxidase as a risk factor for Parkinson's disease. *Mov Disord* 1994;9(3):305–310.

89. Costa P, Checkoway H, Levy D, et al. Association of a polymorphism in intron 13 of the monoamine oxidase B gene with Parkinson disease. *Am J Med Genet* 1997;74(2):154–156.

90. Kurth JH, Kurth MC, Poduslo SE, et al. Association of a monoamine oxidase B allele with Parkinson's disease. *Ann Neurol* 1993;33(4):368–372.

91. Ho SL, Kapadi AL, Ramsden DB, et al. An allelic association study of monoamine oxidase B in Parkinson's disease. *Ann Neurol* 1995;37(3):403–405.

92. Kimpara T, Takeda A, Watanabe K, et al. Microsatellite polymorphism in the human heme oxygenase-1 gene promoter and its application in association studies with Alzheimer and Parkinson disease. *Hum Genet* 1997;100(1):145–147.

93. Wilhelmsen KC, Wszolek ZK. Is there a genetic susceptibility to idiopathic parkinsonism? *Parkinsonism Relat Disord* 1995;1:73–84.

94. Gasser T, Müller-Myhsok B, Supala A, et al. The CYP2D6B-allele is not over-represented in a population of German patients with idiopathic Parkinson's disease. *J Neurol Neurosurg Psychiatry* 1996;61(5):518–520.

95. Takakubo F, Yamamoto M, Ogawa N, et al. Genetic association between cytochrome *P450IA1* gene and susceptibility to Parkinson's disease. *J Neural Transm Genet Sect* 1996;103(7):843–849.

96. Wang J, Liu Z. No association between paraoxonase 1 (PON1) gene polymorphisms and susceptibility to Parkinson's disease in a Chinese population. *Mov Disord* 2000;15(6):1265–1267.

97. Harhangi BS, Oostra BA, Heutink P, et al. *N*-Acetyltransferase-2 polymorphism in Parkinson's disease: the Rotterdam study. *J Neurol Neurosurg Psychiatry* 1999;67(4):518–520.

98. Kruger R, Vieira-Saecker AM, Kuhn W, et al. Increased susceptibility to sporadic Parkinson's disease by a certain combined alpha-synuclein/apolipoprotein E genotype. *Ann Neurol* 1999;45(5):611–617.

99. Whitehead AS, Bertrandy S, Finnan F, et al. Frequency of the apolipoprotein E epsilon 4 allele in a case-control study of early onset Parkinson's disease. *J Neurol Neurosurg Psychiatry* 1996;61(4):347–351.

100. Parsian A, Racette B, Zhang ZH, et al. Mutation, sequence analysis, and association studies of alpha-synuclein in Parkinson's disease. *Neurology* 1998;51(6):1757–1759.

101. Funayama M, et al. A new locus for Parkinson's disease (PARK8) maps to chormosome 12p11.2-q13.1. *Ann Neurol* 2002;51(3):296–301.

102. Pankratz N, et al. Genome screen to identify susceptibility genes for Parkinson disease in a sample without parkin mutations. *Am J Hum Genet* 2002;7(1):124–135.

39

NEUROACANTHOCYTOSIS

JUHA O. RINNE
MYUNG SIK LEE

Acanthocytes are erythrocytes bearing irregular spines and thorny projections over the cell surface (Fig. 39.1). Acanthocytes are not normally present in peripheral blood. Sometimes echinocytes may be erroneously called acanthocytes, but echinocytes have numerous fine uniform spicules distributed equally over the cell surface, whereas acanthocytes have an irregular shape of cell body bearing fewer spicules of variable length (1,2). Acanthocytosis is nonspecific and can be encountered, for instance, in anorexia nervosa, in hypothyroidism, after splenectomy, and in severe hepatocellular disease (2). The basis for the formation of acanthocytes is unclear. However, in abetalipoproteinemia, there is accumulation of apolipoprotein B and triglycerides within erythrocytes, and a mutation of the microsomal triglyceride-transfer protein gene in chromosome 4 has been reported (3). In acanthocytosis with normal lipoprotein levels, alterations of erythrocyte membrane lipid composition have been noted. Changes in the phospholipid content as well as ultrastructural abnormalities of the erythrocyte membrane skeleton and in the degree of membrane protein phosphorylation have been reported (4–8).

These changes are thought to result in reduced erythrocyte membrane fluidity (9).

Many neurologic diseases associated with acanthocytes have been called "neuroacanthocytosis." They can be divided arbitrarily into two groups according to the lipid metabolism status. Neuroacanthocytosis with abnormal lipid metabolism may include Bassen-Kornzweig syndrome (characterized by hypobetalipoproteinemia, progressive ataxia, retinitis pigmentosa, steatorrhea, and vitamins A and E deficiency) and HARP syndrome (a variant form of Hallervorden-Spatz syndrome characterized by hypoprebetalipoproteinemia, acanthocytosis, retinitis pigmentosa, and pallidal degeneration). Another group of neuroacanthocytoses with normal serum lipid levels may include familial amyotrophic chorea (Levine-Critchley syndrome, amyotrophic chorea with acanthocytosis, familial neuroacanthocytosis), McLeod's syndrome, progressive parkinsonism, Hallervorden-Spatz syndrome, MELAS (mitochondrial myopathy, encephalopathy, lactacidosis, and stroke), and spinocerebellar degeneration. In this chapter, we discuss neuroacanthocytosis with normal lipid metabolism.

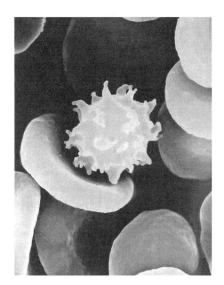 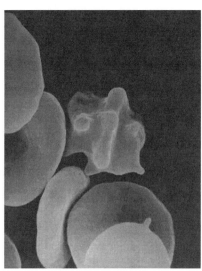

FIG. 39.1. A scanning electron microscopic study shows an irregularly shaped acanthocyte with several spicules of variable length *(left)* and a type III echinocyte bearing many short spicules evenly distributed over the surface of the spherical cell *(right)*.

AMYOTROPHIC CHOREOATHETOSIS WITH ACANTHOCYTOSIS

Clinical Features

Many authors use the term neuroacanthocytosis as a synonym for amyotrophic choreoathetosis with acanthocytosis. Patients suffering from amyotrophic choreoathetosis with acanthocytosis may present with a variety of clinical features, including chorea, tics, orofacial dyskinesia, seizures, cognitive impairment, and peripheral neuropathy (4,8,10–57). No epidemiologic data on the prevalence or incidence of amyotrophic choreoathetosis with acanthocytosis are available. The age at onset has varied from 6 to 62 years, the mean being 31 years. Survival time from disease onset has also varied considerably from 4 to 43 years, with a mean survival time of 13.5 years.

Involuntary movements, typically chorea and orofacial dyskinesia, are the most common initial symptoms (4,8, 10–13,19–57) (Table 39.1). Chorea is generalized but most frequently affects the limbs. Orofacial dyskinesia interferes with speech and swallowing, and can lead to orolingual self-mutilation with tongue and lip biting. These features become increasingly common during the course of the disease. Seizures, gait disturbance, cognitive impairment, psychiatric symptoms, and limb weakness have also been reported as initial symptoms. Dystonia and parkinsonism are rarely seen on initial presentation.

During the disease course, involuntary movements are seen in almost all (95%) cases (Table 39.2). The most commonly observed involuntary movements are chorea and orofacial dyskinesias (in more than 80% of cases; Table 39.2). About one third of patients develop dystonia, but usually later during the clinical course. In some cases, hyperkinesia during the early clinical course is later gradually replaced by akinetic-rigid

TABLE 39.1. INITIAL SYMPTOMS OF AMYOTROPHIC CHOREOATHETOSIS WITH ACANTHOCYTOSIS REPORTED IN THE LITERATURE[a]

Initial Symptom	N	%
Involuntary movement	**41**	**56**
Chorea	18	23
Orofacial dyskinesia	22	29
Tongue biting	4	5
Dystonia	3	4
Parkinsonism	3	4
Motor/vocal tic	4	5
Speech disturbance	**13**	**17**
Dysphagia	**5**	**6**
Gait disturbance	**10**	**13**
Limb weakness	**6**	**8**
Cognitive and behavioral change	**10**	**13**
Behavioral change	8	10
Intellectual impairment	2	3
Seizure	**15**	**19**
Total	**77 cases**	

[a]Includes cases from references 4, 8, 10–13, 19–57.
N, number of cases.

TABLE 39.2. CLINICAL MANIFESTATIONS REPORTED IN AMYOTROPHIC CHOREOATHETOSIS WITH ACANTHOCYTOSIS SEEN AT SOME STAGE OF THE DISEASE COURSE[a]

Symptoms and Signs	N	%
Involuntary movements	99	95
Limb dyskinesia, chorea	85	82
Orofacial dyskinesia	86	83
Tongue biting	43	41
Dystonia	32	31
Parkinsonism	16	15
Motor/vocal tics	48	46
Cognitive and behavioral change	40	38
Cognitive impairment	31	30
Memory impairment	12	11
Learning difficulties	10	10
Inattention/distractibility	3/11	3/11
Personality change	33	32
Irritability/aggression	8/10	8/10
Obsessive-compulsive behavior	5	5
Disinhibition	10	10
Mood disorder	36	35
Depression/apathy	14/8	14/8
Anxiety/agitation	11/5	11/5
Emotional lability	9	9
Speech disturbance	60	58
Swallowing difficulty	51	48
Gait disturbance	56	54
Cerebellar dysfunction	13	13
Neuromuscular manifestation	67	65
Muscle weakness	49	47
Proximal/distal/All	3/13/7	3/13/7
Uex/Lex/All	2/12/9	2/12/9
Hypotonia	24	23
Proximal/distal/All	0/0/14	0/0/13
Uex/Lex/All	0/0/17	0/0/16
Muscle wasting	49	47
Proximal/distal/All	7/14/8	7/14/8
Uex/Lex/All	7/8/20	7/8/20
Hyporeflexia/areflexia	63	61
Sensory abnormality	18	17
Vibration/pinprick	12/5	12/5
Abnormal plantar response	5	2
Bony deformity	11	11
Seizures	38	34
Total	102 cases	

[a]Includes cases from references 4, 8, 10–13, 19–57.
Uex, upper extremity; Lex, lower extremity.

parkinsonism (10,11), or hyperkinesia is present together with akinetic-rigid features from the early clinical phase (12,13). Motor and vocal tics occur in about half of the patients with amyotrophic choreoathetosis. Speech disturbances, swallowing difficulties, and gait disturbances are seen in about half of the patients (Table 39.2). The detailed character of the gait disturbance has rarely been described. The term most frequently used in the earlier literature is "lurching gait." The gait disturbance may be caused by several factors, such as atrophy of the leg muscles (e.g., steppage gait due to atrophy of the anterior tibialis muscle), or difficulty in maintaining balance due to dyskinesias of the limbs, or a combination of these. Cerebellar dysfunction may also be seen (Table 39.2).

Psychiatric symptoms are relatively common. Personality change was reported in one third of patients and included irritability, aggressiveness, obsessive-compulsive behavior, and disinhibition. Depression, apathy, anxiety, agitation and emotional lability are the most common mood changes reported. Cognitive impairment is seen in about one third of cases. Memory impairment and learning difficulties have been reported, and the profile of cognitive impairment may resemble that of Huntington's disease (HD) and subcortical vascular cognitive impairment (14,15), showing executive function deficits consistent with disruption of frontosubcortical circuits.

Muscular weakness and wasting have been reported in almost half of the patients with distal and lower extremity predominance (Table 39.2). Tendon reflexes are commonly absent or diminished. Hypotonia was present in one fourth of the patients. Seizures, most frequently generalized tonic-clonic seizures, were present in slightly more than one third of patients.

Genetics

The genetics of amyotrophic choreoathetosis with acanthocytosis is heterogeneous. Six families with 6 affected members over multiple generations, suggestive of autosomal dominant inheritance, have been reported. Among the 6 families, 2 reported patients from 2 families had parental consanguinity. More than 2 affected siblings in one generation were found in 27 families (53 patients in total). Among the 27 families, 21 reported cases from 10 families had a history of parental consanguinity. Twenty-eight sporadic cases have been reported. Among them, 5 cases had consanguinous parents, suggestive of autosomal recessive inheritance. In 15 cases, no family histories were described.

In 11 families with members affected by amyotrophic choreoathetosis with acanthocytosis, linkage studies found a responsible gene located at chromosome 9q21 (16). Recently, investigators refined the locus region and identified a full-length cDNA encoding a presumably structural protein, which was called chorein (17). A deletion and several mutations have been identified leading to alterations in an evolutionarily conserved protein that is probably involved in protein sorting (17,18).

Neuropathology and Neurochemistry

Neuropathologic findings have been reported in 12 patients with amyotrophic choreoathetosis with acanthocytosis (Table 39.3). The most consistent neuropathologic finding is severe neuronal loss and gliosis in the striatum (19–25,32,42,43). The caudate nucleus is usually more severely affected than the putamen. The globus pallidus is

TABLE 39.3. AUTOPSY FINDINGS OF PATIENTS WITH AMYOTROPHIC CHOREOATHETOSIS WITH ACANTHOCYTOSIS

Autopsy Study							
Reference #	23	20	42	24	21	21	25
Caudate nucleus	NL(ma),G(ma)	NL(ma),G(ma)	NL(ma),G(ma)	NL(ma)	NL(ma),G(ma)	NL,G	NL(ma)
Putamen	NL(mo),G(mo)	NL(mo),G(mo)	NL(mo),G(mo)	NL(ma)	NL(ma),G(ma)	NL,G	NL(ma)
Globus pallidus	NL(mi),G(mi)	normal	NL(mo),G(mi)	Atrophy(mo)	Atrophy	NL,G	Atrophy(mo)
Thalamus	normal	NL(mi),G(mi)	NM	NM	NM	Atrophy(mo)	NM
STN	normal	normal	NM	NM	NM	NM	NM
Substantia nigra	normal	normal	NM	normal	NM	some pallor	normal
Cerebral cortex	normal	normal	normal	NM	NM	NM	normal
Brainstem	normal	NM	normal	NM	NM	NM	normal
Cerebellum	normal	NM	normal	NM	NM	NM	normal
Spinal cord	normal	normal	NL(ant.horn)	NM	NM	NM	NL(ant.horn)
	25	43	34	19	19		
Caudate nucleus	NL	atrophy,NL,G	NL(ma),G(ma)	NL(ma),G(ma)	NL(ma),G(ma)		
Putamen	NL(ma)	atrophy	normal	NL(ma),G(ma)	NL(ma),G(mo)		
Globus pallidus	Atrophy(mo)	NM	normal	NL,G(mo)	NL,G(mo)		
Thalamus	NM	NM	normal	G(mi)	normal		
STN	NM	NM		normal	normal		
Substantia nigra	normal	NM	normal	NL(mi)	NL(ma)		
Cerebral cortex	normal	NM	normal	normal	normal		
Brainstem	normal	NM	normal	normal	normal		
Cerebellum	normal	NM		normal	normal		
Spinal cord	NL(ant.horn)	NM	NL(motor N)	NM	normal		

STN, subthalamic nucleus; NL, neuronal loss; G, gliosis; ma, marked; mo, moderate; mi, mild; ant. horn, anterior horn; nm, not mentioned.

also almost invariably affected with gliosis and a variable degree of neuronal loss. The thalamus has not been studied in detail. Mild neuronal loss and gliosis are seen, but the thalamus has been said to be normal in some cases. It seems that especially the medial thalamus, the nuclei of which project to the striatum, is affected (19–21). The substantia nigra has generally been reported to be normal, although "some pallor" was noted in one case. However, when the number of nigral neurons was quantitatively studied, nerve cell loss was evident in all regions of the substantia nigra, the ventrolateral part being most severely affected (22). The cerebral cortex, pons, medulla, and cerebellum are preserved. In a few cases, there was neuronal loss in the anterior horns of the spinal cord.

Neurochemical changes in amyotrophic choreoathetosis with acanthocytosis have been reported only in a few cases without consistent findings. Postmortem biochemical studies have revealed normal glutamic acid decarboxylase (GAD) levels in the caudate, putamen, and cerebral cortex (23). In contrast, other studies showed decreased (cortex, thalamus, substantia nigra, red nucleus) and increased (putamen, globus pallidus, nucleus accumbens) activity of GAD (24). Choline acetyltransferase (ChAT) activity has been reported to be normal, reduced, or increased (23,24). Dopamine levels are reduced and dopamine D2 receptor number increased in the caudate nucleus and putamen, and elevated noradrenaline (globus pallidus, putamen) levels and reduced substance P concentration (striatum, substantia nigra) have been found (25).

Laboratory Findings

In addition to acanthocytosis in the peripheral blood smear, serum CK levels are elevated in about 80% of the patients with amyotrophic choreoathetosis with acanthocytosis. In the literature, the mean CK level was 567 International Units (range 32–5,000). Otherwise, blood tests, including serum lipoprotein levels are normal.

Neurophysiologic studies have revealed sensory nerve conduction abnormalities (low action potentials, low conduction velocity, or both) in about half of the reported cases, and motor nerve abnormalities (e.g., slow conduction velocity) have been found in 23% of the cases (35,42). Electromyography studies have shown a neurogenic pattern with positive sharp waves and giant motor unit potentials. Fasciculation was present in a few cases. In most patients (17 out of 19 investigated, 89%), muscle biopsy studies show neurogenic and secondary myopathic changes (46,49). Results of nerve biopsy studies have been reported in 18 cases most often showing combined axonal degeneration and demyelination, although both have also been reported in isolation.

Structural brain imaging studies with computed tomography or magnetic resonance imaging (MRI) have revealed atrophy of the caudate nucleus and putamen, along with cerebral atrophy and ventricular enlargement (26–28). Brain MRI may show high signal intensity lesions (in T2-weighted images) both in the caudate nucleus and the putamen (Fig. 39.2). These finding are not specific; they may occur in other degenerative brain

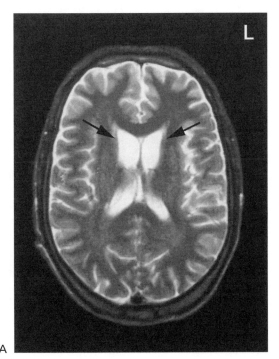
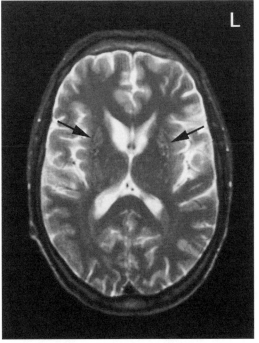

FIG. 39.2. Brain T2-weighted image of a 29-year-old man with amyotrophic choreoathetosis with acanthocytosis. Panel A shows caudate atrophy and enlargement of the horns of the lateral ventricles *(arrows)*, and panel B shows signal change in the putamen *(arrows)*, especially on the left. L, left.

diseases, such as HD. Functional brain imaging with positron emission tomography (PET) shows marked caudate and putaminal hypometabolism (29–31). In addition, striatal and cortical, especially frontal, blood flow and oxygen metabolism are depressed (26,29). Unfortunately, these findings, like those obtained with structural imaging, are nonspecific. [^{18}F]Fluorodopa ([^{18}F]dopa) PET scans reflecting presynaptic dopaminergic function show damage to the ventrolateral nigral projections to the posterior putamen (29,32), which is consistent with the distribution of nigral neuronal loss seen in postmortem pathologic studies. The pattern of presynaptic dopaminergic hypofunction resembles that of idiopathic PD. Dopamine D2 receptors evaluated with [^{11}C]raclopride showed a mean reduction of 65% in the caudate and a 53% loss in the putaminal uptake, indicating striatal degeneration or impaired neuronal function (29). These findings fit the theory that preferential degeneration of the D2 receptor–bearing striatal neurons to the external globus pallidus results predominantly in choreiform syndrome. Damage to the connection between the striatum and the medial globus pallidus, together with the loss of nigrostriatal connections to the posterior putamen, may possibly result in progressive akinetic-rigid syndrome. These findings give a pathophysiologic basis to the chorea and parkinsonism often seen simultaneously in patients with amyotrophic choreoathetosis with acanthocytosis. This is probably too simplistic because there is also widespread pathology in the striatum and pallidum disrupting the function of the cortico-striato-pallido/nigral-subthalamo-pallido-thalamo-cortical loop.

Differential Diagnosis

In amyotrophic choreoathetosis with acanthocytosis, the symptoms are associated with significant acanthocytosis (more than 3% of acanthocytes in peripheral blood smear) and normal serum lipoproteins. Sometimes repeated blood testing is required to detect acanthocytes, which may appear late in the disease course (33); in fact, cases of amyotrophic choreoathetosis without acanthocytes have been reported (34,58). The characteristic clinical picture of amyotrophic choreoathetosis with acanthocytosis, including movement disorders, personality changes, and frontal-lobe cognitive impairment, resembles that of HD. Amyotrophic choreoathetosis with acanthocytosis and HD also share common pathological features. However, HD is an autosomal dominant disorder associated with an excess of trinucleotide repeats (CAG repeats) in chromosome 4, and a diagnostic laboratory test is available.

Since the initial presentation of amyotrophic choreoathetosis with acanthocytosis may vary, acanthocytes should be examined in patients with tic disorders, in atypical cases of dystonia or parkinsonism, seizures, psychiatric disorders, muscle atrophy, or peripheral neuropathy.

Treatment

There is no curative treatment for amyotrophic choreoathetosis with acanthocytosis; therefore, therapy remains symptomatic. However, the response of parkinsonism to levodopa or involuntary movements to drug treatment has been ineffective. Seizures should be managed with appropriate anticonvulsants.

MCLEOD'S SYNDROME

The McLeod phenotype refers to a situation whereby erythrocytes express Kell antigens weakly. It was first described in 1961 and named after the proband (59). In this syndrome, the Kell group of erythrocyte antigens (third most important after ABO and Rhesus systems) is expressed only weakly, whereas the surface marker Kx, thought to stabilize the Kell antigen, is absent (9). The exact mechanism causing acanthocyte formation in McLeod's syndrome is not known, but focal changes in the cytoskeletal structure of the erythrocyte are thought to be responsible (7,9). McLeod's syndrome is an X-linked autosomal recessive disorder. The gene responsible for McLeod's syndrome has been located at the Xp21 region and encodes for a membrane transport protein (60). So far, several separate point mutations have been reported.

In the earlier literature, 34 cases with McLeod's syndrome have been reported (12,54,59,61,62,64–77) (Table 39.4). About one fifth of the patients showed no neurologic manifestations initially. The neurological manifestations of McLeod's syndrome vary (Table 39.5). Systemic features of McLeod's syndrome include hemolytic anemia, splenomegaly, cardiomyopathy, and cardiac arrhythmias. Movement disorder, seizures, or cognitive impairment indicates central nervous system involvement. Clinically, there is a certain overlap between McLeod's syndrome and amyotrophic choreoathetosis with acanthocytosis, and a clinical picture resembling amyotrophic choreoathetosis with acanthocytosis, including orofacial dyskinesias, chorea, seizures, and cognitive impairment, has been reported (61–63). In McLeod's syndrome, brain CT and MRI studies have revealed striatal, especially caudate, and cortical atrophy, as well as signal change in the caudate on T2-weighted images. Functional imaging with PET or single photon emission computed

TABLE 39.4. CLINICAL FEATURES OF REPORTED CASES WITH MCLEOD'S SYNDROME[a]

Age of onset (yr)	Mean 37 (range 22–52)
Gender	31 men, 3 women
Positive family history	27/34 cases (79%)
Acanthocytes	Mean 17% (range 3–80%)
Creatine kinase level	Mean 1,937 IU (range 34–5,292 IU)

[a]Includes cases from references 12, 54, 59, 61, 62, 64–77.

TABLE 39.5. SYMPTOMS AND SIGNS OF 34 REPORTED PATIENTS WITH MCLEOD'S SYNDROME[a]

Symptom/Sign	Present (%)	
	At Onset[b]	At Some Stage
Involuntary movements	25	59
Limb dyskinesia, especially chorea	8	53
Orofacial dyskinesia	21	35
Dystonia	—	12
Parkinsonism	—	3
Tongue biting	8	15
Motor/vocal tics	8	21
Neuromuscular manifestations	21	41
Neuropsychiatric manifestations	14	38
Gait disturbance	11	18
Dysphagia	—	6
Speech abnormality	4	29
Hyporeflexia	—	59
Seizures	14	15
Cardiac symptoms	8	24

[a]Includes cases from references 12, 54, 59, 61, 62, 64–77.
[b]21% of patients were initially asymptomatic and were first identified through blood tests.

tomography shows striatal and cortical, especially frontal, hypometabolism. Striatal dopamine receptors were reported to be normal or decreased. Thus, the neuroimaging studies are nonspecific and not helpful in differentiating patients with McLeod's syndrome from those with amyotrophic choreoathetosis with acanthocytosis. There are, however, some differences in the clinical picture. In amyotrophic choreoathetosis with acanthocytosis, the movement disorder seems to start at an earlier age, and orofacial dyskinesias with lip and tongue biting are more common. Parkinsonism and seizures seem to be more common in amyotrophic choreoathetosis with acanthocytosis than in McLeod's syndrome. About 12% of the patients with the McLeod phenotype have a mild compensatory hemolytic anemia, and cardiomyopathy was reported in 24% of patients. Although cardiomyopathy has been reported in amyotrophic choreoathetosis with acanthocytosis, it is reported more frequently in McLeod's syndrome. In spite of these differences, clinically, McLeod's syndrome is not always distinguishable from amyotrophic choreoathetosis with acanthocytosis, and the rationale for separating them clinically has been questioned (9). However, different views have also been advocated, suggesting that the term amyotrophic choreoathetosis with acanthocytosis should be restricted to cases in which the McLeod phenotype, neuraxonal dystrophy, and lipoprotein disorders have been excluded (64). Regardless of the nomenclature used, individuals with neuroacanthocytosis should have a Kell blood grouping and lipoprotein electrophoresis because the genetics of syndromes associated with acanthocytosis are different and thus have implications for genetic counseling.

ACKNOWLEDGMENTS

The authors thank Dr. S.H. Oh at the Department of Neurology, Youngdong Severance Hospital, Yonsei University College of Medicine (Seoul, Korea) for assisting in the preparation of this chapter. The magnetic resonance image shown in Fig. 39.2 was kindly provided by Prof. Hasse Karlsson and Dr. Mika Hakala (University of Turku). M.S. Lee is supported by the Brain Korea 21 Project for Medicine, Yonsei University.

REFERENCES

1. Hardie RJ. Acanthocytosis and neurological impairment—a review. *Q J Med* 1989;71:291–306
2. Glader BE, Lukens JN. Hereditary spherocytosis and other anemias due to abnormalities of the red cell membrane. In: Lee GR, Foerster J, Lukens J, et al., eds. *Wintrobe's clinical hematology*, 10th ed. Baltimore: Williams & Wilkins, 1999:1132–1152.
3. Narcisi TME, Shoulders CC, Cheste SA, et al. Mutations of the microsomal triglyceride-transfer-protein gene in abetalipoproteinaemia. *Am J Hum Genet* 1995;57:1298–1310.
4. Olivieri O, De Franceschi L, Bordin L, et al. Increased membrane protein phosphorylation and anion transport activity in chorea-acanthocytosis. *Haematologica* 1997;82:648–653.
5. Oshima M, Osawa Y, Asano K, et al. Erythrocyte membrane abnormalities in patients with amyotrophic chorea with acanthocytosis. Part 1. Spin labelling studies and lipid analyses. *J Neurol Sci* 1985;68:147–160.
6. Sakai T, Antoku Y, Iwashita H, et al. Chorea-acanthocytosis: abnormal composition of covalently bound fatty acids of erythrocyte membrane proteins. *Ann Neurol* 1991;29:664–669.
7. Terada N, Fujii Y, Ueda H, et al. Ultrastructural changes of erythrocyte membrane skeletons in chorea-acanthocytosis and McLeod syndrome revealed by the quick-freezing and deep-etching method. *Acta Haematol* 1999;101:25–31.
8. Ueno E, Oguchi K, Yanagisawa N. Morphological abnormalities of erythrocyte membrane in the hereditary neurological disease with chorea, areflexia and acanthocytosis: a study with freeze-fracture electron microscopy. *J Neurol Sci* 1982;56:89–97.
9. Stevenson V, Hardie RJ. Acanthocytosis and neurological disorders. *J Neurol* 2000;248:87–94.
10. Sakai T, Mawatari S, Iwashita H, et al. Choreoacanthocytosis: clue to clinical diagnosis. *Arch Neurol* 1981;38:335–338.
11. Spitz MC, Jankovic J, Killian JM. Familial tic disorder, parkinsonism, motor neuron disease, and acanthocytosis. *Neurology* 1985;35:366–370.
12. Hardie RJ, Pullon HWH, Harding AE, et al. Neuroacanthocytosis: a clinical, haematological, and pathological study of 19 cases. *Brain* 1991;114:13–49.
13. Yamamoto T, Hirose G, Shimazaki K, et al. Movement disorder of familial neuroacanthocytosis syndrome. *Arch Neurol* 1982;39:298–301.
14. Medalia A, Merriam A, Sandberg M. Neuropsychological deficits in choreoacanthocytosis. *Arch Neurol* 1989;46:573–575.
15. Kartsounis LD, Hardie RJ. The pattern of cognitive impairments in neuroacanthocytosis: a frontosubcortical dementia. *Arch Neurol* 1996;53:77–80.
16. Rubio JP, Danek A, Stone C, et al. Chorea-acanthocytosis: genetic linkage to chromosome 9q21. *Am J Hum Genet* 1997;61:899–908.
17. Ueno S, Maruki Y, Nakamura M, et al. The gene encoding a

newly discovered protein, chorein, is mutated in chorea-acanthocytosis. *Nat Genet* 2001;28:121–122.

18. Rampoldi L, Dobson-Stone C, Rubio JP, et al. A conserved sorting-associated protein is mutant in chorea-acanthocytosis. *Nat Genet* 2001;28:119–120.

19. Rinne JO, Daniel SE, Scaravilli F, et al. Neuropathological features of neuroacanthocytosis. *Mov Disord* 1994;9:297–304.

20. Iwata M, Fuse S, Sakuta M, et al. Neuropathological study of chorea-acanthocytosis. *Jpn J Med* 1984;23:118–122.

21. Alonso MaE, Teixeira F, Jimenes G, et al. Chorea-acanthocytosis: report of a family and neuropathological study of two cases. *Can J Neurol Sci* 1989;16:426–431.

22. Rinne JO, Daniel SE, Scaravilli F, et al. Nigral degeneration in neuroacanthocytosis. *Neurology* 1994;44:1629–1632.

23. Bird TD, Cederbaum S, Valpey RW, et al. Familial degeneration of the basal ganglia with acanthocytosis: a clinical, neuropathological, and neurochemical study. *Ann Neurol* 1978;3: 253–258.

24. Sato YA, Ohnishi A, Tateishi J, et al. An autopsy case of chorea-acanthocytosis—special reference of the histopathological and biochemical findings of basal ganglia. *Brain Nerve (Tokyo)* 1984; 36:105–111.

25. De Yebens JG, Brin MF, Mena MA, et al. Neurochemical finding in acanthocytosis. *Mov Disord* 1988;3:300–312.

26. Tanaka MT, Hirai S, Kondo S, et al. Cerebral hypoperfusion and hypometabolism with altered striatal signal intensity in chorea-acanthocytosis: a combined PET and MRI study. *Mov Disord* 1998;13:100–107.

27. Kutcher JS, Kahn MJ, Andersson HC, et al. Neuroacanthocytosis masquerading as Huntington's disease: CT/MRI findings. *J Neuroimaging* 1999;9:187–189.

28. Serra S, Xerra A, Scribano E, et al. Computerized tomography in amyotrophic choreoacanthcytosis. *Neuroradiology* 1987;29: 480–482.

29. Brooks DJ, Ibanez V, Playford ED, et al. Presynaptic and postsynaptic striatal dopaminergic function in neuroacanthocytosis: a positron emission tomographic study. *Ann Neurol* 1991;30: 166–171.

30. Bohlega S, Riley W, Powe J, et al. Neuroacanthocytosis and aprebetalipoproteinemia. *Neurology* 1998;50:1912–1914.

31. Dubinsky RM, Hallett M, Levey R, et al. Regional brain glucose metabolism in neuroacanthocytosis. *Neurology* 1989;39: 1253–1255.

32. Peppard RF, Lu CS, Chu NS, et al. Parkinsonism with neuroacanthocytosis. *Can J Neurol Sci* 1990;17:298–301.

33. Sorrentino G, De Renzo A, Miniello S, et al. Late appearance of acanthocytes during the course of chorea-acanthocytosis. *J Neurol Sci* 1999;163:175–178.

34. Malandrini A, Fabrizi GM, Palmeri S, et al. Choreo-acanthocytosis like phenotype without acanthocytes: clinicopathological case report—a contribution to the knowledge of the functional pathology of the caudate nucleus. *Acta Neuropathol (Berl)* 1993; 86:651–658.

35. Vita G, Serra S, Dattola R, et al. Peripheral neuropathy in amyotrophic chorea-acanthocytosis. *Ann Neurol* 1989;26:583–587.

36. Gross KB, Skrivanek JA, Carlson KC, et al. Familial amyotrophic chorea with acanthocytosis. *Arch Neurol* 1985;42:753–756.

37. Aguilar JL, Berga L, Merino A, et al. A further case of choreo-acanthocytosis. *Acta Hematol* 1988;80:175–176.

38. Villegas A, Moscat J, Calero VF, et al. A new family with hereditary choreo-acanthocytosis. *Acta Hematol* 1987;77:215–219.

39. Vance JM, Pericak-Vance MA, Bowman MH, et al. Chorea-acanthocytosis: a report of three new families and implications for genetic counseling. *Am J Med Gen* 1987;28:403–410.

40. Silvestri R, Raffaele M, Domenico PD, et al. Sleep features in Tourette's syndrome, neuroacanthocytosis, and Huntington's chorea. *Neurophysiol Clin* 1995;25:66–77.

41. Aminoff MJ. Acanthocytosis and neurological disease. *Brain* 1972;95:749–760.

42. Sobue G, Mukai E, Fujii K, et al. Peripheral nerve involvement in familial chorea-acanthocytosis. *J Neurol Sci* 1986;76:347–356.

43. Feinberg TE, Cianci MS, Morrow JS, et al. Diagnostic tests for choreoacanthocytosis. *Neurology* 1991;41:1000–1006.

44. Tsai CH, Chen RS, Chang HC, et al. Acanthocytosis and spinocerebellar degeneration: a new association? *Mov Disord* 1997; 12:456–459.

45. Delecluse F, Deleval JMS, Gerard JM, et al. Frontal impairment and hypoperfusion in neuroacanthocytosis. *Arch Neurol* 1991;48: 232–234.

46. Limos LC, Ohnishi A, Sakai T, et al. "Myopathic" changes in chorea-acanthocytosis. *J Neurol Sci* 1982;55:49–58.

47. Kito S, Itoga E, Hiroshige Y, et al. A pedigree of amyotrophic chorea with acanthocytosis. *Arch Neurol* 1980;37:517.

48. Levine IM, Estes JW, Looney JM. Hereditary neurological disease with acanthocytosis. *Arch Neurol* 1968;19:403–409.

49. Ohnichi A, Sato Y, Nagara H, et al. Neurogenic muscular atrophy and low density of large myelinated fibers of sural nerve in chorea-acanthocytosis. *J Neurol Neurosurg Psychiatry* 1981;44:645–648.

50. Aasly J, Skandsen T, Ro M. Neuroacanthocytosis—the variability of presenting symptoms in two siblings. *Act Neurol Scand* 1999;100:322–325.

51. Bharucha EP, Bharucha NE. Choreo-acanthocytosis. *J Neurol Sci* 1989;89:135–139.

52. Sotaniemi KA. Choreo-acanthocytosis: neurological disease with acanthocytosis. *Acta Neurol Scand* 1983;68:53–56.

53. Schwarz MS, Monro PS, Leigh PN. Epilepsy as the presenting feature of neuroacanthocytosis in siblings. *J Neurol* 1992;239: 261–262.

54. Ishikawa S, Tachibana N, Tabata KI, et al. Muscle CT scan findings in McLeod syndrome and chorea-acanthocytosis. *Muscle & Nerve* 2000;23:1113–1116.

55. Wihl G, Volkmann J, Allert N, et al. Deep brain stimulation of the internal pallidum did not improve chorea in a patient with neuroacanthocytosis. *Mov Disord* 2001;16:572–575.

56. Hirayama M, Hamano T, Shiratori M, et al. Corea-acanthocytosis with polyclonal antibodies to ganglioside G$_{M1}$. *J Neurol Sci* 1997;151:23–24.

57. Critchley EMR, Clark DB, Wikler A. Acanthocytosis and neurological disorder without abetalipoproteinemia. *Arch Neurol* 1968;18:134–140.

58. O'Brien CF, Schwarz J, Kurlan R. Neuroacanthocytosis without acanthocytes. *Mov Disord* 1990;5:98.

59. Allen FH, Krabbe SMR, Corcoran PA. A new phenotype (McLeod) in the Kell blood-group system. *Vox Sang* 1961;6: 555–560.

60. Ho M, Chelly J, Carter N, et al. Isolation of the gene for McLeod syndrome that encodes a novel membrane transport protein. *Cell* 1994;77:869–880.

61. Malandrini A, Fabrizi GM, Truschi F, et al. Atypical McLeod syndrome manifested as X-linked chorea-acanthocytosis, neuromyopathy and dilated cardiomyopathy: report of a family. *J Neurol Sci* 1994;124:89–94.

62. Takashima H, Sakai T, Iwashita H, et al. A family of McLeod syndrome, masquerading as chorea-acanthocytosis. *J Neurol Sci* 1994;124:56–60.

63. Witt TN, Danek A, Reiter M, et al. McLeod syndrome: a distinct form of neuroacanthocytosis. *J Neurol* 1992;239:302–306.

64. Danek A, Tison F, Rubio J, et al. The chorea of McLeod syndrome. *Mov Disord* 2001;16:882–889.

65. Zyskowski LP, Bunch TW, Hoagland C, et al. McLeod syndrome

(hemolysis, acanthocytosis, and increased serum creatine kinase): potential confusion with polymyositis. *Arthritis Rheum* 1983;26: 806–808.

66. Ueyama H, Kumamoto T, Nagao SI. A novel mutation of the McLeod syndrome gene in a Japanese family. *J Neurol Sci* 2000; 176:151–154.
67. Symmans WA, Shepherd CS, Marsh WL, et al. Hereditary acanthocytosis associated with the McLeod phenotype of the Kell blood group system. *Br J Hematol* 1979;42:575–583.
68. Swash M, Schwartz MS, Carter ND, et al. Benign X-linked myopathy with acanthocytes (McLeod syndrome): its relationship to X-linked muscular dystrophy. *Brain* 1983;106:717–733.
69. Jung HH, Hergersberg M, Kneifel S, et al. McLeod syndrome: a novel mutation, predominant psychiatric manifestations, and distinct striatal image findings. *Ann Neurol* 2001;49:384–392.
70. Oechsner M, Buchert R, Beyer W, et al. Reduction of striatal glucose metabolism in McLeod choreoacanthocytosis. *J Neurol Neurosurg Psychiatry* 2001;70:517–520.
71. Kawakami T, Takiyama Y, Sakoe K, et al. A case of McLeod syndrome with unusually severe myopathy. *J Neurol Sci* 1999;166: 36–39.
72. Hanaoka N, Yoshida K, Nakamura A, et al. A novel frameshift mutation in the McLeod syndrome gene in a Japanese family. *J Neurol Sci* 1999;165:6–9.
73. Barnett MH, Yang F, Iland H, et al. Unusual muscle pathology in McLeod syndrome. *J Neurol Neurosurg Psychiatry* 2000;69: 655–657.
74. Marsh WL, Schnipper EF, Johnson CL, et al. An individual with McLeod syndrome and the Kell blood group antigen K (K1). *Transfusion* 1983;23:336–338.
75. Danek A, Witt TN, Stockmann HBAC, et al. Normal dystrophin in McLeod myopathy. *Ann Neurol* 1990;28:720–722.
76. Dotti MT, Battisi C, Malandrini A, et al. McLeod syndrome and neuroacanthocytosis with a novel mutation in the *XK* gene. *Mov Disord* 2000;15:1282–1284.
77. Faillace RT, Kingston WJ, Nanda NC, et al. Cardiomyopathy associated with the syndrome of amyotrophic chorea and acanthocytosis. *Arch Intern Med* 1982;96:616–617.

INFECTIOUS AND TRANSMISSIBLE MOVEMENT DISORDERS

FRANCISCO CARDOSO

Since the previous edition of this book, the literature on movement disorders associated with infectious agents has focused mainly on (a) the impact of highly active antiretroviral therapy (HAART) on the neurologic complications in patients infected with human immunodeficiency virus (HIV) and (b) the role played by β-hemolytic streptococci in the generation of Sydenham's chorea (SC) and other conditions related to basal ganglia dysfunction. The aim of this chapter is to provide an overview on the epidemiology, pathogenesis, phenomenology, diagnosis, and management of AIDS-related movement disorders, SC, human prion diseases, postencephalitic parkinsonism (PEP), subacute sclerosing panencephalitis (SSPE), and other movement disorders associated with infectious agents. Table 40.1 is a summary of the most common transmissible movement disorders.

AIDS-RELATED MOVEMENT DISORDERS

At least 60% of patients with acquired immunodeficiency syndrome (AIDS) develop neurologic complications because of opportunistic infections, direct lesion by human immunodeficiency virus (HIV), or both (1). At the peak of the AIDS epidemic, movement disorders were recognized in 2% to 3% of these patients (2). However, investigations in which patients were prospectively followed up showed that basal ganglia dysfunction, particularly tremor and parkinsonism, is more common than previously appreciated, being recognized in 5% to 44% of patients (3). With the introduction of HAART there is evidence of decline in the incidence of neurologic complications, including movement disorders, in AIDS (4).

Hyperkinetic Movement Disorders

Although epidemiologic studies are lacking, a literature review suggests that hemichorea-hemiballism is the most commonly reported dyskinesia in AIDS patients (2,5). Typ-

ically, hemichorea-hemiballism is an acute complication in patients already diagnosed with AIDS. However, in a few instances this movement disorder may be the presenting symptom of HIV infection (5). In most patients the chorea is focal or involves one half of the body (hemichorea). Tremor is the second most commonly reported hyperkinesia in AIDS patients. Aside from this movement disorder associated with HIV encephalopathy, discussed in the context of parkinsonism related to AIDS, the Holmes tremor (formerly called rubral or midbrain tremor) with rest, postural, and kinetic components is typically seen in AIDS. These patients often present with associated signs of midbrain dysfunction, such as paresis of oculomotor nerve and contralateral hemiparesis. There is growing awareness of the AIDS patient's vulnerability to tremor as a side effect of medications. The list of offending drugs includes not only dopamine receptor–blocking drugs, causing rest tremor and other parkinsonian signs, but also trimethoprim-sulfamethoxazole (6,7). The latter has been described as producing rest or action tremor without parkinsonism (7). Patients with HIV infection may also develop generalized or focal dystonia (8). One of our patients at the Movement Disorders Clinics of the Federal University of Minas Gerais (MDC-UFMG) exemplifies this possibility. A man previously healthy and unknown to be HIV positive suddenly became comatose. On admission, computed tomography (CT) of the head displayed multiple hypodense lesions, particularly in the right basal ganglia region, surrounded by contrast-enhanced ring and edema with severe mass effect. He also had positive HIV and *Toxoplasma gondii* tests. After a few days of treatment with sulfadiazine and pyrimethamine, the patient recovered consciousness, displayed radiologic improvement, but developed dystonia of the right arm characterized by flexion of the fingers and wrist at rest, exacerbated by action. Other hyperkinetic movement disorders described in HIV-positive patients include action cortical myoclonus, spinal myoclonus, and peripheral segmental myoclonus; akathisia; neuroleptic malignant syndrome; oculomasticatory myorhythmia asso-

TABLE 40.1. THE MOST COMMON MOVEMENT DISORDERS ASSOCIATED WITH INFECTIOUS AGENTS

Agent	Movement Disorder	Agent	Movement Disorder
Arboviruses	Parkinsonian syndrome	Measles virus	Myoclonus (subacute sclerosing panencephalitis)
Cytomegalovirus	Chorea		
Enteroviruses	Parkinsonian syndrome		
	Chorea		Parkinsonian syndrome
Epstein-Barr virus	Chorea		Chorea
Herpes simplex viruses	Tics	Paramyxovirus (mumps)	Chorea
	Chorea		
HIV	Tremor	Rubella virus	Chorea
	Parkinsonian syndrome	Varicella-zoster virus	Parkinsonian syndrome
	Myoclonus		Chorea
	Dystonia	Prions	Myoclonus
HIV and *T. gondii*	Hemichorea, hemiballismus		Parkinsonian syndrome
	Midbrain tremor		Choreoathetosis
	Dystonia	*Bordetella pertussis*	Ataxia
	Parkinsonian syndrome	*Corynebacterium diphtheriae*	Chorea
	Akathisia		
HIV and drugs	Tremor	*Legionella* sp	Chorea
	Parkinsonian syndrome	*Mycoplasma pneumoniae*	Parkinsonian syndrome
	Dystonia		Chorea
	Tremor and rigidity (neuroleptic malignant syndrome)		Dystonia
HIV and herpes zoster virus	Myoclonus	Group A *Streptococcus*	Chorea and tics (Sydenham's chorea) (Tourette's syndrome?)
		T. pallidum	Chorea
HIV and *Mycobacterium tuberculosis*	Chorea	*Plasmodium falciparum*	Chorea
		Schistosoma mansoni	Segmental myoclonus
HIV and *T. pallidum*	Chorea	Cysts of *T. solium*	Chorea
Influenza virus	Parkinsonian syndrome (postencephalitic parkinsonism?)		Dystonia
			Parkinsonian syndrome
	Chorea		

ciated with Whipple's disease; and paroxysmal dyskinesias (2,9–12).

Hyperkinesias in AIDS are almost invariably caused by *Toxoplasma gondii* abscess. Alternative causes include *Treponema pallidum*, progressive multifocal encephalopathy, *Cryptococcus neoformans*, drugs, primary lymphoma of the central nervous system (CNS), vacuolar myelopathy, and HIV encephalopathy (2,3,5–7,9,10,13). The opportunistic lesions bring about hyperkinesias by damaging the basal ganglia or their connections. Striking examples are granulomas in the subthalamus causing hemichorea-hemiballism and in the cerebellar outflow pathways producing Holmes' tremor. There is a growing body of evidence indicating that HIV encephalopathy is associated with severe damage of the dopaminergic basal ganglia system. Some of the findings supporting this conclusion are reduced levels of dopamine and homovanillic acid in the cerebrospinal fluid (CSF) and neuronal loss in the pallidum of HIV-positive patients (12,14). These results not only explain the occurrence of movement disorders in AIDS patients with HIV encephalopathy as well but also account for their susceptibility to develop movement disorders when exposed to dopamine receptor–blocking drugs. The mechanism underlying tremor associated with exposure to trimethoprim-sul-

famethoxazole in AIDS patients remains to be determined, but there is speculation that this drug causes disruption of dopamine production as a result of glutathione or tetrahydrobiopterin deficiency (7).

Most patients with AIDS and movement disorders are already known to be HIV positive. However, as discussed above, occasionally hemichorea-hemiballism may be the first manifestation of AIDS. For this reason, all patients with this hyperkinesia should undergo investigation for HIV infection. The investigation of patients suspected of having movement disorders associated with HIV infection is targeted at identifying opportunistic infections. CT or magnetic resonance imaging (MRI) of the head usually shows the typical findings of toxoplasmosis: multiple contrast-enhanced lesions with mass effect and surrounding edema in the contralateral basal ganglia. However, the definite diagnosis of cerebral toxoplasmosis depends on cerebral biopsy findings. That procedure is reserved for patients with negative serology for *T. gondii* or progressive clinical or radiologic deterioration despite empiric antitoxoplamosis therapy for 2 weeks (1). Even the use of anti-*Toxoplasma* prophylaxis has not changed this policy substantially. For example, based on prospective follow-up of 136 AIDS patients with focal brain lesions, Antinori et al. (15)

demonstrated that the chance of cerebral toxoplasmosis is still 59% in a *T. gondii*-seropositive patient undergoing prophylaxis. They recommend polymerase chain reaction (PCR) for Epstein-Barr virus DNA and *T. gondii* in the CSF. If the former is negative and the latter is positive, there is a 0.99 probability of toxoplasmosis, and empiric therapy should be started. In practice, CSF studies are not done in patients with intracranial hypertension because of the high risk of brain herniation. Under these circumstances it is safer to start antitoxoplasmosis treatment and to perform lumbar puncture if the patient fails to respond to these drugs. Investigation of alternative causes is pursued in case the workup indicates that toxoplasmosis is not responsible for the movement disorder. Images similar to those seen in toxoplasmosis can be found in primary lymphoma as well as other opportunistic infections, such as cryptococcosis. HIV encephalopathy often causes a hyperintense signal of the basal ganglia on T2-weighted images.

The most effective treatment of cerebral toxoplasmosis in HIV-positive patients is the combination of sulfadiazine and pyrimethamine. Clindamycin with pyrimethamine, although equally effective for acute treatment, is associated with a higher occurrence of long-term relapses (1). To my knowledge, there is no study addressing HAART in the management of hyperkinesias associated with HIV infection. However, based on preliminary data indicating that neurologic complications in general and motor slowing in particular become less frequent after starting this treatment, one may expect that HAART will reduce the incidence of hyperkinesias associated with HIV infection (4,16).

Symptomatic improvement of hemichorea-hemiballism is often seen after treatment of toxoplasmosis. However, patients who remain disabled may be helped by drugs usually employed in the management of chorea, such as dopamine receptor–blocking drugs, reserpine, tetrabenazine, and valproic acid. However, use of these medications is often complicated by the increased susceptibility of AIDS patients to side effects such as dystonia, parkinsonism, and tremor (1–3,5–7). It is not rare, for instance, to have a patient with hemichorea-hemiballism controlled by neuroleptics to develop parkinsonism on the other side of the body. On the other hand, empiric anti-*Toxoplasma* therapy commonly fails to improve the tremor. Levodopa, anticholinergics, clonazepam, propranolol, primidone, carbamazepine, and isoniazid may help some patients who remain with disabling tremor (17). Unfortunately, no drug is consistently effective for midbrain tremor (18). Of course, the best treatment for drug-induced movement disorders is discontinuation of the offending agent.

Parkinsonism

AIDS patients may develop parkinsonism without opportunistic infections as part of HIV encephalopathy (2,3). These subjects often display a non-levodopa-responsive syndrome characterized by rigidity, bradykinesia, and postural instability without the typical pill-rolling rest tremor. In one study, however, the authors claim that levodopa improves parkinsonism associated with AIDS in children (19). Tremor sharing a pathogenesis with parkinsonism is often seen in HIV. In one study (20) it was estimated that 5.5% of patients with HIV encephalopathy display tremor, although with progression of the disease this figure rises to 44% (21). Typically the movement disorder is an isolated, mild, bilateral, postural tremor; however, rarely patients display an additional kinetic component (17). Seldom HIV-associated tremor is severe enough to require treatment. However, its recognition is important to defining the prognosis. For instance, in a study in the pre-HAART era, Arendt et al. (22) showed that 76% of CDC stage IVA–D patients with this and other movement disorders died during a 2-year follow-up.

The most common cause of parkinsonism and tremor in AIDS patients is HIV encephalopathy associated with damage to basal ganglia resulting in decreased dopaminergic activity (2,3,14,17). As antidopaminergic drugs are associated with at least 50% of reported cases of parkinsonism, one may conclude that even subjects without overt parkinsonian symptoms and signs often have a preclinical dopamine dysfunction (2,3). It remains to be determined what mechanisms are responsible for the dopamine cell loss in HIV encephalopathy; some suggest that excitotoxicity may have a role (23). Toxoplasmosis abscesses and parenchymatous tuberculosis granuloma have also been reported as reversible causes of parkinsonism in AIDS (24,25).

Treatment for HIV-associated parkinsonism is based on management of opportunistic infections, use of antitremor drugs, and HAART. Although reports of effect of levodopa in these patients are not encouraging, a 4-week trial of levodopa/carbidopa 125/12.5 mg three times a day is worth pursuing. Occasionally one finds a patient with a good therapeutic response. As discussed before, the role of HAART in parkinsonism and other movement disorders remains to be determined. However, preliminary data suggest that combination of antiretroviral drugs with action in the CNS (zidovudine, stavudine, lamividine, abacavir, nevirapine, efavirenz, and indinavir) prevents movement disorders and helps their symptomatic management (1,4,16).

SYDENHAM'S CHOREA

In 1686, Thomas Sydenham accurately described the clinical syndrome that we now know as Sydenham's chorea, differentiating it from other movement disorders that were collectively known as Saint Vitus dance. However, it was three centuries later that a causal relationship between streptococcal infection and SC was firmly established (26), and SC is now regarded as a major manifestation of rheumatic fever (RF) (27). Still unclear is why not all subjects with RF develop SC and, conversely, why up to 20% of SC patients not to display any other manifestation of RF. It is also intriguing why the percentage of RF patients with SC varies according to temporal and geographic factors. For instance, Carapetis et al. (28) found SC in 49% of aboriginal people with RF in Australia, and Cardoso et al. (29) in 26% of consecutive RF patients in Brazil.

The improvement in public health conditions in North America and western Europe produced a significant decrease in the incidence of RF until the late 1980s, leading to a decline in the number of SC cases. This is illustrated by the finding that the annual age-adjusted incidence rate of initial attacks of RF per 100,000 children declined from 3 in 1970 to 0.5 in 1980 in Fairfax County, Virginia (30). Furthermore, Nausieda et al. (31) demonstrated that SC accounted for 0.9% of children's admissions to hospitals in Chicago before 1940; this number dropped to 0.2% during the period 1950 to 1980. More recently, though, at least eight outbreaks of RF with occurrence of SC have been identified in the United States (32). Interestingly, most patients belonged to families of high- to middle-income brackets with ready access to medical care, and in four of the outbreaks most patients were adults. However, RF has remained a significant public health problem in developing areas, particularly in the low-income population. The importance of RF in these regions is highlighted by the finding that RF is responsible for 120 of the 274 monthly visits of patients to the Pediatrics Cardiology Clinic of UFMG (Cardoso and Mota, unpublished findings, 1997). The top end of the Northern Territory in Australia, an area predominantly inhabited by aboriginal people, is also plagued by RF. Carapetis et al. (28) recently demonstrated that the annual incidence of RF in this portion of Australia between 1989 and 1993 was 254 per 100,000 aboriginal people aged 5 to 14 years, with a point prevalence of 9.6 per 1,000 in 1995. In these high-prevalence areas, where rheumatic valvular disease may account for up to 40% of all cardiac surgeries, a recent increase in the incidence of SC has been observed (29).

Typically patients develop SC 6 to 8 weeks after an episode of streptococcal pharyngitis. In most series there is a female preponderance, and the usual age at onset of SC is 8 to 9 years, although there are reports of patients developing chorea in the third decade of life (28,29,31,32). The choreic movements spread rapidly, becoming generalized, but up to 20% of patients remain with hemichorea (29,31). The random and continuous flow of contractions typical of chorea produces motor impersistence, particularly noticeable during tongue protrusion and ocular fixation. The muscle tone is usually decreased, and in severe and rare cases this is so pronounced that the patient may be bedridden. The latter form, known as chorea paralytica, has been observed in 2.3% of 130 consecutive SC patients prospectively followed up at the MDC-UFMG. Subjects with SC often display other neurologic and nonneurologic symptoms and signs. Although the distinction between chorea and motor tics may be difficult, motor tics and simple vocal tics are frequently observed in SC. Dysarthria is common, and patients with more severe forms of SC may present a remarkably decreased verbal output reminiscent of what is observed in Huntington's disease. Cardoso et al. (29) recently demonstrated that many patients with active chorea have hypometric saccades, and a few of them also show oculogyric crisis. In the older literature there are also references to papilledema, central retinal artery occlusion, and seizures in a few patients with SC. More recently, attention has been drawn to behavioral abnormalities present in SC. In a study of 30 patients with SC the authors demonstrated that 70% of the subjects presented with obsessions and compulsions whereas 16.7% of them met criteria for obsessive-compulsive disorder (OCD). Of 20 patients with rheumatic fever without chorea, none had obsessions or compulsions (33). These results were replicated by a more recent study, which, however, found that patients with rheumatic fever without chorea had more obsessions and compulsions than healthy controls (34). These findings and the observation that hyperactivity, learning disorders, and other behavioral problems are common in patients with RF and chorea contributed to establish the notion that SC is a model for childhood autoimmune neuropsychiatric disorders (35). Cardiac involvement in SC has been reported in 23% to 84% of patients with RF, whereas the association with arthritis does not exceed 30% (29). The greater proportion of carditis in the latter study may reflect systematic use of echocardiography to investigate patients with SC. This may also reflect ascertainment bias because subjects were seen at a pediatrics cardiology clinic.

The concept of SC as a self-limited condition has recently been challenged by the observation that despite best available treatment up to half of patients remain with active chorea after 2 years of follow-up (36). In the other patients the movement disorder goes into remission after a mean period of 6 to 9 months (29). Recurrences triggered by new bouts of streptococcal infections, pregnancy (*chorea gravidarum*), or oral contraceptives may occur in up to 50% of patients (29,37).

As SC lacks a specific biological marker, diagnosis relies on the recognition of acute chorea and absence of an underlying cause (27,36). Although other manifestations of RF strongly support the hypothesis of SC, their presence is not mandatory for the diagnosis according to the modified Jones criteria (27). Nevertheless, it remains to be determined whether the 10% of cases of acute childhood chorea without other signs of RF represent SC or other undetermined forms of chorea. Tests of acute-phase reactions (erythrocyte sedimentation rate, C-reactive protein, leukocytosis, as well as other blood tests, such as rheumatoid factor, mucoproteins, and protein electrophoresis) and supporting evidence of preceding streptococcal infection (increased antistreptolysin O or other antistreptococcal antibodies; positive throat culture for group A *Streptococcus*; recent scarlet fever) are much less help-ful in SC than in other forms of RF because of the usual long latency between the infection and onset of the movement dis-order. Recently, it was claimed that identification of the B-cell alloantigen D8/17, which indicates increased risk for RF, may help to differentiate SC from other forms of chorea (38). However, although the sensitivity of this test is good, its specificity is low because 17% of controls and 84% of patients with tics and OCD related to streptococcal infection are positive for this marker. CSF analysis is usually normal, but it may show a slightly increased lymphocyte count. CT of the brain invariably fails to display abnormalities in SC. Similarly, head MRI is often normal, although there are case reports of reversible hyperintensity in the basal ganglia area during the activity of the chorea. The study with the largest sample of SC patients showed increased signal in just 2 of 24 patients, although morphometric techniques revealed mean values for the size of the striatum and pallidum larger than controls (39). Unfortunately, these findings afford little help for the diagnosis of SC on an individual basis because there was extensive overlap between controls and patients. PET and single photon emission computed tomography (SPECT) investigations done on SC patients have shown reversible stri-atal hypermetabolism. This finding is in contrast to chorea associated with conditions such as Huntington's disease, neu-roacanthocytosis, nonketotic hyperglycemia, and others in which there is decreased metabolism in the striatum, proba-bly resulting from loss of function of projection neurons of the caudate nucleus and putamen. The authors of one these studies speculate that increased afferent inputs to the striatum resulting from striatal or subthalamic nucleus dysfunction account for the transient hypermetabolism (40).

Although the pathogenesis of SC remains ill defined, a large and growing body of clinical, pathologic, and imaging evidence points to the involvement of basal ganglia. The pres-ence in SC patients of tics, saccadic abnormalities, decreased verbal output, obsessive-compulsive symptoms, and other behavioral abnormalities strengthens the hypothesis of dys-function of this brain region (29,33–35). The few published results of autopsies on SC patients show widespread cell loss in the basal ganglia, frontal cortex, and temporal cortex, with evidence of diffuse vasculitis of small vessels (41). MRI and SPECT studies show increased size of the striatum and pal-lidum and occasional reversible increased signal in this struc-ture as well as hypermetabolism of the striatum (39,40). Improvement of SC with dopamine-blocking or depleting drugs suggests that this neurotransmitter may have a role in its pathogenesis. Although neurochemical studies in SC are scarce and have yielded conflicting results, most of them sug-gest the existence of increased release of dopamine in these patients (42).

The current theory to explain the pathogenesis of SC pro-poses that infection with group A β-hemolytic streptococci in genetically predisposed individuals leads to generation of antibodies that cross-react against antigens on the surface of subthalamic neurons. These antineuronal antibodies (ANABs) cause autoimmune subthalamotomy, leading to disinhibition of neurons of the ventrolateral thalamus result-ing in hyperexcitability of the motor cortex neurons. Husby et al. (43), using an indirect immunofluorescence technique, were the first to find circulating antibodies reacting with sub-thalamic and caudate nuclei neurons in the serum of SC patients. More recently, our group has found positivity for ANABs on an enzyme-linked immunosorbent assay (ELISA) essay in 95%, 56%, 13%, and 0% of, respectively, acute SC patients, chronic/persistent SC patients, RF patients, and normal controls (44). The observation that corticosteroids, plasmapheresis, and intravenous immune immunoglobulin are useful in the management of SC further supports the notion that immune factors mediate the pathogenesis of this condition (45). The final proof of the pathogenic role played by ANABs is the experiment in which SC serum infused in the subthalamus of rats induces circling behavior in these ani-mals when apomorphine is injected intraperitoneally. When these animals were sacrificed, indirect immunohistochem-istry demonstrated antibodies interacting with the surface of subthalamic nucleus neurons (46).

There are no controlled studies of symptomatic treat-ment of SC. The first choice of the author is valproic acid with initial dosage of 250 mg/day increased during a 2-week period to 250 mg three times a day. If the response is not satisfactory the dosage can be gradually increased to 1,500 mg/day. As this drug has a somewhat slow onset of action, I usually wait 2 weeks before concluding that a reg-imen is ineffective. In case the patient fails to respond to this medication, the next option is to prescribe neurolep-tics. Pimozide, a potent dopamine D2 receptor blocker, is usually effective in controlling the hyperkinesia without causing major side effects such as somnolence and parkin-sonism, which are quite common with other drugs like haloperidol. Despite the mention to the possibility of devel-opment of atrioventricular block with use of pimozide, this has not been seen in the more than 100 patients with SC followed at the MDC-UFMG. The usual initial regimen is 1 mg twice a day. If the chorea is still troublesome 2 weeks later, the dosage is increased to 2 mg twice a day. Only rarely do patients fail to respond to this dosage of pimozide. Neuroleptics are the first choice of treatment in the rare patients who present with chorea paralytica. There are no published guidelines on when to discontinue antichoreic agents. My personal policy is to attempt gradual decrease of the dosage (25% reduction every 2 weeks) after the patient has been free of chorea for at least one month. Immuno-suppressive measures, such as corticosteroids, intravenous immunoglobulin, and plasmapheresis, have been reported as efficient treatment for chorea in SC. However, the effi-cacy and safety of valproic acid and antidopaminergic agents in the management of SC, along with the possible complications and high cost of immunomodulatory treat-ment, make it an option of little practical value. At the

MDC-UFMG, pulsotherapy with methylprednisolone for 5 days is reserved for those patients who failed to respond to valproic acid and neuroleptics and remain disabled by chorea. Finally, the most important measure in the treatment of patients with SC is secondary prophylaxis with penicillin or, if there is allergy, sulfa drugs up to age 21 years. If the onset is after this age, the recommendation is to maintain prophylaxis indefinitely (47).

Recent interest in bacterial infections and movement disorders has focused on the concept that basal ganglia dysfunction mediated by immune mechanism triggered by β-hemolytic group A streptococci may result in pediatric autoimmune neuropsychiatric disorders in genetically predisposed individuals (PANDAS) (35). According to this theory, *Streptococcus* infections would account for a subset of patients with Tourette's syndrome (TS), OCD, and other neuropsychiatric disorders. The proponents of the theory have even advanced a set of diagnostic criteria for PANDAS: OCD and/or tic disorder, pediatric onset, episodic clinical course, association with group A β-hemolytic *Streptococcus* infection, and presence of choreiform movements (48). This new concept is supported by the finding of ANABs in patients with TS and OCD; tics, OCD, and other behavioral abnormalities in SC patients; enlargement of the basal ganglia on MRI in some patients with TS and/or OCD; and case reports of improvement of tics and obsessiveness after treatment with penicillin or immunosuppressive measures (49–51). However, some major problems must be overcome before the concept of PANDAS can be fully embraced. For example, the proposed criteria are vague (what do the authors mean by "choreiform movements?"). Evidence of *Streptococcus* infection can be found in up to 80% of children and adolescents, and have not been validated. If the underlying mechanism the same as in SC and RF, it is surprising that carditis has not been reported in TS or that the incidence of tic disorder is not increased in areas where RF is endemic. The only controlled study to test the concept of PANDAS failed to demonstrate that prophylaxis with penicillin improves tic control in TS. Although our own study has shown that 20% of TS patients test positive for ANABs on ELISA, we were not able to clinically separate the positive patients from negative subjects (44,51,52). Right now evidence suggests that ANABs induced by β-hemolytic streptococci likely are a pathogenic factor in a subset of TS patients, but these subjects do not constitute a clinically distinct group. Because of this fact, there are no grounds to justify the routine use of antibiotics or immunomodulatory measures in the management of TS, OCD, and related disorders.

INFECTIOUS PRION DISEASES

The term *prion*, coined by Prusiner (53), designates proteinaceous and infectious particles causing kuru, Creutzfeldt-Jakob disease (CJD), Gerstmann-Sträussler-Scheinker disease (GSS), fatal familial insomnia (FFI), and such animal diseases such as scrapie and bovine spongiform encephalopathy (BSE). Collectively these disorders are labeled spongiform encephalopathies in reference to the common presence of spongiform changes in the brain (54). This terminology has been criticized on the grounds that not all patients display the pathologic change. As all patients are found to have prions, the name *prion diseases* should be used.

Prions are exclusively constituted by an isoform (PrP^{Sc}) of a normally occurring protein (PrP^C) encoded by a gene on chromosome 20p in humans. Although the chemical properties of PrP^C and PrP^{Sc} are identical, the former is rich in α helices, whereas the latter just contains β sheets (54). Prions are generated by the transformation of PrP^C to PrP^{Sc}. This may be accomplished by horizontal transmission of PrP^{Sc}, vertical transmission of mutation in the open reading frame or protein-coding region of the PrP gene, spontaneous conversion of PrP^C to PrP^{Sc}, and somatic mutation of the open reading frame of the PrP gene (54). The first mechanism accounts for kuru and iatrogenic CJD, the infectious forms of human prion diseases. It remains undetermined how the infected PrP^{Sc} induces the host PrP^C to undergo a structural transition from the α-helix structure to the β-sheet structure. It is suggested that this phenomenon occurs at the plasma membrane or along an endocytic pathway to the lysosome and the inoculated PrP^{Sc} acts as a template (53). The second mechanism is responsible for the inherited human prion diseases (FFI, familial CJD, and most cases of GSS), and the others are presumably involved in the pathogenesis of sporadic CJD and GSS. It is beyond the scope of this chapter to discuss inherited and sporadic prion diseases; therefore, the focus will be on infectious forms.

Infectious prion diseases are rare. Until a few decades ago, kuru was common among subjects in the Fore tribe of the highlands of New Guinea, but it has been eliminated with the disappearance of cannibalism (55). The incidence of sporadic CJD is estimated to be one case per million population per year. Iatrogenic CJD, related to corneal and dura mater transplants, inadequately sterilized neurosurgical instruments, and contaminated growth hormone or gonadotropins prepared from cadaveric pituitary tissue, is even rarer, with about 70 published cases in the literature (56). The risk of developing CJD in the treated hypopituitary population is estimated to range from 1 in 100 to 1 in 1,000. Recent evidence indicates that the risk of developing iatrogenic CJD is increased by valine homozygosity at codon 129 of the PrP gene (56).

Typically the onset of sporadic CJD is in the sixth and seventh decades of life with a clinical picture characterized by a rapidly progressive dementia and other behavioral disorders; death ensues in less than a year (56,57). The age at onset of iatrogenic forms is more variable, and the latency ranges from a few months to 10 to 15 years. Shorter latencies are usually observed in surgical cases, whereas patients exposed to contaminated hormones develop CJD after a much longer period (56). In a large series of patients with pathologically verified sporadic CJD, 92% of subjects developed dementia; 91% displayed movement disorders, of whom 81% had multifocal cortical myoclonus; electroencephalographic periodicity was seen in 80% of patients, whereas the more specific periodic triphasic 1- to 2-Hz waves were identified in 55% of them; "extrapyramidal" signs were seen in 66% of subjects, and a similar number had ataxia. Less common findings were visual abnormalities, pyramidal signs, headache, lower motor neuron disease, sensory abnormalities, seizures, vertigo, and other cranial nerve changes. Although not always clearly described in the literature, movement disorders other than myoclonus mentioned in patients with CJD are tremor, rigidity, parkinsonism, chorea, and athetosis (56). Ataxia as a presenting sign of CJD often predicts a more protracted course with less severe cognitive changes, similar to kuru, which was further characterized by a coarse tremor, saccadic abnormalities, and dysphagia (54,56). CJD transmitted by contaminated hormones differs from CJD resulting from surgical contamination. The latter is similar to sporadic CJD, whereas the former closely resembles kuru (56). It is suggested that in patients exposed to hormones, prions are taken up by hypothalamic neurons and transported to the basal ganglia and their cerebellar connections. However, in a recent report on a Japanese patient with CJD acquired from a contaminated dura fragment, the clinical presentation was spastic paraparesis (58).

The characteristic pathologic features of CJD are spongiform degeneration in the cortex with severe neuronal loss, astrocytic gliosis, compact (kuru) amyloid plaques stained by α-PrP antibodies in about 10% of patients, and absence of an inflammatory reaction (54,56). In kuru, compact plaques are invariably present, particularly in the cerebellum, and spongiform changes occur mainly in the thalamus and basal ganglia (56,57). Prusiner and Hsiao (54) emphasize that the pathologic changes in human prion diseases are so variable that they cannot be used as diagnostic markers on an individual basis. Indeed, there are reports of prion dementia without characteristic pathologic changes. Thus, the gold standard for the diagnosis of infectious prion diseases is the detection of PrP^{Sc} in brain tissue by immunologic techniques such as dot blot, Western blot, and staining of cryostat sections with α-PrP antibodies (54). Hsich et al. (59) reported on an assay for detection of the 14-3-3 brain protein in the CSF of patients with prion diseases. Although its sensitivity is high (96% of patients with prion dementia are positive), the specificity is low because, for instance, all patients with viral encephalitis also tested positive. These findings suggest that the 14-3-3 brain protein is a nonspecific marker of neuronal lesion and that the test is just helpful in patients with a history of dementia (59). Hill et al. (60) also developed an immunologic technique to detect PrP^{Sc} in tonsil biopsy material.

New-variant CJD (nvCJD) is the term coined to designate cases of this condition that have been detected in Great Britain as well as in continental Europe in the last decade (57). Unlike classical CJD, the onset of nvCJD is in the third decade of life, the median illness duration is 14 months (range, 8 to 38 months), and the median age at death is 29 years (range, 18 to 53 years). In almost all patients the presenting symptoms are psychiatric, with a combination of anxiety and depression, and sensory, dysesthesias, followed 6 months later by ataxia, cognitive decline, and movement disorder. Besides the typical myoclonus, chorea has been identified in many patients with nvCJD. The usual triphasic 1- to 2-Hz waves on electroencephalogram are seldom seen, but at least half of the patients have bilateral pulvinar high signal on MRI as well as 14-3-3 brain protein in the CSF (61,62). Recently, mounting evidence indicates that the new variant of CJD is related to BSE (mad cow disease). Its infectious nature is supported by features more reminiscent of kuru than CJD, such as onset before age 40, early behavioral symptoms, prominent ataxia, longer clinical course, absence of electroencephalographic findings, formation of PrP plaques in the cerebrum and the cerebellum, and little spongiform change (57,61,63). More importantly, Collinge et al. (64) demonstrated that the molecular characteristics of the PrP isoform associated with the new variant of CJD are distinct from other types of CJD and resemble those of BSE transmitted to mice, domestic cat, and macaque. However, some questions remain, such as how the infection occurs. Interestingly, the beef of animals with BSE is free from infectious PrP. One possible explanation is contamination of products, such as sausages and hamburgers, by brain-derived material rich in PrP. Also unexplained is the preference for young people, unlike classical CJD. A genetic background must certainly play a role in the pathogenesis of nvCJD because almost every patient studied to date has been homozygous for methionine at codon 129 (61). Finally, an extremely important question that remains concerns the size of the epidemics. As of this writing, fewer than 100 cases of nvCJD, almost all of them in Great Britain, have been identified. However, epidemiologists remain uncertain as to the extent of the population distribution of this condition. Conservative estimates indicate the existence of not more than 300 cases, but a more drastic picture comprising thousands of infected patients cannot be ruled out (63).

POSTENCEPHALITIC PARKINSONISM

PEP following encephalitis lethargica or Von Economo's disease is the classic example of an infectious movement disorder (65). All attempts to identify its causative agent have failed so far. The pandemic started in Austria in 1916 and quickly spread to western Europe and the United States. The incidence of the disease abated from 1927, and since 1930 very few new cases have been reported (66).

The acute phase of encephalitis lethargica was characterized by fever, ophthalmoplegia, somnolence, with mildly elevated protein and pleocytosis (50 to 100 lymphocytes) in the CSF. About 40% of affected patients died during the initial phase of the disease, and the autopsy disclosed periventricular and midbrain inflammation. Although a few survivors developed parkinsonism from the outset, the rule was that this complication set in after a variable asymptomatic period. Follow-up of the patients showed that 50% of them developed parkinsonian syndrome in 5 years, and this proportion increased to 80% in 10 years (67). The underlying mechanism responsible for the delayed onset and subsequent progression of the condition has never been elucidated. The parkinsonism in PEP, although levodopa progressive and levodopa responsive, is readily distinguished from idiopathic Parkinson's disease by its coexistence with oculogyric crisis, blepharospasm, palilalia, dystonia, chorea, tics, hiccups, and affective and conduct disorders (67).

The pathologic findings of PEP are neuronal loss in the substantia nigra and other areas of the midbrain with neurofibrillary tangles (NFTs) widespread in the brain. Recently interest in studying the neuropathology of PEP has been renewed by the demonstration of similarities with other degenerative diseases characterized by NFTs: progressive supranuclear palsy, Guam parkinsonism-dementia complex, and Alzheimer's disease. For instance, Geddes et al. (66) failed to identify any histologic feature that could distinguish PEP, progressive supranuclear palsy, and Guam parkinsonism-dementia. Furthermore, Pramstaller et al. (68) proposed that there might be a clinical overlap between PEP and progressive supranuclear palsy. Mizukami et al. (69) demonstrated that NFTs in PEP are immunohistochemically and ultrastructurally similar to those observed in Alzheimer's disease, containing paired helical filaments, tau, and ubiquitin. In conclusion, despite the distinctive clinical features and presumably different causes, the similar findings in Alzheimer's disease, progressive supranuclear palsy, and PEP suggests a common disease mechanism.

Encephalitis caused by arboviruses, enteroviruses, influenza virus, varicella-zoster virus, and encephalitis of unknown cause may be associated with parkinsonism and other movement disorders (70,71). Japanese encephalitis, with 30,000 cases a year in Asia, is most likely the most common viral cause of parkinsonism. For instance, one recent study shows that 80% of patients seen in tertiary centers in endemic areas will develop movement disorders at some point of their disease (71). These clinical features are associated with lesions in basal ganglia, thalamus, and midbrain. Parkinsonism, characterized by rigid-akinetic syndrome, is the most common movement disorder seen in these patients. In at least 10% of patients pure parkinsonian syndrome associated with isolated lesions of the substantia nigra are seen (70). After a 6-month follow-up, most patients with parkinsonism display spontaneous improvement. Dystonia, though less frequently seen, usually carries a more ominous prognosis because many patients remain severely disabled despite best treatment (71).

SUBACUTE SCLEROSING PANENCEPHALITIS

Subacute sclerosing panencephalitis (SSPE) is a progressive degenerative disease caused by persistent measles virus infection of the CNS (72). Estimated to occur in one of 100,000 patients with natural measles, it is two or three times more common in boys than in girls. At least 50% of the affected persons had measles before age 2 years. SSPE has been nearly eradicated in areas where vaccine against measles is used, since the risk of developing SSPE after vaccination is 10% or less of that following natural infection. In recent years there have been reports on large series of patients from India, Saudi Arabia, and Turkey (73,74). Although there is one report of an AIDS patient who developed SSPE, seemingly this is an unusual complication in HIV-positive subjects.

The onset of SSPE occurs a mean of 6 years after the patient had measles. Typically the first symptoms are behavioral and cognitive changes, followed by cortical myoclonus that is usually stimulus sensitive, multifocal, or generalized, and associated with periodic 2- to 3-Hz slow-wave bursts on the electroencephalogram. With progression of the disease myoclonus becomes more severe and often is associated with other extrapyramidal features, such as rigidity and hyperkinesias, including chorea, ballism, and athetosis. Other features often observed are visual changes (chorioretinitis, visual field defects, optic atrophy, cortical blindness, nystagmus), seizures, and focal deficits. At the terminal stages the patient is in a vegetative state, and death usually occurs 1 to 3 years after onset (72,74). Despite the stereotyped course seen in most patients, up to 20% of subjects have a more protracted disease lasting as long as 10 years, not infrequently displaying periods of stabilization and even spontaneous improvement.

MRI often shows high signal areas on T2-weighted images, frequently in the periventricular or subcortical white matter. Basal ganglia, particularly in the putamen, and brainstem lesions are less common. Importantly, the extent and location of the periventricular white matter lesions and cerebral atrophy do not correlate with the neurologic status in many patients. Consistent with these imaging findings, pathologic studies disclose generalized changes characterized by lymphocytic leptomeningeal infiltration, perivascular collections of lymphocytes, proliferation of microglial cells, astrocytosis, and demyelination. However, the hallmark of SSPE pathology is intranuclear and intracytoplasmic inclusion bodies in neurons, astrocytes, and oligodendroglial cells that are measles virus antigens (72–74). Bancher et al. (75) demonstrated that NFTs in the brains of patients with SSPE are not related to measles virus antigens. This finding supports the notion that NFTs are a final outcome of neuronal lesion triggered by different causes (66). Although these pathologic findings firmly establish a causal relationship between measles virus infection and SSPE, the pathogenesis of this condition remains elusive. Presumably a combination of mutations of viral proteins, such as protein M and others, and host failure to raise antibodies against the mutated proteins play a crucial role in the persistence of the infection (72).

To date no treatment has been demonstrated to be consistently effective in halting the progression of SSPE. Among the several antiviral agents tested, isoprinosine is most often regarded as capable of changing the natural history of SSPE. However, this conclusion is based on anecdotal reports and uncontrolled studies. More recent findings suggest that the usefulness of this antiviral agent in SSPE is limited (73). The combined use of oral isoprinosine and intraventricular α-interferon has been reported as inducing remission in 50% and stabilization in 22% of patients. Unfortunately, a long-term follow-up of the 16 patients who had initial benefit demonstrated that 7 died and the 4 remaining deteriorated (73). Finally, the use of intravenous immunoglobulin in a few patients has yielded conflicting results (73).

MISCELLANEOUS INFECTIONS

Encephalitis either related to direct viral invasion or mediated by immune mechanism may cause transient or permanent chorea. This hyperkinesia has been reported as occurring in association with arboviruses, cytomegalovirus, enteroviruses, Epstein-Barr virus, herpes simplex encephalitis, influenza, mononucleosis, mumps, rubella, and even as a postvaccination complication (76–78). Although chorea is the most common movement disorder related to viral encephalitis, other hyperkinesias, such as tics and dystonia, may result from these infections (79). There are case reports of patients with diphtheria, legionnaire's disease, typhoid fever, and whooping cough developing chorea (80). Chorea may also be observed in cerebral malaria and neurosyphilis in HIV-negative patients (81). Rarely, *Mycoplasma pneumoniae* causes basal ganglia damage leading to parkinsonism, chorea, and dystonia (82). Neurocysticercosis (NC), which is infestation of the CNS by encapsulated larvae of *Taenia solium*, is the most common neurologic parasitic disease worldwide (83). This condition, highly prevalent in developing areas, is becoming increasingly common in regions with high rates of immigration from endemic areas. For instance, Scharf (84) diagnosed 238 cases of NC in a California hospital in a 5-year period. Epilepsy and intracranial hypertension due to hydrocephalus are present in up to 92% of NC patients, but the clinical manifestations are protean and may include focal deficits, meningitis, optic neuropathy, stroke, and others (83,84). There are few reports on movement disorders associated with NC. Bhigjee et al. (85) described a South African girl with multiple

cysticerci, some of them in the right striatum, who developed a left hemichorea. There is also a recent report on reversible parkinsonian syndrome complicating cysticercus midbrain encephalitis (86). Recently, a 39-year-old man was evaluated at the MDC-UFMG with a year-long history of right-sided movement disorder. On neurologic examination he displayed right hemichorea with ipsilateral dystonic posturing of the hand. MRI of the brain (Fig. 40.1) showed a large cystic lesion with contrast ring enhancement in the head of the left caudate nucleus. Routine CSF analysis was normal, but ELISA for cysticerci antigen was positive. Treatment with albendazole caused significant improvement of the chorea but no change in the dystonic posturing. At our institution NC has been recognized in 7.3% of 1,129 autopsies done on subjects older than 2 years (87). Surprisingly, NC accounts for only three cases (the case described above plus two additional cases recently diagnosed, one with hemifacial spasm and cysti in the ipsilateral cerebellopontine angle, and the other with parkinsonism and lesions in the midbrain) in a series of 5,000 consecutive subjects seen at the MDC-UFMG in an 8-year period. One possible explanation for the rarity of movement disorders in NC is the slow growth of the cysts, which gradually displace the basal ganglia structures without lesioning them. *Schisto-*

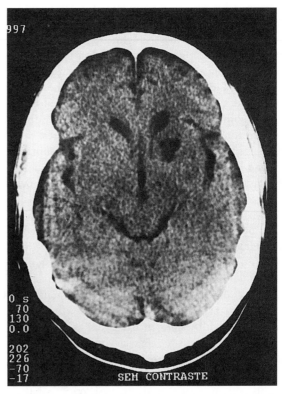

FIG. 40.1. CT scan of the brain of a patient with right hemichorea-dystonia displaying a large cystic lesion in the head of the left caudate nucleus. The patient had positive *Taenia solium* serology in the cerebrospinal fluid.

somiasis mansoni infection is an endemic parasitic disease in developing areas. It is estimated that there are 10 million patients in Brazil. This parasite usually causes intestinal and hepatic lesions. Occasionally, the eggs of the parasite may reach the spinal cord, causing acute myelitis, and rarely there may be cerebral schistosomiasis (88). At the MDC-UFMG we saw one 13-year-old boy who developed transient segmental spinal myoclonus during recovery from schistosomiasis myelitis.

ACKNOWLEDGMENTS

Immunologic study of the CSF and MRI of the patient with neurocysticercosis were done, respectively, by Professor Dr. Antonio Spina-França, Professor Dr. L. A. Ramos-Machado, and Professor Dr. J. Livramento of the University of São Paulo, Brazil; and Professor Dr. Francisco Otaviano Perpétuo of the Federal University of Minas Gerais, Brazil.

REFERENCES

1. Brew BJ. *HIV neurology.* New York: Oxford, 2001.
2. De Mattos JP, Rosso AL, Correa RB, et al. Involuntary movements and AIDS: report of seven cases and review of the literature. *Arquivos de Neuropsiquiatria* 1993;51:491–497.
3. Mirsattari SM, Power C, Nath A. Parkinsonism with HIV infection. *Mov Disord* 1998,13:684–689.
4. Sacktor NC, Skolasky RL, Lyles RH, et al. Improvement in HIV-associated motor slowing after antiretroviral therapy including protease inhibitors. *J Neurovirol* 2000;6:84–88.
5. Piccolo I, Causarano R, Sterzi R, et al. Chorea in patients with AIDS. *Acta Neurol Scand* 1999;100:332–336.
6. Edelstein HE, Chirurgi VA, Gloudeman MW, et al. Adverse reactions to phenothiazine antiemetics in AIDS. *DICP* 1991;25:1007.
7. Van Gerpen JA. Tremor caused by trimethoprim-sulfamethoxazole in a patient with AIDS. *Neurology* 1997;48:537–538.
8. Abbruzzese G, Rizzo F, Dall'Agata D, et al. Generalized dystonia with bilateral striatal computed-tomographic lucencies in a patient with human immunodeficiency virus infection. *Eur Neurol* 1990;30:271–273.
9. Carrazana E, Rossitch E, Martinez J, et al. Unilateral "akathisia" in a patient with AIDS and a toxoplasmosis subthalamic abscess. *Neurology* 1989;39:449–450.
10. Bernstein WB, Scherokman B. Neuroleptic malignant syndrome in a patient with acquired immunodeficiency syndrome. *Acta Neurol Scand* 1986;73:636–637.
11. Jankovic J. Whipple's disease of the central nervous system in AIDS. *N Engl J Med* 1986;315:1029–1030.
12. Mirsattari SM, Berry ME, Holden JK, et al. Paroxysmal dyskinesias in patients with HIV infection. *Neurology* 1999;52:109–114.
13. Teive HA, Troiano AR, Cabral NL, et al. Hemichorea-hemiballism associated to cryptococcal granuloma in a patient with AIDS: case report. *Arquivos de Neuropsiquiatria* 2000;58:965–968.
14. Lopez OL, Smith G, Meltzer CC, et al. Dopamine systems in human immunodeficiency virus-associated dementia. *Neuropsychiatry Neuropsychol Behav Neurol* 1999;12:184–192.
15. Antinori A, Ammassari A, DeLuca A, et al. Diagnosis of AIDS-related focal brain lesions: a decision-making analysis based on clinical and neuroradiologic characteristics combined with polymerase chain reaction assays in CSF. *Neurology* 1997;48:687–694.
16. Maschke M, Kastrup O, Esser S, et al. Incidence and prevalence of HIV-associated neurological disorders since the introduction of highly active antiretroviral therapy (HAART). *J Neurol Neurosurg Psychiatry* 2000;69:376–380.
17. Singer C, Weiner WJ. Tremor in the acquired immune deficiency syndrome. In: Findley LJ, Koller WC, eds. *Handbook of tremor disorders.* New York: Marcel Dekker, 1995:483–489.
18. Remy P, de Recondo A, Defer G, et al. Peduncular "rubral" tremor and dopaminergic denervation: a PET study. *Neurology* 1995;45:472–477.
19. Mintz M, Tardieu M, Hoyt L, et al. Levodopa therapy improves motor function in HIV-infected children with extrapyramidal syndromes. *Neurology* 1996;47:1583–1585.
20. Berger JR, Moskowitz L, Fischl M, et al. The neurologic complications of AIDS: frequently the initial manifestation. *Neurology* 1984;34[Suppl]:134–135.
21. Navia BA, Jordan BD, Price RW. The AIDS dementia complex: I. Clinical features. *Ann Neurol* 1986;19:517–524.
22. Arendt G, Hefter H, Hilperath F, et al. Motor analysis predicts progression in HIV-associated brain disease. *J Neurol Sci* 1994;123:180–185.
23. Kieburtz KD, Epstein LG, Gelbard HA, et al. Excitotoxicity and dopaminergic dysfunction in the acquired immunodeficiency syndrome dementia complex: therapeutic implications. *Arch Neurol* 1991;48:1281–1284.
24. de la Fuente Aguado J, Bordon J, Moreno JA, et al. Parkinsonism in an HIV-infected patient with hypodense cerebral lesion. *Tuberculosis Lung Dis* 1996;77:191–192.
25. Murakami T, Nakajima M, Nakamura T, et al. Parkinsonian symptoms as an initial manifestation in a Japanese patient with acquired immunodeficiency syndrome and *Toxoplasma* infection. *Intern Med* 2000;39:1111–1114.
26. Taranta A, Stollerman GH. The relationship of Sydenham's chorea to infection with group A streptococci. *Am J Med* 1956;20:170.
27. Special Writing Group of the Committee of Rheumatic Fever, Endocarditis, and Kawasaki Disease of the Council on Cardiovascular Disease of the Young of the American Heart Association. Guidelines for the diagnosis of rheumatic fever. *JAMA* 1992;268:2069–2073.
28. Carapetis JR, Wolff DR, Currie BJ. Acute rheumatic fever and rheumatic heart disease in the top end of Australia's Northern Territory. *Med J Aust* 1996;164:146–149.
29. Cardoso F, Santos CE, Mota CC. Sydenham's chorea in 50 consecutive patients with rheumatic fever. *Mov Disord* 1997;12:701–703.
30. Schwartz RH, Hepner SI, Ziai M. Incidence of acute rheumatic fever: a suburban community hospital experience during the 1970s. *Clin Pediatrics* 1983;22:798–801.
31. Nausieda PA, Grossman B J, Koller WC, et al. Sydenham chorea: an update. *Neurology* 1980;30:331–334.
32. Ayoub EM. Resurgence of rheumatic fever in the United States: the changing picture of a preventable illness. *Postgrad Med J* 1992;92:133–136.
33. Asbahr FR, Negrao AB, Gentil V, et al. Obsessive-compulsive and related symptoms in children and adolescents with rheumatic fever with and without chorea: a prospective 6-month study. *Am J Psychiatry* 1998;155:1122–1124.
34. Mercadante MT, Busatto GF, Lombroso PJ, et al. The psychiatric symptoms of rheumatic fever. *Am J Psychiatry* 2000;157:2036–2038.
35. Swedo SE. Sydenham's chorea: a model for childhood autoimmune neuropsychiatric disorders (clinical conference). *JAMA* 1994;272:1788–1791.
36. Cardoso F, Vargas AP, Oliveira LD, et al. Persistent Sydenham's chorea. *Mov Disord* 1999;14:805–807.

37. Cardoso F. Chorea gravidarum. *Arch Neurol* 2002;59:868.
38. Feldman BM, Zabriskie JB, Silverman ED, et al. Diagnostic use of B-cell alloantigen D8/17 in rheumatic chorea. *J Pediatrics* 1993;123:84–86.
39. Giedd JN, Rapoport JL, Kruesi MJP, et al. Sydenham's chorea: magnetic resonance imaging of the basal ganglia. *Neurology* 1995;45:2199–2202.
40. Goldman S, Amrom D, Szliwowski HB, et al. Reversible striatal hypermetabolism in a case of Sydenham's chorea. *Mov Disord* 1993;8:355–358.
41. Colony S, Malamud N. Sydenham's chorea: a clinicopathologic study. *Neurology* 1956;6:672.
42. Naidu S, Narasimhachari N. Sydenham's chorea: a possible presynaptic dopaminergic dysfunction initially. *Ann Neurol* 1980;8:445–447.
43. Husby G, van de Rijn I, Zabriskie JB, et al. Antibodies reacting with cytoplasm of subthalamic and caudate nuclei neurons in chorea and acute rheumatic fever. *J Exp Med* 1976;144:1094–1110.
44. Dale RC, Church A, Cardoso F, et al. Antineuronal antibodies in Sydenham's chorea. *Ann Neurol* 2001;50:588–595.
45. Garvey MA, Swedo SE, Shapiro MB, et al. Intravenous immunoglobulin (IVig) and plasmapheresis as effective treatments of Sydenham's chorea (SC). *Neurology* 1996;46[Suppl 2]:A147.
46. Hallett J, Poskanzer K, Cardoso F. Neuronal dysfunction induced by Sydenham's chorea serum. *Brain* 2002 (in press).
47. Gebremariam A. Sydenham's chorea: risk factors and the role of prophylactic benzathine penicillin G in preventing recurrence. *Ann Trop Paediatrics* 1999;19:161–165.
48. Swedo SE, Leonard HL, Garvey M, et al. Pediatric autoimmune neuropsychiatric disorders associated with streptococcal infections: clinical description of the first 50 cases. *Am J Psychiatry* 1998;155:264–271.
49. Giedd JN, Rapoport JL, Garvey MA, et al. MRI assessment of children with obsessive-compulsive disorder or tics associated with streptococcal infection. *Am J Psychiatry* 2000;157:281–283.
50. Allen AJ, Leonard HL, Swedo SE. Case study: a new infection-triggered, autoimmune subtype of pediatric OCD and Tourette's syndrome. *J Am Acad Child Adolesc Psychiatry* 1995;34:307–311.
51. Perlmutter SJ, Leitman SF, Garvey MA, et al. Therapeutic plasma exchange and intravenous immunoglobulin for obsessive-compulsive disorder and tic disorder in childhood. *Lancet* 1999;354:1153–1158.
51a. Kurlan R. Tourette's syndrome and "PANDAS": will the relation bear out? Pediatric autoimmune neuropsychiatric disorders associated with streptococcal infection. *Neurology* 1998;50:1530–1534.
52. Garvey MA, Perlmutter SJ, Allen AJ, et al. A pilot study of penicillin prophylaxis for neuropsychiatric exacerbations triggered by streptococcal infections. *Biol Psychiatry* 1999;45:1564–1571.
53. Prusiner SB. Novel proteinaceous infectious particles cause scrapie. *Science* 1982;216:136–144.
54. Prusiner SB, Hsiao KK. Human prion diseases. *Ann Neurol* 1994;35:385–395.
55. Gajdusek DC. Unconventional viruses and the origin and disappearance of kuru. *Science* 1977;197:943–960.
56. Brown P. Transmissible human spongiform encephalopathy (infectious cerebral amyloidosis): Creutzfeldt-Jakob disease, Gerstmann-Sträussler-Scheinker syndrome, and kuru. In: Calne DB, ed. *Neurodegenerative diseases.* Philadelphia: WB Saunders, 1994:839–876.
57. Epstein LG, Brown P. Bovine spongiform encephalopathy and a new variant of Creutzfeldt-Jakob disease. *Neurology* 1997;48:569–571.
58. Kimura K, Nonaka A, Tashiro H, et al. Atypical form of dural graft associated Creutzfeldt-Jakob disease: report of a post-mortem case with review of the literature. *J Neurol Neurosurg Psychiatry* 2001;70:696–699.
59. Hsich G, Kenney K, Gibbs CJ, et al. The 14-3-3 brain protein in cerebrospinal fluid as a marker for transmissible spongiform encephalopathies. *N Engl J Med* 1996;335:924–930.
60. Hill AF, Zeidler M, Ironside J, et al. Diagnosis of new variant Creutzfeldt-Jakob disease by tonsil biopsy. *Lancet* 1997;349:99–100.
61. Will RG, Zeidler M, Stewart GE, et al. Diagnosis of new variant Creutzfeldt-Jakob disease. *Ann Neurol* 2000;47:575–582.
62. Bowen J, Mitchell T, Pearce R, et al. Chorea in new variant Creutzfeldt-Jakob disease. *Mov Disord* 2000;15:1284–1285.
63. Bruce ME. "New variant" Creutzfeldt-Jakob disease and bovine spongiform encephalopathy. *Nat Med* 2000;6:258–259.
64. Collinge J, Sidle KC, Meads J, et al. Molecular analysis of prion strain variation and the aetiology of "new variant" CJD. *Nature* 1996;383:685–690.
65. Von Economo C. *Encephalitis lethargica: its sequelae and treatment.* Newman KO (trans). New York: Oxford University Press, 1931.
66. Geddes JF, Hughes AJ, Lees AJ, et al. Pathological overlap in cases of parkinsonism associated with neurofibrillary tangles: a study of recent cases of postencephalitic parkinsonism and comparison with progressive supranuclear palsy and Guamanian parkinsonism-dementia complex. *Brain* 1993;116:281–302.
67. Krusz JC, Koller WC, Ziegler DK. Historical review: abnormal movements associated with epidemic encephalitis lethargica. *Mov Disord* 1987;2:137–141.
68. Pramstaller PP, Lees AJ, Luxon LM. Possible clinical overlap between postencephalitic parkinsonism and progressive supranuclear palsy. *J Neurol Neurosurg Psychiatry* 1996;60:589–590.
69. Mizukami K, Sasaki M, Shiraishi H, et al. A neuropathologic study of long-term, Economo-type postencephalitic parkinsonism with a prolonged clinical course. *Psychiatry Clin Neurosci* 1996;50:79–83.
70. Pradhan S, Pandey N, Shashank S, et al. Parkinsonism due to predominant involvement of substantia nigra in Japanese encephalitis. *Neurology* 1999;53:1781–1786.
71. Kalita J, Misra UK. Markedly severe dystonia in Japanese encephalitis. *Mov Disord* 2000;15:1168–1172.
72. Johnson RT. Slow infections of the central nervous system caused by conventional viruses. *Ann NY Acad Sci* 1994;724:6–13.
73. Anlar B, Yalaz K, Oktem F, et al. Long-term follow-up of patients with subacute sclerosing panencephalitis treated with intraventricular α-interferon. *Neurology* 1997;48:526–528.
74. Yaqub BA. Subacute sclerosing panencephalitis (SSPE): early diagnosis, prognostic factors, and natural history. *J Neurol Sci* 1996;139:227–234.
75. Bancher C, Leitner H, Jellinger K, et al. On the relationship between measles virus and Alzheimer neurofibrillary tangles in subacute sclerosing panencephalitis. *Neurobiology Aging* 1996;17:527–533.
76. Shoulson I. On chorea. *Clin Neuropharmacol* 1986;9[Suppl 2]:S85–S89.
77. Gascon GG, al Jarallah AA, Okamoto E, et al. Chorea as a presentation of herpes simplex encephalitis relapse. *Brain Dev* 1993;15:178–181.
78. Tachi N, Nagata N, Chiba S, et al. Detection of Epstein-Barr virus genome in cerebrospinal fluid from a patient with acquired chorea by the polymerase chain reaction. *J Child Neurol* 1993;8:424–425.
79. Northam RS, Singer HS. Postencephalitic acquired Tourette-like syndrome in a child. *Neurology* 1991;41:592–593.
80. Bamford JM, Hakin RN. Chorea after legionnaire's disease. *BMJ* 1982;284:1232–1233.

81. Jones AL, Bouchier IA. A patient with neurosyphilis presenting as chorea. *Scott Med J* 1993;38:82–84.

82. Brandel JP, Vidailhet M, Noseda G, et al. *Mycoplasma pneumoniae* postinfectious encephalomyelitis with bilateral striatal necrosis. *Mov Disord* 1996;11:333–336.

83. Del Brutto OH, Rajshekhar V, White AC Jr, et al. Proposed diagnostic criteria for neurocysticercosis. *Neurology* 2001;57:177–183.

84. Scharf D. Neurocysticercosis: two hundred thirty-eight cases from a California hospital. *Arch Neurol* 1988;45:777–780.

85. Bhigjee AI, Kemp T, Cosnett JE. Cerebral cysticercosis presenting with hemichorea. *J Neurol Neurosurg Psychiatry* 1987;50:1561–1562.

86. Verma A, Berger JR, Bowen BC, et al. Reversible parkinsonian syndrome complicating cysticercus midbrain encephalitis. *Mov Disord* 1995;10:215–219.

87. Pitella JEH. Neurocysticercosis. *Brain Pathol* 1997;7:649–662.

88. Ferrari TC. Spinal cord schistosomiasis: a report of 231 cases and review emphasizing clinical aspects. *Medicine* 1999;78:176–190.

MAGNETIC RESONANCE IMAGING OF MOVEMENT DISORDERS

MARIO SAVOIARDO
MARINA GRISOLI

Correlations between magnetic resonance (MR) images and pathologic specimens, which are the best way to validate the neuroradiologic diagnosis, are difficult to obtain in neurodegenerative disorders because patients affected by these diseases often have a long course and rarely die in the hospital. Therefore, postmortem studies are rarely obtained, and biopsies are rarely justified during life. However, in the past decade, so much neuroradiologic knowledge, mainly related to MR imaging (MRI), has been accumulated that MRI has become a very useful tool in supporting the clinical diagnosis of a neurodegenerative disorder.

In this chapter, we shall review the most common movement disorders in which MRI studies may be relevant for the diagnosis. We shall therefore describe the neuroradiologic findings that may be observed in Parkinson's disease (PD) and atypical parkinsonian disorders: multiple system atrophy (MSA), both in the form with predominant parkinsonian features (MSA-P) and in the form with predominant cerebellar features (MSA-C); progressive supranuclear palsy (PSP); and corticobasal degeneration (CBD). We shall also review Huntington's chorea, Wilson's disease, and Hallervorden-Spatz disease.

IRON AND PARKINSONIAN SYNDROMES

Interest in MRI studies of parkinsonism was stimulated by the paper published by Drayer on the distribution of iron in the brain and by two articles that appeared in the same issue of *Radiology* dealing with Parkinson-plus syndromes (1) and with Shy-Drager syndrome (2). It had been observed that in T2-weighted images obtained at high field intensity MRI, the distribution of low signal intensity in the basal ganglia and other areas of the brain corresponded to the distribution of iron demonstrated by Perls' stain in brain sections.

In the brain, iron is not present at birth. It gradually accumulates during lifetime with a predilection for basal ganglia, substantia nigra and red nuclei, and dentate nuclei.

Significant amounts of iron are also present in the deep cortical layers. In the basal ganglia, the selective distribution of iron is not uniform; the amount of iron is greater in the pallidum than in the putamen. However, in old people in their seventies or eighties, the amount of iron in the putamina increases and tends to reach the amount seen in the pallida (3,4). Iron is demonstrated by high field intensity MRI because of its magnetic susceptibility effect that shortens T2. Therefore, its presence is demonstrated by low signal intensity (hypointensity) in T2-weighted images. This magnetic susceptibility effect is proportional to the square of the field intensity; this means that the effect on T2-weighted images at 1.5 Tesla (T) is nine times greater than that observed at 0.5 T. This difference accounts for the better demonstration of iron (or, for instance, hemosiderin in old hematomas or in cavernous hemangiomas) in studies done at 1.5 T than at 0.5 T. This fact has to be kept in mind when dealing with certain neurodegenerative disorders; the magnetic susceptibility effects of iron or other paramagnetic substances, well demonstrated in T2-weighted images at 1.5 T, may not be visible in studies done at 0.5 T (5).

The hypointensity caused by iron is more evident in gradient echo images to the point that loss of signal intensity may also be seen in T1-weighted images. However, in this chapter, when we describe hypointensity caused by iron, we refer to signal intensities of T2-weighted images unless otherwise specified.

The interest stirred up by the above-mentioned papers by Drayer (1) and Pastakia (2) was caused by their demonstration of abnormal distribution of iron (or, rather, of low signal intensity in T2-weighted images, probably indicating the presence of iron or other paramagnetic substances) within the basal ganglia in MSA. This observation could help in differentiating parkinsonism not responding to L-dopa therapy from PD.

In agreement with the consensus statement on the diagnosis of MSA (6), we shall not use terms such as Parkinson-plus syndrome or Shy-Drager syndrome, used in the original articles but no longer useful, but instead shall use the terms MSA-P and MSA-C, which have replaced striatoni-gral degeneration (SND) and sporadic olivopontocerebellar atrophy (OPCA), respectively.

PARKINSON'S DISEASE

In PD two pathologic features may be relevant in determining the MRI aspect: (a) progressive atrophy of the substantia nigra caused by the cumulative death of nigrostriatal neurons; and (b) accumulation of iron in the substantia nigra. Iron has been known to be normally present, particularly in the pars reticulata, but some studies have demonstrated that in parkinsonian brains iron selectively increases in the zona compacta (7). Several investigators have examined the MRI findings of patients with PD focusing on the substantia nigra (1,3,8,9). The band of relatively high intensity, normally separating the substantia nigra from the red nucleus, decreases in size in parkinsonian patients; this finding has been attributed to atrophy of the pars compacta or, possibly, to increased iron also in the pars compacta (8) (Fig. 41.1). Another finding, restoration of signal intensity in the dorsal lateral part of the substantia nigra, has suggested either depletion of iron or local cell death that expands the extracellular space, thus increasing the signal intensity which, in turn, overwhelms the effects of iron (3). A feature noted in some of these reports was that occasional putaminal hypointensity was present in patients with PD and in normals, but not as significant as that observed in patients with MSA. A more recent report (9) suggests that it may be possible to demonstrate a correlation of substantia nigra iron-related contrast and some testing of motor performance in PD patients. Accurate MRI studies on the substantia nigra may shed further light on the role of iron

in the pathogenesis of PD; however, in a clinical situation, we believe that in a patient with parkinsonian features it is more important to observe the putamen than the substantia nigra because putaminal changes may indicate a poor prognosis and suggest a diagnosis of MSA (10). Smudging of the substantia nigra hypointensity toward the red nucleus is a frequent observation in PD, but also in other parkinsonian syndromes (Fig. 41.1).

A recent technical advancement may become very useful in the studies on PD. Hutchinson and Raff (11) developed a method for depicting the substantia nigra by using inversion recovery sequences with suppression of the signal from the white matter and from the gray matter. A ratio of these two images allows a very accurate demonstration of the substantia nigra; the radiologic measure of the substantia nigra correlates with the clinical measure of disease severity and has the potential for detecting presymptomatic disease. Hu et al. (12), using inversion recovery MRI, observed that the structural changes seen in the substantia nigra of patients with PD correlate with measures of striatal dopaminergic function using ^{18}F-dopa positron emission tomography (PET), but found that ^{18}F-dopa PET is more reliable than inversion recovery MRI in discriminating PD patients from normal subjects.

Functional MRI (fMRI) studies describing brain activation in patients with PD are just beginning; in akinetic patients, decrease fMRI signal in the rostral part of the supplementary motor area and in the right dorsolateral prefrontal cortex, as previously demonstrated in PET studies, has been shown, accompanied by hyperactivation of several other cortical areas (13). A very recent event-related fMRI study also demonstrated a relative normalization of dysfunctional activation after levodopa administration (14).

A large number of papers should be mentioned that deal with methods that use MRI to identify the target for deep brain stimulation in PD. Most of these papers concern identification of the subthalamic nuclei, coupled with electrophysiologic recording and stimulation (15,16). We shall not expand further on this subject.

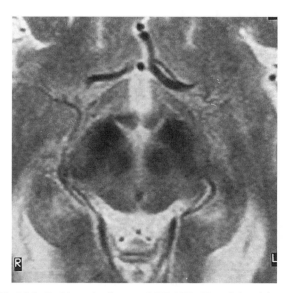

FIG. 41.1. Parkinson's disease. 1.5-T MRI, T2-weighted image. Smudging of the hypointensity in the substantia nigra toward the red nucleus.

MULTIPLE SYSTEM ATROPHY

The first MRI studies of MSA demonstrated abnormalities in the putamen and occasionally in posterior fossa (1). In reports of these studies, the term *multiple system atrophy* (MSA) was used as a synonym for Shy-Drager syndrome (SDS) (2). In MSA, extrapyramidal signs are combined with autonomic failure and cerebellar disturbances, all with different degrees of severity in the various patients. The best way to approach the definition of the MRI features of MSA is to isolate "pure" syndromes, that is, to isolate patients with parkinsonism not responding to therapy (patients with MSA-P) and patients with predominant cerebellar disturbances (patients with MSA-C).

Autonomic failure, which is often associated with parkinsonism not responsive to therapy, does not have a correlative abnormality in MRI studies. In fact, the pathology responsible for the autonomic failure is located in the intermediolateral columns of the spinal cord, where MRI abnormalities have not so far been demonstrated. Patients with pure autonomic failure studied by Brown et al. (17) did not exhibit any brain MRI abnormalities. Positron emission tomography (PET), done in a series of our MSA patients by Perani et al. (18), demonstrated abnormalities that suggest inferior frontal and temporal dysfunction in patients with autonomic failure; MRI was normal in these regions.

We have now seen more than 200 MRI studies done in patients with clinical diagnosis of MSA, with different involvement of the extrapyramidal, autonomic, and cerebellar systems. When moderate to severe involvement of extrapyramidal and cerebellar systems was present, we observed MRI abnormalities both in basal ganglia and in posterior fossa. They were sometimes absent (more frequently the putaminal abnormalities) in early cases with slight clinical involvement. However, the MRI studies often became positive as the disease progressed.

We shall describe separately the MRI findings observed in MSA-P and MSA-C.

MSA-P

The first reports on MSA-P (1,2) did not make a clear distinction between SND and SDS. MSA-P is diagnosed in patients usually presenting with symptoms and signs consistent with PD, who later fail to respond to L-dopa treatment. The most striking pathologic findings are shrinkage and discoloration of the putamina, with neuronal and myelin loss, and gliosis. Loss of pigmented cells is found in the substantia nigra. The 1.5-T MRI abnormalities described in the putamina in the above-mentioned papers are indeed in the putamina, where one can observe significant hypointensity in T2-weighted images consistent with magnetic susceptibility effect of iron or other paramagnetic substances. This hypointensity is equal to or more marked than that normally seen in the pallida (Fig. 41.2B).

Iron, manganese, neuromelanin, and hematin pigments have been demonstrated in the putamina, with ferric iron being the most important determinant of the signal loss (2,9,19,20).

In the most lateral part of the putamen, a tiny line of hyperintensity is often also seen in 1.5-T studies (5). In 0.5-T MRI studies, we observed less significant or absent hypointensity but a larger area of hyperintensity, mostly involving the posterior putamen and fading anteriorly (5,10,21,22). The hyperintensity, consistent with an increased amount of water associated with cell loss and gliosis, simply prevails over the magnetic susceptibility effect of iron, which is poorly appreciable at this field intensity. A constant feature of the putaminal abnormalities is that they mostly involve the posterior lateral part of the putamen, which is most affected in pathologic specimens (19,20,23, 24). In a pathologic case of MSA-P that we reviewed, the dorsolateral and posterior part of the putamen exhibited neuronal loss and astrocytic gliosis in a markedly loose tissue; the amount of iron demonstrated by Perls' stain in the same territory briskly diminished just before the lateral margin of the putamen, leaving a thin rim of loose tissue almost devoid of iron just beneath the external capsule (Fig. 41.3). This find-

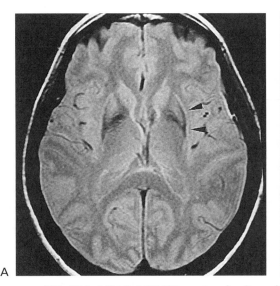
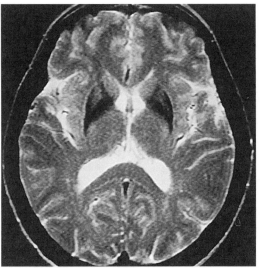

A   B

FIG. 41.2. MSA-P. 1.5-T MRI, proton density and T2-weighted axial sections **(A, B)** in a 57-year-old patient. The marked T2 hypointensity of the putamina, particularly in the lateral posterior part **(B)**, is less evident in proton density image **(A)** which shows better the lateral rim of hyperintensity (*arrowheads* on the left).

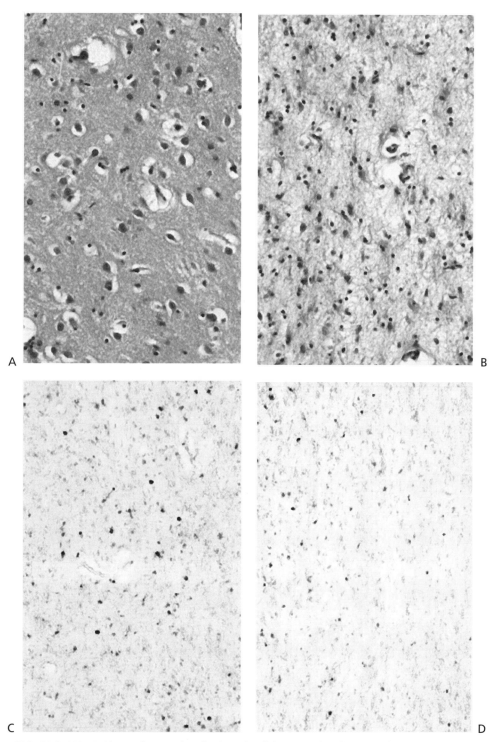

FIG. 41.3. MSA-P. Photomicrographs of striatonigral degeneration, hematoxylin and eosin **(A, B:** original magnification, ×130), Perls' stain **(C, D:** original magnification, ×65). The anterior part of the putamen is normal **(A)**, whereas the posterior lateral part shows spongiform changes with loss of neurons and astrogliosis **(B)**. Iron deposition, which is abundant in this posterior lateral part **(C)**, briskly diminishes close to the external capsule **(D)**; in this area, spongiform changes and gliosis are most severe, thus explaining the lateral rim of hyperintensity on magnetic resonance images. (Courtesy of Dr. G. Giaccone.) (See color section.)

ing may explain the lateral rim of hyperintensity that, in combination with the hypointensity, may add specificity to the MRI findings in MSA-P (25).

Further proof of the reliability of these MRI abnormalities in making the diagnosis of MSA-P is given by the abnormalities observed in very initial cases presenting with hemiparkinsonism; in these patients, minimal signal abnormalities are only found in the contralateral putamen. It is also useful to observe proton density images: when the hyperintense rim is not clearly detectable in T2-weighted images, it may often be seen in proton density images because the hypointensity from the magnetic susceptibility from iron is much less pronounced and, therefore, its masking effect is less marked or negligible (Fig. 41.2A). It should also be known that conventional spin-echo (SE) images should be obtained rather than turbo SE images; turbo SE T2-weighted images are very poor in demonstrating the magnetic susceptibility effects.

A few studies have investigated the sensitivity and specificity of these MRI findings (21,22,26,27). There is general agreement that 1.5-T studies can detect putaminal abnormalities much more than 0.5-T studies; the specificity and positive predictive value are very high, and the sensitivity is lower, ranging from about 50% to 83% in a series studied with 1.5-T MRI (27).

In conclusion, the absence of these putaminal abnormalities does not exclude the diagnosis; however, in most cases, MRI may strongly support the diagnosis of MSA-P.

MSA-C

Pathologic examinations of MSA-C brains demonstrate that the atrophy involves the pons, the middle cerebellar peduncles, and the cerebellum, with the hemispheres more affected than the vermis. These findings of gross pathology are already diagnostic and can be demonstrated in living patients by MRI with T1-weighted images. Atrophy of the pons is better appreciated in the midline sagittal section (Fig. 41.4A), but coronal sections demonstrate the loss of

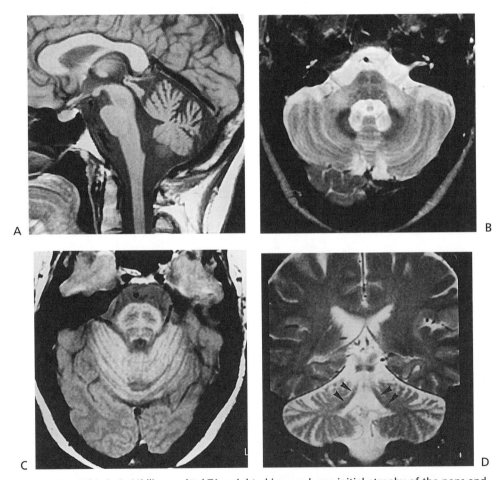

FIG. 41.4. MSA-C. **A:** Midline sagittal T1-weighted image shows initial atrophy of the pons and cerebellum. **B, C:** Axial T2-weighted and proton density images at different levels in a different patient show increased signal intensity of the pontine transverse fibers and middle cerebellar peduncles. The pyramidal tracts retain normal signal intensity. The proton density image at upper pontine level **(C)** demonstrates more clearly hyperintensity of transverse pontine fibers and cerebellar cortex. **D:** Coronal T2-weighted image in another patient shows hyperintensity of the whole cerebellum; superior cerebellar peduncles retain normal signal intensity *(arrowheads)*.

the rounded aspect of the lateral parts of the pons that become pointed because of the atrophy of the middle cerebellar peduncles (28).

However, microscopic examination shows additional findings. There is a loss of neurons in the pontine nuclei and degeneration of their fibers, which run in the pons as transverse pontine fibers. These fibers cross the midline in the raphe, are arranged in bundles mostly in the anterior and posterior part of the basis pontis, and reach the cerebellum through the middle cerebellar peduncles. In the cerebellum there is significant loss of Purkinje cells and degeneration of their fibers to the dentate nuclei; the whole cerebellum becomes gliotic. However, the dentate nuclei do not degenerate; therefore, their fibers, which run through the superior cerebellar peduncles to the red nuclei and thalami, remain intact. The last finding—cell loss and gliosis of the inferior olives—seems to be a secondary phenomenon caused by retrograde degeneration following cortical cerebellar lesions.

MRI demonstrates slight to moderate increase in signal intensity in proton density and T2-weighted images exactly in the same distribution as the pathologic findings, that is, in transverse pontine fibers, middle cerebellar peduncles, and cerebellum. The fiber tracts and areas that do not degenerate (superior and inferior cerebellar peduncles, corticospinal tracts, pontine tegmentum) maintain their normal signal intensity and therefore stand out against the abnormal background (10,28) (Fig. 41.4B–D). In good-quality studies, mild hyperintensity in proton density images may also be recognized in the inferior olives.

Two suggestions regarding diagnosis in early stages of the disease can be made: (a) in midline sagittal section, the first sign of atrophy of the pons is flattening of its inferior part, with loss of its normal bulging over the medulla oblongata (Fig. 41.4A); and (b) when the increased signal intensity of the cerebellum in T2-weighted images is slight or poorly appreciable in transverse sections, one should obtain coronal sections that allow easy comparison with the normal signal intensity of supratentorial structures (10,28) (Fig. 41.4D).

The excellent correlation of atrophy and signal abnormalities distribution (observed now in about 100 cases) with the pathologic changes of MSA-C makes MRI a reliable diagnostic tool. Doubtful MRI findings may of course be seen in initial, clinically suspected cases of MSA-C; in such cases, the findings became clearly abnormal on follow-up studies, together with clinical progression of the disease (10).

The sensitivity and specificity of these posterior fossa abnormalities are high in most studies (21,22,26). In the review made by Schrag et al. (22), 83% of the patients with MSA-C could be classified unequivocally based on these MRI findings. However, specificity may become lower if, in addition to considering patients with sporadic ataxias or atypical parkinsonian disorders, we also include patients with hereditary ataxias. Patients with spinocere-

bellar ataxias type 1, 2, and 3 (SCA1, SCA2, and SCA3 or Machado-Joseph disease) have been reported to present these same findings, generally with milder severity, in a large number of cases (29,30). In fact, there is considerable overlap of the pathologic changes seen in these hereditary diseases and in sporadic MSA-C that MRI, obviously, cannot discriminate. Clinical presentation, family history, the course of the disease, and molecular genetic studies must all be taken into account when the MRI findings are clinically evaluated.

PROGRESSIVE SUPRANUCLEAR PALSY

Pathologic observations of PSP brains demonstrate atrophy of the midbrain; this finding was also recognized in neuroradiologic studies even at the time of pneumoencephalography. Computed tomography (CT) may also demonstrate midbrain atrophy.

Our first series of PSP patients studied with MRI (5) was expanded to 28 cases in a subsequent review (31). The essential MRI features remained unchanged after the addition of cases. However, because of the learning curve, the percentage of patients in whom midbrain atrophy was recognized increased considerably (31).

When slight but unquestionable atrophic changes are included, midbrain atrophy is present in the large majority of the clinically diagnosed PSP cases: 89% in our series published by Soliveri et al. (31), 77% in the series by Schrag et al. (22). Atrophy is more recognizable in sagittal than in transverse sections because it also involves the height of the mesencephalon (Fig. 41.5A). Three characteristic features should be looked for:

1. *Thinning of the cranial part of the midbrain tectum.* More significant atrophy in this region probably correlates with the gaze abnormalities seen in these patients.
2. *Concave aspect of the floor of the third ventricle (i.e., of the upper profile of the midbrain)*, associated with disproportionate enlargement of the third, compared with the lateral ventricles, observed in axial section. This simply demonstrates atrophy of the diencephalon in addition to that of the midbrain.
3. *Hyperextension of the head.* This last aspect sometimes catches the eye of the observer, who can make a brilliant diagnosis by immediately verifying the presence of the other characteristic findings of PSP. As a matter of fact, the head of the patient is normally positioned by the technician but becomes hyperextended during the examination.

Signal abnormalities are very subtle. The most common, which in our series was recognizable in 60% of the cases (31), is a slightly increased signal intensity in proton density and T2-weighted images in the periaqueductal area, where gliosis is present in pathologic specimens (Fig.

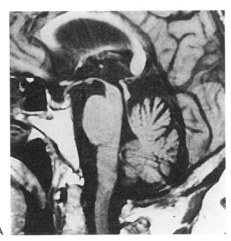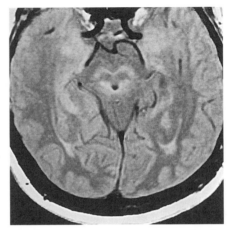

A   B

FIG. 41.5. Progressive supranuclear palsy. **A:** Midline sagittal T1-weighted section shows midbrain atrophy with thinning of the cranial part of the tectum and slightly concave floor of the third ventricle; compare with normal-size midbrain of Fig. 41.4A. **B:** Proton density image shows tectal, periaqueductal hyperintensity.

41.5B). At high field intensity in T2-weighted images, smudging of the hypointensity of the substantia nigra toward the red nucleus can be seen, as in other parkinsonian syndromes (10).

Abnormalities in the putamen are not seen in PSP. Of the 15 patients studied with 1.5-T MRI, only two had significant hypointensity in the putamen. One was 79 years old, and at that age the finding may be normal. The other, a patient of 66, had putaminal hypointensity but without the lateral rim of hyperintensity—a finding that remains characteristic of MSA. In this connection, we would like to mention that in one pathologically proven PSP brain, both Perls' stain and postmortem MRI did not show iron in the putamen (10). Pallidal hyperintensity, sometimes taking on the aspect of the "eye-of-the-tiger" sign, has been reported (22,32).

In PSP, supratentorial diffuse atrophy is present in many patients, mostly in the temporal and frontal lobes (22), but is less severe than that seen in CBD and without asymmetries (31). Some areas of periventricular hyperintensity may also be seen, not in excess to what is usually observed in patients of the same age.

On MR spectroscopy (MRS), *N*-acetylaspartate (NAA) reduction in the lentiform nucleus, predominantly in the pallidum, has been observed (32).

In conclusion, characteristic MRI findings may be observed in PSP patients; with increased experience, slight midbrain atrophy can be detected, so that MRI becomes helpful in establishing the diagnosis in about 80% of the cases (22,31). A simple measurement that may accurately differentiate PSP from PD has recently been proposed (33). Of interest is the fact that a few cases we observed with clinical features pointing in part to MSA and in part to PSP presented mixed MRI abnormalities, possibly indicating the coexistence of the two disorders.

CORTICOBASAL DEGENERATION

Corticobasal degeneration (CBD), first described by Rebeiz et al. in 1968, is a progressive disorder characterized by asymmetrical akinetic-rigid syndrome, apraxia, dysarthria, and dysphagia; the "alien limb" phenomenon is often a very impressive sign. Gross pathology is characterized by cortical atrophy in the posterior frontal and parietal regions, more marked on the side contralateral to the clinically more affected limbs. On microscopic examination, severe neuronal loss is found in the atrophic cortex; microglial proliferation and presence of swollen achromatic cells, similar to those seen in Pick's disease but lacking in Pick bodies, are also found. Neuronal loss and gliosis are also present in the striatum, substantia nigra, red nucleus, midbrain tegmentum, and lateral thalamic nucleus, slightly more marked on the side of the affected cortex.

We have reviewed the MRI findings of 16 patients with clinical diagnosis of CBD (31). All of the patients showed diffuse cerebral atrophy, more marked in the superior frontal and parietal regions, definitely asymmetric, more marked on the side contralateral to clinical symptoms (Fig. 41.6). Particularly the coronal sections showed loss of the bulk of white matter on the atrophic side, with enlargement of the ipsilateral ventricle. Thinning of the cortex was probably present in the atrophic regions, but it appeared definite in only two cases. In six patients, slight hyperintensity in proton density and T2-weighted images in the white matter of the frontoparietal regions of the affected, atrophic hemisphere was observed; signal changes in the atrophic cortex were more difficult to detect and better seen in proton density images. Hyperintensity of the cerebrospinal fluid (CSF) masked a possible hyperintensity in T2-weighted images (Fig. 41.6). Hyperintensity in diffusion-weighted images in the frontopari-

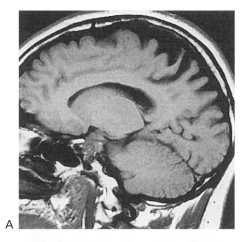

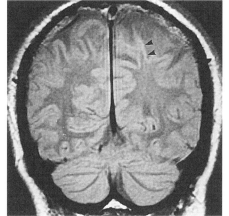

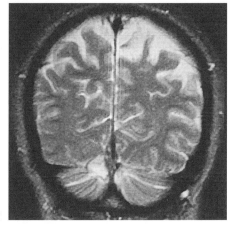

FIG. 41.6. Corticobasal degeneration, with clinical signs on the right side. Sagittal, left paramedian T1-weighted image. **(A)** Posterior frontal and parietal atrophy. Coronal proton density and T2-weighted images. **(B, C,** adjacent sections) Atrophy in left parietal region, with cortical thinning and hyperintensity (*arrowheads,* **B**).

etal white matter, more severe on the affected hemisphere, has been described (34).

We were unable to detect signal abnormalities in the basal ganglia or other regions in 0.5-T MRI studies that were more numerous. In three of the seven studies done with 1.5-T equipment, hypointensity in T2-weighted images was present in the putamina, inferior or equal to that seen in the pallidum; in two of these patients, putaminal hypointensity was slightly more marked on the side contralateral to the more affected limbs. It will be interesting to collect larger series studied with high field intensity MRI to verify the frequency of these findings. It is worth noting that in one 76-year-old clinically diagnosed CBD patient, the eye-of-the-tiger sign in the globi pallidi was observed (35).

Because of the clinical similarities observed in initial cases of CBD and PSP, we paid particular attention to the midbrain; only one patient of this series had mild atrophy of the midbrain (31). Therefore, absence of midbrain atrophy is very important in differentiating CBD from PSP.

It is worth mentioning that asymmetry of the parietal atrophy was not described in the first MRI report of the first cases of this series (36). Only when we became aware of the possible presence of asymmetries were we able to reg-

ularly detect them without knowing the clinically affected side. This fact again demonstrates that in degenerative disorders, in which the MRI findings are often subtle, awareness of the pathologic features of a disease is essential; otherwise MRI abnormalities are easily missed.

HUNTINGTON'S CHOREA

In Huntington's disease there is diffuse cerebral atrophy and even more severe atrophy of the striatum. Atrophy of the head of caudate nucleus causes dilatation of the frontal horns of the lateral ventricles with flattening of their lateral profile. This finding could be detected by neuroradiologists even with pneumoencephalography; CT essentially demonstrated the same findings, whereas MRI may also demonstrate the atrophy of the putamen, which is difficult to recognize on CT scan. Morphometric MRI studies have indeed demonstrated that in Huntington's disease, putaminal atrophy exceeds the caudate atrophy and may identify mutation-positive subjects up to 6 years prior to the estimated age of clinical onset (37).

For several years, signal abnormalities were not mentioned in the literature. Hyperintensity in the neostriatum, head of caudate nucleus, and putamen was first reported by us in the rigid form of the disease (38). The hyperintensity, seen both in proton density and T2-weighted images, was moderate or slight, but always easily recognizable by comparing the signal of the putamen with that of the adjacent insular cortex (Fig. 41.7). Patients with the hyperkinetic form of Huntington's disease had normal signal intensity; no hypointensity was seen even in our more recent cases studied at 1.5 T, whereas hypointensity has been reported by Rutledge et al. (3).

The pathologic findings that correlate with rigidity are controversial; however, it is generally accepted that a more marked neuronal loss is present in the putamen of patients with the rigid variant (39). Because the patients with the rigid form tend to be younger, early onset of the disease may have a role in determining more marked pathologic changes in the neostriatum reflected by the MRI signal abnormalities. In fact, a report on juvenile Huntington's disease (40) describes three patients studied with MRI who had neostriatal atrophy and hyperintensity; two of them had rigidity.

With the increase in the number of cases studied by MRI, patients classified as hyperkinetic with signal abnormalities were found. Our review of 32 subjects with Huntington's disease demonstrated that the 6 rigid patients and 7 of the 26 with the classic form had hyperintensity in the neostriatum (41). Splitting the hyperkinetic group into patients with and patients without signal abnormalities, we found that the patients classified as hyperkinetic with signal abnormalities were significantly different from the patients without signal abnormalities; they had less hyperkinesia and more akinesia and mental deterioration, and were therefore halfway between the rigid and the more hyperkinetic patients.

Atrophy of the putamen has been reported to be greater in the akinetic-rigid form of Huntington's disease (39); increase of bicaudate diameter (i.e., atrophy of the caudate)

was more marked in our rigid versus hyperkinetic patients. We can conclude that neostriatal atrophy and abnormal signal intensity seen in Huntington's patients are the expression of greater anatomic damage that occurs in akinetic-rigid patients and correlates with more severe motor and cognitive impairment (41).

A few investigators have studied metabolic abnormalities in patients with Huntington's disease with proton MRS, demonstrating decreased NAA and increased lactate in the occipital cortex and the striatum (42). An interesting study on presymptomatic gene carriers and advanced akinetic patients with ^{1}H MRS has been reported by Sánchez-Pernaute et al. (43); hyperkinetic patients were deliberately excluded. These investigators found a marked reduction of NAA and creatine in both groups of patients, particularly in the advanced group; however, reduction of the metabolites was also significant in the presymptomatic patients. Creatine reduction, which suggests an impairment of energy metabolism, correlated with performance in cognitive tests and with the length of CAG expansion. The authors propose that the creatine signal be used as a marker for progression in Huntington's disease.

WILSON'S DISEASE

Wilson's disease is an autosomal recessive disease of copper metabolism, in which copper accumulates in several organs, primarily liver and brain. Clinical presentation, when neurologic, usually consists of various movement disorders, but behavioral abnormalities or intellectual deterioration may occasionally mark the onset of the disease. The neuroradiologist might, therefore, be the first physician to propose the correct diagnosis on MRI examination; for this reason, it is very important to be familiar with the characteristic MRI findings of Wilson's disease.

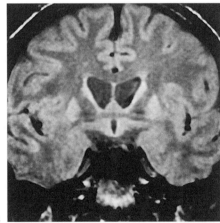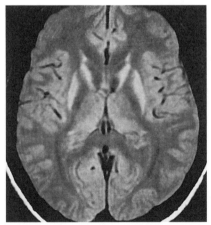

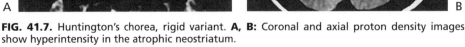

FIG. 41.7. Huntington's chorea, rigid variant. **A, B:** Coronal and axial proton density images show hyperintensity in the atrophic neostriatum.

Pathologic changes consist of shrinkage and a light brown discoloration of the lenticular nuclei where neuronal loss and degeneration of myelinated fibers are present. These changes may also involve the caudate, the substantia nigra, and the dentate nuclei. Marked astrocytic hyperplasia is found in the basal ganglia, thalami, cerebral cortex, brainstem, and cerebellum. In advanced cases, cavitations may develop in the lentiform nuclei, mainly in the putamina. Copper deposition is present in basal ganglia, where microhemorrhages may also occur when destructive changes develop in severely affected cases. Therefore, two main types of signal abnormalities are expected and indeed found on MRI scans of patients with Wilson's disease.

The first and by far the most common type of signal abnormality is high signal intensity in proton density and T2-weighted images in the basal ganglia (mainly in the putamina), lateral part of the thalami, midbrain (substantia nigra, red nuclei, and periaqueductal area), and pons. The involvement of the putamen is often more marked on its outer rim, which appears markedly hyperintense and swollen in T2-weighted images; in a few instances, the external capsule and the claustrum are distinctly involved

(44). The pons, which is the second most commonly involved area (44,45), may be affected either in the basis or in the tegmentum, or both. Cerebral white matter, corpus callosum, corticospinal tracts (particularly at the level of the internal capsule), middle cerebellar peduncles, and dentatorubrothalamic tracts running in the superior cerebellar peduncles are less frequently affected (44,46). These abnormalities are probably caused by neuronal loss, gliosis, degeneration of fibers, and vacuolization that are associated with increased water content of the tissue (Fig. 41.8A, B). In T1-weighted images, these lesions are hypointense and less evident; however, T1 hypointensity is marked if cystic degeneration and cavitations are present.

The second and more unusual type of MRI change has a more limited distribution and consists of decrease or loss of signal intensity in T2-weighted images in the putamen, pallidum, and, even more rarely, in the head of the caudate nucleus, likely caused by deposition of copper or iron (Fig. 41.8C). The pattern of distribution of these signal abnormalities is often characteristic; the loss of signal intensity is located in the central part of the nucleus involved, whereas the border is hyperintense, giving the general appearance of

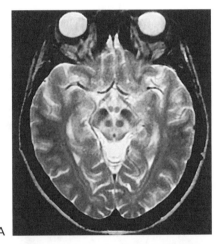

A

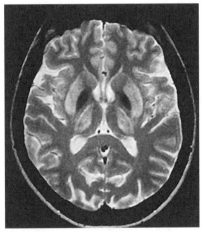

B

C

FIG. 41.8. Wilson's disease. Axial T2-weighted images. **A, B:** Hyperintensity in the midbrain surrounding the red nuclei and, at level of the basal ganglia, in the lateral part of the thalami and putamina. Pallidal hypointensity **(B)** is more marked than that usually seen in a 26-year-old patient. In a different patient, the basal ganglia on a T2-weighted image **(C)** exhibit marked hypointensity in the putamina and heads of the caudate nuclei, probably caused by copper deposition, surrounded by a hyperintense halo *(arrows)*. Mild abnormalities are also present in the lateral parts of the thalami and posterior periventricular white matter. (Courtesy of Dr. N. Colombo, Milano.)

a hyperintense halo surrounding the signal loss (47,48). In other, probably more severely involved cases, the putamen is shrunk and the hypointensity is more irregular and patchy; the hyperintensity always tends to remain more peripheral. The loss of signal intensity, probably related to copper or both copper and iron, is more visible at high field intensity MRI, whereas it may be poorly demonstrated in 0.5-T studies.

Improvement in signal abnormalities after treatment may occur. This improvement mainly regards the hyperintensity; similarly, the hypodensity observed in the putamen on CT scans has been reported to decrease or disappear (49). An interesting observation was made by Engelbrecht et al. (50); after D-penicillamine therapy, the hyperintensity seen on MRI in proton density images in the lentiform nuclei, mostly in the putamina, and in the lateral part of the thalami almost disappeared, whereas the hypointensity of T2-weighted images became more evident and extended to the whole lentiform nuclei. Because clinical improvement was associated with urinary copper excretion, these authors suggested that iron deposition in exchange for copper might explain these findings. However, rarity or absence of T2 hypointensity has been noted in a series of treated patients (44). MRI studies in untreated patients with clinical, imaging, and laboratory follow-up in the course of treatment are needed to possibly clarify the substrate of the signal changes.

Finally, a third type of signal change may be seen in T1-weighted images: hyperintensity in the pallidum, sometimes extending caudally along a tract to the substantia nigra, or more rarely in the thalami (44,45). Pallidal T1 hyperintensity is seen in patients who have severe liver failure and portosystemic shunt. The explanation for this peculiar T1 hyperintensity is not completely clear, although the hyperintensity may be attributable to manganese, because of analogies with other portosystemic encephalopathies and with similar MRI findings observed in patients undergoing long-term parenteral nutrition (51,52). However, a few patients with Wilson's disease who exhibited this finding did not have significant abnormalities in liver function; therefore, the shortened T1 relaxation time of these patients with Wilson's disease has been tentatively attributed to a paramagnetic effect of copper, which may be reversible with removal of copper following treatment (44).

HALLERVORDEN-SPATZ DISEASE

Hallervorden-Spatz disease is a rare neurologic disorder in which the possibility of diagnostic studies with MRI was expected. In fact, since the early descriptions of the disease, it has been known that the pallidum presents a brown pigmentation caused by deposits of iron. Because various disorders that share similar clinical features may be

included, the term Hallervorden-Spatz syndrome has also been used (53).

The disease is inherited as an autosomal recessive trait and starts in late childhood or early adolescence. Dystonia with oromandibular involvement, mental deterioration, pyramidal signs, and retinal degeneration are the main clinical features (54). No biological markers have been found. A gene associated with Hallervorden-Spatz syndrome has been mapped to chromosome 20p12.3-p13 (53). Neuraxonal dystrophy with swollen axon fragments is present in the pallidum but not outside the brain; therefore, skin or conjunctival biopsy is not helpful, as in other neuraxonal dystrophies.

The deposits of iron in the form of granules in the vessel walls or free in the tissue are mainly located in the pallidum, but may be found in lesser amounts in the substantia nigra and red nuclei. Dystrophic axons, residual neurons, and reactive astrocytes have the same distribution but may also be seen in other parts of the basal ganglia (55).

As in other diseases in which magnetic susceptibility effects have an important diagnostic role, MRI again shows different findings at 0.5 and 1.5 T. At both field intensities, the abnormalities are confined to the pallidum: high signal intensity in T2-weighted images in 0.5-T studies, and prevalent marked low intensity in 1.5-T examinations. However, even in the 1.5-T scans, a small area in the medial anterior part of the pallidum remains hyperintense (Fig. 41.9A, B). This finding, called the "eye-of-the-tiger" sign by Sethi et al. (56), is characteristic of Hallervorden-Spatz disease. This peculiar topographic distribution is explained by the pathologic observation that the tissue of the pallidum is not uniformly abnormal in Hallervorden-Spatz disease. The tissue is somewhat "loose," with vacuolization and small amounts of iron in the most medial anterior part, where hyperintensity is seen on MRI; it is more "dense," with no vacuoles and more abundant deposits of iron, in the remaining part, which appears markedly hypointense at high field intensity MRI (55) (Fig. 41.9C).

A "pupil" in the eye-of-the-tiger, that is, a central spot of hypointensity in the hyperintense area, that we observed in three of our cases may be attributed to calcifications. In fact, high-density spots were present on CT in the same position. Marked hypointensity was present in proton density images, with moderate decrease in T2-weighted images, while the surrounding pallidal tissue, where iron is expected to be present, exhibited a dramatic change from proton density to T2-weighted images (55).

In conclusion, even if similar pallidal abnormalities have occasionally been reported in other extrapyramidal syndromes (32,35), we believe that the MRI findings described here coincide so neatly with the distribution and the characteristics of the pathologic changes of Hallervorden-Spatz disease as to become pathognomonic, at least in children and adolescents.

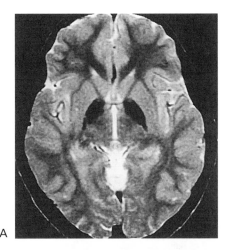
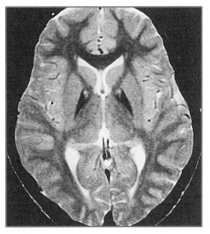

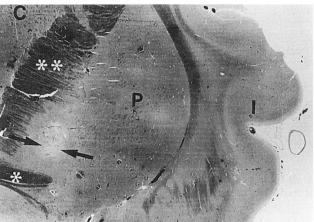

FIG. 41.9. Hallervorden-Spatz disease. **A, B:** Axial, contiguous T2-weighted sections show very marked pallidal hypointensity in a 10-year-old girl. The cranial anteromedial part of the pallidum is hyperintense because of vacuolization and absence of iron. Compare with pallor in this area *(arrows)* in the coronal histologic section **(C)** Heidenhain's myelin stain. P, putamen; I, insula; C, caudate nucleus; *, anterior commissure; **, internal capsule. (From Savoiardo M, Halliday WC, Nardocci N, et al. Hallervorden-Spatz disease: MR and pathologic findings. *Am J Neuroradiol* 1993;14:155–162, with permission.)

CONCLUSION

The MRI findings of movement disorders are often highly characteristic or even pathognomonic; their contribution in establishing a definite diagnosis cannot be dismissed. Even when the diagnosis is established with certainty by genetic studies, variations in the clinical phenotypes may be observed. Together with the clinical phenotype, the "MRI phenotype" should be taken into consideration. By adding this variable, a better and more complete understanding of the patient may be reached.

ACKNOWLEDGMENTS

We are very grateful to Dr. F. Girotti, neurologist, for his innumerable contributions on neurodegenerative disorders and helpful criticism.

REFERENCES

1. Drayer BP, Olanow W, Burger P, et al. Parkinson plus syndrome: diagnosis using high field MR imaging of brain iron. *Radiology* 1986;159:493–498.
2. Pastakia B, Polinsky R, Di Chiro G, et al. Multiple system atrophy (Shy-Drager syndrome): MR imaging. *Radiology* 1986;159:499–502.
3. Rutledge JN, Hilal SK, Silver AJ, et al. Study of movement disorders and brain iron by MR. *Am J Neuroradiol* 1987;8:397–411.
4. Drayer BP. Imaging of the aging brain. Part II. Pathologic conditions. *Radiology* 1988;166:797–806.
5. Savoiardo M, Strada L, Girotti F, et al. MR imaging in progressive supranuclear palsy and Shy-Drager syndrome. *J Comput Assist Tomogr* 1989;13:555–560.
6. Gilman S, Low PA, Quinn N, et al. Consensus statement on the diagnosis of multiple system atrophy. *J Auton Nerv Syst* 1998;74:189–192.
7. Sofic E, Paulus W, Jellinger K, et al. Selective increase of iron in substantia nigra zona compacta of parkinsonian brains. *J Neurochem* 1991;56:978–982.

8. Braffman BH, Grossman RI, Goldberg HI, et al. MR imaging of Parkinson disease with spin-echo and gradient-echo sequences. *Am J Neuroradiol* 1988;9:1093–1099.

9. Gorell JM, Ordidge RJ, Brown GG, et al. Increased iron-related MRI contrast in the substantia nigra in Parkinson's disease. *Neurology* 1995;45:1138–1143.

10. Savoiardo M, Girotti F, Strada L, et al. Magnetic resonance imaging in progressive supranuclear palsy and other parkinsonian disorders. *J Neural Transm* 1994;42[Suppl]:93–110.

11. Hutchinson M, Raff U. Structural changes of the substantia nigra in Parkinson's disease as revealed by MR imaging. *Am J Neuroradiol* 2000;21:697–701.

12. Hu MTM, White SJ, Herlihy AH, et al. A comparison of ^{18}F-dopa PET and inversion recovery MRI in the diagnosis of Parkinson's disease. *Neurology* 2001;56:1195–1200.

13. Sabatini U, Boulanouar K, Fabre N, et al. Cortical motor reorganization in akinetic patients with Parkinson's disease: a functional MRI study. *Brain* 2000;123:394–403.

14. Haslinger B, Erhard P, Kämpfe N, et al. Event-related functional magnetic resonance imaging in Parkinson's disease before and after levodopa. *Brain* 2001;124:558–570.

15. Bejjani B, Dormont D, Pidoux B, et al. Bilateral subthalamic stimulation for Parkinson's disease by using three-dimensional stereotactic magnetic resonance imaging and electrophysiological guidance. *J Neurosurg* 2000;92:615–625.

16. Lang AE. Surgery for Parkinson disease: a critical evaluation of the state of the art. *Arch Neurol* 2000;57:1118–1125.

17. Brown NT, Polinsky RJ, Di Chiro G, et al. MRI in autonomic failure. *J Neurol Neurosurg Psychiatry* 1987;50:913–914.

18. Perani D, Bressi S, Testa D, et al. Clinical/metabolic correlations in multiple system atrophy: a fludeoxyglucose F18 positron emission tomographic study. *Arch Neurol* 1995;52:179–185.

19. Dexter DT, Carayon A, Javoy-Agid F, et al. Alterations in the levels of iron, ferritin, and other trace metals in Parkinson's disease and other neurodegenerative diseases affecting the basal ganglia. *Brain* 1991;114:1953–1975.

20. Goto S, Matsumoto S, Ushio Y, et al. Subregional loss of putaminal efferents to the basal ganglia output nuclei may cause parkinsonism in striatonigral degeneration. *Neurology* 1996;47: 1032–1036.

21. Schrag A, Kingsley D, Phatouros C, et al. Clinical usefulness of magnetic resonance imaging in multiple system atrophy. *J Neurol Neurosurg Psychiatry* 1998;65:65–71.

22. Schrag A, Good CD, Miszkiel K, et al. Differentiation of atypical parkinsonian syndromes with routine MRI. *Neurology* 2000; 54:697–702.

23. Fearnley JM, Lees AJ. Striatonigral degeneration: a clinicopathological study. *Brain* 1990;113:1823–1842.

24. Lang AE, Curran T, Provias J, et al. Striatonigral degeneration: iron deposition in putamen correlates with the slit-like void signal of magnetic resonance imaging. *Can J Neurol Sci* 1994;21:311–318.

25. Kraft E, Schwarz J, Trenkwalder C, et al. The combination of hypointense and hyperintense signal changes on T2-weighted magnetic resonance imaging sequences: a specific marker of multiple system atrophy? *Arch Neurol* 1999;56:225–228.

26. Testa D, Savoiardo M, Fetoni V, et al. Multiple system atrophy: clinical and MR observations on 42 cases. *Ital J Neurol Sci* 1993; 14:211–216.

27. Antonini A, Benti R, Righini A, et al. Sensitivity and specificity of ECD/SPECT and high field (1.5 T) MRI in the differential diagnosis between MSA and Parkinson's disease. *Neurology* 1999; 52[Suppl 2]:A351–A352.

28. Savoiardo M, Strada L, Girotti F, et al. Olivopontocerebellar atrophy: MR diagnosis and relationship to multisystem atrophy. *Radiology* 1990;174:693–696.

29. Bürk K, Abele M, Fetter M, et al. Autosomal dominant cerebellar ataxia type I. Clinical features and MRI in families with SCA 1, SCA 2, and SCA 3. *Brain* 1996;119:1497–1505.

30. Murata Y, Yamaguchi S, Kawakami H, et al. Characteristic magnetic resonance imaging findings in Machado-Joseph disease. *Arch Neurol* 1998;55:33–37.

31. Soliveri P, Monza D, Paridi D, et al. Cognitive and magnetic resonance imaging aspects of corticobasal degeneration and progressive supranuclear palsy. *Neurology* 1999;53:502–507.

32. Davie CA, Barker GJ, Machado C, et al. Proton magnetic resonance spectroscopy in Steele-Richardson-Olszewski syndrome. *Mov Disord* 1997;12:767–771.

33. Warmuth-Metz M, Naumann M, Csoti I, et al. Measurement of the midbrain diameter on routine magnetic resonance imaging: a simple and accurate method of differentiating between Parkinson disease and progressive supranuclear palsy. *Arch Neurol* 2001;58: 1076–1079.

34. Ikeda K, Iwasaki Y, Ichikawa Y. Cognitive and MRI aspects of corticobasal degeneration and progressive supranuclear palsy [letter]. *Neurology* 2000;54:1878.

35. Molinuevo JL, Muñoz E, Valldeoriola F, et al. The eye of the tiger sign in cortical-basal ganglionic degeneration. *Mov Disord* 1999; 14:169–171.

36. Grisoli M, Fetoni V, Savoiardo M, et al. MRI in corticobasal degeneration. *Eur J Neurol* 1995;2:547–552.

37. Harris GJ, Codori AM, Lewis RF, et al. Reduced basal ganglia blood flow and volume in pre-symptomatic, gene-tested persons at-risk for Huntington's disease. *Brain* 1999;122:1667–1678.

38. Savoiardo M, Strada L, Oliva D, et al. Abnormal MRI signal in the rigid form of Huntington's disease. *J Neurol Neurosurg Psychiatry* 1991;54:888–891.

39. Albin RL, Reiner A, Anderson KD, et al. Striatal and nigral neuron subpopulations in rigid Huntington's disease: implications for the functional anatomy of chorea and rigidity-akinesia. *Ann Neurol* 1990;27:357–365.

40. Ho VB, Chuang HS, Rovira MJ, et al. Juvenile Huntington disease: CT and MR features. *Am J Neuroradiol* 1995;16:1405–1412.

41. Oliva D, Carella F, Savoiardo M, et al. Clinical and magnetic resonance features of the classic and akinetic-rigid variants of Huntington's disease. *Arch Neurol* 1993;50:17–19.

42. Jenkins BG, Rosas HD, Chen Y-CI, et al. ^{1}H NMR spectroscopy studies of Huntington's disease: correlations with CAG repeat numbers. *Neurology* 1998;50:1357–1365.

43. Sánchez-Pernaute R, García-Segura JM, del Barrio Alba A, et al. Clinical correlation of striatal ^{1}H MRS changes in Huntington's disease. *Neurology* 1999;53:806–812.

44. King AD, Walshe JM, Kendall BE, et al. Cranial MR imaging in Wilson's disease. *Am J Roentgenol* 1996;167:1579–1584.

45. Saatci I, Topcu M, Baltaoglu FF, et al. Cranial MR findings in Wilson's disease. *Acta Radiol* 1997;38:250–258.

46. van Wassenaer-van Hall HN, van den Heuvel AG, Jansen GH, et al. Cranial MR in Wilson disease: abnormal white matter in extrapyramidal and pyramidal tracts. *Am J Neuroradiol* 1995;16: 2021–2027.

47. Magalhaes ACA, Caramelli P, Menezes JR, et al. Wilson's disease: MRI with clinical correlation. *Neuroradiology* 1994;36:97–100.

48. van Wassenaer-van Hall HN, van den Heuvel AG, Algra A, et al. Wilson disease: findings at MR imaging and CT of the brain with clinical correlation. *Radiology* 1996;198:531–536.

49. Nazer H, Brismar J, Al-Kawi MZ, et al. Magnetic resonance imaging of the brain in Wilson's disease. *Neuroradiology* 1993; 35:130–133.

50. Engelbrecht V, Schlaug G, Hefter H, et al. MRI of the brain in Wilson disease: T2 signal loss under therapy. *J Comput Assist Tomogr* 1995;19:635–638.

51. Inoue E, Hori S, Narumi Y, et al. Portal-systemic encephalopathy: presence of basal ganglia lesions with high signal intensity on MR images. *Radiology* 1991;179:551–555.

52. Mirowitz SA, Westrich TJ, Hirsch JD. Hyperintense basal ganglia on T1-weighted images in patients receiving parenteral nutrition. *Radiology* 1991;181:117–120.

53. Guillerman RP. The eye-of-the-tiger sign. *Radiology* 2000;217:895–896.

54. Angelini L, Nardocci N, Rumi V, et al. Hallervorden-Spatz disease: clinical and MRI study in eleven cases diagnosed in life. *J Neurol* 1992;239:417–425.

55. Savoiardo M, Halliday WC, Nardocci N, et al. Hallervorden-Spatz disease: MR and pathologic findings. *Am J Neuroradiol* 1993;14:155–162.

56. Sethi KD, Adams RJ, Loring DW, et al. Hallervorden-Spatz syndrome: clinical and magnetic resonance imaging correlations. *Ann Neurol* 1988;24:692–694.

Reference Added in Proof

Righini A, Antonini A, Ferrarini M, et al. Thin section MR study of the basal ganglia in the differential diagnosis between striatonigral degeneration and Parkinson disease. *J Comput Assist Tomogr* 2002;26:266–271.

MOVEMENT DISORDERS: FUNCTIONAL IMAGING

DAVID J. BROOKS

Functional imaging provides a sensitive means of detecting and characterizing the regional changes in brain metabolism and receptor binding associated with movement disorders. It can be of diagnostic value and also help to throw light on the pathophysiology underlying parkinsonian syndromes and involuntary movements. Functional imaging also provides a means of detecting subclinical disease in subjects at-risk for degenerative disorders and of objectively following disease progression. There are four main approaches to functional imaging: Positron emission tomography (PET) has the highest sensitivity and currently a resolution of 3 to 5 mm, and allows quantitative in vivo examination of alterations in regional cerebral blood flow (rCBF); glucose, oxygen, and dopa metabolism and brain pharmacology. Single photon emission computed tomography (SPECT), which is less sensitive but more widely available, provides measures of rCBF and receptor binding. Magnetic resonance spectroscopy (MRS) has a lower sensitivity and spatial resolution than the two radioimaging approaches and provides measures at a millimolar level of metabolite levels (N-acetylaspartate (NAA), lactate, phospholipids, ATP). Finally, magnetic resonance imaging (MRI) can detect activation-induced changes in blood oxygenation to brain regions when subjects perform tasks—the so-called BOLD (blood oxygenation level dependent) technique.

The changes in regional cerebral function that characterize the different movement disorders can be examined in two main ways: First, focal changes in resting levels of regional cerebral metabolism, blood flow, and neuroreceptor availability can be measured. Second, abnormal patterns of brain activation can be demonstrated when patients with movement disorders perform motor and cognitive tasks. Because the majority of functional imaging research into brain function in movement disorders has, to date, concerned PET and SPECT, this chapter will concentrate on these techniques but will address functional MRI (fMRI) and proton MRS findings where relevant.

PARKINSON'S DISEASE

The pathology of Parkinson's disease (PD) targets the dopamine cells in the substantia nigra in association with the formation of neuronal Lewy inclusion bodies. Serotonergic cells in the median raphe and noradrenergic cells in the locus ceruleus are also involved as are other pigmented and brainstem nuclei (1). Loss of cells from the substantia nigra in PD results in profound dopamine depletion in the striatum, with the lateral nigral projections to putamen being most affected (2–4). While the pathology of PD targets subcortical nuclei, the anterior cingulate and association cortex are also involved, and currently it remains uncertain whether dementia of Lewy body type and PD represent ends of a spectrum. Dementia of Lewy body type has overlapping features with Alzheimer's disease though is associated with a higher prevalence of fluctuating confusion, hallucinations, early-onset rigidity, and gait difficulties (5).

Presynaptic Dopaminergic System

The function of dopamine terminals in PD can be examined in vivo in several ways: First, terminal dopa decarboxylase (DDC) activity can be measured with ^{18}F-dopa or ^{11}C-dopa PET (6,7). Second, the availability of presynaptic dopamine transporters (DATs) can be assessed with tropane-based PET and SPECT tracers (8,9). Third, vesicle monoamine transporter density in dopamine terminals can be examined with ^{11}C-dihydrotetrabenazine PET (10).

The first reports on striatal ^{18}F-dopa uptake in PD concerned early hemiparkinsonian cases (11). ^{18}F-dopa PET showed normal caudate but bilaterally reduced putamen tracer uptake, with activity being most depressed in the putamen contralateral to the affected limbs. These studies were the first demonstration that subclinical disease could be detected in PD by PET as evidenced by involvement of the "asymptomatic" putamen contralateral to clinically unaffected limbs. These observations were subsequently widely reproduced (6,12,13).

On average, PD patients show a 50% loss of specific putamen ^{18}F-dopa uptake (6) compared with a 60% to 80% loss of ventrolateral nigra compacta cells and 95% loss of putamen dopamine at postmortem examination (3). These findings suggest that striatal dopamine terminal DDC activity is relatively up-regulated in PD, presumably to boost dopamine turnover by remaining neurons. Cases of early PD (Hoehn and Yahr stage 1) show a 40% loss of ^{18}F-dopa uptake in the putamen contralateral to the affected limbs (14), suggesting that this loss of DDC activity may represent the threshold for onset of symptoms.

It is known that the pathology of PD is not uniform, ventrolateral nigral dopaminergic projections to the dorsal putamen being more affected than dorsomedial projections to the head of caudate (4). ^{18}F-dopa PET reveals that in the striatum contralateral to "asymptomatic" limbs in patients with unilateral PD (H&Y stage 1) dorsal posterior putamen dopamine storage is first reduced (14). As all limbs become clinically affected, dorsal posterior putamen ^{18}F-dopa uptake falls further while ventral and anterior putamen and dorsal caudate function now become involved. Only when the disease is well established does ventral head of caudate ^{18}F-dopa uptake start to fall.

More recently, it has become apparent that not all dopamine fibers degenerate in early PD. Along with nigrostriatal dopamine projections there is also a lesser nigropallidal pathway. The striatum is the main input and the globus pallidus interna (GPi) the main output nucleus of the basal ganglia, and dopamine release modulates the function of both structures. Recent PET studies have established that GPi ^{18}F-dopa uptake initially increases in PD but subsequently falls as the disease advances and treatment complications, such as fluctuating responses to levodopa, are manifested (15). The mesofrontal dopamine fibers arise from the midbrain tegmentum and project to the orbitofrontal cortex, anterior cingulate, and amygdala. In early PD both anterior cingulate and amygdala show increases in ^{18}F-dopa uptake that subsequently normalize (16). It is known that lesioning the mesofrontal dopaminergic fibers with 6-hydroxydopamine in nonhuman primates leads to a reciprocal increase in K^+ evoked dopamine release from the caudate (17). It is, therefore, conceivable that, as the nigrostriatal dopaminergic system begins to degenerate in PD, there is an adaptive up-regulation of dopamine turnover in nigropallidal and mesofrontal dopaminergic pathways.

There are now a wealth of tropane-based tracers available for measuring DAT binding on nigrostriatal terminals that can be used to provide a measure of integrity of dopaminergic function in PD. PET tracers include ^{11}C-CFT (18), ^{18}F-CFT (8), and ^{11}C-RTI-32 (19), which bind to both dopamine and noradrenaline reuptake sites. Available SPECT tracers include the tropane analogs ^{123}I-β-CIT (9), ^{123}I-FP-CIT (20), ^{123}I-altropane (21), and ^{99m}Tc-TRODAT-1 (22). ^{123}I-β-CIT gives the highest striatal/cerebellar

uptake ratio of these SPECT tracers; however, it binds nonselectively to dopamine, noradrenaline, and serotonin transporters and has the disadvantage of requiring 24 hours to equilibrate throughout the brain following intravenous injection, so that scanning has to be delayed until the following day. In addition, the low cerebellar reference signal is difficult to quantitate accurately. For this reason, SPECT tracers such as ^{123}I-FP-CIT and ^{123}I-altropane have come into vogue as, despite their lower and time-dependent striatal/cerebellar uptake ratios, a diagnostic scan can be performed within 2 to 3 hours of tracer injection and all appear to differentiate clinically probable PD from normal subjects sensitively. More recently, a technetium-based tropane tracer, ^{99m}Tc-TRODAT-1, has been developed. This gives a lower striatal/cerebellar uptake ratio than the ^{123}I-based tracers and is less well extracted by the brain; however, it also appears to adequately discriminate established PD from normal and has the advantage of being readily available in kit form.

The above PET and SPECT ligands as well as the PET vesicle transporter marker ^{11}C-dihydrotetrabenazine (10) have been shown to discriminate clinically probable PD patients from normal subjects and essential tremor cases with greater than 90% specificity. Their striatal uptake shows an inverse correlation with degree of locomotor disability in PD correlating best with limb bradykinesia and poorly with tremor severity (20,23). Whereas all of these tracers are effective markers of loss of dopamine terminal function relative to the dopamine vesicle transporter marker ^{11}C-dihydrotetrabenazine, in a given PD population it has been shown that putamen ^{18}F-dopa uptake is up-regulated and binding of the DAT marker ^{11}C-methylphenidate down-regulated (24). This finding makes physiologic sense as increased dopamine turnover and decreased reuptake in a dopamine deficiency syndrome would help to preserve synaptic transmitter levels.

Detection of Preclinical Disease

It has been estimated from postmortem studies that for every patient who presents with clinical PD there may be 10 to 15 subclinical cases with incidental brainstem Lewy body disease in the community (25). Surveys of the prevalence of PD will inevitably fail to recognize these cases with subclinical pathology. The most likely subjects to be at risk of developing PD are relatives of patients with this disorder.

Piccini et al. (26) used ^{18}F-dopa PET to study 32 asymptomatic adult relatives in seven kindreds with familial PD. Each of these families contained at least two affected individuals with levodopa-responsive parkinsonism clinically indistinguishable from sporadic PD. In five of these kindreds the pathology was unknown, and the index cases had disease onset from the fourth to the seventh decades. The sixth kindred was subsequently found to have *parkin* gene mutations, whereas the seventh kindred was known to have diffuse Lewy body disease and was characterized by onset of parkinsonism in the fourth decade. Affected individuals from the six non-*parkin* kindreds all showed the typical pattern of reduced striatal ^{18}F-dopa uptake associated with sporadic PD; putamen tracer uptake was more severely reduced than caudate. The *parkin* cases showed a severe loss of both caudate and putamen dopamine storage. Eight of 32 asymptomatic adult relatives scanned showed levels of putamen ^{18}F-dopa uptake reduced more than 2.5 SD below the normal mean. Figure 42.1 shows striatal ^{18}F-dopa uptake for a normal control, a clinically affected member of the *parkin* kindred, and a sibling with preclinical disease. Five years after PET, three of the eight asymptomatic relatives with reduced putamen ^{18}F-dopa uptake had developed clinical parkinsonism.

Based on clinical surveys, a 15% prevalence is normally quoted for the presence of a positive family history in PD, although this approaches 40% if a fully informative history is available (27). Piccini's ^{18}F-dopa PET findings indicate that 25% of asymptomatic adult relatives of index cases with familial parkinsonism (i.e., 50% of the at-risk population) have evidence of dopaminergic dysfunction. This could arise from environmental causes as well as genetic susceptibility if the kindreds were exposed to some common environmental toxin.

The ^{18}F-dopa PET findings for 34 asymptomatic and two clinically concordant cotwins of affected PD patients aged 23 to 67 years have also been reported (28). Eighteen cotwins were monozygotic (MZ) whereas 16 were dizygotic (DZ). Ten (55%) of the 18 MZ and three (18%) of the 16 DZ cotwins had levels of putamen ^{18}F-dopa uptake that were reduced more than 2.5 SD below the normal mean, and all of these were assigned to a PD category by discriminant analysis. The finding of a significantly higher concordance (55% vs. 18%, $p = 0.03$) for dopaminergic dysfunction in MZ compared with DZ cotwins is more in favor of a genetic than an environmental contribution to PD where similar concordances would be expected. Interestingly, when

a subgroup of these cotwins were scanned serially, all 10 of the asymptomatic MZ cotwins (mean age 57.1 ± 13.6 years) scanned showed a progressive decrease in putamen ^{18}F-dopa uptake on repeat scanning; 4.0 ± 1.7 years after the first scan, the mean rate of the loss of putamen ^{18}F-dopa uptake was 4.5% per year. On the basis of their follow-up scans, three additional MZ cotwins were classified as having subclinical PD by discriminant analysis. Nine asymptomatic DZ cotwins (mean age 56.7 ± 15.2 years) were also scanned twice over a period of 4.3 ± 2.2 years but showed a nonsignificant mean reduction in putamen ^{18}F-dopa uptake of 1.0% per year. Only four of the nine DZ cotwins (two with subclinical dopaminergic dysfunction at baseline) showed any individual evidence of progression. The percentage annual loss in putamen ^{18}F-dopa uptake for MZ and DZ cotwins was significantly different ($p = 0.001$). Over the 7 years of follow-up, two MZ cotwins and one DZ cotwin died without developing symptoms, whereas four MZ cotwins became clinically concordant for PD (at 65, 70, 72, and 78 years of age, 14, 2, 9, and 20 years after the onset of PD in their cotwin), resulting in a clinical concordance of 22.2% at follow-up. The clinical concordance within the MZ pairs over 60 years of age was higher (50%; four of eight). None of the DZ twin pairs became clinically concordant and the difference in clinical concordance between the MZ and DZ twin pairs in the 60- to 70-year age group of age was significant ($p = 0.04$; Fisher's exact test).

However, despite the fact that these ^{18}F-dopa PET cotwin data support a genetic susceptibility for PD in apparently sporadic cases, they do not have the power to exclude an environmental cause for PD. Mitochondrial DNA is maternally transmitted and a disorder manifesting this form of inheritance would also be predicted to show equal concordances in MZ and DZ twins. Such an equal concordance has been reported in a study from Cologne where all five DZ and two MZ PD cotwins studied were said to have abnormal ^{18}F-dopa PET findings (29). However, this finding was based on a variety of different analytic approaches and so is somewhat hard to interpret. Piccini's

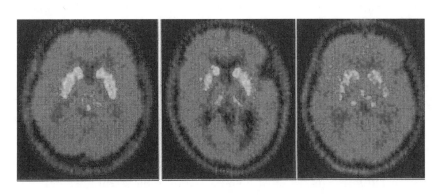

Control   **IPD**   **Parkin**

FIG. 42.1. PET images of striatal ^{18}F-dopa uptake collected 30 to 90 minutes after tracer administration for a normal control, a clinically affected Parkinson's disease patient with *parkin* disease, and his sibling with preclinical disease. (Picture courtesy of Drs. P. Piccini and N. Khan.) (See color section.)

findings cannot fully exclude PD arising from mitochondrial inheritance but, as there is no excess maternal transmission in PD, it seems unlikely that this disorder arises as a primary consequence of a mitochondrial gene defect.

It has long been recognized that PD patients perform poorly on the UPSIT olfactory test battery. In a recent survey, 25 hyposmic and 23 normosmic relatives of PD patients were scanned with β-CIT SPECT to screen for the presence of subclinical dopaminergic dysfunction (30). Four subclinical cases were found, and these are being followed longitudinally.

Neuroinflammation in Parkinson's Disease

Microglia constitute 10% to 20% of white cells in the brain and form its natural defense mechanism. They are normally in a resting state but local injury causes them to activate expressing human leukocyte and other antigens on the cell surface and releasing cytokines. The mitochondria of activated microglia express peripheral benzodiazepine sites which are not evident in their resting state. ^{11}C-PK11195 is an isoquinoline that binds selectively to peripheral benzodiazepine sites and so provides an in vivo PET marker of neuroinflammation.

The degenerative loss of nigral cells in PD is known to be associated with microglial activation (31). Gerhardt and co-workers (32) have used ^{11}C-PK11195 PET to study microglial activation in PD and have detected both increased nigral and pallidal signal (Fig. 42.2). Whereas the nigral ^{11}C-PK11195 uptake probably reflects local degeneration, the pallidal signal may result from excess glutamate release from subthalamic projections following dopamine deficiency (33).

Progression of Parkinson's Disease

Assessing the progression of PD with clinical rating scales can be problematic for several reasons: First, these scales are subjective, nonlinear, consider multiple aspects of the dis-

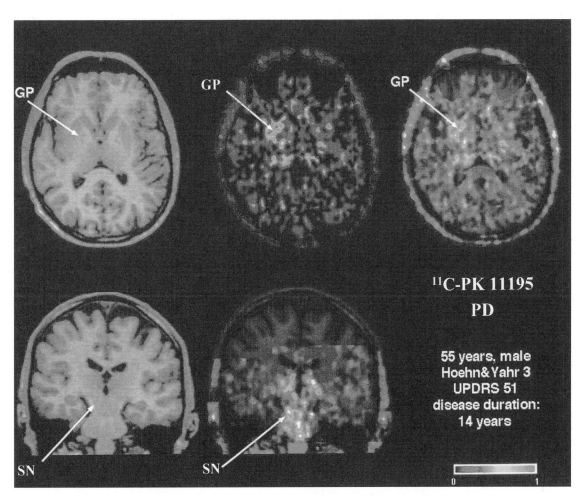

FIG. 42.2. PET images of ^{11}C-PK11195 uptake in a Parkinson's disease patient. Microglial activation can be seen in the nigra and pallidum. (Picture courtesy of Drs. R. Banati and A. Gerhardt.) (See color section.)

order, and are biased toward certain symptoms—bradykinesia in the case of the Unified Parkinson's Disease Rating Scale (UPDRS). Second, symptomatically effective therapy can mask disease progression, and full washouts are difficult to achieve because of poor patient tolerance. Functional imaging provides a biological marker for objectively monitoring disease progression in vivo in PD and avoids the above problems. However, it is limited to providing information concerning one aspect of the condition—generally dopamine terminal function.

Striatal ^{18}F-dopa uptake has been shown to correlate with subsequent postmortem dopaminergic cell densities in the substantia nigra and striatal dopamine levels of patients (200) and of 1-methyl-4-phenyl-1,2,3,6-tetrahydropyridine (MPTP)–lesioned monkeys (34). In principle, ^{18}F-dopa PET can be used as a marker of dopamine terminal function in PD, although it probably overestimates terminal density due to a relative up-regulation of DDC in response to nigral cell loss (24).

Vingerhoets and colleagues (35) were the first to demonstrate that loss of striatal ^{18}F-dopa uptake occurs more rapidly in PD than in age-matched controls. Morrish (36) measured dorsal putamen ^{18}F-dopa influx constants and found a mean 12% annual decline in baseline putamen K_i value for a group of 17 PD patients with a baseline clinical disease duration of 40 months when scanned serially a mean of 18 months apart. Ten controls showed no significant change in putamen ^{18}F-dopa uptake over 3 years. These workers subsequently extended their dataset to a cohort of 32 PD patients and reported a mean 9% annual decline of the baseline-specific putamen ^{18}F-dopa uptake while caudate K_i declined by 3% per annum (37). Extrapolation of levels of putamen ^{18}F-dopa uptake against clinical disease duration suggested a preclinical disease window of 6 ± 3 years and symptom onset after a 30% fall in putamen ^{18}F-dopa uptake from normal levels.

^{123}I-β-CIT, ^{123}I-FP-CIT, and ^{123}I-IPT SPECT have all been used to monitor rate of loss of striatal DATs in PD. Marek and colleagues (38) reported a mean 9% annual loss of striatal ^{123}I-β-CIT uptake in early PD patients. This group also noted that rate of disease progression correlated with initial levels of striatal ^{123}I-β-CIT binding (39). Those PD patients with symptoms for less than 2 years progressed four times faster than those with more established disease—a similar finding to that noted in the Morrish series. In contrast, Schwarz and co-workers (40) reported only a mean 3% annual decline in striatal ^{123}I-IPT binding in 11 PD cases followed over 12 months. However, the Schwarz series contained both early and late cases, and this may have biased their cohort toward a slower rate of loss of dopaminergic function.

As functional imaging can objectively follow PD progression, it provides a potential means of monitoring the efficacy of putative neuroprotective agents such as dopamine agonists, monoamine oxidase B (MAO-B)

inhibitors, free-radical scavengers, and nerve growth factors. Rakshi and co-workers have studied the relative rates of progression of early PD in patients started on the dopamine agonist ropinirole or L-dopa. Forty-five patients with early PD were randomized 2:1 to ropinirole or L-dopa treatment in this double-blind trial (41). Supplementary L-dopa was allowed if there was lack of therapeutic effect. ^{18}F-dopa PET scans were performed at baseline ($n = 45$) and again after 2 years later ($n = 37$). After 2 years, the mean percentage reduction in putamen ^{18}F-dopa uptake (K_i^o) was not significantly different between groups (13% ropinirole, $n = 28$, vs. 18% L-dopa, $n = 9$).

Holloway and colleagues have reported serial ^{123}I-β-CIT findings for a cohort of 82 early PD patients randomized 1:1 to the dopamine agonist pramipexole or levodopa (42). Supplementary L-dopa was allowed if there was lack of therapeutic effect. Patients treated initially with pramipexole ($n = 39$) showed a mean decline of 20.0% in striatal β-CIT uptake compared with a 24.8% decline in subjects treated initially with levodopa ($n = 39$). Again, these progression rates were not significantly different ($p = 0.15$).

Implant Function in Parkinson's Disease

As well as providing a way of following natural disease progression, functional imaging provides a means of examining the function of striatal implants of dopaminergic cells in PD. Possible approaches include fetal mesencephalic cells; transformed cells that secrete dopamine, nerve growth factors, or express anti-apoptotic genes; stem cells; xenografts; and direct striatal infusions of nerve growth factors. Several hundred fetal mesencephalic tissue transplantations have been performed at a variety of centers, but only about 100 patient studies have been reported with detailed serial clinical assessments accompanied by functional imaging.

The Lund group have reported serial clinical and ^{18}F-dopa PET findings over a period of 10 years on two PD patients following implantation of fetal midbrain cells into the putamen contralateral to their more affected limbs (43,44). Both of these patients have maintained a clinical improvement, particularly in "on" time and in dexterity of the limbs contralateral to the engrafted putamen. One has now received bilateral putamen implants, whereas the other does not wish further surgery. It has been demonstrated that the unilateral graft of this second case is capable of releasing normal levels of synaptic dopamine after an amphetamine challenge (Fig. 42.3). Another four unilaterally transplanted PD patients showed PET evidence of graft function one year following surgery (43). Three of these four have responded clinically to transplantation, but the fourth has deteriorated and is now showing signs suggestive of atypical disease.

Clinically successful transplantation of fetal tissue with corroborative serial ^{18}F-dopa PET findings has also been reported for five PD patients in a 2-year follow-up French

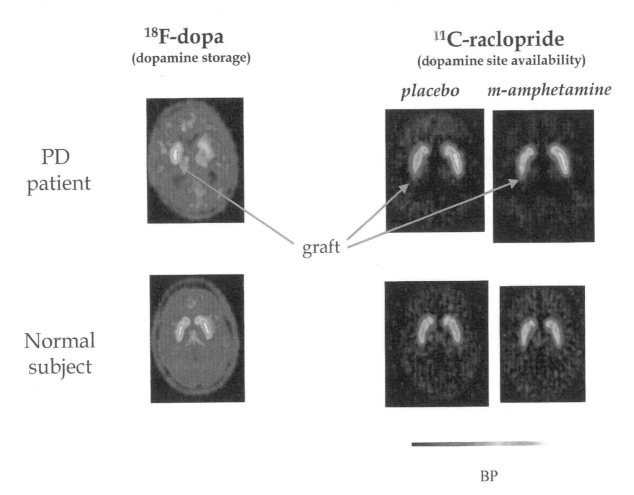

FIG. 42.3. PET images of ¹¹C-raclopride uptake in a Parkinson's disease patient with a putamen implant of fetal dopamine cells. It can be seen that after an amphetamine challenge the grafted putamen shows a normal fall in raclopride binding, indicating an increase in the level of synaptic dopamine. (Picture courtesy of Dr. P. Piccini.) (See color section.)

study (45) and for six PD patients in a 2-year follow-up series from Tampa, Florida (46). In the French study, grafted putamen K_i values were shown to correlate well with percentage time spent "on" during the day and measures of finger dexterity while in the "off" state. Two of the transplanted PD patients in the Florida series subsequently died from an unrelated cause, and at postmortem viable tyrosine hydroxylase staining graft tissue forming connections with host neurons was seen (47,48). This finding confirms that ¹⁸F-dopa PET measures graft function rather than simply reflecting a host reaction to foreign tissue or the presence of blood–brain barrier breakdown.

As a consequence of these pilot data, two major studies on the efficacy of implantation of fetal cells in PD were sponsored by the U.S. National Institutes of Health, and the first of these has been reported (49). Forty patients who were 34 to 75 years of age and had severe PD (mean duration, 14 years) were randomized in a double-blind manner to receive a transplant or undergo sham surgery and were followed for 1 year. In the transplant recipients, mesen-

cephalic tissue from four embryos cultured for up to 1 month was implanted into the putamen bilaterally (two embryos per side). In the patients who underwent sham surgery, holes were drilled in the skull but the dura was not penetrated. Transplanted patients showed a significant mean 18% improvement in motor scores on the UPDRS compared with the sham-surgery group when tested in the morning before receiving medication ($p = 0.04$). This improvement was more evident for patients younger than 60 years (34% improvement, $p = 0.005$). Of 19 transplanted patients, 16 showed an increase in putamen ¹⁸F-dopa uptake (group mean increase 40%). A drawback was that "off" dystonia and dyskinesias developed in 15% of the patients who received transplants in this series, even after reduction or discontinuation of the dose of levodopa.

Fluctuations and Dyskinesias

Patients with fluctuating responses to levodopa have been reported to show significantly lower putamen ¹⁸F-dopa uptake than those with early disease and sustained therapeutic responses (50,51). A confounder when trying to compare pre-synaptic dopamine terminal function in PD patients with and without motor complications is that the former tend to have an earlier age of disease onset, more severe disease, longer disease duration, and a greater cumulative exposure to levodopa. De la Fuente-Fernández and colleagues (52) addressed this problem in two ways: First, they used analysis of covariance (ANCOVA) to factor out effects of age at onset and disease duration in groups of fluctuators and nonfluctuators. Second, they matched subgroups of fluctuators and nonfluctuators for age of onset and disease duration. These workers found that mean putamen ^{18}F-dopa uptake was 28% lower in PD patients with motor complications than in those without but that there was considerable overlap of the two individual ranges. They concluded that, while loss of striatal dopamine terminal function predisposes PD patients to development of levodopa-associated complications, it cannot alone be responsible for determining the timing of onset of fluctuations and involuntary movements.

Dopamine receptors broadly fall into type D1 (D1, D5), which activate adenyl cyclase, and type D2 (D2, D3, D4), which either inhibit or have no effect on this enzyme. The striatum contains mainly D1 and D2 receptor subtypes, and these both play a primary role in modulating locomotor function. PET studies with spiperone-based tracers and ^{123}I-IBZM SPECT series have reported normal levels of striatal D2 binding in untreated PD patients later shown to be levodopa or apomorphine responsive, whereas ^{11}C-raclopride PET studies in de novo PD have shown 10% to 20% increases in D2 site availability in the putamen contralateral to the more affected limbs (53–55). Putamen ^{11}C-raclopride binding inversely correlates with ^{18}F-dopa uptake (56). These findings suggest that in untreated PD putamen D2 availability is mildly up-regulated whereas caudate D2 binding, where dopamine terminal function is relatively preserved, remains normal.

Studies with ^{11}C-methylspiperone PET and ^{123}I-IBZM SPECT have reported normal (57,58) or mildly reduced striatal D2 binding in chronically treated PD (53). Serial ^{11}C-raclopride PET has shown that after months of exposure to levodopa the mildly increased putamen ^{11}C-raclopride binding seen in de novo PD patients normalizes (54,59). Chronically levodopa-exposed PD cases continue to show normal levels of putamen D2 binding while caudate D2 binding is reduced by around 20% (55). These findings are in good agreement with in vitro reports of striatal dopamine D2 receptor binding based on post-mortem material from end-stage patients (60).

^{11}C-SCH23390 is an antagonist at D1 sites, binding reversibly during the time course of PET. In de novo hemiparkinsonian patients, later shown to be levodopa responsive, ^{11}C-SCH23390 PET shows no relative up-regulation of putamen binding contralateral to the affected limbs, suggesting that D1 binding remains at a normal level (61). In contrast, PD patients who have been exposed to levodopa for several years show a 20% reduction in striatal D1 binding (55). As previously discussed, a confounder when trying to compare postsynaptic dopamine receptor function in PD patients with and without motor complications is that the former tend to have an earlier age of onset, more severe disease, longer disease duration, and a greater cumulative exposure to levodopa. Turjanski and co-workers examined striatal dopamine receptor availability in subgroups of eight levodopa-exposed dyskinetic and ten non-dyskinetic patients (55). These subgroups were age matched (dyskinetic 49 to 74 years, non-dyskinetic 42 to 78 years) and had similar clinical disease durations (dyskinetic 3 to 10 years, non-dyskinetic 3 to 9 years). There were nonsignificant trends toward greater disease severity (mean motor UPDRS 19 vs. 13) and higher daily levodopa dosage (560 mg vs. 450 mg) in the dyskinesia subgroup. Mean caudate and putamen D1 and putamen D2 binding were normal for both the dyskinetic and the non-dyskinetic PD subgroups, whereas caudate D2 binding was similarly reduced by around 15%.

Other workers have also reported that striatal dopamine D1 and D2 binding are similar in fluctuating and dyskinetic PD patients when compared with sustained responders (62). In these studies, ANCOVA was used to factor out the confounding effects of differences in age of onset and disease duration between the PD subgroups. These PET studies all suggest that onset of motor complications in PD is not primarily associated with alterations in striatal dopamine receptor availability.

^{11}C-raclopride PET provides an indirect marker of changes in levels of dopamine in the synaptic cleft of the striatum. A challenge with an intravenous bolus of 0.3 mg/kg methamphetamine causes a 24% reduction in putamen ^{11}C-raclopride binding in normal subjects due to the dopamine released (44).

Torstenson and colleagues (63) have used ^{11}C-raclopride PET to examine levodopa-induced fluxes in synaptic dopamine levels in PD. The patients were divided into subgroups with either early hemidisease or with advanced disease exhibiting fluctuating treatment responses and levodopa-induced dyskinesias (LIDs). A total dose of 3 mg/kg levodopa was administered as an intravenous bolus; this resulted in a clinical response in all the PD patients. The early cases showed a mean 10% fall in ^{11}C-raclopride binding in posterior dorsal putamen after levodopa. No effect on ^{11}C-raclopride binding was seen in the asymptomatic putamen contralateral to the unaffected limbs. The advanced PD cases showed 23% and 20% falls in posterior and anterior dorsal putamen ^{11}C-raclopride binding after levodopa. Reductions in putamen ^{11}C-raclopride binding correlated with disease severity assessed off medication with the UPDRS. These findings indicate that severe loss of dopamine terminals in PD leads to excessive levels of synaptic dopamine when exogenous levodopa is administered. This reflects a combination of up-regulation of striatal dopamine synthesis and release by those terminals remaining along with severe loss of DATs preventing dopamine reuptake, This, rather than changes in postsynaptic dopamine D1 and D2 receptor binding, is likely to explain the more rapid response of advanced PD patients to oral levodopa. High swings in synaptic dopamine levels may also lead to excessive dopamine receptor internalization promoting fluctuations.

More recently, De la Fuente-Fernandez and colleagues (64) have examined changes in raclopride binding after an oral levodopa challenge in advanced PD and shown that "off" episodes do not necessarily correlate with low synaptic dopamine levels. This finding is again in favor of fluctuations occurring either due to inappropriate levels of dopamine receptor internalization at times, making them unpredictably unavailable at the cell surface for stimulation, or due to aberrant downstream changes in basal ganglia transmission making the basal ganglia refractory, rather than due to lack of dopaminergic tone at postsynaptic D2 receptors.

The caudate and putamen contain a dense population of medium spiny projection neurons that cotransmit opioids along with γ-aminobutyric acid (GABA) in the pallidum (65). Striatal projections to external globus pallidus (GPe) contain enkephalin, which binds mainly to δ opioid sites and inhibits GABA release in the GPe. Striatal projections to GPi transmit dynorphin, which binds to κ opioid sites and inhibits glutamate release from STN afferents to the GPi. It is thought that phasic firing of striatopallidal projection neurons results primarily in GABA release while more sustained firing causes additional modulatory opioid release. The caudate and putamen also contain high densities of μ, κ, and δ opioid sites. These receptors are located both presynaptically on dopamine, where they regulate dopamine release, and postsynaptically on interneurons and medium spiny projection neurons to pallidum terminals (66).

There is now strong evidence supporting the presence of deranged opioid transmission in the basal ganglia of PD patients both from postmortem studies and lesioned animal models of this disorder. At postmortem, end-stage-treated PD patients show raised levels of pallidal preproenkephalin (67). In rats lesioned with the nigral toxin 6-hydroxy-dopamine there are raised levels of striatal enkephalin and preproenkephalin expression whereas prodynorphin expression is suppressed (65,68). When such animals are made hyperkinetic or frankly dyskinetic after chronic exposure to pulsatile doses of levodopa, further overexpression of striatal preproenkephalin is seen along with raised expression of prodynorphin. Levodopa-naive MPTP-lesioned monkeys have also been reported to show raised striatal enkephalin and reduced substance P mRNA expression (69). Exposure to levodopa for one month failed to normalize striatal preproenkephalin mRNA expression, whereas substance P mRNA expression became elevated.

[11]C-Diprenorphine PET is a nonselective marker of μ, κ, and δ opioid sites and its binding is sensitive to levels of endogenous opioids. If raised basal ganglia levels of enkephalin and dynorphin are associated with LIDs, then PD patients with motor complications would be expected to show reduced binding of ^{11}C-diprenorphine compared to those with sustained treatment responses. Piccini and co-workers studied six PD patients with motor fluctuations and LIDs and seven patients without dyskinesias (70). Mean age, disease and treatment duration, and daily L-dopa dosage were not significantly different. There were significant reductions in ^{11}C-diprenorphine binding in caudate, putamen, thalamus, and anterior cingulate in the dyskinetic patients compared with sustained responders. Individual levels of putamen ^{11}C-diprenorphine uptake correlated inversely with severity of dyskinesia when rated with Part 4 of the UPDRS. These in vivo findings would support the presence of elevated levels of endogenous opioids in the basal ganglia of dyskinetic PD patients and suggest that this, rather than a primary alteration in dopamine receptor binding, is partly responsible for the appearance of involuntary movements.

Resting Brain Metabolism in Parkinson's Disease

PET studies have shown increased levels of resting oxygen and glucose metabolism in the contralateral lentiform nucleus of hemiparkinsonian patients with early disease, whereas PD patients with established bilateral involvement have normal levels of lentiform metabolism (71,72). However, ANCOVA reveals an abnormal profile of relatively raised resting lentiform nucleus and lowered frontal metabolism in PD patients with established disease and the degree of expression of this profile correlates with their disease severity (73).

Nondemented PD patients show normal or mildly decreased cortical metabolism (74). [18]FDG scans of frankly demented PD patients generally show an Alzheimer pattern of impaired brain glucose utilization, with the posterior parietal and temporal association areas being most affected (75). Currently, it remains unclear whether the pattern of glucose hypometabolism in demented PD patients reflects coincidental Alzheimer's disease, cortical Lewy body disease, loss of cholinergic projections, or some other degenerative process. Clinicopathologic series suggest that there is considerable overlap in the cortical FDG PET findings of coincidental Alzheimer's disease and cortical Lewy body disease but that cortical Lewy body disease cases show a greater reduction in resting glucose metabolism of the occipital cortex (76).

Hu and colleagues have recently studied nondemented cases of established PD with FDG PET and ^{31}P nuclear magnetic resonance (NMR) spectroscopy (77). These workers found that around one third of their PD patients showed subclinical resting temporoparietal cortical metabolic dysfunction. Whether these are patients who will go on to dement is still unclear, and a longitudinal study is in process.

Activation Studies in Parkinson's Disease

Studies of resting cerebral blood flow and metabolism only provide partial insight into the pathophysiology of the cerebral dysfunction underlying movement disorders. A more sensitive way of elucidating the nature of the functional disturbance underlying the bradykinesia of PD is to stress the system by asking patients to perform motor or cognitive tasks while measuring the associated changes in rCBF.

When normal subjects made paced movements of a joystick in freely selected directions with their right hand, $H_2^{15}O$ PET showed associated rCBF increases in contralateral sensorimotor cortex (SMC) and lentiform nucleus and bilaterally in anterior cingulate, supplementary motor area (SMA), lateral premotor cortex (PMC), and dorsolateral prefrontal cortex (DLPFC) (78). Self-paced extensions of the index finger resulted in a similar pattern of activation (79). When PD patients, scanned after stopping levodopa for 12 hours, performed the same motor tasks, normal levels of activation of SMC, PMC, and lateral parietal association areas were seen, but there was selectively impaired activation of the contralateral lentiform nucleus and the anterior cingulate, SMA, and DLPFC (cortical areas that receive direct input from the basal ganglia).

It is well recognized that while patients with PD can perform single finger movements efficiently, attempts to perform repetitive or sequences of finger movements results in a rapid fall in amplitude and occasionally motor arrest. A number of groups have investigated patterns of regional cerebral activation in PD during generation of sequential finger movements. Using $H_2^{15}O$ PET, Samuel and colleagues (80) demonstrated underactivity of mesial frontal and deactivation of dorsolateral prefrontal areas when patients perform prelearned sequential opposition finger thumb movements with one or both hands. These workers also now found relative overactivity of lateral premotor and parietal areas, suggesting a switch to a network facilitating externally instructed rather than freely chosen movements (81). In support of this viewpoint, Rascol and co-workers (82) have reported abnormally raised levels of cerebellar rCBF during sequential finger–thumb opposition movements in PD patients.

Functional MRI has also demonstrated underactivity of the anterior SMA and DLPFC and overactivity of lateral premotor and parietal areas in PD during sequential finger movements (83). With this approach overactivity of motor cortex and caudal SMA was also evident. The detection of motor area overactivity may in part reflect a greater sensitivity of the MRI activation approach, but may also reflect

the more complex design of Sabatini's paradigm. In Sabatini's study, the subjects had to perform fist clenching in-between series of finger–thumb opposition movements. In support of the presence of motor cortex overactivation in PD, a second group has reported this finding when patients performed an externally cued reaching task (84).

It is thought that DLPFC plays a crucial role in motor decision making while the SMA prepares and optimizes volitional motor programs once selected (81,85). In contrast, lateral PMC is believed to have a primary role in facilitating motor responses to external visual and auditory stimuli. An inability to activate SMA and DLPFC during freely selected movements could explain the difficulty that PD patients experience in initiating such movements. In contrast, their ability to activate lateral PMC normally allows them to respond well to visual and auditory cues, such as stepping over lines on the floor to aid their walking.

Effects of Medical and Surgical Therapy

If loss of tonic dopaminergic activity is responsible for the impaired activation of striatofrontal projections in PD, then it should be possible to functionally restore such activity by administering a dopaminergic agent. The nonselective dopamine D1 and D2 agonist apomorphine has been subcutaneously administered while PD patients performed paced joystick movements in freely chosen directions (86,87). Reduction of akinesia was associated with significant increases in both SMA and DLPFC blood flow, implicating these areas in the initiation of volitional movements. In separate rCBF studies with ^{133}Xe SPECT, it has also been demonstrated that improvement in SMA flow occurs when PD patients are successfully treated with apomorphine or levodopa (88,89). Event-related fMRI has also shown that mesial frontal activation improves in PD patients performing free-choice joystick movements after taking levodopa (90). Overactivity of motor and lateral PMC was also reduced.

The effects of striatal fetal dopaminergic cell implantation on movement-related premotor and prefrontal activation in PD have been studied (91). Four PD patients who received bilateral human fetal mesencephalic transplants into caudate and putamen were studied with $H_2^{15}O$ PET at baseline and over the 2 years following surgery. Six months after transplantation mean striatal dopamine storage capacity, measured by ^{18}F-dopa PET, was significantly elevated in these patients (putamen 78%, caudate 27%). This was associated with a mean 12-point clinical improvement on the UPDRS but no significant change in cortical activation. At 18 months postsurgery there was a 24-point reduction in UPDRS score despite no further increase in striatal ^{18}F-dopa uptake. SMA and DLPFC activation during performance of joystick movements in freely chosen directions had also significantly improved (Fig. 42.4). These findings

Pre-graft

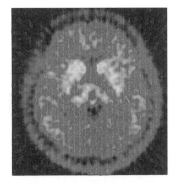

Post-graft

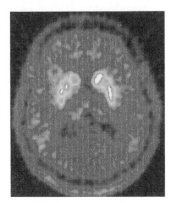

FIG. 42.4. Serial PET images over 20 months of striatal ^{18}F-dopa uptake by a grafted Parkinson's disease patient, alongside a graph showing putamen F-dopa uptake, motor UPDRS scores, and levels of activation-induced supplementary motor area and dorsal prefrontal cortex blood flow change. It can be seen that clinical recovery parallels improved cortical activation rather than graft dopamine storage capacity. (Picture courtesy of Drs. P. Piccini and N. Khan.) (See color section.)

suggest that the function of the graft goes beyond that of a simple dopamine delivery system and that functional integration of the grafted neurons into the host brain is necessary to produce substantial clinical recovery and restore cortical activation in PD.

Current theories on basal ganglia connectivity argue that loss of striatal dopamine in PD is associated with reduced inhibition of the GPi by striatum resulting in excessive inhibitory pallidal output to the ventral thalamus and cortex. It is argued that by inhibiting motor GPi, either by lesioning or high-frequency electrical deep brain stimulation (DBS), this excessive inhibition will be removed so facilitating volitional movements and frontal activation in PD patients. Alternatively, the excitatory glutamatergic input to GPi from the subthalamic nucleus (STN) can be disrupted by STN DBS. It is now well established that pallidotomy, pallidal DBS, and STN DBS all lead to improvements in rigidity and bradykinesia but, paradoxically, the main effect of pallidal inhibition is to abolish levodopa-induced dyskinesias.

Two centers have reported the functional effects of pallidotomy on cerebral activation in PD. Grafton and co-work-ers (92) examined the regional cerebral activation in six PD patients associated with reaching out to grasp lighted targets every 3 seconds while off medication. Despite an absence of change in patient performance, this patient group showed significantly increased SMA and lateral premotor activation after pallidotomy. Subsequently, Samuel and colleagues (93) demonstrated significantly increased activation of SMA, lateral PMC, and dorsal prefrontal cortex in PD patients after pallidotomy when making joystick movements in freely selected directions while off medication. The findings of these activation studies, therefore, lend support to the hypothesis that pallidotomy results in removal of excess pallidal inhibitory drive to frontal association areas in PD.

There have been three $H_2^{15}O$ PET reports on the effects of high frequency electrical pallidal stimulation on regional brain function. In the first study, levels of resting rCBF were measured with the stimulator switched off, switched on at a sub-effective intensity, and switched on at an effective intensity (94). Effective GPi stimulation improved contralateral bradykinesia and rigidity in eight of the nine PD patients when they were assessed while off medication. This was associated with increased resting SMA and putamen/external pallidal rCBF. Stimulation of the GPi at a lower intensity did not lead to clinical improvement or increase SMA rCBF. In two other studies, changes in regional brain activation associated either with moving a joystick in freely chosen directions or with reaching to touch a visual target were measured during pallidal stimulation. In the first report six PD patients were studied while off medication with the GPi stimulator switched off and then again when the stimulator was switched on (95). In this study clinically effective GPi stimulation did not lead to any significant changes in levels of SMA or DLPFC activation during free choice joystick movements. In the second study clinically effective GPi stimulation lead to increased lateral premotor and anterior cingulate activation during the reaching task (96).

There have also been two reports of $H_2^{15}O$ PET activation findings in PD patients before and during STN stimulation. In both studies levels of rCBF were measured in patients with PD when off medication during performance of paced joystick movements in freely selected directions. The first study reported relative increases in activation of rostral SMA lateral premotor and DLPFC during movement when the STN stimulator was switched on, findings similar to those reported following pallidotomy. However, in contrast to pallidotomy, STN stimulation was also associated with reduced motor cortex activation and led to increases in resting thalamic and decreases in resting motor cortex and caudal SMA rCBF (97). The second study also found that STN stimulation in their six PD cases led to increased SMA and DLPFC and decreased motor cortex activation (95). The mechanism causing the decreased motor cortex activation remains unclear, although antidromic stimulation of direct projections to STN may be feasible.

ATYPICAL PARKINSONIAN SYNDROMES
Multiple System Atrophy

Multiple system atrophy (MSA), also known as Shy-Drager syndrome, includes striatonigral degeneration (SND), olivopontocerebellar atrophy (OPCA), and progressive autonomic failure (PAF) within its spectrum. It is characterized pathologically by argyrophilic, α-synuclein positive, inclusions in glia and neurons in substantia nigra, striatum, brainstem and cerebellar nuclei, and intermediolateral columns of the cord. [18]FDG PET studies in levodopa-non-responsive akinetic-rigid patients with clinically probable SND have reported reduced levels of striatal glucose metabolism in contrast to PD where striatal metabolism is preserved (98–100). Eidelberg (100) found that 8 of 10 probable SND patients showed reduced striatal metabolism, while this was normal or raised in levodopa-responsive PD patients. These workers also reported that akinetic-rigid patients with low levels of striatal glucose metabolism, irrespective of levodopa response, show little improvement after pallidotomy (101). De Volder and colleagues (98) studied seven patients with probable striatonigral degeneration, two of whom had additional autonomic failure and cerebellar ataxia and so had the full syndrome of MSA. They found reduced mean levels of putamen and caudate glucose metabolism, and cerebellar metabolism was also reduced in the two patients with ataxia. Otsuka et al. (99) reported significantly reduced striatal glucose metabolism in eight patients with probable SND, whereas striatal glucose metabolism was preserved in eight PD patients. [18]FDG PET, therefore, provides a sensitive means of detecting the presence of striatal dysfunction where atypical parkinsonism is suspected.

Proton magnetic resonance spectroscopy is also a potential means of discriminating SND from PD. NAA is found in high concentrations in neurons and is believed to be a metabolic marker of neuronal integrity. Reduced NAA/creatine ratios in the proton MRS signal from the lentiform nucleus in six of seven clinically probable SND cases has been reported, whereas eight of nine probable PD cases showed normal levels of putamen NAA (102).

In patients with clinically probable SND the function of both the pre- and postsynaptic dopaminergic systems is impaired. As in PD, putamen ^{18}F-dopa uptake is reduced to around 50% of normal levels in established SND and individual levels of putamen ^{18}F-dopa uptake correlate with locomotor status (6,103). In patients with the full syndrome of MSA, mean caudate ^{18}F-dopa uptake is significantly more depressed than in PD though the individual ranges overlap (99,103). This finding suggests that the nigra is more uniformly involved by the pathology of SND

than PD, and pathologic studies corroborate this conclusion (104). However, the pattern of caudate and putamen ^{18}F-dopa uptake only discriminates SND from PD with 70% specificity (105), so that [18]FDG PET and proton MRS are likely to provide more sensitive tools than ^{18}F-dopa PET for this purpose. Recently, Pirker and colleagues (106) examined ^{123}I-β-CIT binding in 18 MSA patients. These workers concluded that, while ^{123}I-β-CIT SPECT reliably discriminated PD and MSA from normal, it could not discriminate between the two parkinsonian conditions.

Striatal dopamine D1 and D2 binding has been studied with PET in SND (107–109). Mild but significant reductions in mean putamen ^{11}C-SCH23390 and ^{11}C-raclopride uptake have been reported, although an overlap between SND, normal, and PD ranges is evident. Striatal D1 and D2 binding, therefore, does not provide sensitive discrimination of SND from PD. In support of this viewpoint, Schwarz et al. found reduced striatal D2 binding with ^{123}I-IBZM SPECT in only 8 of their 12 de novo parkinsonian patients who showed a negative apomorphine response (110). As a significant number of parkinsonian patients who respond poorly to levodopa retain normal levels of striatal D2 binding, it seems likely that degeneration of downstream brainstem and pallidal rather than striatal projections is responsible for their poor response to levodopa. Recently, Seppi and co-workers (111) have used ^{123}I-IBZM SPECT to objectively longitudinally monitor striatal degeneration in a group of early MSA patients. They found an annual 10% loss of striatal D2 binding in their 18-month study and concluded that ^{123}I-IBZM SPECT provides a valid future approach for testing the efficacy of putative neuroprotective agents in MSA.

The basal ganglia are rich in opioid peptides and binding sites, and these are differentially affected in SND and PD (112). ^{11}C-Diprenorphine is a nonspecific opioid antagonist binding with equal affinity to μ, κ, and δ sites. In non-dyskinetic PD patients caudate and putamen ^{11}C-diprenorphine uptake is preserved, whereas putamen uptake is reduced in 50% of patients thought to have SND (113). Druschky and colleagues (114) have recently used ^{123}I-MIBG SPECT to study functional integrity of cardiac sympathetic innervation in PD and MSA. Both these conditions showed a reduction in mediastinal ^{123}I-MIBG signal, but this was significantly greater in PD, even in cases where no clinical evidence of autonomic failure was present. The authors interpreted this finding as demonstrating a greater involvement of postganglionic sympathetic innervation of the heart in PD compared with MSA.

[11]C-PK11195 PET, an in vivo marker of microglial activation, has been used to study neuroinflammatory changes in MSA (32). Widespread subcortical increases in ^{11}C-PK11195 uptake were seen, particularly in nigra, putamen, pallidum, thalamus, and brainstem, in contrast to PD where significant increases were restricted to nigra and pallidum. It remains to be determined whether [11]C-

PK11195 PET will provide sensitive discrimination of MSA and PD.

In order to determine the overlap between pure autonomic failure, OPCA, and SND, groups of these patients have been studied with PET and proton MRS. In a series of seven PAF patients, putamen ^{18}F-dopa uptake was found to be abnormal in two, suggesting that subclinical nigral dysfunction was present (103). One of these patients subsequently developed MSA. In a series of ten sporadic OPCA patients with autonomic failure but no rigidity, seven revealed reduced putamen ^{18}F-dopa uptake whereas four had reduced putamen ^{11}C-diprenorphine binding indicative of the presence of subclinical SND (115). Reduced levels of striatal ^{18}F-dopa uptake (116), striatal glucose hypometabolism (117), and reduced lentiform NAA/creatine signal (102) have also been reported in other series of sporadic OPCA cases. It would seem, therefore, that the majority of sporadic OPCA cases with autonomic failure show functional imaging evidence of subclinical striatonigral dysfunction.

Progressive Supranuclear Palsy

Progressive supranuclear palsy (PSP) is characterized pathologically by neurofibrillary tangle formation and neuronal loss in the substantia nigra, pallidum, superior colliculi, brainstem nuclei, and the periaqueductal gray matter, with lesser cortical involvement. There have been a number of studies of resting regional cerebral glucose metabolism in patients with probable PSP, several of whom later had the diagnosis confirmed at autopsy (118–122). Cortical metabolism is globally depressed and frontal areas are particularly targeted, levels of metabolism correlating with disease duration and performance on psychometric tests of frontal function (119). Hypofrontality is not specific for PSP; it can be seen in PD, SND, Pick's disease, Huntington's disease (HD), and depression. A case of clinically probable PSP with appropriate [18]FDG PET findings has been reported to show progressive subcortical gliosis at postmortem (123).

Basal ganglia, cerebellar, and thalamic glucose metabolism are also depressed in PSP (see Fig. 42.5) distinguishing it from PD where metabolism is preserved. Proton MRS studies have also shown reduced lentiform nucleus NAA/Cr ratios in PSP in contrast to PD (124). Unfortunately, while [18]FDG PET and proton MRS help distinguish PSP from PD, they are less useful for discriminating PSP from SND as striatal and frontal hypometabolism are present in both of these disorders.

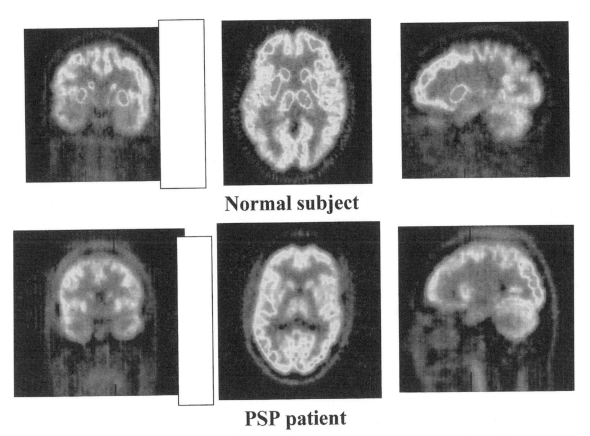

Normal subject

PSP patient

FIG. 42.5. [18]Fluorodeoxyglucose PET images of a normal subject and a progressive supranuclear palsy (PSP) patient. Reduced striatal, thalamic, and frontal metabolism is evident in the PSP case. (Picture courtesy of Dr. P. Piccini.) (See color section.)

The pathology of PSP targets nigrostriatal dopaminergic projections so that, not surprisingly, striatal ^{18}F-dopa uptake in PSP is significantly reduced, the levels correlating with disease duration (6,125,126). However, unlike PD, putamen and caudate ^{18}F-dopa uptake appear to be equivalently affected in PSP, suggesting that the nigra is uniformly involved by the pathology in agreement with postmortem studies (127,128). In practice, ^{18}F-dopa PET can discriminate 90% of PSP from PD cases on the basis of this uniform caudate and putamen involvement (105). There appears to be little correlation between levels of striatal ^{18}F-dopa uptake in PSP and the degree of disability. Unlike PD and SND, where locomotor impairment appears to result primarily from loss of dopaminergic fibers, loss of mobility in PSP is probably more determined by degeneration of pallidal and brainstem projections.

Loss of striatal DAT binding has also been studied in PSP with ^{123}I-β-CIT SPECT. Messa and colleagues (129) have reported a similar loss of putamen ^{123}I-β-CIT uptake in PD and PSP but significantly greater caudate involvement in the latter. However, Pirker et al. (106) found ^{123}I-β-CIT SPECT less able to discriminate between PD and PSP.

Caudate and putamen D2 binding in PSP has been studied with both PET and SPECT. Overall, groups of PSP patients consistently show reductions in mean caudate and putamen D2 binding, though only 50% to 70% of individual patients show significant receptor loss (58,108,130, 131). It is likely that, as in SND, degeneration of downstream pallidal and brainstem projections is in part responsible for the poor L-dopa responsiveness of PSP along with loss of dopamine receptors. One study has examined striatal opioid binding in PSP (113). Striatal ^{11}C-diprenorphine was reduced in all six cases studied and, in contrast to SND, where caudate function was spared, caudate and putamen were equally affected in PSP. Levels of acetylcholinesterase activity have also been measured in PSP with ^{11}C-physostigmine PET (132). Striatal acetylcholinesterase activity was found to be significantly reduced and levels correlated with locomotor disability.

Corticobasal Degeneration

Corticobasal degeneration is also known as corticobasal ganglionic degeneration, corticodentatonigral degeneration, and neuronal achromasia. Patients classically present with an akinetic-rigid, apraxic limb that may exhibit alien behavior. Cortical sensory loss, dysphasia, myoclonus, supranuclear gaze problems, and bulbar dysfunction are also features, but intellect is spared until late. Eventually, all four limbs become involved and the condition is invariably poorly L-dopa responsive. The pathology consists of collections of swollen, achromatic, tau-positive Pick cells in the absence of argyrophilic Pick bodies that target the posterior frontal, inferior parietal, and superior temporal lobes, the substantia nigra, and the cerebellar dentate nuclei (132a).

PET and SPECT studies on patients with the clinical syndrome of CBD have predictably shown greatest reductions in resting cortical oxygen and glucose metabolism in posterior frontal, inferior parietal, and superior temporal regions (133–136). The thalamus and striatum are also involved, and the metabolic reductions are strikingly asymmetric, being most severe contralateral to the more affected limbs. This contrasts with PD patients, who have preserved and symmetric levels of striatal and thalamic glucose metabolism.

Striatal ^{18}F-dopa uptake is also reduced in CBD in an asymmetric fashion, again being most depressed contralateral to the more affected limbs (133). In contrast to PD, caudate and putamen ^{18}F-dopa uptake are similarly depressed in CBD. ^{123}I-β-CIT SPECT also shows an asymmetric reduction in striatal DAT binding in PSP (106), whereas ^{123}I-IBZM SPECT shows a severe asymmetric reduction of striatal D2 binding (137).

The above imaging findings help to discriminate CBD from Pick's disease where inferior frontal hypometabolism predominates from PD where striatal metabolism is preserved and caudate ^{18}F-dopa uptake is relatively spared, and from PSP where frontal and striatal metabolism tend to be more symmetrically involved (138).

INVOLUNTARY MOVEMENT DISORDERS

Huntington's Disease and Other Choreas

Huntington's disease is an autosomal dominantly transmitted disorder associated with an excess of CAG triplet repeats (>38) in the *IT15* gene on chromosome 4. The function of this gene is still uncertain, but the pathology of HD targets medium spiny projection neurons in the striatum. Those patients with predominant chorea show a selective loss of striato-GPe projections that express GABA and enkephalin, whereas those with a predominant akinetic-rigid syndrome show additional severe loss of striato-GPi fibers containing GABA and dynorphine (139). A number of other degenerative disorders can also cause chorea, including neuroacanthocytosis (NA), dentatorubropallidoluysian atrophy (DRPLA), and benign familial chorea (BFC).

Inflammatory diseases such as systemic lupus erythematosus (SLE) and Sydenham's chorea are also associated with chorea, as is tardive dyskinesia (TD). The mechanism underlying TD is uncertain; postmortem studies have found low levels of subthalamic and pallidal glutamate decarboxylase whereas neurochemical studies on a primate TD model have reported severe depletion of subthalamic and pallidal GABA. These findings suggest that TD, like HD, may be associated with deranged GABA transmission.

Clinically affected HD patients show severely reduced levels of glucose and oxygen metabolism of the caudate and lentiform nuclei (140–142). Levels of resting putamen metabolism correlate with locomotor function and caudate metabolism with performance on tests sensitive to frontal lobe function (143,144). In early HD cortical metabolism is preserved, but as the disease progresses and dementia becomes prominent it also declines, the frontal cortex being targeted (145). Caudate hypometabolism is not specific to HD; it is also seen in NA, DRPLA, and some cases of BFC, so that its presence cannot be used to discriminate these degenerative choreiform disorders (146–149). In contrast, striatal glucose metabolism has been reported to be normal or elevated in chorea secondary to SLE (150), Sydenham's chorea (151), and TD (152).

Regional cerebral metabolism in HD has also been studied with proton MRS. NAA levels in the basal ganglia are reduced in affected patients whereas lactate levels in the basal ganglia and cortex are elevated, suggesting that mitochondrial dysfunction is a feature of this disorder (153). If the pathology of HD arises due to mitochondrial dysfunction one might expect to be able to find raised lactate levels in asymptomatic adult gene carriers. To date, lactate levels have been reported to be normal in asymptomatic gene carriers, which is more in favor of mitochondrial dysfunction representing an associated disease phenomenon rather than being the cause of the degenerative process.

It has also been suggested that the pathology of HD may arise from abnormal sensitivity of striatal neurons to glutamate, a naturally occurring excitotoxic amino acid. This hypothesis has arisen from the observation that kainic acid, ibotenic acid, and quinolinic acid (all glutamate agonists) cause a loss of medium spiny neurons when injected into striatum (154). A recent proton MRS study has reported that the GLX peak from the lentiform nuclei of affected HD patients is increased (155). This peak contains proton resonances from both glutamate and glutamine moieties, so that the exact interpretation of this finding is not yet clear. However, it is compatible with abnormal compartmentalization of basal ganglia glutamate occurring in HD and adds support to the excitotoxic hypothesis.

The medium spiny striatal neurons that degenerate in HD express D1, D2, opioid, and benzodiazepine receptors. PET studies with spiperone-based tracers and ^{123}I-IBZM SPECT have all confirmed that striatal D2 binding is severely reduced in affected HD patients (53). Karlsson et al. (156) have studied affected HD patients with ^{11}C-SCH23390 PET and demonstrated reduced D1 binding in both striatum and temporal cortex. Turjanski and colleagues (157) used ^{11}C-SCH23390 and ^{11}C-raclopride PET to study both D1 and D2 binding in HD. They found a parallel reduction in striatal binding to these receptor subtypes, with the levels of binding correlating with severity of rigidity rather than chorea. Striatal opioid and benzodiazepine binding have also been shown to be reduced in clinically affected HD patients (158,159). However, reductions are relatively small (20%) in comparison with the mean 60% loss of dopamine receptor binding.

The finding of reduced striatal dopamine receptor binding in patients with degenerative chorea is, again, not spe-

cific for HD as a mean 70% reduction of striatal ^{11}C-raclopride binding has been reported in neuroacanthocytosis (160). In contrast, normal striatal D2 binding has been reported in SLE chorea (157) and TD (161,162). This finding argues against the hypothesis that TD results from striatal D2 receptor supersensitivity following prolonged exposure to neuroleptics and suggests that the finding of downstream reductions in pallidal and subthalamic GABA levels may be of greater relevance.

Mildly affected HD patients show at least a 30% loss of striatal glucose metabolism and dopamine receptor binding, suggesting that ^{18}FDG, ^{11}C-SCH23390, and ^{11}C-raclopride PET should all be capable of detecting subclinical dysfunction when present in asymptomatic *HD* gene carriers. Reduced caudate glucose metabolism has been reported in 9 of 12 (163) and 3 of 8 (164) asymptomatic adult *HD* gene carriers in two different series. Weeks et al. (165) showed a significant parallel loss of striatal D1 and D2 binding in 4 of 8 asymptomatic adults with the HD mutation (Fig. 42.6). The rate of progression of HD has also been followed with PET. Grafton and colleagues (166) found that caudate glucose metabolism annually declined by 3.1% in their cohort of HD patients, whereas Antonini reported an annual 6% change in striatal D2 binding (167). Andrews and colleagues have reported an annual fall in striatal D1 and D2 binding of 3% to 4% in symptomatic *HD* gene carriers and 6% in asymptomatic *HD* gene carriers with active subclinical disease (168).

These findings suggest that functional imaging provides an objective means of following HD progression.

Transplantation of Huntington's Disease

Experimental grafting of fetal mesencephalic cells into the striatum of adults with PD has been reported to produce significant clinical improvements in the majority of younger patients (169). Transplantation of embryonic striatal tissue into the degenerated striatum of rat and primate models of HD has been shown to be safe, and has demonstrated good graft survival with differentiation and integration of striatal grafts into host striatum (170–172). Small-animal ^{11}C-raclopride PET has been able to detect recovery of striatal dopamine D2 binding in rats and marmosets lesioned with ibotenic acid after implantation of fetal striatal, but not fetal cortical, tissue (173–175). In primate models, recovery of skilled motor and cognitive performance has been reported within two months of grafting, and improvements in dystonia scores within 4 to 5 months (176). No improvement in cognitive or motor function was seen in three sham-operated monkey controls. Physiologic, neurochemical, and anatomic studies have shown that partial restoration of striatal input and output circuitry by implanted striatal neurons does occur, but the time course of this in primates and humans remains unclear.

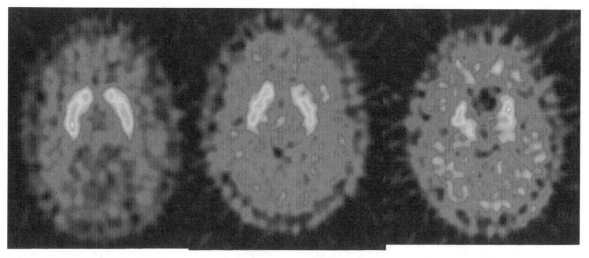

gene negative   **gene carrier**   **HD patient**

FIG. 42.6. PET images of ^{11}C-raclopride uptake in *HD* gene–negative and positive subjects. It can be seen that significant loss of striatal dopamine D_2 binding has occurred in the asymptomatic *HD* gene carrier. (Picture courtesy of T. Andrews.) (See color section.)

Groups in the United States, France, and England have now begun clinical studies of the possible therapeutic effects of striatal allografts in patients with HD. Recently, Bachoud-Levi and co-workers (177,178) have reported the preliminary [18]FDG PET findings for five HD patients implanted with striatal cells from 8- to 9-week gestation fetuses. Three subjects were felt to have improved over the course of 12 months in this series, whereas two deteriorated. In those three that clinically improved it was possible to detect striatal graft function, as evidenced by loci of increased glucose utilization seen with [18]FDG PET, but not in the two patients who subsequently deteriorated.

Dystonia

Dystonia is characterized by involuntary posturing and muscle spasms. The primary torsion dystonias (PTDs) range from severe, young-onset, generalized disorders to late-onset focal disease. The most common familial form of generalized PTD, DYT1 dystonia, has early onset and is an autosomal dominant disorder with around 40% penetrance. Onset is usually in childhood involving a limb, though onset in adulthood is occasionally seen. All cases of DYT1 dystonia identified have a common mutation—a GAG deletion within the coding region of the *DYT1* gene on chromosome 9q34, which codes for torsin A, an ATP-binding protein of unknown function. A second generalized PTD locus has been mapped to chromosome 8p *(DYT6)* and affected individuals have adult-onset generalized dystonia with craniocervical disease or focal dystonia. A third PTD gene *(DYT13)* has been mapped to chromosome 1p and has a phenotype of craniocervical and upper limb involvement with occasional generalization.

Postmortem studies have shown that DYT1 mRNA is highly expressed in dopaminergic neurons of the substantia nigra pars compacta, suggesting possible abnormal dopaminergic neurotransmission in dystonia. However, pathologic studies have failed to identify consistent structural or neurotransmitter abnormalities in idiopathic torsion dystonia (ITD). Regions often affected by causes of secondary dystonia include caudate, putamen, globus pallidus, and posterior thalamus (179). It has been suggested that ITD arises due to a reduced inhibitory output from the basal ganglia to ventral thalamus and frontal association areas causing these to become inappropriately overactive.

There have been a number of [18]FDG PET studies on resting levels of regional cerebral glucose metabolism in dystonia. A problem in interpreting the findings of earlier studies arises due to the heterogeneity of the patient groups recruited: familial, sporadic, and acquired dystonia have all been considered together and patients with focal or hemidystonia have been favored in order to provide side-to-side comparisons of basal ganglia function. As a consequence, the relevance of some of these PET findings to PTD is uncertain. In addition, some of these patients were clearly experiencing active muscular spasms while supposedly at rest. Resting lentiform nucleus metabolism in dystonia has been variously reported to be increased (180,181), normal (182–184), and decreased (185).

Covariance analysis of [18]FDG PET findings in *DYT1* carriers has produced more consistent and interpretable findings. In a series of reports, Eidelberg and colleagues (186) have shown an abnormal inverse relationship in *DYT1* carriers between resting levels of lentiform nucleus and frontal metabolism, the former being relatively reduced and the latter raised. This pattern is seen whether gene carriers are clinically affected or asymptomatic and is a pattern opposite to that seen in PD. A study on dystonic patients during sleep has also shown preservation of this abnormal pattern of resting glucose metabolism and confirmed that it is not movement related (187). These findings would support the concept of hyperexcitable frontal circuitry in dystonic patients even in the absence of movement.

Cerebral activation studies in PTD have suggested an imbalance between sensorimotor and PMC function. If dystonia patients perform paced joystick movements with their right hands in freely selected directions they show significantly increased levels of contralateral putamen, rostral SMA, lateral PMC, and dorsolateral prefrontal area activation (188,189). In contrast, there is impairment of activation of contralateral SMC and caudal SMA, that is, those cortical executive areas that send direct pyramidal tract projections to the spinal cord. Using a vibrotactile stimulator, Tempel and Perlmutter (190,191) also found impairment of SMC and caudal SMA activation in PTD and focal dystonia. The pattern of activation in dystonia is, therefore, very different from the pattern associated with PD where striatal, SMA, and prefrontal areas underfunction while primary motor cortex activation is normal or increased.

It would seem, therefore, that dystonic limb movements in PTD are associated with inappropriate overactivity of basal ganglia–frontal association area projections. Patients with acquired hemi- or focal dystonia due to basal ganglia and thalamic lesions also show increased levels of mesial and lateral PMC and dorsolateral prefrontal area activation during arm movement (192). In contrast to the PTD patients, acquired dystonia patients show raised rather than reduced primary motor cortex activation. This finding suggests that the pathology of PTD may have a direct inhibitory effect on primary motor cortex function.

The question arises, what is the significance of the frontal association area overactivity that is evident in both idiopathic and acquired dystonia? Three possibilities can be envisaged: First, the overactivity represents a primary dysfunction of motor planning circuitry. Second, the functional deficit in dystonia is at an executive level and the prefrontal cortex becomes overactive as the individual makes a conscious attempt to suppress the unwanted movements. Third, the frontal overactivity simply represents a secondary phenomenon reflecting primary basal ganglia overactivity.

Against the first hypothesis is the observation that ITD patients and normal subjects activate dorsolateral prefrontal and rostral SMAs equivalently when simply imagining joystick movements in freely chosen directions, but not performing them (193). This suggests that the primary functional deficit in idiopathic dystonia must lie at an executive rather than planning level. However, whether the frontal association area overactivity is simply secondary to primary basal ganglia overactivity or represents an adaptive phenomenon in a conscious attempt to suppress the syndrome remains unclear. In order to investigate this further, writer's

cramp patients were studied while writing before and after treatment with botulinum toxin (194). These patients again demonstrated premotor overactivity and sensorimotor underactivity while writing continuously, and this pattern did not reverse after relief of the associated forearm cramp with botulinum toxin. This would suggest that the frontal overactivity seen in dystonics is part of the pathophysiology of the syndrome and not simply an adaptive phenomenon to the presence of involuntary muscle spasms.

PET reports on dopaminergic function in dystonia have also suffered from inclusion of heterogeneous groups of patients. The only study to assess striatal ^{18}F-dopa uptake in purely familial PTD was by Playford and co-workers (195). These workers found that 8 of 11 PTD patients had normal striatal tracer uptake but that three with severe disease taking high doses of anticholinergics showed mild impairment of putamen ^{18}F-dopa uptake. The authors concluded that dopamine terminal function was normal in the majority of PTD patients. Two asymptomatic obligate gene carriers were studied and both had normal striatal ^{18}F-dopa uptake.

Martin et al. (196) examined three PTD dystonic subjects with ^{18}F-dopa PET. One of these had normal and two reduced striatal ^{18}F-dopa uptake. In contrast, Otsuka and colleagues (183) found a mildly raised level of mean striatal ^{18}F-dopa uptake in eight patients with ITD. Most recently, a ^{123}I-β-CIT SPECT study reported normal striatal uptake in ten patients with torticollis (197). Combining the findings of these studies, it would appear likely that striatal dopamine terminal function is normal in the majority of ITD cases.

Striatal D2 binding has also been studied in dystonia. A recent ^{18}F-spiperone PET study reported reduced putamen D2 binding in patients with Meige's syndrome and writer's cramp, but there was a wide overlap with the normal binding range (198). A similar finding was reported in an ^{123}I-epidepride SPECT study involving ten torticollis cases (197). The authors speculated that reduced striatal D2 binding could result in inappropriate activity of the indirect striatopallidal pathway similar to that seen in HD, resulting in involuntary movements.

Dopa-Responsive Dystonia and Dystonia-Parkinsonism

Dominantly inherited dopa-responsive dystonia (DRD) is related to GTP-cyclohydrolase 1 deficiency in the majority of cases, the genetic defect being located on chromosome 14. This enzyme constitutes part of the tetrahydrobiopterin synthetic pathway; tetrahydrobiopterin is the cofactor for tyrosine hydroxylase. Patients are unable to manufacture dopa, and hence dopamine, from endogenous tyrosine but can convert exogenous levodopa to dopamine. DRD patients generally present in childhood with diurnally fluctuating dystonia and later develop background parkinsonism. Occasionally, the condition presents as pure parkinsonism in adulthood. ^{18}F-dopa PET findings are normal in the majority of DRD patients (199,200), which can help to distinguish this condition from early-onset dystonia-parkinsonism where severely reduced putamen ^{18}F-dopa uptake is found (200,201). One might predict that striatal D2 binding would be raised in dopa-naive DRD patients in response to the chronically low levels of striatal dopamine present, and this has been reported to be the case (202). Treated DRD patients appear to have normal striatal D2 binding.

CONCLUSION

This chapter details the ways in which functional imaging has been used to demonstrate and distinguish the characteristic patterns of derangement of regional resting cerebral metabolism and neuropharmacology in the different parkinsonian, choreiform, and dystonic syndromes. Both PET and SPECT provide an objective means of detecting and discriminating parkinsonian syndromes. They also enable PD and HD progression to be objectively monitored and already have a role in evaluating the efficacy of putative neuroprotective and restorative agents, such as implants of fetal cells. In addition, PET has been able to detect subclinical functional abnormalities in at-risk subjects for PD and HD and has provided strong support for a role of inheritance in the former.

PET activation studies have helped to establish that the akinesia of PD is associated with selective underfunctioning of the SMA and dorsal prefrontal cortex, whereas inappropriate overactivity of these areas is associated with dystonia. Ligand activation approaches can now be used to measure levels of synaptic dopamine release and have shown that (a) parkinsonian off periods do not correlate well with basal ganglia synaptic dopamine levels (2), and (b) implants of fetal tissue can release normal amounts of dopamine after amphetamine challenge.

It is likely that changes in release of other neurotransmitters during parkinsonism and involuntary movements will become measurable and that the immune response to different movement disorders will be quantifiable.

REFERENCES

1. Jellinger K. The pathology of parkinsonism. In: Marsden CD, Fahn S, eds. *Movement disorders 2*. London: Butterworths, 1987:124–165.
2. German DC, Manaye K, Smith WK, et al. Midbrain dopaminergic cell loss in Parkinson's disease: computer visualization. *Ann Neurol* 1989;26:507–514.
3. Fearnley JM, Lees AJ. Ageing and Parkinson's disease: substantia nigra regional selectivity. *Brain* 1991;114:2283–2301.
4. Kish SJ, Shannak K, Hornykiewicz O. Uneven pattern of dopamine loss in the striatum of patients with idiopathic Parkinson's disease. *N Engl J Med* 1988;318:876–880.
5. McKeith I, Fairbairn A, Perry R, et al. Neuroleptic sensitivity in patients with senile dementia of Lewy body type. *BMJ* 1992; 305:673–678.
6. Brooks DJ, Ibañez V, Sawle GV, et al. Differing patterns of striatal ^{18}F-dopa uptake in Parkinson's disease, multiple system atrophy, and progressive supranuclear palsy. *Ann Neurol* 1990; 28:547–555.
7. Tedroff J, Aquilonius S-M, Hartvig P, et al. Cerebral uptake and utilisation of therapeutic [b-^{11}C]-L-dopa in Parkinson's disease measured by positron emission tomography: relations to motor response. *Acta Neurol Scand* 1992;85:95–102.
8. Rinne JO, Bergman J, Ruotinnen H, et al. Striatal uptake of a novel PET ligand, [^{18}F]b-CFT, is reduced in early Parkinson's disease. *Synapse* 1999;31:119–124.
9. Seibyl JP, Marek KL, Quinlan D, et al. Decreased single-photon emission computed tomographic [^{123}I]b-CIT striatal uptake correlates with symptom severity in Parkinson's disease. *Ann Neurol* 1995;38:589–598.
10. Frey KA, Koeppe RA, Kilbourn MR, et al. Pre-synaptic monoaminergic vesicles in Parkinson's disease and normal aging. *Ann Neurol* 1996;40:873–884.
11. Nahmias C, Garnett ES, Firnau G, et al. Striatal dopamine distribution in parkinsonian patients during life. *J Neurol Sci* 1985;69:223–230.
12. Leenders KL, Salmon EP, Tyrrell P, et al. The nigrostriatal dopaminergic system assessed in vivo by positron emission tomography in healthy volunteer subjects and patients with Parkinson's disease. *Arch Neurol* 1990;47:1290–1298.
13. Martin WRW, Adam MJ, Bergstrom M, et al. In vivo study of DOPA metabolism in Parkinson's disease. In: Fahn S, Jenner P, Marsden CD, et al., eds. *Recent developments in Parkinson's disease*. New York: Raven Press, 1986:97–102.
14. Morrish PK, Sawle GV, Brooks DJ. Regional changes in [^{18}F]dopa metabolism in the striatum in Parkinson's disease. *Brain* 1996;119:2097–2103.
15. Whone AL, Moore RY, Piccini P, et al. Compensatory changes in the globus pallidus in early Parkinson's disease: An F-18-dopa PET study. *Neurology* 2001;56[Supp 3]:A72–A73.
16. Rakshi JS, Uema T, Ito K, et al. Frontal, striatal, and midbrain dopaminergic function in early and advanced Parkinson's disease: a 3D ^{18}F-dopa PET study. *Brain* 1999;122:1637–1650.
17. Roberts AC, Desalvia MA, Wilkinson LS, et al. 6-hydroxy-dopamine lesions of the prefrontal cortex in monkeys enhance performance on an analog of the Wisconsin Card Sort Test: possible interactions with subcortical dopamine. *J Neurosci* 1994; 14:2531–2544.
18. Frost JJ, Rosier AJ, Reich SG, et al. Positron emission tomographic imaging of the dopamine transporter with ^{11}C-WIN 35,428 reveals marked declines in mild Parkinson's disease. *Ann Neurol* 1993;34:423–431.
19. Guttman M, Burkholder J, Kish SJ, et al. [^{11}C]RTI-32 PET studies of the dopamine transporter in early dopa-naive Parkinson's disease: implications for the symptomatic threshold. *Neurology* 1997;48:1578–1583.
20. Benamer HTS, Patterson J, Wyper DJ, et al. Correlation of Parkinson's disease severity and duration with I-123-FP-CIT SPECT striatal uptake. *Mov Disord* 2000;15:692–698.
21. Morris ED, Bonab AA, Alpert NM, et al. Concentration of dopamine transporters: to B-max or not to B-max? *Synapse* 1999;32:136–140.
22. Mozley PD, Schneider JS, Acton PD, et al. Binding of [Tc-99m]TRODAT-1 to dopamine transporters in patients with Parkinson's disease and in healthy volunteers. *J Nucl Med* 2000; 41:584–589.
23. Vingerhoets FJG, Schulzer M, Caine DB, et al. Which clinical sign of Parkinson's disease best reflects the nigrostriatal lesion? *Ann Neurol* 1997;41:58–64.

24. Lee CS, Samii A, Sossi V, et al. In vivo positron emission tomographic evidence for compensatory changes in presynaptic dopaminergic nerve terminals in Parkinson's disease. *Ann Neurol* 2000;47:493–503.

25. Golbe LI. The genetics of Parkinson's disease: a reconsideration. *Neurology* 1990;40[Suppl 3]:7–16.

26. Piccini P, Morrish PK, Turjanski N, et al. Dopaminergic function in familial Parkinson's disease: a clinical and ^{18}F-dopa PET study. *Ann Neurol* 1997;41:222–229.

27. Lazzarini AM, Myers RH, Zimmerman TRJ, et al. A clinical genetic study of Parkinson's disease: evidence for dominant transmission. *Neurology* 1994;44:499–506.

28. Piccini P, Burn DJ, Ceravalo R, et al. The role of inheritance in sporadic Parkinson's disease: evidence from a longitudinal study of dopaminergic function in twins. *Ann Neurol* 1999;45:577–582.

29. Holthoff VA, Vieregge P, Kessler J, et al. Discordant twins with Parkinson's disease: positron emission tomography and early signs of impaired cognitive circuits. *Ann Neurol* 1994;36:176–182.

30. Berendse HW, Booij J, Francot CMJE, et al. Subclinical dopaminergic dysfunction in asymptomatic Parkinson's disease patients' relatives with a decreased sense of smell. *Ann Neurol* 2001;50:34–41.

31. McGeer PL, Itagaki S, Boyes BE, et al. Reactive microglia are positive for HLA-DR in the substantia nigra of Parkinson's and Alzheimer's disease brains. *Neurology* 1988;38:1285–1291.

32. Gerhardt A, Banati RB, Cagnin A, et al. In vivo imaging of activated microglia with [C-11]PK11195 positron emission tomography (PET) in idiopathic and atypical Parkinson's disease. *Neurology* 2001;56[Supp 3]:A270 (abstr).

33. Olanow CW, Jenner P, Brooks D. Dopamine agonists and neuroprotection in Parkinson's disease. *Ann Neurol* 1998;44[Suppl 1]:S167–S174.

34. Pate BD, Kawamata T, Yamada T, et al. Correlation of striatal fluorodopa uptake in the MPTP monkey with dopaminergic indices. *Ann Neurol* 1993;34:331–338.

35. Vingerhoets FJG, Snow BJ, Lee CS, et al. Longitudinal fluorodopa positron emission tomographic studies of the evolution of idiopathic parkinsonism. *Ann Neurol* 1994;36:759–764.

36. Morrish PK, Sawle GV, Brooks DJ. An [^{18}F]dopa PET and clinical study of the rate of progression in Parkinson's disease. *Brain* 1996;119:585–591.

37. Morrish PK, Rakshi JS, Sawle GV, et al. Measuring the rate of progression and estimating the preclinical period of Parkinson's disease with [^{18}F]dopa PET. *J Neurol Neurosurg Psychiatry* 1998;64:314–319.

38. Marek KL, Seibyl J, Fussell B, et al. 123I b-CIT: assessment of progression in Parkinson's disease. *Neurology* 1997;48[Suppl 2]:A207.

39. Marek KL, Innis R, Seibyl J. b-CIT/SPECT assessment of determinants of variability in progression of Parkinson's disease. *Neurology* 1999;52[Suppl 2]:A91–A92 (abstr).

40. Schwarz J, Tatsch K, Linke R, et al. Measuring the decline of dopamine transporter binding in patients with Parkinson's disease using 123I-IPT and SPECT. *Neurology* 1997;48[Suppl 2]:A208.

41. Rakshi JS, Bailey DL, Uema T, et al. Is ropinirole, a selective D$_2$ receptor agonist, neuro-protective in early Parkinson's disease? An [^{18}F]dopa PET study. *Neurology* 1998;50[Suppl 4]:A330 (abstr).

42. Holloway R, Shoulson I, Kieburtz K, et al. Pramipexole vs levodopa as initial treatment for Parkinson disease—a randomized controlled trial. *JAMA* 2000;284:1931–1938.

43. Wenning GK, Odin P, Morrish PK, et al. Short- and long-term survival and function of unilateral intrastriatal dopaminergic grafts in Parkinson's disease. *Ann Neurol* 1997;42:95–107.

44. Piccini P, Brooks DJ, Bjorklund A, et al. Dopamine release from nigral transplants visualised *in vivo* in a Parkinson's patient. *Nat Neurosci* 1999;2:1137–1140.

45. Remy P, Samson Y, Hantraye P, et al. Clinical correlates of [^{18}F]fluorodopa uptake in five grafted parkinsonian patients. *Ann Neurol* 1995;38:580–588.

46. Hauser RA, Freeman TB, Snow BJ, et al. Long-term evaluation of bilateral fetal nigral transplantation in Parkinson disease. *Arch Neurol* 1999;56:179–187.

47. Kordower JH, Freeman TB, Snow BJ, et al. Neuropathological evidence of graft survival and striatal reinnervation after the transplantation of fetal mesencephalic tissue in a patient with Parkinson's disease. *N Engl J Med* 1995;332:1118–1124.

48. Kordower JH, Freeman TB, Chen EY, et al. Fetal nigral grafts survive and mediate clinical benefit in a patient with Parkinson's disease. *Mov Disord* 1998;13:383–393.

49. Freed CR, Greene PE, Breeze RE, et al. Transplantation of embryonic dopamine neurons for severe Parkinson's disease. *N Engl J Med* 2001;344:710–719.

50. Leenders KL, Palmer AJ, Quinn N, et al. Brain dopamine metabolism in patients with Parkinson's disease measured with positron emission tomography. *J Neurol Neurosurg Psychiatry* 1986;49:853–860.

51. Staffen W, Mair A, Unterrainer J, et al. Measuring the progression of idiopathic Parkinson's disease with [I-123] beta-CIT SPECT. *J Neural Transm* 2000;107:543–552.

52. De la Fuente-Fernández R, Pal PK, et al. Evidence for impaired presynaptic dopamine function in parkinsonian patients with motor fluctuations. *J Neural Transm* 2000;107:49–57.

53. Playford ED, Brooks DJ. In vivo and in vitro studies of the dopaminergic system in movement disorders. *Cerebrovasc Brain Metab Rev* 1992;4:144–171.

54. Rinne JO, Laihinen A, Rinne UK, et al. PET study on striatal dopamine D2 receptor changes during the progression of early Parkinson's disease. *Mov Disord* 1993;8:134–138.

55. Turjanski N, Lees AJ, Brooks DJ. PET studies on striatal dopaminergic receptor binding in drug naive and L-dopa-treated Parkinson's disease patients with and without dyskinesia. *Neurology* 1997;49:717–723.

56. Sawle GV, Playford ED, Brooks DJ, et al. Asymmetrical presynaptic and postsynaptic changes in the striatal dopamine projection in dopa-naive parkinsonism: diagnostic implications of the D$_2$ receptor status. *Brain* 1993;116:853–867.

57. Hagglund J, Aquilonius SM, Eckernas SA, et al. Dopamine receptor properties in Parkinson's disease and Huntington's chorea evaluated by positron emission tomography using 11C-N-methyl-spiperone. *Acta Neurol Scand* 1987;75:87–94.

58. Brucke T, Podreka I, Angelberger P, et al. Dopamine D2 receptor imaging with SPECT: studies in different neuropsychiatric disorders. *J Cereb Blood Flow Metab* 1991;11:220–228.

59. Antonini A, Schwarz J, Oertel WH, et al. [^{11}C]raclopride and positron emission tomography in previously untreated patients with Parkinson's disease: influence of L-dopa and lisuride therapy on striatal dopamine D$_2$-receptors. *Neurology* 1994;44:1325–1329.

60. Guttman M, Seeman P, Reynolds GP, et al. Dopamine D2 receptor density remains constant in treated Parkinson's disease. *Ann Neurol* 1986;19:487–492.

61. Rinne JO, Laihinen A, Nagren K, et al. PET demonstrates different behaviour of striatal dopamine D1 and D2 receptors in early Parkinson's disease. *J Neurosci Res* 1990;27:494–499.

62. Kishore A, De la Fuente-Fernández R, Snow BJ, et al. Levodopa-induced dyskinesias in idiopathic parkinsonism (IP): a simultaneous PET study of dopamine D1 and D2 receptors. *Neurology* 1997;48:A327(abstr).

63. Torstenson R, Hartvig P, Långström B, et al. Differential effects

of levodopa on dopaminergic function in early and advanced Parkinson's disease. *Ann Neurol* 1997;41:334–340.

64. De la Fuente-Fernández R, Lu JQ, Sossi V, et al. Biochemical variations in the synaptic level of dopamine precede motor fluctuations in Parkinson's disease: PET evidence of increased dopamine turnover. *Ann Neurol* 2001;49:298–303.

65. Henry B, Brotchie JM. Potential of opioid antagonists in the treatment of levodopa-induced dyskinesias in Parkinson's disease. *Drugs Aging* 1996;9:149–158.

66. Murrin LC, Coyle JT, Kuhar MJ. Striatal opiate receptors: pre- and postsynaptic localisation. *Life Sci* 1980;27:1175–1183.

67. Nisbet AP, Foster OJF, Kingsbury, A et al. Preproenkephalin and preprotachykinin messenger-RNA expression in normal human basal ganglia and in Parkinson's disease. *Neuroscience* 1995;66:361–376.

68. Jolkkonen J, Jenner P, Marsden CD. L-Dopa reverses altered gene expression of substance P but not enkephalin in the caudate-putamen of common marmosets treated with MPTP. *Mol Brain Res* 1995;32:297–307.

69. Lavoie B, Parent A, Bedard PJ. Effects of dopamine denervation on striatal peptide expression in parkinsonian monkeys. *Can J Neurol Sci* 1991;18:373–375.

70. Piccini P, Weeks RA, Brooks DJ. Opioid receptor binding in Parkinson's patients with and without levodopa-induced dyskinesias. *Ann Neurol* 1997;42:720–726.

71. Miletich RS, Chan T, Gillespie M, et al. Contralateral basal ganglia metabolism is abnormal in hemiparkinsonian patients: an FDG-PET study. *Neurology* 1988;38:S260.

72. Wolfson LI, Leenders KL, Brown LL, et al. Alterations of regional cerebral blood flow and oxygen metabolism in Parkinson's disease. *Neurology* 1985;35:1399–1405.

73. Eidelberg D, Moeller JR, Dhawan V, et al. The metabolic topography of parkinsonism. *J Cereb Blood Flow Metab* 1994;14:783–801.

74. Peppard RF, Martin WRW, Guttman M, et al. The relationship of cerebral glucose metabolism to cognitive deficits in Parkinson's disease. *Neurology* 1988;38[Supp 1]:364.

75. Kuhl DE, Metter EJ, Benson DF, et al. Similarities of cerebral glucose metabolism in Alzheimer's and parkinsonian dementia. *J Cereb Blood Flow Metab* 1985;5:S169–S170(abstr).

76. Bohnen NI, Minoshima S, Giordani B, et al. Motor correlates of occipital glucose hypometabolism in Parkinson's disease without dementia. *Neurology* 1999;52:541–546.

77. Hu MTM, Taylor-Robinson SD, Chaudhuri KR, et al. Cortical dysfunction in non-demented Parkinson's disease patients: a combined ^{31}phosphorus MRS and ^{18}FDG PET study. *Brain* 2000;123:340–352.

78. Playford ED, Jenkins IH, Passingham RE, et al. Impaired mesial frontal and putamen activation in Parkinson's disease: a PET study. *Ann Neurol* 1992;32:151–161.

79. Jahanshahi M, Jenkins IH, Brown RG, et al. Self-initiated versus externally-triggered movements: measurements of regional cerebral blood flow and movement-related potentials in normals and Parkinson's disease. *Brain* 1995;118:913–933.

80. Samuel M, Ceballos-Baumann AO, Blin J, et al. Evidence for lateral premotor and parietal overactivity in Parkinson's disease during sequential and bimanual movements: a PET study. *Brain* 1997;120:963–976.

81. Thaler DE, Passingham RE. The supplementary motor cortex and internally directed movement. In: Crossman AR, Sambrook M, eds. *Neural mechanisms in disorders of movement.* London: Libby, 1989:175–181.

82. Rascol O, Sabatini U, Fabre N, et al. The ipsilateral cerebellar hemisphere is overactive during hand movements in akinetic parkinsonian patients. *Brain* 1997;120:103–110.

83. Sabatini U, Boulanouar K, Fabre N, et al. Cortical motor reor-

ganization in akinetic patients with Parkinson's disease—a functional MRI study. *Brain* 2000;123:394–403.

84. Thobois S, Dominey P, Decety J, et al. Overactivation of primary motor cortex is asymmetrical in hemiparkinsonian patients. *Neuroreport* 2000;11:785–789.

85. Mushiake H, Inase M, Tanji J. Selective coding of motor sequence in the supplementary motor area of the monkey cerebral cortex. *Exp Brain Res* 1990;82:208–210.

86. Brooks DJ, Jenkins IH, Passingham RE. Positron emission tomography studies on regional cerebral control of voluntary movement. In: Mano N, Hamada I, DeLong MR, eds. *Role of the cerebellum and basal ganglia in voluntary movement.* Amsterdam: Excerpta Medica, 1993:267–274.

87. Jenkins IH, Fernandez W, Playford ED, et al. Impaired activation of the supplementary motor area in Parkinson's disease is reversed when akinesia is treated with apomorphine. *Ann Neurol* 1992;32:749–757.

88. Rascol O, Sabatini U, Chollet F, et al. Supplementary and primary sensory motor area activity in Parkinson's disease: regional cerebral blood flow changes during finger movements and effects of apomorphine. *Arch Neurol* 1992;49:144–148.

89. Rascol O, Sabatini U, Chollet F, et al. Normal activation of the supplementary motor area in patients with Parkinson's disease undergoing long-term treatment with levodopa. *J Neurol Neurosurg Psychiatry* 1994;57:567–571.

90. Haslinger B, Erhard P, Kampfe N, et al. Event-related functional magnetic resonance imaging in Parkinson's disease before and after levodopa. *Brain* 2001;124:558–570.

91. Piccini P, Lindvall O, Bjorklund A, et al. Delayed recovery of movement-related cortical function in Parkinson's disease after striatal dopaminergic grafts. *Ann Neurol* 2000;48:689–695.

92. Grafton ST, Waters C, Sutton J, et al. Pallidotomy increases activity of motor association cortex in Parkinson's disease—a positron emission tomographic study. *Ann Neurol* 1995;37:776–783.

93. Samuel M, Ceballos-Baumann AO, Turjanski N, et al. Pallidotomy in Parkinson's disease increases SMA and prefrontal activation during performance of volitional movements: an H$_2^{15}$O PET study. *Brain* 1997;120:1301–1313.

94. Davis KD, Taub E, Houle S, et al. Globus pallidus stimulation activates the cortical motor system during alleviation of parkinsonian symptoms. *Nat Med* 1997;3:671–674.

95. Limousin P, Greene J, Polak P, et al. Changes in cerebral activity pattern due to subthalamic nucleus or internal pallidum stimulation in Parkinson's disease. *Ann Neurol* 1997;42:283–291.

96. Eidelberg D, Nakamura T, Mentis M, et al. Brain activation responses with internal pallidal stimulation in Parkinson's disease. *Neurology* 1999;52[Suppl 2]:A176(abstr).

97. Ceballos-Baumann AO, Boecker H, Bartenstein P, et al. A positron emission tomographic study of subthalamic nucleus stimulation in Parkinson disease–enhanced movement-related activity of motor-association cortex and decreased motor cortex resting activity. *Arch Neurol* 1999;56:997–1003.

98. De Volder AG, Francard J, Laterre C, et al. Decreased glucose utilisation in the striatum and frontal lobe in probable striatonigral degeneration. *Ann Neurol* 1989;26:239–247.

99. Otsuka M, Ichiya Y, Hosokawa S, et al. Striatal blood flow, glucose metabolism, and ^{18}F-dopa uptake: difference in Parkinson's disease and atypical parkinsonism. *J Neurol Neurosurg Psychiatry* 1991;54:898–904.

100. Eidelberg D, Takikawa S, Moeller JR, et al. Striatal hypometabolism distinguishes striatonigral degeneration from Parkinson's disease. *Ann Neurol* 1993;33:518–527.

101. Eidelberg D, Moeller JR, Ishikawa T, et al. Regional metabolic correlates of surgical outcome following unilateral pallidotomy for Parkinson's disease. *Ann Neurol* 1996;39:450–459.

102. Davie CA, Wenning GK, Barker GJ, et al. Differentiation of

multiple system atrophy from idiopathic Parkinson's disease using proton magnetic resonance spectroscopy. *Ann Neurol* 1995;37:204–210.

103. Brooks DJ, Salmon EP, Mathias CJ, et al. The relationship between locomotor disability, autonomic dysfunction, and the integrity of the striatal dopaminergic system, in patients with multiple system atrophy, pure autonomic failure, and Parkinson's disease, studied with PET. *Brain* 1990;113:1539–1552.

104. Fearnley JM, Lees AJ. Striatonigral degeneration: a clinico-pathological study. *Brain* 1990;113:1823–1842.

105. Burn DJ, Sawle GV, Brooks DJ. The differential diagnosis of Parkinson's disease, multiple system atrophy, and Steele-Richardson-Olszewski syndrome: discriminant analysis of striatal ^{18}F-dopa PET data. *J Neurol Neurosurg Psychiatry* 1994;57:278–284.

106. Pirker W, Asenbaum S, Bencsits G, et al. [I-123]beta-CIT SPECT in multiple system atrophy, progressive supranuclear palsy, and corticobasal degeneration. *Mov Disord* 2000;15:1158–1167.

107. Shinotoh H, Aotsuka A, Yonezawa H, et al. Striatal dopamine D$_2$ receptors in Parkinson's disease and striato-nigral degeneration determined by positron emission tomography. In: Nagatsu T, Fisher A, Yoshida M, eds. *Basic, clinical, and therapeutic advances of Alzheimer's and Parkinson's diseases,* Vol 2. New York: Plenum Press, 1990:107–110.

108. Brooks DJ, Ibanez V, Sawle GV, et al. Striatal D$_2$ receptor status in Parkinson's disease, striatonigral degeneration, and progressive supranuclear palsy, measured with ^{11}C-raclopride and PET. *Ann Neurol* 1992;31:184–192.

109. Shinotoh H, Inoue O, Hirayama K, et al. Dopamine D$_1$ receptors in Parkinson's disease and striatonigral degeneration: a positron emission tomography study. *J Neurol Neurosurg Psychiatry* 1993;56:467–472.

110. Schwarz J, Tatsch K, Arnold G, et al. ^{123}I-Iodobenzamide-SPECT predicts dopaminergic responsiveness in patients with de-novo parkinsonism. *Neurology* 1992;42:556–561.

111. Seppi K, Donnemiller E, Riccabona G, et al. Disease progression in PD vs. MSA: a SPECT study using 123-I IBZM. *Parkinsonism Relat Disord* 2001;7:S24(abstr).

112. Goto S, Hirano A, Matsumoto S. Met-enkephalin immunoreactivity in the basal ganglia in Parkinson's disease and striatonigral degeneration. *Neurology* 1990;40:1051–1056.

113. Burn DJ, Rinne JO, Quinn NP, et al. Striatal opioid receptor binding in Parkinson's disease, striatonigral degeneration, and Steele-Richardson-Olszewski syndrome: an ^{11}C-diprenorphine PET study. *Brain* 1995;118:951–958.

114. Druschky A, Hilz MJ, Platsch G, et al. Differentiation of Parkinson's disease and multiple system atrophy in early disease stages by means of I-123-MIBG-SPECT. *J Neurol Sci* 2000;175:3–12.

115. Rinne JO, Burn DJ, Mathias CJ, et al. PET studies on the dopaminergic system and striatal opioid binding in the olivopontocerebellar atrophy variant of multiple system atrophy. *Ann Neurol* 1995;37:568–573.

116. Otsuka M, Ichiya Y, Kuwabara Y, et al. Striatal ^{18}F-dopa uptake and brain glucose metabolism by PET in patients with syndrome of progressive ataxia. *J Neurol Sci* 1994;124:198–203.

117. Gilman S, Koeppe RA, Junck L, et al. Patterns of cerebral glucose metabolism detected with positron emission tomography differ in multiple system atrophy and olivopontocerebellar atrophy. *Ann Neurol* 1994;36:166–175.

118. D'Antona R, Baron JC, Samson Y, et al. Subcortical dementia: frontal cortex hypometabolism detected by positron emission tomography in patients with progressive supranuclear palsy. *Brain* 1985;108:785–799.

119. Blin J, Baron JC, Dubois P, et al. Positron emission tomography

120. Foster NL, Gilman S, Berent S, et al. Cerebral hypometabolism in progressive supranuclear palsy studied with positron emission tomography. *Ann Neurol* 1988;24:399–406.

121. Goffinet A, DeVolder AG, Gillain C, et al. Positron tomography demonstrates frontal lobe hypometabolism in progressive supranuclear palsy. *Ann Neurol* 1989;25:131–139.

122. Otsuka M, Ichiya Y, Kuwabara Y, et al. Cerebral blood flow, oxygen and glucose metabolism with PET in progressive supranuclear palsy. *Ann Nuc Med* 1989;3:111–118.

123. Foster NL, Gilman S, Berent S, et al. Progressive subcortical gliosis and progressive supranuclear palsy can have similar clinical and PET abnormalities. *J Neurol Neurosurg Psychiatry* 1992;55:707–713.

124. Davie CA, Barker GJ, Machado C, et al. Proton magnetic resonance spectroscopy in Steele-Richardson-Olszewski syndrome. *Mov Disord* 1997;12:767–771.

125. Leenders KL, Frackowiak RS, Lees AJ. Steele-Richardson-Olszewski syndrome: brain energy metabolism, blood flow, and fluorodopa uptake measured by positron emission tomography. *Brain* 1988;111:615–630.

126. Bhatt MH, Snow BJ, Martin WRW, et al. Positron emission tomography in progressive supranuclear palsy. *Arch Neurol* 1991;48:389–391.

127. Jellinger K, Riederer P, Tomananga M. Progressive supranuclear palsy: clinicopathological and biochemical studies. *J Neural Transm* 1980;[Suppl 16]:111–128.

128. Kish SJ, Chang LJ, Mirchandani LJ, et al. Progressive supranuclear palsy: relationship between extrapyramidal disturbances, dementia, and brain neurotransmitter markers. *Ann Neurol* 1985;18:530–536.

129. Messa C, Volonte MA, Fazio F, et al. Differential distribution of striatal [^{123}I]b-CIT in Parkinson's disease and progressive supranuclear palsy, evaluated with single-photon emission tomography. *Eur J Nucl Med* 1998;25:1270–1276.

130. Baron JC, Maziere B, Loc'h C, et al. Loss of striatal (76Br)bromospiperone binding sites demonstrated by positron tomography in progressive supranuclear palsy. *J Cereb Blood Flow Metab* 1986;6:131–136.

131. Wienhard K, Coenen HH, Pawlik G, et al. PET studies of dopamine receptor distribution using [18F]fluoroethylspiperone: findings in disorders related to the dopaminergic system. *J Neural Transm* 1990;81:195–213.

132. Pappata S, Traykov L, Tavitian B, et al. Striatal reduction of acetylcholinesterase in patients with progressive supranuclear palsy (PSP) as measured in vivo by PET and ^{11}C-physostigmine (^{11}C-PHY). *J Cereb Blood Flow Metab* 1997;17[Suppl 1]:S687.

132a. Feaney MB, Ksiezakreding H, Liu WK, et al. Epitope expression and hyperphosphorylation of tau protein in corticobasal degeneration–differentiation from progressive supranuclear palsy. *Acta Neuropathologica* 1995;90:37–43.

133. Sawle GV, Brooks DJ, Marsden CD, et al. Corticobasal degeneration: a unique pattern of regional cortical oxygen metabolism and striatal fluorodopa uptake demonstrated by positron emission tomography. *Brain* 1991;114:541–556.

134. Eidelberg D, Dhawan V, Moeller JR, et al. The metabolic landscape of cortico-basal ganglionic degeneration: regional asymmetries studied with positron emission tomography. *J Neurol Neurosurg Psychiatry* 1991;54:856–862.

135. Blin J, Vidhailhet M-J, Pillon B, et al. Corticobasal degeneration: decreased and asymmetrical glucose consumption as studied by PET. *Mov Disord* 1992;7:348–354.

136. Markus HS, Lees AJ, Lennox G, et al. Patterns of regional cerebral blood flow in corticobasal degeneration studied using

study in progressive supranuclear palsy. *Arch Neurol* 1990;47:747–752.

HMPAO SPECT—comparison with Parkinson's disease and normal controls. *Mov Disord* 1995;10:179–187.

137. Frisoni GB, Pizzolato G, Zanetti O, et al. Corticobasal degeneration: neuropsychological assessment and dopamine D-2 receptor SPECT analysis. *Eur Neurol* 1995;35:50–54.

138. Nagahama Y, Fukuyama H, Turjanski N, et al. Cerebral glucose metabolism in corticobasal degeneration: comparison with progressive supranuclear palsy and normal controls. *Mov Disord* 1997;12:691–696.

139. Albin RL, Reiner A, Anderson KD, et al. Striatal and nigral neuron subpopulations in rigid Huntington's disease: implications for the functional anatomy of chorea and rigidity-akinesia. *Ann Neurol* 1990;27:357–365.

140. Kuhl DE, Phelps ME, Markham CH, et al. Cerebral metabolism and atrophy in Huntington's disease determined by ^{18}FDG and computed tomographic scans. *Ann Neurol* 1982;12:425–434.

141. Hayden MR, Martin WRW, Stoessl AJ, et al. Positron emission tomography in the early diagnosis of Huntington's disease. *Neurology* 1986;36:888–894.

142. Leenders KL, Frackowiak RSJ, Quinn N, et al. Brain energy metabolism and dopaminergic function in Huntington's disease measured in vivo using positron emission tomography. *Mov Disord* 1986;1:69–77.

143. Young AB, Penney JB, Starosta-Rubinstein S, et al. PET scan investigations of Huntington's disease: cerebral metabolic correlates of neurological features and functional decline. *Ann Neurol* 1986;20:296–303.

144. Berent S, Giordani B, Lehtinen S, et al. Positron emission tomographic scan investigations of Huntington's disease: cerebral metabolic correlates of cognitive function. *Ann Neurol* 1988;23:541–546.

145. Kuwert T, Lange HW, Langen KJ, et al. Cortical and subcortical glucose consumption measured by PET in patients with Huntington's disease. *Brain* 1990;113:1405–1423.

146. Dubinsky RM, Hallett M, Levey R, et al. Regional brain glucose metabolism in neuroacanthocytosis. *Neurology* 1989;39:1253–1255.

147. Hosokawa S, Ichiya Y, Kuwabara Y, et al. Positron emission tomography in cases of chorea with different underlying diseases. *J Neurol Neurosurg Psychiatry* 1987;50:1284–1287.

148. Kuwert T, Lange HW, Langen KJ, et al. Normal striatal glucose consumption in two patients with benign hereditary chorea as measured by positron emission tomography. *J Neurol* 1990;237:80–84.

149. Suchowersky O, Hayden MR, Martin WRW, et al. Cerebral metabolism of glucose in benign hereditary chorea. *Mov Disord* 1986;1:33–45.

150. Guttman M, Lang AE, Garnett ES, et al. Regional cerebral glucose metabolism in SLE chorea: further evidence that striatal hypometabolism is not a correlate of chorea. *Mov Disord* 1987;2:201–210.

151. Weindl A, Kuwert T, Leenders KL, et al. Increased striatal glucose consumption in Sydenham chorea. *Mov Disord* 1993;8:437–444.

152. Pahl JJ, Mazziotta JC, Cummings J, et al. Positron emission tomography in tardive dyskinesia and Huntington's disease. *J Cereb Blood Flow Metab* 1987;7:1253–1255.

153. Jenkins BG, Koroshetz WJ, Beal MF, et al. Evidence for impairment of energy metabolism in vivo in Huntington's disease using localised ^{1}H NMR spectroscopy. *Neurology* 1993;43:2689–2695.

154. Beal MF. Does impairment of energy metabolism result in excitotoxic neuronal death in neurodegenerative illnesses? *Ann Neurol* 1992;31:119–130.

155. Taylor-Robinson SD, Weeks RA, Sargentoni J, et al. Proton MRS in Huntington's disease: evidence in favour of the glutamate excitotoxic theory? *Mov Disord* 1996;11:167–173.

156. Karlsson P, Lundin A, Anvret M, et al. Dopamine D1 receptor number—a sensitive PET marker for early brain degeneration in Huntington's disease. *Eur Arch Psychiatry Clin Neurosci* 1994;243:249–255.

157. Turjanski N, Weeks R, Dolan R, et al. Striatal D_1 and D_2 receptor binding in patients with Huntington's disease and other choreas: a PET study. *Brain* 1995;118:689–696.

158. Weeks RA, Cunningham VJ, Piccini P, et al. ^{11}C-Diprenorphine binding in Huntington's disease: a comparison of region of interest analysis and statistical parametric mapping. *J Cereb Blood Flow Metab* 1997;17:943–949.

159. Holthoff VA, Koeppe RA, Frey KA, et al. Positron emission tomography measures of benzodiazepine receptors in Huntington's disease. *Ann Neurol* 1993;34:76–81.

160. Brooks DJ, Ibanez V, Playford ED, et al. Presynaptic and postsynaptic striatal dopaminergic function in neuroacanthocytosis: a positron emission tomographic study. *Ann Neurol* 1991;30:166–171.

161. Andersson U, Eckernas SA, Hartvig P, et al. Striatal binding of ^{11}C-NMSP studied with positron emission tomography in patients with persistent tardive dyskinesia: no evidence for altered dopamine receptor binding. *J Neural Transm* 1990;79:215–226.

162. Blin J, Baron JC, Cambon H, et al. Striatal dopamine D2 receptors in tardive dyskinesia: PET study. *Neurology* 1989;39:274.

163. Grafton ST, Mazziotta JC, Pahl JJ, et al. A comparison of neurological, metabolic, structural, and genetic evaluations in persons at risk for Huntington's disease. *Ann Neurol* 1990;28:614–621.

164. Hayden MR, Hewitt J, Martin WRW, et al. Studies in persons at risk for Huntington's disease. *N Engl J Med* 1987;317:382–383.

165. Weeks RA, Piccini P, Harding AE, et al. Striatal D_1 and D_2 dopamine receptor loss in asymptomatic mutation carriers of Huntington's disease. *Ann Neurol* 1996;40:49–54.

166. Grafton ST, Mazziotta JC, Pahl JJ, et al. Serial changes of cerebral glucose metabolism and caudate size in persons at risk for Huntington's disease. *Arch Neurol* 1992;49:1161–1167.

167. Antonini A, Leenders KL, Spiegel R, et al. Striatal glucose metabolism and dopamine D-2 receptor binding in asymptomatic gene carriers and patients with Huntington's disease. *Brain* 1996;119:2085–2095.

168. Andrews TC, Weeks RA, Turjanski N, et al. Huntington's disease progression: PET and clinical observations. *Brain* 1999;122:2353–2363.

169. Lindvall O. Cerebral implantation in movement disorders: state of the art. *Mov Disord* 1999;14:201–205.

170. Brasted PJ, Robbins TW, Dunnett SB. Distinct roles for striatal subregions in mediating response processing revealed by focal excitotoxic lesions. *Behav Neurosci* 1999;113:253–264.

171. Brasted PJ, Watts C, Robbins TW, et al. Associative plasticity in striatal transplants. *Proc Natl Acad Sci USA* 1999;96:10524–10529.

172. Brasted PJ, Watts C, Torres EM, et al. Behavioural recovery following striatal transplantation: effects of postoperative training and P-zone volume. *Exp Brain Res* 1999;128:535–538.

173. Fricker RA, Torres EM, Hume SP, et al. The effects of donor stage on the survival and function of embryonic striatal grafts in the adult rat brain. II. Correlation between positron emission tomography and reaching behaviour. *Neuroscience* 1997;79:711–722.

174. Kendall L, Rayment D, Aigbirhio F, et al. In vivo PET analysis of the status of striatal allografts in the common marmoset. *Eur J Neurosci* 1998;10:15604.

175. Torres EM, Fricker RA, Hume SP, et al. Assessment of striatal graft viability in the rat *in vivo* using a small diameter PET scanner. *Neuroreport* 1995;6:2017–2021.

176. Palfi S, Conde F, Riche D, et al. Fetal striatal allografts reverse cognitive deficits in a primate model of Huntington's disease. *Nature Med* 1998;4:963–966.

177. Bachoud-Levi A, Remy P, Nguyen JP, et al. Motor and cognitive improvements in patients with Huntington's disease after neural transplantation. *Lancet* 2000;356:1975–1979.

178. Bachoud-Levi AC, Bourdet C, Brugieres P, et al. Safety and tolerability assessment of intrastriatal neural allografts in five patients with Huntington's disease. *Exp Neurol* 2000;161:194–202.

179. Bhatia KP, Marsden CD. The behavioural and motor consequences of focal lesions of the basal ganglia in man. *Brain* 1994;117:859–876.

180. Chase T, Tamminga CA, Burrows H. Positron emission studies of regional cerebral glucose metabolism in idiopathic dystonia. *Adv Neurol* 1988;50:237–241.

181. Eidelberg D, Dhawan V, Cedarbaum J, et al. Contralateral basal ganglia hypermetabolism in primary unilateral limb dystonia. *Neurology* 1990;40[Suppl 1]:399.

182. Gilman S, Junck L, Young AB, et al. Cerebral metabolic activity in idiopathic dystonia studied with positron emission tomography. *Adv Neurol* 1988;50:231–236.

183. Otsuka M, Ichiya Y, Shima F, et al. Increased striatal ^18F-dopa uptake and normal glucose metabolism in idiopathic dystonia syndrome. *J Neurol Sci* 1992;111:195–199.

184. Stoessl AJ, Martin WRW, Clark C, et al. PET studies of cerebral glucose metabolism in idiopathic torticollis. *Neurology* 1986;36: 653–657.

185. Karbe H, Holthoff VA, Rudolf J, et al. Positron emission tomography demonstrates frontal cortex and basal ganglia hypometabolism in dystonia. *Neurology* 1992;42:1540–1544.

186. Eidelberg D, Moeller JR, Antonini A, et al. Abnormal metabolic brain networks in DYT-1 dystonia. *Neurology* 1997;48 [Suppl 2]:A62.

187. Eidelberg D, Moeller JR, Antonini A, et al. Functional brain networks in DYT1 dystonia. *Ann Neurol* 1998;44:303–312.

188. Playford ED, Passingham RE, Marsden CD, et al. Increased activation of frontal areas during arm movement in idiopathic torsion dystonia. *Mov Disord* 1998;13:309–318.

189. Ceballos-Baumann AO, Passingham RE, Warner T, et al. Overactivity of rostral and underactivity of caudal frontal areas in idiopathic torsion dystonia: a PET activation study. *Ann Neurol* 1995;37:363–372.

190. Tempel LW, Perlmutter JS. Abnormal vibration-induced cerebral blood flow responses in idiopathic dystonia. *Brain* 1990; 113:691–707.

191. Tempel LW, Perlmutter JS. Abnormal cortical responses in patients with writer's cramp. *Neurology* 1993;43:2252–2257.

192. Ceballos-Baumann AO, Passingham RE, Marsden CD, et al. Overactivity of primary and accessory motor areas after motor reorganisation in acquired hemi-dystonia: a PET activation study. *Ann Neurol* 1995;37:746–757.

193. Ceballos-Baumann AO, Marsden CD, Passingham RE, et al. Cerebral activation with performing and imagining movement in idiopathic torsion dystonia (ITD): a PET study. *Neurology* 1994;44[Suppl 2]:A338(abstr).

194. Ceballos-Baumann AO, Sheean G, Marsden CD, et al. Botulinum toxin does not reverse the cortical dysfunction associated with writer's cramp. *Brain* 1997;120:571–582.

195. Playford ED, Fletcher NA, Sawle GV, et al. Integrity of the nigro-striatal dopaminergic system in familial dystonia: an ^18F-dopa PET study. *Brain* 1993;116:1191–1199.

196. Martin WRW, Stoessl AJ, Palmer M, et al. PET scanning in dystonia. *Adv Neurol* 1988;50:223–229.

197. Naumann M, Pirker W, Reiners K, et al. Imaging the pre- and postsynaptic side of striatal dopaminergic synapses in idiopathic cervical dystonia: a SPECT study using [^123I]Epipride and [^123I]b-CIT. *Mov Disord* 1998;13:319–323.

198. Perlmutter JS, Stambuk MK, Markham J, et al. Decreased [F-18] spiperone binding in putamen in idiopathic focal dystonia. *J Neurosci* 1997;17:843–850.

199. Sawle GV, Leenders KL, Brooks DJ, et al. Dopa-responsive dystonia: [^18F]-dopa positron emission tomography. *Ann Neurol* 1991;30:24–30.

200. Snow BJ, et al. Human positron emission tomographic [^18F]fluorodopa studies correlate with dopamine cell counts and levels. *Ann Neurol* 1993;34:324–330.

201. Turjanski N, Bhatia K, Burn DJ, et al. Comparison of striatal ^18F-dopa uptake in adult-onset dystonia-parkinsonism, Parkinson's disease, and dopa-responsive dystonia. *Neurology* 1993;43: 1563–1568.

202. Kunig G, Leenders KL, Antonini A, et al. D-2 receptor binding in dopa-responsive dystonia. *Ann Neurol* 1998;44: 758–762.

BOTULINUM TOXIN IN MOVEMENT DISORDERS AND SPASTICITY

CHARLES H. ADLER

Botulinum toxins are the most potent neurotoxins known. There are multiple antigenically distinct botulinum toxins, and all act by inhibiting the release of acetylcholine from nerve terminals. Harnessing this neurotoxic effect by reducing neuromuscular transmission and reducing glandular secretions has led to numerous neurologic and nonneurologic applications for this toxin in clinical medicine. Disorders such as dystonia, tremor, spasticity, sialorrhea, achalasia, excessive sweating, and even wrinkles have all been responsive to these treatments. This chapter will give an overview of botulinum toxins as the field is quite vast with books written on this topic alone (1).

HISTORICAL PERSPECTIVE

Botulinum toxins are neurotoxins produced by the anaerobic bacteria *Clostridium botulinum,* as well as *C. butyricum, C. baratii,* and *C. argentinense* (2). Botulism can occur following ingestion of contaminated food or from a wound infection. Clinical signs of botulism include limb paralysis, facial weakness, ophthalmoplegia, dysarthria, dysphagia, dyspnea progressing to respiratory arrest, constipation progressing to ileus, and urinary retention (3). *C. botulinum* produces seven antigenically (immunologically) distinct neurotoxins: A, B, C1, D, E, F, and G. These neurotoxins all block neuromuscular transmission resulting in both skeletal and smooth muscle paralysis. They also block neuroendocrine transmission involved in glandular secretion but have no effect on sensory neurons.

Studies using botulinum toxin type A (BTX-A) to block skeletal muscle action in monkeys led to trials in humans for strabismus, then blepharospasm (4). In December 1989, the U.S. Food and Drug Administration approved the use of BTX-A (Botox) for use in strabismus, blepharospasm, hemifacial spasm, and other disorders of the seventh cranial nerve in patients 12 years of age or older. Further clinical research has led to the approval of Botox for the management of cervical dystonia or torticollis, and a second botu-linum toxin, BTX-B (Myobloc), has also recently been approved for the management of cervical dystonia. Concurrently, a second BTX-A, Dysport, has been developed and marketed outside of the United States.

MECHANISM OF ACTION

BTXs are all inactive single-polypeptide chains of approximately 150 kd. Activation occurs when they are cleaved into a 100-kd heavy chain and 50-kd light chain by trypsin or other enzymes that remain linked by a disulfide bond. The C terminus of the heavy chain binds to the presynaptic acetylcholine nerve terminal, and it is proposed that there are different receptors, possibly gangliosides, for each BTX type (5). Following endocytosis of the toxin complex, the light chain passes from the endosome into the cytosol via a channel formed through the membrane by the N terminus of the heavy chain (6). While much of the toxin is not homologous, the light chains are all zinc endopeptidases that cleave the synaptic proteins critical to exocytosis, and it is this portion of the toxin that is most homologous (7).

All BTXs inhibit acetylcholine release by disrupting exocytosis at the nerve ending. Exocytosis requires the interaction of multiple proteins that are embedded in the vesicle membrane, the cytosol, and the nerve terminal membrane. These proteins are responsible for the attachment of the vesicle to the presynaptic membrane to facilitate exocytosis. Each toxin cleaves one of these proteins at a different location. BTX-B, D, and F cleave synaptobrevin, also known as VAMP (vesicle-associated membrane protein), a protein embedded in the acetylcholine-containing vesicle membrane (6,7). BTX-A and E cleave SNAP-25, a cytosolic protein attached to the presynaptic membrane, and BTX-C cleaves syntaxin, a cytosolic protein that is embedded in the presynaptic membrane (6,7). BTX-A cleaves nine residues from the carboxy terminus of SNAP-25, whereas BTX-E cleaves 26 residues.

It is acetylcholine release that is critical for neuromuscular transmission and control of muscle (skeletal and smooth) contractions. By inhibiting the release of acetylcholine BTXs block neuromuscular transmission and thus block the input for the muscle to contract, resulting in muscle paralysis. When used for its clinical effects, the dosage of BTX can be titrated to reduce but not completely block neuromuscular transmission.

PREPARATION AND DOSING ISSUES

There are two commercially available types of botulinum toxins in most parts of the world: BTX-A (Botox, Dysport) and BTX-B (Myobloc) (Table 43.1). Two different companies produce BTX-A: Botox is made by Allergan, whereas Dysport is made by Speywood. Although they are both type A toxin preparations, they differ in dosing. All three of these formulations are produced by fermentation of the bacteria followed by purification of the toxin. BTX-A is lyophilized then freeze-dried, whereas BTX-B is kept in a solution. The unit of measure for all three toxins is the "unit," with one unit of each toxin being the mouse LD_{50} following intraperitoneal injection. However, due to species variability, toxin complex variability, amount of albumin in the vial, and other factors, in humans, not only does the number of units needed to treat the same human muscle differ between the BTX-A and BTX-B preparations, but even the two type A preparations, Botox and Dysport, have different effects in humans on a unit-to-unit basis (8,9). Thus, treating physicians must be extremely aware of which drug they are injecting and which guidelines they are referring to when establishing the dosage.

Since both BTX-A preparations come as a freeze-dried powder, prior to injection they must be diluted with preservative-free saline, and they should be used within 4 hours of reconstitution. There are conflicting data regarding whether freezing or refrigerating the toxin, following reconstitution, results in degradation and loss of potency (10,11). However, the labeling from the companies, and the practice of most clinicians is to dilute the 100-U vial with 1 to 4 mL of saline, for a concentration of 2.5 to 10 U/0.1 mL, and use the toxin immediately. The procedure for BTX-B toxin is much simpler as it is already in solution with pH of 5.6,

and at a concentration of 5,000 U/ml. BTX-B toxin must be kept in the refrigerator rather than the freezer, and is used undiluted (unless lower concentrations are needed).

In terms of dosing in humans, care must be given to identifying which drug is being used. A number of studies have been conducted to determine equivalency for the different agents. Most have shown that for the BTX-A preparations, 1 U of Botox is equivalent to 2 to 6 U of Dysport (9). This is a fairly big range, so care must be taken when reading the literature or treating a patient. In terms of comparisons for Botox with Myobloc, very few data are available but the preliminary results suggest that about 1 U of Botox is equivalent to 25 to 50 U of Myobloc (12,13). It is critical to understand that this is not a hard and fast recommendation, just an estimate in terms of the starting ratios between the various drugs, and this is based on data for patients with torticollis and not other types of dystonia or disorders. No data are available comparing Dysport with Myobloc as of yet. The best recommendation at this time is to consider the drugs independently; when starting with a specific formulation, use the recommended dosage for that formulation and don't try to convert one drug dosage to another.

CLINICAL USE OF BOTULINUM TOXINS

The clinical use of the botulinum toxins is based on directly injecting BTX into a hyperactive muscle and partially or completely paralyzing that muscle (Table 43.2). By adjusting the dosage it is possible to weaken the muscles enough to relieve the involuntary contractions but to possibly leave some voluntary muscle control. The goal when using BTXs for the management of movement disorders is to reduce the involuntary movement without necessarily stopping voluntary movements. That is because movement disorders patients have involuntary movements in body parts that normally remain important for voluntary movement as well. Thus, injecting facial muscles or the vocal cords for a movement disorder requires finding the dose needed to reduce the involuntary movement without fully paralyzing the muscle, which might result in profound facial weakness or a breathy voice. This is in contrast to spasticity patients,

TABLE 43.1. CLINICALLY AVAILABLE BOTULINUM TOXINS

Botulinum toxin type A
  Botox (Allergan)
  Dysport (Speywood)
Botulinum toxin type B
  Myobloc (Elan)

TABLE 43.2. USES FOR BOTULINUM TOXINS

Dystonias
  Blepharospasm, cervical, oromandibular, laryngeal, limb,
    trunk, spasmodic dysphonia
Hemifacial spasm
Tremor
Tics
Myoclonus
Tardive dyskinesia
Spasticity

who usually do not have good voluntary control over the region being injected. The injections for spasticity can therefore be aimed specifically at reducing the spasms.

All patients who are being considered for BTX treatment must be carefully examined to determine the anatomy of the disorders. It is critical to determine which muscles are hyperactive and causing the involuntary movement, as opposed to which muscles may be acting in a compensatory fashion. In a patient with torticollis with head turning to the right, usually it is the left (or contralateral) sternocleidomastoid, not the right, that is involved. The dose of BTX used should be based on muscle mass, muscle location, potential adverse effects if the muscle is overly weakened, and degree of hyperactivity. Small muscles need smaller doses of BTX than large muscles. A discussion of various disorders that can be managed with BTXs follows.

DYSTONIAS

Dystonias are a group of disorders characterized by involuntary twisting, turning, and posturing of a specific body part. The movements can be tonic or phasic but always involve a period of posturing. The dystonias can be classified by the distribution (focal, segmental, multifocal, or generalized), with focal or segmental dystonias being those usually treated with BTX. In some cases of generalized dystonia, the use of BTX to treat one or two body regions, such as the vocal cords, the eyes, or the neck, may be appropriate.

Blepharospasm

Dystonic closure of the eyes, known as blepharospasm, was one of the initially approved indications for BTX-A. Involuntary activity of the orbicularis oculi leads to eye closing, and there can be involvement of the frontalis and the corrugator muscles in the forehead as well. Multiple open-label and double-blind, placebo-controlled trials of BTX-A have shown efficacy in up to 90% of patients treated, with an onset of action of about 3 to 5 days (8,14). The average duration of response is 3 to 4 months, and the most common side effects are ptosis, lagophthalmos, change in tearing, localized pain, and bruising. There is one case report of acute angle-closure glaucoma (15). Headache and facial pain may be associated with blepharospasm and may be responsive to BTX injections as well (16). If the orbicularis oculi is somewhat overweakened patients may have difficulty closing the eye while awake, and even when trying to go to sleep; these patients must be counseled to use lubricants liberally to avoid corneal abrasion.

The technique used to inject patients with blepharospasm varies by physician. Consensus now exists that injections of the upper eyelid should be done medially and

laterally, and injectors should avoid the central portion of the upper eyelid where the levator palpebrae inserts, so as to avoid ptosis as a side effect. Some physicians inject the lower eyelid only laterally, whereas others inject quite medially as well. Most inject lateral to the lateral canthus. Injections into the frontalis and/or corrugator muscles of the forehead should be done only if there is obvious involvement of those regions on examination. Injections into the pretarsal region of the orbicularis oculi are usually recommended because they appear to be more effective and have a reduced incidence of ptosis (17).

Blepharospasm is often accompanied by eyelid opening apraxia, a disorder characterized by the inability to open the eyes (thought due to inhibition of the levator palpebrae muscle) rather than involuntary eyelid closures. This disorder may also respond to BTX injections (17). Although there have been reports of response to both BTX-A and BTX-F, no reports of treatment with BTX-B have been published.

Dosing of BTX-A should be carefully considered. Using Botox the overall starting dose should be about 5 to 10 U per eye, whereas with Dysport the dose is higher (8). The concentration for Botox can be from 2.5 to 10 U/0.1 ml depending on doses being used at each site injected. In all likelihood there is less spread of the drug if it is more concentrated, and this may reduce side effects. Dosing of Myobloc has yet to be published, but studies are ongoing.

Cervical Dystonia/Torticollis

The most common movement disorder managed with BTX by most neurologists is cervical dystonia. Patients with cervical dystonia may have a variety of head postures, including torticollis (head turn), laterocollis (head tilt), anterocollis (neck flexion), and retrocollis (neck extension). The posturing may be phasic or tonic, and there may be associated features such as pain, tremor, shoulder elevation, and/or anterior deviation. Limitation of neck range of motion is common and can be a major factor in the disability associated with this disorder. The dystonic movements occur as a result of involuntary contractions of cervical muscles, and determining the combination of muscles involved in individual patients is the art of managing cervical dystonia.

Torticollis is usually caused by contractions of the contralateral sternocleidomastoid along with the ipsilateral splenius capitis, splenius cervicis, and some of the deeper posterolateral neck muscles ipsilateral to the head turn. Laterocollis often involves the ipsilateral splenius muscles as well as the levator scapulae, which is also involved in shoulder elevation and anterior deviation. Retrocollis may involve the bilateral splenius capitis, trapezius, and deep posterior cervical muscles, whereas anterocollis involves both sternocleidomastoid, scalene muscles, and anterior intervertebral muscles. One cannot emphasize enough the importance of determining which muscles are causing the involuntary movements, as often there are muscles that appear involved yet are only acting to compensate for the actual involuntary movement.

The methodology used to inject patients with cervical dystonia varies based on the physician injecting. Some injectors use electromyographic (EMG) guidance with a hollow monopolar needle, localize the muscle that is contracting, and inject the BTX through the needle. Others use palpation of the neck to localize the muscles involved and then inject without EMG guidance. Controlled studies using both techniques and with all BTX types have shown efficacy (12,13,18–21). Approximately 75% to 85% of all cervical dystonia patients injected will get some relief, and the degree of relief may vary from 50% to 95% by subjective criteria. Pain is often one of the most responsive symptoms to BTX injection, and whether it is a direct action of BTX on pain or a reduction in the muscle spasms that relieves the pain is unclear. Response usually lasts for 10 to 16 weeks, and repeated injections remain beneficial in most cases. There may be some shift in the pattern of dystonia over time, so that careful examination of the patient at each visit is critical (22). In addition, there have been reports of up to 5% to 10% of cervical dystonia patients treated with Botox developing a secondary nonresponsiveness to the drug (23). For this reason it is recommended that dosage be the minimal effective one and that injections be spaced a minimum of 3 months apart. Although the development of secondary nonresponsiveness to Botox has resulted in patients' no longer getting benefit, many of these patients will benefit from injections of BTX-B (Myobloc) (13). Whether secondary nonresponsiveness will develop in these patients or in patients treated exclusively with Myobloc is unclear. Currently, determining loss of response to Botox is best done clinically by injecting the corrugator muscle on one side of the forehead with 10 to 15 U of Botox and checking for weakening of forehead frowning on that side 1 to 2 weeks later (24). Alternatively, 5 to 10 U of Botox can be injected into two sites of one forehead; then assessment of eyebrow elevation can be checked in 1 to 2 weeks. Patients who do not respond to these injections are secondarily nonresponsive, and treatment with Myobloc can be initiated. A similar type of clinical test to evaluate maintenance of response to Myobloc and Dysport can be done, although guidelines for the correct test doses have not yet been published.

In terms of dosage, many papers have been written about dosing the various BTX preparations for cervical dystonia, and an exhaustive review is beyond the scope of this chapter. With all of the drugs the goal should be to use the lowest effective dose in the majority of affected muscles. The overall dose of Botox averages 150 to 250 U per injection session (19), for Dysport the average is about 400 to 1,000 U (8), while for Myobloc the pivotal trials have used 5,000 to 10,000 U (20).

The side effect profile of BTX injections for cervical dystonia is quite good. The majority of adverse effects are localized to the area treated and include injection site pain, bruising, neck weakness, and dysphagia (19). There appears to be a higher incidence of dry mouth in patients receiving BTX-B (20). Systemic effects have been reported including flu-like symptoms and generalized weakness. Also, there is evidence that injections in the neck or face can result in remote neuromuscular effects in the limbs (25). These remote effects were determined electrophysiologically, using single-fiber electromyography, and none of the patients had remote effects by clinical criteria. A systemic botulism-like reaction, including bulbar weakness, occurred in a patient injected multiple times for torticollis, and the symptoms resolved over several weeks (26).

Oromandibular Dystonia

Oromandibular dystonia (OMD) involves the mouth, jaw, and/or tongue. Multiple combinations of movement may occur including jaw closing, jaw opening, jaw deviation, lip pursing, etc. OMD in combination with upper facial spasms is called cranial dystonia or Meige's syndrome. BTX-A can be very effective for oromandibular dystonia, with a 35% to 75% improvement in function and 10- to 16-week duration of benefit (27,28). Secondary loss of responsiveness to BTX-A has recently been reported, and some of these patients have responded to other BTX types, including BTX-B (Myobloc) (29).

As in cervical dystonia, the critical issue when treating oromandibular dystonia is to understand the anatomy. Jaw-opening dystonia requires injections of the digastric muscles (anterior or posterior bellies) and, in some cases, the lateral pterygoids. Jaw-closing dystonia usually involves the masseter and temporalis muscles bilaterally, but in some cases, injections of the medial pterygoid are also required (21,27). Some cases may involve the geniohyoids and the mylohyoids. Jaw protrusion and lateral deviation involves the lateral pterygoids, and tongue protrusion involves the genioglossus and hyoglossus muscles (27). Initial dosing should be conservative, with about 20 U of Botox in the masseter, temporalis, and tongue muscles, 10 to 15 U in the pterygoids, and 5 to 10 U in the digastrics (27). These doses can be increased as needed. The mean dosage of Botox for jaw-closing dystonia in one series was 54.2 U in the masseter and 28.6 U in the submentalis complex (21). The technique of injection varies, with some using EMG guidance and others not. Dosage guidelines for BTX-B (Myobloc) have not yet been established.

The side effects of BTX injections for OMD are mainly local and include dysphagia, chewing problems, dysarthria, dyspnea, and biting of the inside of the cheek (21). Dysphagia must be watched carefully as aspiration can occur. Injections into the tongue itself can be quite dangerous, with overweakness resulting in the tongue dropping posteriorly and blocking the airway as the major concern.

Spasmodic Dysphonia—Adductor and Abductor

Spasmodic dysphonias are disorders of the larynx/vocal cords, with the adductor type characterized by a choked, strained voice with voice arrests, and the abductor type characterized by a breathy voice. The adductor type is often accompanied by a vocal tremor. Response to BTX-A is outstanding, with 90% to 95% of patients treated achieving an 80% to 100% improvement in voice quality and in the effort required to speak (30,31). Injections are done directly into the vocal cords (vocalis muscle) with some groups using a percutaneous technique through the cricothyroid membrane with EMG guidance, whereas others use direct laryngoscopic guidance (30,32). Dosing of BTX-A for adductor spasmodic dysphonia is usually very low with doses of 0.75 to 2.5 U (Botox) and 3.0 to 3.75 U (Dysport) per vocal cord (30,31). Some physicians inject these patients bilaterally, while others advocate unilateral injections; no study has proven that one method should be used and not the other (30,33). Side effects include transient dysphagia and hypophonic, whispering speech (33).

Management of abductor spasmodic dysphonia is more complicated because the muscles involved are usually the posterior crycoarytenoids. The injections must either be done through the lateral neck musculature or through the cricothyroid membrane and then through the cricoid cartilage, both requiring EMG guidance (34,35). Some patients benefit from unilateral injections whereas others require bilateral injections, and benefits can be expected in 70% of patients lasting around 10 to 14 weeks (35). Side effects in these patients are not too common, with exertional wheezing/stridor and dysphagia being the major concerns (34). Dosing needs to be well monitored as there is a danger of severe stridor, which could necessitate tracheostomy.

Limb Dystonia

Usually beginning as a task-specific dystonia of the hand in adults (writer's or musician's cramp), dystonia can be present at rest and can involve the foot and leg, especially in children. The dystonic movements can interfere with activities, be disabling, and be painful, especially in the foot. BTX-A has been very effective in the management of these types of dystonia, with approximately 70% to 80% of patients improving (36,37). Patients must be observed carefully to determine which muscles are involuntarily active. Individual fingers may flex or extend, and the wrist may also move involuntarily, but often hand and wrist movements may be compensating for the abnormal posturing, so observation is critical. Injections into the target muscles can then be done, either by palpating the muscle or by using

EMG guidance, with doses of BTX-A (Botox) being higher for finger and wrist flexors than extensors (36,37). The main issue is being able to titrate the dose so that the improvement in the dystonia is not outweighed or offset by weakening of the hand muscles (not as much of a problem with foot/leg injections).

In leg dystonia, BTX-A is effective at reducing the movement as well as reducing the pain component. Most patients have either dystonic foot plantar extension, plantar flexion, inturning, or toe movements. Injections must target various muscle groups, including the gastrocnemius and soleus muscles, tibialis anterior, tibialis posterior, toe extensors, or flexors (36). These injections can be done by palpation (especially the gastrocnemius and soleus muscles) or with EMG guidance. Doses of BTX-A range from 50 to 200 U (Botox) and from 200 to 500 U (Dysport) in each muscle group because these are generally large, powerful muscles. Benefit is usually delayed by 3 to 10 days and lasts for 2 to 4 months for all limb dystonias (36,38).

Truncal Dystonia

Truncal dystonia usually involves the paraspinal muscles and other muscles of the back, such as the latissimus dorsi, side, and abdomen. The spasms result in involuntary bending, twisting, and tilting of the trunk, often associated with pain, and with some patients being mistaken as having scoliosis. Treatment should be targeted to the muscles that are overactive, and benefit can be significant (38,39).

HEMIFACIAL SPASM

Hemifacial spasm, usually the result of vascular compression of the facial nerve, is characterized by involuntary twitching of both upper and lower facial muscles. This can result in involuntary eye closures, mouth movements, and twitching of the platysma. Studies have demonstrated good benefit with BTX-A: 80% to 90% of patients improve significantly (40). The duration of benefit is usually 3 to 5 months, and an equivalent efficacy can be maintained even after multiple treatment sessions.

Injections of BTX-A must be tailored to the sites that are in spasm in patients with hemifacial spasm, and this differs from patient to patient. It is reasonable to begin with injecting around the orbicularis oculi only, since some patients will have satisfactory relief of eye closure and not need lower facial injections. Doses range from 1.25 to 2.5 U (Botox) (slightly higher for Dysport) into the medial and lateral superior eyelid, the lateral (and sometimes medial) lower eyelid, and lateral to the lateral canthus. Currently, recommendations for dosing with BTX-B (Myobloc) have not yet been published but anecdotal reports suggest that it is efficacious. If relief of the eye-closing spasms is not sufficient to reduce the rest of the facial spasms, BTX can be injected into other facial muscles, including frontalis, corrugator, risorius, zygomaticus major, orbicularis oris, and platysma. The treatment strategy may change with time, with some patients avoiding lower facial injections initially and then trying these injections in the future.

As with blepharospasm, the main side effects when injecting around the eye are ptosis, lagophthalmos, change in tearing, localized pain, and bruising. Lower facial injections can result in facial droop, drooling, and mild dysarthria.

TREMOR DISORDERS

Essential tremor is one of the most common movement disorders, most often involving the hands but also the head and voice. Various oral medications have moderate benefit, and surgical intervention by thalamotomy or thalamic stimulation may be beneficial but quite invasive. Tremor may also occur in patients with dystonia, multiple sclerosis, or other neurologic disorders. There have been a number of studies evaluating BTX treatment for tremor disorders, mainly essential or dystonic tremors. In a double-blind, placebo-controlled study of BTX-A (Botox) for essential tremor of the hands, a modest benefit was found for postural tremor but not kinetic tremor, and no clear improvement for motor tasks or functional measures was found (41). A dose-dependent grip/hand weakness was found. Other studies have found similar modest benefits that must be weighed against the mild hand weakness that usually occurs (42). On the other hand, head tremor and vocal tremor have both been effectively managed with BTX-A (Botox, Dysport) with minimal side effects (43,44). Benefit has also been achieved in patients with palatal tremor/palatal myoclonus (45).

TICS

Tics are rapid movements that can result in a motor movement or vocalization. These movements often appear purposeful, which underscores the need to carefully titrate dosing to avoid inhibiting not only the involuntary movement but voluntary movements as well. BTX-A is effective in treating patients with dystonic tics (46–48). Treatments of eye closure tics, neck and shoulder tics, and vocal tics (injecting the vocal cords) have all been successful (46–48). Injecting the vocal cords of patients with malignant coprolalia due to Tourette's syndrome has also been of benefit (49). Doses of BTX-A are the same as used in the dystonias described above. BTX-B treatment of tics has not yet been reported.

OTHER MOVEMENT DISORDERS

Any movement disorder may potentially respond well to BTX injections. Myoclonic jerks will respond as will dyski-

netic movements around the mouth due to tardive dyskinesia. These disorders require the treating physician to understand the anatomy of the movement and the potential adverse reactions to weakening the muscles involved. Around the mouth one must be concerned about changes in speech, swallowing, facial symmetry, and drooling. As for drooling, some disorders have this as a symptom, including Parkinson's disease and amyotrophic lateral sclerosis. Although not really treating the movement disorder per se, studies have shown that injecting the parotid and submandibular glands with BTX-A (Botox) results in a marked reduction in saliva production without side effects (50).

SPASTICITY

The goal when using BTXs to manage spasticity is to reduce or abolish involuntary spasms of a specific body region. Treatment with BTXs may be indicated to reduce pain caused by the muscle spasms, as well as prophylactically be used to prevent contractures at certain joints. In other cases the spastic region moves involuntarily, which can be annoying and sometimes dangerous. Since the body region being injected is usually already paretic or plegic, there is little concern for possibly excessively weakening that body region. Therefore, unlike the treatment of movement disorder patients, where a balance of weakness and maintenance of voluntary activity is important and desired, spasticity patients usually do not have good voluntary control over the region being injected. The injections for spasticity can therefore be aimed specifically at reducing the spasms.

A number of studies have shown that BTX-A treatment results in benefit for upper and lower extremity spasticity due to multiple sclerosis, traumatic brain injury, spinal cord injury, stroke, and cerebral palsy (51–53). In patients with multiple sclerosis, BTX-A (Botox and Dysport) improved leg adductor spasticity and resulted in ease of nursing care/hygiene in comparison with placebo (54). Spasticity due to cerebral palsy also improves with BTX-A (Botox) injections (55). Dosing of BTX-A (Botox) has been well outlined in a review article (56).

A systemic botulism-like reaction, including bulbar weakness, has occurred in a patient injected one time for spasticity, and symptoms resolved over several weeks (26). This is the paper that also reported a similar reaction in a patient with torticollis (see above).

CONTRAINDICATIONS

There are no absolute contraindications to using BTX treatment but relative contraindications include pregnancy, neuromuscular junction (NMJ) disorders, and concomitant use of aminoglycosides. As BTXs act by inhibiting acetylcholine release at the NMJ, patients who already have NMJ disorders (myasthenia gravis, Lambert-Eaton syndrome) or motor neuron diseases (amyotrophic lateral sclerosis) may have exacerbation of their symptoms following BTX. The treating physician must decide if the potential decrease in NMJ activity is outweighed by the potential improvement in the disorder being treated. The majority of patients with NMJ disorders treated with BTX have not had any problem, but there are reports of remote weakness developing in some cases (57). Motor neuron disease patients with sialorrhea have received BTX-A in the salivary glands with good response and no systemic weakness. Injection of BTX in women who are pregnant is not recommended, but there are no reports of adverse events despite anecdotal reports of injections being done during pregnancy. One pregnant woman developed botulism from contaminated food at week 23 of gestation, and despite 2 months on ventilator support, there was no obvious abnormality when the baby was born (58).

LACK OF OR LOSS OF RESPONSE TO BTX

Most patients being treated for any of the disorders discussed above will respond in some manner to BTX injections. The main reason for a lack of response after the first series of injections is that either the dose used was not sufficient to weaken the targeted muscles or the targeted muscles were not the correct group of muscles to inject. All patients should be told when first being treated that it may take two or three series of injections to determine the optimal dose and muscle combinations needed to improve their disorder. This is usually simpler for disorders such as adductor spasmodic dysphonia (only one muscle injected) as compared with complicated cervical dystonia (multiple muscles must be injected with different doses).

There may be a very small percentage of patients who will never respond to BTX injections. Causes for this can include having immunity to BTX and having contractures. A contracture at a joint indicates that the joint cannot be fully or partially moved, and this is an abnormality of the joint and not of muscle contractions moving the joint (although that may have led to the contracture). Once a contracture has developed BTX will not be effective (59). It is also possible that previous exposure to BTX infection or even vaccination could lead to a loss of response when BTXs are tried for therapeutic indications.

The phenomenon of secondary nonresponsiveness to BTX injections implies that the patient has responded to treatment initially and then over time has lost the response. In most cases this is thought to be secondary to an immune response to the BTX used. Thus, if injected with BTX-A then the immune response is to BTX-A as the different types of BTX are antigenically distinct, and thus treatment with a different type of BTX has been shown to be beneficial (13,60). The reasons for the development of an immune response are likely multiple and are beyond the scope of this chapter. These appear to include issues regarding the protein content of the drug formulation, the dose being injected, and the frequency of injections; the higher the dose and the more frequent the injections, the greater the chance of an immune response (61). The development of antibodies to a specific BTX is likely not the only cause of secondary nonresponsiveness, and research is currently ongoing trying to determine other factors (61). Some patients who have been secondarily nonresponsive have subsequently responded to repeat injections, so retreatment in the future should be considered.

REFERENCES

1. Jankovic J, Hallett M. *Therapy with botulinum toxin.* New York: Marcel Dekker, 1994.
2. Johnson EA. Biomedical aspects of botulinum toxin. *J Toxicol Toxin Rev* 1999;18:1–15.
3. Davis LE. Botulinum toxin: from poison to medicine. *Western J Med* 1993;158:25–29.
4. Schantz EJ, Johnson EA. Botulinum toxin: the story of its development for the treatment of human disease. *Perspect Biol Med* 1997;40:317–327.
5. Schengrund CL. What is the cell surface receptor(s) for the different serotypes of botulinum neurotoxin? *J Toxicol Toxin Rev* 1999;18:35–44.
6. Brin MF, Hallett M, Jankovic J. *Scientific and therapeutic aspects of botulinum toxin.* Philadelphia: Lippincott Williams & Wilkins, 2002.
7. Schiavo G, Benfenati F, Poulain B, et al. Tetanus and botulinum-B neurotoxins block neurotransmitter release by proteolytic cleavage of synaptobrevin. *Nature* 1992;359:832–835.
8. Bigalke H, Wohlfarth K, Irmer A, et al. Botulinum A toxin: dysport improvement of biological availability. *Exp Neurol* 2001; 168:162–170.
9. First ER, Pearce LB, Borodic GE. Dose standardization of botulinum toxin. *Lancet* 1994;343:1035.
10. Gartlan MG, Hoffman HT. Crystalline preparation of botulinum toxin type A (Botox): degradation in potency with storage. *Otolaryngol Head Neck Surg* 1993;108:135–140.
11. Sloop RR, Cole BA, Escutin RO. Reconstituted botulinum toxin type A does not lose potency in humans if it is refrozen or refrigerated for 2 weeks before use. *Neurology* 1997;48:249–253.
12. Brashear A, Lew MF, Dykstra DD, et al. Safety and efficacy of NeuroBloc (botulinum toxin type B) in type A-responsive cervical dystonia. *Neurology* 1999;53:1439–1446.
13. Brin MF, Lew MF, Adler CH, et al. Safety and efficacy of NeuroBloc (botulinum toxin type B) in type A-resistant cervical dystonia. *Neurology* 1999;53:1431–1438.
14. Durif F. Clinical bioequivalence of the current preparations of botulinum toxin. *Eur Neurol* 1995;2:17–18.
15. Corridan P, Nightingale S, Mashoudi N, et al. Acute angle-closure glaucoma following botulinum toxin injection for blepharospasm. *Br J Ophthalmol* 1990;74:309–310.
16. Johnstone SJ, Adler CH. Headache and facial pain responsive to botulinum toxin: an unusual presentation of blepharospasm. *Headache* 1998;38:366–368.
17. Aramideh M, Ongerboer de Visser BW, Brans JWM, et al. Pretarsal application of botulinum toxin for treatment of blepharospasm. *J Neurol Neurosurg Psychiatry* 1995;59:309–311.
18. Comella CL, Buchman AS, Tanner CM, et al. Botulinum toxin injection for spasmodic torticollis: increased magnitude of benefit with electromyographic assistance. *Neurology* 1992;42:878–882.
19. Comella CL, Jankovic J, Brin MF. Use of botulinum toxin type

A in the treatment of cervical dystonia. *Neurology* 2000;55[Suppl 5]:S15–S21.

20. Lew MF, Brashear A, Factor S. The safety and efficacy of botulinum toxin type B in the treatment of patients with cervical dystonia: summary of three controlled clinical trials. *Neurology* 2000;55[Suppl 5]:S29–S35.

21. Tsui JK, Eisen A, Stoessl AJ, et al. Double-blind study of botulinum toxin in spasmodic torticollis. *Lancet* 1986;2:245–246.

22. Gelb DJ, Yoshimura DM, Olney RK, et al. Change in pattern of muscle activity following botulinum toxin injections for torticollis. *Ann Neurol* 1991;29:370–376.

23. Borodic G, Johnson E, Goodnough M, et al. Botulinum toxin therapy, immunologic resistance, and problems with available materials. *Neurology* 1996;46:26–29.

24. Hanna PA, Jankovic J, Vincent A. Comparison of mouse bioassay and immunoprecipitation assay for botulinum toxin antibodies. *J Neurol Neurosurg Psychiatry* 1999;66:612–616.

25. Girlanda P, Vita G, Nicolosi C, et al. Botulinum toxin therapy: distant effects on neuromuscular transmission and autonomic nervous system. *J Neurol Neurosurg Psychiatry* 1992;55:844–845.

26. Bakheit AMO, Ward CD, McLellan DL. Generalized botulism-like syndrome after intramuscular injections of botulinum toxin type A: a report of two cases. *J Neurol Neurosurg Psychiatry* 1997; 62:198.

27. Brin MF, Blitzer A, Herman S, et al. Oromandibular dystonia: treatment of 96 patients with botulinum toxin type A. In: Jankovic J, Hallet M, eds. *Therapy with botulinum toxin.* New York: Marcel Dekker, 1994:429–435.

28. Tan EK, Jankovic J. Botulinum toxin A in patients with oromandibular dystonia: long-term follow-up. *Neurology* 1999;53: 2102–2107.

29. Adler CH, Factor SA, Brin MF, et al. Secondary nonresponsiveness to botulinum toxin type A in oromandibular dystonia. *Mov Disord* 2001 *(in press).*

30. Brin MF, Blitzer A, Stewart C. Laryngeal dystonia (spasmodic dysphonia): observations of 901 patients and treatment with botulinum toxin. In: Fahn S, Marsden CD, DeLong M, eds. *Dystonia 3.* Advances in neurology, vol 78. Philadelphia: Lippincott–Raven Publishers, 1998:237–252.

31. Whurr R, Lorch M, Fontana H, et al. The use of botulinum toxin in the treatment of adductor spasmodic dysphonia. *J Neurol Neurosurg Psychiatry* 1993;56:526–530.

32. Rhew K, Fiedler DA, Ludlow CL. Technique for injection of botulinum toxin through the flexible nasolaryngoscope. *Otolaryngol Head Neck Surg* 1994;111:787–794.

33. Zwirner P, Murry T, Woodson GE. Perceptual-acoustic relationships in spasmodic dysphonia. *J Voice* 1993;7:165–171.

34. Blitzer A, Brin MF, Stewart C, et al. Abductor laryngeal dystonia: a series treated with botulinum toxin. *Laryngoscope* 1992;102: 163–167.

35. Meleca RJ, Hogikyan ND, Bastian RW. A comparison of methods of botulinum toxin injection for abductory spasmodic dysphonia. *Otolaryngol Head Neck Surg* 1997;117:487–492.

36. Pullman SL, Greene P, Fahn S, et al. Approach to the treatment of limb disorders with botulinum toxin A: experience with 187 patients. *Arch Neurol* 1996;53:617–624.

37. Turjanski N, Pirtosek Z, Quirk J, et al. Botulinum toxin in the treatment of writer's cramp. *Clin Neuropharmacol* 1996;19: 314–320.

38. Quirk JA, Sheean GL, Marsden CD, et al. Treatment of nonoccupational limb and trunk dystonia with botulinum toxin. *Mov Disord* 1996;11:377–383.

39. Comella CL, Shannon KM, Jaglin J. Extensor truncal dystonia:

40. Yoshimura DM, Aminoff MJ, Tami TA, et al. Treatment of hemifacial spasm with botulinum toxin. *Muscle Nerve* 1992;15: 1045–1049.

41. Brin MF, Lyons KE, Doucette J, et al. A randomized, double masked, controlled trial of botulinum toxin type A in essential hand tremor. *Neurology* 2001;56:1523–1528.

42. Jankovic J, Schwartz K, Clemence W, et al. A randomized, double-blind, placebo-controlled study to evaluate botulinum toxin type A in essential hand tremor. *Mov Disord* 1996;11:250–256.

43. Pahwa R, Busenbark K, Swanson-Hyland EF, et al. Botulinum toxin treatment of essential head tremor. *Neurology* 1995;45:822–824.

44. Wissel J, Masuhr F, Schelosky L, et al. Quantitative assessment of botulinum toxin treatment in 43 patients with head tremor. *Mov Disord* 1998;12:722–726.

45. Varney SM, Demetroulakos JL, Fletcher MH, et al. Palatal myoclonus: treatment with *Clostridium botulinum* toxin injection. *Otolaryngol Head Neck Surg* 1996;114:317–320.

46. Adler CH, Zimmerman R, Lyons M, et al. Perioperative use of botulinum toxin in patients with movement disorder–induced cervical spine disease. *Mov Disord* 1996;11:79–81.

47. Jankovic J. Botulinum toxin in the treatment of dystonic tics. *Mov Disord* 1994;9:347–349.

48. Kwak CH, Hanna PA, Jankovic J. Botulinum toxin in the treatment of tics. *Arch Neurol* 2000;57:1190–1193.

49. Scott BL, Jankovic J, Donovan DT. Botulinum toxin injection into vocal cord in the treatment of malignant coprolalia associated with Tourette's syndrome. *Mov Disord* 1996;11:431–433.

50. Friedman A, Potulska A. Quantitative assessment of parkinsonian sialorrhea and results of treatment with botulinum toxin. *Parkinsonism Relat Disord* 2001;7:329–332.

51. Bakheit AM, Thilmann AF, Ward AB, et al. A randomized, double-blind, placebo-controlled, dose-ranging study to compare the efficacy and safety of three doses of botulinum toxin type A (Dysport) with placebo in upper limb spasticity. *Stroke* 2000;31:2402–2406.

52. Grazko M, Polo KB, Jabbari B. Botulinum toxin A for spasticity, muscle spasms, and rigidity. *Neurology* 1995;45:712–717.

53. Simpson DM. Clinical trials of botulinum toxin in the treatment of spasticity. *Muscle Nerve* 1997;20[Suppl 6]:S169–S175.

54. Hyman N, Barnes M, Bhakta B, et al. Botulinum toxin (Dysport) treatment of hip adductor spasticity in multiple sclerosis: a prospective, randomized, double blind, placebo controlled, dose ranging study. *J Neurol Neurosurg Psychiatry* 2000;68:707–712.

55. Gooch JL, Sandell TV. Botulinum toxin for spasticity and athetosis in children with cerebral palsy. *Arch Phys Med Rehabil* 1996;77:508–511.

56. Brin MF, Group atSS. Dosing, administration, and a treatment algorithm for use of botulinum toxin A for adult-onset spasticity. *Muscle Nerve* 1997;20[Suppl 6]:S208–S220.

57. Tarsy D, Bhattacharyya N, Borodic G. Myasthenia gravis after botulinum toxin A for Meige syndrome. *Mov Disord* 2000;15: 736–738.

58. Polo JM, Martin J, Berciano J. Botulism and pregnancy. *Lancet* 1996;348:195.

59. Greene P, Fahn S, Diamond B. Development of resistance to botulinum toxin type A in patients with torticollis. *Mov Disord* 1994;9:213–217.

60. Greene PE, Fahn S. Response to botulinum toxin F in seronegative botulinum toxin A–resistant patients. *Mov Disord* 1996;11: 181–184.

61. Jankovic J, Schwartz K. Response and immunoresistance to botulinum toxin injections. *Neurology* 1995;45:1743–1746.

SURGERY FOR PARKINSON'S DISEASE AND HYPERKINETIC MOVEMENT DISORDERS

JOACHIM K. KRAUSS
ROBERT G. GROSSMAN

Neurosurgical management of Parkinson's disease (PD) and other movement disorders has become an important therapeutic strategy within the past few years. There has been tremendous progress in movement disorders surgery along with advances in neurophysiology, neurobiology, neurology, neurosurgery, neuroimaging, and medical technology. With contemporary methods, symptomatic and functional benefit is achieved at a low risk in appropriately selected patients. Current models of functional basal ganglia organization allow better understanding of the pathophysiology underlying movement disorders and also of the effects of functional stereotactic surgery (1–3). New insights into functional anatomy have led to the introduction of new targets such as the subthalamic nucleus (STN), which is the target most frequently used for treatment of PD in most centers nowadays (4,5).

Various surgical procedures are available for the management of PD and hyperkinetic movement disorders. The goal of functional stereotactic surgery is to modulate the activity in the basal ganglia circuitry. Long-term deep brain stimulation (DBS) has replaced radiofrequency lesioning in many places. With regard to its adaptability and reversibility, it allows the clinician to explore new indications at a low risk. Neurotransplantation differs fundamentally from functional stereotactic neurosurgery, in the way that it attempts to repair the primary defect underlying the development of a movement disorder such as PD. Long-term DBS and neurotransplantation are dealt with elsewhere in this volume. Here we will survey the principles of movement disorders surgery, the results of ablative functional stereotactic neurosurgery, central and peripheral denervation procedures, and the use of intrathecal drug therapy.

HISTORY OF MOVEMENT DISORDERS SURGERY

Before the basal ganglia became recognized as a target for surgical treatment of movement disorders, various opera-

tions on the peripheral and central nervous system and on other organs were performed (6,7). Lesions in the sensory systems were made by posterior rhizotomy, posterior or anterolateral cordotomy, sympathetic ramisectomy, and ganglionectomy. However, most procedures directly targeted the motor system and involved excision of the motor cortex, ablation or undercutting of the premotor cortex, and destruction of the pyramidal tract at various levels (e.g., by subcortical pyramidotomy, mesencephalic pedunculotomy, or high cervical cordotomy). In general, alleviation of the movement disorder was achieved only at the cost of hemiparesis. Other side effects, such as delayed appearance of spasticity, were common and long-term relief was rare in patients with preserved motor function.

Surgery of the basal ganglia circuitry for treatment of movement disorders was not performed until Meyers, in 1939, pioneered his innovative techniques (8). Previously, it was generally thought that such an approach would be impossible because it might result in enduring coma. Among others, Dandy had hypothesized that vegetative centers and the center of consciousness were located in the basal ganglia. Meyers performed techniques such as transventricular section of pallidothalamic pathways, and extirpation of the head of the caudate nucleus and the globus pallidus interna (GPi). Parkinsonian symptoms were improved in about 60% of patients; however, these procedures were burdened with high morbidity and a mortality rate of 12% (9). The next step in the development of functional neurosurgery for movement disorders included electrocoagulation of the pallidofugal pathways via subfrontal or transsylvian approaches (10).

The introduction of stereotactic neurosurgery revolutionized the surgical treatment of movement disorders. The first stereotactic frame was constructed in 1908 by the neurosurgeon Horsley and the mathematician Clarke for use in animal studies to investigate cerebellar physiology. However, it was not until 1947 that his technique was applied to humans. Spiegel and Wycis performed dorsomedial thalamotomies and pallidotomies with the goal to modify "afferent stimuli and emotional reactions" in patients with choreic and athetotic syndromes (11,12). Subsequently, the method was used also in PD patients by neurosurgeons and neuroscientists worldwide. The first ventrolateral thalamotomy for treatment of parkinsonian motor symptoms was performed in 1952 by Mundinger in Freiburg in collaboration with Hassler and Riechert (13). Erroneously, the development of stereotactic pallidotomy and thalamotomy have been attributed to Cooper. In 1952, Cooper accidentally severed the anterior choroidal artery during pedunculotomy for parkinsonian tremor. However, postoperative improvement of the tremor, which was thought to be related to pallidal infarction, led him to the use of anterior choroidal artery ligation and only later to pallidotomy. Likewise, when Cooper reported unexpected striking improvement when a planned pallidal lesion was misdirected to the thalamus in the late 1950s, thalamotomies had already been done in many other centers.

In the early period of functional stereotactic surgery lesions were created using leucotomes, injection of alcohol and procain oil, inflation of balloons, ultrasound, implantation of radioactive pellets, cryosurgery, and electrocoagulation. Later, all these techniques were almost completely replaced by radiofrequency lesioning. In the early and mid-1960s, most surgeons abandoned pallidotomy in favor of thalamotomy for the treatment of movement disorders. The subthalamic region was approached via campotomy and via lesions directed to the zona incerta (14). It was estimated that by 1965, more than 25,000 functional stereotactic procedures for parkinsonism had been performed worldwide. However, the number of functional stereotactic operations dropped rapidly after the introduction of levodopa in clinical routine. Subsequently, in the late 1970s and 1980s few centers continued to perform thalamotomies, particularly for management of tremor and hyperkinetic movement disorders.

The interest in surgical therapy arose again when the limitations of levodopa therapy became apparent in PD, in particular the gradual loss of efficacy with development of motor fluctuations and dyskinesias. Increased attention was focused on surgery for PD when the first results of autologous transplantation of adrenal medullary tissue to the striatum were reported in 1987. The rediscovery of pallidotomy by Laitinen had a major impact on the further development of functional stereotactic surgery for movement disorders (15). Scientific progress had a fast pace within the past few years. While neurotransplantation is still considered experimental, radiofrequency lesioning and DBS have become clinical routine nowadays for many conditions.

CONTEMPORARY PRINCIPLES OF MOVEMENT DISORDERS SURGERY
Functional Anatomy and Targets

The current model of basal ganglia organization is based primarily on animal models of neurodegenerative diseases

and is explained in detail elsewhere in this volume. It allows an explanation of both the occurrence of parkinsonism and hyperkinetic movement disorders. A major principle of basal ganglia organization is the idea that striatal projections are segregated into discrete pools on the basis of their projection targets. At present, it is thought that striatal output to the GPi involves both a direct pathway, which is GABAergic, and an indirect pathway via the globus pallidus externa (GPe) and the STN. The STN is thought to play a pivotal role by regulating the output of the GPi. Although this simplified model has often been criticized, it permits at least a partial explanation of the effect of basal ganglia surgery. The GPi has an inhibitory GABAergic projection to the ventrolateral thalamic nucleus (VL), also referred to as the motor thalamus. Until recently, Hassler's nomenclature subdividing the VL into the nucleus ventralis anterior (V.o.a) and ventralis posterior (V.o.p) was the terminology most commonly used (16,17). The nucleus ventralis intermedius (V.im) is located just posteriorly to the V.o.p. The pallidofugal fibers reach the thalamus via the ansa and the fasciculus lenticularis and are directed to the V.o.a, whereas the V.im receives afferents from dentatothalamic pathways. Recently, a major reclassification of thalamic nuclei has been proposed by Jones (18). This new terminology facilitates unification of the different nomenclatures used thus far in monkeys and humans (Fig. 44.1). According to Jones, Hassler's V.o.p is a region in which islands and fingers of cells proper to the V.o.a and the V.im interdigitate. Therefore, it has been suggested that V.o.p has no standing as an independent nucleus and that an equivalent name in monkey and human would not be needed. On these grounds, it has been proposed to rename Hassler's V.o.a as the anterior ventrolateral nucleus (VLa) and to rename the V.im as the posterior ventrolateral nucleus (VLp). The subthalamic area is composed of the zona incerta, the STN, and white matter containing the fields of Forel (Fig. 44.2). The STN is connected to the GPe and the GPi via pathways that traverse the internal capsule. The zona incerta is the ventral extension of the nucleus reticularis thalami. Its rostral part is situated just dorsal to the STN. The fasciculus lenticularis runs in Forel's field H2 between the STN and the zona incerta, and then curves upward in Forel's field H to form the fasciculus thalamicus in Forel's field H1 before it enters the VLa.

The choice of the target structure depends on the presentation of the patient with a specific movement disorders but also on the surgeon's preference. Nowadays the range of targets that are used is much more limited than before. In summary, contemporary targets for management of movement disorders include the V.im (or VLp according to Jones) for tremor, the GPi and the STN for parkinsonian symptoms, and the GPi for chorea and ballism. Both the GPi and thalamic targets other than the VLp are used for treatment of patients with dystonia. Thalamic subnuclei show a clear somatotopic organization. Basically, the concept of Hassler's thalamic homunculi is still valid today

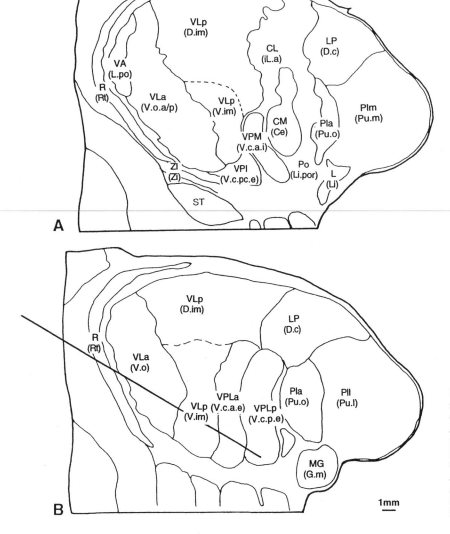

FIG. 44.1. Camera lucida tracings of parasagittal sections of a human thalamus. Nomenclature of the thalamic nuclei according to Jones, with the original names of Hassler in parentheses (A is medial to B). (From Jones EG. Morphology, nomenclature, and connections of the thalamus and basal ganglia. In: Krauss JK, Jankovic J, Grossman RG, eds. *Surgery for Parkinson's disease and movement disorders.* Philadelphia: Lippincott Williams & Wilkins, 2001:24–47, with permission.)

(Fig. 44.3). The leg is presented more lateral in the thalamic VLp than the arm. Therefore, the x coordinate in a patient with tremor undergoing thalamic surgery differs depending on whether the patient also has prominent tremor of the leg. The somatotopy of the GPi is less clear than that of the thalamic VLp (19,20). With microelectrode techniques, investigators have shown that one cell may often respond to movement of multiple joints. Some investigators have found that most of the neurons in patients with PD responsive to passive manipulation or active movements of the limbs were in the lateral portion of the GPi with the upper limb and the axial body presented more frequently further lateral and in the ventral one third, and the lower limb in the dorsal one third. There is no clear somatotopy in the vertical axis for the distribution of tremor-related cells. Microelectrode recording studies in the STN have shown that all neurons with sensorimotor responses were in the dorsolateral region of the STN with arm-related neurons

lateral to leg-related neurons, and presentation of the oromandibular musculature in the middle of the sensorimotor region, ventral to the arm and leg (21).

Techniques in Functional Stereotactic Neurosurgery

The principles of stereotactic surgery include the acquisition of data from various imaging modalities and their transfer to a cartesian coordinate system (22). In functional stereotactic surgery these coordinates are generally referenced to the stereotactic frame that is rigidly fixed to the patient's head. *Stereotaxis* has been derived from the Greek, meaning *three-dimensional arrangement*. The cartesian coordinate system implies that any point in space can be determined by three coordinates (x, y, and z), which are defined with regard to three intersecting orthogonal planes. These three planes—the abscissa, the ordina, and the applicata—intersect at one

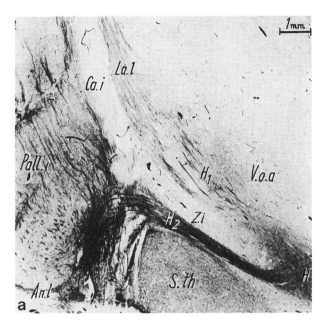

FIG. 44.2. Morphology of the subthalamic area. Coronal section through the anterior thalamus of an 8-month-old fetus. An.l, ansa lenticularis; Ca.i, internal capsule; H, H1 and H2, Forel's fields; La.l, lamella lateralis thalami; Pall.i, globus pallidus interna; S.th, subthalamic nucleus; V.o.a, ventralis oralis anterior; Z.i, zona incerta. (From Hassler R, Mundinger F, Riechert T. *Stereotaxis in Parkinson syndrome.* New York: Springer-Verlag, 1979, with permission.)

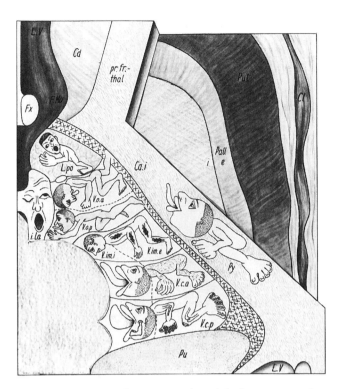

FIG. 44.3. Somatotopic representation of the human ventrolateral and ventrocaudal thalamus. The homunculi demonstrate the somatotopic representation of different thalamic nuclei: L.p, lateropolaris; V.o.a, ventro-oralis anterior; V.o.p, ventro-oralis posterior; V.im.i and V.im.e, ventralis intermedius (internal and external); V.c.a and V.c.p, ventralis caudalis (anterior and posterior). Ca.i, internal capsule; Cd, caudate; Cl, claustrum; F.Mo, foramen of Monro; Fx, fornix; L.V, lateral ventricle; Pall e and i, external and internal segment of globus pallidus; Pu, pulvinar; Put, putamen; Py, pyramidal tract. (Modified from Hassler R, Mundinger F, Riechert T. *Stereotaxis in Parkinson syndrome.* New York: Springer-Verlag, 1979, with permission.)

point, which is commonly defined as zero. By convention, the x coordinate defines the distance to the midsagittal plane (right to left), the y coordinate defines the distance to a reference point along the rostrocaudal axis (anterior to posterior), and the z coordinate defines the distance to a reference point in the coronal plain (superior to inferior). Because stereotactic positive-contrast ventriculography was the method of choice in functional stereotactic neurosurgery long before the advent of contemporary imaging methods, it has been generally accepted to refer the coordinates of a target in the basal ganglia or in the thalamus to anatomic landmarks in the third ventricle. Commonly, the interconnecting line between the anterior commissure (AC) and the posterior commissure (PC), the intercommissural line, is used for this purpose. The general acceptance of the AC and PC as landmarks has resulted in the generation of stereotactic atlases, such as the Schaltenbrand-Bailey atlas and its newer edition, the Schaltenbrand-Wahren atlas (23,24). These atlases contain series of myelin-stained brain sections 1 to 4 mm thick in each of the three orthogonal planes. The atlas coordinates should be corrected in patients with shorter or longer intercommissural lines or widening of the third ventricle. Because these coordinates do not account for individual spatial variability, intraoperative physiologic confirmation and refinement of the target is necessary (25).

Functional stereotactic neurosurgery for management of movement disorders is performed using local anesthesia with few exceptions. Communication with the patient and neurologic assessment are essential during neurophysiologic confirmation of the target. Usually, any drugs for treatment of the movement disorders are withheld preoperatively. In almost all centers, PD patients are operated in the "off" state. This allows the surgeon more ease in monitoring the efficacy of stimulation on parkinsonian target symptoms, such as rigidity, tremor, and bradykinesia, which may guide the decision of whether an electrode should be repositioned or a lesion should be enlarged or additional lesions be made. Furthermore, dyskinesias that can be provoked during target definition are considered useful hints at good surgical outcome in both the GPi and the STN. Careful intraoperative and perioperative monitoring of the patient's blood pressure is helpful for immediately recognizing and counteracting hypertension and hypotension. Monitored care by an anesthesiologist experienced in functional stereotactic surgery has proved to be very valuable in our practice.

It is important when attaching the frame to the patient's head to avoid any rotation or tilt of the head relative to the frame axes. Several methods are available for stereotactic imaging. For decades stereotactic ventriculography was used to identify the AC and the PC. To avoid parallax effects, ventriculography was ideally performed with fixed x-ray tubes with long projection lines (teleradiology). Nowadays ventriculography has largely been replaced by stereotactic computed tomography (CT) or magnetic resonance imaging (MRI). It has been demonstrated that CT- and MRI-guided localization of the commissures is accurate and is even superior to ventriculography (26–28). CT is considered the most geometrically accurate imaging modality for stereotactic localization. In comparison with MRI, CT has the relative disadvantage of being inferior in the display of anatomic details. The geometric accuracy of MRI can be comparable to that of CT scanning when gradient and magnetic field inhomogeneities are corrected. Under optimized conditions, the average difference between CT and MRI stereotactic coordinates of external fiducials, intracerebral target points, and anatomic landmarks is in the order of 1 pixel size. With both stereotactic CT and MRI it is important to obtain 1-mm or at least 2-mm axial scans through the third ventricle and the basal ganglia region. The imaging data can be transferred to a workstation where the axial scans are displayed simultaneously with coordinated reformatted sagittal and coronal images. The simultaneous and multiplanar display allows visualization and accurate confirmation of the localization of the commissures in three planes. Misalignment of the intercommissural line with regard to the three orthogonal axes of the stereotactic frame has to be considered and corrected appropriately (29).

The basal ganglia and thalamic targets are reached usually through a frontal approach. The trajectory can be determined on the stereotactic imaging data to avoid the ventricles or cortical vessels. The cranial opening may be made with a twist drill or a burr hole. The dura is coagulated and incised in a cruciate fashion. A guiding cannula that allows passing of microelectrodes, macroelectrodes, and DBS electrodes is inserted into the brain at the crown of a gyrus. Microelectrode recording is a very efficient and elegant technique, and it offers a unique opportunity for the electrophysiologic study of the basal ganglia. The issue of whether microelectrode recording is necessary to enhance the precision and safety of targeting thalamic and basal ganglia nuclei in movement disorders surgery is a matter of debate. In our experience, microelectrode recording is very useful in clinical routine and it adds little to operative time. Most microelectrodes have impedance from 0.3 to 1.5 Mohm. Microelectrode recording allows detailed mapping of the target region and the trajectory to the target region (19–21,30). Furthermore, by active and passive movements of the patient's extremities, the sensorimotor regions of the target can be refined. We think that microelectrode recording is particularly helpful in GPi and STN surgery (Fig. 44.4). It allows precise definition of the nuclear borders.

The number of pathways with a microelectrode depends on the preference of the surgeon and the quality of the signals. A technical variant is to obtain five parallel trajectories with the electrode tips spaced by 1.5 to 2 mm. Microelectrode recording may be supplemented by microstimulation via the electrodes in situ. This technique may be used to determine thresholds for motor responses or stimulation of structures in the immediate vicinity of the electrode tip.

The target can also be confirmed and further refined with macrostimulation via the lesion-making electrode or via the DBS electrode. Upon insertion of the macroelectrode, a so-called *setzeffekt* consisting of temporary improvement of the movement disorder of the contralateral extremity may occur. This effect is most pronounced in thalamic surgery for tremor, and may result in complete and prolonged disappearance of contralateral tremor. Macrostimulation is used to assess thresholds both for intrinsic responses (effects within the target) and extrinsic responses (effects on neighboring structures). Macrostimulation is typically performed at frequencies of 5 Hz and then at 100 or 130 Hz. The voltage is increased incrementally from 0 V until a response is elicited. The occurrence of intrinsic and extrinsic responses is monitored and protocolled. According to the responses obtained, the electrode may be relocated, and the stimulation may be repeated at the new chosen target.

Nowadays the technique of thermocontrolled radiofrequency lesioning is used almost exclusively. Lesioning electrodes are available in many different sizes and configurations. Radiofrequency electrodes used in movement disorders surgery most commonly have a diameter of 1 to 2 mm and a 1- to 4-mm uninsulated tip. There are numerous variations in how the lesions in thalamotomy or pallidotomy are created by different surgeons. We prefer to space lesions 1.5 to 2 mm apart along the same trajectory by subsequently withdrawing the electrode in pallidotomy. The lesions are created with the temperature controlled at 75°C for 60 seconds. However, other temperatures and times are being used. It is pivotal during lesioning to monitor strength and mobility of the patient's extremities, speech, and visual fields. For the STN, smaller lesioning electrodes are helpful. The predictability of radiofrequency lesions has been shown in experimental lesioning studies in egg white. However, although the lesion may be predicted accurately by such models, there is some variation in the size of the final lesion in clinical functional stereotactic surgery. The technical aspects of chronic DBS are in Chapter 46.

PARKINSON'S DISEASE

Thalamotomy for Parkinson's Disease

Thalamotomy has been the mainstay in movement disorders surgery for PD for decades (31–33). Nowadays it is performed only rarely. Significant improvement or aboli-

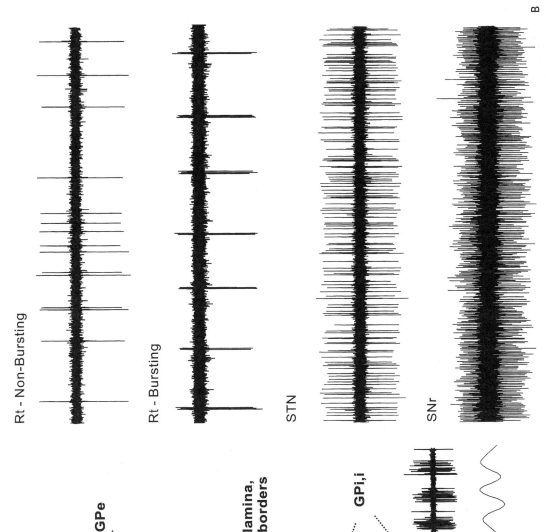

FIG. 44.4. Microelectrode recording in Parkinson's disease surgery. **A:** Typical recordings of "signature" cell types in segments of globus pallidus. Bor, border cell; HFD, high-frequency discharge; LFD-B, low-frequency discharge with bursts; SFD-B, slow-frequency discharge with pauses; TC, tremor cell. The trace below TC is the accelerometer attached to the dorsum of the contralateral hand. **B:** Typical recordings of cell types encountered in trajectories targeting the subthalamic nucleus. Rt, thalamic reticular nucleus; STN, subthalamic nucleus; SNr, substantia nigra pars reticulata. The traces are 2 seconds in duration. (From Hutchison WD. Techniques of microelectrode recording in movement disorders surgery. In: Krauss JK, Jankovic J, Grossman RG, eds. *Surgery for Parkinson's disease and movement disorders.* Philadelphia: Lippincott Williams & Wilkins, 2001:24–47, with permission.)

tion of contralateral tremor is usually achieved in 80% to 90% of patients with VLp thalamotomy (Fig. 44.5). In general, if there is no relapse of tremor in the first few months, the effect of thalamotomy is long-lasting and may persist even with progression of the disease. Lesions that extend into the V.o.a (or the VLa according to Jones) also have an effect against rigidity. There is no effect on bradykinesia, however, and axial symptoms are also not improved. Contralateral dyskinesias often are eliminated by thalamotomy (34). Other studies have demonstrated that PD patients develop fewer or no dyskinesias contralateral to previous thalamotomy (31). When the results of unilateral thalamotomy were evaluated in a blinded fashion at a mean follow-up of 10.9 years, significant reduction of upper extremity tremor was observed contralateral to the stereotactic lesion when compared with the ipsilateral extremity (35). Usually there is no significant reduction of levodopa medication or total equivalent dose. Side effects of unilateral thalamotomy have been reported in a wide range from 0.4% to 23% of patients (36). Complications generally resolve rapidly during the postoperative period. Persistent side effects may include hemiparesis, facial weakness, paresthesias, numbness, and delayed onset of dystonia. The rate of complications may vary enormously from team to team.

In the past, bilateral thalamotomies either were done in the same operative session or were staged. Bilateral abolition or improvement of tremor and rigidity was achieved in about 70% of patients, but considerable variations were reported. The major problem with bilateral thalamotomy is the high occurrence of side effects. In particular, dysarthria has been described to be worsening in 18% to 60% of

patients even when done during an interval of several months (36). Long-term DBS has been shown to be considerably safer in bilateral surgery.

Often with the typical rest tremor of PD there is little postoperative improvement in functional disability. Nevertheless, patients may benefit remarkably in social performance. Nowadays thalamic surgery is indicated only in a minority of PD patients. One of the major reasons is that it has been found that surgery in the STN and the GPi also has a profound antitremor effect. Thalamic DBS and thalamotomy were shown to be equally effective for the suppression of tremor, but thalamic stimulation had fewer adverse effects (37,38). The ideal candidate for thalamotomy would be an elderly PD patient with a long history of markedly asymmetric tremor with little or no effect of medication who does not display other parkinsonian features such as bradykinesia and gait disturbance.

Pallidotomy for Parkinson's Disease

Since its reintroduction in 1992, unilateral pallidotomy probably has been the most commonly performed procedure in movement disorders surgery around the world (15,39). Pallidotomy improves all cardinal PD symptoms, but to a variable extent. Differences in outcome among different series are due to variations in patient selection, assessment of outcome criteria, medical therapy, and surgical technique (40). Improvements have been seen most consistently in the off state, whereas there were wide variations in the on state (41–46). The most immediate effect of pallidotomy is the abolition or marked improvement of contralateral and to a certain extent also of ipsilateral dyskine-

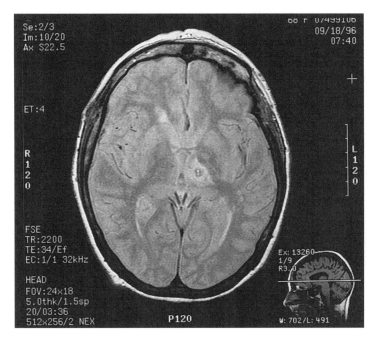

FIG. 44.5. Axial FSE 2200/34 magnetic resonance scans obtained 2 days after a left-sided VLp thalamotomy. Right-sided tremor at rest and intention tremor was completely abolished in this 68-year-old woman with Parkinson's disease and essential tremor.

sias. Usually there is no significant change of levodopa medication or total equivalent dose in the long term.

When the results of several larger studies on unilateral pallidotomy were summarized, bradykinesia was improved by 19% to 43% according to the Unified Parkinson's Disease Rating Scale (UPDRS) (40). There may be mild to moderate ipsilateral improvement, which is usually transient. In a study of 41 patients with advanced PD, objective improvement of bradykinesia contralateral to pallidotomy at 3 months postoperatively was shown by significant improvement of both movement and reaction times (47). The improvement of rigidity on the side contralateral to pallidotomy ranged from 25% to 60% in most studies (40). The improvement of tremor at rest generally ranged from 30% to 70%, although the magnitude in reduction of tremor varied widely between different groups. Unilateral pallidotomy also improves axial symptoms of PD, such as gait disturbance and postural instability, in the off state. Generally, maximal improvement of postural control is seen at 3 months after pallidotomy, with many variables remaining significantly improved at 12 months (48). Fluctuations are improved, and an increase in the time spent by patients in the on state is reported by most groups. In particular, the relation of the percentage of on time without dyskinesias is altered as compared to the percentage of on time with dyskinesias. The improvement of dyskinesias is striking. Along with the reduction of dyskinesia there is improvement of dyskinesia-related disability and pain (49). Complications of unilateral pallidotomy include visual field defects, hemiparesis, and facial weakness. The frequency of persistent side effects may range from 4% to 14% among different groups. Most studies investigating neuropsychological outcome after unilateral pallidotomy have found minimal cognitive changes as compared with the robust improvements in motor function (50–52). There were generally mild to moderate declines in frontal lobe functioning and memory. In some studies, left-sided lesions were associated with impaired verbal learning and phonemic fluency, whereas right-sided lesions caused transient decreases in visuospatial abilities.

Bilateral pallidotomy has been performed much more rarely (53). The additional benefit of a second, contralateral pallidotomy is usually less than that of the initial procedure if the two procedures are staged. The occurrence of complications is clearly higher than that associated with unilateral pallidotomy. Side effects of bilateral pallidotomy include changes in personality, behavior, executive functions and increased dysphagia, dysarthria, and falling. In a report on 12 unilateral and 8 bilateral (simultaneous) pallidotomies, significant declines in mean articulation rate and phonemic fluency were only found in the patients who underwent bilateral procedures (54).

The efficacy of unilateral pallidotomy has been confirmed in a randomized single-blinded multicenter trial (55). A recent meta-analysis of the contemporary literature on pallidotomy for PD revealed that at 1 year postoperatively, the mean improvement in the UPDRS motor score during off periods was 50.3%, and the mean improvement in contralateral dyskinesias during on periods was 86.4% (39). Major adverse events, including intracerebral hemorrhages, contralateral weakness, and visual field defects, occurred in 5.3% of patients. Long-term studies have shown that reduction in limb dyskinesias and off-state tremor scores persisted on the side contralateral to pallidotomy at the end of 3 years, whereas other measures tended to result in deterioration (56). In another study, significant early improvements in off-period contralateral parkinsonism symptoms were sustained for up to 5.5 years (57). Consistent improvement has been described in single patients even up to 10 years, with some recurrence of bradykinesia and an increase in gait freezing (58). Increasing symptoms on the nonoperated side may become an important source of disability.

The role of pallidotomy in the management of PD has changed tremendously within the past few years. In particular, the option of DBS to perform simultaneous bilateral surgery has changed the concept about who should be considered an ideal candidate for unilateral pallidotomy. In most centers, bilateral pallidotomies are not performed. One possible option is to perform pallidotomy on one side and at a later stage of the disease contralateral pallidal stimulation (59). The combination of unilateral pallidotomy with STN DBS later on may be problematic with regard to the need to reduce medication with STN stimulation (60). Pallidal surgery for PD, in general, may be indicated in patients with severe dyskinesias who show poor tolerance for the reduction of levodopa medication because of depression and anhedonia. Most likely, pallidotomy will have more limited application in the future.

Subthalamotomy for Parkinson's Disease

The STN had not been considered a target for lesioning due to the fear of the occurrence of hemiballism/hemichorea until recently. The occurrence of hemiballism or hemichorea as a complication of functional stereotactic surgery had been known since the early pre-levodopa era. However, analysis of the literature of the classic period of functional neurosurgery showed that only a small number of parkinsonian patients with hemiballism/hemichorea had a lesion involving the STN (61). Most patients with PD who developed hemiballism or hemichorea after STN lesioning showed only mild or transient hemiballism. It was hypothesized that the threshold for hemiballism/hemichorea might be higher in parkinsonian conditions than in the normal state (62). Thus, STN inactivation is thought to be less likely to induce hemiballism/hemichorea in PD patients.

Preliminary studies on subthalamotomy for management of PD have become available. Like in STN DBS, it appears that the dorsolateral STN is the most appropriate target for radiofrequency lesioning. In a study on 11 patients with unilateral subthalamotomy, marked improvement in motor function was observed, which was maintained during the follow-up period up to 1 year, and in some patients up to 24 months (62). Improvement was more striking contralateral to the lesion. Levodopa equivalent daily intake was unchanged in most of the patients during the first 12 months. In general, dyskinesia scores did not change postoperatively. One patient developed a large infarction due to the operation and suffered from hemiballism/hemichorea, which was alleviated by a pallidotomy later on. There are few reports on bilateral lesioning of the STN (63,64). The risk profile of a bilateral STN lesioning is unclear at this time, and it is difficult to predict whether it will be performed more widely. Recently, it was shown that subthalamotomy reduces basal ganglia output through the GPi and the substantia nigra pars reticularis, and also influences downstream neural activity in the pons and ventral thalamus (65).

TREMOR DISORDERS

In contrast to PD tremor, considerations must be given to quite different aspects in patients with other types of tremor. Tremor is frequently an isolated neurologic symptom in essential tremor (ET). However, in patients with tremor after severe craniocerebral trauma, multiple sclerosis, or stroke, tremor is usually only one of many symptoms, and the patient's functional abilities are limited by other neurologic and psychological disturbances as well. In ET, no morphologic cerebral lesions are present per definition, whereas widespread damage may be found in the other tremor groups. Taking these considerations into account, it is obvious that the indications for surgery, the goals to be achieved, the nature and frequency of side effects, and the prospects of symptomatic and functional improvement differ considerably. Unfortunately, many reports on stereotactic surgery in the past have grouped all these heterogeneous entities in series under the general heading of intention tremor. This approach often precludes accurate assessment of the different types of tremor and does not allow comparison among different series and methods in the past. Nowadays thalamic targets are used exclusively in functional stereotactic surgery for ET and other tremors.

Essential Tremor

Although ET is a common tremor disorder, it is disabling only in a small percentage of patients. Patients with disabling tremor who do not experience adequate relief with medication or who do not tolerate medication are candidates for functional stereotactic surgery. The relief of ET after thalamic surgery has been thought to be related to disruption of abnormal thalamocortical synchronization.

The first thalamotomy for ET was reported in the early 1960s (66). Generally, the VLp has been used (32,67).

Some surgeons have extended their lesions into the region of the zona incerta (68). Tremor control is achieved almost always in the short term. Studies on the long-term outcome are sparse. Mohadjer et al. reported good long-term improvement, defined as more than 50% benefit, in 69% of a larger population of patients at a mean follow-up of 8.6 years (68). Transient side effects were noted in 33% of patients. The cumulative frequency of persistent side effects was 9%. Persistent side effects, in general, were mild and included hypotonia, gait disturbance, and dysdiadochokinesis. In another recent report, ET was completely abolished in four of six patients at a mean follow-up of 5.9 years (32). Improvement of voice tremor was noted in 71% of patients in one series (67), and improvement of head tremor was found in 80% of patients in another series. In almost all studies, improvement of tremor was paralleled by improvement in functional disability. As in thalamotomy for PD tremor, bilateral thalamotomy in ET patients is burdened with a high risk of persistent dysarthria.

Unilateral VLp thalamotomy produces good long-term tremor control among patients with ET. It may carry a slightly higher risk of permanent neurologic deficits than DBS, as has been shown in the study of Schuurman and colleagues (37). Chronic DBS is clearly the preferred procedure when bilateral procedures are required.

Posttraumatic Tremor

Severe, incapacitating, predominantly postural and kinetic tremors are commonly associated with posttraumatic midbrain syndromes (69,70). Tremor usually manifests with a delay of weeks or months after the accident. Occasionally, tremor may also be present at rest. The coarse jerking 2.5- to 4-Hz tremor can be extremely violent and disabling, with amplitudes of more than 12 cm. Tremors are bilateral in about one third of patients. The mean age in this group of patients is much lower than that of patients with other types of tremor; the majority of patients are adolescents. The history of deceleration trauma and associated clinical findings indicate that most patients with posttraumatic tremor had suffered diffuse axonal injury. Therefore, usually a variety of other symptoms, such as psychological and cognitive deficits, oculomotor disturbances, and truncal and appendicular ataxia, are present. Medical treatment of posttraumatic tremor is notoriously difficult. Thalamotomies were first performed in the early 1960s for posttraumatic tremor. Larger series with longer follow-up periods were published in the 1980s and 1990s (71–75). The data of a total of 128 patients who were reported to have undergone ablative stereotactic surgery for posttraumatic tremor since 1960 are summarized in Table 44.1. Overall, immediate intraoperative or postoperative improvement of tremor was obtained in almost all cases. Amelioration of the tremor on follow-up examination was reported in 81 of 92 instances (88%). However, few studies have assessed true long-term

TABLE 44.1. ABLATIVE FUNCTIONAL STEREOTACTIC SURGERY FOR POSTTRAUMATIC TREMOR: LITERATURE REVIEW

Author(s) and Year	Target	Cases	Immediate Improvement	Long-term Follow-up	Last Follow-up, Mean Yr (Range)	Symptomatic Improvement (%)	Functional Improvement (%)	Persistent Side Effects
Cooper, 1960+	VL	2	2	1	1.3	1/1	1/1	NA
Spiegel et al., 1963	STR	1	1	1	NA	0/1	NA	NA
Fox and Kurtzke, 1966	VL	1	1	1	0.5	1/1	1/1	0/1
Samra et al., 1970	VL	5	5	NA	NA	5/5 (100)	NA	NA
Van Manen, 1974*	VL	2	2	2	7	½	NA	½
Eiras and Garcia, 1980	GP, Vop	1	1	1	2.5	1/1	1/1	0/1
Andrew et al., 1982	VL	8	8	NA	NA	8/8 (100)	8/8 (100)	5/8 (63)
Kandel, 1982*	VL, STR, CP	10	NA	NA	NA	NA	NA	NA
Niizuma et al., 1982*	VIM, Sub-VIM	3	3	NA	NA	NA	NA	1/8 (13)
Ohye et al., 1982	VIM	8	8	NA	NA	NA	NA	NA
Hirai et al., 1983	VL	5	4	NA	NA	NA	NA	0/5
Bullard and Nashold, 1984	VL	7	7	7	1.5 (0.2 to 3)	7/7 (100)	6/7 (86)	3/7 (43)
Bullard and Nashold, 1988**	VL	10	10	8	1.3 (0.2 to 3)	8/8 (100)	7/8 (90)	4/8 (50)
Iwadate et al., 1989	VL	3	2	NA	NA	2/3 (66)	NA	NA
Richardson, 1989	VL	1	1	NA	NA	1/1	NA	NA
Goldman and Kelly, 1992	VL	4	4	4	3 (1.4 to 4.5)	3/4 (75)	3/4 (75)	0/4 (0)
Marks, 1993	VIM	7	6	NA	NA	6/7 (86)	NA	1/7 (14)
Taira et al., 1993	Vop, VIM	3	1	3	0.5	1/3 (33)	NA	2/3 (66)
Krauss et al., 1994	VL, ZI	35	35	32	10.5 (0.5 to 24)	28/32 (88)	26/29 (90)	12/32 (38)
Jankovic et al., 1995	VIM	6	6	6	4	6/6 (100)	3/6 (50)	3/6 (50)
Shahzadi et al., 1995*	VIM	11	11	NA	NA	NA	NA	6/11 (55)
Louis et al., 1996	VL	2	2	2	0.3 and 4	2/2	NA	NA
Total		128	113/118 (96%)	68 (53%)		81/92 (88%)	56/65 (86%)	38/103 (37%)

Stereotactic targets: AL, ansa lenticularis; CP, caudate and putamen; IC, internal capsule; pall (med, lat); pallidum (medial, lateral); SN, substantia nigra; SR, subthalamic region; VIM, ventralis intermedius thalami; VL, ventrolateral thalamus; ZI, zona incerta.
Technique: chem, injection of toxin; cryo, cooling via inserted probe; DBS, chronic deep brain stimulation; EC, electrocoagulation; mech, mechanical lesion.
*, information not available; **, only summarized/no detailed information available; +, the series of Cooper includes the cases of Gioino et al.
From Krauss JK, Jankovic J. Head injury and posttraumatic movement disorders: topic review. *Neurosurgery* 2002;50:927–939 (see for complete list of references), with permission.

follow-up, and in many cases the duration of follow-up was unclear or was limited to 0.5 to 3 years postoperatively. Functional improvement, in general, paralleled the reduction of the kinetic tremors and was described in 56 of 65 patients in whom it was assessed (86%). Both transient and persistent side effects were reported frequently. Transient side effects included worsening of preoperative dysarthria and dysphagia, gait disturbance, and contralateral motor deficits. In the multipatient studies on posttraumatic tremor, the frequency of transient side effects varied from 50% to 90%. Worsening of dysarthria was observed in 70% of patients in the early postoperative period in the series of Bullard and Nashold (73). Decreased velopharyngeal functioning, a decrease in the oronasal pressure differential, and decreased range of motion of the tongue were characteristic findings. Although many patients have a subsequent improvement of adverse effects in the first few weeks or months after the operation, postoperative morbidity tends to persist in a considerable proportion of patients. Overall, persistent side effects have been reported to occur in 37% of the patients, with a range between 0% and 66% in different studies. In the series of 35 patients reported by Krauss et al., the primary target was the contralateral zona incerta alone in 12 patients and in combination with the basis of the VLp in 23 patients (71). In that study persistent improvement of tremor was found in 88% of the patients on long-term follow-up at a mean of 10.5 years. Tremor was absent or significantly reduced in 65% of the patients. Improvement of functional disability on long-term follow-up was seen in all except 4 patients. Persistent side effects were observed in 38% of patients. These side effects consisted mainly in the aggravation of preoperative symptoms, with increased dysarthria in 11 patients (34%) and increased truncal ataxia in 3 patients (9%). Two patients developed postoperative hemiballism. Seven patients with preoperative dystonic postures had an increase in dystonia on long-term evaluation, and seven other patients developed dystonic postures or hemidystonia during follow-up. It was unclear whether this effect was related to the surgical procedure or whether it presented a delayed aftermath of the trauma. Previous investigators observed that in cases

with severe kinetic tremors, larger thalamic lesions were required to control the movement disorder than for other types of tremor (74). Stereotactic lesions in the zona incerta and in the basal VLp offer the advantage of keeping efficient lesions smaller in these patients (Fig. 44.6). Reduction of the lesion size may also minimize the risk of side effects.

VLp thalamotomy or lesioning of the subthalamic area is a highly effective treatment option for persons with disabling persistent posttraumatic tremor. However, these patients seem particularly prone to present with postoperative side effects. This predisposition is probably related to the presence of widespread cerebral damage secondary to diffuse axonal injury. The experience with DBS is limited; nevertheless, DBS appears to be associated with fewer side effects than radiofrequency lesioning in posttraumatic tremor, and its effect can be titrated to balance between improvement of tremor and the induction of stimulation-induced increases in the patients' neurologic deficits (70). More knowledge about the long-term outcome in these patients is needed.

Tremor in Multiple Sclerosis

The use of functional stereotactic surgery for kinetic tremor in patients with multiple sclerosis presents several difficulties. These patients often are severely disabled; various neurologic symptoms are present, and the disease progresses insidiously.

According to a review from 1992 on the effect of thalamotomy in a total of 131 patients pooled from different series, there was immediate postoperative improvement of tremor in 94% of cases (75). Good results were noted to persist on follow-up examinations in 65%; however, long-term follow-up was only exceptionally available. In 29% of patients, the tremor recurred. Persistent new postoperative deficits or worsening of preoperative symptoms were found in 22% of patients. Due to progression of the underlying disease, functional improvement was observed in only 44% of patients. In a recent prospective case-control study, significant improvements in contralateral upper limb postural and kinetic tremors, spiral scores, and head tremor were

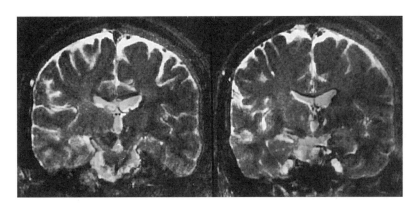

FIG. 44.6. Coronal T2-weighted magnetic resonance images after functional stereotactic surgery for posttraumatic tremor. The images at 3 years postoperatively demonstrate the topographic localization of the small lesion at the base of the ventrolateral thalamus and the zona incerta, and its relationship to the adjacent nuclei. (From Krauss JK, Mundinger F. Functional stereotactic surgery for hemiballism. *J Neurosurg* 1996;85:278–286, with permission.)

detected at 3 months and at 12 months after unilateral thalamotomy (76). Tremor-related disability and finger tapping speed were also significantly better 12 months after surgery, the latter having significantly worsened for the control group. A 3-Hz "filter" for postural upper limb tremor was detected by accelerometry and spectral analysis above which tremor was always abolished but below which some residual tremor invariably remained. However, both patients with and without surgery showed significant deterioration in the expanded disability systems scores.

Patients with multiple sclerosis presenting with kinetic tremor should be carefully evaluated before being considered as candidates for thalamotomy. Notably, symptomatic improvement of tremor will not always translate into functional improvement. Long-term DBS has been used more and more frequently in this group of patients.

DYSTONIA

Surgical management of dystonia is undergoing a renaissance similar to that of surgical management of PD some years ago (77). When considering a surgical approach to dystonia various issues must be taken into account. The indications for different methods and the goals to be achieved depend on the distribution of dystonia, severity, etiologic factors, presence of other neurologic symptoms, and the patient's age. In particular, the choice of the method depends also on whether a patient presents with hemidystonia, focal dystonia, or generalized dystonia. Hemidystonia, which is frequently secondary to contralateral caudatoputaminal lesions, may be stable after delayed onset and progression over several years, whereas idiopathic dystonia may still progressively spread to other body parts later on, thus limiting the benefit of surgery. Current surgical options include lesioning and DBS of the GPi and the thalamus for hemidystonia and generalized dystonia, and intrathecal delivery of baclofen for severe truncal and generalized dystonia. These strategies will be discussed in the following two sections. The outlines of surgical therapy for cervical dystonia (CD), the most common form of focal dystonia, are given in separate sections later in this chapter. It should also be noted that a therapeutic option for severe blepharospasm that is refractory to botulinum toxin injection is surgical orbicularis oculi myectomy.

Functional Stereotactic Surgery for Dystonia

In the past, both thalamotomy and pallidotomy were used in the management of dystonia (78–81). It had been the impression that pallidal targets are more suited for idiopathic dystonia whereas thalamic targets are more suitable for secondary dystonia, and this appears to be confirmed by more recent studies on radiofrequency lesioning and DBS

(82,83). The focus on the management of dystonia these days has shifted more and more to DBS, again because of the lower risk of performing bilateral surgery in one session.

The target for thalamotomy for management of dystonia has been much more variable among different surgeons than thalamic targets for tremor. Thalamotomy has involved the V.o.p, the V.o.a, the nucleus ventro-oralis internus, the V.im, the subthalamic region, the centrum medianum/nucleus parafascicularis complex, and the pulvinar thalami. The comparison of the symptomatic and functional outcome of the reported series of thalamotomy is limited because of the heterogeneity of patients, variations of the target, differences in evaluation of outcome, and variable length of follow-up. Immediate postoperative improvement is less striking than in other movement disorders, such as PD or ET. Often, further amelioration can be observed within months after the operation. In general, postoperative improvement has been reported in 25% to 80% of patients with generalized dystonia and in 33% to 100% of patients with hemidystonia (78,79,82). Andrew and colleagues found moderate or significant overall improvement in 25% of patients with generalized dystonia and in 100% of patients with hemidystonia; the benefit was more significant in secondary dystonia than in primary dystonia (78). Tasker and associates reported that 68% of patients with secondary dystonia had more than 25% clinical improvement, whereas such improvement was seen in only 50% of patients with primary dystonia (79). Patients with secondary dystonia also appeared to have more sustained improvement than patients with primary dystonia with thalamotomy. In the series of Tasker et al., 65% of patients with primary dystonia, but only 31% of patients with secondary dystonia, gradually lost the initial postoperative benefit. Immediate postoperative side effects were described in 7% to 47% of patients in different series. Transient side effects most commonly included confusion and contralateral weakness; similar to that with PD, postoperative speech impairment has been observed more frequently after bilateral thalamotomies. Long-term follow-up has been rarely available. Cardoso et al. reported moderate or significant improvement in 50% of patients with secondary dystonia at a mean follow-up of 41 months and in 43% of patients with primary dystonia at a mean of 33 months (81). Krauss et al. observed sustained moderate improvement in three of six patients with posttraumatic hemidystonia at a mean follow-up of 18 years (80).

Pallidotomy has been reintroduced for management of dystonia only within the past few years (82–84). Our results are generally consistent with those seen in other centers. In 16 patients with generalized dystonia or hemidystonia undergoing pallidotomy at Baylor College of Medicine, 14 patients demonstrated meaningful improvement. Eleven of these patients had bilateral procedures, staged in three and concurrent in eight instances. Patients with genetic dystonias (both DYT-1 positive and DYT-1 negative) consistently demonstrated marked improvement, whereas improvement in secondary dystonias tended to be less dramatic and less consistent. It is difficult to compare the efficacy of unilateral as opposed to concurrent bilateral procedures, as the decision was clinically based on the anatomic distribution of the dystonia. Even more than after thalamotomy, improvement of dystonia is delayed. Whereas improvement of phasic dystonic movements may be seen early after surgery, tonic dystonic postures improve over much longer time. At a mean of 1.5 years follow-up, improvement was sustained (82). Persistent side effects were uncommon. Pallidotomy has been shown also to improve symptomatic dystonia resulting from other neurodegenerative diseases, such as Hallervorden-Spatz disease and Huntington's disease (85,86). The response of dystonia patients to pallidotomy may depend on cause, according to the recent experience of different centers. It appears that patients with primary dystonia respond well to pallidotomy, whereas patients with secondary dystonia without structural lesions enjoy moderate improvement, whereas patients with secondary dystonia and structural brain lesions often have only minimal benefit (87). Nevertheless, some patients with secondary dystonia may gain substantial benefit from pallidal surgery (88). In conclusion, the response of patients with secondary hemidystonia to pallidal surgery (both lesioning and DBS) appears to be somewhat unpredictable. Whereas a minority of patients may improve, most patients appear not to benefit.

Due to the relatively small number of patients with dystonia undergoing lesioning procedures, the variations in surgical methods, and the inconsistent outcome assessments, no definite recommendations about the best surgical options and ideal targets can be made at this time. DBS is being explored more extensively at many centers. The most problematic aspect is the high voltage needed in dystonia patients requiring early replacement of the pulse generators.

Intrathecal Baclofen Delivery

The mechanisms of actions by which intrathecal baclofen treatment alters dystonia may involve both spinal and cranial levels. Intrathecal baclofen has been used for a decade in patients with generalized dystonia (89,90). Patients may be screened with bolus injections of baclofen via lumbar puncture or by continuous infusion via an external micropump and an intrathecal catheter. When the dystonia responds to the testing, a programmable subcutaneous pump is implanted and connected to an intrathecal catheter. This treatment modality results in reduction of dystonia and associated pain. Possible side effects include infection and lethargy. In contrast to patients with spasticity, dystonia patients are more likely to respond to continuous infusion than to bolus injections. They require higher dosages, are more likely to become resistant to the treatment, and are less likely to experience substantial improvement in function than individuals being treated for spasticity.

CERVICAL DYSTONIA (SPASMODIC TORTICOLLIS)

The goals of treatment for CD are improvement of abnormal neck posture and associated pain, and prevention of secondary complications such as development of contractures, cervical myelopathy, and radiculopathy (91). Medical treatment with anticholinergics and muscle relaxants often has limited benefit, and patients are frequently burdened by side effects. The treatment of choice for CD undoubtedly is the local injection of botulinum toxin type A into the dystonic muscles (92). The estimated frequency of primary nonresponders to botulinum toxin injections is 6% to 14% of patients with CD, and this approach loses its efficacy with continued use because of the development of immunoresistance in about another 3% to 10% of patients. Patients with secondary immunoresistance may benefit from newer types of botulinum toxin. Surgical treatment should be considered both in primary and in secondary nonresponders to botulinum toxin. It may also be considered an alternative in selected patients after years of successful trials with botulinum toxin because it can provide more permanent relief of the movement disorder.

Surgical Approaches and Strategies

Currently, surgery is performed mainly in patients who are primary or secondary nonresponders to botulinum toxin injections. Surgical treatment, in general, is indicated in those patients with functional disability caused by the dystonic movement disorder. Restriction of social activities because of embarrassment related to CD is also a major driving force, particularly in younger patients, to seek more invasive therapies. Surgical management of CD can be used also as an adjunct to conservative management to reduce drug dosages. Surgical options for patients with otherwise intractable CD are gaining increased attention and acceptance. The operations most commonly used today aim at selectively weakening the dystonic muscles by nerve sectioning or myotomy. An alternative that has been reexplored is modification of basal ganglia activity. One of the crucial points of contemporary surgery for CD is tailoring the approach to the specific pattern of the individual patient, and this may involve several successive operative steps as well as the use of different surgical techniques. In the past, operative procedures for management of CD were often performed as "standard" procedures, not taking into account the specific pattern of dystonic activity in the individual patient.

Nowadays extradural procedures and, to a lesser extent, intradural nerve sectioning procedures are performed with the greatest frequency. The primary goal of these techniques is to reduce the increased muscle tone. The denervation of muscles that are not involved in the production of dystonia should be avoided. The basic difference between intradural anterior cervical rhizotomy and extradural posterior rami-sectomy is shown in Fig. 44.7. Myotomies and myectomies are rarely used as a first step in patients with CD, but these techniques can be used as an adjunct to selective denervation or for management of dystonic activities in muscles that cannot be denervated completely with ease (91,93). Such muscles include the scalene muscles, the levator scapulae, and the omohyoid muscle. In patients who present with painful dystonic activity of the trapezius muscle resulting in elevation and protraction of the shoulder or contributing to ipsilateral head tilt, partial myotomy and myectomy of the upper portion of the trapezius muscle can be performed with an asleep–awake–asleep operative technique (93).

Microvascular decompression (MVD) of the spinal accessory nerve for management of CD has been used in analogy to the therapeutic benefit of this procedure in other cranial neuropathies, such as hemifacial spasm (94,95). The existence of two pathogenetically different types of CD has been suggested by proponents of MVD. The first is CD of "central" origin and the second is "spasmodic torticollis of 11th nerve origin." However, it is difficult to understand how MVD of the spinal accessory nerve should work, regarding both the pathophysiologic concept of MVD and the fact that almost always muscles other than the sternocleidomastoid are involved in dystonic activity. Outcome data of MVD for treatment of CD are very limited. Often, nerve sectionings were performed in addition to MVD (96). Jho and Jannetta claimed a cure of CD in 65% of their patients (13 of 20 patients), improvement considered as significant in four patients (20%), as moderate in one patient (5%), and as minimal in two patients on long-term

follow-up between 5 and 10 years after MVD (94). In some series, high rates of surgical morbidity were described.

Intradural Section of Nerve Roots

Intradural anterior cervical rhizotomy was the most common operation for CD in the past (97,98). The standard procedure includes bilateral intradural sectioning of the C1-3 anterior roots and of the caudal rootlets of the spinal accessory nerves. As mentioned above, more restricted and selective sectioning is advisable to avoid postoperative side effects. For example, in a patient with rotational CD, unilateral anterior rhizotomy combined with contralateral spinal accessory nerve section may be sufficient. In general, denervation with this approach is limited downward to the anterior root of C3 if it is performed bilaterally. The C4 root may be sectioned on one side, but that approach endangers functioning of the diaphragm.

Both the reported results and the complication rates in different series are highly variable. Most studies claimed useful postoperative improvement in 60% to 90% of their patients (97,98). However, other series have reported only very modest results (99). Most often, it is unclear whether symptomatic amelioration of the abnormal postures or movements translated into improvement in functional disability with regard to the relatively high number of side effects. Postoperative mortality ranges between 0% and 1% in most series. Bilateral rhizotomies are associated with a higher rate of postoperative neck weakness and dysphagia. Transient neck weakness has been estimated to occur in about 40% of patients and transient dysphagia in about

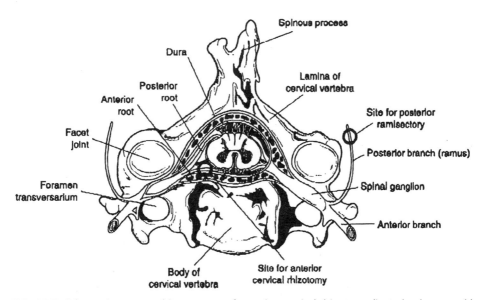

FIG. 44.7. Schematic topographic anatomy of anterior cervical rhizotomy (intradural approach) and posterior ramisectomy (extradural approach). (From Krauss JK, Grossman RG. Principles and techniques of movement disorders surgery. In: Krauss JK, Jankovic J, Grossman RG, eds. *Surgery for Parkinson's disease and movement disorders.* Philadelphia: Lippincott Williams & Wilkins, 2001:74–109, with permission.)

30% (100). A high variability of other complications has been described, including cerebrospinal fluid fistulas, brainstem infarction, and infection.

Posterior Ramisectomy and Peripheral Denervation

Extradural sectioning of the posterior primary division of the cervical nerve roots is also known as ramisectomy. Bertrand coined the term *selective peripheral denervation* for the combination of sectioning of the peripheral branch of the spinal accessory nerve to the sternocleidomastoid muscle combined with posterior ramisectomy from C1 to C6 (101). In contrast to anterior rhizotomy, there is no need for laminectomy and opening of the dura in posterior ramisectomy. With this technique, denervation of laryngeal and pharyngeal muscles is largely avoided. The approach can be performed either unilaterally or bilaterally, depending on the pattern of dystonia. Beneficial results have been reported in the range of 70% to 90% of patients in most series, with a few persistent side effects (101–103). Side effects may include infection, paresthesias and hypesthesia in the territory of the major occipital nerve, pain, and transient dysphagia (104). In most studies, head tremor and phasic dystonic movements are improved to a lesser extent than dystonic postures. Recently, it was demonstrated that patients with no or minimal degenerative changes of the cervical spine had significant improvement in pain and severity of CD after selective denervation, whereas no difference was found in those with moderate or severe changes (105). Thus, it was concluded that effective early treatment of CD had a protective effect. A recent prospective study showed that reinnervation is not uncommon after initially successful selective peripheral denervation (103). Occasionally, selective denervation can be useful in patients with fixed dystonic postures, with the goal not to correct the head position but to alleviate accompanying pain (106).

Within the past few years, the concept of posterior ramisectomy and selective peripheral denervation has gained more widespread acceptance. In many institutions it has replaced intradural anterior rhizotomy. It appears that the efficacy of both procedures is comparable but that side effects are much rarer and less severe with posterior ramisectomy.

Combination of Different Techniques

Surgical treatment combining several approaches and techniques can be successfully applied to patients with CD (107). We have evaluated the symptomatic and functional outcome in a retrospective series of 46 consecutive patients with independent assessment using the Toronto Western Spasmodic Torticollis Rating Scale (TWSTRS). In this group, 76 surgical procedures were performed, including intradural denervation in 33 instances, extradural denerva-

tion in 21 instances, and muscle sections in 22 instances. Global improvement at long-term follow-up at a mean of 6.5 years postoperatively was rated as excellent in 21% of patients, as marked in 27%, as moderate in 21%, as mild in 21%, and as nil in 11%. Almost all mean TWSTRS subscores for severity of CD, functional disability, and pain were significantly improved. Mild transient side effects were present in 10% of the patients and included swallowing difficulties, severe neck pain or headaches, psychotic decompensation, and cellulitis at the site of the skin incision. However, persistent side effects occurred only in one patient. In this series, there were no significant differences in the distribution of outcome scores between patients with idiopathic and secondary dystonia, nor were significant differences reported between patients who primarily did not respond to botulinum toxin injections and those who had developed secondary immunoresistance. There was a significant difference, however, with regard to the number of procedures performed. Patients with an excellent outcome had a higher number of surgical procedures on average than patients who had achieved no benefit.

Functional Stereotactic Surgery for Cervical Dystonia

Functional stereotactic surgery for CD was performed in several centers in the past. However, with the refinement of peripheral techniques and the widespread use of botulinum toxin injections, this treatment modality was largely abandoned. The experience with pallidal surgery for dyskinesias and dystonia in patients with PD, the beneficial effect in dystonic movement disorders, and review of the history of functional stereotactic surgery of CD has also prompted reevaluation of the potential of basal ganglia surgery for management of CD. Between 1960 and the early 1980s, approximately 300 patients with CD were reported to have undergone functional stereotactic surgery (108). Overall, postoperative improvement was claimed in about 50% to 70% of patients in most studies. A delay in improvement varying between a few weeks and 2 years postoperatively was often described. Various thalamic nuclei were targeted according to different pathophysiologic concepts in an attempt to account for the specific phenomenology of CD.

There is evidence that there is bilateral involvement in patients with CD regardless of the specific pattern of CD. Positron emission tomography (PET) investigations have shown higher glucose metabolism bilaterally in the lentiform nucleus in CD patients without significant differences concerning the laterality, the specific pattern or severity of CD in individual cases (109). Bilateral basal ganglia involvement has also been suggested by recent single photon emission computed tomography (SPECT) studies. Also, bilateral rather than unilateral surgery is supported by accumulated knowledge on the innervation of neck muscles. Bilateral pallidal DBS has been shown to be promising in patients with severe complex CD as well as in patients with cervical dyskinesias who undergo spinal surgery (110,111). Results have been stable more than 2 years postoperatively.

HEMIBALLISM AND HEMICHOREA

Hemiballism and hemichorea are relatively rare movement disorders. Hemiballism secondary to stroke most often has a favorable prognosis with spontaneous improvement over a few weeks. On the other hand, persistent hemiballism is well recognized. Surgical treatment is indicated in this subset of patients. In general, it should not be considered until 6 months after the onset of the movement disorder, except in patients with extremely violent hemiballism or in patients who do not tolerate medical therapy.

Early surgical treatment of hemiballism included several drastic measures, such as paralyzing limbs by alcohol injections, "stretching" of the brachial plexus, and even amputation of affected limbs. Over several decades, the mainstay of surgical treatment was manipulation of the motor cortex and the corticospinal tract. Such methods are only used

exceptionally nowadays. Cervical cordotomy may be considered a last resort for patients who are not considered candidates for other treatment modalities.

Functional stereotactic surgery for treatment of hemiballism has been performed in a limited number of patients (81,112,113). We have identified a total of 60 patients in reports published between 1950 and 1999 in whom the diagnosis of hemiballism could be verified (114). Since the 1980s, only thalamic and pallidal targets have been used for treatment of hemiballism. Overall, immediate postoperative improvement was achieved in most patients, and for those patients in whom long-term follow-up was available improvement has been sustained, in general (Table 44.2). In a more recent report, symptomatic and functional outcome was analyzed in a series of 14 patients with persistent hemiballism operated on over a period of 25 years (113). In 7 patients concomitant hemichorea was present. Radiofrequency lesions were placed into the contralateral zona incerta combined with lesions in the basis of the VL in 13 patients. In 2 patients the GPi was targeted. Hemiballism was abolished or was considerably improved in the early postoperative period after 14 of 15 procedures. Lasting improvement at a mean of 11 years postoperatively was

TABLE 44.2. FUNCTIONAL STEREOTACTIC SURGERY FOR HEMIBALLISM: LITERATURE REVIEW

Author(s) and Year	No. of Cases	Stereotactic Targets	Technique	Improvement in Hemiballism (Early Postop)	Improvement in Hemiballism (Follow-up >1 yr)	Complications
Talairach et al., 1950	1	GP, IC, CP, AL	EC	1/1	1/1	1/1
Roeder and Orthner, 1956	1	GPi, AL	EC	1/1	*	0/1
Gurny, 1957	1	GP	Chem	1/1	*	*
Velasco-Suarez, 1957	1	GP, IC	Chem, mech	0/1	*	1/1
Martin and McCaul, 1959	1	VL	Chem	1/1	*	1/1
Andy, 1962	4	GPi, IC, SR	EC	4/4	1/1	2/4
Yasargil, 1962**	3	GPi, or VL, IC	EC	3/3	*	*
Spiegel et al., 1963	1	SN	EC	1/1	*	*
Gioino et al., 1966	5	GPi, or VL, SR	Chem	5/5	3/3	3/5
Cooper, 1969***+	(4 + 5) 9	GPi, or VL, SR	Chem	**	**	*
Mundinger et al., 1970**	11	GPi, or VL, ZI	RF	*	7/11	*
Tsubokawa and Moriyasu, 1975	2	GPe	RF, chem	2/2	2/2	*
Kandel, 1982**	3	GPi, or VL, SR	Cryo	*	*	*
Levesque, 1992	1	VL	RF	1/1	*	1/1
Siegfried and Lippitz, 1994	1	VIM	DBS	1/1	1/1	*
Tsubokawa et al., 1995	2	VL, VIM	DBS	2/2	2/2	0/2
Cardoso et al., 1995	2	VL, VIM	RF	2/2	1/1	2/2
Krauss and Mundinger, 1996	14	VL, ZI, or GPi	RF	13/14	12/13	3/13
Suarez et al., 1997	1	GPi	RF	1/1	*	1/1
Vitek et al., 1999	1	GPi	RF	1/1	1/1	0/1

Stereotactic targets: AL, ansa lenticularis; CP, caudate and putamen; IC, internal capsule; pall (med, lat); pallidum (medial, lateral); SN, substantia nigra; SR, subthalamic region; VIM, ventralis intermedius thalami; VL, ventrolateral thalamus; ZI, zona incerta.
Technique: chem, injection of toxin; cryo, cooling via inserted probe; DBS, chronic deep brain stimulation; EC, electrocoagulation; mech, mechanical lesion.
*, information not available; **, only summarized/no detailed information available; +, the series of Cooper includes the cases of Gioino et al.
From Krauss JK, Mundinger F. Surgical treatment of hemiballism and hemichorea. In: Krauss JK, Jankovic J, Grossman RG, eds. *Surgery for Parkinson's disease and movement disorders.* Philadelphia: Lippincott Williams & Wilkins, 2001:397–403 (see for complete list of references), with permission.

found in 12 of 13 patients (92%) available for long-term follow-up. Seven of those patients (54%) were free of any hyperkinesias, and 5 (39%) had minor residual predominantly hemichoreic hyperkinesias. In 6 patients who had presented preoperatively with hemichorea in addition to hemiballism, hemichorea was completely abolished in 3 in the long term, whereas mild choreic movements persisted in the other 3 patients. Early postoperative side effects were present following 7 of the 15 procedures (47%). In general, these side effects were mild and included lateropulsion on walking, increase of preoperative hemiparesis, and confusion. Persistent morbidity was found in 3 patients. Two patients had mild dystonia in the extremities that had been affected by hemiballism previously, and 1 patient had a mild hemiparesis. There was a highly significant reduction of functional disability on long-term follow-up. The Huntington's disease Activities of Daily Living Scale was reduced from a preoperative mean of 83% of maximal disability to a mean of 30%. Residual disability was most often related to cardiovascular disease in older patients. Pallidotomy has been used more recently to effectively abate hemiballism (112). Bilateral ballism may be completely incapacitating and may require bilateral basal ganglia surgery. Under such circumstances, bilateral thalamotomy may be useful. Functional stereotactic surgery, in general, is not indicated for choreic dyskinesias in patients with Huntington's disease. Most patients tend to be more disabled by their behavioral and cognitive problems than by the choreic movement disorder. Several patients with Huntington's disease underwent pallidotomies in the 1950s and 1960s. Frequently, beneficial results with regard to the movement disorder were achieved. However, symptomatic improvement often was not paralleled by similar functional improvement. In a recent report, a 40-year-old man with Huntington's chorea experienced complete relief of right-sided hemichoreoathetosis after a left pallidotomy; nevertheless, there was little overall benefit because of the accompanying dementia (115).

Functional stereotactic surgery is a rewarding treatment modality in patients with persistent disabling hemiballism. Contemporary experiences with pallidal and thalamic ablative surgery have shown lasting symptomatic and functional improvement at a low frequency of mostly mild side effects. The question of which is the best target for hemiballism—the pallidum, the subthalamic region including the zona incerta, or the thalamus—cannot be settled based on the available data.

TICS AND TOURETTE'S SYNDROME

In most patients with tics and Tourette's syndrome, the symptoms can be satisfactorily controlled, if necessary, with pharmacologic therapy and adjunct measures such as botulinum toxin injections. Few patients continue to be severely disabled by their motor and vocal tics or the concomitant behavioral

disorder. Surgery might be considered primarily to alleviate severe tics or to improve obsessive-compulsive disorder (OCD) or self-injurious behavior (116). The evaluation of the effect of surgery, particularly in the long term, has difficulties with regard to variability as well as to waxing and waning of symptoms that occur spontaneously. The experience with functional stereotactic surgery for motor and vocal tics is limited. Encouraging results were reported in single case studies, whereas in other studies overall functional disabilities declined because of side effects. Hassler and Dieckmann reported their experience in 15 patients on whom they had operated for Tourette's syndrome in the 1970s (117). Multiple lesions were made in the rostral interlaminar and medial thalamic nuclei, often bilaterally, in a staged fashion. Follow-up in 9 patients showed that tics in 4 were thought to be improved between 90% and 100%, whereas in the other 5 patients they were improved by 50% to 80%. Some patients suffered severe adverse side effects, such as hemiparesis and personality changes. A review of the experiences with 17 consecutive patients treated between 1970 and 1998 in Freiburg was published recently (118). Eleven of 17 patients were available at a mean follow-up of 7 years. Lesions were placed in the zona incerta, the VL, and the thalamic lamella medialis. Patients underwent unilateral surgery based on asymmetry of tics, with second-stage contralateral surgery later on in some instances. Alleviation of vocal tics was more significant than that of motor tics. Both vocal and motor tics were relieved on long-term follow-up. Transient complications consisting of dysarthria, hemiparesis, hemiballism, and dystonia occurred in 68% of patients. One permanent complication was registered in the six patients followed-up after unilateral surgery, whereas two of five patients had permanent disabling side effects after bilateral surgery.

For treatment of OCD in patients with Tourette's syndrome, several ablative surgical procedures have been used, including anterior cingulotomy, limbic leucotomy, and anterior capsulotomy (116). In general, such procedures have been described as effective in 33% to 61% of patients with OCD. Interestingly, although improvement of OCD in Tourette's syndrome was reported in several case reports after psychiatric surgery, the effect on tics has been more variable (120,121).

Surgical management of Tourette's syndrome may be considered a treatment option in certain patients with severe disabling symptoms that are refractory to medical treatment. Surgery in such cases should be considered only a part of an entire treatment plan and should be followed by appropriate neuropsychiatric programs. Recent experiences with thalamic DBS have shown promise (122).

SPASTICITY AND CHOREOATHETOSIS

Spasticity is a common sequelae of neurologic diseases. Although in some patients spasticity is useful in compensating lost motor strength, in many other patients it may hinder useful function and can be associated with severe pain. When not controllable by physical therapy, medication, or botulinum toxin injections, spasticity can be improved by various surgical measures such as neurostimulation, intrathecal pharmacotherapy, or selective ablative procedures. The choice of the procedure depends on the underlying pathology, associated symptoms, distribution and pattern of spasticity, degree of accompanying paresis, and the prospects for functional recovery.

Epidural spinal cord stimulation has been described to be useful for treatment of moderate degrees of spasticity. This method offers the possibility of a percutaneous trial of stimulation to assess whether there is a positive response or not. If relief occurs, the system can be internalized. The procedure involves chronic implantation of electrodes in the spinal epidural space via small partial laminectomies or percutaneous techniques, and subcutaneous implantation of a programmable system for neurostimulation. The electrodes may be placed at the level of the injury in patients with spinal cord trauma or over the upper spinal cord in children with spastic cerebral palsy. A meta-analysis of several published series including patients with different pathologies yielded good or very good results for reductions of spasticity in 40% of patients, fair results in 24%, no improvement in 36%; good or very good improvement of motor function was reported in 37% of patients, fair improvement in 14%, and no change in 49%; amelioration of bladder function was judged as good or very good in 48% of patients, fair in 17%, and was not seen in 35% (123). Although these data indicate efficacy of spinal cord stimulation in a certain proportion of patients with spasticity, a prospective double-blind study with a limited number of cases, consisting of eight children with spastic cerebral palsy, failed to show significant improvement with this treatment modality (124). The most frequent complications consist of lead fracture and electrode displacement occurring in about 10% of patients, and infections occurring in about 5% of patients (123). Several mechanisms have been proposed to explain the effect of spinal cord stimulation, including activation of inhibitory long-loop reflexes.

In patients with severe generalized spasticity, intrathecal application of baclofen via an implanted programmable pump may be considered (125). The efficacy of intrathecal baclofen infusion has been demonstrated in randomized, double-blind, crossover studies (126). Before a pump is internalized, trials are performed with lumbar injections or infusion of baclofen. Large variations in efficacy thresholds have been observed between patients. Implantation of the pump is performed under general or local anesthesia. The pump is placed in a subcutaneous pocket in the abdomen and connected to an intrathecal silicon catheter inserted via lumbar puncture. The pump needs refilling every 2 to 3 months. In a study on 59 patients with severe spasticity of spinal origin, the mean Ashworth score, which measures the degree of

hypertonicity, decreased significantly (127). Catheter-related problems occurred 19 times in 15 patients. The dose of baclofen had to be doubled in about 1 year. Pharmacologic tolerance can be managed with drug holidays. The most common adverse drug reactions include obstipation, dizziness, drowsiness, and muscular hypotonia. Drug overdose can be managed with intravenous physostigmine.

Selective lesioning can be performed at the level of peripheral nerves, spinal roots, spinal cord, or dorsal root entry zone (DREZ) (128). Peripheral neurotomies are indicated when spasticity is localized to muscles or muscular groups supplied by a single or few peripheral nerves that are easily accessible. Neurotomies of the tibial nerve at the popliteal region for the so-called spastic foot and of the obturator nerve just below the subpubic canal for spastic flexion-adduction deformity of the hip are the most frequently performed peripheral procedures. Neurotomies are also performed for spasticity in the upper limb, including selective fascicular neurotomies in the musculocutaneous nerve as well as in the median and ulnar nerves. Occasionally, neurotomies of brachial plexus branches have been performed for treating the spastic shoulder. Posterior rhizotomies are performed in children with cerebral palsy. There are several technical variants, such as selective posterior rhizotomy, sectorial posterior rhizotomy, partial posterior rhizotomy, or functional posterior rhizotomy. Overall, about 75% of the patients have nearly normal muscle tone at 1 year postoperatively. Most children demonstrated improved stability in sitting or improvement of walking. In cases of fixed contractures, complementary orthopedic surgery was sometimes necessary. Longitudinal myelotomy is only rarely performed nowadays (129). Although it has been shown to have a good effect on spasticity, a harmful effect on bladder function was present in 27% of patients. Lesioning of the DREZ is helpful both for severe spasticity and for associated pain (130). A refinement of this method, termed microDREZotomy, attempts to interrupt small nociceptive and large myotactic fibers while sparing lemniscal fibers (128). DREZotomy can be performed for the lower limbs or for the upper limbs. Percutaneous techniques for rhizotomies have been described. Complementary orthopedic surgery may be necessary when deformities have become irreducible.

Functional ablative stereotactic surgery has been used in the past for choreoathetosis in children with cerebral palsy. The reported results have been highly variable, which may have partially been related to the methodologic assessment. Although some degree of improvement with targets in the VL and the subthalamic region was observed in the majority of patients, wide variations in outcome were reported. Significantly improved outcome has been described ranging between 18% and 73% in different studies (131,132). The dentate nuclei have been advocated as a target for lesioning or chronic stimulation in the past for the management of spasticity and choreoathetosis. Nowadays cerebellar targets have been almost completely abandoned. In a recent series of 33 pallidotomies in 24 patients with cerebral palsy, 67% of patients had subjective improvement, and 42% had subjective and objective improvement (133). Many of those patients enjoyed functional gains, such as the ability to feed themselves or to maneuver their wheelchairs. The complication rate was 50% and included swallowing and speech difficulties. The permanent complication rate was 17.5%. Again, pallidal DBS is being explored as an alternative.

OTHER MOVEMENT DISORDERS

Hemifacial Spasm

Botulinum toxin injection is the therapeutic option that is most frequently employed nowadays. The alternative which renders permanent relief of hemifacial spasm is MVD of the facial nerve via a lateral suboccipital approach. This technique was elaborated and refined by Jannetta for management of cranial nerve root compression. Exposure of the root exit zone is achieved with microneurosurgical techniques. After the offending vessel has been identified, it is mobilized and repositioned with small implants of Teflon or other nonresorbable materials placed between the facial nerve and the vessel. The integrity of both the facial nerve and the vessel are preserved. In patients with typical or so-called classic hemifacial spasm, the causative vessel is usually found to be compressing the nerve from a caudadand anterior direction. Usually, the causative vessel is identified as the posterior inferior cerebellar artery. The anterior inferior cerebellar artery may be involved in more than one third of cases. In patients with so-called atypical hemifacial spasm (progression of the spasm from the lower face to the upper face), the side of compression appears to be rostrad and posterior to the nerve and the root exit zone.

Complete or near-complete resolution of hemifacial spasm is reported in 80% to 90% of patients in more recent series (134,135). Recurrences were observed in 1% to 10% of patients in the long term. In a large series of 703 patients reported by Barker and Jannetta, excellent results, defined as complete or near-complete abolition of spasms, were obtained in 86% of patients at 1 month postoperatively and in 79% at 10-year follow-up. Including patients who had reoperations for recurrence, the figure for excellent improvement at 10-year follow-up increased to 84% of patients, whereas partial improvement was achieved in 7% and failures occurred in 9%. Operative mortality was 0.1%, and operative complications included brainstem infarction in 0.3%, cerebellar hematoma in 0.5%, deafness in 2.7%, permanent facial weakness in 1.5%, and mild transient complications in 4.5%. The pattern of hemifacial spasm is an important predictor of operative success. Overall, only 70% of patients with atypical hemifacial spasm have immediate relief of spasm. Also, long-term results of atypical hemifacial spasms are less gratifying. At 10 years postoper-

atively, only 59% of patients report excellent relief of symptoms. Sometimes resolution of hemifacial spasm may be gradual (136).

Stiff-Man Syndrome

Stiff-man syndrome and progressive encephalomyelitis with rigidity and myoclonus (PERM) can be managed with intrathecal baclofen, if there is no sufficient relief by oral medication (137,138). Similar to what is done for patients with spasticity or dystonia, intrathecal test boluses are given before pump implantation. Maintenance doses of baclofen vary greatly among patients. Particular in patients with PERM, requirements may increase rapidly. In a series of 15 patients, 11 patients before intrathecal baclofen were either wheelchair bound or bedridden. Five patients achieved the ability to walk with crutches, whereas three other patients walked freely. Symptoms of autonomic dysfunction were also alleviated after administration of intrathecal baclofen. Complications of intrathecal baclofen therapy for patients with stiff-man syndrome or PERM differ from patients with spasticity. Patients may experience severe sedation. Drug withdrawal may result in severe consequences. Only hours after drug administration is reduced or stopped, spasms may develop, occasionally associated with massive vegetative symptoms such as diaphoresis, tachycardia, tachypnea, and hyperthermia. Clinically, the picture may resemble that of myocardial infarction or gram-negative sepsis. In particular, because of these risks intrathecal baclofen is the last resort alternative to oral treatment in these patients.

Myoclonus

The experience with functional ablative surgery for myoclonus is very limited. Patients with familial essential myoclonus may benefit from thalamic surgery. Such surgery should also be considered a therapeutic alternative in patients with disabling drug-refractory essential myoclonus (139).

CONCLUSION

Major progress has been achieved in the surgical treatment of patients with Parkinson's disease and other movement disorders within the past few years (140,141). All surgical therapies used for the management of movement disorders nowadays have their relative advantages and disadvantages, and it is hard to predict which methods and targets will have the greatest impact in the next few years. Long-term stimulation techniques have furthered and expanded considerably the options of movement disorders surgery. In particular, it is possible to perform bilateral contemporaneous surgery, which is not useful with lesioning procedures.

While the combination of clinical symptoms may favor one approach in an individual patient, in many instances different alternatives can be taken into consideration.

ACKNOWLEDGMENTS

The authors thank Margot Meckesheimer for her assistance in the preparation of the manuscript.

REFERENCES

1. Alexander GE, Crutcher MD, Delong MR. Basal ganglia thalamocortical circuits: parallel substrates for motor, oculomotor, "prefrontal" and "limbic" functions. *Prog Brain Res* 1990;85:119–146.
2. Marsden CD, Obeso JA. The functions of the basal ganglia and the paradox of stereotaxic surgery in Parkinson's disease. *Brain* 1994;117:877–897.
3. Mink JW. Basal ganglia motor control before and after surgery. In: Krauss JK, Jankovic J, Grossman RG, eds. *Surgery for Parkinson's disease and movement disorders.* Philadelphia: Lippincott Williams & Wilkins, 2001:56–73.
4. Guridi J, Luquin MR, Herrero MT, et al. The subthalamic nucleus: a possible target for stereotaxic surgery in Parkinson's disease. *Mov Disord* 1993;8:421–429.
5. Limousin P, Krack P, Pollak P, et al. Electrical stimulation of the subthalamic nucleus in advanced Parkinson's disease. *N Engl J Med* 1998;339:1105–1111.
6. Gildenberg PL. The history of stereotactic and functional neurosurgery. In: Gildenberg PL, Tasker RR, eds. *Textbook of stereotactic and functional neurosurgery.* New York: McGraw-Hill, 1998:5–19.
7. Krauss JK, Grossman RG. Historical review of pallidal surgery for treatment of parkinsonism and other movement disorders. In: Krauss JK, Grossman RG, Jankovic J, eds. *Pallidal surgery for the treatment of Parkinson's disease and movement disorders.* Philadelphia: Lippincott–Raven, 1998:1–23.
8. Meyers R. The modification of alternating tremor, rigidity, and festination by surgery of the basal ganglia. *Res Publ Assoc Res Nerv Ment Dis* 1942;21:602–665.
9. Meyers R. The surgery of the hyperkinetic disorders. In: Vinken PJ, Bruyn GW, eds. *Handbook of clinical neurology,* vol 6. Amsterdam: North Holland, 1968:844–878.
10. Fenelon F. Essais de traitement neurochirurgical du syndrome parkinsonien par intervention directe sur les voies extrapyramidales immediatement sous striopallidales (ou lenticulaires). *Rev Neurol* 1950;83:437–440.
11. Spiegel EA, Wycis HT. Thalamotomy and pallidotomy for treatment of choreic movements. *Acta Neurochir* 1952;2:417–422.
12. Spiegel EA, Wycis HT, Marks M, et al. Stereotaxic apparatus for operations on the human brain. *Science* 1947;106:349–350.
13. Hassler R, Riechert T. Indikationen und Lokalisationsmethode der gezielten Hirnoperationen. *Nervenarzt* 1954;25:441–447.
14. Mundinger F, Riechert T. Die stereotaktischen Hirnoperationen zur Behandlung extrapyramidaler Bewegungsstörungen (Parkinsonismus und Hyperkinesen) und ihre Resultate. *Fortschr Neurol Psych* 1963;31:1–66, 69–120.
15. Laitinen LV, Bergenheim AT, Hariz MI. Leksell's posteroventral pallidotomy in the treatment of Parkinson's disease. *J Neurosurg* 1992;76:53–61.
16. Hassler R. Architectonic organization of the thalamic nuclei. In: Schaltenbrand G, Walker AE, eds. *Stereotaxy of the human brain.* Stuttgart: Thieme Medical, 1982:140–180.
17. Hassler R, Mundinger F, Riechert T. *Stereotaxis in Parkinson syndrome.* New York: Springer-Verlag, 1979.
18. Jones EG. Morphology, nomenclature, and connections of the thalamus and basal ganglia. In: Krauss JK, Jankovic J, Grossman RG, eds. *Surgery for Parkinson's disease and movement disorders.* Philadelphia: Lippincott Williams & Wilkins, 2001:24–47.
19. Taha JM, Favre J, Baumann TK, et al. Characteristics and somatotopic organization of kinesthetic cells in the globus pallidus of patients with Parkinson's disease. *J Neurosurg* 1996;85:1005–1112.
20. Guridi J, Gorospe A, Ramos E, et al. Stereotactic targeting of the globus pallidus internus in Parkinson's disease: imaging versus electrophysiological mapping. *Neurosurgery* 1999;45:278–287.
21. Rodriguez-Oroz MC, Rodriguez M, Guridi J, et al. The subthalamic nucleus in Parkinson's disease: somatotopic organization and physiological characteristics. *Brain* 2001;124:1777–1790.
22. Krauss JK, Grossman RG. Principles and techniques of movement disorders surgery. In: Krauss JK, Jankovic J, Grossman RG, eds. *Surgery for Parkinson's disease and movement disorders.* Philadelphia: Lippincott Williams & Wilkins, 2001:74–109.
23. Schaltenbrand G, Bailey P. *Introduction to stereotaxis with an atlas of the human brain.* Stuttgart: Thieme Medical, 1959.
24. Schaltenbrand G, Wahren P. *Atlas for stereotaxy of the human brain.* Stuttgart: Thieme Medical, 1977.
25. Kelly PJ, Derome P, Guiot G. Thalamic spatial variability and the surgical results of lesions placed with neurophysiologic control. *Surg Neurol* 1978;9:307–315.
26. Di Pierro CG, Francel PC, Jackson TR, et al. Optimizing accuracy in magnetic resonance image-guided stereotaxis: a technique with validation based on the anterior commissure–posterior commissure line. *J Neurosurg* 1999;90:94–100.
27. Holtzheimer PE III, Roberts DW, Darcey TM. Magnetic resonance imaging versus computed tomography for target localization in functional stereotactic neurosurgery. *Neurosurgery* 1999;45:290–297.
28. Schuurman PR, de Bie RMA, Majoie CBL, et al. A prospective comparison between three-dimensional magnetic resonance imaging and ventriculography for target-coordinate determination in frame-based functional stereotactic neurosurgery. *J Neurosurg* 1999;91:911–914.
29. Krauss JK, King DE, Grossman RG. Alignment correction algorithm for transformation of stereotactic anterior commissure/posterior commissure–based coordinates into frame coordinates in image-guided functional neurosurgery. *Neurosurgery* 1998;42:806–812.
30. Hutchison WD. Techniques of microelectrode recording in movement disorders surgery. In: Krauss JK, Jankovic J, Grossman RG, eds. *Surgery for Parkinson's disease and movement disorders.* Philadelphia: Lippincott Williams & Wilkins, 2001:110–118.
31. Kelly PJ, Gillingham FJ. The long-term results of stereotaxic surgery and L-dopa therapy in patients with Parkinson's disease. *J Neurosurg* 1980;53:332–337.
32. Jankovic J, Cardoso F, Grossman RG, et al. Outcome after stereotactic thalamotomy for parkinsonian, essential, and other types of tremor. *Neurosurgery* 1995;37:680–687.
33. Linhares MN, Tasker RR. Microelectrode-guided thalamotomy for Parkinson's disease. *Neurosurgery* 2000;46:390–395.
34. Narabayashi H, Yokochi F, Nakajima Y. Levodopa-induced dyskinesias and thalamotomy. *J Neurol Neurosurg Psychiatry* 1984;471:831–839.
35. Diederich N, Goetz CG, Stebbins GT, et al. Blinded evaluation confirms long-term asymmetric effect of unilateral thalamotomy or subthalamotomy on tremor in Parkinson's disease. *Neurology* 1992;42:1311–1314.
36. Tasker RR. Movement disorders. In: Apuzzo MLJ, ed. *Brain*

surgery: complication avoidance and management. New York: Churchill Livingstone, 1993:1509–1524.

37. Schuurman PR, Bosch DA, Bossuyt PM, et al. A comparison of continuous thalamic stimulation and thalamotomy for suppression of severe tremor. *N Engl J Med* 2000;342:461–468.

38. Tasker RR. Deep brain stimulation is preferable to thalamotomy for tremor suppression. *Surg Neurol* 1998;49:145–153.

39. Alkhani A, Lozano AM. Pallidotomy for Parkinson's disease: a review of contemporary literature. *J Neurosurg* 2001;94:43–49.

40. Payne BR, Bakay RAE, Vitek JL. Pallidotomy for treatment of Parkinson's disease. In: Krauss JK, Jankovic J, Grossman RG, eds. *Surgery for Parkinson's disease and movement disorders.* Philadelphia: Lippincott Williams & Wilkins, 2001:161–169.

41. Baron MS, Vitek JL, Bakay RA, et al. Treatment of advanced Parkinson's disease by posterior GPi pallidotomy: 1-year results of a pilot study. *Ann Neurol* 1996;40:355–366.

42. Johansson F, Malm J, Nordh E, et al. Usefulness of pallidotomy in advanced Parkinson's disease. *J Neurol Neurosurg Psychiatry* 1997;62:125–132.

43. Lang AE, Lozano AM, Montgomery E, et al. Posteroventral medial pallidotomy in advanced Parkinson's disease. *N Engl J Med* 1997;337:1036–1042.

44. Kondziolka D, Bonaroti E, Baser S, et al. Outcomes after stereotactically guided pallidotomy for advanced Parkinson's disease. *J Neurosurg* 1999;90:197–202.

45. Krauss JK, Desaloms M, Lai EC, et al. Microelectrode-guided posteroventral pallidotomy for treatment of Parkinson's disease: postoperative magnetic resonance imaging findings. *J Neurosurg* 1997;87:358–367.

46. Lai EC, Jankovic J, Krauss JK, et al. Long-term efficacy of posteroventral pallidotomy in the treatment of Parkinson's disease. *Neurology* 2000;55:1218–1222.

47. Ondo WG, Jankovic J, Lai EC, et al. Assessment of motor function after stereotactic pallidotomy. *Neurology* 1998;50:266–270.

48. Roberts-Warrior D, Overby A, Jankovic J, et al. Postural control in Parkinson's disease after unilateral posteroventral pallidotomy. *Brain* 2000;123:2141–2149.

49. Jankovic J, Lai E, Ben-Arie L, et al. Levodopa-induced dyskinesias treated by pallidotomy. *J Neurol Sci* 1999;167:62–67.

50. Perrine K, Dogali M, Fazzini E, et al. Cognitive functioning after pallidotomy for refractory Parkinson's disease. *J Neurol Neurosurg Psychiatry* 1998;65:150–154.

51. Trépanier LL, Saint-Cyr JA, Lozano AM, et al. Neuropsychological consequences of posteroventral pallidotomy for the treatment of Parkinson's disease. *Neurology* 1998;51:207–215.

52. Rettig GM, York MK, Lai EC, et al. Neuropsychological outcome after unilateral pallidotomy for the treatment of Parkinson's disease. *J Neurol Neurosurg Psychiatry* 2000;69:326–336.

53. Ghika J, Ghika-Schmid F, Fankhauser H, et al. Bilateral contemporaneous posteroventral pallidotomy for the treatment of Parkinson's disease: neuropsychological and neurological side effects—report of four cases and review of the literature. *J Neurosurg* 1999;91:313–321.

54. Scott R, Gregory R, Hines N, et al. Neuropsychological, neurological, and functional outcome following pallidotomy for Parkinson's disease: a consecutive series of eight simultaneous bilateral and twelve unilateral procedures. *Brain* 1998;121:659–675.

55. De Bie RMA, Schuurman PR, Bosch DA, et al. Outcome of unilateral pallidotomy in advanced Parkinson's disease: cohort study of 32 patients. *J Neurol Neurosurg Psychiatry* 2001;71:375–382.

56. Pal PK, Samii A, Kishore A, et al. Long-term outcome of unilateral pallidotomy: follow up of 15 patients for 3 years. *J Neurol Neurosurg Psychiatry* 2000;69:337–344.

57. Fine J, Duff J, Chen R, et al. Long-term follow-up of unilateral pallidotomy in advanced Parkinson's disease. *N Engl J Med* 2000;342:1708–1714.

58. Hariz MI, Bergenheim AT. A 10-year follow-up review of patients who underwent Leksell's posteroventral pallidotomy for Parkinson disease. *J Neurosurg* 2001;94:552–558.

59. Merello M, Starkstein S, Nouzeilles MI, et al. Bilateral pallidotomy for treatment of Parkinson's disease induced corticobulbar syndrome and psychic akinesia avoidable by globus pallidus lesion combined with contralateral stimulation. *J Neurol Neurosurg Psychiatry* 2001;71:611–614.

60. Merello M. Subthalamic stimulation contralateral to a previous pallidotomy: an erroneous indication? *Mov Disord* 1999;14:890.

61. Guridi J, Obeso JA. The subthalamic nucleus, hemiballismus and Parkinson's disease: reappraisal of a neurosurgical dogma. *Brain* 2001;124:5–19.

62. Alvarez L, Macias R, Guridi J, et al. Dorsal subthalamotomy for Parkinson's disease. *Mov Disord* 2001;16:72–78.

63. Gill SS, Heywood P. Bilateral dorsolateral subthalamotomy for advanced Parkinson's disease. *Lancet* 1997;350:1224.

64. Barlas O, Hanagasi HA, Imer M, et al. Do unilateral ablative lesions of the subthalamic nucleus in parkinsonian patients lead to hemiballism? *Mov Disord* 2001;16:306–310.

65. Su PC, Ma Y, Fukuda M, et al. Metabolic changes following subthalamotomy for advanced Parkinson's disease. *Ann Neurol* 2001;50:514–520.

66. Guiot G, Brion S, Fardeau M, et al. Dyskinesie volitionelle d'attitude supprimee par la coagulation thalamocapsulaire. *Rev Neurol* 1960;102:220–229.

67. Goldman MS, Ahlskog JE, Kelly PJ. The symptomatic and functional outcome of stereotactic thalamotomy for medically intractable essential tremor. *J Neurosurg* 1992;76:924–928.

68. Mohadjer M, Goerke H, Milios E, et al. Long-term results of stereotaxy in the treatment of essential tremor. *Stereotact Funct Neurosurg* 1990;54:125–129.

69. Krauss JK, Wakhloo AK, Nobbe F, et al. MR pathological correlations of severe posttraumatic tremor. *Neurol Res* 1995;17:409–416.

70. Krauss JK, Jankovic. Head injury and posttraumatic movement disorders. *Neurosurgery* 2002;50:927–939.

71. Krauss JK, Mohadjer M, Nobbe F, et al. The treatment of posttraumatic tremor by stereotactic surgery. *J Neurosurg* 1994;80:810–819.

72. Andrew J, Fowler CJ, Harrison MJG. Tremor after head injury and its treatment by stereotaxic surgery. *J Neurol Neurosurg Psychiatry* 1982;45:815–819.

73. Bullard DE, Nashold BS Jr. Stereotaxic thalamotomy for treatment of posttraumatic movement disorders. *J Neurosurg* 1984;61:316–321.

74. Hirai T, Miyazaki M, Nakajima H, et al. The correlation between tremor characteristics and the predicted volume of effective lesions in stereotaxic nucleus ventralis intermedius thalamotomy. *Brain* 1983;106:1001–1018.

75. Goldman MD, Kelly PJ. Symptomatic and functional outcome of stereotactic ventralis lateralis thalamotomy for intention tremor. *J Neurosurg* 1992;77:223–229.

76. Alusi SH, Aziz TZ, Glickman S, et al. Stereotactic lesional surgery for the treatment of tremor in multiple sclerosis: a prospective case-controlled study. *Brain* 2001;124:1576–1589.

77. Jankovic J. Re-emergence of surgery for dystonia. *J Neurol Neurosurg Psychiatry* 1998;65:434.

78. Andrew J, Fowler CJ, Harrison MJG. Stereotaxic thalamotomy in 55 cases of dystonia. *Brain* 1983;106:981–1000.

79. Tasker RR, Doorly T, Yamashiro K. Thalamotomy in generalized dystonia. *Adv Neurol* 1988;50:615–631.

80. Krauss JK, Mohadjer M, Braus DF, et al. Dystonia following

head trauma: a report of nine patients and review of the literature. *Mov Disord* 1992;7:263–272.

81. Cardoso F, Jankovic J, Grossman RG, et al. Outcome after stereotactic thalamotomy for dystonia and hemiballismus. *Neurosurgery* 1995;36:501–508.

82. Ondo WG, Desaloms M, Krauss JK, et al. Pallidotomy and thalamotomy for dystonia. In: Krauss JK, Jankovic J, Grossman RG, eds. *Surgery for Parkinson's disease and movement disorders.* Philadelphia: Lippincott Williams & Wilkins, 2001:299–306.

83. Yoshor D, Hamilton WJ, Ondo W, et al. Comparison of thalamotomy and pallidotomy for the treatment of dystonia. *Neurosurgery* 2001;48:818–826.

84. Ondo WG, Desaloms JM, Jankovic J, et al. Pallidotomy for generalized dystonia. *Mov Disord* 1998;13:693–698.

85. Justesen CR, Penn RD, Kroin JS, et al. Stereotactic pallidotomy in a child with Hallervorden-Spatz disease. *J Neurosurg* 1999; 90:551–554.

86. Cubo E, Shannon KM, Penn RD, et al. Internal globus pallidotomy in dystonia secondary to Huntington's disease. *Mov Disord* 2000;15:1248–1251.

87. Alkhani A, Khan F, Lang AE, et al. The response to pallidal surgery for dystonia is dependent on the etiology (abst). *Neurosurgery* 2000;47:504.

88. Loher TJ, Hasdemir MG, Burgunder JM, et al. Long-term follow-up study of chronic globus pallidus internus stimulation for posttraumatic hemidystonia. *J Neurosurg* 2000;92:457–460.

89. Albright AL. Intrathecal baclofen for treatment of dystonia. In: Krauss JK, Jankovic J, Grossman RG, eds. *Surgery for Parkinson's disease and movement disorders.* Philadelphia: Lippincott Williams & Wilkins, 2001:316–322.

90. Albright AL, Barry MJ, Shafton DH, et al. Intrathecal baclofen for generalized dystonia. *Dev Med Child Neurol* 2001;43: 652–657.

91. Krauss JK, Grossman RG, Jankovic J. Treatment options for surgery of cervical dystonia. In: Krauss JK, Jankovic J, Grossman RG, eds. *Surgery for Parkinson's disease and movement disorders.* Philadelphia: Lippincott Williams & Wilkins, 2001:323–324.

92. Jankovic J, Hallett M. *Botulinum toxin treatment.* New York: Marcel Dekker, 1994.

93. Krauss JK, Koller R, Burgunder JM. Partial myotomy/myectomy of the trapezius muscle with an asleep–awake–asleep anesthetic technique for treatment of cervical dystonia. *J Neurosurg* 1999;91:889–891.

94. Jho HD, Jannetta PJ. Microvascular decompression for spasmodic torticollis. *Acta Neurochir* 1995;134:21–26.

95. Shima F, Fukui M, Kitamura K. Pathogenesis of spasmodic torticollis of 11th nerve origin (abst). *J Neurosurg* 1990;72: 335A–336A.

96. Freckmann N, Hagenah R, Herrmann HD, et al. Bilateral microsurgical lysis of the spinal accessory nerve roots for treatment of spasmodic torticollis. *Acta Neurochir* 1986;83:47–53.

97. Hamby WB, Schiffer S. Spasmodic torticollis: results after cervical rhizotomy in 50 cases. *J Neurosurg* 1969;31:323–326.

98. Friedman AH, Nashold BS Jr, Sharp R, et al. Treatment of spasmodic torticollis with intradural selective rhizotomies. *J Neurosurg* 1993;78:46–53.

99. Hernesniemi J, Keränen T. Long-term outcome after surgery for spasmodic torticollis. *Acta Neurochir* 1990;103:128–130.

100. Colbassani HJ Jr, Wood JH. Management of spasmodic torticollis. *Surg Neurol* 1986;25:153–158.

101. Bertrand CM. Selective peripheral denervation for spasmodic torticollis: surgical technique, results, and observations in 260 cases. *Surg Neurol* 1993;40:96–103.

102. Braun V, Richter HP. Selective peripheral denervation for the treatment of spasmodic torticollis. *Neurosurgery* 1994;35:58–63.

103. Munchau A, Palmer JD, Dressler D, et al. Prospective study of selective peripheral denervation for botulinum-toxin resistant patients with cervical dystonia. *Brain* 2001;124:769–783.

104. Munchau A, Good CD, McGowan S, et al. Prospective study of swallowing function in patients with cervical dystonia undergoing selective peripheral denervation. *J Neurol Neurosurg Psychiatry* 2001;71:67–72.

105. Chawda SJ, Munchau A, Johnson D, et al. Pattern of premature degenerative changes of the cervical spine in patients with spasmodic torticollis and the impact on the outcome of selective peripheral denervation. *J Neurol Neurosurg Psychiatry* 2000;68: 465–471.

106. Weigel R, Rittmann M, Krauss JK. Spontaneous craniocervical osseous fusion resulting from cervical dystonia. *J Neurosurg (Spine)* 2001;95:115–118.

107. Krauss JK, Toups EG, Jankovic J, et al. Symptomatic and functional outcome of surgical treatment of cervical dystonia. *J Neurol Neurosurg Psychiatry* 1997;63:642–648.

108. Krauss JK, Pohle T. Historical review of functional stereotactic neurosurgery for treatment of cervical dystonia. *Mov Disord* 1998;13[Suppl 2]:134.

109. Magyar-Lehmann S, Antonini A, Roelcke U, et al. Cerebral glucose metabolism in patients with spasmodic torticollis. *Mov Disord* 1997;12:704–708.

110. Krauss JK, Pohle T, Weber S, et al. Bilateral stimulation of globus pallidus internus for treatment of cervical dystonia. *Lancet* 1999;354:837–838.

111. Krauss JK, Loher TJ, Pohle T, et al. Pallidal deep brain stimulation in patients with cervical dystonia and severe cervical dyskinesias with cervical myelopathy. *J Neurol Neurosurg Psychiatry* 2002;72:249–256.

112. Suarez JI, Verhagen Metman L, Reich SG, et al. Pallidotomy for hemiballismus: efficacy and characteristics of neuronal activity. *Ann Neurol* 1997;42:807–811.

113. Krauss JK, Mundinger F. Functional stereotactic surgery for hemiballism. *J Neurosurg* 1996;85:278–286.

114. Krauss JK, Mundinger F. Surgical treatment of hemiballism and hemichorea. In: Krauss JK, Jankovic J, Grossman RG, eds. *Surgery for Parkinson's disease and movement disorders.* Philadelphia: Lippincott Williams & Wilkins, 2001:397–403.

115. Laitinen LV, Hariz MI. Movement disorders. In: Youmans JR, ed. *Neurological surgery,* 4th ed. Philadelphia: WB Saunders, 1996:3575–3609.

116. Rauch SL, Baer L, Cosgrove GR, et al. Neurosurgical treatment of Tourette's syndrome: a critical review. *Compr Psychiatry* 1995; 36:141–156.

117. Hassler R, Dieckmann G. Traitement stereotaxique des tics et cris inarticules ou coprolalique consideres comme phenomene d'obsession motrice au cours de maladies de Gilles de la Tourette. *Rev Neurol* 1970;123:89–106.

118. Babel TB, Warnke PC, Ostertag CB. Immediate and long term outcome after infrathalamic and thalamic lesioning for intractable Tourette's syndrome. *J Neurol Neurosurg Psychiatry* 2001;70:666–671.

119. Spangler WJ, Cosgrove GR, Ballantine HT, et al. Magnetic resonance image-guided stereotactic cingulotomy for intractable psychiatric disease. *Neurosurgery* 1996;38:1071–1078.

120. Kurlan R, Kersun J, Ballentine HT Jr, et al. Neurosurgical treatment of severe obsessive-compulsive disorder associated with Tourette's syndrome. *Mov Disord* 1990;5:152–155.

121. Baer L, Rauch SL, Jenike MA, et al. Cingulotomy in a case of concomitant obsessive-compulsive disorder and Tourette's syndrome. *Arch Gen Psychiatry* 1994;51:73–74.

122. Vandewalle V, van der Linden C, Groenewegen HJ, et al. Stereotactic treatment of Gilles de la Tourette syndrome by high frequency stimulation of thalamus. *Lancet* 1999;353:724.

123. Gybels J, van Roost D. Spinal cord stimulation for spasticity. In:

Sindou M, Abbott R, Keravel Y, eds. *Neurosurgery for spasticity.* New York: Springer-Verlag, 1991:73–81.

124. Hugenholtz H, Humphreys P, McIntyre WMJ, et al. Cervical spinal cord stimulation for spasticity in cerebral palsy. *Neurosurgery* 1988;22:707–714.

125. Ochs G, Struppler A, Meyerson BA, et al. Intrathecal baclofen for long-term treatment of spasticity: a multi-centre study. *J Neurol Neurosurg Psychiatry* 1989;52:933–939.

126. Penn RD, Savoy S, Corcos D, et al. Intrathecal baclofen for severe spinal spasticity. *N Engl J Med* 1989;320:1517–1521.

127. Ordia JI, Fischer E, Adamski E, et al. Chronic intrathecal delivery of baclofen by a programmable pump for the treatment of severe spasticity. *J Neurosurg* 1996;85:452–457.

128. Sindou MP, Mertens P. Ablative surgery for treatment of spasticity. In: Krauss JK, Jankovic J, Grossman RG, eds. *Surgery for Parkinson's disease and movement disorders.* Philadelphia: Lippincott Williams & Wilkins, 2001:421–436.

129. Laitinen LV, Singounas E. Longitudinal myelotomy in the treatment of spasticity of the legs. *J Neurosurg* 1971;35:536–540.

130. Sindou M, Jeanmonod D. Microsurgical DREZ-otomy for the treatment of spasticity and pain in the lower limbs. *Neurosurgery* 1989;24:655–670.

131. Narabayashi H. Stereotaxic surgery for athetosis of the spastic state of cerebral palsy. *Confin Neurol* 1962;22:364–367.

132. Broggi G, Angelini L, Bono R, et al. Long term results of stereotactic thalamotomy for cerebral palsy. *Neurosurgery* 1983;12:195–202.

133. Teo C. Functional stereotactic surgery of movement disorders in cerebral palsy. In: Krauss JK, Jankovic J, Grossman RG, eds. *Surgery for Parkinson's disease and movement disorders.* Philadelphia: Lippincott Williams & Wilkins, 2001:410–420.

134. Barker FG, Jannetta PL, Bissonette DJ, et al. Microvascular decompression for hemifacial spasm. *J Neurosurg* 1995;82:201–210.

135. Payner TD, Tew JM. Recurrence of hemifacial spasm after microvascular decompression. *Neurosurgery* 1996;38:686–691.

136. Ishikawa M, Nakanishi T, Takamiya Y, et al. Delayed resolution of residual hemifacial spasm after microvascular decompression operations. *Neurosurgery* 2001;49:847–856.

137. Meinck HM, Tronnier V, Marquardt G. Surgical treatment of stiff man syndrome with intrathecal baclofen. In: Krauss JK, Jankovic J, Grossman RG, eds. *Surgery for Parkinson's disease and movement disorders.* Philadelphia: Lippincott Williams & Wilkins, 2001:393–396.

138. Meinck HM, Tronnier V, Rieke K, et al. Intrathecal baclofen treatment for stiff-man syndrome: pump failure may be fatal. *Neurology* 1994;44:2209–2210.

139. Grimes DA, Lozano AM, Lang AE. Vim thalamotomy for familial essential myoclonus. *Mov Disord* 1998;13[Suppl 2]:236.

140. Lozano AM, ed. *Movement disorder surgery.* Basel: Karger, 2000.

141. Krauss JK, Jankovic J, Grossman RG, eds. *Surgery for Parkinson's disease and movement disorders.* Philadelphia: Lippincott Williams & Wilkins, 2001.

45

NEURAL AND STEM CELL TRANSPLANTATION

OLLE LINDVALL
PETER HAGELL

The basic principle of cell therapy is very simple: to restore brain function that has been lost due to damage or disease by replacing dead cells with new healthy cells through transplantation. Given the complexity of human brain structure and function, this prospect may seem remote. However, if cell replacement will work in the human brain, it could provide radical new therapies for severe neurodegenerative disorders like Parkinson's disease (PD) and Huntington's disease (HD). Whether it will work or not depends on, first, whether the grafted neurons can survive and form connections in the patient's brain and, second, whether the patient's brain can integrate and use the grafted neurons.

It is important to underscore, not least in the perspective of the emerging technology of neural stem cells, that convincing preclinical data are a prerequisite for clinical application of any cell replacement therapy. These data should demonstrate functional efficacy in an animal model resembling the human disease and also reveal the biological mechanism underlying the observed functional recovery. The cell replacement strategy in PD is based on such a well-defined biological mechanism, namely, the recovery of function by restoration of dopamine (DA) neurotransmission in the striatum. It was demonstrated more than 20 years ago that embryonic mesencephalic DA-rich tissue implanted in a rat model of PD reinnervated the denervated striatum and ameliorated some functional deficits. Extensive animal studies have subsequently shown that the grafted DA neurons display many of the morphologic and functional characteristics of intrinsic DA neurons: they reinnervate the denervated striatum and form synaptic contacts with host neurons, are spontaneously active and release DA, and receive afferent inputs from the host (1). Reinnervation by the grafts is accompanied by significant amelioration of several aspects of the DA deficiency syndrome both in rodents and in monkeys (1,2).

Based on these animal experimental data, trials with transplantation of human embryonic mesencephalic tissue to the striatum in patients with PD were initiated in 1987. From the clinical point of view, there is definitely a need for new therapeutic approaches in this disorder. The cell replacement strategy is also particularly suitable to explore in PD because the main pathology is a rather selective degeneration of the nigrostriatal DA system, that is, of a specific neuronal population in a restricted area of the brain. The dopaminergic deficit in PD should, therefore, be easier to correct by transplantation than, say, the more widespread loss of many different cell types in Alzheimer's disease.

Clinical application of neural transplantation also seems justified in patients with HD. Many of the symptoms in this disorder result from the loss of striatal GABAergic neurons. These inhibitory neurons form an essential link in the corticostriatopallidal circuitry and have an important role in both motor and cognitive processes. In animal models of HD, created by intrastriatal injections of excitotoxins or systemic injections of metabolic toxins, intrastriatal grafts of embryonic striatal neuroblasts form a striatum-like structure at the site of implantation and restore some of the essential efferent and afferent striatal connections (3). Thus, cells in the grafts differentiate into mature striatal projection neurons, establishing a functional connection with the host globus pallidus and receiving regulatory afferent inputs from the host brain (e.g., from the cerebral cortex) (3). This level of reconstruction of the circuitry is sufficient to reverse deficits in both motor and cognitive behavior, not only in rats but also in the larger and more complex striatal system of monkeys (4,5).

In this chapter, we will first argue, based on the experiences with neural transplantation in patients with PD and HD performed so far, that cell replacement can work in the diseased human brain. In this perspective, we will then discuss the possible role of the stem cell technology for the further development of cell therapies in movement disorders, particularly in PD.

CLINICAL EXPERIENCES WITH NEURAL TRANSPLANTATION IN PARKINSON'S DISEASE

Short- and Long-term Graft Survival and Growth

So far, about 350 patients with PD have received grafts of primary embryonic tissue of human or porcine origin. It is well established that the human embryonic mesencephalic DA neurons can survive transplantation into the brain of PD patients. Significant increase of [^{18}F]fluorodopa uptake in the grafted striatum has been shown using positron emission tomography (PET) in more than 40 PD patients (6–17). In one patient, fluorodopa uptake in the putamen was normalized after transplantation (12,18). Histopathologic studies have confirmed the survival of dopaminergic grafts and demonstrated reinnervation of the striatum in two parkinsonian patients who died after transplantation (19–21). Between 80,000 and 135,000 dopaminergic neurons had survived on each side. The neuritic outgrowth from the grafted neurons extended up to approximately 7 mm within the putamen. With six tracts, placed 5 mm apart, confluent reinnervation of 24% to 78% of the designated target area in the postcommissural putamen could be obtained, although in the patient with the densest reinnervation the putamen was shrunken (20). The dopaminergic innervation occurred in a patch-matrix pattern, and electron microscopy revealed synaptic connections between graft and host. There was no evidence that sprouting had occurred from the patients' own DA neurons.

Grafts of human mesencephalic tissue can exhibit long-term survival despite an ongoing disease process and continuous antiparkinsonian drug treatment. In two patients, who were transplanted unilaterally in the putamen, the fluorodopa uptake in the grafted structure was still high at 6 and 10 years after surgery (12,18). In contrast, there had been a progressive fall of tracer uptake in nongrafted striatal regions, indicating degeneration of the patient's own DA neurons. Immunologic rejection of the grafts has not been reported in any PD patient, even several years after withdrawal of immunosuppression.

Magnitude of Clinical Improvement

Several clinical research groups have demonstrated therapeutic improvement associated with graft survival (6–18,22–24). In the most successful cases, patients have been able to withdraw L-dopa treatment during several years after transplantation (12,13,16). For a more detailed account of clinical observations, including constrains and morbidity, following neural transplantation in PD, see (24) and (25).

Table 45.1 summarizes the magnitude of the overall clinical benefit at 10 to 24 months postoperatively in four series of patients who were grafted bilaterally with human embryonic mesencephalic tissue (13,14,16,17). In the three open-label trials, patients were grafted bilaterally with primary human embryonic mesencephalic tissue from about three to five donors into each putamen. In some cases, tissue was also implanted in the caudate nucleus. According to the Unified Parkinson's Disease Rating Scale (UPDRS) (26) motor score during practically defined "off" (i.e., in the morning, at least 12 hours after the last dose of antiparkinsonian medication), the overall symptomatic relief at 10 to 24 months postoperatively was between 30% and 40%. In addition, there was a decrease (by 43% to 59%) of the average daily time spent in the "off" phase. The mean daily L-dopa requirements were reduced by 16% to 45% (13,14,16). It is interesting to note that in these three studies, even if the patients showed increased fluorodopa uptake (by about 60%) in the puta-

TABLE 45.1 AMOUNT OF GRAFT TISSUE AND MAGNITUDE OF POSTOPERATIVE CHANGES OF PUTAMINAL FLUORODOPA UPTAKE AND MOTOR FUNCTION IN FOUR SERIES OF PATIENTS WITH IDIOPATHIC PD AT 1024 MONTHS AFTER BILATERAL INTRASTRIATAL IMPLANTATION OF HUMAN EMBRYONIC MESENCEPHALIC TISSUE

	Hauser et al. (Ref. 14) (n=6)	Hagell et al. (Ref. 13) (n=4[a])	Brundin et al. (Ref. 16) (n=5)	Freed et al. (Ref. 17) (n=19)
Number of VM/putamen	3–4	4.9	2.8[b]	2
Fluorodopa uptake (putamen):				
Preop[c]	34%	31%	31%	n.r.
Postop[c]	55%	52%	48%	n.r.
Δ	+61%	+69%	+55%	+40%
UPDRS motor score in "off" (Δ)[d]	–30%	–30%	–40%	–18%
Daily time in "off" phase (Δ)	–43%	–59%	–43%	n.r.
Daily L-dopa dose (Δ)	–16%	–37%	–45%	n.r.

[a]Excluding one patient with possible multiple system atrophy.
[b]The graft tissue was treated with the lazaroid tirilazad mesylate.
[c]Mean percent fluorodopa uptake compared to the normal mean as measured in healthy volunteers.
[d]As assessed during practically defined "off."
Abbreviations: VM, ventral mesencephalon; Δ, mean postoperative change (%) from baseline; Preop, preoperatively; Postop, postoperatively; UPDRS, Unified Parkinson's Disease Rating Scale; n.r., not reported.

men, indicating graft survival, the uptake after transplantation was still only about 50% of the normal mean. This probably explains the incomplete functional recovery and indicates that there is room for considerable improvement.

A recent double-blind, placebo-controlled study (17) demonstrated a more modest clinical response with 18% reduction of UPDRS motor score in "off" at 12 months after bilateral putaminal grafts, but no improvement in the sham-operated group. In patients younger than 60 years, the improvement of UPDRS score was 34%. These data are important because they provide the first direct evidence of a specific graft-induced improvement, distinguishable from a placebo effect. In this trial less tissue was implanted than in the open-label trials and, in agreement, the increase of fluorodopa uptake was lower (only 40% as compared with 60%). In two patients who died after grafting, the number of dopaminergic neurons in each putamen was only between 7,000 and 40,000 (17), whereas in the two patients in one of the open-label trials, the dopaminergic cell counts ranged from 80,000 to 135,000 (19–21). One important explanation to the low cell number is probably that the tissue was stored in cell culture for up to 4 weeks before implantation. In agreement, the postoperative clinical improvement was smaller than that reported in the other patient series. These findings provide further support for the notion that the number of viable implanted DA neurons is of fundamental importance for the magnitude of symptomatic relief (27).

Dyskinesias develop in the "off" phase after transplantation in some patients (23,24). Freed et al. (17) reported that 15% of their patients experienced severe dyskinesias. These

were proposed to be due to a continued fiber outgrowth from the graft resulting in a relative DA excess. However, in the patients analyzed by Hagell et al. (28), the dyskinesias were not of such dramatic severity and only rarely constituted a clinical therapeutic problem. The severity of dyskinesias was not related to the magnitude of graft-derived dopaminergic reinnervation or symptomatic relief (Fig. 45.1). Thus, there was no evidence of a dopaminergic overgrowth. The data of Hagell et al. (28) demonstrate that effective DA neuron replacement and major recovery of motor function are not coupled to the development of severe dyskinesias. The occurrence of severe dyskinesias is not a characteristic feature of DA cell replacement per se and therefore should not impede the further development of a cell therapy for PD.

Mechanisms of Graft Function

The clinical observations discussed above demonstrate that the grafts can survive, store DA, and give rise to symptomatic relief in PD patients. Recent studies also provide evidence that grafts of primary human embryonic mesencephalic tissue can restore regulated release of DA in the striatum and that they can become functionally integrated into the neural circuitries in the patient's brain.

One patient who was transplanted unilaterally in the putamen showed major clinical improvement and, in agreement, fluorodopa uptake in the grafted putamen was normalized at 3 years with no further change at 10 years postoperatively (Fig. 45.2) (18). In contrast, the nongrafted putamen exhibited a progressive decrease of fluorodopa uptake, which at 10 years after surgery was only about 10% of the normal level.

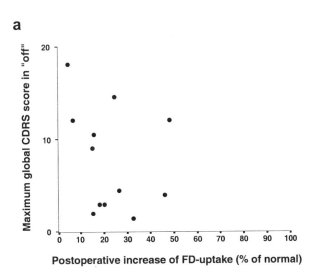
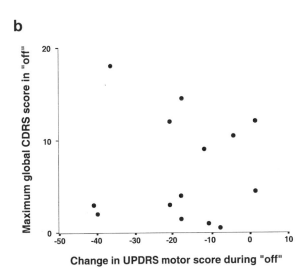

FIG. 45.1. "Off" phase dyskinesias following neural transplantation are not linked to effective dopamine (DA) cell replacement and major clinical improvement. Scatterplots of the relationship between the maximum postoperative global Clinical Dyskinesia Rating Scale (CDRS) scores in practically defined "off" and the change in fluorodopa uptake **(A)**, expressed as a percentage of normal mean, and in the Unified Parkinson's Disease Rating Scale (UPDRS) motor score **(B)** at the time of maximal postoperative "off" phase CDRS scores.

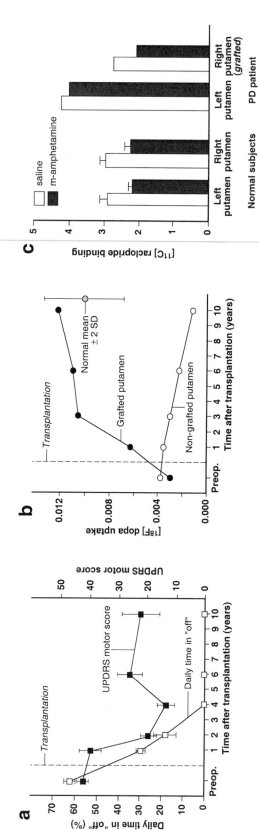

FIG. 45.2. Neural grafts can restore dopamine (DA) storage and release in the striatum to normal levels and give major symptomatic relief for more than a decade in patients with PD. **A:** Percentage of the day spent in the "off" phase (*open squares*) and UPDRS motor score (*filled squares*) in the practically defined "off" phase preoperatively and at various time points after transplantation of human embryonic mesencephalic tissue unilaterally into the right putamen. Data are mean ± 95% confidence interval. Dashed vertical line indicates time of transplantation. **B:** Fluorodopa uptake in the grafted (*filled circles*) and nongrafted (*open circles*) putamen in the same patient. Comparative data (mean ± 2 SD) are given for a group of 16 healthy volunteers (*shaded circle with error bars*). Dashed vertical line indicates time of transplantation. **C:** Basal and drug-induced DA release as assessed using [¹¹C]raclopride PET to measure DA D2 receptor occupancy by the endogenous transmitter. In the baseline condition (saline infusion; *open bars*), [¹¹C]raclopride binding is increased in the nongrafted putamen in the patient, whereas it is normal on the grafted side (right putamen). After amphetamine administration (*filled bars*), the binding reduction in the grafted putamen is similar to that seen in the putamen of normal subjects, whereas it is negligible in the nongrafted putamen. (Data from Piccini P, Brooks DJ, Björklund A, et al. Dopamine release from nigral transplants visualized in vivo in a Parkinson's patient. *Nat Neurosci* 1999;2:1137–1140.)

Dopamine release was quantified at 10 years using [^{11}C]raclopride and PET to measure DA D2 receptor occupancy by endogenous DA (18). Both basal and amphetamine-induced DA release was normal in the grafted putamen, whereas the release in the contralateral, nongrafted putamen was very low (Fig. 45.2). It seems highly likely that the efficient restoration of DA release in large parts of the grafted putamen underlies the patient's major clinical improvement.

The activation of two frontal cortical areas associated with movements, the supplementary motor area (SMA) and the dorsolateral prefrontal cortex (DLPFC), was analyzed using regional cerebral blood flow measurement with PET

(29) in four patients grafted bilaterally in the caudate and putamen. The SMA and DLPFC are known to be important in the preparation and selection of voluntary movements, their function is influenced by the basal ganglia–thalamocortical neural circuitries, and their impaired activation is believed to underlie parkinsonian akinesia. Preoperatively, there was only a small activation of the SMA and no significant activation of the DLPFC (Fig. 45.3). No significant differences in activation were observed in these patients at 6.5 months after grafting in comparison with preoperatively, whereas at 18.3 months there was significantly increased activation of both the SMA and

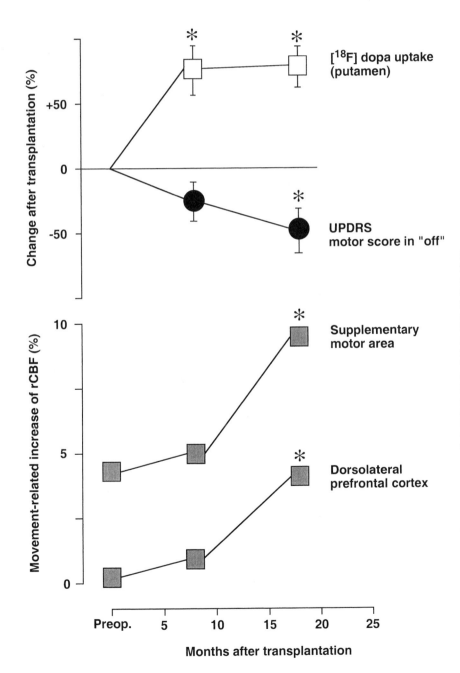

FIG. 45.3. Evidence for functional integration of dopaminergic grafts in Parkinson's disease (PD) patients. Changes of fluorodopa uptake in the putamen and UPDRS motor score in the "off" phase *(upper panel)* and movement-related increases of regional cerebral blood flow compared to resting condition in the supplementary motor area (SMA) and dorsolateral prefrontal cortex (DLPFC) *(lower panel)*, preoperatively and at 6.5 and 18.3 months after bilateral implantation of human embryonic mesencephalic tissue into the putamen and caudate nucleus in four PD patients. Putaminal fluorodopa uptake is significantly elevated already at 6.5 months after transplantation with no further changes thereafter. In contrast, the symptomatic relief is only partial at 6.5 months and substantial clinical improvement, as measured by the UPDRS motor score, does not occur until the second postoperative year. The gradual and delayed symptomatic relief is paralleled by the recovery of movement-related cortical activation. Data are mean ± SD. *$p < 0.001$, compared to preoperatively, *t* test. Putaminal [^{18}F]dopa uptake, *open squares*; UPDRS motor score in "off," *filled circles*; SMA, *black squares*; DLPFC, *shaded squares*. (Modified from Piccini P, Lindvall O, Björklund A, et al. Delayed recovery of movement-related cortical function in Parkinson's disease after striatal dopaminergic grafts. *Ann Neurol* 2000;48:689–695.)

DLPFC. The time course of clinical improvement paralleled that of the increase of cortical activation, with partial recovery after 6.5 months and substantial improvement at 18.3 months (Fig. 45.3). In contrast, striatal fluorodopa uptake was significantly elevated at 6.5 months, with no further change at 18.3 months after grafting (Fig. 45.3). Taken together, these findings indicate that successful grafts in patients with PD, by improving striatal dopaminergic neurotransmission, can restore movement-related cortical activation, which probably is necessary to induce substantial clinical improvement. They also provide new evidence that the functional effects of the grafted neurons go beyond those of a simple DA delivery system. Restoration of non-regulated DA release, as in the early stages of graft maturation, when fluorodopa uptake is already significantly elevated, seems to be insufficient to improve cortical activation during movement and to induce maximal clinical recovery. In order to increase basal ganglia–thalamocortical neurotransmission and movement-related cortical activation, the grafted DA neurons probably need to establish both efferent and afferent synaptic connections with the host brain.

Strategies to Increase Survival of Grafted Dopamine Neurons

Although the clinical grafting trials in PD have provided proof of concept for the cell replacement strategy, it seems unlikely that transplantation of human embryonic central nervous system tissue can be developed into therapies for large numbers of patients. First, the availability of human embryonic tissue is very limited; second, there is a clear problem with the standardization, purity, and viability of the graft tissue; and, third, there are ethical concerns about the need for a continuous supply of large amounts of human embryonic tissue. A major problem is that the survival of grafted DA neurons is low, only 5% to 20%, and therefore tissue from six to eight donors is needed for each PD patient in order to induce significant clinical improvement. In animal experiments, the survival of grafted mesencephalic DA neurons can be increased two- to fourfold by exposure of the graft to growth factors, and compounds that reduce oxidative stress or inhibit caspases (for review, see 30). The only compounds that have been tested clinically are the lazaroid, tirilazad mesylate, and glial-derived neurotrophic factor (GDNF) (15,16). These clinical studies provide evidence that both tirilazad mesylate and GDNF (administered to the graft tissue during a 6 days pre-grafting storage) may improve survival of grafted DA neurons in PD patients.

Xenografts

In the initial attempts with porcine xenografts in PD patients, the survival of DA neurons was poor with questionable clinical benefits (31,32). Major concerns with porcine xenografts, apart from immunologic rejection and transfer of virus, are, first, that a very large number of porcine donors and many implant sites may be needed to effectively reinnervate the human striatum, and, second, that the porcine DA neurons may have a lesser capacity to integrate functionally into the patient's brain as compared with human DA neurons.

CLINICAL EXPERIENCES WITH NEURAL TRANSPLANTATION IN HUNTINGTON'S DISEASE

Although several clinical trials with neural transplantation in HD have been undertaken or are ongoing, the available data on graft survival and clinical effects emanate mainly from two studies. Bachoud-Levy et al. described five patients with HD who received intrastriatal grafts bilaterally, with a year's interval between the two grafts (33). Striatal tissue from 7- to 9-week-old human embryos was used for the grafts. Tissue from one or two donors was injected into each caudate nucleus and putamen along four or five needle tracks. Immunosuppressive therapy was given until 12 months after the second transplantation. Measurement of $[^{18}F]$fluorodeoxyglucose uptake using PET showed that, compared with preoperatively, three of the five patients had either increased or stable metabolic activity throughout the striatum, and higher activity in some small areas, at 1 year after the second grafting. These data are consistent with the survival of metabolically active neural grafts. A cohort of 22 patients with HD who were assessed in parallel showed worsening of chorea and performance in most neuropsychological tests. By contrast, the patients with presumed surviving grafts had stable or even improved neuropsychological test results, improvement in activities of daily living, and reductions in severity of chorea and bradykinesia. Two of these patients had improvements in somatosensory evoked potentials, which were not found in the untreated patients. In support of the possibility that survival of the grafts accounted for the observed clinical benefit in three patients, the decreased metabolic activity in the striatum postoperatively in the other two patients was accompanied by deterioration of cognitive and motor function.

In a parallel study, Freeman et al. using histopathologic techniques confirmed surviving grafts with morphologic features of developing striatum in a patient with HD who died 18 months after transplantation (34). The striatum-like part of the grafted tissue, which occupied about 50% of the graft volume, was innervated by dopaminergic fibers from the host brain. No clinical observations were reported.

The findings in these clinical trials are encouraging, despite the low number of grafted patients, and provide evidence that neuronal replacement can also work in HD. However, whether cell therapy can be developed into a clinically useful treatment for HD patients remains unclear. First, the impact of intrastriatal grafts on the course of the

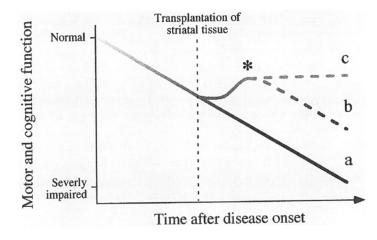

FIG. 45.4. Effects of intrastriatal neural grafts on the course of Huntington's disease (HD) are unknown. Three possible scenarios are depicted here: (a) worsening of functional impairment in the nongrafted patient for comparison; (b) stability or improvement in some functional variables at an early time point after transplantation (*), which is followed by progressive deterioration due to degeneration of the graft, the host corticostriatal circuitry, or both; (c) stability over many years because the grafts have taken over the function of the patient's own striatum, and the grafts and the host corticostriatal circuitry are not destroyed by the disease process. Only if this state is achievable can cell therapy be of major therapeutic value for patients with HD.

disease is unknown (Fig. 45.4). The ability of the graft to maintain a stable condition over a long time will be essential for its therapeutic value. Since follow-up data after bilateral transplantation thus far are limited to 1 year, it remains to be determined whether the striatal transplants can survive and function long enough to prevent further clinical deterioration. It is also unknown to what extent striatal transplants can counteract the concurrent degenerative processes in the host brain. Reconstruction of the striatal circuitry alone may be insufficient because the progressive degeneration in the neocortex seen in patients with HD is unlikely to be caused by retrograde changes secondary to neuronal loss in the striatum. Indeed, intrastriatal mesencephalic grafts in PD have not been able to retard the degeneration of the intrinsic DA neurons caused by the disease process (18). Second, since the primary mode of action of the grafts is to replace lost striatal neurons, the total number of surviving grafted striatal neurons is likely to be critical for the magnitude of the therapeutic effect. In the study of Bachoud-Levy et al. (33), it is not clear how much of the normal volume of the striatum was replaced by the grafts. In Freeman and colleagues' study (34), the total volume of the surviving grafts corresponded to only 8% to 10% of the volume of the remaining caudate-putamen. These data suggest that the size of the surviving grafts may have to be increased to obtain maximal therapeutic effects.

STEM CELL TRANSPLANTATION IN MOVEMENT DISORDERS

It seems highly likely that stem cell–based therapies will be tested first in patients with PD. One major reason is that there is already good evidence that a cell replacement strategy can work in this disorder. It is also conceivable that with stem cell approaches the best chances of success are in diseases in which clinical efficacy is determined by a single, defined biological mechanism, such as restoration of DA transmission in PD. In principle, there are two ways of using

immature progenitors for grafting in PD. The first way is for the cells to be predifferentiated in vitro to dopaminergic neurons prior to transplantation. Thus, stem cells could become an almost unlimited source for the generation of DA neurons. The cell preparations could be standardized and quality controlled with respect to viability and purity. The second alternative is for the progenitors to be differentiated in vivo to dopaminergic neurons following implantation in the striatum or substantia nigra. These neurons may integrate better than primary embryonic neurons and, in the ideal scenario, reconstruct the nigrostriatal pathway. However, whether this will be possible is presently unknown. It will require that the mechanisms to instruct the immature progenitors to differentiate into the missing DA neurons operate also in the PD patient's brain. Some support for this strategy was given by the recent report (35) that undifferentiated mouse embryonic stem cells, implanted in low numbers into the DA-denervated rat striatum, proliferated and a proportion of them differentiated into cells expressing several markers of mesencephalic dopaminergic neurons. The grafts ameliorated drug-induced rotational asymmetry, but their capacity to reinnervate the striatum and release DA, as well as to improve behavioral deficits resembling the symptoms in PD, is unclear.

Based on the results from the clinical trials as well as from studies in animal models, a set of requirements can be identified that must be fulfilled for a graft to induce marked and clinically valuable improvement in patients with PD: (a) The grafted cells have to express the complete cellular machinery for DA synthesis and release, and possess the properties of fully mature mesencephalic DA neurons, both morphologically and electrophysiologically. (b) At least 100,000 grafted DA neurons should survive long-term in each putamen. (c) The grafted DA neurons should reestablish a dense, functional, DA-releasing terminal network in large parts of the striatum. (d) The grafts have to become functionally integrated into host basal ganglia–thalamocortical circuitries. (e) When tested preclinically in animal models of PD, the cells must be functional not only in tests of drug-induced behavior but also in tests of spontaneous motor behavior (akinesia and limb-use tests).

Hypothetically, DA neurons could be made from stem cells of four different sources: embryonic stem cells from the fertilized egg, neural stem cells from the embryonic or adult brain, or stem cells in other tissues. Of course, the crucial question is if those neurons will become functional DA neurons, fulfilling the criteria described above. Another unresolved issue is whether nondopaminergic neurons and glial cells normally present in the primary mesencephalic grafts used so far in PD patients are important for the differentiation and function of the DA neurons. If this is the case, an enriched population of predifferentiated DA neurons may not be the optimal preparation.

The possibility to generate DA neurons for transplantation from stem cells or neuronal precursors has been explored using several approaches. Figure 45.5 schematically illustrates five different alternatives.

In one approach, Studer and co-workers (36) expanded committed mesencephalic DA neuron precursors from rat embryos in culture. Upon removal of the mitogen, basic fibroblast growth factor (bFGF), part of the cells differen-

tiated into tyrosine hydroxylase (TH)–positive, presumed dopaminergic neurons. The expanded cells survived transplantation to the rat striatum but the survival of the grafted TH-positive cells was poor. In more recent studies, McKay, Studer, and collaborators have reported that the presence of ascorbic acid promotes dopaminergic differentiation when the mesencephalic precursors are proliferated or passaged for extended periods in vitro (37). In another investigation, Studer et al. reported that when the predifferentiation of the precursors was carried out in cultures with low oxygen, both proliferation and dopaminergic differentiation were enhanced (38). It is not yet known, though, whether ascorbic acid and low oxygen will increase the yield of surviving dopaminergic neurons after transplantation in vivo.

In the second approach, mesencephalic progenitors from rat embryos were expanded under epidermal growth factor stimulation in neurosphere cultures (39–41). The cells could subsequently be differentiated into a dopaminergic phenotype in response to signals provided by a combination of cytokines, mesencephalic membrane fragments, and striatum-conditioned medium. The generated cells survived

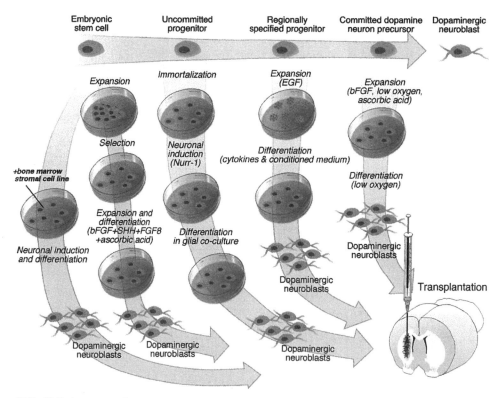

FIG. 45.5. Large numbers of cells with characteristics of dopamine (DA) neurons can be generated from in vitro expanded progenitors. The use of stem cells and immature progenitors for grafting in Parkinson's disease probably necessitates predifferentiation of the cells into dopaminergic neurons prior to implantation. This strategy has been explored using mouse embryonic stem cells; genetically engineered, immortalized mouse neural stem cells; in vitro expanded, regionally specified rat mesencephalic progenitors; and committed mesencephalic DA neuron precursors from rat embryos.

transplantation to the rat striatum but the survival was clearly lower than that in grafts of primary embryonic mesencephalic DA neurons.

In the third approach, Arenas and co-workers (42) induced a dopaminergic phenotype in an immortalized multipotent neural stem cell line by overexpression of Nurr-1, in combination with as yet unidentified factors derived from type 1 astrocytes of ventral mesencephalic origin. Nurr-1 is a transcription factor that is likely to play a critical role in development of mesencephalic DA neurons. Most of the Nurr-1 transduced cells expressed the TH enzyme as well as two other markers of mesencephalic DA neurons. The engineered neurons survived transplantation to the mouse striatum but the yield was very low.

In the fourth approach, DA and serotonin neurons were generated in high yield from mouse embryonic stem cells in vitro (43). The undifferentiated stem cells were expanded and central nervous system stem cells selected and then expanded in the presence of bFGF. By removal of the mitogen, the cells were differentiated to TH-positive neurons, which produced DA. Transplantation of these cells was not performed.

In a fifth approach, Sasai and collaborators also used mouse embryonic stem cells (44). When the embryonic stem cells were cocultured with various cell lines, it was discovered that a bone marrow–derived stromal cell line was a potent inducer of neuronal differentiation. After coculture, almost all cultures contained differentiated neurons and there was a significant yield of TH-positive neurons. These cells produced DA and showed substantial short-term survival (at 2 weeks) after transplantation to the mouse striatum.

Although these data are promising and support the notion that it will be possible to generate DA neurons from stem cells for transplantation purposes, there are still several unresolved issues. One problem is that the survival of these predifferentiated DA neurons after transplantation in animal models, when it has been tested, has been poor in most cases. Virtually nothing is known about long-term survival. It is also unclear if these cells display the functional characteristics of fully mature mesencephalic DA neurons after grafting, which is probably crucial if they are to work in a clinical setting. Also, relatively little is known about human cells because most studies have used cells of rodent origin.

The finding that the adult human brain also contains neural stem cells has raised the possibility that the patient's own neural stem cells could be used to generate, say, DA neurons for transplantation. The cells would then be taken out, predifferentiated in vitro, and reimplanted. One major advantage could be the lack of any immune reaction. However, several problems with this approach might be envisaged. First, it will probably involve extra surgery in an already diseased brain. Second, it is not known if these human cells can be expanded in sufficient numbers and if

they can be differentiated into specific neurons, such as DA neurons. Finally, in a patient with a chronic neurodegenerative disorder, these cells may be functionally impaired due to age, disease process, or long-term drug treatment.

CONCLUSION

The most important scientific conclusion from the clinical trials with neural transplantation in PD and also to some extent in HD is that cell replacement can work in the diseased human brain. However, with the development of new effective treatments for patients with advanced PD, such as deep brain stimulation (see Chapter 46), it is necessary to ask whether it is justified to expend further effort to develop cell-based therapies for this disorder. In our opinion, cell therapy, if successful, offers several unique features and distinct advantages over other treatment strategies. Cell therapy aims to restore DA transmission in the striatum (i.e., in the precise area that has lost its intrinsic DA afferent innervation). In successful cases, this has given rise to major clinical improvements and allowed the patient to stop antiparkinsonian medication, without major side effects. The grafted neurons are not destroyed by the disease process up to at least 10 years after surgery, indicating that the symptomatic relief can be maintained for many years.

Stem cell technology may become the scientific breakthrough that will turn cell replacement strategies into useful treatments for large numbers of patients with movement disorders. But we need to learn much more about the mechanisms of cell differentiation, regeneration, and functional recovery. At present, we do not know the best stem cell source for generating new neurons for implantation into the human brain. Therefore, research on embryonic stem cells and stem cells from embryonic or adult brain or other tissues should be pursued in parallel. It is important, however, to emphasize that the biological problems that must be solved before stem cell–based therapies for movement disorders can be developed are complex and should not be underestimated. Scientists and clinicians must proceed with caution.

ACKNOWLEDGMENTS

Our own work was supported by grants from the Swedish Medical Research Council, the Kock Foundation, the Wiberg Foundation, the King Gustav V and Queen Victoria Foundation, and the Söderberg Foundation.

REFERENCES

1. Brundin P, Duan WM, Sauer H. Functional effects of mesencephalic dopamine neurons and adrenal chromaffin cells

grafted to the rodent striatum. In: Dunnett SB, Björklund A, eds. *Functional neural transplantation.* New York: Raven Press, 1994:9–46.

2. Annett LE. Functional studies of neural grafts in parkinsonian primates. In: Dunnett SB, Björklund A, eds. *Functional neural transplantation.* New York: Raven Press, 1994:71–102.

3. Dunnett SB, Nathwani F, Björklund A. The integration and function of striatal grafts. *Prog Brain Res* 2000;127:345–380.

4. Kendall AL, Rayment FD, Torres EM, et al. Functional integration of striatal allografts in a primate model of Huntington's disease. *Nat Med* 1998;4:727–729.

5. Palfi S, Condé F, Riche D, et al. Fetal striatal allografts reverse cognitive deficits in a primate model of Huntington's disease. *Nat Med* 1998;4:963–966.

6. Lindvall O, Brundin P, Widner H, et al. Grafts of fetal dopamine neurons survive and improve motor function in Parkinson's disease. *Science* 1990;247:574–577.

7. Lindvall O, Sawle G, Widner H, et al. Evidence for long-term survival and function of dopaminergic grafts in progressive Parkinson's disease. *Ann Neurol* 1994;35:172–180.

8. Sawle GV, Bloomfield PM, Björklund A, et al. Transplantation of fetal dopamine neurons in Parkinson's disease: PET [^{18}F]6-L-fluorodopa studies in two patients with putaminal implants. *Ann Neurol* 1992;31:166–173.

9. Peschanski M, Defer G, N'Guyen JP, et al. Bilateral motor improvement and alteration of L-dopa effect in two patients with Parkinson's disease following intrastriatal transplantation of foetal ventral mesencephalon. *Brain* 1994;117:487–499.

10. Remy P, Samson Y, Hantraye P, et al. Clinical correlates of [^{18}F]fluorodopa uptake in five grafted parkinsonian patients. *Ann Neurol* 1995;38:580–588.

11. Freeman TB, Olanow CW, Hauser RA, et al. Bilateral fetal nigral transplantation into the postcommissural putamen in Parkinson's disease. *Ann Neurol* 1995;38:379–388.

12. Wenning GK, Odin P, Morrish P, et al. Short- and long-term survival and function of unilateral intrastriatal dopaminergic grafts in Parkinson's disease. *Ann Neurol* 1997;42:95–107.

13. Hagell P, Schrag A, Piccini P, et al. Sequential bilateral transplantation in Parkinson's disease: effects of the second graft. *Brain* 1999;122:1121–1132.

14. Hauser RA, Freeman TB, Snow BJ, et al. Long-term evaluation of bilateral fetal nigral transplantation in Parkinson disease. *Arch Neurol* 1999;56:179–187.

15. Mendez I, Dagher A, Hong M, et al. Enhancement of survival of stored dopaminergic cells and promotion of graft survival by exposure of human fetal nigral tissue to glial cell line–derived neurotrophic factor in patients with Parkinson's disease. *J Neurosurg* 2000;92:863–869.

16. Brundin P, Pogarell O, Hagell P, et al. Bilateral caudate and putamen grafts of embryonic mesencephalic tissue treated with lazaroids in Parkinson's disease. *Brain* 2000;123:1380–1390.

17. Freed CR, Greene PE, Breeze RE, et al. Transplantation of embryonic dopamine neurons for severe Parkinson's disease. *N Engl J Med* 2001;344:710–719.

18. Piccini P, Brooks DJ, Björklund A, et al. Dopamine release from nigral transplants visualized in vivo in a Parkinson's patient. *Nat Neurosci* 1999;2:1137–1140.

19. Kordower JH, Freeman TB, Snow BJ, et al. Neuropathological evidence of graft survival and striatal reinnervation after the transplantation of fetal mesencephalic tissue in a patient with Parkinson's disease. *N Engl J Med* 1995;332:1118–1124.

20. Kordower JH, Rosenstein JM, Collier TJ, et al. Functional fetal nigral grafts in a patient with Parkinson's disease: chemoanatomic, ultrastructural, and metabolic studies. *J Comp Neurol* 1996;370:203–230.

21. Kordower JH, Freeman TB, Chen EY, et al. Fetal nigral grafts survive and mediate clinical benefit in a patient with Parkinson's disease. *Mov Disord* 1998;13:383–393.

22. Lindvall O, Widner H, Rehncrona S, et al. Transplantation of fetal dopamine neurons in Parkinson's disease: 1-year clinical and neurophysiological observations in two patients with putaminal implants. *Ann Neurol* 1992;31:155–165.

23. Defer GL, Geny C, Ricolfi F, et al. Long-term outcome of unilaterally transplanted parkinsonian patients: I. Clinical approach. *Brain* 1996;119:41–50.

24. Lindvall O, Hagell P. Clinical observations after neural transplantation in Parkinson's disease. *Prog Brain Res* 2000;127:299–320.

25. Lindvall O. Rationales and strategies of fetal neural transplantation in Parkinson's disease. In: Krauss JK, Jancovic J, Grossman RG, eds. *Surgery for Parkinson's disease and movement disorders.* Philadelphia: Lippincott Williams & Wilkins, 2001:194–209.

26. Fahn S, Elton RL, members of the UPDRS Development Committee. Unified Parkinson's Disease Rating Scale. In: Fahn S, Marsden CD, Calne DB, et al., eds. *Recent developments in Parkinson's disease,* vol 2. Florham Park: Macmillan Healthcare Information, 1987:153–163.

27. Hagell P, Brundin P. Cell survival and clinical outcome following intrastriatal transplantation in Parkinson's disease. *J Neuropathol Exp Neurol* 2001;60:741–752.

28. Hagell P, Piccini P, Björklund A, et al. Dyskinesias following neural transplantation in Parkinson's disease. *Nat Neurosci* 2002;5:627–628.

29. Piccini P, Lindvall O, Björklund A, et al. Delayed recovery of movement-related cortical function in Parkinson's disease after striatal dopaminergic grafts. *Ann Neurol* 2000;48:689–695.

30. Brundin P, Karlsson J, Emgård M, et al. Improving the survival of grafted dopaminergic neurons: a review over current approaches. *Cell Transplant* 2000;9:179–195.

31. Deacon T, Schumacher J, Dinsmore J, et al. Histological evidence of fetal pig neural cell survival after transplantation into a patient with Parkinson's disease. *Nat Med* 1997;3:350–353.

32. Schumacher JM, Ellias SA, Palmer EP, et al. Transplantation of embryonic porcine mesencephalic tissue in patients with PD. *Neurology* 2000;54:1042–1050.

33. Bachoud-Lévi AC, Rémy P, Nguyen JP, et al. Motor and cognitive improvements in patients with Huntington's disease after neural transplantation. *Lancet* 2000;356:1975–1979.

34. Freeman TB, Cicchetti F, Hauser RA, et al. Transplanted fetal striatum in Huntington's disease: phenotypic development and lack of pathology. *Proc Natl Acad Sci USA* 2000;97:13877–13882.

35. Björklund LM, Sánchez-Pernaute R, Chung S, et al. Embryonic cells develop into functional dopaminergic neurons after transplantation in a Parkinson rat model. *Proc Natl Acad Sci USA* 2002;99:2344–2349.

36. Studer L, Tabar V, McKay RDG. Transplantation of expanded mesencephalic precursors leads to recovery in parkinsonian rats. *Nat Neurosci* 1998;1:290–295.

37. Yan J, Studer L, McKay RDG. Ascorbic acid increases the yield of dopaminergic neurons derived from basic fibroblast growth factor expanded mesencephalic precursors. *J Neurochem* 2001;76:307–311.

38. Studer L, Csete M, Lee SH, et al. Enhanced proliferation, survival, and dopaminergic differentiation of CNS precursors in lowered oxygen. *J Neurosci* 2000;20:7377–7383.

39. Ling Z, Potter ED, Lipton JW, et al. Differentiation of mesencephalic progenitor cells into dopaminergic neurons by cytokines. *Exp Neurol* 1998;149:411–423.

40. Potter ED, Ling Z, Carvey PM. Cytokine-induced conversion of mesencephalic-derived progenitor cells into dopamine neurons. *Cell Tissue Res* 1999;296:235–246.

41. Carvey PM, Ling ZD, Sortwell CE, et al. A clonal line of mesencephalic progenitor cells converted to dopamine neurons by hematopoietic cytokines: a source of cells for transplantation in Parkinson's disease. *Exp Neurol* 2001;171:98–108.

42. Wagner J, Åkerud P, Castro DS, et al. Induction of a midbrain dopaminergic phenotype in Nurr1-overexpressing neural stem cells by type 1 astrocytes. *Nat Biotechnol* 1999;17:653–659.

43. Lee SH, Lumelsky N, Studer L, et al. Efficient generation of midbrain and hindbrain neurons from mouse embryonic stem cells. *Nat Biotechnol* 2000;18:675–679.

44. Kawasaki H, Mizuseki K, Nishikawa S, et al. Induction of midbrain dopaminergic neurons from ES cells by stromal cell–derived inducing activity. *Neuron* 2000;28:31–40.

DEEP BRAIN STIMULATION

RAJEEV KUMAR

Functional neurosurgery for the management of movement disorders has markedly increased in the past decade due to a greater understanding of the functional organization of the basal ganglia and the impact of nigral degeneration and striatal dopamine deficiency on normal physiology, and improved neuroimaging of the basal ganglia with magnetic resonance imaging (MRI). The observation that high-frequency intraoperative stimulation of the thalamus was predictive of the results of thalamotomy led to the development of a permanently implantable deep brain stimulation (DBS) system. DBS has now become a widely performed procedure for the management of advanced medication–refractory movement disorders, including Parkinson's disease (PD), dystonia, and various forms of tremor. DBS has been applied to the ventralis intermedius (VIM) nucleus of the thalamus, globus pallidus interna (GPi), and subthalamic nucleus (STN).

VIM DBS has been shown to markedly improve all forms of tremor in a fashion similar to that achieved with thalamotomy, but with fewer persistent adverse effects (1–3b). Although VIM DBS can markedly improve parkinsonian tremor, this form of therapy does not significantly improve other features of parkinsonism (2,3). However, STN DBS and GPi DBS can markedly improve all levodopa-responsive motor features of parkinsonism (4–8c). This is consistent with the classic model of basal ganglia functioning because these procedures should decrease the abnormal hyperactivity of the STN or GPi seen in parkinsonism. Although worldwide experience with GPi DBS for dystonia is quite limited, several case series clearly demonstrate that many patients (especially with idiopathic dystonia) can obtain dramatic improvement (9–13d).

MECHANISM OF DEEP BRAIN STIMULATION

How DBS exerts its clinical effects is unknown (14). Since the main clinical effects mimic those of lesioning the target structure, it has been hypothesized that high-frequency stimulation results in reversible inhibition. The effects of DBS are clearly frequency dependent, with stimulation at more than 100 Hz needed to induce a major symptomatic improvement. Relatively low currents are used with relatively small current spread; therefore, the benefit is likely due to a highly localized effect of stimulation. Physiologic studies by Ashby and others suggest that the clinical effects are mediated by true stimulation of large myelinated axons rather than cell bodies and not by direct inhibition or creation of a depolarization blockade. For thalamic stimulation, activated axons may excite neurons in the reticular nucleus of the thalamus, resulting in inhibition of corticothalamic neurons. Further studies also suggest that GPi stimulation may activate axons that produce GABAergic inhibition of GPi neurons. It has also been hypothesized that high-frequency nonphysiologic stimulation may result in neuronal jamming with an uninterpretable signal sent to afferent structures.

Upon discontinuation of stimulation, the clinical effects of DBS are reversible over seconds (in the case of VIM DBS for tremor) to hours (with STN DBS for parkinsonian freezing of gait). Occasional patients with parkinsonian tremor undergoing VIM DBS may develop tremor rebound upon discontinuation of stimulation, as described above; however, this state can typically be temporarily reversed if stimulation is discontinued for 1 or 2 days (15). Patients with severe essential tremor (ET) who develop tolerance to stimulation require increasingly higher stimulation settings to suppress tremor (15). As with tremor rebound, a stimulation holiday can often reverse tolerance and resensitize patients to a lower stimulation voltage. Postmortem examination of patients who have undergone chronic stimulation reveals that there is no significant brain lesion and only minimal gliosis surrounding the stimulating electrode. Therefore, the persistence of some of the effects of DBS after discontinuation of stimulation suggests that some degree of downstream central nervous system plasticity is induced with chronic stimulation.

PERIOPERATIVE AND INTRAOPERATIVE PATIENT MANAGEMENT

Electrode implantation is generally performed with the patient awake to facilitate feedback as to the beneficial and adverse clinical effects of microstimulation and macrostimulation. However, in patients with severe generalized dystonia who are unable to tolerate awake surgery, electrode implantation is commonly performed under general anesthesia (especially with younger children).

In patients with tremor, antitremor medications should be tapered and discontinued prior to surgery to maximize tremor during surgery. Similarly, in patients with PD, interventions that maximize off-period parkinsonism and reduce the chance of intraoperative confusion may be valuable because they may facilitate detection of improvement in parkinsonian signs during stimulation and validity of patient reports of adverse effects. Preoperative reduction in anti-Parkinson medication can achieve both goals.

With the exception of the final stage of either electrode implantation or radiofrequency lesioning, the intraoperative methodology is similar for both DBS and ablative stereotactic neurosurgery. First, the target structure is identified with neuroimaging. T1-weighted MRI with the patient in a stereotactic head frame allows identification of the anterior and posterior commissures, and T2-weighted MRI facilitates identification of the STN or GPi target. Individual thalamic subnuclei cannot be visualized at present with MRI. Some groups also use computed tomography (CT)/MRI image fusion or ventriculography to help compensate for image distortion related to magnetic field inhomogeneities. Physiologic identification of the target site using microelectrode recording (MER), microstimulation, and/or macrostimulation is an important second step given the inherent imprecision of the surgical technique and the possibility of intraoperative brain shift. Single-unit MER permits precise identification of characteristic neuronal discharge patterns in the target structure including movement- and tremor-synchronous discharges and the boundaries of the target. Multiple sequential or simultaneous microelectrode recording tracts may be used to map the target region. The intraoperative clinical effects of microstimulation and/or macrostimulation are used to select the final site for electrode implantation because these are predictive of the effects obtained with chronic stimulation. A neurologist must assess the stimulation-induced improvements in tremor, bradykinesia, and rigidity in addition to the threshold for induction of adverse effects such as paresthesias, tonic motor contraction, eye deviation, dysarthria, photopsias, and vegetative or affective symptoms (e.g., sensations of heat or sweating, depression, or euphoria). The target signs that must be repeatedly assessed during different sites and amplitudes of stimulation need to be individualized depending on the patient's specific clinical features. An optimal site for electrode implantation results in marked stimulation-induced clinical improvement with a large therapeutic window before the induction of adverse effects. The DBS electrode is then implanted using x-ray control (either fluoroscopy using a C-arm, or teleradiography and correlation of intraoperative x-ray images with the preoperative imaging) with the middle of the electrode positioned over the area resulting in the greatest therapeutic benefit. There are two models of DBS electrodes (Medtronic, Minneapolis, MN) that may be implanted each of which has four contacts. Each contact measures 1.5 mm in length and may be separated by either 0.5 mm (Model 3389) or 1.5 mm (Model 337). The electrode is then fixed to the skull using a plastic cap, a metal plate, or cement (Fig. 46.1). Where concern exists regarding the location of the

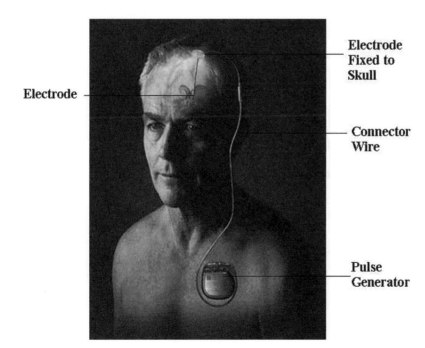

Electrode

Electrode Fixed to Skull

Connector Wire

Pulse Generator

FIG. 46.1. Deep brain stimulation hardware (see text for details).

implanted electrode because of inadequate response to intraoperative stimulation or other technical factors, externalization of the DBS electrode via a percutaneous extension may be advisable for a period of test stimulation using an external stimulator. Such test stimulation may be carried out using a hand-held stimulator (Medtronic Model 3625 or 3628) or an electrically isolated constant-current stimulator. If acceptable results are obtained from intraoperative stimulation, no period of test stimulation is needed. Under general anesthesia, the electrode is connected to an extension cable (Extension Kit 7495), which is buried underneath the scalp and skin of the neck and finally attached to an implantable pulse generator (IPG) (Fig. 46.1).

Elderly patients with PD sometimes develop postoperative confusion following bilateral STN electrode implantation, which may last from 1 day to 2 weeks (5,6). In general, only supportive therapy is required, and anti-Parkinson medication can usually be reinstituted during this period though at a reduced dose compared with preoperatively. In rare cases of prolonged confusion accompanied by psychotic features, such as hallucinations, the use of atypical neuroleptics such as clozapine may be helpful. Many patients with GPi electrode implantation alone will note improvement in both off-period parkinsonism and dyskinesias as a result of the micropallidotomy effect (Table 46.1) (16). STN electrode implantation may reduce dyski-

TABLE 46.1. COMPARISON OF CLINICAL EFFECTS OF GLOBUS PALLIDUS INTERNA, SUBTHALAMIC NUCLEUS, AND VENTRALIS INTERMEDIUS DEEP BRAIN STIMULATION IN PARKINSON'S DISEASE

	GPi DBS	STN DBS	VIM DBS
Overall clinical effects of bilateral DBS	Mean improvements in rating scales: off-period parkinsonism 30–50%; on-period parkinsonism 0–25%; on-period dyskinesias reduced 66–90%; off-period dystonia usually improved.	Mean improvements in rating scales: off-period parkinsonism 45–65%; on-period parkinsonism improved 10–30%; on-period dyskinesias reduced 67–83%; off-period dystonia usually markedly reduced.	Tremor improved 90%. Minor improvement in rigidity. ADLs not improved.
Overall clinical effects of unilateral DBS	Mean improvements: off-period parkinsonism 10–35%; on-period parkinsonism not improved; on-period dyskinesias reduced 70–80%; off-period dystonia usually reduced.	Mean improvements: off-period parkinsonism 25–30%; effects on on-period parkinsonism and dyskinesias not studied; off-period dystonia usually reduced.	Contralateral limb tremor improved 90%. Minor improvement in axial and ipsilateral tremor. Minor improvement in rigidity. ADLs not improved.
Microlesion effect	Minor beneficial improvement in off-period parkinsonism measurable at least 3 months; moderate anti-dyskinetic effect that may last 6 months or more.	Mild beneficial effects on off-period parkinsonism. Effect on dyskinesias is variable (may be pro-dyskinetic in some and anti-dyskinetic in other patients).	Significant reduction in contralateral tremor measurable for at least 3 mo. Occasional patients with marked persistent tremor reduction not requiring stimulation.
Regional stimulation within the nucleus	Dorsal electrodes—greater antiparkinsonian effect and can produce contralateral stimulation-induced dyskinesias. Ventral electrodes—greater anti-dyskinetic effect and may block the beneficial effects of levodopa on bradykinesia and gait.	Stimulation-induced laughter and mania due to current spread to limbic portion of STN or adjacent hypothalamus. Acute stimulation-related depression with electrode inferior to STN in SNr.	None.
Mechanism of effects on levodopa-induced dyskinesias	Anti-dyskinetic effect of microlesion and direct anti-dyskinetic effect of stimulation.	Mainly due to reduction in drug dosage. In some patients, microlesion effect directly reduces dyskinesias (possibly due to lesion of lenticular fasciculus). STN stimulation has a pro-dyskinetic effect with no direct anti-dyskinetic effect of stimulation. Stimulation above the STN in the zona incerta or below the STN in the SNr may directly suppress dyskinesias similar to GPi DBS.	Electrodes placed within or adjacent to CM/Pf or Voa/Vop may markedly suppress contralateral dyskinesias.

(continued)

TABLE 46.1. *(continued)*

	GPi DBS	STN DBS	VIM DBS
Stimulation-induced dyskinesias	Onset within 1–2 min. Contralateral. Similar form and distribution to the patient's preoperative peak dose levodopa-induced dyskinesias (though usually milder). Usually abates in minutes or hours with chronic stimulation.	Onset usually within 5 min, but occasionally delayed onset up to 2 d with chronic stimulation. Tends to improve with time. Contralateral or even ipsilateral. Two different forms: hemiballistic/hemichoreic and sometimes very different from the patient's preoperative peak-dose levodopa-induced dyskinesias (often resembling diphasic dyskinesias); or dyskinesias resembling the patients preoperative peak dose dyskinesias. Both types may occur in the same individual: type 1 at low amplitude stimulation and type 2 at high amplitudes. Levodopa and STN DBS have a synergistic effect in promoting dyskinesias; therefore, drug reduction is necessary to reduce dyskinesias and allow the use of higher stimulation parameters.	None. Current spread ventrally to the cerebellothalamic fibers may result in stimulation-induced ataxia. Rebound tremor with discontinuing stimulation due to physiologic adaptation.
Postoperative drug management	Usually no change. Occasional patients with severe preoperative dyskinesias may tolerate higher levodopa doses.	Mean reduction in drug dosage 50% (range 0%–100%).	Usually no change. Occasional patients with severe tremor and very mild bradykinesia may reduce anti-Parkinson medication.
Timing of anti-Parkinson effects	Tremor improvement almost immediate. Most other features of parkinsonism improve within 1 min rapidly escalating to maximal effect in <5 min.	Tremor improvement almost immediate. Other features of parkinsonism improve within 1 min, but slower escalation to maximal benefit compared to GPi DBS and slower offset: perhaps 15 min, but possibly up to several hours (for effects on gait and bradykinesia).	Tremor improvement almost immediate.

GPi, globus pallidus interna; STN, subthalamic nucleus; VIM, ventralis intermedius; DBS, deep brain stimulation; ADLs, activities of daily living; SNr, substantia nigra pars reticulata; CM, centromedian; Pf, parafascicularis; Voa/Vop, ventralis oralis anterior/ventralis oralis posterior.
Adapted from ref. 62 and Kumar R. Methods for programming and patient management with deep brain stimulation of the globus pallidus for the treatment of advanced Parkinson's disease and dystonia. *Mov Disord* 2002;17[Suppl 3]:198–207.

nesias possibly due to lesioning of the pallidal outflow (especially the lenticular fasciculus) or more commonly may improve off-period parkinsonism and reduce the threshold for anti-Parkinson medication to induce dyskinesias (probably as a result of lesioning the STN itself) (6). In the latter case, it is often necessary to temporarily reduce anti-Parkinson medication to reduce dyskinesias. Mild chorea may occasionally occur following STN electrode implantation. Generally this subsides within 48 hours. If significant chorea is present, a temporary reduction in levodopa dosage by 50% or more is prudent until the chorea resolves. If the patient is lucid postoperatively and there are no dyskinesias resulting from electrode insertion, no change in drug dosage is immediately necessary.

STIMULATION PARAMETERS: BASIC PRINCIPLES OF DEEP BRAIN STIMULATION PROGRAMMING

Stimulation settings are programmed by means of a console programmer (Model 7432, MemoryMod HF Software Cartridge Model 7458) attached to a transducer head that is applied over the IPG. The currently available single-channel IPG for movement disorder applications in the United States is the Soletra, whereas in Europe the Kinetra, a dual-channel IPG, is also available. With the Soletra, the patient can be instructed to turn the stimulator on or off using a magnet (Control Magnet Model 7452) applied over the IPG (Fig. 46.1) or using a hand-held patient programmer. The Kinetra comes with an Access Therapy Controller that allows the patient to turn the stimulator on and off electronically and also to modify the stimulation amplitude within a given set of parameters determined by the physician.

With the Soletra or Kinetra, a number of stimulation variables must be selected, including the following: choice of active stimulation contacts including monopolar versus bipolar stimulation, frequency, pulse width, and amplitude. Determining the most effective contact(s) for stimulation is the first and most important task during stimulation programming. Monopolar stimulation is always tested first with the pulse generator case itself set as the anode (i.e., +) with a single contact on the lead set as the cathode (i.e., −). Any of the four contacts on the lead may be set as the cathode. For any given stimulation voltage or amplitude, monopolar stimulation results in a wide distribution of current spread of approximately 1 to 1.5 mm diameter per milliampere (14). Although generally one contact is used as the cathode, it is occasionally useful to activate two adjacent contacts for a broader field of current diffusion. Bipolar stimulation involves using two contacts on the lead: one as the anode and the other as the cathode. This results in a narrower field of current spread compared with monopolar stimulation and thus more focused effects. Monopolar stimulation is most commonly used since the greater current spread typically allows lower stimulation settings in comparison with bipolar stimulation. In contrast, bipolar stimulation may be especially useful when adverse effects due to current spread limit stimulation efficacy.

With an increase in stimulation amplitude, current spread increases linearly. However, Soletra battery consumption increases abruptly with an increase in stimulation from 3.6 V to 3.7 V due to a "doubling circuit" in which a second capacitor is switched into the system. Similarly, the battery drain also jumps when amplitude is increased to above 7.3 V. As a result, efforts should be made to obtain optimal clinical results using an amplitude less than or equal to 3.6 V. If greater current spread and clinical effects are required with a given electrode combination, stimulation pulse width may be increased and voltage reduced to more economically achieve this end. For the Kinetra, battery consumption is linear across the entire amplitude range.

The Soletra and Kinetra produce square-wave pulses of 60 to 450 μs duration. Changing stimulation pulse width can alter the neural elements affected by DBS—longer pulse width has a greater effect on cell soma whereas shorter pulse width preferentially affects axons (14). Typically, a pulse width of 60 to 120 μs is used in DBS, but much longer pulse widths may be required in dystonic patients undergoing GPi stimulation. The Soletra is capable of stimulating at 0 to 185 Hz and the Kinetra at rates up to 250 Hz. VIM stimulation has been shown to have frequency-dependent effects: tremor improvement begins at approximately 100 Hz, plateaus at 130 Hz, and only mild further benefit is obtained with increases up to 185 Hz in selected

cases (17). Similar effects on bradykinesia and rigidity have been noted with STN DBS in PD. Increasing stimulation frequency does not increase current spread but does reduce battery life. Therefore, for VIM and STN stimulation 130 Hz is used initially; frequency is only increased to 185 Hz if suboptimal benefit is achieved and an increase in pulse width or amplitude results in adverse effects due to current spread. Most reports suggest that GPi DBS for PD has the greatest effects at very high stimulation frequencies, so that 185 Hz is routinely used (16,18,19). Stimulation at rates greater than 185 Hz has not been shown to increase clinical benefit. Stimulation frequencies have been more variable in dystonia, but with few exceptions most groups have employed frequencies similar to those used in PD.

Battery life varies greatly depending on the chronic stimulation settings and the average daily use. Most patients with thalamic stimulation for tremor are able to turn stimulation off at night and on only during waking hours in order to reduce battery drain. Most patients undergoing STN or GPi DBS for PD use stimulation 24 hours per day because turning the stimulators off at night often compromises nocturnal mobility; therefore, the average Soletra battery life with STN or GPi DBS is typically 3 to 5 years. Many patients with dystonia use the maximal pulse width of the pulse generator, which markedly shortens battery life and necessitates yearly battery replacement. Battery replacement can be delayed until the battery has been completely depleted, but this may result in marked worsening of symptoms. In PD patients who have substantially decreased their anti-Parkinson drug dosage, acute deterioration of parkinsonism may occur, and there is a theoretical risk of a neuroleptic malignant-like syndrome that may necessitate a temporary increase in drug dose. Similarly, patients with severe generalized dystonia may develop status dystonicus and rhabdomyolysis; however, unlike PD, acute administration of most antidystonia medications is unlikely to quickly resolve this state. Pulse generator batteries typically fail gradually over several days; therefore, patients should be advised to contact their physician if they notice a waning of the effects of stimulation so that this possibility can be evaluated by checking the pulse generator current drain and the battery may be replaced expediently if necessary. In select patients who live far from a tertiary care center, prophylactic battery replacement according to the forecasted life span of the battery may be advisable.

LONG-TERM STIMULATION, MEDICATION, AND PATIENT MANAGEMENT

The time required to optimally set stimulation parameters may at times be substantial. Although this time is highly variable among individual patients, a few DBS programming sessions are usually required to optimize stimulation settings. The clinical effects and complexity of response to DBS varies with the site of stimulation in PD (Table 46.1).

Ventralis Intermedius Deep Brain Stimulation for Tremor

Patients should withhold antitremor and/or anti-Parkinson medication at least overnight prior to the initial programming session. Usually a concentrated period of 1 to 3 hours is adequate to determine the most effective antitremor settings in the vast majority of patients. For patients with VIM DBS, stimulation parameters remain fairly stable by 1 month postoperatively, and only very minor adjustments, such as slightly increasing the amplitude, may be necessary beyond 3 months. However, up to 10% to 25% of patients undergoing long-term VIM DBS for ET may develop tolerance to stimulation requiring progressively higher voltages to maintain the same degree of effectiveness (15,20, 21). Instructing patients to discontinue stimulation at night may reduce the development of tolerance. In those with established tolerance, limiting daytime stimulation to times when optimal motor control is required, such as when writing, may reduce tolerance. In rare cases where tolerance is severe and markedly limits the usefulness of DBS, radiofrequency lesioning of the thalamus via the DBS electrode may eliminate tremor and tolerance (22,23). Tolerance has not been reported with VIM DBS for PD, but some patients may develop rebound increase in tremor when turning stimulation off at night (15). As a result, some PD patients must keep stimulation on at night to permit sleep.

Many ET patients with complete or near-complete tremor suppression may be able to reduce or discontinue all antitremor medications. Although the majority of patients with PD undergoing VIM DBS require little or no change in medication, patients taking large doses of levodopa to suppress tremor may be able to reduce medication somewhat (Table 46.1) (2,3).

Parkinson's Disease

For GPi DBS or STN DBS for PD, most DBS programming is performed with patients off medication, and ideally sessions should be scheduled in the morning after overnight drug withdrawal. Assessment of the effects of DBS on drug-induced dyskinesias is often best performed in the afternoon once patients have taken more than one dose of levodopa prior to attending the clinic since dyskinesias commonly exhibit a diurnal pattern, mild in the morning with worsening in the afternoon and evening.

Subthalamic Nucleus Deep Brain Stimulation

STN DBS has a synergistic effect with dopaminergic medication for the induction of dyskinesias (Table 46.1). The presence of stimulation-induced dyskinesias in the drug-off state is an excellent sign and suggests that parkinsonism can be maximally improved (24). With drug reduction and continuous STN stimulation, the threshold for induction of dyskinesias gradually increases, allowing a corresponding

increase in stimulation. This process typically takes several weeks, with the majority of patients reaching their final stimulation parameters by 3 months postoperatively. The maximal anti-Parkinson effect of STN stimulation correlates with that achievable by high-dose levodopa therapy, with the exception that tremor may be improved more by stimulation (5,6). Therefore, the preoperative "best on" can only slightly be improved by the combination of STN stimulation and anti-Parkinson drug therapy (24). In contrast, if a direct anti-dyskinetic effect of stimulation is noted, one is likely stimulating the substantia nigra pars reticulata (SNr) below the STN or the zona incerta above the STN (25a,b).

If stimulation-induced adverse effects prevent optimal improvement, then changing stimulation to an adjacent contact or bipolar stimulation should be considered. If optimum improvement is still not achievable, the electrode is likely suboptimally positioned and dopaminergic therapy should be increased. An average reduction of 50% of dopaminergic therapy is achieved at 1-year follow-up (5) with STN DBS. Approximately 5% to 10% of patients can be optimally improved and remain off all anti-Parkinson medication 1 to 2 years after surgery; 30% remain off levodopa but take dopamine agonists, whereas the majority of patients take low-dose levodopa (24,25b). Nevertheless, we prefer to first reduce and discontinue levodopa while maintaining continuous dopaminergic stimulation if needed with long-acting dopamine agonists that are less likely to induce dyskinesias and usually do not result in perceptible motor fluctuations.

Reduction in dopaminergic medication may unmask symptoms of restless legs syndrome in patients who previously never complained of such symptoms (26a). More severe cases may be accompanied by dyskinesias during the day resembling periodic limb movements of sleep. Although an increase in stimulation may improve these symptoms somewhat, as has been previously reported with pallidotomy, in our experience this usually results in inadequate symptom relief and drug therapy is needed (26a). Reintroduction of controlled-release levodopa or dopamine agonists may be very helpful but may significantly increase dyskinesias. In such cases, use of benzodiazepines or opiates can improve restless legs syndrome symptoms without inducing dyskinesias.

Overly aggressive reduction in anti-Parkinson medication should be avoided because levodopa also improves nonmotor symptoms of PD. A levodopa withdrawal syndrome of abulia, anhedonia, and depression may result (24,25b). Reinstitution of levodopa up to the threshold that produces mild nondisabling dyskinesias usually quickly improves these symptoms. For persistent symptoms or when disabling dyskinesias limit levodopa therapy, the use of selective serotonin reuptake inhibitors can be helpful (25b). Depression due to drug withdrawal must be differentiated from acute stimulation-induced depression due to unintentional stimulation of the SNr below the level of the STN (27). In such cases, depression immediately improves with discontinuation of stimulation and greater improvement in parkinsonism is achieved stimulating through a more proximal contact.

Postoperative hypomania or mania may occur with STN stimulation that is highly effective for the motor features of parkinsonism and mimics the euphoria-inducing effects of levodopa (28). Rapid reduction in dopaminergic therapy and, if necessary, stimulation will commonly improve this behavior. Similarly, laughing spells associated with the appropriate affect have been induced by high-stimulation settings and accompanied by stimulation-induced dyskinesias (29,30).

Preoperative levodopa-refractory postural instability is unlikely to be substantially improved with STN stimulation. As a result of significant improvement in bradykinesia and speed of gait, falls may actually become more frequent postoperatively. Although this may sometimes be improved with physiotherapy, many patients require a walker.

Globus Pallidus Interna Deep Brain Stimulation

Two groups have reported on the apparent functional differences between dorsal and ventral globus pallidus stimulation (Fig. 46.1) (18,19). Dorsal stimulation has a marked anti-Parkinson effect, may induce rather than suppress dyskinesias (similar to STN stimulation), and may actually be due to stimulation of the globus pallidus externa (GPe) (31). Ventral simulation may exacerbate akinesia and block the beneficial effects of levodopa on bradykinesia and gait, while improving rigidity and markedly suppressing dyskinesias. As a result, the middle of the pallidum is probably the optimal site for globus pallidus stimulation taking advantage of these two divergent effects. Therefore, GPi DBS has an anti-dyskinetic effect and anti-Parkinson medication is usually not altered postoperatively (Table 46.1). In patients with marked levodopa sensitivity and disabling dyskinesias preoperatively, the anti-dyskinetic effects of GPi stimulation may allow higher levodopa doses; patients taking hourly liquid levodopa can usually be converted to a simpler medication regimen. As with thalamic stimulation, parameters remain fairly stable by 1 month postoperatively and only very minor adjustments, such as slightly increasing the stimulation amplitude, may be necessary beyond 3 months.

Dystonia

The worldwide experience with GPi DBS for dystonia is limited in comparison to that with PD and is marked by considerable heterogeneity with respect to the type of patients operated and the stimulation settings used. A response to stimulation may occur abruptly within seconds or may be delayed and progressive over weeks or months, with mobile forms of dystonia tending to respond more quickly than fixed abnormal posturing and gait disorders. A specific pattern of clinical effects correlating with stimulation in different parts of the GPi has not been described in patients with dystonia. However, empirically many groups have begun with stimulation in the ventral part of the GPi just above the optic tract (since this region has been shown to have anti-dyskinetic effects in PD) with a long pulse width, high frequency, and amplitude just below that for adverse effects (9). These groups have then awaited a delayed response before considering changing site of stimulation. As a result, it is generally quite useful to allow at least 24 hours of continuous stimulation on any one setting before assessing the efficacy of stimulation. In patients who do not exhibit a relatively quick response, sessions can be relatively brief, with assessment of current settings and institution of new settings to be assessed during the next session. Patients with marked improvement in dystonia with GPi DBS are often able to reduce or discontinue anti-dystonia medications, such as anticholinergics.

DEEP BRAIN STIMULATION VERSUS LESIONING

Thalamic lesioning and DBS are of approximately the same efficacy for tremor, and data in PD suggest that lesioning of the STN or GPi also has beneficial effects similar to those of stimulation (1). However, DBS has fewer central adverse effects than lesioning because much less tissue is destroyed with electrode implantation alone as confirmed by the recent randomized trial performed by Schuurman et al. (1). Stimulation is also adjustable in order to maximize benefit and minimize adverse effects. Unlike lesions, the hardware for DBS is quite costly and may be problematic, with both immediate and delayed complications relating to hardware infection, breakage, and battery changes (21,24,32). Case series in which patients have been followed in the long term suggest that these complications occur in 5% to 40% of patients. Surgical exploration and replacement of damaged hardware is often necessary to correct these problems. Electrode repositioning may also be necessary if the electrode has been suboptimally positioned initially. Many follow-up visits are often necessary to adjust stimulation settings (especially with STN DBS for PD), and a large effort by physicians and patients is required (8). This may not be practical in patients who live in geographically isolated locations far from surgery centers. Tolerance to VIM DBS in patients with ET may not be uncommon; this phenomenon is not seen with thalamotomy. Many patients often express a preference for one or another treatment modality. As a result, the choice of stimulation or lesioning must be individualized depending on resources available at the surgical center and a number of patient-specific factors.

PATIENT SELECTION: GENERAL PRINCIPLES

A multidisciplinary team comprising a neurologist, a neurosurgeon, a neuropsychologist, and, often, a psychiatrist is usually needed to comprehensively evaluate a patient's suitability for surgery. There are a number of criteria typically used by experienced surgical centers to select patients for surgery that are common to all movement disorders stereotactic surgery (Kumar R, Lang AE. Patient selection for movement disorders surgery. In: Tarsy D, et al., eds. *Surgical treatment of Parkinson's disease and other movement disorders.* Humana 2002 [in press]).

1. Given that the risks of stereotactic surgery include a 1% to 2% risk of hemorrhage with severe permanent disability, patients must have significant disability in performance of activities of daily living or tasks necessary for employment, despite appropriate maximal drug therapy.
2. Patients should be in reasonable general health without specific contraindications to the neurosurgical procedure and have the physical and mental stamina to provide appropriate feedback during a lengthy and demanding procedure. Patients who are generally ill or debilitated or who have unstable or severe cardiac, pulmonary, renal, hepatic disease, uncontrolled hypertension, or cancer are poor candidates for surgery.
3. The patient's biological age and life expectancy and, as a result, expected duration of benefit should justify the risks of surgery. Some groups restrict surgery to those with a biological age of less than 70 years.
4. Patients and their families should have reasonable expectations about the effects of surgery (e.g., patients with PD should not expect to be "cured" or be relieved of symptoms that generally are unaffected by surgery).
5. Patients should have a good understanding of the risks of surgery, including the risk of hemorrhage, which may result in serious neurologic disability or death.
6. There should be absence of significant uncontrolled psychiatric illness, especially anxiety or mood disorders, which may result in intraoperative patient decompensation, compromising the quality of patient feedback necessary to obtain optimal results. PD patients with untreated depression undergoing STN DBS may be predisposed to severe worsening postoperatively and even suicide in the face of motorically successful surgery (BP Bejjani, unpublished observations) (33).
7. Patients must not be demented or have significant cognitive disability. Demented patients may be unable to provide appropriate intraoperative feedback. Such patients with DBS may be difficult to program because they lack insight into their own motor status or may be unable to manage their own stimulation (i.e., learning to turn the stimulators on and off when appropriate). Surgery may also significantly worsen cognition in patients with preexisting cognitive problems, especially

patients with PD (33,34). Neuropsychological evaluation and, if necessary, psychiatric evaluation are mandatory in all cases of surgery for PD and often useful in surgery for tremor and dystonia (33). Although a discussion of the specific psychometric instruments that may be used is beyond the scope of this chapter, recommendations for screening, clinical, and research evaluations have recently been published (33). Cognitive abnormalities in keeping with the underlying diagnosis of PD or dystonia should not lead one to advise against surgery, but significant abnormalities not normally seen in uncomplicated PD (such as markedly impaired naming and verbal fluency) should lead one to question the patient's suitability for surgery (33).
8. Emotional support must be available from family or other caregivers to help the patient adjust postoperatively to his new role, with increased physical capabilities and less physical dependence. Patients who have been dependent for many years may have psychological problems learning to cope with a new, independent life (24). Family members should also be fully aware of the need to adapt to the changes experienced by the patient. Caregivers must be available to assist patients requiring multiple and frequent physician visits for DBS programming, especially PD patients who may need to attend clinic visits after anti-Parkinson drug withdrawal and when they have extremely poor mobility.
9. Preoperative MRI should not reveal severe cerebral atrophy or extensive white matter T2 signal changes which may increase the risk of intracerebral hemorrhage (24).

Parkinson's Disease: Patient Selection and Clinical Effects

Surgery should be considered for PD in patients who have severe medication-refractory motor fluctuations and levodopa-induced dyskinesias, disabling medication-refractory tremor, or marked medication intolerance making medical management unsatisfactory. (Caution should be exercised with the latter criteria with respect to hallucinations or other psychiatric symptoms occurring on low doses of dopaminergic drugs since this is often a forewarning of subsequent dementia.) Nondopaminergic problems and nonmotor symptoms should not be the major source of disability as these are not markedly improved with surgery, though one group has preliminarily reported an improvement in nonmotor symptoms of parkinsonism with bilateral STN DBS (35).

Although surgery for PD is effective late in the disorder, the timing of surgery should be gaged with respect to when the advantages of surgery outweigh the risks of surgery and the risks of medical treatment. Patient quality of life, based on personal, professional, and social factors, is an important gage that the patient must use to judge the risk/benefit ratio of surgery. However, surgery should not be delayed until the patient loses his or her job because of physical disability and there is marked loss of independence and loss of ability to effectively participate in society or family affairs. There has been speculation that STN DBS or lesioning might alter the course of PD by potentially reducing excitotoxic glutamatergic outflow from the STN to a number of targets, but especially to the substantia nigra pars compacta (36). If this were the case, there would be significant justification for moving surgery to a much earlier stage of the disease. Although there are supportive data in animal models of PD, there are no convincing clinical data in humans that STN surgery is neuroprotective. Indeed, STN DBS might actually increase glutamate release. Therefore, at this time hope for neuroprotection should not influence one's decision regarding surgery.

Some groups have found that older patients (especially those older than 70 years) tend to benefit less from pallidotomy and DBS, though this has not been confirmed by other surgical teams (24). This may reflect greater levodopa-resistant symptoms seen in the elderly. Elderly patients are less tolerant of surgery and more frequently may have intraoperative or postoperative confusion, especially when undergoing bilateral STN DBS. Persistent postoperative decline is also more common in elderly patients with STN DBS, especially if there is any preoperative cognitive dysfunction (34).

Very little has been published on the subject of surgery for atypical parkinsonian syndromes. Patients with multiple system atrophy (MSA) may initially respond well to levodopa, but this response typically wanes within a few years. It is possible that such patients might have some short-term benefit from GPi or STN surgery. One case of non-levodopa-responsive MSA and one case of vascular parkinsonism have been reported with failure to improve following STN DBS (24,37). Nevertheless, it may be appropriate to consider surgery for levodopa-related dystonia or dyskinesias in MSA patients with a clearly preserved levodopa response. On the other hand, patients with *parkin* gene mutations, as opposed to idiopathic PD, reportedly have had an excellent response to STN DBS, in keeping with their young age of onset, excellent levodopa response, prominent and early levodopa-induced dyskinesias, and pathology typically restricted to the substantia nigra (24).

Previous surgery for PD does not contraindicate additional surgery if the patient is otherwise an appropriate surgical candidate. There are reports of successful bilateral STN DBS in patients with prior unilateral thalamotomy, unilateral or bilateral thalamic DBS, unilateral pallidotomy, and unilateral or bilateral GPi DBS who benefited from initial surgery but subsequently developed additional disability, despite aggressive medical therapy (24,38).

The response to levodopa is predictive of the response to STN DBS and pallidotomy on off-period features of parkinsonism (7,39). Similarly, lentiform nucleus hypermetabolism on fluorodeoxyglucose PET scanning correlates with the response to pallidotomy and also correlates with levodopa response (40). Therefore, the levodopa challenge test after overnight withdrawal of all anti-Parkinson medication, using a supramaximal dose of levodopa, is an important part of the evaluation to determine the degree of benefit obtainable with surgery. This process also educates the patient and family regarding appropriate expectations from surgery. Most symptoms resistant to a supramaximal levodopa dose fail to respond to surgery, though one report suggests that bilateral STN DBS in combination with levodopa may be able to slightly improve persistent preoperative on-period axial disability (41). However, persistent on-period tremor can often be improved more with surgery than with levodopa (6,24). How severe the motor signs of parkinsonism must be in the off period to justify surgery is a highly subjective determination; however, some groups have arbitrarily set a minimum cutoff of 30/108 on the Unified Parkinson's Disease Rating Scale (UPDRS) motor section (though most patients with PD for 10 to 20 years have a score of 40 to 80), except for tremor-dominant patients who may have a lower total score (24). Similarly, determining what degree of expected improvement justifies surgery is difficult, and some groups believe that a suprathreshold dose of levodopa should improve parkinsonism by at least 50% before proceeding with surgery (24). Nevertheless, it may be reasonable to judiciously consider surgery in carefully selected patients with significant persistent on-period disability who may only be modestly improved by surgery. On the other hand, operating on patients who have very poor on-period postural stability with frequent falls preoperatively may put such patients at an even higher risk of falls and injury due to reduced bradykinesia and a faster gait; furthermore, such patients may fracture or displace their hardware due to falls if they receive DBS (unpublished observations).

More severe dyskinesias and motor fluctuations do not predict a poorer response on off-period parkinsonism, with either GPi or STN surgery both of which markedly reduce dyskinesias, though by different mechanisms (Table 46.1) (4). As a result, patients with significant disability due to severe motor fluctuations are likely to benefit more with surgery than those without such motor complications. As mentioned above, significant cognitive abnormalities on detailed neuropsychological testing are a contraindication to surgery. Simple cognitive screening tools that can be used in the clinic may be helpful to screen out some patients before even referring them for detailed testing. The Grenoble group excludes patients with a Mini-Mental Status Examination score ≤24/30 or with a Mattis Dementia Rating Scale score ≤130/144 (24). Drug-induced hallucinations and psychosis in patients with PD may markedly worsen intraoperatively, resulting in confusion and agitation, which may persist for several days postoperatively, and so such patients should be excluded from surgery (33,34). It is an open question as to whether all patients with any history of drug-induced hallucinations should be excluded from surgery. If such patients pass detailed neuropsychological testing and can be managed temporarily preoperatively on a reduced but suboptimal dose of anti-Parkinson medication without neuroleptic therapy, surgery can be successfully performed without significant postoperative cognitive decline (R. Kumar, unpublished observations). However, as mentioned previously, preoperative occurrence of hallucinations is a strong predictor for the subsequent development of dementia, and the increased probability of severe cognitive decline developing in the future needs to be taken into account. On the other hand, in highly select cases surgery might be considered in patients with the combination of mild preoperative cognitive abnormalities and severe motor disability, where the potential for worsening cognition with surgery is outweighed by the possibility of improvement in motor disability, functionally improving the patient's ability to carry out activities of daily living and making it easier for the caregiver to care for the patient (42).

Thalamic Deep Brain Stimulation

VIM DBS in PD results in virtually complete suppression of off-period contralateral tremor and mild improvement in rigidity (Table 46.1) (2,3). However, electrode placement in the centromedian/parafascicularis (CM/Pf) nucleus of the thalamus or anterior to the VIM [i.e., in the ventralis oralis anterior/ventralis oralis posterior (Voa/Vop)] may also suppress levodopa-induced dyskinesias (43). Thalamic surgery does not significantly improve bradykinesia or gait disorders, which are commonly the greatest sources of disability. Reports of improvement in bradykinesia probably are artifactual due to reduction in tremor-related interference with tasks used to measure bradykinesia (3). Quality of life may be improved with thalamic DBS, but activities of daily living, measured by the UPDRS, are generally unchanged (1–3). Because bradykinesia and gait are not improved, several patients initially treated with thalamic DBS for tremor-dominant PD have subsequently undergone STN DBS for other symptoms of parkinsonism that have become more pronounced over time (24). Furthermore, the antitremor effects of STN DBS seem comparable to those of thalamic DBS. As a result, thalamic surgery can no longer be recommended in PD.

Subthalamic Nucleus and Globus Pallidus Internus Deep Brain Stimulation

A summary and comparison of the specific clinical effects of STN and GPi DBS in PD is presented in Table 46.1. The total effect of DBS is achieved as a result of the microlesion caused by electrode implantation (minor effect) and the direct effect of stimulation (major effect). Commonly, the benefit achieved with microlesioning is maximal immediately post-operatively and declines over several weeks as the

edema surrounding the implanted electrodes resolves. Nevertheless, some microlesion effects may be noticeable for at least six months (16). A dramatic and beneficial effect of both STN and GPi DBS has been consistently observed. STN and GPi surgery can improve all of the cardinal features of PD, including tremor, bradykinesia, and rigidity, in addition to improving levodopa-induced dyskinesias (4). Both interventions result in significant improvements in motor fluctuations and dyskinesias as measured by patient home diary assessments: in a large multicenter study, on time without dyskinesia during the waking day increased from 25% to 30% at baseline to 65% to 75% 6 months postoperatively, and in a complementary fashion these interventions markedly decreased off time and on time with dyskinesia (4). Although some preliminary results have suggested that STN DBS may be a superior intervention, no large randomized trial of STN and GPi DBS has been conducted, and it remains unknown as to whether STN or GPi DBS is more efficacious for the management of advanced PD. Patient selection criteria for surgery at either site are quite similar since it is unknown what preoperative factors may suggest that a patient would have a better response to one surgery than another (e.g., severe dyskinesias, prominent axial disability, etc.). The STN may be an easier physical target in that it is small and easily seen on MRI (Fig. 46.2), has low spatial variability between patients, and has reliable effects with response to intraoperative stimulation predictive of final benefit (24). Unlike GPi surgery, bilateral STN DBS allows a marked reduction in anti-Parkinson medication (4). Average anti-Parkinson drug reduction is approximately 50% (4–6). This is particularly favorable in patients unable to tolerate adequate doses of anti-Parkinson medication because of somnolence, severe nausea and vomiting despite domperidone and other antiemetics, or psychiatric adverse effects in the absence of cognitive impairment. Levodopa and dopamine agonists may actually worsen on-period freezing in some patients. Therefore, STN DBS might actually improve on-period freezing by allowing a reduction in levodopa dose. If levodopa is toxic to nigral neurons, then the levodopa sparing effect of STN surgery may also be neuroprotective. Less medication is less expensive and less inconvenient for patients (especially if the number of drug doses per day is reduced). Likely because the STN is a smaller target, DBS parameters are generally lower than for the GPi, and this results in longer battery life and fewer battery changes in the long run (7). However, bilateral STN DBS, in comparison with GPi DBS, requires much more frequent follow-up with complex adjustments of stimulation parameters and anti-Parkinson medication. In addition, other postoperative management problems are more common, including stimulation-induced dyskinesias, mood changes, hypophonia, stimulation-induced dysarthria and sialorrhea (8).

Cognitively, both bilateral GPi DBS and bilateral STN DBS are well tolerated in younger patients, including lack

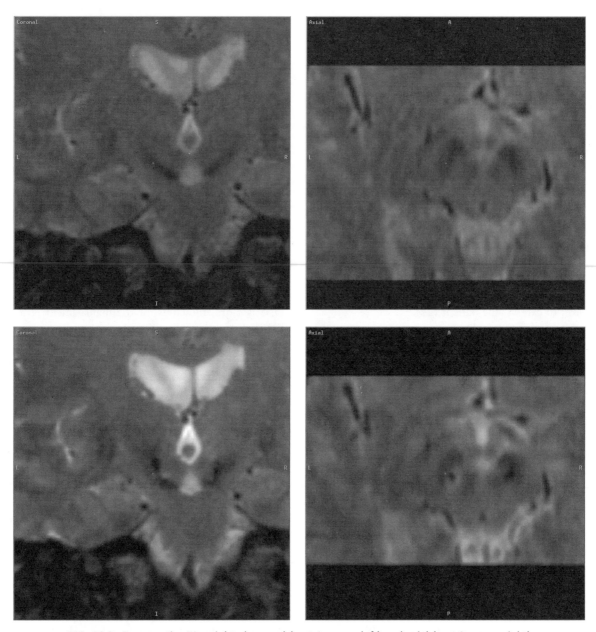

FIG. 46.2. Preoperative T2-weighted coronal (part 1, upper left) and axial (part 2, upper right) magnetic resonance images of the subthalamic nucleus (STN) coregistered to postoperative coronal (part 3, lower left) and axial (part 4, lower right) magnetic resonance images in a patient with Parkinson's disease who has undergone bilateral STN deep brain stimulation. Localization of each electrode contact is based on the postoperative magnetic resonance artifact and is then mapped onto the preoperative magnetic resonance image to verify the position of each contact with respect to the center of the STN. Centl, center of left STN; centr, center of right STN; 0l, most distal contact of left electrode; 0r, most distal contact of right electrode; 1l, second most distal contact of left electrode; 1r, second most distal contact of right electrode.

of detrimental effects on executive function. Both interventions result in mild decline in lexical fluency. STN DBS may result in mild improvement in working memory and psychomotor speed, not seen with GPi DBS (44–46). On the other hand, bilateral STN DBS may adversely affect frontal executive function in patients older than 69 years, and patients with borderline cognitive status risk postoperative decompensation including development of a progressive supranuclear palsy–like syndrome (34).

GPi DBS may be performed unilaterally or bilaterally. Bilateral surgery has more pronounced anti-Parkinson and anti-dyskinetic effects. Unilateral surgery may be considered most appropriate in patients with highly asymmetric parkinsonism and levodopa-induced dyskinesias or dystonia. Although no overall cognitive decline has been reported with GPi DBS, a subgroup of elderly individuals using high doses of levodopa may be at risk (33,47). Although most case series have included only patients who have not undergone surgery, our clinical experience suggests that GPi DBS applied contralaterally to a prior unilateral pallidotomy may be an effective strategy in patients who have significant residual disability due to levodopa-induced dyskinesias and parkinsonism ipsilateral to the lesion (48). Bilateral pallidotomy is associated with a high incidence of bulbar dysfunction, including dysarthria, hypophonia, dysphagia, and drooling. A severe dysexecutive syndrome has also been reported in isolated cases. As a result, bilateral pallidotomy cannot be recommended, and either bilateral GPi DBS or unilateral pallidotomy with contralateral GPi DBS is preferred. We have also found that bilateral STN DBS may also be a useful intervention in patients who have undergone unilateral pallidotomy or GPi DBS and subsequently present with persistent or recurrent disability.

As with GPi surgery, bilateral STN DBS results in greater improvement than unilateral STN DBS, with not only marked bilateral improvement in parkinsonism but also greater improvement in parkinsonism on each side (49). As a result, bilateral GPi or STN surgery is preferred in most patients with advanced PD. Unilateral STN surgery may also result in problems balancing the effects of drugs and stimulation because the stimulated side requires less anti-Parkinson medication and may become dyskinetic without drug reduction, whereas drug reduction may result in undertreatment of the unstimulated side (a similar situation applies to unilateral STN stimulation combined with contralateral GPi DBS). Although this has been our experience with unilateral STN DBS, other investigators report less difficulty in achieving the appropriate balance (J. Vitek, personal communication). Nevertheless, we have found that unilateral STN DBS may be effectively applied in patients with highly asymmetric tremor-dominant parkinsonism, including patients with a prior thalamotomy or unilateral thalamic DBS.

Although progression of predominately non-levodopa-responsive axial symptoms has been reported on long-term follow-up of patients who have undergone STN DBS, most of the benefit has been maintained (24,26). Ghika has reported decreased efficacy of bilateral GPi DBS after more than 12 months of follow-up, requiring additional anti-Parkinson medication and partial loss of the anti-dyskinetic effect (50). There are very few additional data reported on the long-term effects of bilateral GPi DBS. However, several patients who experienced waning benefit with bilateral GPi DBS have subsequently undergone bilateral STN DBS with significant benefit (38).

Tremor: Patient Selection and Clinical Effects

Severe nonparkinsonian tremor is a common cause of severe disability, requiring DBS of the motor thalamus—usually the VIM nucleus, Vop nucleus, and, occasionally, the zona incerta. Such patients typically have ET, multiple sclerosis

(causing cerebellar tremor), dystonic tremor, or Holmes' tremor (usually due to head trauma or brainstem infarction). Thalamic stimulation markedly improves most forms of tremor, may reduce dystonia associated with dystonic tremor, but does not improve and may even exacerbate ataxia in cerebellar tremor. In general, thalamic DBS is preferable to thalamotomy because of the increased rate of adverse effects with unilateral thalamotomy, including alteration in speech in approximately 30% of patients and possibly a greater improvement in quality of life with VIM DBS (1).

Essential Tremor

Essential tremor is the most common cause of tremor, and VIM DBS is considered the surgical treatment of choice for patients who are disabled despite optimal medical therapy (53a–c). Although ET is manifest predominantly as postural tremor, a high proportion of patients also have significant kinetic or intention tremor. This subgroup has higher tremor-related disability and is more likely to require surgery. Prior to consideration of surgery, patients should have significant tremor-related disability despite optimal medical therapy. All patients should receive an adequate trial of first-line antitremor drugs—propranolol (240 to 350 mg/day), primidone (250 to 750 mg/day), and possibly gabapentin (1,800 to 3,600 mg/day)—alone and/or in combination (53a). If first-line therapy fails, trials of additional medications are not mandatory and may result in unnecessary delay in surgery, since there is relatively little chance of marked improvement with second line (clonazepam, alprazolam, and mirtazepine) and third line (clonidine, acetazolamide, flunarizine, and theophylline) agents (53a).

Thalamic DBS almost uniformly markedly improves or abolishes distal postural tremor, though treatment for intention tremor and severe proximal arm tremor is less efficacious. Patients with marked intention tremor have only approximately 50% to 75% long-term benefit with thalamic DBS (17). Patients with severe bilateral tremor are best treated with bilateral VIM DBS because bilateral thalamotomy is associated with a high rate of bulbar and cognitive adverse effects. Patients who have previously undergone unilateral thalamotomy and who have developed significant tremor ipsilateral to the lesion should be treated with contralateral thalamic DBS (17). Although patients with prominent head, vocal, and trunk tremor may note some improvement with unilateral DBS, a better response is seen in these axial signs with bilateral DBS (53d). In contrast to patients with severe bilateral PD in whom bilateral STN or GPi DBS is most often performed simultaneously, bilateral thalamic surgery is frequently staged.

Cerebellar Tremor

Cerebellar tremor is most commonly problematic in patients with multiple sclerosis (MS), with relatively few patients with posttraumatic tremor, spinocerebellar ataxia, or the cerebellar subtype of MSA referred for surgery. Disabling tremor is seen in approximately 5% to 10% of MS clinic patients (51). Cerebellar tremor is characterized by unilateral or bilateral intention tremor (though postural tremor may also be present) that is less than 5 Hz. Head and trunk titubation are common and may be the most disabling form of axial tremor. Medical therapy is rarely successful with typical agents such as carbamazepine, clonazepam, L-5-hydroxytryptophan, and buspirone (51,52). Occasionally, patients may have mild improvement with high-dose propranolol. Superimposed ataxia often makes it difficult to determine which component of the disability is due to ataxia and which is due to tremor. Deuschl has suggested simple inspection to assess this, examining the regularity of the movements when patients make typical movements that cause disability (53). For example, during examination of a patient attempting to drink from a cup, the examiner must decide if the disability is primarily due to rhythmic or arrhythmic movements. Physiologic assessment may help to predict those most likely to benefit from surgery. Upper extremity postural tremor frequency analysis using accelerometry was predictive in one series of VIM DBS, with patients with tremor greater than 3 Hz experiencing tremor ablation but those with tremor less than 3 Hz not improving with surgery (52). Frequency analysis during a wrist tracking task may also be predictive of response of action tremor to thalamotomy, with 80% tremor reduction in those patients with just one frequency peak in the spectra and only 30% tremor reduction in those with multiple frequency peaks (54).

MS patients also have multiple other nervous system lesions, resulting in other neurologic deficits. The effect of these deficits on the potential for surgery to improve tremor must also be considered. Patients with marked sensory impairment in the target limb, excessive arm weakness (less than grade 4/5), or marked truncal weakness resulting in a bed-bound state should not be offered surgery because significant functional improvement would not be achieved even if tremor were eliminated (52).

There have been several recent studies of VIM DBS for MS-associated cerebellar tremor. Of these most have noted significant reduction in tremor, though overall disability was only mildly improved probably because of the presence of other neurologic deficits (1,55,56). Additional important issues include increased risk of adverse effects from surgery given the presence of multiple coexistent brain lesions and a possible negative effect on disease progression, including postoperative exacerbation of MS due to breach of the blood–brain barrier (52).

Dystonia

Dystonia is a highly heterogeneous disorder with both primary (genetically defined and idiopathic) and secondary etiologies, variable distribution (generalized, hemidystonia, segmental, and focal), and variable age at onset. There are no controlled studies of surgery for dystonia and the optimal target (GPi, thalamus, or other) has not been determined. There are no predictive clinical tests comparable to levodopa response in PD. As a result, conclusions about appropriate patient selection for various surgeries for dystonia must be tempered in light of the gaps in the current state of knowledge. Furthermore, there has been no systematic study of the cognitive effects of surgery for dystonia. As with PD, surgery for dystonia should be restricted to those patients with significant functional disability despite maximal medical therapy.

Thalamic Deep Brain Stimulation

Only a handful of cases of dystonia managed by thalamic DBS have been reported. Sellal et al. noted improvement with DBS of the ventroposterolateral nucleus of the thalamus in a patient with symptomatic hemidystonia who preoperatively noted reduction in dystonic posturing with superficial sensory stimulation (57). The Grenoble group has performed VIM DBS on ten patients with a variety of forms of dystonia with mild to moderate improvement in about half. Some of these patients have gone on to subsequently receive GPi stimulation with greater benefit (10). A patient with severe tardive dystonia undergoing simultaneous implantation bilateral into GPi and VIM obtained benefit only with GPi DBS and no additional improvement with concurrent VIM stimulation (58). In comparison with PD, higher stimulation pulse width and voltage has been required, necessitating frequent battery changes.

Globus Pallidus Internus Deep Brain Stimulation

GPi DBS for dystonia is typically restricted to those with severe generalized or segmental dystonia who continue to be disabled despite drug therapy (9–11). Several small case series have been reported demonstrating dramatic benefits in both children and adults (9,10). Patients with longstanding dystonia may be improved to the same degree as those with relatively shorter disease duration, and improvement in longstanding orthopedic deformities can be seen after long-term stimulation (10). More recently, bilateral GPi DBS has also been successfully employed in those with complex cervical dystonia who have responded inadequately to botulinum toxin injections or have become resistant to botulinum toxin (12,13). Although the majority of operated patients have had primary dystonia, with the best results reported in those who possess mutations in the torsin A gene (DYT-1) (9,10), there are increasing reports of significant improvement in patients with secondary dystonia (59,60). The most consistent improvements have been noted in children with DYT-1 mutations, with reduction in Burke-Fahn-Marsden (BFM) rating scale movement scores commonly exceeding 75% (9). Lesser improvements are noted in adults and patients with non-DYT-1 primary dystonia (9,10). Follow-up for 1 to 4 years in children with DYT-1 dystonia suggests sustained improvement and reduction or discontinuation of antidystonia medication (9). Both axial and limb dystonia is improved with bilateral GPi DBS. GPi DBS may also be valuable in patients with secondary dystonia without focal brain lesions (e.g., postanoxic states). Abnormal MRI result seems to reduce the likelihood of an optimal response (10,59). Recent reports suggest that evaluation of this therapy in individuals with metabolic diseases, such as Hallervorden-Spatz syndrome (NBIA [neurodegeneration with brain iron accumulation] type 1) and glutaric acidemia, is warranted even though preliminary results have been highly variable. The value of this therapy in patients with dystonia due to focal lesions (especially symptomatic hemidystonia) is less certain and has not been successful in our hands (unpublished data).

GPi DBS may be employed unilaterally or bilaterally depending on the distribution of the patient's dystonia. As with PD, unilateral GPi DBS has been successful when used contralaterally to a prior unilateral pallidotomy (61). Although this surgical approach seems to be the most promising, additional investigations are necessary to explore the effects of surgery on other targets because GPi surgery is clearly not effective in all patients, especially those with secondary dystonia. Indeed, STN stimulation has recently been combined with GPi stimulation, resulting in some additional benefit in a case of neurodegeneration with brain accumulation type 1 (10).

CONCLUSION

The ability to perform DBS allows neurologists and neurosurgeons to effectively manage movement disorders that previously could not be adequately improved and as a result markedly improve the quality of life of the most disabled patients. Obtaining optimal results from DBS requires knowledge of the technical aspects of stimulation in addition to detailed knowledge of basal ganglia anatomy and the clinical pharmacology and medical management of tremor, PD, and dystonia. The indications for DBS are rapidly evolving and expanding such that it is likely that these techniques will be applied earlier in the course of neurodegenerative disorders such as PD, as well as in a more widespread fashion in the case of nonmotor basal ganglia disorders such as severe obsessive-compulsive disorder or even affective disorders such as depression.

ACKNOWLEDGMENTS

Supported in part by the Colorado Neurological Institute and the National Parkinson Foundation (Miami, FL).

REFERENCES

1. Schuurman PR, Bosch DA, Bossuyt PM, et al. A comparison of continuous thalamic stimulation and thalamotomy for suppression of severe tremor. *N Engl J Med* 2000;342:461–468.
2. Koller W, Pahwa R, Busenbark K, et al. High frequency unilateral thalamic stimulation in the treatment of essential and parkinsonian tremor. *Ann Neurol* 1997;42:292–299.
3. Limousin P, Speelman JD, Gielen F, et al., and the study collaborators. Multicentre European study of thalamic stimulation in parkinsonian and essential tremor. *J Neurol Neurosurg Psychiatry* 1999;66:289–296.
3a. Krauss JK, Jankovic J, Grossman RG, eds. *Surgery for Parkinson's disease and movement disorders.* Philadelphia: Lippincott Williams & Wilkins, 2001:1–449.
3b. Jankovic J. Surgery for Parkinson's disease and other movement disorders: benefits and limitations of ablation, stimulation, restoration, and radiation. *Arch Neurol* 2001;58:1970–1972.
4. The Deep-Brain Stimulation for Parkinson's Disease Study Group. Deep-brain stimulation of the subthalamic nucleus or the pars interna of the globus pallidus in Parkinson's disease. *N Engl J Med* 2001;345:956–963.
5. Limousin P, Krack P, Pollak P, et al. Electrical stimulation of the subthalamic nucleus in advanced Parkinson's disease. *N Engl J Med* 1998;339:1105–1111.
6. Kumar R, Lozano AM, Kim YJ, et al. Double-blind evaluation of subthalamic nucleus deep brain stimulation in advanced Parkinson's disease. *Neurology* 1998;51:850–855.
7. Krack P, Pollak P, Limousin P, et al. Subthalamic nucleus or internal pallidal stimulation in young onset Parkinson's disease. *Brain* 1998;121:451–457.
8. Volkmann J, Allert N, Voges J, et al. Safety and efficacy of pallidal or subthalamic nucleus stimulation in advanced PD. *Neurology* 2001;56:548–551.
8a. Lanotte MM, Rizzone M, Bergamasco B, et al. Deep brain stimulation of the subthalamic nucleus: anatomical, neurophysiological, and outcome correlations with the effects of stimulation. *J Neurol Neurosurg Psychiatry* 2002;72:53–58.
8b. Valldeoriola F, Pilleri M, Tolosa E, et al. Bilateral subthalamic stimulation monotherapy in advanced Parkinson's disease: long-term follow-up of patients. *Mov Disord* 2002;17:125–132.
8c. Vingerhoets FJ, Villemure JG, Temperli P, et al. Subthalamic DBS replaces levodopa in Parkinson's disease: two-year follow-up. *Neurology* 2002;58:396–401.
9. Coubes P, Roubertie A, Vayssiere N, et al. Treatment of DYT1-generalised dystonia by stimulation of the internal globus pallidus. *Lancet* 2000;355:2220–2221.
10. Vercueil L, Pollak P, Fraix V, et al. Deep brain stimulation in the treatment of severe dystonia. *J Neurol* 2001;248:695–700.
11. Kumar R, Dagher A, Hutchison WD, et al. Globus pallidus deep brain stimulation for generalized dystonia: clinical and PET investigation. *Neurology* 1999;53:871–874.
12. Krauss JK, Pohle T, Weber S, et al. Bilateral stimulation of globus pallidus internus for treatment of cervical dystonia. *Lancet* 1999;354:837–838.
13. Parkin S, Aziz T, Gregory R, et al. Bilateral internal globus pallidus stimulation for the treatment of spasmodic torticollis. *Mov Disord* 2001;16:489–493.
13a. Brin MF, Germano I, Danisi F, et al. Deep brain stimulation in the treatment of dystonia. In: Krauss JK, Jankovic J, Grossman RG, eds. *Surgery for Parkinson's disease and movement disorders.* Philadelphia: Lippincott Williams & Wilkins, 2001:307–315.
13b. Bereznai B, Steude U, Seelos K, et al. Chronic high-frequency globus pallidus internus stimulation in different types of dystonia: a clinical, video, and MRI report of six patients presenting

with segmental, cervical, and generalized dystonia. *Mov Disord* 2002;17:138–144.

13c. Ghika J, Villemure JG, Miklossy J, et al. Postanoxic generalized dystonia improved by bilateral Voa thalamic deep brain stimulation. *Neurology* 2002;58:311–313.

13d. Krauss JK, Loher TJ, Pohle T, et al. Pallidal deep brain stimulation in patients with cervical dystonia and severe cervical dyskinesias with cervical myelopathy. *J Neurol Neurosurg Psychiatry* 2002;72:249–256.

14. Ashby P. What does stimulation in the brain actually do? *Prog Neurolog Surg* 2000;15:236–245.

15. Hariz MI, Shamsgovara P, Johansson F, et al. Tolerance and tremor rebound following long-term thalamic stimulation for parkinsonian and essential tremor. *Sterotact Funct Neurosurg* 1999;72:208–218.

16. Kumar R, Lang AE, Rodriguez MC, et al. Deep brain stimulation of the globus pallidus pars interna in advanced Parkinson's disease. *Neurology* 2000;55[Suppl 6]:S34–S39.

17. Benabid AL, Pollak P, Gao DM, et al. Chronic electrical stimulation of the ventralis intermedius nucleus of the thalamus as a treatment of movement disorders. *J Neurosurg* 1996;84,203–214.

18. Bejjani B, Damier P, Arnulf I, et al. Pallidal stimulation for Parkinson's disease: two targets? *Neurology* 1997;49:1564–1569.

19. Krack P, Pollak P, Limousin P, et al. Opposite motor effects of pallidal stimulation in Parkinson's disease. *Ann Neurol* 1998;43:180–192.

20. Kumar R, Lang AE, Sime E, et al. Late failure of thalamic deep brain stimulation in Parkinson's disease and essential tremor. *Neurology* 1999;52[Suppl 2]:A457.

21. Koller WC, Lyons KE, Wilkinson SB, et al. Long-term safety and efficacy of unilateral deep brain stimulation of the thalamus in essential tremor. *Mov Disord* 2001;16:464–468.

22. Oh MY, Hodaie M, Kim SH, et al. Deep brain stimulator electrodes used for lesioning: proof of principle. *Neurosurgery* 2001;49:363–367.

23. Kumar R, McVicker JM. Radiofrequency lesioning through an implanted deep brain stimulating electrode: treatment of tolerance to thalamic stimulation in essential tremor. *Mov Disord* 2000;15[Suppl 3]:69.

24. Pollak P. Deep Brain Stimulation. Annual Course of the American Academy of Neurology, Innovative surgical treatment of movement disorders 3AC.0006. San Diego 2000.

25a. Kumar R, Kedia S, McVicker JH. Chronic electrical stimulation of the zona incerta and fields of Forel in Parkinson's disease: implications for the mechanism of deep brain stimulation. *Mov Disord* 2001;16:991.

25b. Volkmann J, Fogel W, Krack P. Postoperative neurological management: stimulation of the subthalamic nucleus. *Akt Neurol* 2000;27[Suppl 1]:S23–S29.

26. Rodriguez-Oroz MC, et al. Deep brain stimulation of the subthalamic nucleus and globus pallidus pars interna in Parkinson's disease: a 4-year follow-up. *Neurology* 2001;56[Suppl 3]:A273.

26a. Kumar R, Kramer RE. Emergence of restless legs syndrome (RLS) during subthalamic nucleus deep brain stimulation (STN DBS) for Parkinson's disease (PD). *Parkinsonism and Rel Disord* 2001;7:S80.

27. Bejjani BP, Damier P, Arnulf I, et al. Transient acute depression induced by high-frequency deep-brain stimulation. *N Engl J Med* 1999;340:1476–1480.

28. Ghika J, Vingerhoets F, Albanese A, et al. Bipolar swings in mood in patient with bilaterak subthalamic nucleus deep brain stimulation (DBS) free of anti-Parkinson medication [abst.]. *Parkinsonism Rel Disord* 1999;5[Suppl 1]:104.

29. Kumar R, Krack P, Pollak P. Transient acute depression-induced by high-frequency deep-brain stimulation [letter]. *N Engl J Med* 1999;341:1003–1004.

30. Krack P, Kumar R, Ardouin C, et al. Mirthful laughter induced by subthalamic nucleus stimulation. *Mov Disord* 2001;16:867–875.

31. Yelnik J, Damier P, Bejjani BP, et al. Functional mapping of the human globus pallidus: contrasting effect of stimulation in the internal and external pallidum in Parkinson's disease. *Neuroscience* 2000;101:77–87.

32. Lyons KE, Koller WC, Wilkinson SB, et al. Surgical and device-related complications with deep brain stimulation. *Neurology* 2001;56[Suppl 3]:A147.

33. Saint-Cyr JA, Trepanier LL. Neuropsychologic assessment of patients for movement disorder surgery. *Mov Disord* 2000;15:771–783.

34. Saint-Cyr JA, Trepanier LL, Kumar R, et al. Neuropsychological consequences of chronic bilateral stimulation of the subthalamic nucleus in Parkinson's disease. *Brain* 2000;123:2091–2108.

35. Witjas T, Kaphan E, Azulay JP, et al. Effects of subthalamic nucleus (STN) deep brain stimulation (DBS) on non-motor fluctuations (NMF) on Parkinson's disease. *Neurology* 2001;56[Suppl 3]:A274.

36. Rodriguez MC, Obeso JA, Olanow CW. Subthalamic nucleus-mediated excitotoxicity in Parkinson's disease: a target for neuroprotection. *Ann Neurol* 1998;44[Suppl 1]:S175–S188.

37. Krack P, Dowsey PL, Benabid AL, et al. Ineffective subthalamic nucleus stimulation in levodopa-resistant postischemic parkinsonism. *Neurology* 2000;54:2182–2184.

38. Houeto JL, Bejjani PB, Damier P, et al. Failure of long-term pallidal stimulation corrected by subthalamic stimulation in PD. *Neurology* 2000;55:728–730.

39. Bonnet AM, Welter M-L, Houeto J-L, et al. Subthalamic stimulation in Parkinson's disease: perioperative predictive factors. *Neurology* 2001;56[Suppl 3]:A277.

40. Kazumata K, Antonini A, Dhawan V, et al. Preoperative indicators of clinical outcome following stereotaxic pallidotomy. *Neurology* 1997;49:1083–1090.

41. Bejjani BP, Gervais D, Arnulf I, et al. Axial parkinsonian symptoms can be improved: the role of levodopa and bilateral subthalamic stimulation. *J Neurol Neurosurg Psychiatry* 2000;68:595–600.

42. Wheelock VJ, King DS, Levine DK, et al. Efficacy of pallidotomy and thalamotomy in cognitively impaired Parkinson disease patients. *Neurology* 2001;56[Suppl 3]:A277–A278.

43. Caparros-Lefebvre D, Blond S, Feltin MP, et al. Improvement of levodopa induced dyskinesias by thalamic deep brain stimulation is related to slight variation in electrode placement: possible involvement of the centre median and parafascicularis complex. *J Neurol Neurosurg Psychiatry* 1999;67:308–314.

44. Ardouin C, Pillon B, Peiffer E, et al. Bilateral subthalamic or pallidal stimulation for Parkinson's disease affects neither memory nor executive functions: a consecutive series of 62 patients. *Ann Neurol* 1999;46:217–223.

45. Jahanshahi M, Ardouin CM, Brown RG, et al. The impact of deep brain stimulation on executive function in Parkinson's disease. *Brain* 2000;123:1142–1154.

46. Pillon B, Ardouin C, Damier P, et al. Neuropsychological changes between "off" and "on" STN or GPi stimulation in Parkinson's disease. *Neurology* 2000;55:411–418.

47. Vingerhoets G, van der Linden C, Lannoo E, et al. Cognitive outcome after unilateral pallidal stimulation in Parkinson's disease. *J Neurol Neurosurg Psychiatry* 1999;66:297–304.

48. Galvez-Jimenez N, Lozano A, Tasker R, et al. Pallidal stimulation in Parkinson's disease patients with a prior unilateral pallidotomy. *Can J Neurol Sci* 1998;25:300–305.

49. Kumar R, Sime E, Halket E, et al. Comparative effects of unilateral and bilateral subthalamic nucleus deep brain stimulation. *Neurology* 1999;53:561–566.

50. Ghika J, Villemure JG, Fankhauser H, et al. Efficiency and

safety of bilateral contemporaneous pallidal stimulation (deep brain stimulation) in levodopa-responsive patients with Parkinson's disease with severe motor fluctuations: a 2-year follow-up review. *J Neurosurg* 1998;89:713–718.

51. Alusi SH, Worthington J, Glickman S, et al. A study of tremor in multiple sclerosis. *Brain* 2001;124:720–730.

52. Alusi SH, Aziz TZ, Glickman S, et al. Stereotactic lesional surgery for the treatment of tremor in multiple sclerosis: a prospective case-controlled study. *Brain* 2001;124:1576– 1589.

53. Deuschl G, Raethjen J, Lindemann M, et al. The pathophysiology of tremor. *Muscle Nerve* 2001;24:716–735.

53a. Louis ED. Clinical practice: essential tremor. *N Engl J Med* 2001;345:887–891.

53b. Pahwa R, Koller WC. Thalamic stimulation for treatment of essential tremor. In: Krauss JK, Jankovic J, Grossman RG, eds. *Surgery for Parkinson's disease and movement disorders.* Philadelphia: Lippincott Williams & Wilkins, 2001:278–281.

53c. Ondo W, Vuong K, Almaguer M, et al. Thalamic deep brain stimulation: effects on the nontarget limbs and rebound phenomenon. *Mov Disord* 2001;16:1137–1142.

53d. Taha JM, Janszen MA, Favre J. Thalamic deep brain stimulation for the treatment of head, voice, and bilateral limb tremor. *J Neurosurg* 1999;91:68–72.

54. Liu X, Aziz TZ, Miall RC, et al. Frequency analysis of involuntary movements during wrist tracking: a way to identify ms patients with tremor who benefit from thalamotomy. *Stereotact Funct Neurosurg* 2000;74:53–62.

55. Montgomery EB Jr, Baker KB, Kinkel RP, et al. Chronic thalamic stimulation for the tremor of multiple sclerosis. *Neurology* 1999;53:625–628.

56. Geny C, Nguyen JP, Pollin B, et al. Improvement of severe postural cerebellar tremor in multiple sclerosis by chronic thalamic stimulation. *Mov Disord* 1996;11:489–494.

57. Sellal F, Hirsch E, Barth P, et al. A case of symptomatic hemidystonia improved by ventroposterolateral thalamic electrostimulation. *Mov Disord* 1993;8(4):515–518.

58. Trottenberg T, Paul G, Meissner W, et al. Pallidal and thalamic neurostimulation in severe tardive dystonia. *J Neurol Neurosurg Psychiatry* 2001;70:557–559.

59. Roubertie A, Cif L, Vayssiere N, et al. Symptomatic generalized dystonia: neurosurgical treatment by continuous bilateral stimulation of the internal globus pallidus in eight patients. *Mov Disord* 2000;15[Suppl 3]:156.

60. Loher TJ, Hasdemir MG, Burgunder J-M, et al. Long-term follow-up study of chronic blobus pallidus internus stimulation for post-traumatic hemidystonia [case report]. *J Neurosurg* 2000;92:457–460.

61. Vitek JL, Evatt M, Zhang J-Y, et al. Pallidotomy and deep brain stimulation as a treatment for dystonia. *Neurology* 1999;52[Suppl 2]:A294.

62. Kumar R. Methods for programming and patient management with deep brain stimulation. In: Tarsy D, et al., eds. *Surgical treatment of Parkinson's disease and other movement disorders.* Humana 2002 (in press).

SUBJECT INDEX

Page numbers in *italic* denote figures; those followed by a *t* denote tables.